THIS BOOK BELONGS TO:

S0-AGV-962

PSYCHIATRIC/ MENTAL HEALTH NURSING

The Therapeutic Use of Self

The skills of psychiatric nurses merit celebration. They have been honed over centuries of development. . . . Psychiatric nurses (today) have a remarkable opportunity to use their skills to provide a separate and/or complementary alternative form of treatment for psychiatric patients.

(Peplau H: Tomorrow's World. Nursing Times 83:29, 32; 1987)

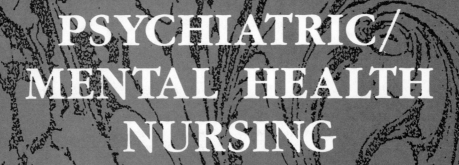

PSYCHIATRIC/ MENTAL HEALTH NURSING

The Therapeutic Use of Self

LORETTA M. BIRCKHEAD

R.N., B.S. (University of Richmond); B.S.N.
(Medical College of Virginia); M.S. (Rutgers
University Graduate Program in
Psychiatric/Mental Health Nursing); Ed.D.
(Boston University)

*Associate Professor, Department of Nursing
California State University, Los Angeles;
Private Practice
Los Angeles, California*

with contributors

J. B. Lippincott Company Philadelphia

Cambridge   New York   St. Louis   San Francisco   •   London   Singapore   Sydney   Tokyo

Acquisition/Sponsoring Editor: Nancy Mullins
Developmental Editor: David Carroll
Coordinating Editorial Assistant: Ellen Campbell
Manuscript Editor: Virginia Barishek
Indexer: Ann Blum

Interior Designer: Susan Hess Blaker
Cover Designer: Anita Curry
Production Coordinator: Pamela Milcos
Compositor: TAPSCO, Inc.
Printer/Binder: The Murray Printing Company

Copyright © 1989, by J. B. Lippincott Company. All rights reserved. No part of this book may be used or reproduced in any manner whatsoever without written permission except for brief quotations embodied in critical articles and reviews. Printed in the United States of America. For information write J. B. Lippincott Company, East Washington Square, Philadelphia, Pennsylvania 19105.

1 3 5 6 4 2

Library of Congress Cataloging-in-Publication Data

Psychiatric/mental health nursing: the therapeutic use of self/
 [edited by] Loretta M. Birckhead; with 36 contributors.
      p. cm.
    Includes bibliographies and index.
    ISBN 0-397-54412-X
    1. Psychiatric nursing.   2. Nurse and patient.   I. Birckhead,
Loretta M.
    [DNLM: 1. Nurse-Patient Relations.   2. Psychiatric Nursing.   WY
160 P97207]
RC440.P728   1989
610.73'68—dc19
DNLM/DLC
for Library of Congress   88-39647
                                                             CIP

Any procedure or practice described in this book should be applied by the health-care practitioner under appropriate supervision in accordance with professional standards of care used with regard to the unique circumstances that apply in each practice situation. Care has been taken to confirm the accuracy of information presented and to describe generally accepted practices. However, the authors, editors, and publisher cannot accept any responsibility for errors or omissions or for consequences from application of the information in this book and make no warranty, express or implied, with respect to the contents of the book.

Every effort has been made to ensure drug selections and dosages are in accordance with current recommendations and practice. Because of ongoing research, changes in government regulations, and the constant flow of information on drug therapy, reactions, and interactions, the reader is cautioned to check the package insert for each drug for indications, dosages, warnings, and precautions, particularly if the drug is new or infrequently used.

*In appreciation of psychiatric/mental health nurses and their
demonstrated efforts in promoting the well-being of clients.*

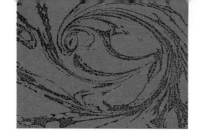

CONTRIBUTORS

Ira Trail Adams, D.P.H., R.N.
Dean, College of Nursing and Allied Health Sciences
The University of Tulsa
Tulsa, Oklahoma

Donna Aguilera, R.N., Ph.D., F.A.A.N.
Private Practice/Consultant
Los Angeles, California

Lorna Mill Barrell, Ph.D., R.N.
Associate Professor and Chairperson
Department of Community and Psychiatric Nursing
Virginia Commonwealth University
Richmond, Virginia

Loretta M. Birckhead, R.N., B.S., B.S.N., M.S., Ed.D.
Associate Professor, Department of Nursing
California State University, Los Angeles;
Private Practice
Los Angeles, California

Wilma Bradley, R.N., B.S.N., O.C.N.
Clinical Educator
Charter Suburban Hospital
Los Angeles, California

Vivian Brown, Ph.D.
Chief Executive Officer
Prototypes: A Center for Innovation in Health, Mental
    Health, and Social Services
Los Angeles, California

Gerald L. Cipkala-Gaffin, Ph.D.
Staff Psychologist
Coordinator of Psychology Internship Training Program
Cigna Health Plans
Los Angeles, California

Janet A. Cipkala-Gaffin, R.N., M.N.
Clinical Nurse Specialist, Bone Marrow Transplant/
    Mental Health
Children's Hospital of Los Angeles
Los Angeles, California

Susan Cramer, R.N., M.N.
Private Practice
Los Angeles, California

Kathleen Delaney, D.N.Sc., R.N.
Department of Psychiatric Nursing
Rush-Presbyterian St. Luke's Hospital
Chicago, Illinois

Nancy K. English, R.N., M.S.N.
Professor, Nursing Education
Golden West College
Huntington Beach, California

Jacquelyn H. Flaskerud, R.N., Ph.D., F.A.A.N.
Associate Professor, School of Nursing
University of California
Los Angeles, California

Margaret L. Franks, R.N., M.A.
Professor Emeritus
Cypress College
Cypress, California

Joy Dan Graves, R.N., Ph.D.
Licensed Clinical Psychologist
Los Angeles, California

Judith F. Karshmer, R.N., Ph.D.
Associate Professor, Department of Nursing
New Mexico State University
Las Cruces, New Mexico

Sally Knorr-Newman, R.N., M.A.
Clinical Nurse Specialist
Adult Day Treatment Services
UCLA Neuropsychiatric Institute
Los Angeles, California

Jill Ione Lomax, R.N., M.N.
Evening Nursing Supervisor
Kaiser Permanente Mental Health Center
Los Angeles, California

Marcia Luna-Raines, R.N., M.N., C.S.
Mental Health Clinical Nurse Specialist
Surgical/Obstetrical Division of Nursing
UCLA Medical Center
Los Angeles, California

Ronda Mintz, R.N., M.N.

Instructor, School of Nursing
University of California;
Private Practice
Los Angeles, California

Margaret L. Mitchell, R.N., M.N., M.Div., M.A.

Deacon, LaCañada Presbyterian Church;
Senior Mental Health Counselor,
Director, Psychiatric Mobile Response Team
San Fernando Valley Crisis Center
Van Nuys, California

Jean M. Moore, R.N., M.N.

Director, State Health Service Corps
New York State Department of Health;
Adjunct Instructor
Junior College of Albany
Albany, New York

Madeline A. Naegle, Ph.D., R.N.

Chairperson, American Nurses' Association Committee
    on Impaired Nursing Practice;
Psychotherapist in Private Practice;
Associate Professor, Division of Nursing
New York University
New York, New York

Roberta Nicholson, R.N., M.N.

Program Manager, Psychiatric Services
Torrance Memorial Hospital Medical Center
Torrance, California

Maryann H. Ogonowski, R.N., M.N.

Assistant Clinical Professor, Nursing Administration
Virginia Commonwealth University
Richmond, Virginia;
Director of Nursing
Central State Psychiatric Hospital
Petersburg, Virginia

Elizabeth Ojala, R.N., Ph.D.

Private Practice
Redondo Beach, California

Diana E. Olson, R.N., M.S.N.

Clinical Professor
Cypress College
Cypress, California

Kathy Patusky, R.N., M.A.

Private Practice
San Diego, California

Elizabeth C. Poster, R.N., Ph.D.

Director, Nursing Research and Education
UCLA Neuropsychiatric Institute;
Assistant Clinical Professor,
UCLA School of Medicine and School of Nursing
Los Angeles, California

Daya Rao, R.N., M.S.N.

Patient Care Coordinator
Riverside Hospice
Riverside, California

Jane A. Ryan, R.N., M.N., C.N.A.A.

Director of Nursing Systems
UCLA Neuropsychiatric Institute;
Assistant Clinical Professor, School of Nursing
University of California
Los Angeles, California

Shirl A. Scheider, R.N., Ph.D.

Consultant in Holistic Nursing
Newburg, Oregon

JoAnna Shear, R.N., M.N.

Psychiatric Clinical Specialist, Emergency Room
Cedars-Sinai Medical Center
Los Angeles, California

Gwen Marram Van Servellen, R.N., Ph.D., F.A.A.N.

Associate Professor, School of Nursing
University of California
Los Angeles, California

Rebecca A. Van Slyke-Martin, Ph.D.

Health Care Consultant
Newburg, Oregon

Rose A. Vasta, R.N., Ph.D., C.S.

Psychoanalyst
Beverly Hills, California;
Lecturer, School of Nursing
University of California
Los Angeles, California

Jean F. Wyman, Ph.D., R.N.

Assistant Professor and Director
Graduate Program in Gerontological Nursing
Department of Community and Psychiatric Nursing
Virginia Commonwealth University
Richmond, Virginia

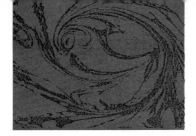

PREFACE

The profession of nursing has seen dramatic changes from the days of Nightingale to today's advanced technology. Within each specialty of nursing the scientific knowledge base has expanded, clinical practice has evolved, and skill requirements have increased. Similar to other specialties, psychiatric/mental health nursing has also undergone many changes since its beginning in the 1800s. Developmental theories have expanded the knowledge base of human behavior; advances in pharmacotherapeutics have dramatically altered the prognosis for many clients who were considered "hopeless;" and nursing research has demonstrated the efficacy of nurse/client interactions.

Yet, with all the advances that have taken place, one factor has remained constant: the practice of psychiatric/mental health nursing continues to focus on nurses' interactions with clients. Professional psychiatric/mental health nurses enter into interpersonal relationships with clients in order to assist clients in overcoming emotional or behavioral problems, and to promote the growth of clients and the achievement of optimum levels of mental health.

While other nursing specialties focus on health or illness concerns of particular age groups of health problems, psychiatric/mental health nursing is concerned with all age groups and the achievement of mental health for all clients, regardless of their physical health. Psychiatric/mental health nursing is a key aspect of all nursing care, not strictly with clients who have behavioral or emotional problems.

The objective of this text is to provide nursing students with the knowledge base necessary to intervene with all clients in order to promote mental health, identify mental health problems, and assist clients in their recovery from problems. It provides the necessary foundation for students who will practice psychiatric/mental health nursing after graduation, as well as those who choose to work in other specialties of nursing. The book presents the practice of psychiatric/mental health nursing from a clinical perspective, since nurses interact with clients in a variety of psychiatric and nonpsychiatric settings.

The Conceptual Framework

It would be ideal if psychiatric/mental health nurses could base their practice on one set of principles that would guide all of their interactions with clients. However, every client is unique and has a different biological, familial, social, environmental, and cultural background. Because of the uniqueness of each person, a number of developmental and psychological theories have been proposed to explain human behavior. The conceptual framework of this text integrates these theories and organizes them into the following elements that appear throughout the text.

The Therapeutic Use of Self. Since nurses' interpersonal interactions with clients form the basis of psychiatric/mental health nursing, nurses have a responsibility to work with clients in ways that promote mental health and foster client growth. This concept, which is based on Peplau's interpersonal theory provides clinical direction for effecting useful relationships with clients who have psychological concerns. By understanding one's own self, and with the use of developmental theories, and basic principles of human behavior, nurses can interact therapeutically to assist clients in resolving mental health problems and achieving optimum mental health.

Systems Theory. Individuals do not exist in isolation, but are in constant interaction with other people and objects in their environment. Systems theory enables nurses to focus on the biological, psychological, environmental, societal, and cultural aspects that are unique to each client.

Levels of Prevention. Nurses work with clients at different points along the health-illness continuum. Therefore, it is important for nurses to understand and implement appropriate interventions for clients at each level of prevention. Clients who are healthy can benefit from early case finding and from gaining a better understanding of psychological principles that will enable them to attain higher levels of mental health and psychological well-being. Clients with psychological problems can benefit from therapeutic interactions with nurses. Psychiatric/mental health nurses do not accept the label "chronic," but believe that human beings are capable of growth if they are provided with an opportunity to facilitate that growth.

The Nursing Process. Since the nursing process is the framework within which nursing care is delivered, it is used as the organizational structure, where appropriate. Mental health problems are organized and discussed in terms of nursing assessment, diagnosis, planning, intervention, and evaluation.

Structure of the Text

The text begins with general background material essential to understanding the current contexts of psychiatric/mental health nursing practice. Part I includes a historical overview of the practice of psychiatric/mental health nursing, as well as a discussion of the contemporary role of the nurse in mental health practice. The process of working with other disciplines is includes, as are the issues of accountability, autonomy, and authority in clinical nursing practice.

Part I also begins the focus on clinical work in psychiatric/mental health nursing. Communication, a key concept in therapeutic interaction, is presented, as are nurses' attitudes that promote therapeutic interactions with clients.

Part II focuses on the delivery of psychiatric/mental health nursing care, and includes chapters on the nursing process and the therapeutic use of self. All aspects of the nursing process are specifically applied to psychiatric/mental health nursing. Nursing diagnoses are considered in detail, including the diagnoses developed by the North American Nursing Diagnosis Association (NANDA), as well as the recently issued American Nurses' Association taxonomy of nursing diagnoses for psychiatric/mental health nursing.

This part concludes with a chapter on the therapeutic use of self: the nature of nurse–client interactions that are established by nurses to facilitate mental health and growth in clients. The therapeutic use of self is enhanced by a discussion of the nature of the Self of the client, the Others who are significant to the client, and the Relationship between the Self and Others. This chapter also focuses on the emotional life of the client, especially anxiety. Other sections of this chapter present interviewing skills used in psychiatric/mental health nursing, the phases of the nurse–client relationship, and the process of empathy.

Part III presents the theoretical frameworks that guide nurses in clinical practice. Harry Stack Sullivan's work on interpersonal relationships is included, and provides background for the development of Peplau's principles of psychiatric/mental health nursing. Other discussions include the psychoanalytic model, the ideas of Carl Rodgers, ego psychology, object relations theory, and learning theory.

Other chapters in Part III present major theorists from a life span perspective; stress as a precipitating factor in the development of psychological problems; and emotional responses to illness. This chapter includes an important section on family responses to illness.

Part IV presents the intervention modalities in which care is provided. These modalities include individual relationship intervention (the nurse and the client working together); group work; family therapy; crisis intervention; and milieu therapy. Topics such as the change process and resistance to change; short-term therapy; and ethical issues in working with clients are discussed in these chapters. Throughout Part IV professional nurses are viewed as individuals who *intervene* with clients, not as observers of the work of other disciplines.

Part V focuses on responses to the illness processes of depression and mania, thought disorders (schizophrenia), learning and developmental disorders, psychophysiological disturbances, personality disorders, substance abuse, and family violence. All chapters in Part V include a nursing intervention focus, with clinical examples and nursing care plans. A discussion of levels of prevention is provided in each chapter.

Part VI provides a discussion of psychiatric/mental health interventions across the life span. Specific chapters provide information on mental health counseling of children, adolescents, adults, and older adults. Intervention guidelines specific to each age group are provided, and a separate chapter is devoted to nursing interventions in human sexuality. Additional topics considered in Part VI include working with families, women's health concerns, problems related to AIDS, and elder abuse.

Part VII presents an overview of the mental health care delivery system. Separate chapters discuss nursing administration in mental health care facilities, the inpatient system, aftercare and day care treatment programs, and home care. One chapter discusses psychiatric liaison nursing, and the role of nurses working in nonpsychiatric settings, such as medical-surgical units. The final chapter in Part VII focuses on community mental health, a topic of current interest.

The last four chapters focus on special considerations in psychiatric/mental health nursing, including spirituality; legal aspects; political, social, and economic influences on psychiatric nursing practice; and the impact of research on psychiatric/mental health nursing practice. Each of these chapters emphasizes the role of the professional nurse in interactions with clients, other professionals, and other systems that impact on psychiatric/mental health nursing practice.

Special Features

The major feature of this text is its emphasis on *clinical practice*. The roles of professional nurses in working with clients in the mental health system are clearly delineated, and suggested interventions are provided.

Nursing care plans are provided in pertinent chapters to suggest appropriate nursing interventions for use in working with clients who have mental health problems. Care plans are reinforced with *introductory vignettes,* and are supplemented with numerous *clinical examples.*

Each chapter begins with clearly stated *learning objectives* and a *chapter outline* that provide students with an overview of the expectations of the chapter. Content is reinforced with tables and boxes that highlight important concepts. A *chapter summary* and current *references* complete each chapter.

The most current nursing diagnoses approved by the North American Nursing Diagnosis Association (NANDA) are included throughout the text. In addition, the American Nurses' Association's *Taxonomy for the Classification of Human Responses of Concern for Psychiatric/Mental Health Nursing* are included. Where appropriate, diagnoses from the American Psychiatric Association's *Diagnostic and Statistical Manual of Mental Disorders, Third Edition—Revised* (1987) have been included.

Recent psychiatric/mental health research is integrated throughout the text. *Relevant Research* boxes demonstrate principles presented in the text discussions.

Rather than present all psychopharmacology in one chapter, it has been integrated into the discussions where pharmacologic treatment modalities are indicated. Special *drug card* boxes are included to emphasize properties of commonly encountered drugs and nursing care associated with these particular drug therapies. In addition, a comprehensive psychotropic drug table has been included in the Appendix.

Another unique feature of the text is the appendix covering *Psychiatric Emergencies.* This quick reference section includes appropriate interventions for working with clients experiencing a wide variety of psychiatric crises. It can easily be located by the blue border on the top edge of the page at the back of the text.

It is the hope of the author and the contributors that students will be able to share in the special joy of working in the area of psychiatric/mental health nursing. The challenges and struggles of learning about and working with mental health problems are great, but the rewards are far greater.

Special acknowledgment is made of the opportunities to work on this text provided by Gwen Marram Van Servellen, R.N., Ph.D. A special thanks to Nancy Mullins and Dave Carroll of J. B. Lippincott Company for their professionalism, skill, and encouragement. Appreciation is extended for the time and consideration offered by Teri Stanford, Carol Dearborn, Pam Rahn, John Overton, and Tom Mullen.

Loretta M. Birckhead, R.N., C.S., Ed.D.

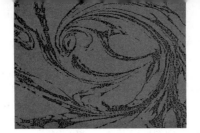

INTRODUCTION TO THE PSYCHIATRIC/MENTAL HEALTH NURSING PROFESSION

A number of questions and uncertainties arise when students first study and practice psychiatric/mental health nursing. These questions may include "How is psychiatric/mental health nursing different from, and similar to, other nursing specialties?" "What are nurses attempting to do in their interactions with clients?" "What are the legitimate boundaries and limitations to the psychiatric/mental health nurse's role?" "What interventions contribute to effective nurse–client relationships and coordinated interdisciplinary efforts?" More personal uncertainties may also come up, for example, "How will I be affected by this practice?" and "How will I affect clients and my co-workers?"

Although answers to these questions may be subjective and changeable, it is important that students address them using authoritative opinions that express the state of the art and science of psychiatric/mental health nursing. It is hoped that a foundation of concepts and authoritative opinions will assist students in the discovery of their potential as psychiatric/mental health nurses.

It is particularly useful to have a conceptual framework from which to approach these questions. A conceptual framework can help to achieve clarity and reduce ambiguity. At a minimum, a framework should provide a way of looking at the client as a "person," a way of looking at health and wellness, and a way of looking at nursing care within the scope of psychiatric/mental health nursing.

The following discussion introduces the conceptual framework of this book, from which basic premises and philosophies of the text are derived. This framework of concepts and theories is illustrated throughout the book using actual clinical practice examples and case vignettes.

Systems Theory

Clients in nursing and health care are currently viewed as unique human beings whose behavior, emotions, and thoughts are the products of the interaction between clients and their environments. This basic premise, addressed throughout the text, is the principle of general systems theory.

General systems theory proposes that individuals are not isolated entities, but are affected by various factors in their environments. Rather than addressing one aspect of the client, for example, genetic predisposition or psychological vulnerability to stress and illness, nurses should analyze *the system:* the *interaction* of multiple variables that affect clients. It should be emphasized that while clients' lives are the outcomes of the interdependent nature of individuals and their environments, this premise does not rule out individuals' abilities to direct their lives. Each person is viewed as unique and, as such, has the potential to exercise *freedom of choice* and the *freedom to change.* Individuals have freedom to choose among alternatives and, in this way, direct the unique aspects of their life patterns. However, individuals can become sufficiently burdened with concerns that they become unable to make choices.

In keeping with the premises of general systems theory, *illness-maintaining responses* may be seen as the result of clients' needs to cope with certain internal and external forces. For example, when a client remains "sick" under optimal therapeutic conditions, the client may be attempting to maintain some sense of permanence; although this is not "healthy," this adjustment is adaptive for the client. Other clients do not yet have sufficient internal or external resources to overcome psychological problems. For example, they may not have access to professional help to assist them in working with their problems and conflicts.

Others, who do not have illness-maintaining responses and who are on the "healthy" end of the health–illness continuum, can alternate between difficult periods and periods marked by a sense of well-being. Childbirth, for example, is a "normal" event. It may involve difficulties of life patterning, such as the accompanying role changes that occur in the family after delivery. These difficulties, however, may be followed by periods of well-being, which may then be followed by a difficult period, and so on. At the healthy end of the health–illness continuum one experiences a definite sense of well-being, though difficulties that require attention do occur in the person's life.

To further illustrate the client from both a predeterministic and self-deterministic viewpoint, it is useful to employ a specific theoretical framework. This theoretical framework focuses on the interdependent concepts of a client's *biological* and *psychological* makeup, as well as the influence of *environmental, cultural,* and *social* phenomena. A systems framework transcends a focus on a single theory of life circumstances (such as the psychological), and provides a more integrated approach. A systems orientation allows the nurse to look beyond a specific focus (for example, the psychological vulnerability of the client) in order to analyze the client in the context of dynamic interaction with what is outside the person (such as the environment), yet in interaction with the person.

These parts are conceived as interdependent regions. The *psychological* region represents the client's internal experiences, including thoughts and feelings. The *societal* unit of analysis describes the nature of the client's relationship with others. This region draws attention to the fact that an essential aspect of our nature includes a tendency to be social and to form groups. Families and significant others are examples of the societal region. The *cultural* aspect calls attention to the fact that individuals are members of a collective group with a characteristic belief system and patterns of living. The *environment* includes the elements of the external work that are relevant to the client or group (such as physical space or air pollutants). The *biological* unit of analysis includes one's physical well-being.

The parts of the client system are in a dynamic interplay because one or more parts (in any combination) can affect the well-being of the client at any one time. One, two, three, four, or all five system parts may be of particular importance at any one time. Similarly, at any one time the nurse may have to consider from one to five aspects of the person in order to formulate the most appropriate actions to care for a particular client.

For example, consider a client who has cancer and is depressed. The family (societal unit) and emotional state (psychological unit) of analysis may be the areas of primary focus. The nurse may assess that other aspects of the client's experience (environmental, cultural, and biological units), although important, are not currently influencing the client's health status to any degree. The units of analysis, however, *may shift.* At some later point in working with the client and the client's family, the biological aspect may become a priority concern.

This shifting phenomenon makes psychiatric/mental health nursing challenging, stimulating, and difficult. In many instances there is no easy answer to the question: "What am I dealing with as a psychiatric nurse in respect to this client?" Nurses must use *all* of their skills to focus their work on facilitating growth for clients.

In keeping with the general systems philosophy of

viewing the person from this perspective, all subsystems or parts should be considered at all times, since all parts operate simultaneously. The total system is said to be in *dynamic interaction,* since more than one part is influencing the client at one time, and the parts that exert significant effects of the person can change.

This condition of dynamic interaction is directed by two phenomena: (1) the individual's need to maintain a state of equilibrium and (2) the individual's need to exercise freedom of choice.

Nursing interventions may *not* be successful if they are directed only at a segment of the problem. For example, a nurse may be working with a depressed Hispanic immigrant to the United States. The client is married and has seven children. The client may state that she feels overwhelmed, listless, and unable to concentrate, and wishes that her husband would help her with the care of the children. The nurse should not quickly conclude that a mere change in child care would significantly relieve the client's depression. A more dynamic analysis is needed.

In this example the nurse should examine the *biological* and the *psychological* dynamics of the client's depression *and* the *societal, environmental,* and *cultural* variables that play a role. To emphasize only the psychological aspects of the client without viewing the societal, environmental, and cultural forces operating in the family would not bring about a change in family functioning.

Important variables that the nurse may find in this case might include the beliefs of the client's extended family about her proper *cultural* role as mother; the client's *biological* status (would medications for depression help?); and the effect of *environmental* variables (the neighborhood and climate may be very different from what the client is used to).

To focus on *only* one part of the client's system is to work with only part of the client's reality. The work of the nurse and client may then become distorted. If the nurse focuses on only one factor, such as agreeing with the client and blaming the husband, the client will still feel alienated from her husband and hopeless.

The Self, the Other, and the Relationship of Self and Other

The client is viewed as a person (a *Self*) who interacts with *Others,* who are significant to the client. These Others can be the nurse, family members, other clients, or a variety of other individuals. The client also maintains *Relationships* with these significant Others. The relationships may be minimal, but few individuals live as true hermits. Humans are fundamentally interpersonal beings—they want others to be near and want to engage with them in day-to-day life.

The ideas of *Self, Other,* and the *Relationship* of Self and Other (S/O/R) are used in concert with the other constructs in the conceptual framework. The S/O/R construct serves to give a more detailed description of the psychological aspects of human nature. The idea of the therapeutic use of self focuses on how best to assist clients. The nursing process offers a problem-solving method to follow in providing care. Systems theory provides general rules to understand how a collection of parts of a system (such as parents and children) may function together. The S/O/R construct offers a more detailed look at core elements of psychological functioning. It provides some idea of the nature of the Self—the primary psychological unit with which the mental health disciplines work.

Tenets of S/O/R include the following principles:

1. Each person can be placed at some point on the continuum of awareness of his or her own thoughts, feelings, and actions.

2. The person can be placed at some point on the continuum of awareness of another person's (the Other's) thoughts, feelings, and actions.

3. Each person can be placed at some point on the continuum of awareness of what occurs in the Relationship of Self and Other.

In much of what occurs in an individual's psychological life, the person is concerned with awareness of Self, the Other, or the Relationship of Self and Other. In other words, much of how well we feel psychologically depends on the clarity with which we perceive our own selves; others around us who are, or have been, important to us; and the relationship, or what happens between ourselves and our significant others.

Some of the elements of the S/O/R construct are as follows:

1. A client may change the focus of concern. For example, at one point a client may be attempting to clarify his or her own feelings, and at another time what occurs in the client's Relationship with his or her spouse. The nurse deals with issues in the client's psychological life as well as problems in the client's Relationships.

2. Mental illness comes, in part, from a lack of clarity of one's S/O/R. Perhaps a parent abused the client. The client may, as a child or as an adult, have a distorted idea (thought) about the parent. The child may not have been sufficiently psychologically mature to understand what was occurring during the abuse, or the child may have been so anxious during the abuse that the child could not clearly perceive the situation.

3. One goal of mental health is concerned with the individual's sense of well-being regarding one's Self, one's idea of the Other, and one's Relationship with the Other. People are aware, or can become aware, of their understanding of S/O/R. An individual has a certain perception of the Other. Self and Other may have to discuss and work on this perception in their Relationship, if it is to remain conflict-free. Many problems occur in Relationships wherein each member has an inaccurate perception of the Other. The Other is not given his or her "full due," so to speak, as a total person. They are seen only in part, or seen to be something the client wishes to occur rather than how the Other really is.

4. The nurse enters into the professional relationship with the client in order to assist the client to change. The nurse becomes an "Other" to the client and a Relationship exists between the two. The nurse and client can work on any lack of clarity on the part of the client about the nurse. The client, for example, may perceive the nurse as "all good" and "perfect" and the client as "all bad." This perception, no doubt, is one displayed by the client in many of his or her relationships. The client can achieve much by clarifying such perceptions with the nurse.

In summary, psychiatric/mental health nursing is a specialization in nursing practice that, although it deals particularly with psychological problems in clients, reflects the orientation of the whole of nursing. In this way, psychiatric/ mental health nursing is both similar to, and different from, other areas of concentration. These similarities and differences will become even more apparent as the student becomes familiar with psychiatric/mental health clients, settings, and the theories of mental health intervention.

The Nursing Process

In psychiatric/mental health nursing, as in nursing in general, nurses are concerned simultaneously with promoting health and preventing illness by attending to actual and potential health problems. The nurse's role also includes efforts to support the resources of individuals, families, and groups in order to modify the disabilities and handicaps that can arise from impairment.

The *nursing process* is central to this role. The nursing process is viewed as a deliberate, problem-solving activity, consisting of five major components that direct the nature of the relationship of the nurse with the client or client group. These components are assessment, diagnosis, planning, intervention, and evaluation.

Assessment is a systematic collection and interpretation of data relating to the psychological, biological, social, cultural, and environmental aspects of the client. Assessment is accomplished by observation, interviewing, history-taking, physical assessment, and the examination of records.

A *nursing diagnosis* is a nursing conclusion about the health or illness potential. It results from a critical analysis of the data obtained during the nursing assessment. In this text nursing diagnoses are derived from two sources: nursing diagnoses recognized by the North American Nursing Diagnosis Association (NANDA), and those developed by the American Nurses' Association.[1]

Diagnoses from the *Diagnostic and Statistical Manual, Third Edition—Revised* (DSM-III-R)[3] are also included. These diagnoses were developed by the American Psychiatric Association and serve as psychiatric (medical) diagnoses. The DSM-III-R offers a useful summary of major psychiatric diagnoses and relevant signs and symptoms. Reference to DSM-III-R diagnoses are made, in part, because other disciplines in mental health care use these diagnoses. Because nurses work with other disciplines they need to know the diagnostic "language" of these disciplines. Nursing diagnoses complement the symptom-based diagnoses of illness (DSM-III-R). Together, these perspectives provide guidelines for nurses whose focus goes beyond illness, but whose knowledge base must also include illness nomenclature.

Planning represents the third phase of the nursing process. In this phase objectives and goals for nursing actions are set and prioritized in order to give specific direction for nursing actions.

Intervention is defined as the execution of the nursing plan using diagnostic, therapeutic, or educational nursing actions. These actions include, but are not limited to, providing emotional support, anticipatory guidance, health education, psychotherapeutic intervention, and physical care and comfort.

Evaluation is the nurse's assessment of the degree of effectiveness of the actions taken to resolve existing or potential health problems. Such an evaluation could include interviews and observations of clients, interviews with the client's significant others, physical and mental status examinations, record review, and conferences with other health care personnel who are directly involved with the client.

It should be mentioned that psychiatric/mental health nursing maintains the same general philosophy and commitment to the nursing process as other nursing specialties. There are specific elements, however, that address the commonalities and potential differences, and these are worth noting.

Psychiatric nursing, more than any other specialty, has adopted a humanistic philosophy and a perspective that emphasizes the meaning or interpretation of experiences to individuals. Inherent in this philosophy are several basic premises: (1) nurses view individuals as having the potential to grow, and (2) the major impact on clients is in the common ground of negotiated *meaning* between individuals. That is to say, the nurse must view the client's behavior within its social context. Through the process of discovering and respecting each client's individual experience (and the meaning attached to it) the nurse comes closer to a true therapeutic interchange. For nurses, humanism yields a systems view of mind/body relations; a collaborative decision-making model; an expanded role for nurses, and a general posture of negotiation and advocacy in relation to clients in social and political, as well as medical, areas.

In an attempt to clarify the intent of psychiatric/mental health nursing practice, the ANA Division on Psychiatric and Mental Health Nursing Practice[2] provided specific interpretations of the role of the psychiatric/mental health nurse. These interpretations and a brief explanation follow.

1. The nursing profession is committed to health and to the fullest possible utilization of human potential. "Psychiatric/mental health nurses have a particular responsibility to speak out on behalf of the public's need for holistic and humane services."[2]

    Respect for the humanity of each client is an inherent aspect of psychiatric/mental health nursing, with strong roots in the history of psychiatric/mental health nursing practice. Respect is warranted regardless of the condition or status of the client. This respect reflects a strong orientation toward the self-actualizing potential of the client. While intervening at the client's current interpersonal and intellectual competency level, the nurse is always concerned with the client's potential for higher levels of competence.

2. Nursing care is defined and developed by nurses who assume responsibility and authority for its quality. Elements unique to nursing that distinguish it from other disciplines are "(a) a holistic approach to people, and (b) a crisis orientation."[2]

    Nurses strive to promote wellness, rather than simply the absence of illness. This orientation includes a perspective on the reality of clients' experiences as they understand it. Clients perceive that nurses understand their total experiences, and are "with" clients in all facets of this experience.

3. In psychiatric/mental health nursing the interpersonal relationship of the client and nurse is the means used to bring about change and growth.

    Clients use the relationship with nurses in many ways: as a reference point to view their own self-worth; as a model for future relationships in which mutual respect predominates; and in a corrective manner, to heal the wounds inflicted by previously damaging relationships with significant others. The primary tool of the nurse is not a stethoscope, a syringe, or monitor; it is the *therapeutic use of the "self."* In this manner, the personal maturity, sensitivity, insights, and capacity for empathy of the nurse enter into the nurse–client relationship. In psychiatric/mental health nursing the growth and change of the client is often based on the growth and maturity of the nurse. The art and science of the use of self in interpersonal relationships with clients is a major focus of this text.

4. The recipient of care is not only the individual client, but the "family, social group and/or community in which the client interacts."[2]

    It is not possible to conceive of clients in isolation from their families, and social and cultural contexts. In truth, interventions intended for the client can have beneficial consequences for others. The nurse must simultaneously consider both the client and the client's living group(s).

The Therapeutic Use of Self: A Way of Looking at Psychiatric/ Mental Health Nursing

A current research study will be used to introduce the idea of the therapeutic use of self—an important concept in this text. This research,[6,7] done in Vermont, studied 269 clients, who in the early 1960s, were labeled "profoundly ill, severely disabled, and long-stay" (schizophrenic). The purpose of the study was to determine their current status. The research is the longest and best-documented study of its kind.

One half to two thirds of the former clients were greatly improved or fully recovered 25 to 32 years after release from the psychiatric hospital. Forty-five percent displayed no psychiatric symptoms at all, and half of these used no medication. Sixty-eight percent of the former schizophrenic clients were socially and psychologically functional.

The researchers stated that the view once held in the mental health sciences that such clients were hopeless is an artifact of old biases. Indeed, the term "chronic" may be a damaging self-fulfilling prophecy. If family members are told to expect little from the clients, and if mental health care staff offer little true treatment for the clients, it is natural for the clients also to adopt a hopeless attitude.

Clients in the Vermont research had been part of an early 1960s study on the effects of a new medication, chlorpromazine, on backward, "hopeless" mental patients. The clients studied were the "failures," or the ones the medication did not help. Of the original 269 subjects, 168 were studied in (or around) 1986. In 1985, the subjects ranged from 38 to 83 years of age.

When asked what had aided them in their recovery they responded that food, clothing, and housing were primary. They had also wanted to know ways to manage their own symptoms, and wanted mental health services graded to their unique needs.

The most important element in recovery, however, was that "someone believed" in them. As stated by one client, "someone thought I could get well."[4] That someone was a nurse.

Nurses assist with or perform many functions with clients. Food, housing, and clothing are important, as are carefully monitored medications. Clients need to understand their symptoms and how they can manage their symptoms. Clients are capable of partial or total self-care when offered the guidance they need.

Yet, there is another important ingredient. Nurses make use of their own attitudes, intellect, emotions, and self-awareness to guide clients to graded steps of competencies. Nurses *approach* clients with an attitude of assisting clients to attain graded levels of intellectual and interpersonal competencies. Nurses do *not* approach clients with the attitude that they are "hopeless" or too severely ill to make use of anything another person could offer. The most important aspects of the nurse's approach to the client are that:

- The nurse believes in the client.
- The client perceives the nurse's belief.
- The nurse's gestures of respect and verbal assistance offered through the nurse–client interviews encourage the client to sustain the movement toward health and to achieve interpersonal and intellectual competencies.

The above description is the core of what is termed the nurse's *therapeutic use of self.* Most of this text is concerned with describing the therapeutic use of self as

nurses work with the unique aspects of clients to assist in their growth.

While it may not be apparent to a beginning clinician, the exact nature of the nurse–client interchange is purposeful. Nurses use a frame of reference or theory in their approach with clients. Though the issues with psychiatric clients are in many instances emotional, nurses apply professional practice skills to maintain a focus on clients' growth, not merely on their emotions. This type of caring provides an interpersonal environment for clients to attain competency rather than dependence and enmeshment with a professional person, who will not always be a part of the client's life.

In order to bring about an effective therapeutic use of self, nurses use their skills to recognize clients' patterns of behavior that need attention; select the interventions that are most conducive to fostering changes in these patterns; communicate; express themselves competently to clients; demonstrate interpersonal and intellectual astuteness; assist clients in reordering perceptions; offer sustained interventions over time to effect change in long-standing problems. The psychiatric nurse performs these skills with precision and certainty.

The quote by Hildegard Peplau in the beginning of this text highlights several aspects of the practice of psychiatric/mental health nursing. "The skills of psychiatric nurses merit celebration. They have been honed over centuries of development. . . . Psychiatric nurses (today) have a remarkable opportunity to use their skills to provide a separate and/or complementary alternative form of treatment for psychiatric patients."[9]

The skills of psychiatric/mental health nurses are outstanding. Many psychiatric/mental health nurses know the sense of pride and heightened comradeship that comes from working well with clients. Such skills in psychiatric nursing care have been "honed over centuries of development." Peplau, the founder of psychiatric/mental health nursing, has examined the skills of the psychiatric nurse in the therapeutic use of self with clients.

Peplau stated that the skills of psychiatric/mental health nurses are needed now more than ever. "Mental health problems seem to be increasing in scope, kinds, and numbers." Skills, in this sense, are defined as "having a learned power of doing a thing completely: a developed or acquired aptitude or ability. Skill performance is done with knowledge; practice, and an examination of the effect of that practice; aptitude; understanding; and discernment."[9]

Peplau stated that "nursing is a service for people that enhances healing and health by methods that are humanistic and primarily non-invasive."[9] This value is being put to the test. "With the increasing biomedicalization of psychiatry, psychiatric nurses have a remarkable opportunity to use their skills to provide a separate and/or complementary alternative form of treatment for psychiatric patients."[9] In other words, psychiatric nurses can bring to fruition the use of their refined skills in mental health/illness care. They can exert their separateness and complementarity with psychiatry and other disciplines to achieve greater access to clients who need their care.

Although the therapeutic use of self is a core process

in psychiatric/mental health nursing, it does not describe all that a nurse needs to know in order to guide clients with psychological problems. Hence, this text covers a number of additional constructs to provide nurse clinicians with a foundation of understanding of the field of psychiatric/mental health nursing.

Levels of Prevention

While this text considers caring for ill individuals, it also discusses the *prevention* of psychological illness. Psychiatric/mental health nursing focuses on the *health–illness continuum*. Caplan[5] has addressed the continuum in his work on the levels of prevention.

The *primary level* is prevention of health problems. The psychiatric/mental health nurse acts to promote wellness and to provide individuals with internal and external resources in order to stay well. For example, a nurse may meet with a family with a member who has been admitted to a psychiatric hospital. Such a meeting can offer the family an opportunity to ask questions about mental illness and what can be expected, thereby lessening family stress.

The nurse works at the *secondary level* of prevention by doing early case finding and prompt referral and treatment. Finding cases of potential child abuse in families at risk is an example of where nurses can function to protect children and their families from developing injurious patterns.

The *tertiary level* of prevention involves restoring ill people to their maximum level of functioning. The focus of this level is on the scientific principles that guide psychiatric/mental health nursing interventions and are used with clients who have psychological problems or conflicts.

Across all levels of prevention nurses must know what constitutes mental health and mental illness. The difficulties inherent in defining mental health have led to ambiguity. Because of these difficulties, the definition of mental health and illness has been a professional and political battleground.

One significant attempt to define mental health and mental illness was made by the President's Commission on Mental Health. Aware of the many controversies that surround a definition, and in an attempt to unify diverse forces, the Commission adopted a broad definition of mental health. Acknowledging the mental and emotional impact of problems such as alcoholism, drug abuse, child abuse, learning disabilities, mental retardation, and physical handicaps, the commission reported:

> America's mental health problems cannot be defined only in terms of disabling mental illnesses and identified psychiatric disorders. They must include the damage to mental health associated with unrelenting poverty and unemployment and the institutionalized discrimination that occurs on the basis of race, sex, class, age, and mental or physical handicaps. . . . It is not to suggest that those working in the mental health field can resolve far-reaching social issues. We are firmly convinced,

however, that mental health services cannot adequately respond to the needs of the citizens of this country unless those involved in the planning, organization, and delivery of those services fully recognize the harmful effect that a variety of social, environmental, physical, psychological, and biological factors can have on the ability of individuals to function in society, develop a sense of their own worth, and maintain a strong and purposeful self-image.[10]

The definition provided by the President's commission reflects the attitude of the general population. People expect and want to be able to achieve freedom from undue stress and worry, an ability to function in their customary roles, and a sense of well-being and happiness. Combining these ideas, mental health can be defined as a state of well-being in which a person is able to function comfortably within society, and in which personal achievements and characteristics are satisfying.

The absence of health could designate a less than optimal state and/or the presence of mental illness. Like mental health, mental illness can be a difficult concept to define. DSM-III-R addresses the difficulty in defining mental illness and mental disorder. Essentially, the DSM-III-R provides a system of diagnosis based upon statistically significant symptom clusters. Major depression, for example, is said to consist of a specific group of symptoms that include changes in sleeping and eating (weight loss), ability to concentrate, and suicidal ideation. However, definitive guidelines for what constitutes an illness or a disease process are still somewhat elusive. The manual reports that there is no satisfactory definition that specifies precise boundaries for the concept "mental disorder." This is also true for concepts such as physical disorder and mental and physical health. Nevertheless, it is important to understand the many phenomena that, when viewed together, represent the essence of disorder and dysfunction by the consensus of the psychiatric–mental health profession.

Mental disorder as defined by the DSM-III-R is "a clinically significant behavioral or psychological syndrome or pattern that occurs in a person and that is associated with present distress (a painful symptom) or disability (impairment in one or more important areas of functioning) or with a significantly increased risk of suffering death, pain, disability, or an important loss of freedom."[3] This syndrome, in order to be considered a mental illness, must not be an "expectable response to a particular event" (such as the death of a spouse). Deviant behavior (legal, sexual, or religious, or conflicts between an individual and society) is also not considered a mental illness.

Psychiatric disorders, or mental illness, include all of the behavioral or psychological syndromes or patterns listed in the DSM-III-R. The DSM-III-R framework for viewing mental illness is referred to as an absolute paradigm of mental functioning. That is to say, the framework defines when illness is present or absent. With the exception of "hard-and-fast" medical models, most current mental illness theories are based on the recognition of two important phenomena: (1) mental health and mental illness are dynamic processes that can be charted along a

A CONCEPTUAL FRAMEWORK FOR THE PRACTICE OF PSYCHIATRIC/MENTAL HEALTH NURSING*

The Client comes to the nurse–client relationship with:

1. System components, including
   a. A level of psychological functioning
   b. A level of biological functioning
   c. A societal background (family)
   d. A cultural background (beliefs)
   e. An environment in which the client lives
2. Responses to being ill
3. Responses to stress

   In the *Nurse–Client Relationship* the client receives respect, caring, and professional guidance to achieve an increased sense of well-being.

The Nurse comes to the nurse–client relationship with:

1. An awareness of self
2. An understanding of
   a. The therapeutic use of self
   b. Different modalities of care (individual, family, group, milieu)
   c. Different settings of care (inpatient, home care, community)
   d. Nursing management and leadership
   e. Communication
   f. The nursing process
   g. Levels of prevention
   h. Theories of psychological development and illness
   i. Societal impingements on the nurse's role
   j. Legal and ethical issues
   k. Research in the field

   * All concepts mentioned in this box are represented by chapters or parts of chapters in this text.

continuum, and (2) the label "mental illness" is highly contingent upon societal prescriptions and the perceptions of those assigned to judge the presence of illness and health.

It is hoped that this brief introduction will direct the student in a beginning exploration of the key issues that influence nursing practice in the psychiatric/mental health nursing field. The accompanying box summarizes the elements of the conceptual framework used in this text.

References

1. American Nurses' Association: Taxonomy for the Classification of Human Responses of Concern for Psychiatric/Mental Health Nursing. Kansas City, American Nurses' Association, 1986
2. American Nurses' Association Division on Psychiatric and Mental Health Nursing Practice: Statement on Psychiatric and Mental Health Nursing Practice. Kansas City, American Nurses' Association, 1982
3. American Psychiatric Association: Diagnostic and Statistical Manual III-R. Washington, D.C., American Psychiatric Association, 1987
4. Brain/Mind Bulletin: Chronic-Schizophrenia Label a Self-Fulfilling Prophecy? 13:6, 1988
5. Caplan G: Principles of Preventive Psychiatry. New York, Basic Books, 1964
6. Harding C, Brooks G, Ashikaga T, et al: The Vermont Longitudinal Study of Persons with Severe Mental Illness, I: Methodology, Study Sample, and Overall Status 32 Years Later. Am J Psychiatry 144:718, 1987
7. Harding C, Brooks G, Ashikaga T, et al: The Vermont Longitudinal Study of Persons with Severe Mental Illness, II: Long-Term Outcome of Subjects Who Retrospectively Met DSM-III Criteria for Schizophrenia. Am J Psychiatry 144:727, 1987
8. Kim M, McFarland G, McLane S: Classification of Nursing Diagnoses: Proceedings of the Fifth National Conference. St. Louis, C. V. Mosby, 1984
9. Peplau H. Tomorrow's world. Nursing Times 83:29, 1987
10. President's Commission on Mental Health: Final Report. Washington, D.C., U.S. Government Printing Office, 1978

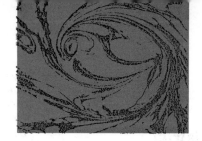

CONTENTS

PSYCHIATRIC/ MENTAL HEALTH NURSING

The Therapeutic Use of Self

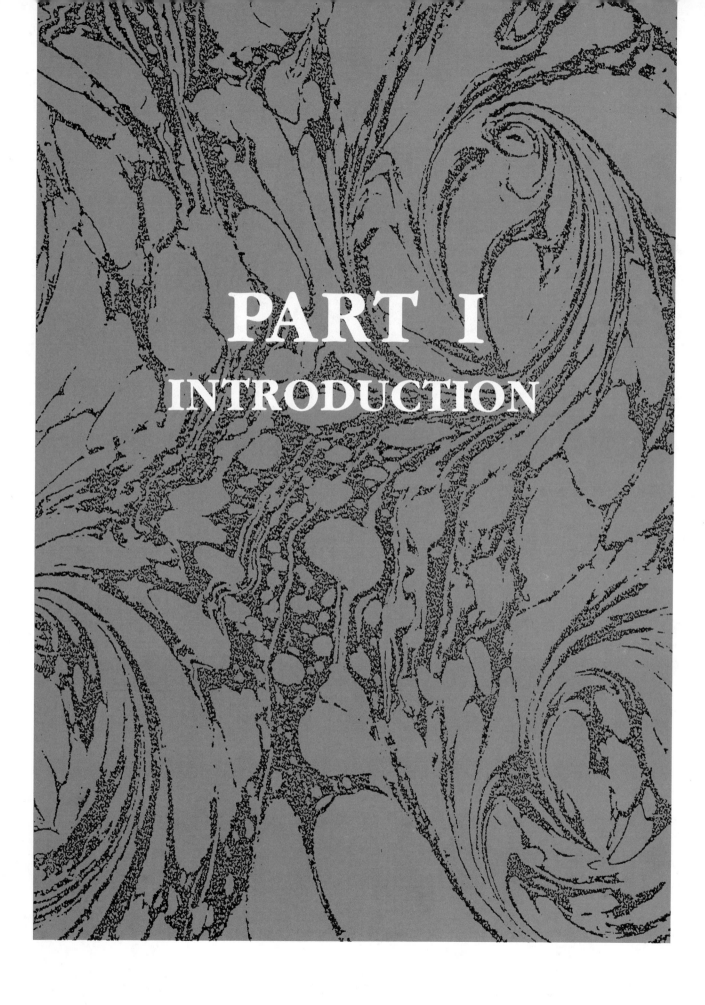

PART I
INTRODUCTION

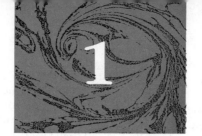

IRA TRAIL ADAMS

THE EVOLUTION OF PSYCHIATRIC/MENTAL HEALTH NURSING

Learning Objectives

Upon completion of this chapter the student should be able to do the following:
1. Identify key historical developments in psychiatric/mental health nursing practice.
2. Compare and contrast the development of psychiatric/mental health nursing and the development of psychiatry in general.
3. Describe how nursing education and research have affected the roles and functions of the psychiatric/mental health nurse.
4. Identify major events in the evolution of specialization in psychiatric nursing practice.
5. Identify two ways in which the role of the psychiatric/mental health nurse has been expanded to include more autonomous yet collaborative aspects.

Introduction

In the last 50 years, conditions and treatment in the management of mental disorders have changed radically. Psychiatric/mental health nursing has been profoundly influenced by these changes, as well as by education and research. For decades, psychiatric/mental health nurses have given primary care in hospitals, clinics, and private practice. Today other roles have emerged in family practice and community mental health centers. A historical perspective on the development of psychiatric/mental health nursing and treatment of mental illness can increase understanding of psychiatric/mental health nursing today. Table 1-1 highlights many important events in mental health/illness care.

The Birth of Modern Psychiatric Treatment

During the 18th century, mentally ill people were shackled in "mad-houses." These individuals were thought to be "hopelessly insane," "dangerous," or "possessed by demons." They were isolated, chained, beaten, and frightened by methods thought to "bring them to their senses." Bedlam Hospital (as it was commonly known) in London was a typical institution. Patients in these institutions were thought to be devoid of human feeling, and their management was indifferent, if not brutal.

The birth of modern psychiatry may be traced to Philippe Pinel (1745–1826), who was appointed Physician in Chief of Bicetre Hospital for the Insane in Paris. Dr. Pinel removed the chains from the inmates, and the era of humane treatment began. Jean-Etienne Esquirol (1772–1826), a student of Pinel, established that there is an emotional basis for psychiatric disturbances. Several years later, Benjamin Rush (1745–1813) published the first textbook of psychiatry in the United States. An attempt to label disturbances occurred when Benedict-Augustin Morel (1809–1873) labeled schizophrenia "dementia praecox;" Ewald Hecker (1843–1909) identified a disturbance as "hebephrenia;" and Karl Kahlbaum (1828–1899) called another "catatonia." These physicians opened the way for Emil Kraepelin (1856–1926) to formulate an elaborate system of psychiatric classification that is still in use. Eugen Bleuler (1857–1930) described the symptoms of schizophrenia as "autism, apathy, ambivalence, and associative looseness." During this era of descriptive psychiatry, however, few contributions to treatment emerged. Care for the mentally ill continued to be more custodial than therapeutic.

Despite the progress being made in the diagnosis and symptomatic descriptions of mentally ill people and their behavior, more than half a century passed in the United States before Dorothea Dix (1802–1887) began her personal crusade for change in the 1840s. Dix, a retired schoolteacher, became shocked at what she saw in the care of the mentally ill. Patients were locked up in filthy cells and often neglected. Dix's activities in the United States, Canada, and Europe, through various government agencies, led to widespread reforms. In this country, 20 states built or enlarged mental hospitals as a result of her efforts. Although these pioneering humanitarian efforts improved conditions for patients, state-supported facilities were built far from families and friends. The mental hospitals were kept from public scrutiny, and patients were often victims of maltreatment and neglect.[17,19]

Beginning Education for the Psychiatric Nurse

Education for psychiatric nurses in the United States began in 1882 when the first school of nursing specifically for the care of the mentally ill opened at McLean Hospital, a private psychiatric hospital in Belmont, Massachusetts. Influencing this development was Linda Richards (1841–1930), who is considered America's first trained nurse. Richards graduated in 1873 from a one-year program at New England's Hospital for Women and Children. After graduation, she went to England to study the methods of Florence Nightingale. Nursing for the physically and mentally ill was based on Nightingale's "sanitary principles." Nightingale was concerned with crowded conditions in the big cities, poverty, filth, infectious diseases, and high infant mortality rates. On returning to the United States, Richards organized nursing service and nursing education programs at Boston City Hospital and at McLean Hospital. These were two-year programs. Using trained nurses was accepted as an economical way to staff hospitals, clean them up, make them safe for mentally ill people, and at the same time provide free, apprentice-type "training" for young women in a safe, supervised environment. This was a period of custodial care for the mentally ill. Based on Nightingale's sanitary principles for the physically ill, the primary emphases for the mentally ill were on clean wards, personal hygiene, fresh air, exercise, adequate food, sleep, and kindness to the patient.

As mental hospitals became overcrowded, it became evident to the medical staff that the "trained" nurses' skills needed to be used for other than menial tasks. Administrative psychiatrists, who were considered superintendents of psychiatric hospitals, relieved the nurses of the menial tasks to assist doctors in what were considered more therapeutic measures. Psychiatric aides were hired to do many of the housekeeping tasks of the nurses.[25] Santos and Stainbrook (1949) have stated that by the end of the century the therapeutic nature of the role of the psychiatric nurse was in place. Psychiatric nurses' duties included assisting physicians with procedures such as administering sedative drugs and carrying out hydrotherapeutic measures such as wet sheet packs, hot and cold douches, and showers. While these duties upgraded the status of the "trained" nurse, the primary emphasis of nursing care continued to be on the general physical needs of the patient. The only psychological skill used

TABLE 1-1.
TIMELINE: IMPORTANT LANDMARKS IN THE EVOLUTION OF MODERN PSYCHIATRIC TREATMENT
AND PSYCHIATRIC/MENTAL HEALTH NURSING PRACTICE

DATE	EVENT
1700	St. Mary of Bethlehem (Bedlam) Hospital, London, where the mentally ill were cruelly treated, was founded.
1795	Philippe Pinel began humane treatment of the mentally ill.
1800	Esquirol proposed an emotional basis for mental illness.
	Rush published the first textbook in psychiatry in the U.S.
1850	Social reformers and nurses, such as Dix, Richards, and Nightingale, improved the treatment of clients.
1830 to 1930	Psychiatric disturbances were labeled by Morel, Kraepelin, Bleuler, and others.
1882	McLean Hospital opened the first school of nursing for psychiatric nurses.
1893 to present	The science of mental health/illness was expanded by:
	Charcot (the first modern physician to make a serious attempt to treat emotional disorders)
	Freud (developed ideas of the unconscious and the tripartite view of the psyche)
	Jung (developed ideas concerning the collective unconscious)
	Rogers, Carl (developed a humanistically-oriented psychotherapy approach)
	Sullivan, Harry S. (began the interpersonal school of psychiatry)
	Kohut, Heinz (began the self-psychology school of thought)
	Davanloo, H. (developed a dynamic short-term psychotherapy approach)
1910 to 1960	Literary works raised public consciousness of the needs of the mentally ill:
	A Mind that Found Itself[4]
	The Snake Pit[30]
	The Shame of the States[7]
	I Never Promised You a Rose Garden[10]
	One Flew Over The Cuckoo's Next[15]
1949	The National Institute of Mental Health (NIMH) was established
1930 to present	Somatotherapies were developed:
	Psychiatric medications (*e.g.,* tranquilizers)
	Electroshock therapy
1960 to present	Genetic/biological studies of the occurrence of mental illness were carried out.
1950 to present	Psychiatric/mental health nurses developed clinical approaches:
	Hildegard Peplau
	Dorothy Gregg
	Gwen Tudor
1950 to present	Psychiatric/mental health nurses developed clinical research.
1950	Milieu therapy fostered client care.
1952	The National League for Nursing developed curriculum guides for psychiatric nursing education.
1960	NIMH funds became available to nurses for special training in psychiatric/mental health nursing.
1965	Legislation was passed supporting development of community mental health (CMH) centers and clinical specialty roles at the graduate level.
1970	Private practice alternatives for the clinical nurse specialist (CNS) developed.
1980	Certification of psychiatric nurse generalists and clinical specialists began.
	New programs for the homeless mentally ill, child psychiatric nursing, geriatric psychiatry, and alcohol and drug abuse developed.
1986	The taxonomy of diagnoses for psychiatric/mental health nursing by the American Nurses' Association was released.
1987	The American Psychiatric Nursing Association was formed.

by the nurse was that of maintaining a kind, tolerant, humane attitude toward the patient.[25]

The Emergence of Psychotherapeutic Approaches

In 1908, Clifford Beers, a former mental patient, published *A Mind That Found Itself,*[4] a book that gave an account of what he had endured as a mental patient. This book aroused considerable public concern; subsequently, with the support of many prominent people, Beers organized the Connecticut Society for Mental Hygiene. Less than a year later, Beers organized the Committee for Mental Hygiene in New York City and was instrumental in organizing the National Association for Mental Health in 1909.

By the time Beers began his public agitation, a new scientific psychology, *dynamic psychiatry,* was emerging. This concept revealed some of the mechanisms by which forces within the environment were thought to have an effect on individual behavior and adjustment. Sig-

SOCIETY'S EVOLVING IDEA OF THE MENTALLY ILL

DATE	IDEA
18th century	The mentally ill are dangerous and should be shut away.
19th century	The mentally ill deserve to be treated as "human."
	They have identifiable problems.
	They should be kept away from others.
	They can be neglected.
20th century	The mentally ill are not to be "warehoused." Some can be neglected.
	They can be placed in physical closeness to others.
	They may be emotionally distant from others because of the stigma of mental illness or because of the client's own fears/anxieties about personal closeness.
	Many can get assistance for food, clothing, and shelter in the mental health care system.
	Some seem to be unreachable, but require sophisticated care, available to only a few.

mund Freud (1856–1939) initiated the concept of psychoanalysis. The concept emphasized internal drives as major determinants of psychiatric symptoms, and led to increasing awareness of the *unconscious* and *defense mechanisms* as primary factors in the development of mental disorders. It can be said that psychoanalysis was born when Freud learned about posthypnotic suggestions from Jean-Martin Charcot (1825–1893) and about the *talking cure* (free association), transference, and catharsis from Joseph Breuer (1842–1925). With the advent of psychoanalysis, the transition from physiogenic to psychogenic explanation of mental problems was enhanced.

From the early 1900s to 1950, there was a burst of activity that culminated in new and innovative approaches to the treatment of the mentally ill. Those who figured prominently in the field were Carl Jung (1875–1961), who highlighted unconscious processes common to all people; Alfred Adler (1870–1937), who emphasized individual psychology (the drive for superiority vs the feeling of community); and Harry Stack Sullivan (1892–1949), who emphasized the ways in which interpersonal relationships affect one's sense of security or anxiety.

Other theorists formed the *third force* in psychology, so called because they discussed ideas not included in either behaviorism or psychoanalysis. Abraham Maslow (1908–1970), for example, described the individual as involved in meeting needs that are arranged hierarchically, ranging from lower needs for food and shelter to higher needs for self-actualization.

Carl Rogers (1902–1987), another third-force clinician/theorist, described the person as capable of valuing or of deciding questions of belief by the self. Rogers also emphasized the need to be aware of one's feelings and to seek a sense of genuineness about one's self.

Dynamic psychiatry evolved as a plan of one-to-one communication between the psychiatrist and the patient. Concepts such as infantile sexuality, the Oedipal complex, and the origin of anal aggressive behavior shocked lay people and professionals alike. In the beginning, psychoanalytic treatment took place in the private offices of psychiatrists, but it soon became the treatment mode in private mental hospitals and eventually in large public mental hospitals. Psychoanalytic theory became part of the curriculum in medical schools and teaching hospitals.

Important steps in the treatment of mental disorders were *somatic therapies*. The use of these medical treatments met with wide acceptance in the 1930s. They included deep sleep therapy (1930), insulin shock therapy (1935), Metrazol shock therapy (1935), electroshock therapy (1937), and psychosurgery (1935–1936). In addition, sedation was used to reduce subjective distress, and tranquilizers were used to reduce anxiety and tension. Antidepressant, antiexcitement, and antihallucinatory preparations were introduced. Soon came the unanticipated conclusion that somatotherapy did not cure mental disorders, but rather made patients more amenable to and accessible for psychotherapy. Psychotherapy was used to reinforce somatotherapy.[14]

The Beginning of the Role of Psychiatric Nurses

During the era of psychoanalysis (dynamic psychiatry), there appeared to be no role for the nurse. The one-to-one relationship between psychiatrist and patient was tightly maintained, and the psychiatrist guarded this relationship. Nurses working in mental institutions soon recognized both their limitation in caring for psychiatric patients and the need for theoretical concepts on which to base nursing practice.

A major step in psychiatric nursing education came in 1893, when the American Society of Superintendents of Training Schools for Nurses in the United States and Canada was formed. Its purpose was to standardize and improve education for nurses. In 1912, the organization's name was changed to the National League for Nursing Education. Originally planned for nurses only, the organization changed its policies to include lay members, and by 1952 had changed its name to the National League for Nursing (NLN). The organization issued curriculum guides for schools of nursing that included courses in psychiatric nursing.

During the next 20 years, following the emergence of curricula designed by the NLN, several plans were developed to educate nurses to care for the mentally ill. These plans included giving weekly courses in proce-

THE EVOLUTION OF PSYCHIATRIC/
MENTAL HEALTH NURSING

DATE	EVENT
19th to early 20th centuries	Psychiatric/mental health (P/MH) nursing was focused on a clean, safe environment for the mentally ill. Clients received kindness and adequate food.
Middle 20th century	Nurses were educated in the scientific principles of mental illness. P/MH nurses perceived themselves as having an active role in their interpersonal work with clients to promote the client's recovery.
Late 20th century	Research in the role of P/MH nursing by nurses fosters the nurse's role. P/MH nurses have a primary role in mental health care. Hildegard Peplau develops the first substantial theory for use by P/MH nurses. P/MH nurses receive Master's and doctoral degrees in their specialty.
Early 21st century (the future)	P/MH nurses in private practice gain admitting privileges to psychiatric hospitals. Increased numbers of P/MH nurses serve as program administrators. Increased numbers of P/MH nurses work in organizations providing mental health care in the home. Additional substantive theories are developed for application to P/MH nursing. Greater emphasis on the clients' spiritual belief systems becomes a part of care. More clinical emphasis is placed on practice in the community with groups of individuals who share the same living space. Increased research is done in the practice of P/MH nursing, especially in the areas of mental *health*, and *all* aspects of the person as a system (societal, environmental, psychological, etc.). Greater emphasis is placed on women's oppression (family violence, incest, rape). Political influence increases toward improving working conditions for nurses. Involvement of P/MH nursing in substance abuse treatment increases. There is increased specialization within P/MH nursing. The development of the taxonomy of P/MH nursing diagnoses continues. The American Psychiatric Nurses' Association (founded in 1987) has a significant impact on P/MH nursing.

dures for using somatic therapy, and building knowledge of such concepts as conflict, normal and abnormal behavior, and mental mechanisms. By 1910, nursing educators recognized the need to extend training beyond the narrow specialization of the psychiatric and general hospitals. Affiliations were established whereby nurses in training programs in psychiatric hospitals spent at least two months in general hospitals and nurses in training programs in general hospitals spent two months in psychiatric hospitals. In addition, many psychiatric hospitals offered postgraduate study for nurses who had completed their training but were interested in acquiring knowledge and skills in the nursing of people with mental disorders. By 1934, psychiatric nursing information and skills had become a standard part of nursing programs.[11]

National Recognition of Mental Illness as a Problem

World War II and the problems of returning veterans stimulated further public interest in mental illness, which became recognized as a national problem.

The mass media became interested and a number of exposés swept the United States and Canada, such as Albert Deutsch's *The Shame of the States*[7] (1948) and Jan Ward's *The Snake Pit*[30] (1946). Newspapers and popular journals continued to write articles about psychiatric institutions and treatments, decrying the inhumane conditions and procedures.

Since the founding of the United Nations in 1945, the concept of mental health has achieved international recognition. The constitution of the World Health Organization (WHO) defined *health* as a state of complete physical, mental, and social well-being, and not merely the absence of disease or infirmity. The term *mental health* was seen as representing a variety of human aspirations: prevention of mental disorder, rehabilitation of the mentally disturbed, reduction of tension, and attainment of a state of well-being in which the individual functions at a level consistent with mental and physical potentials. At the same time, the role of nursing evolved from that of custodian, apprentice, and keeper to that of psychiatric nurse. An increasing awareness of the extent of mental illness as a national health problem has focused on the magnitude of the emotional needs of all people and the obligation of all health workers to understand human behavior.[19]

National Institute of Mental Health and Nursing Education

The National Mental Health Act, passed by Congress in 1946, made possible the creation of the National Institute of Mental Health (NIMH) in 1949 within the Department of Health, Education, and Welfare (now called the Department of Health and Human Services). State hospitals received increased budgets, and significant federal funds were made available for research, training, and facilities. NIMH is the major funding resource in the U.S. for applied research in mental health and the behavioral sciences, for demonstration projects, and for the training of mental health professionals. Through funds from NIMH, psychiatric nursing was able to develop as a discipline in accredited college and university programs at both undergraduate and graduate levels.

When NIMH funds were made available for training professional psychiatric personnel, nursing education took advantage of this opportunity to prepare psychiatric nursing teachers and to integrate psychiatric nursing principles into school curricula. These funds allowed nursing students to acquire the knowledge and skills necessary to meet the psychological needs of patients in psychiatric units and hospitals, in general hospitals, and in community agencies. Psychiatric nursing principles began to be applied to patients of all ages throughout the students' education.

Collegiate schools responded to the challenge. Most noteworthy was the experiment at Skidmore College.[26] The purpose of this study was to investigate and demonstrate how the nursing department's resources could be used to foster students' awareness of psychiatric concepts and techniques, and to help students apply them to the nursing care of all patients. The integration of psychiatric nursing principles and concepts into medical/surgical nursing care enhanced the role of the psychiatric nurse. Stress and anxiety, sensory overload, and sensory deprivation are but a few of the concepts that psychiatric nurses have taught other nurses in general practice to understand as they cared for patients with acute and chronic illnesses.

The Contribution of the Behavioral Sciences to Psychiatric Nursing Theory

The increasing recognition by psychiatric nursing educators of a need for a conceptual and theoretical framework on which to base practice prompted an interest in the behavioral sciences as disciplines from which roles and functions for psychiatric nurses could be brought into focus. The disciplines of psychology, sociology, and anthropology were chosen as foundations for psychiatric nursing practice. Empirical investigations by these behavioral sciences into human personality, behavior, and identification of individuals as unique "systems", capable of influencing their own perceptions of health and illness, assisted psychiatric nursing in developing guidelines for psychiatric nursing practice.

Perhaps the most influential nurse educator to define a conceptual framework for psychiatric nursing practice is Hildegard Peplau (born in 1909). Peplau's work involves two basic assumptions: (1) the nurse's behavior makes a substantial difference in what clients learn as they are nursed through their experiences, and (2) it is the function of nursing and nursing education to foster personality development in the direction of maturity. Peplau emphasizes the need for improved interpersonal relations skills—the nurse must be able to observe keenly what goes on in the life of a client and respond expertly.[22]

Gwen Tudor also contributed to the advance of psychiatric nursing by describing the use of *nurse–patient* or *nurse–client relationship* therapy. Tudor demonstrated the value of the nurse's acceptance, instead of condemnation or rejection, of the patient's behavior. When the nurse shows acceptance, more therapeutic measures can be instituted. Since the publication of Tudor's paper, many articles have appeared in the literature describing this kind of therapy.[28]

Nurse–client relationship therapy became as accepted in psychiatric nursing as the psychoanalytic doctor–patient relationship was accepted in psychiatry. Psychiatric nurses now had a professional role in which they assisted clients in their social interactions with others. The nurses' acceptance of the clients' strengths and weaknesses helped in the development of the clients' potential for more effective patterns of behavior with others.[14]

Psychiatrists accepted this role for nursing care of the patient, and began to confer with the nurse as a member of the treatment team. The roles of psychiatrist and nurse complement each other because both professionals use their particular form of knowledge and skills in the care of the client.

The Therapeutic Community as the Cultural Norm in the Psychiatric Ward

Because of the shortage of personnel and the increased client population in psychiatric hospitals, a new method for dealing with patients' behavioral problems was proposed by Jones in 1953. Jones viewed the "therapeutic community" as a favorable environment in which treatment could take place. He saw this as essential to attaining successful outcomes.[13] He determined that all personnel (*e.g.,* doctors, nurses, aides, housekeepers) were responsible for interactions in a healthy community life. The "health" and cultural norm of the community (psychiatric ward or unit) were the responsibility of all staff. Limits were set to protect the community from antisocial people. In short, normalcy was the frame of reference for interactions.

The psychiatric nurse in this community served as the *clarifier* and *interpreter* of the norms for both clients and staff, and assisted in transmitting the hospital culture to them. The resulting healthy environment produced a stable, secure, and friendly community in which treatment could take place and clients would improve in their functioning.

The Psychiatric Nurse Clinical Specialist

The next important event in the development of psychiatric/mental health nursing was the initiation of clinical specialist programs. NIMH funds were used to develop graduate programs in psychiatric nursing at major colleges and universities in the United States. With these funds, traineeships and stipends enabled nurses to devote full-time efforts to education and training. Professionals emerged from these programs with more advanced knowledge and skills. Graduate programs began to require a thesis, so these nurses were able to test principles and concepts related to understanding human behavior and to develop theories on which to base their practice. In addition, these students received preparation as teachers, consultants, and administrators in psychiatric nursing. This resulted in a new level of nursing, at which nurses could respond to the research, teaching, consulting, administrative, and clinical skill needs of psychiatric nursing.[5]

Because baccalaureate-prepared nurses are generalists, the need for advanced specialization in psychiatric nursing was met by graduate education at the master's degree level. The unique expertise required of the nurse in a psychiatric setting is considered the source of the impetus for developing the nurse *clinical specialist* role. The formalization of the clinical specialist role occurred in May 1958, when the Western Council on Higher Education in Nursing (WCHEN) delineated the clinical content necessary to be taught at the master's degree level. The primary role of the psychiatric nurse clinical specialist was defined as carrying out psychotherapy utilizing nurse–client relationship therapy in the care of the mentally ill client. A group of psychiatric nursing faculty headed by Fujiki (1969) stated that additional nursing roles included the application of relevant theories as a basis for clinical practice, the acquisition of clinical expertise before teaching or supervising others, and the ability to apply psychiatric nursing concepts and principles in any setting in which psychiatric services are needed.[9]

The norm for preparation of the psychiatric nurse clinical specialist became the development of knowledge about, and skills in therapeutic interventions with individuals, groups and families, the ability to utilize interpersonal relationships through understanding of clients' problems, the ability to teach and supervise other nursing personnel, and the ability to create and maintain a nurse-client relationship. In addition, skills in clinical research for the improvement of nursing interventions were required of the clinical specialist.

Practice Areas Within Psychiatric/Mental Health Nursing

Today there are many potential practice areas for the psychiatric/mental health nurse. Psychiatric nurses practice in a wide variety of settings. While some settings are in traditional hospitals, others are found in the community, schools, and workplace. Some of the roles more frequently found are described here.

The Child Psychiatric Nurse

The child psychiatric nurse assists emotionally disturbed children, usually in a residential treatment center. The nurse's role was initially that of surrogate mother in a therapeutic, nonthreatening environment in which psychotherapy takes place. Setting limits appropriate to the age of the child, participating as a member of the treatment team, and assisting in interpersonal relationship therapy were, and remain, a part of the nursing role. The nurse generalist and the clinical specialist in child psychiatric nursing work on child psychiatric units. The clinical specialist usually has the advanced role of coordinating the clinical program or clinical supervision. The role of the psychiatric nurse working with children is further discussed in Chapters 22 and 23.

The Geriatric Psychiatric Nurse

The geriatric psychiatric nurse works with the elderly, usually by providing supportive therapy in multiservice community centers or in homes for the elderly. The goal is to enhance self-esteem, self-confidence, and emotional security during old age. The aim of therapy is to support the individual's strengths and reinforce the client's beliefs in internal resources. As in the case of the child psychiatric nurse, the clinical specialist working with the older adult typically performs a clinical management role. Home care programs, however, employ the generalist nurse prepared at the baccalaureate level to administer psychiatric care for the home-bound client. Chapter 26 explores the specific nursing roles used in working with the elderly.

The Psychiatric Nurse as a Consultation/Liaison Nurse

The consultation/liaison nurse works both with clients having illnesses derived from an emotional cause and those who have physical ailments that carry emotional consequences. Emotions and personality maladjustments can produce physiological dysfunction that can be seen occasionally in health problems such as hypertension, ulcerative colitis, and bronchial asthma. Formerly called *psychosomatic illnesses* (a term that is now in disfavor),[18] these problems appear to stem, in part, from some emotional influence. Similarly, physical problems can have emotional consequences. For example, viral infections can produce some level of depression, clients may have difficulty adjusting to changes in body image following surgery, or the threat of impending death can result in normal or abnormal grief responses.

Psychiatric liaison nurses can serve as consultants to nurses working in hospitals for clients with medical problems. Psychiatric nursing concepts can help other nurses to assess the meaning to the client of the illness, and to change the attitudes of nurses in caring for clients who suffer from physiological conditions with strong emotional consequences. The psychiatric consultation/liaison nurse is based in a medical hospital and, because of the complex nature of the role, usually has a master's degree as a clinical specialist. The role of the psychiatric/liaison nurse is further discussed in Chapter 31.

The Psychiatric Nurse in Suicide Prevention

Due to the large number of suicides in California, Farberow and Schneidman developed suicide prevention centers there in 1958.[8] Suicide continues to be a national problem.

Psychiatric nurses work in these centers dealing with people *at risk*. They assess the call from the potentially suicidal person, establish rapport, evaluate the potential for actual carry-out of the threat, and decide on a course of action. The purpose is to prevent the suicide until someone can arrive at the scene. Referrals are usually made to general hospitals, nurse psychotherapists, physicians, psychiatrists, clergy, or other community agencies. Follow-up is essential to the success of these programs. Presently there are suicide prevention centers in various areas of the country.

The Psychiatric Nurse in Crisis Intervention

The aim of the nurse in crisis intervention is to provide intensive, short-term intervention to assist clients in resolving immediate problems. The psychiatric nurse is especially well-equipped to deal with clients with a problem-oriented focus. The nurse assesses the situation, identifies the precipitating event, and determines why existing coping mechanisms are no longer sufficient for the client. The nurse then helps the client use alternate coping mechanisms through a better cognitive awareness of the problem, and encourages the individual to express emotions more effectively, thus reducing the tension of the moment.

Crisis intervention provided by health professionals in community mental health centers is widely advocated

as an alternative to longer-term psychiatric inpatient hospitalization.[3] Some crisis units briefly hospitalize the person in crisis (usually for not more than three days), and provide intensive therapy with the client's support system outside the hospital. Both nurse generalists and clinical specialists work with clients in crisis.

Community Mental Health Treatment Facilities

Federal legislation passed in 1963 provided for the establishment of *community mental health centers*.[29] Prior to this, many clients remained in psychiatric hospitals because there were no provisions for treatment in the community. The movement toward deinstitutionalization prompted the establishment of halfway houses, daycare centers, nightcare centers, and community mental health clinics. The use of somatotherapies (*e.g.,* medications) allowed for early discharge from hospitals and made possible aftercare in the community facilities. In addition, two new illnesses were recognized by mental health care providers. Drug addicts and alcoholics were now being treated for their disease rather than being punished for their addictions.

The focus in these centers is prevention and rehabilitation. The aim is to preserve the clients' personal relationships with families and the local community. Successful treatment depends on the support of the client by the family or the person (psychiatrist, nurse, social worker, or psychologist) in the community center. Adequate provision must be made for immediate care in a crisis situation. The emphasis is on the health of the client and returning the client to a productive lifestyle. The nurse doing psychotherapy in such a setting is frequently prepared at the master's degree level.

Despite the trend toward deinstitutionalization and the goal of maintaining the client in the community, recent criticisms point to the inadequacy of this plan. Currently there is much discussion about the need for community mental health centers to meet the demands of the community. Much has been written about the plight of the homeless mentally ill. It appears that in some cases no outreach programs exist to meet the needs of this growing population. The goal of federal and county mental health centers to maximize the health of clients while they reside more comfortably in familiar surroundings is difficult to attain.

Expanding the Role of Psychiatric Nurse to That of Psychiatric/Mental Health Nurse

With the emphasis on community mental health centers, many psychiatric nurses moved from employment in state hospitals to practice in local communities. With this change came the addition of the role of *mental health* (meaning community-focused) nurse to that of *psychiatric* nurse (meaning hospital-based).

It soon became evident that the baccalaureate nurse, prepared as a generalist, was not always prepared for the complexity of care required for nursing in the community. Many public health nurses, prepared at the baccalaureate level, were aware of the need for additional preparation for caring for the emotionally disturbed people in the community. Thus, training of the psychiatric clinical specialist in the knowledge and skills of community organization, community consultation and mental health administration, and social change theory was needed. In addition, psychiatric clinical specialists had to reexamine their own roles and value systems. Moving from a carefully defined structure to a loosely structured community presented many problems for the psychiatric clinical specialist,[27] among which were new-found autonomy and even greater needs for collaboration with the mental health team.

In 1967, the National Institute of Mental Health funded several post-master's degree programs in community mental health nursing to meet these needs. Two of these programs were at the University of Maryland and the Langley Porter Institute at the University of California, San Francisco. The Maimonides Community Mental Health Center training program in New York was developed in 1969, under the tutelage of Florence Williams and Rose Davidites.[6] The curriculum provided students with theory and principles essential for community mental health practice. Content included courses in group and family dynamics, the epidemiology of mental illness, dynamics of human behavior, normal growth and development, social psychology, and role theory. Good clinical supervision and the availability of consultation were also stressed. Using this theoretical background, students were expected to develop skills in community organization assessment, in institutional planning (as community mental health administrators), in mental health consultation, and in decision-making with peers, clients, professionals, and nonprofessional personnel. They served in community groups as leaders and co-leaders, identifying and analyzing psychological, biological, and sociological factors that influence human behavior.[6]

Another important factor in the expansion of the role of the psychiatric/mental health nurse is the concept of the *multidisciplinary team* approach to treatment. In this approach, the care team may be led by any member, rather than strictly by the psychiatrist or physician (as is usually the case in hospitals). Leadership and case management roles are based on individual skills and experience. Further, the same therapist provides, and is responsible for, the total treatment of the client. This primary therapist is responsible for continuity of care in all areas of client need that develop, from diagnosis to rehabilitation.

In this new capacity, the psychiatric/mental health nurse may assume the role of psychotherapist, mental health consultant, mental health community worker, mental health teacher, and/or mental health administra-

tor. The nurse may also supervise nursing students.[31] This expanded role makes the nurse a more autonomous, yet collaborative, practitioner in the mental health care of individuals, families, and community groups. A psychiatric/mental health nursing diagnosis taxonomy[1] has been formulated, which parallels the taxonomy for psychiatric (medical) diagnoses.[2]

The Psychiatric/Mental Health Nurse as Private Practice Clinician

Perhaps the most challenging and most recent expansion of the role of the nurse is in private practice. Individual nurses or groups of nurses have established private caseloads of patients, sometimes in association with physicians, hospitals, and clinics. This expansion of the role represents the highest level of autonomy, authority, and accountability experienced by the psychiatric/mental health nurse to date. Private practice skills include individual, family, and group therapy approaches. Crisis intervention or short-term dynamic psychotherapy orientations are frequently a characteristic of these nurses' practice approaches.

The various roles of the psychiatric nurse described above require a theory base. This body of understanding serves as a guide to enable the nurse to work with the client with a sense of knowledge and direction. In psychiatric nursing this knowledge comes from the biological and behavioral sciences as well as from nursing frameworks. The knowledge bases developed by nurses are described below.

Psychiatric Nursing Models

In 1986, Murphy and Hoeffer[20] conducted a survey of course offerings in psychiatric/mental health nursing programs. The authors also asked program directors about critical issues or problems facing the specialty. The issues most frequently mentioned concerning knowledge development were the need for theory development and research in psychiatric and mental health nursing.

There are currently two developments in the knowledge base of psychiatric/mental health nursing. One is the elaboration of nursing models developed in the medical/surgical specialty of nursing that pertain to psychiatric nursing. Another development is the description of nursing models specifically for psychiatric/mental health nursing.

Models applied to psychiatric nursing are Rogers's *unitary man model,* King's *systems model,* Orem's *self-care model,* Roy's *adaptation model,* and Johnson's *behavioral system model.* These models will be discussed on the following pages.[9] Models presented by Peplau and Birckhead are discussed more extensively in other chapters of this text.

Rogers's unitary man model[23] is based on the concept of the interaction between the person and the environment. In this interaction, there occurs increasing complexity of the interaction and of the parts (person and environment) themselves. Rogers believes, for instance, that one person–environment interaction of increasing complexity is a longer life span for individuals.

Rogers presents a systems view of the person—a framework also used in this book. Just as there is no separation of mind and body in an individual, behavior cannot be predicted by the behavior of parts of the system taken separately.

In this model the person is viewed as an *open system,* which means that the person exchanges matter and energy with the environment. The person is also characterized by the capacity to abstract; to use imagery, language, and thought; and to sense and feel.

The applicability of Rogers's approach to psychiatric/mental health nursing includes the focus on the development across the life span. For example, this model supports the work done with geriatric clients. These clients are viewed as having the capacity for understanding their psychological problems and for further growth. Also, the family, using this model, is viewed as an *open system* that can engage in exchanges with the environment (since it can accept the help offered by the psychiatric nurse, and it can be affected by different cultural practices in its neighborhood).

King's systems model[16] includes the concepts of the person, perception (meaning observation through the senses, such as hearing), interpersonal relations, social systems, and health and illness. The person is viewed as *evolving* in biological, psychological, and social aspects. The person's perceptions of experiences influence the interaction with the environment.

King defines "health" as an adaptation to stress through the beneficial use of one's resources. Nursing is a process of interaction with the client to help the client move toward health. The nurse assesses the client's personal, interpersonal, and social aspects. Health is affected by biological, economic, ethnic, religious, emotional, and intellectual elements of the person. In health, these elements are in harmony.

King's model also applies to psychiatric/mental health nursing because it focuses on the person as a system within other systems. For example, the nurse working with a family to assist them in resolving interaction problems could apply King's focus on the interaction of parts in a system. Ethnic and spiritual aspects of the person are also seen as important for providing care. This text discusses these concepts as relevant to psychiatric care.

Orem's self-care model[21] concerns the person's environment, health, and self-care. The person's state of health is seen as a reflection of the integrity of the whole. Orem states that when individuals need assistance with self-care activities to maintain integrity, nursing intervention is needed.

To Orem, the person functions biologically, symbolically, and socially. Functioning is linked to the environment, and the person and the environment both form an integrated system. The person has a need for self-care in biological, symbolic, and social spheres of functioning. For example, people perform, on their own behalf, self-care practices of forming relations with others, eating, making decisions, and so on. Self-care activities are related to one's culture. This model is applicable to psychiatric nursing because it provides a positive view of the person who needs or wants self-care. This provides for a health- and hope-focused approach to psychiatric care. The model also encourages further theory development in the areas of (1) the needs of some psychiatric clients to have others take care of them, and (2) the needs for competency attainment (as in the development of interpersonal relationships) in those who have lost skills because of prolonged isolation.

Roy's adaptation model[24] focuses on the health–illness continuum, adaptation, and the person–environment system. The person's place on the health–illness continuum is seen as a function of the individual's ability to adapt to the environment. The function of nursing care is to promote effective adaptation responses.

The person demonstrates adaptation in the areas of physiology, self-concept, role function, and interdependence; these areas also affect each other. For example, one's positive self-concept can affect one's physiological functioning.

Problems in adaptation occur when the person has inadequate resources to meet demands made of the person. The nurse assists the client to identify the problem areas of functioning, to diagnose the adaptation problem, and to select methods to alter the stimuli causing the problem.

The applicability of this model to psychiatric nursing includes a focus on self-concept. A person's negative self-appraisal, for example, is viewed as a symptom of psychological trouble. The focus on adaptation itself is also useful because it promotes a positive view of the person as having the capacity to adapt effectively, even if the assistance of a professional person, such as a nurse, may be needed to maximize this capacity.

In formulating the *Johnson behavioral system model,*[12] Dorothy Johnson relied heavily on systems theory. She believed that a person seeks to maintain a behavioral system balance by adjusting to forces impinging on the individual.

The behavioral system is a purposeful way of acting that is specific to each person. The behavioral system establishes the relationship of the person to the environment.

Johnson defined seven behavioral subsystems. These include the affiliative, the dependency, the ingestive, the eliminative (relating to bodily waste products), the sexual, the aggressive, and the achievement subsystems.

Johnson stated that medicine focuses on the biological system, whereas nursing focuses on the behavioral system. Furthermore, nursing diagnosis is concerned with characteristics of the subsystems, or an insufficiency or discrepancy in behavioral subsystems.

Johnson's model emphasizes the psychological aspects of the person. However, the model is, as yet, insufficient to provide an elaborate description of psychiat-

CONCEPTS IN NURSING MODELS APPLICABLE TO PSYCHIATRIC/MENTAL HEALTH NURSING

MODEL	CONCEPTS
Unitary man model (by M. Rogers)	The person is a whole composed of *more than* simply the sum of the parts (such as one's psychology, environment, etc.).
	The person is *increasing* in complexity/development.
	There is *hope* in the capability of the person.
Systems model (by I. King)	The person is seen as a *system* composed of observation skills, *interpersonal relations*, and other parts.
	The nurse assists the client to move toward *health*.
	Spiritual concerns of the client are considered.
	The *complexity* of the client and the client's environment is viewed *realistically*.
Self-care model (by D. Orem)	Nursing practice involves promoting the client's ability for *self-care*.
	The client's *dignity* and ability to use at least some talents for self-care are preserved.
Adaptation model (by Sister C. Roy)	The client's position on the *health–illness continuum* is a function of *adaptation* to demands placed on the individual.
	Self-concept can affect one's physiology and vice versa.
	Nursing needs to be *concerned with, or provide for*, missing client resources.
Behavioral systems model (by D. Johnson)	Nursing's focus is on the person's *behavioral system*.
	The behavioral system is composed of affiliative, dependency, ingestive, eliminative, sexual, aggressive, and achievement parts.
	The individual attempts to maintain a sense of *equilibrium*.
	The nurse acts *to preserve* the integration of the client's behavior.
	The behavior of the client is in keeping with the *social and cultural* group.
	One utility of the model is that it focuses on *observable* client behaviors.
Interpersonal relations model (by H. Peplau)	The nurse and client come together and form an *interpersonal* relationship.
	Through the interpersonal relationship the client gains *interpersonal* and *intellectual skills* with which to attain a sense of well-being.
	The self-system of the client is an organized network of ideas, feelings, and actions that every person has as a consequence of interactions with others.
	Anxiety can decrease the client's likelihood of *learning* about life and relationships with others.
	The person goes through *developmental stages* (infancy through old age) in which specific competencies of living are learned.
	The process of cure through the nurse–client interpersonal relationship is recognized.
The Self/Other/Relationship model (by L. Birckhead)	The *Self* is a central phenomenon with which the psychiatric/mental health nurse works.
	The *Other* is described as a person who is significant to the client.
	The Other must be known to the Self *realistically*, rather than the way the Self would like the Other to be.
	The *Relationship* of the Self and the Other is a necessary part of human existence.
	Psychological *well-being* is determined in part by the ability to maintain an awareness of the nature of one's Self, the Other, and the Relationship of the Self and the Other.
	Intimacy (love) occurs when one experiences the need to be with another person as well as a true recognition of the nature of the other person.
	There is a recognition of the process of cure through personal resolution of the anxiety of the *opposing* qualities and needs of one's Self compared with those of one's Relationship(s) with Others.

ric/mental health nursing. Health, for example, is not well defined. Also, because behaviors are the focus of the model, feelings and thoughts may receive insufficient attention.

There are other models that focus more specifically on psychiatric nursing. This text highlights Peplau's interpersonal model of nursing and Birckhead's Self/Other/Relationship model.

Hildegard Peplau[22] is considered the founder of modern psychiatric nursing. Her work focuses on the cli-

ent's interpersonal life with the family and with the nurse. Central concepts of Peplau's framework include learning, the stages of the nurse–client relationship, anxiety, and nurse–client rapport. Peplau's ideas serve as the basis for much of the content of this text.

Loretta Birckhead's work builds on the work of Peplau and H. S. Sullivan, an American psychiatrist. Birckhead's model termed the *Self/Other/Relationship framework*, focuses on the need to understand both one's personal identity (Self) as well as the nature of Others with whom the person relates. The framework also includes a discussion of the nature of the Self as a changing process rather than a set personality. This framework is described further in this work.

New Directions

Psychiatric/mental health nursing began as a custodial role, but today psychiatric/mental health nurses practice in a number of treatment settings and use various techniques. Some psychiatric/mental health nurses have training in exercise and biofeedback and assist clients with stress management. Others lead group therapy and/or family therapy on inpatient units and with outpatients. Many nurses work in substance abuse treatment programs, where they mesh the treatment for the psychosocial concerns of the client with treatment for the disease process of substance abuse. Similarly, nurses are employed in treatment programs for eating disorders and for victims of sexual abuse.

Although the theory and research base formed within psychiatric/mental health nursing are not yet of great depth and breadth, the development of such theory and research is inevitable. As theory development and research continue to evolve in psychiatric/mental health nursing, the roles and responsibilities of psychiatric/mental health nurses will continue to expand.

Summary

1. The history of psychiatric nursing has developed parallel, to some degree, with the history of psychiatry.
2. Psychiatric nursing's prevailing norms and values reflect its historical background and the current social, economic, and political forces that govern health care practice.
3. Psychiatric/mental health nursing began with a focus on providing a protective environment for clients. Today psychiatric/mental health nursing provides psychotherapeutic care through various roles to assist the client in attaining the highest possible level of health.

References

1. American Nurses' Association: Taxonomy for the Classification of Human Responses of Concern for Psychiatric/Mental Health Nursing Practice. Kansas City, American Nurses' Association, 1986
2. American Psychiatric Association: Diagnostic and Statistical Manual-III-R. Washington, DC, American Psychiatric Association, 1987
3. Aquilera D, Messick J: Crisis Intervention: Theory and Methodology. St Louis, CV Mosby, 1986
4. Beers C: A Mind that Found Itself. Garden City, New York, Doubleday, 1948
5. Colbert L: The Psychiatric Nurse Clinical Specialist Works With Nursing Service. J Psychiatr Nurs 9:21, 1971
6. Davidites R, Williams F: The Training Program. In Stokes G (ed): The Role of the Psychiatric Nurse in Community Mental Health Practice: A Giant Step. Brooklyn, Faculty Press, 1969
7. Deutsch A: The Shame of the States. New York, Hill & Wang, 1948
8. Farberow N, Shneidman E (eds): The Cry for Help. New York, McGraw-Hill, 1961
9. Fujiki S, Clayton B, Estes N et al: Defining Clinical Content in Graduate Nursing Programs: Psychiatric Nursing. Boulder, CO, Western Council on Higher Education in Nursing, 1969
10. Green H: I Never Promised You A Rose Garden. New York, New American Library, 1964
11. Gregg D: The Psychiatric Nurse's Role. Am J Nurs 54:848–851, 1954
12. Johnson D: The Behavioral System Model for Nursing. In Riehl J, Roy C (eds): Conceptual Models for Nursing Practice. East Norwalk, CT, Appleton-Century-Crofts, 1980
13. Jones M: Beyond the Therapeutic Community. New Haven, Yale University Press, 1968
14. Kalkman M, Davis A: New Dimensions in Mental Health/Psychiatric Nursing. New York, McGraw-Hill, 1980
15. Kesey K: One Flew Over the Cuckoo's Nest. New York, Penguin Books, 1962
16. King I: A Theory for Nursing: Systems, Concepts, Process. New York, John Wiley & Sons, 1981
17. Lewis N: American Psychiatry from Its Beginning to World War II. In Arieti S (ed): American Handbook of Psychiatry, Vol I. New York, Basic Books, 1959
18. Lidz T: General Concepts of Psychosomatic Medicine. In Arieti S (ed): American Handbook of Psychiatry, Vol I. New York, Basic Books, 1959
19. Lippitt D: Psychiatry. In Medical and Health Annual. Chicago, Encyclopedia Britannica, 1981
20. Murphy S, Hoeffer B: Results of the 1986 National Survey About Specialty/Subspecialty Course Offerings. Seattle, University of Washington, 1986
21. Orem D: Nursing: Concepts of Practice. New York, McGraw-Hill, 1985
22. Peplau H: Interpersonal Relations in Nursing. New York, GP Putnam, 1952
23. Rogers M: The Theoretical Basis of Nursing. Philadelphia, FA Davis, 1970
24. Roy Sister C: Introduction to Nursing: An Adaptation Model. Englewood Cliffs, NJ, Prentice-Hall, 1984
25. Santos E, Stainbrook E: A History of Psychiatric Nursing in the Nineteenth Century. J Hist Med Allied Sci 4:48, 1949
26. Schmahl J: Experiment in Change: An Interdisciplinary Approach to the Integration of Psychiatric Content in Baccalaureate Nursing Education. New York, Macmillan, 1966
27. Stokes G: The Role of Psychiatric Nurses in Community Mental Health Practice: A Giant Step. Brooklyn, Faculty Press, 1969
28. Tudor G: A Sociopsychiatric Nursing Approach to Intervention in a Problem of Mutual Withdrawal on a Mental Hospital Ward. Psychiatry 15:193, 1952
29. U.S. Department of Health, Education, and Welfare: Community Mental Health Act of 1963, Title II, Public Law 88-164. The Federal Register, May 1964, 5951
30. Ward J: The Snake Pit. Cutchogue, NY, Buccaneer Books, 1946
31. Williams F: The Role of the Psychiatric Nurse in Secondary Prevention. In Stokes G (ed): The Role of Psychiatric Nurses in Community Mental Health Practice: A Giant Step. Brooklyn, Faculty Press, 1969

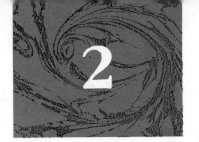

LORETTA M. BIRCKHEAD

THE DEVELOPMENT AND DIFFERENTIATION OF THE PROFESSIONAL ROLE OF THE NURSE

Learning Objectives

Upon completion of this chapter the student should be able to do the following:

1. Describe the role expected of the first nurses in psychiatric/mental health nursing.
2. Describe the effect of an apprenticeship style of learning on nursing practice.
3. Describe the implications for nurses when they are expected to be custodians or controllers of clients. Describe the implications for clients.
4. List some of the early events paving the way for the beginning of professional practice.

5. Describe how a client is treated based on the principles and beliefs of psychiatric/mental health nurses.
6. Describe the implications for nurses of current trends in psychiatric/mental health nursing.
7. List the distinguishing characteristics of psychiatric/mental health nurses.
8. Describe how interdisciplinary team functioning is attained.
9. Explain role strain.
10. Explain the effects of accountability on clinical practice.

Introduction

Individual nurse leaders have been courageous pathfinders whose humanitarianism and intellectualism have prevailed. These leaders have worked within a society that has little knowledge of the capabilities of the professional nurse and in a mental health care system troubled by inadequate funding and competition among health care professionals for time with the client.

Church[11] described the emergence of psychiatric/mental health nursing in the United States as a "noble reform." Nurses have continually proposed working with clients in ways that reinforce the *dignity* of the clients. This reform first occurred at a time when the mentally ill were considered evil or not worthy of care.

This chapter will discuss the historical development of the professional role of the psychiatric/mental health nurse. A general outline of the progression of content over time is provided by Peplau,[19] the founder of modern psychiatric/mental health nursing. Other authors who have contributed to knowledge about this historical progression in the nurse's role development are also included.

A discussion is presented of the differentiation of the psychiatric/mental health nurse from other professionals in the mental health care setting, as well as of the types of relationships that occur among these professionals. The final sections include concepts of the professional role and accountability that dictate how psychiatric nursing is practiced.

Historical Evolution

Beginnings—Apprenticeship (1882–1906)

By 1882 there were many public psychiatric hospitals and a smaller number of private psychiatric hospitals in which clients received custodial care. Psychiatric/mental health nursing began as an organized course of study in 1882 when Dr. Edward S. Cowles, superintendent of McLean Psychiatric Hospital in Massachusetts, established a school for nurses.[19] Although it was common practice to establish "training schools" for nurses as an economical way to staff general hospitals, this was the first school for

nurses in a psychiatric hospital. Such preparation allowed young women to receive an education, minimal pay, and room and board—all useful benefits for women from poor immigrant families.

Cowles's preparation of the nurse took the form of an *apprenticeship*. This apprenticeship meant that the nurse was "bound" to the physician for a period of time, during which content was absorbed by the learner in unquestioning fashion. Until 1965, hospital-based schools served as the means of educating nurses.[4]

The first elementary education of psychiatric/mental health nurses in the hospital training programs occurred at the expense of the nurse. The "development of the nursing profession could not be achieved in an atmosphere where control over the nurse's education resided in the hands of those who wished to exploit her for her labor."[4]

Peplau described this period in psychiatric nursing as one in which information taught to nursing students was patterned on what had been taught to attendants.[20] It was not unusual for attendants and nurses to have classes together. The curriculum included housekeeping, first aid, handling destructive client behaviors, and providing practical advice. Nurses were taught a system of descriptive behaviors in which the focus was on the peculiar traits of the client. Such a system promoted a "labeling" role for the nurse, in which she simply kept track of the behaviors demonstrated by the clients and reported this information to the physician. The nurse's role *did not* include elements of the nursing process (assessment, diagnosis, planning, intervention, and evaluation).

The Nurse as Custodian and Controller (1906–1932)

During the years 1906–1932, the stigma associated with mental illness was still very great. The public feared mental patients, and believed that anyone who worked with such clients was peculiar.[20] Mental patients were no longer kept at home in the community, but were placed in psychiatric hospitals built in remote places. With the advent of diagnostic manuals used by psychiatrists, unusual behavior was labeled as an illness and families could remove ill members from the home and place them in hospitals without feeling guilt about abandoning them.

More psychiatric nurses were needed to care for these clients in the hospitals. By 1915 there were 41 nursing schools in mental hospitals; by 1936 the number peaked at 67. Thus, the increase in nursing schools was partially due to an increase in the number of psychiatric hospitals. In 1920, the first textbook on psychiatric nursing, by Harriet Bailey, was published.[10] This work was the standard text in psychiatric nursing for 20 years. Interestingly, the text was concerned with psychiatric nursing care but contained material about the nurse in industry and child welfare nursing. Bailey also continued to foster a model of nursing focused, in a simplistic manner, on a description of symptoms. Psychiatric nursing was still waiting for other leaders to determine the intricacies of the role of the psychiatric nurse that included all components of the nursing process.

As early as 1936, Bailey contributed to the idea of nurses doing *research.* She conducted a descriptive study of nursing schools in psychiatric hospitals. In her report she described the care provided in the hospitals and condemned the excessive hours demanded of nursing students on the units. She decried the poor staff–client ratios and blamed the clients' poor behavior on the minimal care they received.

Peplau[20] described this period as one in which the emphasis in psychiatric nursing curricula changed from "character development" of the nurse to "rules." Such rules concerned the use of restraints to control patients and how to count medications and sharp objects such as silverware. The nurse's role was that of custodian and controller rather than that of a scientist providing professional care.

At the same time, several developments served to promote the professional role of the nurse. The National League of Nursing Education (later to become the National League for Nursing [NLN]), the American Nurses' Association (ANA), and the Asylum Workers Association began a discussion about problems related to the mentally ill. In 1906, the American Psychiatric Association began a program for the standardization of nursing schools in psychiatric hospitals. There were also discussions of the need for general hospital experiences for nursing students in psychiatric hospitals, as well as psychiatric hospital experience for students in general hospitals. Also, concepts such as conflict, the childhood causation of mental illness, and mental mechanisms such as defense mechanisms began to be considered relevant to psychiatric care. The *American Journal of Nursing* emphasized the need for an eight-hour day rather than the draining twelve-hour days. Thus nurses were taking active stances concerning their practice, stances that promoted the development of the professional role rather than merely the custodial/mothering role.[19]

Growth of Academia (1932–1958)

In the beginning of the period from 1932 to 1958, nurses in psychiatric hospitals were still providing exclusively custodial care. The nurse used "tact, persuasion, coaxing, and praise" as strategies as the nurse bathed, dressed, and cared for the client.[19] The emphasis was on housekeeping, cleanliness, and economy in the use of materials.

Before 1940, nurses in psychiatric service must have been confused about the nature of their role. Were they:

- Custodians?
- Surrogate mothers?
- Informers?
- Friends of the clients?
- Housekeepers?
- Physicians' helpers?
- Police?
- Trainers?
- Public guardians?

An important movement began in 1937, however, when the NLN published curriculum guides advocating an affiliation in psychiatric nursing for all nursing students, and 60 to 80 classroom hours on behavior and its meaning. In 1943, three universities offered graduate programs in psychiatric/mental health nursing. In 1946, the Mental Health Act was passed, which provided educational funds for students interested in graduate study. In 70 years, preparation in psychiatric/mental health nursing moved from apprenticeship to academia. This movement was a major thrust toward the development of the professional role of the psychiatric nurse. Through graduate study every aspect of the professional role could be studied: a description of the professional role, concepts relevant to client care, theoretical frameworks for care, and so on. Nurses were directing their own role preparation. The role would have their unique stamp.

In 1948, Peplau began to direct the graduate program in psychiatric nursing at Teachers College, Columbia University.[19] Peplau worked with students who provided care for individual patients at Brooklyn State Hospital. The students wrote verbatim notes of what was said in the interviews. Peplau's review of these notes led her to the development of the "interpersonal theory of psychiatric/mental health nursing." Through this study the role of the nurse took definite form: the nurse helped the client understand interpersonal relationships with others, because it is within the context of interpersonal relationships that difficulties in living arise and are perpetuated. A range of concepts to study are present in these relationships, including such concepts as mutual withdrawal, conflict, anxiety, and distortion. (See Chaps. 3 and 5.)

In the 1950s, the term *psychiatric/mental health nursing,* was created[14] to describe the combination of two groups of nurses: those who worked with the mentally ill in hospitals, and those whose base of practice was in the community. This broader term denotes the combined focus on: (1) the mentally ill, as in a hospital setting, (2) clients functioning in the community, and (3) the practice of the nurse's role as consultant to other professionals in the community.

Toward Professionalism (1958–Present)

From 1958 to 1988, the number of psychiatric/mental health nurses holding master's degrees increased from a few to hundreds. As of 1988, more than 100 psychiatric nurses held doctoral degrees.[18] There is now a cadre of nurses prepared at the advanced level of psychiatric/ mental health nursing practice who can further define and expand our understanding of the professional role of the psychiatric/mental health nurse. Psychiatric/mental health nurses now publish their research and other writings in four journals specifically oriented to the work of the psychiatric nurse: *Perspectives in Psychiatric Care, The Journal of Psychosocial Nursing and Mental Health Services, Issues in Mental Health Nursing,* and the *Archives of Psychiatric Nursing.*

Statements from the professional nursing organizations have contributed to the description of the professional role of the psychiatric/mental health nurse. The *Statement on Psychiatric and Mental Health Nursing Practice,* first published in 1967 by the ANA and revised in 1976, delineates the role of the nurse within the mental health system.[2] It defines psychiatric/mental health nursing and the scope of practice.

Because this statement of the ANA has provided a major contribution to the development of nursing practice, the major points are discussed in the box below. The *principles* of psychiatric/mental health nursing described in the *Statement* are listed. Relevant to these principles is the concept that psychiatric nurses are aligned with the client in defining and resolving the client's mental health care needs. The box at the right lists certain *beliefs* discussed in the *Statement* that underlie psychiatric/mental health nursing practice. The distinctive *contributions* of nurses to mental health care, as outlined in the *Statement,* are included in a third box, below. Recent trends in psychiatric/mental health nursing and the implications of these trends for nursing are given in Table 2-1.

The principles, beliefs, and contributions outlined above point to the unique place the psychiatric/mental health nurse has in the care setting. The nurse's role includes more than psychological concerns in working with clients. The *Relevant Research* on page 20 demonstrates the impact that culturally sensitive care can have on clients in need of mental health services.

The psychiatric nurse also considers environmental concerns. Crosby[12] stated that, because of their emphasis

---

BELIEFS OF PSYCHIATRIC/ MENTAL HEALTH NURSES

1. Each person has an inherent capacity for change.
2. Each person as an integrated whole performs various functions. Instances of viewing particular behaviors of an individual as the totality of the person are dehumanizing.
3. Differences exist in individuals' values and potential for change. Professionals in the health care field recognize the individual's right to exercise free choice.
4. The nurse and client enter into a professional relationship while relying on acknowledged roles for each. The nurse's professional role carries with it specific qualifications and competencies.
5. The person is more than an internally-driven entity. A person is affected by societal, environmental, and cultural surroundings.

(Data from American Nurses' Association: Statement on Psychiatric and Mental Health Nursing Practice. Kansas City, American Nurses' Association, 1976)

PRINCIPLES OF PSYCHIATRIC/ MENTAL HEALTH NURSING

1. Comprehensive health care involves services for individuals, families, and society.
2. The purpose of comprehensive health care service include:
   a. Promotion and maintenance of health
   b. Prevention, detection, and treatment of illness
   c. Restoration to the highest possible levels of health
3. Nursing has a particular responsibility to speak out on behalf of consumer needs for holistic and humane services.
4. Nursing care is defined and developed by nurses.
5. Nurses are accountable for the quality of care.

(Data from American Nurses' Association: Statement on Psychiatric and Mental Health Nursing Practice. Kansas City, American Nurses' Association, 1976)

THE DISTINCTIVE CONTRIBUTIONS OF PSYCHIATRIC/MENTAL HEALTH NURSES

1. The provision of care that incorporates societal, psychological, environmental, physical, and cultural characteristics of the client
2. The provision of continuous personal care
3. The development of research concerning the various elements mentioned in #1 above
4. The use of the nursing process as systematic steps for the provision of care
5. Skill in crisis intervention
6. Skill in working with severely ill clients
7. Understanding human nature in responding to the needs of the client

(Data from American Nurses' Association: Statement on Psychiatric and Mental Health Nursing Practice. Kansas City, American Nurses' Association, 1976)

TABLE 2-1.
TRENDS IN PSYCHIATRIC/MENTAL HEALTH NURSING PRACTICE, WITH IMPLICATIONS

TRENDS	NURSING IMPLICATIONS
Community-based care	Increased career opportunities in community-based settings rather than in psychiatric hospitals
	Increased need for the psychiatric nurse to understand and assess the community, as well as to identify community resources
	Need for increased skills in working with the families and support groups of clients
	Willingness to have less "control" of the client than when the client is hospitalized
	Ability to establish rapport with the client so that the client maintains contact with community-based staff
	Ability to work with various cultural groups in the community
Short-term care	Need for nurses who can focus quickly and effectively on client concerns
	Need for an "active" approach rather than offering client time for unfocused topic discussion
	Involvement in research to discover which approaches work with various client problems
	Development of a shared community plan of care for particular clients hospitalized at different times in various hospitals
Emphasis on quality of care	Nursing participation on quality assurance committees.
	Need for awareness of ANA's *Standard of Practice*
Emphasis on clients' rights	Need for awareness of laws pertaining to rights of clients, such as the right to adequate treatment
	Ability to explain laws to clients
	Participation in ethics-related studies to weigh need for treatment of client vs. client's rights to refuse treatment
The provision of psychiatric nursing care based on scientific principles tied to nursing's tradition	Development or elaboration of principles of care unique to psychiatric nurses. Systematic testing of such principles of care
	Greater numbers of psychiatric nurses in private practice
	More varied types of private practice, such as therapy of client with both family and relevant community members present
	Practice incorporating societal, cultural, environmental principles related to mind/body
	Admitting privileges at psychiatric hospitals
	Recognition for nursing practice that is seen as relevant to the felt concerns of the client

(Data from American Nurses' Association: Statement on Psychiatric and Mental Health Nursing Practice. Kansas City, American Nurses' Association, 1976)

on *care,* psychiatric nurses should be the key professionals to provide care for the chronically mentally ill, who are often homeless and not amenable to "cure." This care must include, among other things, housing, physical proximity of professional health care workers, and a social structure that provides expectations of appropriate adaptation on the part of the mentally ill individual.

Other developments from 1958 to the present include the publication by the ANA of *Standards of Psychiatric and Mental Health Nursing Practice.*[1] This work provides the standards for quality of care in psychiatric/mental health nursing. Standards provide guidance in achieving excellence in care.

The performance of psychotherapy, by master's degree-prepared clinical specialists in psychiatric/mental health nursing, in an independent practice, is a present reality. Such therapy includes individual psychotherapy as well as group and family psychotherapy.

Certification procedures were created by the American Nurses' Association as a means of recognizing those in advanced practice who meet specific standards. Certification in some states is required to receive insurance reimbursement for providing psychotherapy to clients in private practice. If psychiatric/mental health nurses are not acknowledged by law as eligible to receive insurance reimbursement for providing psychotherapy, many clients will simply go to those professionals who *are* eligible.

The work of clinical specialists in community mental health centers in new forms of practice, including providing play therapy for children, psychodrama, and other special aspects of care, is now recognized.[19]

Differences and similarities have developed between the roles of psychiatric/mental health nurses and those of other mental health professionals, including psychiatrists, social workers, and psychologists. Defining the role of the psychiatric/mental health nurse helps to establish:

1. Professional pride
2. Directions for theory development and refinement
3. Directions for research
4. Substantiation to the consumer and to other professionals that psychiatric/mental health nurses control their own practices and are accountable and responsible for their practice
5. Control by psychiatric/mental health nurses over their own practices in every setting
6. Client access to the unique practice viewpoint of the nurse

RELEVANT RESEARCH

An audit was performed on 100 randomly-selected charts of clients seen in a mental health clinic in California. Of the 100 clients, 61 had not previously received mental health care and 45 were self-referred. No other help had been sought by these 45 clients prior to coming to the clinic. Eighty-six of the 100 clients spoke Spanish only. Typically, the clients studied were traditional Hispanics, not acculturated to the United States. They had an average of six years of education.

All professionals working in the clinic spoke Spanish and were members of the Latin American culture. Because the majority of the clients were self-referred and had no prior history of mental health care, it is evident that traditional Hispanics do recognize mental illness, and want mental health care tailored to their cultural circumstances. Nurses and other health care professionals can facilitate access of clients to such culturally-sensitive care.

(Reeves K: Hispanic utilization of an ethnic mental health clinic. J Psychiatr Nurs 24:23, 1986)

Finally, nursing stresses a continuing commitment to treat all patients, regardless of their placement on the health–illness continuum. Psychiatric/mental health nurses may treat clients with long histories of mental illness, as well as clients receiving mental health services in order to use existing strengths to gain new understandings (as in support groups for single parents). The nurse's goal for all clients is to help them reach the highest quality of life possible, regardless of the initial level of mental health.

The Future

The psychiatric/mental health nursing profession has a strong tradition of clinical service and scientific publications. In continuing this tradition, several trends are important. The nurse must develop increasingly strong bonds between nurse and client in which the client is a partner in efforts to attain a higher quality of life. To foster this trend, the client and nurse should:

1. Set mutually agreed-on goals.
2. Act in ways that reach beyond the clinical setting. For example, the nurse may meet with the client's employer and the client to clarify the client's problems at work.
3. Discuss the rationale for the work the psychiatric/mental health nurse is doing with the client. In the past, clinicians have at times remained distant figures to clients, working in ways clients could not understand. The client acted "on faith" that the clinician was acting on behalf of the client. In some instances, clients were kept in ineffective treatment needlessly or were even exploited.

Psychiatric nurses have shown increased involvement in legislative efforts to strengthen their rights to practice. These legislative efforts include working to establish the right of the nurse to receive reimbursement for services and the right to admit clients to psychiatric hospitals when the need arises. Another legislative effort concerns the right of clients receiving medicare and medicaid to obtain the services of a psychiatric/mental health nurse rather than only of a psychiatrist.

While psychiatric diagnoses have been developed and classified in the *Diagnostic and Statistical Manual of Mental Disorders-III-R* (DSM-III-R),[3] work continues on the development of nursing diagnoses, particularly in the area of psychiatric/mental health nursing. The nurse cannot ignore the DSM-III-R, which was developed by psychiatry and other disciplines to label psychopathology, and is widely used. However, the DSM-III-R does not provide all elements of the classification that a nurse would use. For example, a client may experience a pervasive sense of powerlessness, yet this diagnosis is not included in the DSM-III-R. Further discussion of diagnoses can be found in Chapter 4.

An expanded role has developed to include the nurse who provides theoretical and research-based insight into broad issues facing the public. The consumer needs nursing's voice in matters such as:

1. Alienation of individuals in our technologically-oriented society
2. Self-care in mental health
3. Violence
4. Women's health care
5. Child abuse
6. Care for the underprivileged
7. Developing appropriate expectations of mental health care services

Differentiation From Other Mental Health Care Professionals

The ANA Council on Psychiatric and Mental Health Nursing Practice defined psychiatric/mental health nursing as a specialized area of nursing practice using the theory of human behavior as its science and the therapeutic use of self as its art.[2] It is directed toward the prevention of mental illness, as well as the achievement of the highest possible level of wellness in individuals and communities.

ACTIVITIES OF THE PSYCHIATRIC/MENTAL HEALTH NURSE

1. Providing a therapeutic milieu, concerned largely with the sociopsychological aspects of clients' environments
2. Working with clients concerning the here-and-now living problems they confront
3. Accepting and using roles
4. Detecting and caring for somatic aspects of clients' health problems, including responses to drugs and other treatments
5. Teaching, with specific reference to emotional health as evidenced by various behavioral patterns
6. Assuming the role of social agent concerned with improvement of recreational, occupational, and social competence
7. Providing leadership and clinical assistance to other nursing personnel and generic health care workers
8. Conducting psychotherapy
9. Engaging in social and community action roles related to mental health

(American Nurses' Association: Statement on Psychiatric and Mental Health Nursing Practice. Kansas City, American Nurses' Association, 1976)

The activities of the psychiatric/mental health nurse, as defined by the Council on Psychiatric and Mental Health Nursing Practice, are listed in the box above. In the section of the ANA Statement that lists these activities, there is no stated differentiation in activities performed by baccalaureate and master's degrees prepared psychiatric/mental health nurses.

The following discussion expands on the activities of the psychiatric/mental health nurse. Because professionals from other mental health disciplines perform some of the same activities, they are discussed as well, in order to improve understanding of how each contributes within the health care setting.

Nursing Activities

Establishing the Milieu

The *therapeutic milieu* is the social setting of an inpatient or day treatment unit in which clients are treated. The emphasis of the therapeutic milieu is on the emotional quality of the setting: how the setting, patients, staff, and treatment program all interact with each other to produce an environment that promotes health.

Nurses manage this milieu. They are present when

interactions occur among clients on the unit. Other professionals often have offices *off the unit,* and they are removed from the daily occurrences of the clients. The long period of contact the nurse has with clients is rewarding, because the nurse is present when clients display the behaviors that promote their mental illness. For example, a client may become angry at a nurse when his family leaves the unit after a visit. If the client does not have the competency to share this anger directly with the family, the nurse can help the client develop this competency.

Working With Here-and-Now Living Problems

Typically, the nurse is the only professional person available to help the client understand behavior *at the moment* it occurs. This is one of the most effective times to gain insight. The nurse is present when clients return to the psychiatric unit from their first pass to visit their families, when clients have difficulty sleeping, and at other significant points. Nurses learn through education and practice to deal with client responses to health and illness in such moments, and to search for ways by which the client may alter or strengthen those responses.

Using Roles

At times nurses must also fill a substitute or surrogate role. This does not mean that the nurse promotes dependency on the part of the client or creates an illusory figure in the client—by calling an older male client "Dad," for example. The nurse provides care and direction for the client while helping the client gain the competencies needed to perform desired behaviors. Clients who *can* perform activities of daily living may distort the nurse's role, seeking inappropriate dependence on the nurse. The nurse helps the client to clarify these distortions.

In providing care within many roles, the nurse makes use of the most important therapeutic tool, the *therapeutic use of self*—the person of the nurse. Chapter 5 in this text describes both the cognitive and the affective aspects of the therapeutic use of self.

Caring for Somatic Needs

Many clients are required to take medications to help combat their emotional difficulties. In working with clients receiving medications, the nurse must be familiar with the medications and their interactions with other medications and food. The nurse must also work with the client to resolve practical issues such as paying for medications and the adjustments involved in taking medications for extended periods of time.

Working with clients and their medications is not always a simple matter. A client may be agitated and yet may not want to take medication. The nurse may have to administer a medication to calm the client against the client's wishes. The nurse may see that a client becomes sleepy after taking medications, thus preventing the client from discussing the original problems that created the agitation. The existential issues of free will and choice mentioned in the Introduction can arise. The nurse should talk frequently with other professionals about whether the medications help to improve the quality of life of the client, or whether they serve to control the client solely to fit the needs of others, such as staff or family.

The psychiatric assessment presented in Chapter 4 includes a list of physical body systems. Such a listing is in keeping with the systems approach of this text: the psychological, societal, environmental, cultural, and physical aspects of the person cannot be separated. In addition, assessing and intervening with the physical component can indicate to clients that: (a) they are being cared for in their totality, thereby increasing the overall effectiveness of treatment; (b) all of their true concerns are understood, rather than only the part that the clinician wishes to see; and (c) they are being helped to talk, since discussing physical problems is easier for some clients than talking about psychological concerns.

Teaching

The psychiatric/mental health nurse teaches others about mental health and mental illness principles. Peplau[19] stated that part of the nurse's responsibility is to inform the client about the nature of emotional well-being. For example, the nurse can teach a client about anxiety: what it is, how it feels, and what can be done about it.

Working as a Social Agent

The nurse facilitates the client's improvement in the areas of recreational, occupational, and social competence, understanding that the client is not simply a person who has emotional difficulties. A distorted picture occurs when the client is seen *only* in the confines of a room where the client and nurse converse. The nurse should be comfortable stepping outside this isolated setting. Flaskerud summarizes a number of research studies that indicate that psychiatric nurses feel comfortable visiting clients in the clients' homes and, indeed, believe such a practice contributes a comprehensiveness to care.[15]

Leading Other Staff

At times the psychiatric/mental health nurse gives clinical and administrative direction to others on the treatment staff. The nurse gains much information concerning particular clients as well as the total treatment setting. The nurse can mesh such perspectives with the particular views of staff from other disciplines. For example, a psy-

chiatrist may need to alter the client's medications when told by the nurse that the client is sleeping rather than participating in hospital activities. The social worker may need to speed up work in finding a community placement for a hospitalized client when the client has benefited as much as possible from hospitalization. The nurse makes many observations concerning the ability of clients to make use of the treatment setting.

Conducting Psychotherapy

The Master's degree-prepared psychiatric/mental health nurse can conduct psychotherapy. Nurses with a baccalaureate degree, however, are expected to have skills necessary to perform up to 16 hours of intervention with individuals or groups (including families). Such intervention is different from psychotherapy, and this difference is described further in Chapter 10.

The Stages of Prevention: Promoting Mental Health

The nurse participates in activities related to fostering mental health in the community. In this role the nurse works with clients at any stage of health or illness requiring primary, secondary, or tertiary prevention. *Primary prevention* refers to the promotion of mental health. *Secondary prevention* concerns early case finding and treatment, and *tertiary prevention* refers to rehabilitation. The client may be at any one of these stages; the nurse is not biased toward or against those who are healthy or those who are ill. The stages of prevention are discussed further in Chapter 3.

Other Activities

Although not emphasized by the Council on Psychiatric and Mental Health Nursing Practice, psychiatric/mental health nurses are responsible for a number of other activities, including:

1. *Clinical case management.* The psychiatric/mental health nurse is in a key position to ensure the formulation (developed with the client), implementation, and evaluation of a treatment plan that is suited to the client's needs.[22]
2. *Client advocacy.* The psychiatric/mental health nurse is "responsible and accountable for ensuring that the staff works on behalf of the client's best interest."[22]

The Disciplines

There is considerable overlap in activities among the disciplines involved in mental health. These disciplines include nursing, psychiatry, social work, and psychology. Nurses who practice psychiatric nursing have college or university degrees, as do social workers. Psychologists practicing in the mental health care system typically have doctoral degrees, and psychiatrists are medical doctors.

Nurses and social workers with master's degrees, psychologists, and psychiatrists may all practice psychotherapy, direct clinics, conduct research, perform psychiatric emergency assessments, and work in the community to gain support for mental health care. Specific activities for each discipline are defined by state legislatures. Some nurses, for example, can admit clients to psychiatric hospitals, while others cannot.

There are several unique functions in each discipline, yet, these functions are only tendencies, and role-blurring occurs. The characteristics listed below are also those that individual disciplines have emphasized in the growth of their science.

Psychiatry

The psychiatrist prescribes medications and works with clients who have organic pathology as well as psychopathology. An example of such a client would be an anorexic client experiencing electrolyte imbalance.

Psychology

Psychologists are proficient in performing psychological tests with clients. Some psychologists use behavior therapy techniques with clients in the tradition of B. F. Skinner.

Social Work

Mullaney, Fox, and Liston[18] studied the definitions of the role that psychiatric/mental health clinical nurse specialists and clinical social workers attribute to their respective career activities. The researchers sent questionnaires to schools of social work and nursing, as well as to individuals with social work or nursing careers. The results of the study indicated that the activities of the social worker included:

1. Interpreting social policies pertaining to financial support of clients, such as welfare
2. Assisting clients in applying for support services, such as welfare or job training
3. Assisting clients to obtain appropriate housing
4. Assisting clients to obtain health care-related appliances, equipment, and drugs
5. Arranging for homemaker services for clients
6. Arranging for client transportation
7. Arranging for nursing home placement

Psychiatric Nursing

Psychiatric nursing emphasizes the view that the person is a system. In order to provide care, the nurse assesses the client's psychological, societal, cultural, environmen-

tal, and physical status to determine what influences the client's health status. The nurse considers the client's spiritual aspects as a part of the client's cultural beliefs. This multidimensional view of the client is one of nursing's distinctive aspects.

Psychiatric nursing also emphasizes the importance of crisis theory and works with clients in crisis.

Role Overlap

Regardless of the ability to list discrete activities for each professional group, in the arena of practice overlap of activities occurs among the professional groups and there is competition for the client. For instance, each discipline involved with a mental health unit may want to claim the role of assigning a particular client on a unit to certain groups judged by that professional person to be appropriate. Which discipline performs which activities?

Weiss[24] studied the differentiation of nurses' and doctors' activities by personal interviews and questionnaires administered to nurses, physicians, and consumers of health care in a variety of settings, including mental health practice. While she found no unique nursing activities, a substantial percent of responsibilities in nursing and medicine overlapped. This study demonstrated that distinctions among the activities expected of the various disciplines within the health care system are blurred. Weiss also made the point that even nurses were not clear about activities expected of their own discipline.

For example, a nurse, a social worker, and a psychologist may each wish to discuss a difficult client–family interaction that took place while the client's family visited the mental health unit. The nurse also has an obligation to speak to the client on behalf of the discipline of nursing, and has the right to provide nursing care in such situations.

Regardless of the attempt by professional groups to claim unique responsibility for certain activities, as in the example just mentioned, the psychiatric/mental health nurse needs to keep several principles in mind. The box on p. 24 lists guidelines for role integrity that should be employed in practice by the psychiatric/mental health nurse.

It is important for the psychiatric/mental health nurse to accept only the definition of activities coming from fellow nurses. As mentioned earlier in this chapter, the psychiatric profession initially demanded that nurses be custodians of clients, perform housekeeping chores, control the behavior of clients, and carry out other custodial duties. Although today's nurse may have to perform similar duties at times, these activities are not the primary role of the nurse. Many were originally based on the needs of other professionals. For instance, with reference to the task of behavior control, at times clients need to express what they feel rather than to cover their feelings. Whose needs are being met when clients are told to control their feelings?

Guideline 4 indicates that not just any activities can be performed by the nurse, but that each state has a Nurse

GUIDELINES FOR ROLE INTEGRITY IN PSYCHIATRIC/ MENTAL HEALTH NURSING

1. Accept only *nursing's* definition of the nursing role, not the definitions of other disciplines.
2. Inform other disciplines of the necessary *nursing* activities to be performed.
3. Do not wait for other disciplines to assign *nursing* activities to be performed.
4. Perform the *nursing* activities allowed by the state's Nurse Practice Act.
5. Maintain a nursing perspective (such as a holistic view of the client) in the activities that are performed.

Practice Act that describes the activities performed by the professional nurse. The California State Nurse Practice Act, for example, states that the nurse should obtain statements by nursing's professional groups,[8] such as the ANA, that list activities expected of the psychiatric/mental health nurse. Fortunately, many Nurse Practice Acts and statements by other professional nursing groups are *general,* thus allowing a variety of activities and the expanded activities of the future. Individual counseling, for instance, is included in the broad wording of many Nurse Practice Acts, although the word "counseling" per se does not occur in the acts.

Guideline 5 emphasizes the importance of maintaining a nursing perspective in the practice arena. This accomplishes a number of goals, including:

1. The differentiation of nursing from other disciplines.
2. The promotion of psychiatric/mental health nursing science by advocating for and using the nursing science.
3. The provision of good quality care to the client. Many times the nurse offers what other disciplines do not: a humanistic perspective; a belief in the ability of the client to grow regardless of the severity of the illness; and a systems perspective that includes viewing all aspects of the client and the client's environment.

Interdisciplinary Teams in Mental Health Care

According to Benfer,[6] the development of psychiatric team work is relatively new. It was not until World War II that the early doctor/nurse team was expanded to include other team members. At that time, the large number of psychiatric casualties resulting from the war pointed to the high occurrence of mental health problems in the nation as a whole. Federal legislation made funds available to improve mental health programs. Psy-

chiatric nursing was designated as one of the four mental health disciplines eligible for training funds. The four disciplines (nursing, psychiatry, social work, and psychology) began working together in multidisciplinary teams.

Because nurses are frequently required to work in teams with other health care providers, it is important to understand more about the nature of teams, how they function, and the steps commonly found in the development of teams.

Different types of teams include:

1. *Unidisciplinary:* composed of members of one discipline, such as nursing
2. *Multidisciplinary:* includes members from each of the four disciplines. Each provides discipline-specific services to the same client.
3. *Interdisciplinary:* includes members from each of the four disciplines. These members communicate meaningfully to determine how best to accomplish the task at hand. While each member may provide discipline-specific services, the emphasis is more on the teamwork required to accomplish the task.

In order to function efficiently as a team, the team must establish its effectiveness. This is true whether the team is an administrative team, a clinical treatment team, or any other team in mental health care. Given the professional obligations of each of the disciplines and the potential for overlap among the activities of the different disciplines, it is common and expected that differences of opinion may occur among team members. Professional nurses no longer accept dictates from other disciplines, nor do people in the other disciplines. Differences must be discussed and resolved rather than ignored. Through such dialogue team members establish their *interdisciplinary function.*

Benfer[6] describes two phases through which team members progress toward reaching the goal of interdisciplinary functioning: dependence and interdependence. These two phases, along with their characteristics, are summarized in Table 2-2.

It is difficult to describe the sense of unity, felt by team members as they work together to attain common goals of improved patient care while, *at the same time,* maintaining individual autonomy. This state is not reached easily. Naive members may believe that if they, as individuals, are sufficiently dedicated or knowledgeable, all will go well on a team. This is not the way effective team functioning is attained. A high level of team functioning is reached by working through each phase or issue the group experiences until the phase is reached that meshes the duality of individual autonomy and group cohesiveness. This requires that each member have a strong individual identity, trust, knowledge, and skills to withstand challenges among team members. In addition to contributing to more efficient care for clients, it is personally gratifying to work in an environment in which team members have attained this level of performance with each other.

TABLE 2-2.
PHASES IN TEAM FUNCTIONING

PHASE/CHARACTERISTICS	TEAM PROBLEMS/RESOLUTIONS
DEPENDENCE PHASE	
Team members debate issues of dependence vs. independence. Team members may gravitate to one "camp" or philosophy.	Dependent members rely on others for decisions (common in new members). Independent members dictate decisions. Team members may 1. Advocate consensus 2. Advocate noncompliance with standard philosophies 3. Continue working on the task
There is an "appearance" of team functioning.	Team members may 1. Become detached from each other 2. Intellectualize (for example, dependent members may expect others to develop their care plans) 3. Test each other 4. Seek praise for their individual contributions
A sense of purpose develops.	Independent members challenge dependent members until consensus is attained. Ambiguity and vagueness in the team's objective may arise. Hostility may be present among members.
RELEASE PHASE	
Independent members try to resolve team's turmoil.	Resolution of the turmoil is largely dependent on the maturity of the team members.
Members adopt a rational view or power and authority.	Group goals are developed. Members become more autonomous.
INTERDEPENDENT PHASE	
Members focus on cooperating with one another.	Harmony must be preserved. Members struggle for equal affection rather than power. Differences are not discussed and issues are not resolved.
Members strive to be close.	Members may perceive a loss of individual identity; rejection; or abandonment. Mature members may ask team for assistance, giving the group a new sense of purpose.
Members develop a team goal approach, resulting in improved client care.	Particular strengths of team members are recognized. Team cohesiveness occurs.

Role and Role Strain

As described, psychiatric/mental health nurses must understand their expected professional activities and demonstrate their abilities in a setting in which many disciplines practice (Fig. 2-1). At times they will experience difficulties in managing the expression and acceptance of their roles.[23]

All nurses experience some role strain in performing their professional roles. Role strain and role conflict have been described by many nursing authors. Carser[9] states that role concerns are common in professional practice, as is anxiety related to role concerns. The anxiety stems from values and beliefs nurses have about their roles. Other professionals around the psychiatric/mental health nurse may also experience anxiety as they are asked by the nurse (if only by the nurse's actions) to en-

gage in professional practice alongside the nurse. If care givers do not verbalize such anxiety, the "feelings become covert issues expressed in systems problems and intra-staff conflict."[9] The covert issues may also be expressed in a chaotic atmosphere in the workplace, poor communication in team meetings, factions among staff groups, and a depleted team spirit.

Role Theory

A useful manner of analyzing role difficulties is through the use of "role theory." Roles can be defined as "the actual and intangible forms that the self takes."[17] A person functioning in a certain way takes on a role at that specific moment and in that specific situation. The description of

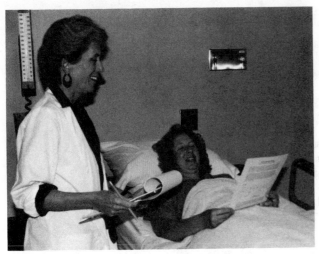

Figure 2-1. A nurse in the role of researcher gathers data for a clinical study.

the role is given (usually automatically, in nonverbal fashion) by both the actor of the role and the others perceiving the enactment of the role. The description of the role given by the self (the actor of the role) and the others observing the role is culturally, socially, and environmentally determined. Psychiatric/mental health nurses may have to explain their role and act in the role for a period of time before other professionals and clients who have never been exposed to the professional role of the nurse (an environmental issue) adapt to the nurse. Others observing the role enactment by the nurse may have to revise their cultural beliefs about nurses (most of whom are women). Others must be made aware that the nurse is sufficiently capable of performing the complex role activities that psychiatric/mental health nursing requires. The others may also have to alter the professional team membership (the societal or group factor) to allow the psychiatric/mental health nurse a place on the treatment team.

Lambert[16] described roles from two viewpoints. One viewpoint is concerned with "status" or "position." Here roles in a system (as in a hospital system) are seen as interrelating. Rules and norms are attributed by individuals or groups for specific roles. For example, each discipline in an institution may have specific norms for behaviors of their own, as well as for other professional groups.

Another viewpoint considers how individuals regulate their own role behaviors according to what is expected of them by others. This perspective studies role "enactments" or role-taking, a process in which individuals organize their behavior with each other (the "interaction") so that roles are "taken." When some roles are taken, remaining roles are taken by others. Other individuals in one's environment may be taken into consideration when deciding on particular behaviors to enact in the role. Most of this behavior is automatic and individuals are unaware of it.

For the psychiatric/mental health nurse, role enactment is complex. It is common for the nurse to experi-

ence stress or "role strain" associated with role enactment. *Role strain* is a general term that incorporates the concepts of role conflict, role discontinuity, role overload, and role ambiguity.

Role conflict occurs when the "person is subjected to two or more contradictory expectations that the person cannot simultaneously satisfy."[16] Role conflict arises when the individual's internal values or beliefs are mutually incompatible, or when internal values or beliefs oppose an external demand placed on the nurse. For example, the nurse wants a professional relationship with other team members so that each collaborates or cooperates with the others, yet the nurse must discuss the removal of clients from group therapy by another team member for private, individual sessions.

Role discontinuity refers to a lack of integration among the different roles an individual is called on to perform. For example, the nurse administers antianxiety medication to a client because there will not be time to guide the client through relaxation exercises after the current activity is completed, and all other staff members are busy.

Role ambiguity occurs when the expectations of a particular role are incomplete, so that the person enacting the role does not know how to perform the role. For example, a Vietnamese client has just been admitted to a mental health unit. The admitting nurse is not familiar with Vietnamese culture, and does not know which members of the family to interview.

Role overload occurs when the demands of the various nursing roles are too numerous or complex. For example, the nurse wants to discuss a client's recent family visit but there are two impending admissions, and a group to lead. The nurse is expected to support clients, nursing administration, and other professional groups in their work, but feels little personal support.

All professionals experience role strain. The health care setting and the interaction of the setting with clients are exciting and complex; however, this atmosphere is conducive to role strain. Role strain is not necessarily a signal to perform the role differently, for to do so may compromise professional standards. By being aware of role strain, the nurse can minimize its effects on work relationships, thereby becoming more effective.

When the nurse becomes aware of the anxiety of role strain, and does not let the anxiety go unanswered, the skill and dedication of the nurse are tested. Peer support, role models, assertiveness training, and administrative support are a few of the creative solutions for the nurse experiencing role strain. Each solution must be cultivated so that role strain becomes manageable.

Obligations of Professional Practice

Boshier[7] presents a rather stark quote from Senator Inouye of Hawaii:

You nurses, you can have whatever you want, you can control the health care system, you have more power than any other group, including all the oil lobbyists, but you will go to your graves with 'docile' written on your tombstones.

Individual nurses must promote the role of the nurse. Nurses are no longer handmaidens to others—they are guided by their own accountability. Each individual nurse should have a sense of obligation and commitment to accountability; nursing cannot grow without it.

In a descriptive study, Batey and Lewis[5] systematically reviewed the literature and interviewed 12 directors of nursing service in the Pacific Northwest to define and elaborate on the concepts of responsibility, authority, and autonomy. They defined the three concepts as preconditions for accountability.

Responsibility

A *responsibility* is a charge for which one is answerable. The focus in this definition is on the "charge" or duty aspect, not on the person to whom one answers concerning the fulfillment of the duty. Responsibilities can come from external or internal sources. Internal sources of responsibility come from nursing itself. All too often in the past, nursing has accepted responsibilities from external sources regardless of the appropriateness of the charge for nursing.

For example, nurses on a mental health unit may not accept the responsibility for care of a client who is violent and belongs in a protected jail environment. In such a situation, the nurses need to state what their appropriate charges or responsibilities are. These statements are needed, because nurses are the only professionals with extended contact with the client.

Nurses do not blindly serve the needs of other disciplines. Batey and Lewis stated that critical incongruence between the expectations of nursing and the expectations of others in the health care setting (hospital administrators, physicians, and clients) can contribute to negative consequences for client care.[5] A responsibility is a charge; it is a noun. Being responsible, however, is a verb; it denotes the acceptance (or nonacceptance) of a responsibility or a charge. Being responsible also denotes choice or the use of free will on the part of the nurse. By stating the nature of nursing responsibility, the *nurse* controls *nursing* practice and takes a part in planning and executing health care.

Authority

Authority is the rightful power to fulfill a charge (responsibility). Authority denotes that the nurse exercises the command to fulfill a responsibility. Authority denotes the fact that there is no one in a position "above" the nurse to assume the authority. For example, the nurse has a professional responsibility to help clients learn about their mental health/illness, and the authority to carry out such a responsibility. In emergency situations, however, the

typical lines of authority may not hold. The rightful power to perform responsibilities is accorded to those present.

In another example, the nurse may act on the "delegated" authority of others. Here the nurse does not act on her own authority. The nurse may administer a medication, but this action occurs as a result of the delegated authority of a nurse practitioner, physician, or pharmacist.

A nurse may be responsible for but have no authority to perform the duty or responsibility. In most states, nurses cannot discharge a psychiatric client from the hospital; only the physician has this authority. In some states, however, nurses do admit and discharge clients from psychiatric hospitals and have the authority over their case load to do so. Lewis and Batey state that "nursing has been reluctant to assert the rightful power" of authority that their knowledge base authorizes.[5]

Autonomy

Autonomy means the "freedom to make discretionary and binding decisions consistent with one's scope of practice and freedom to act on those decisions."[5] If authority is the rightful power to assume a responsibility, then autonomy is the freedom to exercise that rightful power. Discretionary decisions are not the mere performance of standard protocols. Discretionary decisions involve *judgment* in complex health care decisions, such as those of the psychiatric nurse.

Autonomy is "confined to that for which the professional holds authority derived from "their knowledge base and research of the discipline and their individual position (as in the administrative hierarchy).[5] Batey and Lewis stated that nurses can do more to gain autonomy. Nurses are unwilling at times "to assert their decisions and to act on decisions appropriate to their clients."[5] For example, a psychiatric nurse formulated an idea for a group on a psychiatric hospital unit and then asked the physician if the idea was suitable, thus not exercising autonomy. A better approach would have been to discuss the suggestion with the team.

Autonomy "is neither absolute independence nor a state of functioning in isolation from others."[5] It exists as a freedom to act in a professional manner so that client care is enriched.

Accountability

The consequence of autonomy is *accountability*. If the nurse accepts the freedom to act (autonomy), the nurse must be held accountable to others for the actions. Batey and Lewis define accountability as "the fulfillment of a formal obligation to disclose to referent others the purposes, principles, procedures, results, income, and expenditures for which one has authority."[5] The disclosure occurs so that decisions and evaluations can be performed.

Accountability includes the systematic and periodic disclosure of one's responsibilities. Initiating the disclosure is the responsibility of only the one who is accountable. Accountability does not carry the connotation of error. Accountability involves a disclosure at scheduled intervals.

The nurse discloses information to those who must make decisions because of their position or situation. For example, clients need disclosure concerning the benefits of participating in their treatment planning so that they can decide in what ways they will participate.

Accountability denotes the acceptance of the need to disclose and the willingness to work with the effects of the disclosure. Professional nurses are answerable for what they have done; nurses must stand behind and believe in what they have done.

Accountability has been a cornerstone of professional nursing practice for decades. Team members from each discipline should be expected to assume behaviors indicating professional accountability.

Summary

1. The role of the psychiatric/mental health nurse developed initially from the needs of another discipline—medicine.

2. The nursing role initially took the form of housekeeping and the control of others.

3. The development of the professional role of the psychiatric/mental health nurse took place as nurses themselves saw the *client-based need* for care based on scientific principles. The formation of established curricula in psychiatric/mental health nursing, and the more humane treatment of clients in general, assisted in the development of the role.

4. The role was also fostered by the establishment of standards of practice by national nursing governing bodies, as well as the work of leaders in the field of psychiatric/mental health nursing to build nursing's body of knowledge through research and scholarly publication.

5. Currently there are four major disciplines working with mental health clients: nursing, psychiatry, psychology, and social work.

6. There is considerable role overlap among the disciplines working in mental health care.

7. Both cooperation and aggressive competition exist among the professionals working in mental health.

8. Nurses today are accountable for their own performance in the health care field. Psychiatric/mental health nurses define their own practice and function in an interdisciplinary fashion.

References

1. American Nurses' Association: Standards of Psychiatric and Mental Health Nursing Practice. Kansas City, American Nurses' Association, 1982
2. American Nurses' Association: Statement on Psychiatric and Mental Health Nursing Practice. Kansas City, American Nurses' Association, 1976
3. American Psychiatric Association: Diagnostic and Statistical Manual of Mental Disorders-III-R. Washington, DC, American Psychiatric Association, 1987
4. Ashley JA: Hospital Paternalism and the Role of the Nurse. New York, Teachers College Press, 1976
5. Batey M, Lewis F: Clarifying autonomy and accountability in nursing service, parts I and II. J Nurs Adm 12:13, 1982
6. Benfer B: Defining the role and function of the psychiatric nurse as a member of the team. Perspect Psychiatr Care 18:167, 1980
7. Boshier M, Boshier L: Professional Issues. In Critchley D, Maurin J (eds): The Clinical Specialist in Psychiatric/Mental Health Nursing. New York, John Wiley & Sons, 1984
8. California Board of Registered Nursing: Laws Relating to Nursing Education, Licensure, Practice. Sacramento, Board of Registered Nursing, 1980
9. Carser D: Primary nursing in the milieu. J Psychosoc Nurs Ment Health Serv 19:35, 1981
10. Church O: Harriet Bailey—a psychiatric nurse pioneer. Perspect Psychiatr Care 18:62, 1980
11. Church O: That Noble Reform: The Emergence of Psychiatric Nursing in the United States, 1882–1963. Ph.D. dissertation, University of Illinois at the Medical Center, 1982
12. Crosby R: Community care of the chronically mentally ill: A theory for practice. J Psychiatr Nurs 25:33, 1987
13. De Leo D, Magni G, Vallerini A et al: Assessment of anxiety and depression in general and psychiatric nurses. Psychol Rep 52:335, 1983
14. Fagin C: Psychiatric nursing at the crossroads: Quo vadis? Perspect Psychiatr Care 19:99, 1981
15. Flaskerud J: The distinctive character of nursing psychotherapy. Issues Ment Health Nurs 6:19, 1984
16. Lambert V: Role theory and the concept of powerlessness. J Psychosoc Nurs Ment Health Serv 19:12, 1981
17. Moreno J: The role concept: A bridge between psychiatry and sociology. Am J Psychiatry 118:518, 1961
18. Mullaney J, Fox R, Liston M: Clinical nurse specialist and social worker—clarifying the roles. Nurs Outlook 22:712, 1974
19. Peplau H: Psychiatric Nursing: Past, Present, and Future. Presented at the Neuropsychiatric Institute, Los Angeles, University of California, November 1, 1982
20. Peplau H: Some reflections on earlier days in psychiatric nursing. J Psychosoc Nurs Ment Health Serv 20:19, 1982
21. Reeves K: Hispanic utilization of an ethnic mental health clinic. J Psychiatr Nurs 24:23, 1986
22. Romoff V, Kane I: Primary nursing in psychiatry: An effective and functional model. Perspect Psychiatr Care 20:74, 1982
23. Stuart W: Role strain and depression: A causal inquiry. J Psychosoc Nurs Ment Health Serv 19:22, 1981
24. Weiss S: Role differentiation between nurse and physician: Implications for nursing. Nurs Res 32:133, 1983

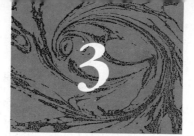

RONDA MINTZ AND LORETTA M. BIRCKHEAD

COMMUNICATION IN PSYCHIATRIC/MENTAL HEALTH NURSING

Learning Objectives

Upon completion of this chapter the student should be able to do the following:

1. Define communication and explain its importance in psychiatric/mental health nursing.
2. Compare the major theories of communication, including the pragmatic, mechanistic, psychological, and interactionist perspectives.
3. Describe how communication techniques differ among the primary, secondary, and tertiary levels of prevention.
4. Differentiate between the following pairs of terms: verbal and nonverbal communication, content and process of communication; therapeutic and social communication.
5. Explain ways in which nurses can effectively communicate with clients from other cultures or races.
6. Identify four listening and four action-oriented communication techniques.
7. Describe the attitudes of nurses that promote therapeutic interactions.
8. Identify three ways in which nurses participate in the process of communication among staff members in the clinical setting.

Introduction

Communication is an integral part of the interchange among family members and friends, as well as between nurses and clients. Communication is easy, or is it? Do we *say* what we mean; do we mean what we say? Do we *hear* responses? What are we saying nonverbally? Do we assume we know what the other person means, or do we clarify the meaning? Do we approach topics openly, without passing judgment, or do we reject thoughts, ideas, or opinions that differ from our own? Communication may appear simple at first, but it is a very complex exchange. Because communication is one of the primary tools of the psychiatric nurse, understanding communication is essential.

Communicating with clients is a skill that must be learned and perfected, much like the techniques of learning to apply sterile dressing or assisting as a scrub nurse in the operating room. Often, nurses assume that they know how to talk and listen and don't concentrate on perfecting therapeutic communication by practice, as they do other nursing interventions. The techniques of therapeutic communication are presented in this chapter, along with concepts of prevention and adaptation of communication to the illness severity level of the client. Theories explaining communication are also discussed.

Theories of Communication

A number of theorists have developed explanations of communication. These theories seek to answer questions concerning the mechanisms through which people communicate, as well as the nature (or description) of the information that is exchanged. A study of communication theories allows the nurse to understand the communication occurring between the nurse and the client, as well as to select the communication techniques that promote client change.

The Pragmatic Perspective

Watzlawick, Beavin, and Jackson[22] studied communication not "as a one-way phenomenon (from speaker to listener)" but as an interaction process. By not limiting the study of communication to the sender, the authors widened the "range of observation" of interaction so that the context or the environment of the sender is included in the observation. They viewed communication from a systems perspective, including the following components in the study of interaction:

1. Communication of the message, verbally or nonverbally
2. The effects of the message on others
3. Others' reaction to it
4. The context in which steps 1, 2, and 3 occur.

The inclusion of these parts of communication indicates that the "system" of communication is important, be-cause all of these parts are related. The relationship between the sender and the receiver(s) is of concern, not merely "the mind" of the sender of the message.

Watzlawick, Beavin, and Jackson also discussed the behavioral effects of communication. They considered the terms *communication* and *behavior* synonymous. The close tie between communication and behavior occurs because of the sender's body language and other behavioral cues, such as tone of voice, that carry much of the message to the receiver.

The authors described the important concept of *feedback*. Feedback occurs when part of the system's output is reintroduced into the system as information about the output. Either positive or negative feedback may occur. Positive feedback leads to change, while negative feedback promotes stability. The terms "positive" and "negative" feedback do not indicate a right or wrong event or experience, but rather the tendency for a particular message to promote, or to discourage, change in a system. Positive and negative feedback are depicted in the following figures.

The authors also explored the process of *metacommunication,* an important concept in psychiatric/mental health care. The authors stated that there is a need to metacommunicate, or communicate about communication. An example of metacommunication occurs when a nurse finds an individual in a room, alone, during group therapy time and asks the client what is occurring. Although nonverbally, the client is communicating that some stressor is present. The nurse attempts to determine the reason for the isolation by communicating (the verbal statement made to the client) about the client's communication (the nonverbal behavior of isolation).

The purposes of metacommunication are numerous, and include:

1. In many instances, individuals do not communicate what should be communicated. For example, a person may nag a spouse as a way of handling fears that the spouse does not care about the individual. The individual does not tell the spouse about the fear because the individual does not have the skill to talk about personal experiences or because the spouse, indeed, does not care about the relationship and this lack of caring has been communicated nonverbally to the person.

   Metacommunication can serve as a means to discuss with others what is occurring in their experience. If the individuals do not want to talk specifically about particular experiences, they can at least acknowledge that unclear communication is occurring.

2. Individuals from different cultures attribute different meanings to behaviors. Metacommunication offers a means to clarify different meanings. Cultural aspects of communication will be discussed further in a later section.

3. At times individuals are not aware of their true experiences, and may not be able to label their feelings. By observing nonverbal behaviors, nurses can meta-

Message Sender	Message	Message Receiver

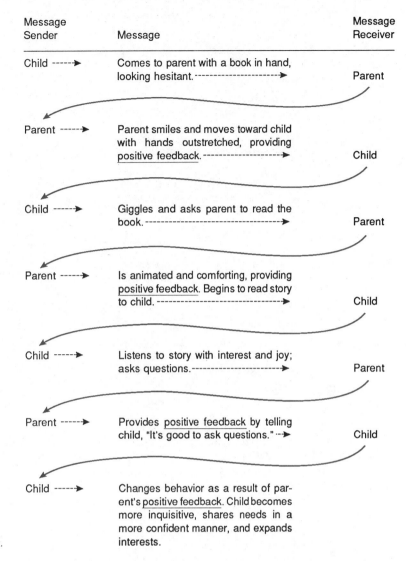

Child ----→ Comes to parent with a book in hand, looking hesitant. -----------→ Parent

Parent ----→ Parent smiles and moves toward child with hands outstretched, providing positive feedback. ---------→ Child

Child ----→ Giggles and asks parent to read the book. ----------------→ Parent

Parent ----→ Is animated and comforting, providing positive feedback. Begins to read story to child. --------------→ Child

Child ----→ Listens to story with interest and joy; asks questions. -----------→ Parent

Parent ----→ Provides positive feedback by telling child, "It's good to ask questions." --→ Child

Child ----→ Changes behavior as a result of parent's positive feedback. Child becomes more inquisitive, shares needs in a more confident manner, and expands interests.

Figure 3-1. An example of positive feedback.

communicate by telling clients what is happening in order to get clients to express their feelings verbally.

The authors also described several axioms of communication, including:

1. "One cannot NOT behave." Both verbal and nonverbal behaviors (even silence) have "message values" because they influence others.

2. "Any communication implies a commitment and thereby defines the relationships." This defining aspect of communication refers to "what sort of message it is to be taken as." For example, one person may say to another, "Of course you're important to me—just let me finish reading the paper." This relationship is defined (at least by one member of the relationship) as one in which the value the person places on the other is uncertain. Watzlawick, Beavin, and Jackson stated that "Relationships are only rarely defined deliberately or with full awareness." To the authors, "Sick relationships are characterized by a constant struggle about the nature of the relationship."

3. "The nature of a relationship is contingent upon the punctuation of the communicational sequences between the communicants." Punctuations serve "to organize common and important interactional sequences." For example, a husband may say to his wife, "You need to express yourself more." The wife responds, "I can't express myself because you are always talking." The husband retorts, "I talk because you don't." This sequence could continue endlessly. The husband would punctuate the interchange as beginning with the wife's silence. The wife would punctuate the interchange differently, by organizing it or describing it as starting with her husband's incessant talking.

4. Human communication can be referred to as digital or analogic. *Digital communication* refers to the specific words used to name something. The word "cat," for example, names a particular animal.

   Analogic communication refers to an individual's "posture, gesture, facial expression, voice inflection, the sequence, rhythm, and cadence of the words themselves, and any other nonverbal behavior

Message Sender	Message	Message Receiver

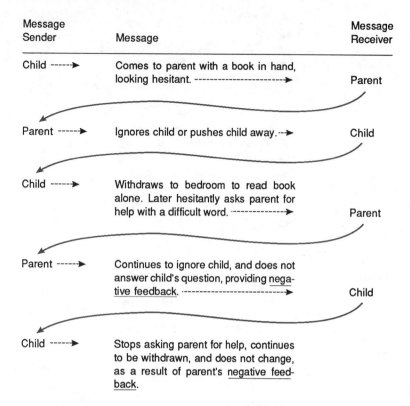

Child ------> Comes to parent with a book in hand, looking hesitant. ----------------------> Parent

Parent ------> Ignores child or pushes child away. --> Child

Child ------> Withdraws to bedroom to read book alone. Later hesitantly asks parent for help with a difficult word. -------------> Parent

Parent ------> Continues to ignore child, and does not answer child's question, providing negative feedback. -------------------------> Child

Child ------> Stops asking parent for help, continues to be withdrawn, and does not change, as a result of parent's negative feedback.

Figure 3-2. An example of negative feedback.

of the organism." In relationships, we rely almost exclusively on an analogic communication to define the nature of the relationship.

5. "All communicational interchanges are either symmetrical or complementary, depending on whether they are based on equality or on difference." In one exchange the emphasis is on the symmetry of the participants, with each participant equal to the others and any differences among them minimized. For example, in a symmetrical "good" relationship, each person takes the other's interests into account and attempts to provide open communication. In a "bad" symmetrical relationship, all members of a group engage in antisocial behavior. In a complementary relationship, there are always two different positions, such as superior–inferior, one-up and one-down, and strong–weak. Each partner behaves in a manner that "presupposes, while at that same time provides reasons for, the behavior of the other."

Watzlawick, Beavin, and Jackson provided other basic understandings about communication, including the following points:

1. Although an individual "cannot not communicate," a person may *attempt* not to communicate. This attempt can be made in the following ways:

   a. A person may reject the communication offered by another. For example, an individual may say, "I do not want to talk." Such a statement is not without repercussions in the relationship. However, an embarrassing silence may occur, so that a relationship with the other has *not* been avoided.

   b. An individual may accept unwanted communication from another. However, the individual may think less of self for doing so, and resent the message-sender.

   c. A person may adopt the defense of "disqualification." The person may "communicate in a way that invalidates communication. Disqualifications include inconsistencies, subject switches, tangentializations, incomplete sentences, misunderstandings, an obscure style of speech," and others. Many of these operations are particularly destructive to individuals and to relationships. For example, while sitting on a bench near a busy street, an abusive parent says to the child, "Go play anywhere you want." The meaning here is obscure. Is the parent protective of the child, as is expected of parents, or is the parent being abusive by telling the child to play in the street? Communicative defenses are very difficult to untangle to reach clarity.

2. The authors described communication theory from a systems perspective. While the systems perspective of this text is discussed in Chapter 7, one component described by Watzlawick, Beavin and Jackson needs further comment: the principle of *equifinality*. This is an important principle used to examine interpersonal behavior. The "principle of equifinality means that the same results may spring from different origins." In an "open system," "different initial conditions yield the same final result and different results may be produced by the same causes." In terms of interpersonal relationships, the specifics of cause or

result are "not nearly so important as the ongoing organization of interaction."

For example, a husband may believe that his wife's bad mood is due to the fact that the wife believes that the husband is "not good" in some way. The husband feels rejected, and an argument begins. However, the husband finds that the wife has a back pain, has had a difficult day at work, and does not wish to attend a necessary meeting that evening.

The initial organization of this interaction was difficult. The wife was in a bad mood, and the husband believed that he was the cause of this bad mood. This sequence of events was not clarified until the argument began. In reality, there were several causes for the bad mood. In interpersonal terms, the important part of the situation was the ongoing organization of how the wife "shared" the bad mood; how the husband interpreted the mood; and how the two people did, or did not, talk about their interaction.

Many individuals find relief in communicating in ways that assume the operation of equifinality. They attempt to verify their assumptions about another's behavior. In many cases, they find that their presumed causes are negative (not true in light of the complexity of the relationship) and hamper the relationship.

Trenholm[21] summarized other perspectives on human communication that broadened the understanding of communication, as described in the sections below.

The Mechanistic Perspective

The *mechanistic perspective* on communication describes communication as a behavioral transfer from one place to another. "A affects B, affects C, and so forth." To study an object properly, it is necessary to isolate the subsystems of the object. Hence, the way to study communication is to reduce the communicative behavior to small units, such as words or gestures. This model assumes that individual objects (people) can be isolated one from another, and that the total collection of people is the sum of the parts. The whole system is NOT seen as more than the sum of the parts, as it is in systems theory.

According to this model, any "feature not intended" by the originator of communication is considered "noise" in the channel of communication. The goal of communication is to transmit a message from the sender to the receiver with as little noise as possible. "The extent to which the message relates its integrity at various points along the channel is called fidelity."

The Psychological Perspective

The *psychological perspective* locates "communication as within the mental processes" of those communicating. Within individuals, "neuro-motor responses are acquired," and meaning is developed. Communication "arises out of the need to reduce uncertainty and to act

effectively." Meaning is "given" to the stimuli rather than "received." In other words, each person develops his or her own meaning for stimuli.

The psychological perspective shares many concepts with learning theory, which "views human behavior as a series of stimulus–response chains." Human beings are affected by stimuli. People respond as a result of processing the stimuli. One assumption of this perspective is that human beings "exist independently within stimulus fields that they both process and produce."

The concept of "mental set" is a part of the psychological perspective. A mental set is a group of "expectations," derived from past experiences, that are used to evaluate present situations. Individuals act according to their evaluations of these experiences.

The human being, however, is an active information processor and can make choices. The capacity to actively select responses separates the psychological perspective from the behavioral perspective.

The psychological perspective promotes research that considers how "drives, needs, goals, and attitudes" affect "message construction and reception." Another focus of study is on the similarity in meanings individuals give to stimuli. Most research in communication, until recently, used either the mechanistic or the psychological perspective.

The Interactionist Perspective

The *interactionist perspective* comes from a body of knowledge termed *symbolic interactionism*. This perspective differs from the psychological perspective in its belief that individuals cannot be thought of in isolation from others in society. Symbolic interactionism suggests that objects in the world are "neither material entities (as in the mechanistic view), nor stimuli (as in the psychological perspective)." Rather, objects are things to which individuals relate in the form of a symbol. In this perspective, "an object becomes significant when it is named, as when an arbitrary symbol is attached to it." Symbols, in turn, are "significant because they are shared" with others in the culture.

According to the symbolic interactionist perspective, the individual uses symbols to designate self. The self is symbolized as an "I" or as a "Me." The "I" is the self who acts and initiates actions. The "Me" is the individual looking at the self as an object. For example, people observe their own actions.

The interactionist perspective differs from the psychological in that the latter views the "self as an independent subject filtering experiences through enduring mental structures." In the interactionist perspective, the "individual constructs the experiences of self by acting toward the self as if it were a social object, thereby designating it symbolically." The "self is constructed symbolically."

Individuals create shared meanings by exchanging significant symbols. Individuals have the ability to assume the perspective of others because they share a common culture. Theorists who adopt the interactionist perspective emphasize "role-taking," or adopting the perspective of others. "Communication is centered in this role-taking process." It is not centered in the individual's perceptual filters, as in the psychological perspective. In the interactionist perspective, "Communication occurs, not as a product of sequential actions between two people, but as individuals experience each other."

The interactionist perspective states that individuals have "not one self (as implied by the psychological perspective), but multiple selves depending on those around them." In this way, we "are the product of others."

To interactionist theorists, effective communication involves sharing meanings among individuals. To those of the mechanistic perspective, effectiveness is an attempt to "minimize information loss by increasing fidelity." To interactionists, it is a product of "mental structure similarity" or shared meanings. Those of the pragmatic perspective do not define effective communication, but seek to describe the development of behavioral patterns among people.

Trenholm[21] states that the interactionist perspective is currently growing in validity, especially among those interested in language development and social-cognitive processing. The recognition that communication affects and is affected by social reality comes from an interactionist perspective.

Comparing the four perspectives, the pragmatic and interactionist perspectives do not focus on individual senders and receivers but on the relationship of behaviors among people. The other two models (the psychological and the mechanistic) focus on the individual. The pragmatic perspective, for example, examines behaviors, and looks for repeated patterns of behavior occurring among people rather than for individual personality traits.

Nurses may use one or more of the perspectives described above. A psychiatric nurse on a child/adolescent unit may participate in a "token economy" program that rewards appropriate behaviors. Such a program is based on a mechanistic perspective. Other nurses, visiting the homes of psychiatric clients (and their families), may use the pragmatic perspective. Peplau's interpersonal theory of nursing is based generally on the interactionist perspective. The Self/Other/Relationship model described in this work is developed from the psychological, pragmatic, and interactionist perspectives.

The Art and Science of Communication

Just as nursing is described as a combination of art and science, therapeutic communication is also an art and a science. Becoming an effective communicator requires practice, willingness to experiment with new styles or ideas, and an openness to receiving constructive criticism and recommendations from respected mentors and supervisors.

In this text, *communication* is defined as *the interchanges among individuals through which they define and change their awareness of Self and their relationships with Others.* While there are numerous definitions of communication, each focusing on various aspects of the communication process, this definition highlights the following points:

1. As communication occurs among people, the individuals change, as do their Relationships with each Other. As shown in Figure 3-3, the three components—the Self, the Other, and the Relationship between the Self and the Other—are continually changing as time progresses. This change is denoted by the changing configurations inside the circles and boxes, although part of the Self/Other and their Relationship does stay the same, as noted by the continuing circle and box shapes. The word "Other" (or significant other) is used to refer to another person or persons with whom an individual (the Self) relates. The Self/Other/Relationship framework itself will be discussed in Chapter 5.

2. Although communication results in a definition of or change in Self, Other, or the Relationship of Self and Other, the definition or change may not happen immediately once communication occurs. For example, many clients must examine a particularly troublesome pattern of behavior many times before they can actually define or understand it.

Communication and the Levels of Prevention

A major principle of effective communication is that it is suitable for the level of prevention required. The word "prevention" denotes stopping a threat before it occurs. Caplan[6] used the phrase "preventive psychiatry." Caplan wrote about prevention in mental health care as much more than the stereotyped idea of hospital programs for the mentally ill. He described a form of social and political action that relates to people at any point on the health–illness continuum. Individuals receiving mental health care can be healthy, moderately ill, or severely mentally ill.

One of the primary tenets of psychiatric/mental health nursing is that *the nurse's communication is tailored to the preventive program needed by the client.* Specific communication practices for the various levels of prevention will be discussed after further description of the levels of prevention.

Preventive mental health/illness care programs are designed according to different levels of prevention. The first level is *primary prevention,* which involves planning and carrying out programs for reducing "the incidence of mental disorders of all types" in the community. *Secondary prevention* practices seek to decrease "the duration of a significant number of those (mental) disorders that do occur." Fostering "improvement that may result from" mental disorders is *tertiary prevention.*[6]

One important principle of preventive health care is that when a health care worker has an opportunity to provide care it is done according to the level of care required, and each level of care is important. This role of practice is reflected in the definition of nursing found in the ANA's *Nursing: A Social Policy Statement:* "Nursing is the diagnosis and treatment of human response to actual or potential health problems."[1] Actual health problems include the care of the mentally ill in hospitals, similar to tertiary prevention. Care for potential health problems (primary prevention) includes providing time for family members to talk about the changes in their lives as a result of the birth of a child.

Human responses to health problems "are often multiple, episodic, or continuous, fluid, and varying, and are less discrete or circumscribed than medical diagnostic categories tend to be."[12] The varying nature of human responses dictates that nurses predicate their communication on the nature of client responses as well as on the nurses' understanding of what can promote mental illness in healthy individuals or populations at risk.

Table 3-1 describes several expected client responses and nurse behaviors at the various levels of prevention. It emphasizes that nurses communicate with clients where *actual* or *potential* health problems exist. The table demonstrates many opportunities for nurse-client communication. Table 3-2 lists several characteristics of effective nurse responses based on client behaviors.

In summary, prevention of mental illness is an important responsibility of psychiatric/mental health nursing. Pothier[18] reported that 11.8% of youths under the age of 18 have some mental disorder, but only 7% receive care for these problems. Psychiatric nurses with "their highly specialized preparation are not being fully utilized in the provision of mental health services for children and families who are in need of such care." Research on the use of early detection and intervention indicates that these nursing actions "can prevent more serious mental illness." However, psychiatric nurses are "not sufficiently recognized by their interdisciplinary colleagues as a group of professionals who are highly qualified to implement preventive interventions."[11] Pothier described the practice of psychiatric nurses in community-based preventive psychiatric care (for example, home care, as described in Chapter 30) as being on the "cutting edge of the nursing profession."[18]

The Nature of Communication

Verbal and Nonverbal Communication

Communication can be either verbal or nonverbal. Verbal communication includes spoken and written words transmitted between people. The nurse cannot assume that spoken words reflect the true meaning of what was

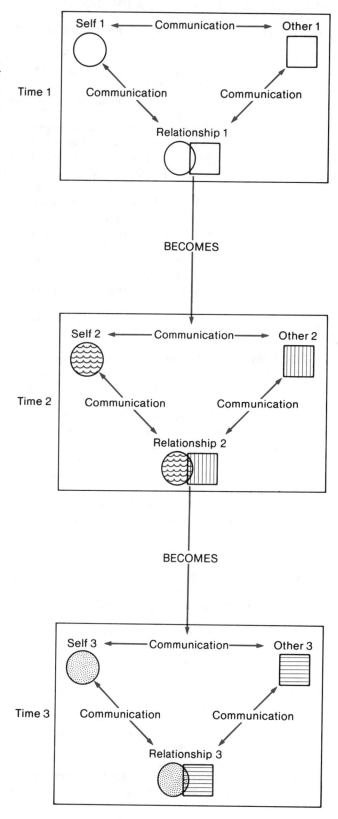

Figure 3-3. Changes in Self, Other, and the Relationship of Self and Other as a result of communication.

TABLE 3-1.
NURSE–HEALTH CARE RECIPIENT BEHAVIORS

LEVEL OF PREVENTION	HEALTH CARE RECIPIENT CHARACTERISTICS	NURSE RESPONSE
Primary	A client is at risk for developing health problems. *Example:* A teenager lives at home with a depressed parent.	Facilitate family discussions about mental illness and changes occurring in the family as a result of the illness.
	A client's developmental stage may increase stressors. *Example:* A client is pregnant.	Provide opportunities for discussion and sharing of feelings, *e.g.,* about body changes, emotional needs.
Secondary	A client develops a disorder for the first time. *Example:* The nurse sees a change in behavior [severe withdrawal] in an adolescent whose father has a Primary Thought Disorder.	Discuss with the father the need to assess the adolescent. Ask the adolescent to attend a family session to introduce the idea of meeting with the adolescent individually.
	A client experiences a crisis and cannot cope. *Example:* A woman is raped and refuses to be examined in the emergency room.	Reassure the client that a woman will remain with her. Sit with the client and allow her to calm down.
Tertiary	A client has a lowered capacity to participate in occupational and social life in the community. *Example:* A veteran has explosive outbursts at work and gets fired.	Refer the client for counseling. Discuss with the client the benefit of therapy groups for veterans. Discuss common veteran responses to combat in order to facilitate assessment.
	A client is admitted to a psychiatric treatment facility.	Provide individual intervention, group therapy, family therapy. Focus on the client's repeated patterns of behavior that cause concern.

said. Sullivan,[20] a psychiatrist who developed the interpersonal theory of psychiatry, stated that in psychiatric care the clinician tries to find the *meaning* of what is occurring, or has occurred, with the client. To Sullivan, much of the work in care involves "improving on earlier approximations of understanding" that the client and clinician have of what has occurred. Sullivan noted that "often the statements that misled (him) would have misled anyone who was paying attention only to what these (the client's) statements presumably meant." There is much more to be understood about the life of a psychiatric client than what is stated verbally. The following box lists a few of the reasons that clients do not state what they truly mean.

Nonverbal communication includes:

Sound patterns, including voice tone, rhythm, and intensity
Bodily movements or facial expressions
Posture or body angle (facing other people while talking to them or turning one's back toward them)
Touch
Space (the distance between those communicating)
Adornments (dress, hairstyle, jewelry)

TABLE 3-2.
CHARACTERISTICS OF EFFECTIVE COMMUNICATION AT THE VARIOUS LEVELS OF PREVENTION

LEVEL OF PREVENTION	CLIENT CHARACTERISTICS	EFFECTIVE NURSE BEHAVIORS
Primary	Client can be identified as part of a population at risk for developing mental health problems. *Example:* A woman with three small children has a husband who has just battered her.	Engage clients in discussion about their mental health. Serve as a role model for assessing stressors in life. Be assertive in confronting stressors. Be positive in discussing potential problems.
Secondary	Client experiences a psychological problem but is undiagnosed. *Example:* A college student with no history of mental illness experiences an episode of a language and thought disorder.	Be open to the clients' description of their true concerns. Take a nonjudgmental approach. Be willing to take action. Serve as a resource person. Effectively identify problems and interventions focused on the problems.
Tertiary	Client functions at a level below capabilities. *Example:* An adult survivor of incest lives an isolated, lonely life.	Present a sense of hope. Be patient in performing interventions repeatedly. Tailor communication so that it can be understood by the client. Do not demonstrate disgust with the client. Provide sufficient limit-setting while not becoming autocratic. Hold appropriate expectations while believing that change is possible.

RELEVANT RESEARCH

This study describes clients' ideas of what helps or hinders recovery from a major mental illness, and the effect of the treatment philosophy on recovery. Thirty-four articles, published between 1856 and 1985, were reviewed to identify factors that foster recovery, from the clients' perspective. The final sample included 20 articles, all authored by clients who described their recoveries from long-term mental illnesses (such as schizophrenia) or major affective disorders. The 20 articles were divided into three time periods: those written prior to 1950, before the use of psychotherapeutic medications; those written between 1950 and 1969, when medications were used but deinstitutionalization was not practiced; and those written between 1970 and 1985, when deinstitutionalization was practiced.

According to the clients' articles:

1. As time has progressed, clients have assumed a more active role in their own care. Provision of care has moved from passive activities (providing rest) to active approaches (encouraging client interaction).

2. The articles written from 1976 to 1985 revealed the clients' sense of terror during the illness, and the horror clients endured while waiting for medications. The horror described was similar to that related by clients receiving insulin shock therapy decades ago.

Other clients described their nurse as an "oasis of caring and sanity." Clients reported the benefits of having others communicate support, a hopeful attitude, understanding, and acceptance. Clients voiced their desire to have clinicians establish trust and explain the care being provided.

3. Another finding relates to the levels of prevention. Clients at the "early stages of recovery need to understand what is happening to them now, whereas in later stages of recovery they need to know how to cope with and anticipate the future." Throughout the illness, clients may move back and forth along the continuum of primary, secondary, and tertiary levels of prevention. Early interventions in the course of illness (at the secondary level of prevention) must focus on "routine, structure, and protection." However, as individuals recover (within the secondary level), "interventions must also reflect a move toward increasing flexibility, freedom, and challenge."

(Plum K: How patients view recovery: What helps, what hinders. Arch Psychiatr Nurs 1:285, 1987)

Body type (muscular or emaciated, fat or thin)
Time (pauses in conversation or promptness in arriving for an appointment)[10]

Proxemics is the study of space in communication. The study of body movements in communication is termed *kinesics*.

EXPLANATIONS OF THE CLIENT'S UNCLEAR VERBALIZATIONS

1. The client is presently anxious.
2. The client was anxious at the time of an event, which leads to unclear memories.
3. The client says what will please the therapist, not what is true.
4. The interviewer is unclear or anxious.
5. The client has not learned, or has temporarily lost, the competency of self-expression.
6. The client does not have sufficient mental imagery or concepts to describe what is occurring.
7. The client fears the clinician's reactions to the client's statements.
8. The client sees no benefit in talking, and minimizes the concerns.
9. The client fears that telling will produce some imaginary, terrible insights about the client.

Edwards and Brilhart[11] listed the functions of nonverbal behavior:

"Supplementary verbal signals (including complementing and repeating, contradicting, and emphasizing the verbal communication); substituting for verbal signals; displaying affect; relating; and regulating"

Two of these functions need particular mention: substituting for verbal signals and displaying affect.

Substituting nonverbal communication for verbal communication is common in clients with mental health problems. Many clients have never acquired, or have lost, the competency of verbal expression. They may be afraid to speak, or may be unclear about the true nature of their feelings. The lack of a verbal expression may also denote depression (the person does not have the energy to speak) or preoccupation. Some individuals believe that sharing verbally with others is not appropriate because personal experiences should be kept private, or because the others would not understand. Some clients believe that speaking to other clients is below their status.

Psychiatric nurses can describe the nonverbal cues they observe. In this process of observation, nurses must first understand the present *environment* or context. They take a systems perspective on the client and thereby understand, from knowing the context, what are appropriate expectations for the moment. This process is based on the symbolic interactionist perspective mentioned earlier. Part of the communication process is having mutual expectations of what is typical behavior in particular situations.

For example, if a client on a psychiatric unit begins to shout loudly in an uncontrolled fashion, the nurse would expect other clients to be frightened. The nurse would then observe facial expressions, movements of clients to get away from the shouting, requests from clients for the nurse to "do something about the shouting," and voice tones indicating fear. This is the *assessment* phase of the nursing process.

Based upon the assessment, the nurse then *plans for care.* The nurse would determine from assessing the shouting client (or from talking with staff) the likelihood that the shouting will continue or that the shouting could progress to other types of aggression. Based upon the plan of care, the nurse intervenes.

Intervening in nonverbal behavior that substitutes for verbal behavior is one of the most difficult aspects of psychiatric nursing to grasp. Obviously, the clients in the example above are not stating how they feel. Some clients have this skill, while others do not. The nurse's *therapeutic use of self* involves using a sense of judgment to know how to adjust verbal and nonverbal behavior to assist the clients.

In the above example, one client calmly goes to her room during the shouting. While assessing how clients are dealing with the shouting, the nurse could say to this client, "How are you reacting to the shouting?"

To another client who easily becomes angry and has a difficult time discussing anger, the nurse may not want to ask immediately for reactions that may include feelings (anger in this example), but rather may state what is occurring and what staff expectations are. For example, the nurse could say, "Mr. Adams is upset and shouting. It is important that others avoid the situation until it is over." The nurse would then wait for the client's response. If the client verbally and nonverbally indicated a calm adjustment to the shouting, the nurse could go on to other tasks. The client may indicate, *only* nonverbally, that he is not adjusting, and is becoming angry. He may, for example, have a tight, drawn facial expression. The nurse could say, "I would like to take you to the library or activity room for half an hour until Mr. Adams is calm. Which would you prefer?"

This intervention is based *only on assessing nonverbal behavior.* Using nonverbal cues possibly allows the nurse to prevent a second client from becoming aggressive. The nurse elects to avoid dealing with the client's anger because the environment (which included the shouting) would not promote a verbal discussion of this client's pattern of dealing with anger. The nurse presents expectations for the client and allows the client to select where he wishes to spend the next half-hour.

The nurse would then *evaluate* the interventions. The angry client could indicate nonverbally that his anger is decreasing (by a calmer facial expression, for example).

Displaying affect is also an important function in mental health care. In this function, nonverbal cues indicate feeling states and may serve as indications of what is not being said. DeVito[10] stated that, when verbal and nonverbal messages differ, a person should believe the nonverbal message. Also, nonverbal cues convey 90% of the meaning in communication. Over half of a message

is communicated by facial expressions. Much more is communicated by clients and nurses than by spoken words. The more understanding the nurse has of nonverbal messages, the better will be the ability to make sense of "silent," but important, messages.

Content and Process

To respond as effectively as possible, the nurse must always be aware of the two *levels of communication* in an interaction: content and process. *Content* encompasses the spoken words, or overt messages, exchanged in an interaction. *Process* describes the ambiance, or aura, surrounding the interaction. Process is "what actually is occurring" in an interaction. It includes nonverbal behavior, the client's covert message(s), the way the client reacts to the nurse (which may be guided by the client's past experiences), and the deeper feelings or thoughts that cannot be spoken.[12]

Process-oriented statements are made by the nurse to direct attention to true concerns. The process-oriented statements bring the client to a deeper level of awareness and understanding of the inner self, and thus to the client's motives, drives, and needs that guide behavior, thoughts, and emotions. Process statements can link the here-and-now with the past, in an attempt to improve the client's future. Knowing a client for a period of time is helpful in using process statements.

Example

1. Client: I have nothing to say today (looks anxious while fidgeting).
2. Nurse: It seems difficult to think of something to talk about.
3. Client: Yeah, I guess. Nothing comes to mind.
4. Nurse: You know, the last few sessions have been really hard for you. As we've talked more about your family and your childhood, tears and sadness have come forth. Perhaps this is why you are having a difficult time right now.
5. Client: Yeah, I've been feeling really embarrassed in here. You know, like exposed or found out or something.
6. Nurse: Found out? I'm not sure I know what you mean.
7. Client: Like my cover has been blown. I can't hide anymore because it is out in the open.
8. Nurse: You mean your past is out in the open? The pain of your childhood has surfaced, and there is no escaping?

Statement 2 is a *content* statement. The nurse restates what the client says, but adds an emotional component by addressing the difficulty that the client has in beginning to talk. Statement 4 is a *process* statement. The nurse refers to the last few sessions that have been tearful and painful for the client. The nurse links the past with the present by hypothetically stating that perhaps the difficulty today is related to the last few sessions. The client responds by referring to embarrassment and being found out. Statement 6 is a *content* statement in which the nurse attempts to clarify specifically what "being found out" means to the client. Statement 8 is a *process* statement in which the nurse relates the feeling of being "exposed" or "found out" to the emotional release of childhood feelings.

The example above illustrates how useful process comments can be in facilitating the client's deeper level of awareness as the past and present are linked together in the session. From a psychoanalytic perspective, the linking of the past to the present (and specifically to the interaction with the therapist) provides the primary curative factor for the client.[14] While process statements can be useful, there are limits to their use in therapeutic interventions. Some clients are unable to benefit from a process statement because they are: (1) experiencing a crisis and need supportive, calming interventions; (2) severely disturbed (psychotic or extremely depressed) and cannot follow the logic of a process statement; (3) not ready to confront the past or see its influence on the present; or (4) emotionally or mentally unable to connect the past with the present.

In another example, demonstrated in the Peanuts cartoon, Lucy needs a compliment. She first provides a hint to elicit one—"I think I have a very cute smile." Lucy then resorts to asking directly for a compliment. Schroeder, for whatever reason, does not give a compliment. His reply is so extreme ("the cutest smile of anyone since the world began") that it is not believable. Lucy senses that Schroeder's comment is not a true compliment and notes that, although he says she has a cute smile, his statement is so extreme he could not intend to give a compliment.

Therapeutic vs. Social Communication

Therapeutic and social communication have certain elements in common, since both include speaking and listening. Therapeutic speaking or interviewing, however, is different from social communication because it focuses on the client's thoughts, feelings, behaviors, conflicts, and confusions.[9] Talking with friends, colleagues, family members, or significant others is a two-way sharing and exchanging of thoughts and feelings, with active participation from both parties. Therapeutic speech is client-focused, with minimal spontaneous, personal sharing from the listener (nurse or clinician). The following example shows the differences between talking with a client and talking with a friend.

Example

Client: I really don't like my roommate. He gets on my nerves. He sings to himself at night, if you can believe it.

Nurse: It sounds like you are uncomfortable around him, and he stirs up some feelings in you. What are the feelings?

Client: He reminds me of the brother I never got along with; he was always the favorite at home.

Nurse: So perhaps you feel some anger or frustration right now from past experiences with your brother.

Example

Friend: I really don't like my roommate. He gets on my nerves. He sings to himself at night, if you can believe it.

Nurse: No kidding! (laughs) I remember a college roommate I had who could only wake up in the morning if the alarm clock was on full blast. People and their quirks, huh?

Friend: Yeah, I know. But what's worse is this guy reminds me of my younger brother—you know, I've told you about Jason before, the favorite at home.

Nurse: Sure, I remember. The one who could do no wrong.

Although the client's statements are somewhat similar, the nurse's responses are quite different. With the client, the nurse identifies feelings and connects previous experiences with the present. With the friend, the nurse shares and interacts without identifying and clarifying the friend's feelings. When the nurse stays in the therapeutic mode and attempts to interact with the friend like a client, the results can be problematic, as seen in this example:

Example

Friend: I really don't like my roommate. He gets on my nerves. He sings to himself at night, if you can believe it.

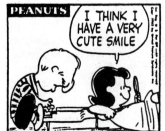 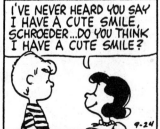 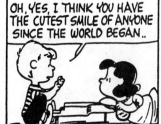 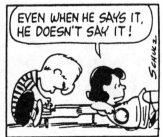

Figure 3-4. The content and process of communication. (© 1963 United Feature Syndicate, Inc.)

Nurse: You seem to be uncomfortable around him. He is stirring up some feelings in you.

Friend: Yeah, well, whatever. He just reminds me of my younger brother, the favorite when I was growing up.

This type of interchange is very common when clinicians attempt to practice therapeutic communication skills on friends and family members. Unfortunately, it is not helpful or positive. Therapeutic communication skills are for client interactions and are dictated by the nurse–client relationship. Friends do not want therapeutically-oriented communication, but usually prefer conversation with a two-way interaction.

Table 3-3 delineates the differences between therapeutic and social communication. It is important to remember these differences when interacting with either a client or a friend.

Cultural Factors

Sue[19] reported that, for effective communication, "the counselor and client must be able to appropriately and accurately send and receive both verbal and nonverbal messages." Communication among individuals from the same culture can be difficult, but the problem of maintaining appropriate communication among people of different racial or ethnic backgrounds is even more of a problem. "Misunderstandings that arise from cultural variations in communication may lead to alienation and/or an inability to develop trust and rapport."[19]

According to Sue, three cultural factors hinder the formation of effective clinician–client relationships:

1. Language barriers
2. Class-related values (many counselors are from the middle class)
3. Culture-bound values with which the clinician assesses health and illness

Sue[19] reported several interviewer and/or client traits that may hinder the counseling relationship. These factors are typically found in relationships between white middle-class interviewers and Third World clients.

TABLE 3-3.
THERAPEUTIC COMMUNICATION VS. SOCIAL CONVERSATION

THERAPEUTIC COMMUNICATION	SOCIAL CONVERSATION
1. Client-focused	1. Two-way talking and listening
2. Client expresses and shares.	2. Mutual expression and sharings
3. Nurses use specific techniques to facilitate clients' expressions.	3. Techniques are rarely used.
4. Goal-oriented	4. Goal-oriented
5. Planned, organized, with specific interventions	5. Spontaneous, mutual talking; nonintervention-focused
6. Professional relationship	6. Friendship

1. Interviewers often expect clients to "exhibit some degree of openness" and be able to discuss intimate psychological concerns. To many Asian-Americans, silence denotes respect for others; there is also restraint about demonstrating feelings.
2. The interviewer–client relationship is one-way. Clients talk about their lives and interviewers listen and provide feedback about the clients' communication. Black persons, however, often have a sense of kinship with others rather than being individually centered.
3. The therapy experience is often ambiguous. To some degree, the interviewing situation is "unstructured and it forces the client to be the primary active participant." Many Hispanics prefer a "concrete, tangible, and structured approach."
4. Therapists often promote long-range goals for clients. Native Americans often prefer working on immediate, short-range goals.
5. Clinicians generally speak standard English. Third World and poor clients may be bilingual and/or speak in little or nonstandard English or in dialect unfamiliar to the clinician.
6. Therapists may distinguish between physical and emotional events. Native Americans may use supernatural explanations for the physical and emotional aspects of the person.
7. Clinicians emphasize cause-and-effect relationship. Native Americans usually emphasize "creative, experimental, intuitive, and nonverbal" views of the world.

In many instances differences between counselor and client can lead to a poor counseling outcome. According to Sue, a minority client's "brief, different, or 'poor' verbal response may lead many counselors to input inaccurate characteristics or motives to" the client.[19]

Bradley and Edinberg[5] pose a question that nurses can ask themselves while counseling clients from different racial or ethnic backgrounds: "How can I (the nurse), with my values, perceptions, background, and role, communicate effectively with a person from a different group with his or her values, perceptions, background, and role as a client?" The authors encourage nurses to maintain the client's sense of self-worth and dignity. Nurses must also respect the client's cultural identity. In many instances, clients will talk about their needs based on their cultural beliefs, if asked in a noncondescending manner. The nurse can also be sensitive to cultural preferences concerning the sick role (or cultural beliefs concerning appropriate behaviors when ill); the role of the family when caring for the sick member; and needs regarding diet and the inclusion of culture-specific healing remedies or practices.

Also, Sue[19] proposes that a culturally-skilled interviewer can do the following:

1. Maintain awareness of one's own cultural beliefs. "Other cultures are seen as being equally valuable as (one's) own."

2. Avoid prejudice. The clinician can avoid holding pre-conceived ideas about a particular culture, and participate in ongoing education or supervision to provide a check on the clinician's cultural perceptions.

3. Understand the current treatment of minorities in the United States. Sue states that it is especially valuable to know the "role cultural racism plays in the development of identity and world views among minority groups."

4. Maintain the ability to recognize a client as different and, at the same time, worthy of respect. The client is not "bad" for being different from the clinician.

5. Develop goals with the client that are consistent with the culture of the client.

6. Base communication on an understanding of the cultural cues given by the client. "A traditional Asian client for whom subtlety is a highly prized art may be offended by a confrontive counselor who sends a clear/accurate message but in a blunt manner."[17]

7. Generate a number of different verbal and nonverbal responses to allow for communication with clients from cultures other than one's own. For example, expressions of respect and warmth vary according to cultural group.

Therapeutic Communication Techniques

The *therapeutic use of self* of the nurse involves making appropriate communicative responses to the client that facilitate the client's growth. Often the focus on being therapeutic is too narrow, necessitating a search for the correct response to a client. The process of therapeutic communication is much more complicated than finding exact words. The box on this page summarizes a few of the ingredients of effective communication.

As the material in the box indicates, *there is no one communication ingredient that is more important than another*. A statement made by a nurse whose nonverbal

---

CHARACTERISTICS OF EFFECTIVE THERAPEUTIC COMMUNICATION

1. Contains words that can be understood by the client
2. Is clear in meaning
3. Allows for a response from the client
4. Deals with the cognitive and emotional aspects of the client
5. Is consistent; the communication implies the same message through time
6. Is repeated by the clinician as required by the client
7. Is direct; the communication reflects pertinent problems and is transmitted to the client with tact

---

communication indicates concern is more effective than a noncaring statement made with correct wording.

It is important to understand how to use the therapeutic techniques that have been found effective in working with clients. Therapeutic communication includes many of the elements in the previous box. All elements work together. Communicators who understand the theories of human behavior, as well as of communication, and are able to deal with emotions offer much to clients.

There are eight common therapeutic responses that can be used by nursing students when interviewing a client. Four are termed *listening* responses, and four are considered *action* responses.[8] The listening responses help clients describe fully what they are thinking and feeling (Fig. 3-5).

Listening Responses

Reflecting. *Reflecting* focuses on the feelings of the client, enabling the client to express more, to become aware of the emotional feeling experience, and/or to separate a cluster of feelings into distinct ones. Although

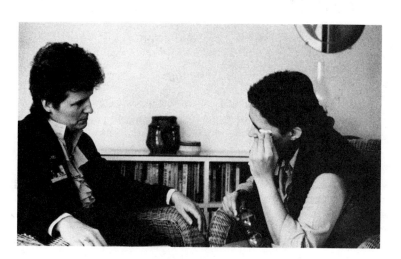

Figure 3-5. A psychiatric nurse listens to the concerns of the client.

reflection is usually thought of as rephrasing what the client has just stated, it should involve different, feeling-oriented words. Lead-in words such as "It seems as if. . . .", or "It appears to me. . . .", or "I'm hearing a lot of. . . ." are good beginnings to reflective interventions.

Example

Client: I don't even know who I am anymore. I'm changing and I don't know what I'm changing into.

Nurse: I hear a lot of confusion about who you are.

or

Nurse: It sounds confusing and scary not to know what's happening to you right now.

Paraphrasing. *Paraphrasing* focuses on the *content* of what a client is saying in order to call attention to something that is unclear or, perhaps, noteworthy. The three lead-ins mentioned above can be used appropriately with paraphrasing, as well. Using the same example above, the nurse might paraphrase as follows:

Nurse: It sounds like your identity is shifting and you're wondering about it all.

or

Nurse: It seems as if you're experiencing a change from the way that you have been in the past.

Clarifying. *Clarifying* most often uses a question to verify what the client has said or to interpret an ambiguous statement or expression of feeling. When using clarification, it is important to refrain from beginning the question with "why." "Why" questions often make the client feel defensive or judged by the nurse. Beginning a question with "Tell me . . .", or "I do not understand" is much more effective. Using the example above, a clarification might be:

Nurse: Tell me more about what you are feeling.

or

Nurse: Describe this experience.

Summarizing. *Summarizing* is most often used at the end of a session to pull together the theme(s) or topics discussed into a few sentences. Usually summarization entails two or more reflections and paraphrases combined together. Using the example above once again, a summarization might be:

Nurse: As we have explored your feelings and thoughts, it seems as if you aren't sure who you are anymore, or what you are becoming. It appears that your identity is shifting, and this feels scary to you.

In summary, therapeutic listening can be described as hearing what the other person is saying without becoming judgmental or defensive. Although this may sound easy, it can be challenging, especially when a client expresses dissatisfaction or anger toward the nurse. However, psychiatric nurses need to remember that clients express anger or dissatisfaction at "the nurse" and the role the nurse represents to the client; the anger is not usually directed specifically at the nurse receiving the outburst. Very often, clients have never had an empathic or sympathetic listener, but rather have had a family member or lover who was judgmental and defensive toward the client. Allowing a client to express emotion with a supportive look and statement can ease the client's distress and discomfort. Compare the following two examples of listening:

Example 1

Client: I'm sick of this place. And I'm sick of you always in my face trying to help. Just leave me alone!!

Nurse: You sound really angry right now. It's so hard to allow yourself to receive help, especially at times when it seems like you are hurting the most.

Client: Why do you have to be so damn nice? Why aren't you like all the rest? Everybody I've ever known has treated me like garbage. Never listening, never asking, never being there. (Begins to cry.)

Nurse: We are all here for you, and we do care about you. It hurts to think about others in your past. Your tears are telling you something. Do you know what it is?

Client: (tearful) That I deserve to be cared for? That it's okay to count on people in here? Why does it hurt so bad then?

In this example, the nurse responded to the hurt and pain underlying the anger and the client responded by becoming tearful and in touch with feelings and past experiences. Compare that with the next example:

Example 2

Client: I'm sick of this place. And I'm sick of you always in my face trying to help. Just leave me alone!!

Nurse: I'm just trying to help you. If you want to be left alone, then go to your room. This dayroom is for clients who want to be with others peacefully.

Client: Fine. I'm going NOW!! *#&%$**#*#!! (Client throws over the dayroom table as he leaves.)

Nurse: Destruction of property! Okay, Tom, that's seclusion room for you. Come on, staff, we need to escort Tom to the seclusion room. He is obviously out of control.

In example 2, the nurse escalated the client's emotions to the point at which he needed to release his emotions physically rather than express feelings verbally. The nurse inadvertently provoked the client toward violence by repeating the type of verbal interaction the client was accustomed to: not being heard or supported. Unfortunately, Tom had to take responsibility for his physically aggressive response to an unempathic response by the nurse. As treatment continues, Tom will hopefully gain control over aggressive reactions, and will verbalize his disappointment or confusion at the nurse's responses.

Action Responses

Action responses attempt to *move* a client toward some change, hence the term *action* response. Instead of responding to the client from the client's point of view, as in listening responses, action responses move beyond the client's viewpoint to state the interviewer's perspective.

Probing. In *probing,* the nurse asks *open-ended questions* to encourage the client to elaborate or provide examples in order to further clarify content. Using the example above, in probing, the nurse might say:

Nurse: Give me an example of when you feel you don't know who you are.

Information-Giving. *Information-giving* provides the client with needed data. Information-giving helps to decrease a client's anxiety, especially if the client feels uncomfortable or bizarre. The nurse can also use information-giving to share appropriate ideas or alternatives. The technique should not be used if it hinders self-expression. With the above example, a nurse using information-giving might say:

Nurse: It is not uncommon for clients in therapy to feel the way you do right now.

or

Nurse: It is not uncommon for clients to experience a shift in their identity as they begin to look more closely at their behaviors and feelings.

Confronting. *Confronting* is most often used to point out a discrepancy in the client's words and actions, verbal and nonverbal behaviors, or feelings and thoughts. Confrontation can also be useful to clarify a mixed or unusual message that seems inappropriate at the time. When confrontation is used, statements are made in an empathic, caring way, rather than in a critical, condemning manner. With the example above, a confrontation might be:

Nurse: I hear you say that you feel a change in your identity, but you are laughing while you say this.

or

Nurse: At the beginning of the session, you stated that you felt secure in who you were. Now you say that you are unclear.

Interpreting. *Interpreting* is a sophisticated means of presenting the client with a connection or reason behind a statement or feeling. Nurses are able to interpret clients' statements or feelings when they know the clients well and have trusting, empathic relationships with the clients. With the above example, an interpretation might be:

Nurse: I wonder if you feel a shift in your identity because you will be visiting your parents this weekend? You and I have talked about how controlling and domineering your mother can be with you.

or

Nurse: Perhaps you feel unsure of your self or your identity in therapy as you and I talk about uncomfortable thoughts and feelings.

While not fitting into the classification of action or listening responses, the following additional communication techniques can be useful in working with clients.

The Use of Silence

Bernstein and Bernstein[3] point out that "Traditionally, health professionals tend to associate helpfulness with" making verbal statements. When pauses occur, clinicians believe they are not doing enough for the client. In general, the appropriateness of client silence depends on the context of the interview situation. Some instances are listed below according to whether the silence is allowed to continue.

Client silence is not interrupted when:

- The client uses the quiet time to formulate thoughts or feelings.
- The client attempts to understand what the clinician or another client (in a group) has said.
- The client would not learn the skill of initiating or continuing to probe a topic if the clinician talks.

Client silence is interrupted when:

- The client is not accustomed to therapy and does not know where to begin.
- The client indicates, nonverbally, that something is happening. For example, the client seems angry, yet does not mention it. The nurse could say, "I notice your fists are clenched. What are you thinking? . . . What are you feeling?"
- The client experiences anxiety to the extent that the client's thoughts are blocked. The nurse should provide some structure for the client, such as, "You stopped talking. What are you feeling?" Chapter 5 contains a further description of anxiety.

Facilitating Emotional Awareness and Experience

A common stereotype of therapy is that therapeutic sessions involve an emotional release by clients prompted by the clinician's statement, "Talk about your feelings." Sue[19] described Asian-Americans as "more restrained in their feelings." A clinician treating such a client would not expect an emotional catharsis from the client. Some clients can benefit, however, from a focus on what is emotionally painful in their life. This is different from an emotional catharsis, and focuses on the cognitive identification of an emotional (or "painful") experience. Some clients do not have a cultural preference for an emotional experience or reliving an event in the therapeutic session.

Other clients can benefit from the therapist's encouragement to experience the emotions that are present. As the client releases emotion, the energy devoted to the client's experiences is released or decreased so that the client can get beyond the barriers of such painful emotions. The nurse could say, "What are you feeling?" or "Tell me more about your feelings," or "Stay on the topic of your feelings," or "Allow yourself to experience your feelings now."

Role-Playing

In *role-playing,* the client acts out a specific scenario, designed by the client and clinician, that is either similar to a difficult situation experienced previously by the client, or a new behavior to be tested by the client.[8] Not all clients are suited to role-playing. A trauma victim, for example, who becomes extremely anxious when discussing the trauma, should not be asked to role-play a traumatic experience.

The role-play experience can be reviewed after it is completed for elements such as client tension during the role-play, the client's difficulty or ease with the behaviors enacted in the role-play, and new insights gained as a result of role-playing.

Therapist's Attitudes Promoting a Therapeutic Interaction

Certain clinician attitudes foster an atmosphere of trust and caring in a therapeutic interchange. Some clinicians weight their responses to the client toward being warm and accepting. Others focus on responding to the immediate concerns of the client and offer help in this manner. Several helping attitudes are discussed below.

Genuineness

Genuineness means "being oneself without being phony or playing a role."[8] Clinicians who are genuine are comfortable to be around and do not exaggerate their own role. The clinicians' verbal and nonverbal behaviors are congruent. The clinicians do not look disgusted while trying to adopt a verbal tone of empathy. They are spontaneous and clear about expectations and roles of themselves and of clients.

Positive Regard

Positive regard includes the ability to "value the client as a person with worth and dignity."[8] In demonstrating positive regard, the clinician has a commitment to follow through with what the clinician has said would be done. The clinician tries to help and to understand the client, thus indicating that the client is important. The clinician accepts the client: there is an attitude of concern, and not disgust, toward the client.

Warmth

Many clients respond well to a clinician who is warm or caring. Warmth is demonstrated through the clinician's tone of voice, eye movement, and in other ways. It serves as a way to reach out to the client to comfort and to indicate that help is available within the clinician–client relationship.[8] Warmth also helps to decrease the client's anxiety.

Honesty

Honesty is the ability to relate one's perception of what is true in an experience or situation. Stating the truth, however, is not done to hurt others. Honesty includes the traits of sincerity, fairness, and straightforwardness.

When clinicians want to help clients, it takes courage to maintain an attitude of honesty and make truthful statements. In these instances, honesty is more effective in the long term than saying what seems helpful at the moment.

For example, a client may say to a nurse, "You aren't mentally ill. How can you help me?" The nurse can respond, "No, I am not ill and there may be some problems that I will not fully understand. I can understand some of your experiences, and you and I can talk about times when you believe I do not understand you." Many clients can model the direct and honest, yet caring, responses of the nurse. To some extent, if the nurse is honest and intent on understanding, the client will be equally honest and focused.

Immediacy

Immediacy "is a characteristic of a counselor's verbal response."[8] When the clinician has an attitude of immediacy, the clinician seeks to provide assistance when it is needed, and as soon as possible. The nurse does not rush the client, yet the nurse also does not withhold information that could be useful.

Immediacy can be used to talk about something that has not been directly discussed because the client is hesitant, for whatever reason, to discuss the matter. The clinician can initiate a discussion of the concern in a thoughtful manner. This is a difficult skill. In many instances it may seem easier to overlook something occurring in the therapy rather than to deal with it directly. Once the norm of immediacy has been established, however, an atmosphere of trust can be established in which many difficult topics can be discussed (Fig. 3-6).

Empathy

While all of the above-mentioned attitudes are important in the practice of psychiatric/mental health nursing, certainly empathy is one of the attributes most discussed. Briefly, *empathy* is the ability to be aware of the emotions of the other in the pursuit of altruistic purposes, wherein the client experiences the empathic attitude of the clinician. The client is understood by the clinician, and the client *has the positive benefit of feeling understood.* The ability of nurses to place themselves in the frame of refer-

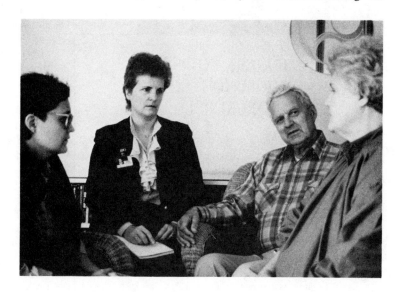

Figure 3-6. A psychiatric nurse confers with the family to understand better their immediate stressors and communication patterns.

ence of the client is communicated to the client. This important concept will be discussed at length in Chapter 5.

Ethics

Johnson[13] reported that there "are serious ethical issues involved in deliberately attempting to influence the attitude acquisition and change of other people." The nurse carries the social responsibility of working for, not against, the welfare of the client. Possibilities exist for "manipulating, exploiting, or brainwashing others for one's own needs and satisfactions."

Johnson also described several ingredients of ethical practice. These points include:

1. Ethical concerns enter the clinical work at the very first nurse–client meeting. The clinician's name, the professional qualifications of the clinician (such as R.N. or student), the number of sessions, the theoretical framework of the clinician, and the objective of the sessions should be discussed.

2. "To attempt to help a person when one is ignorant of how to help is both unethical and irresponsible." As stated by Johnson, the clinician practices according to a body of knowledge and not casual hunches. Nursing students may begin their work with clients using many social skills from their everyday lives, but they must base interventions on what promotes the client's welfare, as well as on a beginning theoretical understanding of psychiatric care. Students also have access to expert clinicians and instructors who facilitate their scientific understanding.

3. "Knowledge is not enough; there must also be trained skills and competencies." Clinicians (including nursing students) have an obligation to obtain clinical training and supervision to ensure the translation of theory into practice.

4. The clinician must maintain an awareness of how the clinician affects the client. Negative effects should be avoided.

5. The clinician maintains the confidentiality of the client(s).[4]

6. The help offered should be within the competencies of the clinician. The clinician should refer clients for needed services that are outside the understanding of the clinician (such as emergency services).[13]

The following box contains the American Nurses' Association[2] guidelines for carrying out nursing responsibilities in a manner consistent with the ethical obligations of the profession. As noted in the Code, the nurse's sense of social responsibility calls for providing care regardless of specific traits of the client. The client is worthy of respect regardless of economic status, religious or cultural beliefs, or degree of illness. The nurse maintains competent clinical skills, both personally and in the agency in which the nurse works. The nurse also promotes the welfare of the client by being an advocate for the client.

A variety of interventions can be used with clients, but how does a nursing student know which technique will be most effective with a client at any specific time? For most clients, there is no one right or wrong response. As long as nurses know the purpose of the communication, and what they are trying to help the client express, many techniques will elicit the same results.

The main distinction is with clients experiencing a crisis, or who are severely psychiatrically disabled at the time of the interview. These clients respond better to reflection and paraphrasing than to other techniques. Because they are able to tolerate only a limited amount of therapeutic communication, clients experiencing a crisis are least able to tolerate interpretations or confrontations. Their thoughts and emotions are so distressing and confusing to them that they are unable to comprehend, or even to hear, the best or most accurate interpretation. The nurse should be available, supportive, and empathic.

Most therapeutic techniques can be used with recovering and more active clients. If clients react negatively to a technique, the nurse should try another technique.

AMERICAN NURSES' ASSOCIATION CODE FOR NURSES

1. The nurse provides services with respect for human dignity and the uniqueness of the client, unrestricted by considerations of social or economic status, personal attributes, or the nature of health problems.

2. The nurse safeguards the client's right to privacy by judiciously protecting information of a confidential nature.

3. The nurse acts to safeguard the client and the public when health care and safety are affected by the incompetent, unethical, or illegal practice of any person.

4. The nurse assumes responsibility and accountability for individual nursing judgments and actions.

5. The nurse maintains competence in nursing.

6. The nurse exercises informed judgment and uses individual competence and qualifications as criteria in seeking consultation, accepting responsibilities, and delegating nursing activities to others.

7. The nurse participates in activities that contribute to the ongoing development of the profession's body of knowledge.

8. The nurse participates in the profession's efforts to implement and improve standards of nursing.

9. The nurse participates in the profession's efforts to establish and maintain conditions of employment conducive to high quality nursing care.

10. The nurse participates in the profession's effort to protect the public from misinformation and misrepresentation and to maintain the integrity of nursing.

11. The nurse collaborates with members of the health professions and other citizens in promoting community and national efforts to meet health needs of the public.

(American Nurses' Association: Code for Nurses with Interpretive Statements. Kansas City, American Nurses' Association, 1985)

Usually, the action techniques, aside from an initial probing question, are used later in the session or after many sessions, once a therapeutic relationship has been built. Often hospitalized psychiatric clients just want someone to listen, to care, to reaffirm that they are not "crazy" or "scary" to people because they have a mental disorder. Nurses represent the non-psychiatrically impaired, and can humanize the experience of the psychiatric client by being supportive and nonjudgmental and by understanding how best to work with the client to achieve a higher level of intellectual and interpersonal competency.

Professionalism

The nurse must maintain a professional quality or character in working with clients. In doing so, the nurse focuses activities on assisting the client to achieve the goals of care. While it is easy to become distracted, and often clients intentionally try to distract the nurse, it is imperative that the nurse maintain a professional attitude.

Psychiatric nurses must also adopt an attitude of neutrality.[17] "The nurse scrupulously avoids responding to any of the client's efforts to evoke approval, disapproval, dominance, or indifference, and maintains a strict neutrality toward all clients." For example, some clients are extremely sensitive. If a nurse leading a group therapy session "caters to one client in the group, the nurse loses all the others."[17] The nurse should say, "When there is silence in the group, any group member can say what he or she is thinking," instead of, "John is the only client who talks and contributes to the group."

Nurses must also use praise carefully. Some clients are over-dependent on the approval of others and feel a sense of well-being only when receiving another's approval. Some clients who are depressed have a low sense of self-worth and will reject or not hear praise. As described by Peplau, "If you tell a person who thinks he's worthless that he is a great man, he is apt to go to great lengths to prove you're wrong."[17]

Barriers to Therapeutic Communication

A nurse and a client may both speak the same language and may both clearly express the need to communicate effectively, yet both may find communication a difficult task. Unintentionally, communication between the nurse and the client may become confused, or not properly received, because of *barriers to communication*. Several of these barriers are included in Table 3-4. It would be very uncommon for *some* barriers to communication not to exist between the nurse and the client.

While the interventions mentioned above are understandable, it is often difficult to put them into practice. It may be easier to intervene appropriately if the clinician adopts a sense of immediacy about the interview. For example, if the clinician believes that the client is experiencing something other than what is being talked about, then the nurse should say so.

This technique of assisting the client to talk about what is really occurring can be anxiety-provoking for the client. The client has had a lot of practice in talking about issues that are NOT of true importance to the client. Breaking this pattern will be stressful, but immeasurably useful.

Clinical Communication

In psychiatric nursing, the details of nursing care are shared with other team members in the form of the assessment, nursing diagnosis, plan of care, and moment-to-moment communication about what is occurring in

RELEVANT RESEARCH

The purpose of this study was to provide a detailed analysis of the interpersonal process of communication between nurse practitioners (NPs) and their clients. It is thought that a better understanding of such communication can lead to improved education of NPs and better client care.

A sample of pediatric nurse practitioners (PNPs) was randomly selected from lists of certified NPs obtained from the American Nurses' Association. Of the 35 PNPs who participated in the study, 19 had masters' degrees, 9 had baccalaureate degrees, and 7 had diplomas or associate degrees. The average length of time they had worked as PNPs was 6.5 years, and their average work week was 33.1 hours. Each nurse submitted audiotapes of one infant and one preschool well-child appointment. More than 70% of their clients were low-income individuals.

The tapes were analyzed using the Pediatric Nurse Practitioner Interpersonal Behavior Constructs (IBC) tool. This assessment analyzes interactions and contains 17 categories of behavior. The IBC results in a frequency total for each behavior for 5-minute interval periods. The 17 categories are combined into 5 main verbal dimensions, including positive or negative affect statements, information-eliciting, and giving or responding to information. In addition to the IBC analysis, the tapes were reviewed for items such as whether the PNP asked if the mother had any questions, or if the PNP responded to concerns expressed by the mother.

Mean overall interrater agreement was estimated. The reliability was 70% for all PNP behaviors and 90% for mother behaviors.

In the data analysis, 10 tapes, lasting less than 15 minutes, were excluded from the study. Data revealed that 96% of the PNPs elicited the mothers' concerns and 3% never assessed whether the mothers had concerns about their children. The PNPs spent half of the visit time asking mothers questions about their family and child. Seventy-five percent of these questions were factual and pertained to family background (such as family history of allergies). Eleven of the questions were closed or negative (such as "Your child doesn't have sleep problems, does he?"). Mothers asked a mean number of 1.7 questions.

In 60% of the interventions by the PNPs, no rationale was offered. Most often, advice was offered for physical or cognitive development, but it was rarely given for family or child behavior problems. Reflective statements acknowledging the mother's feelings or reactions were seldom used by PNPs. Few PNPs praised or supported the mothers' efforts.

PNPs conducted comprehensive assessments and offered educational information. However, the interviews were dominated by PNP questions and commands, and the communication rarely focused on the emotional aspects of child care.

Although the study analyzed only audio- and not videotapes, and the audio taping may have hindered PNP communication, it is thought that PNPs have less skill in the area of mutuality of communication. The authors encouraged the inclusion of "process" courses related to communication and counseling techniques.

(Webster-Stratton C, Glascock J, McCarthy A: Nurse practitioner–patient interactional analyses during well-child visits. Nurs Res 4:247, 1986)

treatment. Much information is recorded in the client's chart. Recording client information serves a number of purposes:

1. As professionals, nurses document care. The documentation is part of a legal statement of what was done in providing care for the client.
2. Documentation informs other team members of what is occurring in treatment with a client. It provides a direction for treatment.
3. Documentation provides a means for future reference. The nurse can review documentation to determine if the care plan is still being implemented.
4. Documentation serves as a way of observing the progress of the client. The written assessment can make the growth of the client apparent.

Several methods of clinical communication are described below.

The Interdisciplinary Treatment Plan

In some facilities an interdisciplinary treatment plan replaces the nursing care plan. A staff member first does the assessment. Typically, this assessment is shared with the staff and a diagnosis is made. In most facilities the client will have a medical (psychiatric) diagnosis. The nurse supplements this diagnosis with nursing diagnoses if the nurse senses that an additional nursing care plan will provide better care for the client. The interdisciplinary team treatment plan may look like the treatment plans found in Part V of this book.

The team decides on a treatment plan. This planning is important because staff must be consistent in their approach with the client. At this time decisions are also made concerning who will carry out what part of the plan. Periodic interdisciplinary team meetings are held to review the current appropriateness of the plan. The Joint Commission on Accreditation of Healthcare Organizations *requires* such meetings.[16]

Interdisciplinary treatment team meetings also accomplish other goals. Team members can become discouraged about the lack of progress of a particular client, or even of the client group as a whole. When this happens, team members act as a support system for one another. Also, information from other team members concerning the client can help to provide a degree of objectivity about the client.

TABLE 3-4.
BARRIERS TO EFFECTIVE COMMUNICATION

BARRIERS TO THERAPEUTIC COMMUNICATION	NURSING INTERVENTIONS
ENVIRONMENTAL BARRIERS *Examples:* Noise, other people, furnishings in the room (too much or too little furniture), inadequate space (if the smallness of the room places the nurse and client in too close proximity)	Prepare the environment prior to talking with a client. Ask others to be quiet. Explain to the client the peculiarities of the environment (for example, "I raised the window to let in some air. Let me know if you become cold.")
CLIENT BARRIERS 1. Resistance or unwillful avoidance of painful emotional issues. *Example:* The client discusses tangential issues.	1. Initiate a discussion of the avoidance behavior (such as, "What was going on that you changed the topic?"). If the client is anxious because it is difficult to talk about a painful topic, help the client deal with the anxiety. (See Chap. 5.)
2. The client's distortion of the nurse (transference) or misperception of the nurse (or other people) based on previous interpersonal experiences *Example:* The client tells you that she doesn't want to attend the group meeting and says that you remind her of her mother.	2. Determine the painful interpersonal patterns the client has had with others in the client's life. Observe when the client repeats such a pattern. Discuss the pattern with the client. Assist the client to develop new ways of responding appropriately to others that are not based on how the client behaved with others the client has known in the past.
NURSING BARRIERS 1. The nurse's distortion of the client (countertransference) or misperception of the client (or other people) based on previous painful interpersonal experiences *Example:* The nurse replies to the client regarding group attendance, "Don't call me your mother, just do as I say."	1. Attend a clinical supervision meeting with peers in which cases are reviewed and personal reactions to clients are discussed. Understand your own past and that your interpersonal patterns are based on the earlier experiences. Be aware of issues that are personally sensitive for you, such as weight, age, height, and others. Understand that when clients make remarks about the nurse's "weaknesses" they are not being purposefully punitive, but simply repeating old, dysfunctional patterns of relating. Maintain a sense of openness about discussing distortions of others. Avoid venting feelings on the client (such as hostility). Review uncomfortable reactions to clients and determine a course of action. Do not simply leave the client alone or abandon the client.
2. Placing inappropriate limitations on the client's potential for growth. *Examples:* The nurse may belittle, control, or make inappropriate demands on the client. The nurse may hurt the client's sense of self-esteem or become parental with the client, thereby limiting the client's freedom.	2. Understand the client's interpersonal and intellectual competency or ability level. Intervene at the level of understanding of the client, not above the client's level. Maintain a respect for human dignity regardless of how society may stereotype characteristics of the client (such as appearance). Treat the client as an individual who is entitled to the benefits offered to any other person. (For example, the nurse should not ask the client to run errands for the nurse.)
3. Prejudice *Example:* A client is admitted to a mental health unit who has severe facial burn scars. The nurse assigned to work with the client has not met with the client and makes inappropriate excuses for not doing so.	3. Understand your own belief systems concerning others who are different in some way. Get to know the other person. Ask the other person about his or her experience. Discuss your thoughts and feelings about the client (especially negative ones) with other staff.

Nursing Notes

Nursing notes serve as a shift-by-shift account of the status of the client and the progress toward a resolution of the client's problems or needs.[15] Nursing notes contain the following information:

1. **Client routines**

    Sleep. Is the client maintaining a normal (for the client) sleep pattern? Was the client restless? Did the client ask for a sleeping medication? Did the client feel rested upon awakening? Were other problems present, such as early morning awakening, too much sleep, or trouble falling asleep?

    Food intake. Does the client eat an appropriate diet? Are unusual meal patterns observed, such as not eating with other clients or taking other clients' food?

    Exercise. Does the client exercise? What is the client's exercise pattern at home? Are medications interfering with mobility?

    Activities of daily living. Does the client provide for daily concerns of living such as bathing, washing clothes, and combing hair? Does the client need assistance with these activities? Is the client's pattern of providing for daily needs similar to the client's behavior at home? Does the (outpatient) client know how to use laundry facilities or how to find the appropriate resources to accomplish the activities of daily living?

Daily interests. How does the client spend time? Is the client self-motivated in undertaking activities? Are the activities solitary or do they involve others? Do the activities seem repetitive and narrow in scope?

2. **Therapeutic data**

Mood. What is the client's mood? What promotes a change in mood?

Deviations in behavior. Is the client behaving in a manner different than usual? For example, is the client suddenly asking for passes to leave the hospital unit? What does the deviation in behavior mean?

Manifested behavior. What is the observed behavior of the client? How does the client react to visitors, other clients, staff? What is the quality of the client's interpersonal relations with others?

Affect. What affect is present? Does this affect represent a change?

Themes present in discussions with the client. What are the client's concerns?

Discussions with staff. What does the client mention as concerns? What is the client doing about these concerns? Has the client engaged in conversation with staff or other professional people (such as lawyers)?

Teaching. What teaching did the client receive? What was the client's reaction or understanding?

Reactions to medications. Were any adverse reactions noted? How is the client affected by the medications?

Nursing notes should reflect discharge planning from the day of admission to the unit. Do arrangements need to be made immediately for a place for the client to live after discharge? Does treatment need to occur with both the client and the family in order to prevent future admissions? Does the client need vocational rehabilitation or help completing financial assistance forms? All of these arrangements need to be accomplished prior to discharge, while the client has professional support and assistance for such activities.

Nursing Rounds

One mechanism for ensuring the performance of the evaluation step is nursing rounds: meetings of the nursing staff during which each client is discussed. The client may or may not be present. Nursing rounds focus on such topics as the nursing diagnosis, other parts of the nursing care plan, or family responses to the client's illness. Nursing staff can also request a consultation with a psychiatric/mental health clinical nurse specialist. This request would be made when concerns about the nursing care of the client cannot be clarified by the nursing staff.

Change-of-Shift Report

The change-of-shift report is a meeting of staff from one shift, who are completing their work time on the unit, with the group of staff coming to work on the unit. The change-of-shift report ensures continuity of care. It is important for *all* staff to hear from the staff finishing work the report concerning *all* clients. In emergency situations, for example, a staff member may have to work with a client to whom the staff person was not assigned. It is also useful for the departing staff to review the current treatment plans so that recommended approaches are used. Evaluation of the nursing care plans can be done at this time.

It is important when giving a report to other staff that the client's name, room number, age, date of admission, nursing diagnosis, and medical diagnosis be stated. It may seem awkward to repeat this information when the client has been on the unit for a week, but new staff (or staff returning from several days off) will need to be reminded of this information. Information similar to that given in nursing notes should be reported.

There are many ways to handle change-of-shift report. The report can be audiotaped so that staff can listen to the report at any time during the initial part of their workday. It is best if the charge nurse on the unit tapes the report. This practice will assist in maintaining a professional tone and focus.

The Problem-Oriented Record

Carnevali stated that the nursing care planning system requires "records so that information, decisions, actions, and outcomes are predictably locatable."[7] The record of care also makes it possible to see client progress over a period of time. The record is a legal document protecting the client's right and the staff's right to have a record of the professional actions and client responses.

The recording style used in many facilities is the problem-oriented record. This style of record-keeping originated in medicine, and was called the problem-oriented *medical* record. Today, health team members call the style "problem-oriented *health* record."

Problem-oriented charting means that statements entered into the record concerning the client are entered according to problems listed. While some physicians want to maintain the problem-oriented health record *only* for their notes, each health care team should have equal access to the form for recording. In addition to reporting on the problem-oriented health record, nurses also record tasks performed with the client, such as medications administered. This recording is usually done in a check-off list.

Notes are included on the problem-oriented health record at the frequency required by the situation of each client or the institution. Thus, the frequency of recording can vary from more than once during a shift to once a month. However, there must be a periodic review of the problem-oriented health record in order to update the required information.

Marriner described problem-oriented charting as composed of "(1) the collection of a data base through an assessment, (2) formulation of a problem list, (3) a plan for management of each problem, and (4) plans for follow-up accompanied with progress notes."[15]

The data base has been described in Chapter 4 as the psychiatric assessment. The problem list can include a medical or nursing diagnosis. SOAP is an acronym suggested to guide the development of ongoing plans for management of the problems: S for subjective data (the client's view of the situation); O for objective data (what can be observed); A for assessment changes noted; and P for the plan of intervention.[7] An example of a problem-oriented health record in the SOAP format is included in the box below.

Also included as part of problem-oriented charting is a flow sheet describing progress on each problem identified for the client. Specific problems are documented as "resolved" when they are no longer a client concern.

Clinical communication takes a number of forms. It can include written treatment plans, or it can take place in statements made about clients by staff members. Regardless of the exact type of communication, many important events happen when there is dialogue.

Staff members exchange ideas about the client and the client's care in order to better assist the client. One staff member's hopeful attitude about care can be communicated to other staff members while engaging in a dialogue, thereby renewing the staff's efforts toward helping the client. While communicating, staff indicate their own "process" about their work in the manner in which they converse, whether it is caring, laissez-faire, frustrated, angry, empathic, hopeless/helpless, or concerned. Making communication pertinent and caring can result in improved client care as well as in a more satisfactory working environment.

Summary

1. Communication is an interchange among individuals through which they define and change their awareness of Self and their Relationships with Others.
2. The interpersonal process or pragmatic theory of communication emphasizes the "systems" nature of interchanges and includes concepts such as feedback and metacommunication.
3. Other theories of communication include the mechanistic perspective, the psychological perspective, and the interactionist model.
4. Communication from the nurse to the client is based on the level of prevention required by the client as well as on the client's ability to understand and respond to the communication.
5. Nurses base their interventions on both the verbal and the nonverbal messages of the client.
6. Nurses can affect the clients' communication by their own behaviors.
7. A variety of communication techniques can be adapted to individual situations in order to foster client growth.
8. Effective communication among staff members promotes care of high quality.

PROBLEM-ORIENTED HEALTH RECORD

Client: Michael Allen
Problem: Abandonment feelings
Date of onset: January 5
Date of completion of SOAP: February 7
S: "Hasn't wanted to go outside the house, no appetite, teary, can't sleep."
O: Affect depressed. Ruminates about wife's death one month ago.
A: Client is experiencing uncomplicated bereavement associated with death of wife. Has no friends or hobbies.
P: Nurse will see client in brief therapy to assist in grieving process (12 sessions), beginning in three days.
Referral to senior services center
Session with client's sister and nurse to provide for someone to stay with the client for four days. Arrangement for regular visits with family after that time
Client to follow daily schedule of activities beginning today. (See attached sheet with schedule.)

References

1. American Nurses' Association: Nursing: A Social Policy Statement. Kansas City, American Nurses' Association, 1980
2. American Nurses' Association: Code for Nurses with Interpretive Statements. Kansas City, American Nurses' Association, 1985
3. Bernstein L, Bernstein R: Interviewing: A Guide for Health Professionals. New York, Appleton-Century-Crofts, 1980
4. Bloch S, Chodoff P: Psychiatric Ethics. New York, Oxford University Press, 1981
5. Bradley J, Edinberg H: Communication in the Nursing Context. Norwalk, Connecticut, Appleton-Century-Crofts, 1986
6. Caplan G: Principles of Preventive Psychiatry. New York, Basic Books, 1964
7. Carnevali D: Nursing Care Planning: Diagnosis and Management. Philadelphia, JB Lippincott, 1983
8. Cormier W, Cormier L: Interviewing Strategies for Helpers. Monterey, California, Brooks/Cole, 1985
9. Cushman D, Cahn D: Communication in Interpersonal Relationships. Albany, State University of New York Press, 1985
10. DeVito J: The Interpersonal Communication Book. New York, Harper & Row, 1980

11. Edwards B, Brilhart J: Communication in Nursing Practice. St Louis, CV Mosby, 1981

12. Enelow A: Elements of Psychotherapy. New York, Oxford University Press, 1977

13. Johnson D: Attitude Modification Methods. In Kanfer F, Goldstein (eds): Helping People Change. New York, Pergamon Press, 1980

14. Kernberg O: Severe Personality Disorders: Psychotherapeutic Strategies. New Haven, Yale University Press, 1984

15. Marriner A: The Nursing Process. St Louis, CV Mosby, 1983

16. Parsons P: Building better treatment plans. J Psychosoc Nurs Ment Health Serv 24:8, 1986

17. Peplau H: Basic Principles of Patient Counseling. New Braunfels, TX, PSF Productions, 1978

18. Pothier P: The issue of prevention in psychiatric nursing. Arch Psychiatr Nurs 1:143, 1987

19. Sue D: Counseling the Culturally Different. New York, John Wiley & Sons, 1981

20. Sullivan H: The Psychiatric Interview. New York, WW Norton, 1954

21. Trenholm S: Human Communication Theory. Englewood Cliffs, NJ, Prentice-Hall, 1986

22. Watzlawick P, Beavin J, Jackson D: Pragmatics of Human Communication. New York, WW Norton, 1967

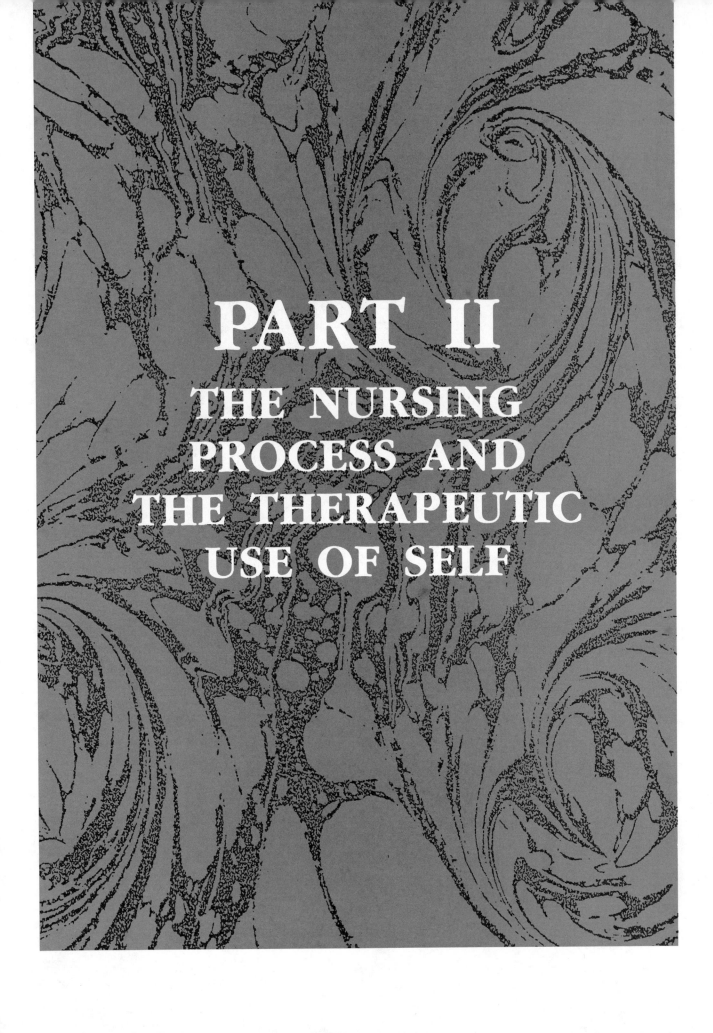

PART II
THE NURSING PROCESS AND THE THERAPEUTIC USE OF SELF

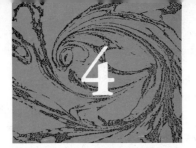

LORETTA M. BIRCKHEAD

THE NURSING PROCESS

Learning Objectives

On completion of this chapter the student should be able to do the following:

1. Describe how the steps of the nursing process follow the progression of thinking and actual care given by the nurse in order to promote client change.
2. Define patterns of concern the psychiatric/mental health nurse and client label as a focus for nursing care.
3. Identify the basic questions that guide a psychiatric assessment.
4. Explain why the evaluation step of the nursing process is more difficult in psychiatric/mental health nursing.
5. Describe five ways in which staff members can communicate with each other and with the client concerning the client's progress.

Introduction

The psychiatric/mental health nurse promotes change in the client by means of the "therapeutic use of self." Here the nurse brings an understanding of human behavior, the nurse's own set of beliefs and values, and the nurse's own emotions to the interchange with the client. Similarly, clients have their own set of beliefs, and their own emotions and behaviors. The amount of information contained in this interchange is immense. How does the nurse obtain a sense of direction in nursing care with so many elements of the nurse–client interchange occurring?

The process of directing care is accomplished by means of *the nursing process.* This problem-solving method of delivering client care establishes an order for the judgments of the nurse in working with clients. Using all the data gathered about the client, the nurse makes a determination about how to best assist the client's growth. The nursing process includes the steps of gathering data, making a diagnosis based on the data, planning care, providing care, and evaluating the results of the care given. Each of these steps will be discussed in this chapter.

Using the nursing process in any area of nursing requires diligence in deriving the best method of providing care, and a sense of judgment in the decision-making involved in each step. Not only is there an immense amount of client data, but other factors enter into nursing care in psychiatric/mental health nursing. One such factor is the interpersonal nature of the exchange with the psychiatric client. The nursing role is no longer seen as doing something "to" the client, but as doing something "with" the client. There is no physical object to give to the client to promote change, such as providing a bandage for a client with a wound. The nurse–client interpersonal exchange required is not so easy to arrange.

When the psychiatric nurse provides care "with" the client, the nurse's own personality can be called in question. Can a nurse who is angry and aggressive help clients to learn about, and change, their patterns of handling anger? Can a nurse who has difficulty in handling emotions help clients who cannot handle their own emotions?

Another factor in providing care to clients is the finding that many clients do not want to change, or that some clients who state that they want to change find it difficult to accomplish this change. The client who needs a bandage probably wants the bandage. The client who needs an alteration in psychological functioning may not want to change, may find it too difficult to accomplish change, or may not know how to accomplish the desired change. The hesitancy to change is not always conscious. Typically, the client does not willfully seek emotional pain or attempt to negate the nurse's efforts.

Much of the resistance to change in psychiatric clients is understandable. Problematic behavior, although it may have caused the individual or family great emotional pain for a number of years, is often like a familiar nuisance that an individual does nothing about. Part of the role of the psychiatric/mental health nurse is to design a way to facilitate change. The steps involved in designing care are described in the nursing process. The "art" of psychiatric/mental health nursing is described as the therapeutic use of self. The combined use of the nursing process and therapeutic use of self serves as a statement of hope to the client that there is an alternate way of living that involves much less emotional pain for the client.

Professional Guidelines for Practice

The American Nurses' Association views the nursing process as the scientific method of delivering care. The *Standards of Psychiatric and Mental Health Nursing Practice*,[5] formulated by the Division on Psychiatric and Mental Health Nursing Practice of the American Nurses' Association, provide a means of assessing and improving the quality of care. The Standards reflect the current understanding of the function of the psychiatric/mental health nurse.

The Standards are written according to the components of the nursing process, and list the components as *data collection, diagnosis, planning, treatment, and evaluation.* Students learn how to plan for client care by using the nursing process. For example, currently there is an effort to define desired client outcomes of nursing intervention. Part of this effort is triggered by the professional nurse's need to evaluate the effects of nursing actions (client outcome measures). The nursing process challenges us to get to know the client, to collect and analyze pertinent data about the client in a scientific man-

ner, to arrive at specific nursing diagnoses, to develop and implement a systematic plan of treatment to assist the client with problems, and to evaluate the results of the treatment.

The Therapeutic Use of Self

This chapter focuses on the nursing process as a problem-solving approach that the nurse uses to meet the needs of the client. In a very narrow sense, perhaps the nursing process is simply a problem-solving guide. It defines the steps to use in gathering data about a client, defining problems or concerns, and describing interventions to use in solving the problems. While the nursing process involves orderly steps, it is not a mechanical operation that the psychiatric nurse does "to" the client.

In working "with" the client, the nursing process is applied in the context of the *therapeutic use of self.* This context is important. For a suicidal client, placing the client in a protective environment, such as a psychiatric hospital, is only the beginning of a difficult, emotionally painful process of cure. The concerns of the client involve much more than the immediate problem of self-injury. The psychiatric nurse must find a way to assist the client to learn about the life circumstances prompting the suicidal intent and to practice other ways of dealing with self-destructive urges. This assistance may be offered to a client who has selected in the past not to learn alternative behaviors. The way the nurse establishes this professional relationship with the client, and fosters it to the benefit of the client, is the therapeutic use of self.

The Nursing Process

Marriner[10] stated that "the proper utilization of the 'nursing process' largely determines the degree of effectiveness and efficiency of nursing intervention." The process is a *method* of doing things that involves a systematic progression of activities to reach a result or goal.

Various names have been applied to the steps of the nursing process, so names may differ in the settings in which the nurse functions. Typically, the nursing process involves five steps: *assessment, diagnosis, planning, intervention,* and *evaluation.* These steps are described below, and a case study is provided that details the five steps.

Assessment

Before providing care, the nurse determines the nature of the client as a system by surveying the elements of the client's psychological, societal, environmental, physical, and cultural life. The assessment phase begins with the collection of data relevant to these five elements, and leads to the nursing diagnosis, a statement of the client's problem.

Information is gathered from the client and, in many settings, the client's family. The institution in which the nurse works may have a standardized assessment format used by professionals from a variety of disciplines. Some professionals may want to add information gathered from the client that is of particular interest to the professional's own discipline. Some nurses prefer to gather data in the client's home setting, where the client and the client's environment, cultural beliefs, and family can be observed and assessed.

The assessment stage of the nursing process allows for personalized nursing care by identifying the specific needs of the client. The written assessment reads in a manner that recognizes the client as an individual.

The Psychiatric Assessment

The psychiatric assessment is the process of gathering information pertinent to the evaluation of the client's mental health/illness status. The assessment is usually divided into two parts, the psychiatric history and the mental status examination. Unlike a physical examination, in which much of what is described can be observed (such as skin color), in the psychiatric assessment much of what is described cannot be observed directly.

The assessment is performed by a staff member at the time of the client's admission to the institution or facility in which the client is treated. This professional person may be a psychiatric nurse, a psychologist, or some other member of the treatment team. The team member doing the assessment must be familiar with what data should be collected. Because some areas of the psychiatric assessment require special knowledge (for example, the ability of the clinician to differentiate mood from affect), the treatment team may want to designate one staff member to specialize in learning the meaning of the various parts of the assessment form and in remaining aware of current writings and research on various parts of the assessment.

The initial data gathered may be minimal if the client is uncommunicative. The assessment will then include information based only on the nurse's observations rather than also including the client's responses to statements made by the nurse. As the client becomes able to communicate verbally with the nurse, the assessment is completed.

In doing the psychiatric assessment, the psychiatric nurse uses the communication techniques described in the previous chapter. Special techniques are needed with some clients. A schizophrenic client, for example, may make a series of statements that have no logical connection. Particular communication techniques required of the psychiatric nurse for special populations will be discussed in Chapters 15 through 21.

The Psychiatric History.   Components of the psychiatric history include identifying data and the history of the client. In each facility treating mental health clients, one member of the nursing staff should become proficient in the preparation and understanding of the psychi-

atric history in order to serve as a resource person for the rest of the staff. The following box outlines the components of the psychiatric history:

The Mental Status Examination.   The mental status examination includes details of the client's psychological functioning. It is more focused on mental functioning than is the psychiatric history. However, much information about the client's mental status can be gained during all parts of the interview. For example, one part of the mental status examination concerns the client's sense of judgment. If the client describes in the psychiatric history episodes of reckless driving, the nurse would have good reason to question the client's sense of judgment. Also, not every question listed needs to be asked of every client. A client who is obviously oriented to time, place, and person does not need to be asked these questions.

Many of the terms included in the mental status examination are listed in the Glossary at the back of the book. However, some need additional explanation, which is included below:

Memory, both remote and recent, can be assessed from the manner in which the client responds to questions in the psychiatric history.

Retention and recall can be assessed by asking the client to repeat three words or phrases provided by the nurse, such as "purple," "steamship," and "1240 East Road." The client is then asked to repeat the words again in five minutes. The client can also be asked to repeat a series of numbers in forward or reversed order after having the nurse read the series to the client. The numbers should be read at the rate of one per second. Most adults can repeat five to eight correct digits forward and four to six correct digits backward. Fewer correct than five forward or three in reverse order indicates impairment of some type.[7]

Visual retention and recall can be assessed by asking the client to copy three figures on a piece of paper. The nurse presents individual pictures of common objects, such a pencil, a chair, and a lamp—one picture every three seconds. The pictures are then placed out of sight, and the client is asked to draw each picture at this point and again in five minutes. The inability to perform such tasks may denote organic impairment.

Abstraction is the ability to apply labels or give theoretical meanings to things or events that go beyond a mere counting of a singular, observable event. For example, the proverb "Two heads are better than one" means that problems can be solved more easily with the ideas of two people rather than of just one. The proverb "People who live in glass houses shouldn't throw stones" means that an individual should not criticize others for doing things that the individual does. Concrete interpretation of the proverbs could include responses such as, "Some people may ask to have two heads," or "Throwing stones at glass can break it."

The nurse can also ask the client to describe how two objects are alike or similar. An axe and a saw are both alike because they both cut wood. A more concrete inter-

THE PSYCHIATRIC HISTORY[12,16]

I. *Identifying Data*

Name, age, sex, marital status, occupation, race, place of birth

II. *History*

A. *Chief complaint and reasons for admission*

What are client's chief complaints and what were the circumstances that led to client's admission to the hospital? Did client seek help voluntarily or was hospitalization instigated by relatives, friends, or others?

B. *Chronological account of onset and course of illness up to the present time*

What was going on in client's life when illness began? Was onset acute or insidious? Were there previous occurrences of the illness? If so, how were they treated and how did client cope with the treatment?

C. *Changes in client's life before onset of illness*

Describe client's life situation. Where and with whom living—married, divorced, or living with a significant other (nature of the relationship, client's role in the relationship, satisfaction in the relationship)? Working or unemployed (old or new job, job lost, or client unable to work)? Illnesses or deaths in the family? Emotional satisfactions and stresses present in client's life before symptoms?

D. *Family history*

Describe client's family situation. Family incidence of mental or other illness, including description of parents? Parents living or dead? Home into which client was born—economic and social status, family background, degree of success of parents? Parental marriage at time of client's birth? If so, how long married? Previous children? Attitude of client's parents, both mother and father, toward client, pregnancy of client and of client's siblings? Compatibility of parents? Others living in home in addition to parents and siblings? In what ways was client's birth a happy event and what stresses and strains did it involve?

E. *Personal developmental history*

1. *Birth:* Date and place of birth, medical data about delivery and about newborn baby? Parental attitudes toward new baby, including any sex preference? Reactions of older siblings to new baby?

2. *Infancy:* Breast or bottle fed? Feeding problem? Schedule or demand feeding? Weaning problem? Weight gain? Activity (vigorous, quiet)? Sleep patterns? Physical or sexual abuse?

3. *Early childhood (preschool):* Role of client in family group? Type of attachment to each parent and to other family members? Number and kind of playmates and attitudes toward them? Favorite play activities? Dislikes of people or activities? Developing ability to share and to tolerate frustration? Friendly? Shy? Possessive? Rebellious? Fearful? Lonely? Techniques for getting own way, getting attention? Early methods of dealing with problems, seeking help from others? Taking care of problems without help? Unable to accept help? Turned to whom for help? Reaction to guidance or discipline? Reaction to family events, such as deaths, illnesses, new home, or separation of family? Physical, sexual, emotional abuse?

4. *Childhood:* What was client like as a child?

a. *School.* Age started and feelings about it; went how far, age when left school, reason for leaving? Scholastic standing and explanation for changes? Special likes and dislikes in school subjects? Extracurricular activities and interests, *e.g.*, art, hobbies, organizations, social activities, sports? Ambitions in school? Interference with schooling by illnesses, accidents, or trouble at home? Attitudes and attachments to teachers and classmates?

b. *Further personality development.* Changing feelings toward parents and home, and relation to extrafamily activities? Friendly? Brought friends into home? What kind of friendships? Shy? Outgoing or seclusive? Fearful? Concealed feelings? Aggressive? Passive? Daydreamer? Sought help or rejected help? Attitudes about competition, irresponsibility, frustration, pleasure, and self-sacrifice? Psychosexual developments, *e.g.*, modesty, curiosity, relations with opposite and same sex, exhibitionism, masturbation? Reactions to any family events, *e.g.*, births, deaths, illnesses, separations? Toilet-training problems? Lying, cheating, fighting? Cleanliness? Bowel and eating habits? Rebelliousness or conformity? Physical, sexual, emotional abuse?

c. *Health.* Illnesses, accidents, operations, and reactions to them?

(Continued)

pretation would be that they are both made of metal. Clients with language and thought disorders may have difficulty abstracting, as may clients with organic impairment.

Calculation and concentration are assessed by asking the client to perform subtraction and multiplication exercises. "Serial sevens" is an exercise frequently used in the mental status examination. The client is asked to subtract seven repeatedly from one hundred. The typical time taken in performing serial sevens is 90 seconds.[7]

The Physical Component of the Person as a System

Just as the psychological, social, cultural, and environmental aspects of the client need to be assessed, the phys-

(Text continues on p. 62.)

THE PSYCHIATRIC HISTORY[12,16] (CONTINUED)

5. *Adolescence:* what was client like as an adolescent?
   a. *Health and development.* Illness, operations, accidents? Reactions to body change during this period? Effect on social activities of bodily changes?
   b. *Psychosexual development.* Attitudes to opposite and same sex, crushes, dating, petting, masturbation, wet dreams, sexual fears? Menarche—age, reaction to first and subsequent periods, emotional and physical changes during periods? Interest in sex literature, guilt feelings, withdrawal from sexual contacts, parties, dancing? Homosexual interests, experiences?
   c. *Family.* Rebellion against family and parents? Continuation of family life? Changes in role in family? Disciplinary problems? Trouble with authorities? Arrest? Physical, sexual, emotional abuse?
   d. *Religion.* Training, interests, activities, changes in them?
   e. *Habits.* Smoking, drinking, drugs, sleeping, eating, recreation, social activities?
   f. *Interests.* Hobbies, music, reading, art, sports, collections, philosophical preoccupations, and others?
   g. *Personality.* Changes in disposition and temperament? Moodiness, fantasies, asceticism? Pleasure-seeking? Conscientiousness? Need for recognition? Competitiveness? Friendliness? Shyness? Social anxieties, seclusiveness?

6. *Cultural factors:*
   a. *Development.* Emphasis placed on spirituality and cultural roots in client's family? Did client as a child or adolescent agree with cultural norms of family?
   b. *Spirituality.* Are religious beliefs a contributing factor in the development of client's illness? Are religious concerns a symptom of a deeper conflict? Is there a religious concern present, and does it serve as a defense of the person to prevent further decompensation? Are client's religious behavior and thinking realistic and comforting?
   c. *Current status.* Is client proud of family's cultural roots? Conflicts between the client's current lifestyle and cultural expectations? Cultural traditions maintained? Does client's culture have a particular belief about mental health services? Does such a belief affect client's use of such services? Do the cultural beliefs bring about problems of assimilation in the United States?

7. *Adult adjustment before illness:*
   a. *Occupation.* Age started to work, type of jobs? How long held? Quit? Fired? Pay? Ambitions and relation of jobs to them?
   b. *Psychosexual.* If in marriage or long-term relationship, age when it began? How long courtship? Children? List by ages. Reactions to pregnancies and children? Age of partner and what kind of person? Sexual relations, frequency, contraceptive methods, reactions to sex relations? Divorced? Why? If client is single, nature of sexual activities and relationships? Uses contraceptives?
   c. *Family.* Nature of continued relations with parental family? Dependence on family? Contributions to support of relatives?
   d. *Military record.* Dates of service, combat experience, army hospitalization, medical discharge, pension? Rank in service, promotions, demotions, disciplinary actions?
   e. *Social adjustment.* Organizations, community activities, antisocial activities, criminal record if any, political interests and activities? Number, customs, and sex preference of friends? Aware of the nature of relationships with others?
   f. *Habits.* Smoking, drinking, drugs? Sleeping, eating habits?
   g. *Interests.* Hobbies, music, reading, art, sports, collections, and others?
   h. *Environment.* Physical safety of living environment, such as crime, pollution, availability of transportation and social/cultural activities?
   i. *Personality and character structure.* How does client describe self? How accurate is the description? Is client like either parent? Would client describe self as calm, easygoing, quick-tempered, impulsive, irritable, moody, unemotional, cold, cheerful, rigid, conscientious, eager for sympathy, affectionate? Any sudden or gradual change in personality before appearance of illness?
   j. *Strengths of client.* What strengths does client describe? What strengths help, or could help, client manage problems? Specify: effective verbal communication, effective coping in relationships, adequate diversional activity, freedom from fear, appropriate grieving, adequate management of provision for necessities of life, knowledge, compliance, appropriate parenting, an adequate sexual relationship, spirituality, appropriate reasoning.

THE MENTAL STATUS EXAM[12]

I. *Appearance*
   A. Dress
      1. Appropriate   2. Inappropriate
   B. Grooming, hygiene (situation and age appropriate?)
      1. Appropriate   2. Inappropriate
   C. Age appearance
      1. Stated   2. Younger   3. Older

      Remarks: _____

      _____

II. *Behavior*
   A. Manner of relating
      1. Cooperative
      2. Indifferent
      3. Withdrawn
      4. Defensive

      Remarks: _____

      _____

   B. Psychomotor activity
      1. Appropriate to situation   6. Posture
      2. Hyperactivity   a. Normal b. Abnormal
      3. Retardation   7. Gait and station
      4. Tremor   a. Normal b. Abnormal
      5. Purposeless activity   8. Repetitive behaviors

      Remarks: _____

      _____

   C. Speech, language
      1. Intensity   6. Deviations
         a. Normal b. Loud c. Soft   a. None   e. Stammering
      2. Pitch   b. Aphasia   f. Clanging
         a. Normal b. Monotone c. Wide swings   c. Neologisms   g. Verbigeration
      3. Rate   d. Echolalia   h. Perseveration
         a. Normal b. Pressured c. Slow   7. Vocabulary, diction, syntax
         d. Halting   a. Appropriate to socioeducational background
      4. Spontaneity, productivity   b. Not appropriate to socioeducational background
         a. Normal b. Intrusive c. Decreased
      5. Relevance, coherence
         a. Normal b. Incoherent c. Irrelevant

      Remarks: _____

      _____

III. *Affect*
      1. Appropriate to content   4. Shallow
      2. Apathetic   5. Blunted
      3. Inappropriate   6. Flattened

      Remarks: _____

      _____

IV. *Mood*
      1. Normal   4. Happy, elated
      2. Anxious   5. Worried, perplexed
      3. Sad, depressed   6. Labile

      Remarks: _____

      _____

(Continued)

THE MENTAL STATUS EXAM[12] (CONTINUED)

V. *Thinking*
   A. Thought
      1. Form
         a. Normal   d. Illogical
         b. Concrete   e. Scattered
         c. Referential
      2. Progression
         a. Normal   d. Loose associations
         b. Circumstantial   e. Flight of ideas
         c. Tangential   f. Blocking

      3. Content
         a. Normal, appropriate   f. Obsessive thoughts
         b. Persecutory trends   g. Phobias
         c. Paranoia, delusions   h. Depressive trends
         d. Hypochondriacal trends   i. Poverty of thought
         e. Grandiosity

      Remarks: _____
      _____

   B. Perception
      1. Normal
      2. Hallucinations
         a. Olfactory   d. Auditory
         b. Visual   e. Tactile
         c. Gustatory   f. Visceral

      Remarks: _____
      _____

   C. General knowledge and information
      1. Tests:
         a. Last five Presidents: _____
         _____

         b. Capitals:
            i.   California: _____
            ii. France: _____
            iii. Canada: _____
            iv. India: _____
         c. Four large U.S. cities:
            i.   _____
            ii. _____
            iii. _____
            iv. _____

         d. Population of U.S.: _____
         e. Population of world: _____
         f. Years of W.W. II (U.S.): _____
         g. Direction and distance:
            i. L.A. to S.F.: _____
            ii. N.Y. to Paris: _____
      2. Conclusion
         a. Normal for socioeducational background
         b. Not normal for socioeducational background

      Remarks: _____
      _____

   D. Sensorium and intellectual function
      1. Orientation
         a. Time _____

         b. Place _____

         c. Person _____

         d. Situation _____

(Continued)

THE MENTAL STATUS EXAM[12] (CONTINUED)

2. Memory
  a. Remote
    i. Normal   ii. Impaired
  b. Recent
    i. Normal   ii. Impaired
  c. Specific abnormalities
    i. Amnesia   iii. Paramnesia
    ii. Hypermnesia   iv. Confabulation

3. Retention and recall   *Immediate*   *5 Min.*
  a. Auditory
    i. "Purple" _____ _____
    ii. "Steamship" _____ _____
    iii. "1240 E. Road" _____ _____
  b. Digit span
    i. *Forward:*   *Responses*
    372 _____
    4916 _____
    82574 _____
    3961528 _____
    ii. *Reversed:*   *Responses:*
    419 _____
    5372 _____
    19386 _____
    359164 _____
  c. Visual   *Immediate*   *5 Min.*
    i. "Pencil" _____ _____
    ii. "Chair" _____ _____
    iii. "Lamp" _____ _____

(Continued)

ical aspects must also be reviewed. It is easy to overlook the physical needs of the psychiatric/mental health client, so the nurse must continually reassess the physical as well as the mental health status in order to provide comprehensive care. The physical and psychiatric assessments should be done twice weekly to ascertain changes in the client's condition. Some clients, such as a person with a history of heart disease or an older adult, may need to be referred to a nurse practitioner or physician.

The components of the physical assessment should include at least the following:

Overall: Weight changes, a feeling of being tired, changes in body temperature, weakness, dizziness
Skin: Color changes, contour changes, itching
Head: Headache, injury
Eyes: Vision changes, excess tearing, eye disease, pain, observable changes
Ears: Hearing changes, pain, discharge
Nose and sinuses: Colds, allergies, blockage, nosebleeds
Mouth and throat: Pain, observable physical changes, discharges, speech changes
Neck: Changes in contour, pain
Breasts: Changes in contour, pain, discharge
Respiratory: Discharge, known respiratory diseases/problems, cough
Cardiac: Known heart problems, any swelling in extremities, pain, felt changes in heart beat, breathing difficulties
Gastrointestinal: Changes in food intake, bowel movements, gas, pain, burning sensation, nausea, vomiting, known gastrointestinal disease
Urinary: Changes in urination frequency, pain
Genitoreproductive: Genital sores, unusual discharges, pain, changes in contour, sexual problems. *Female:* regularity of menstrual periods, changes in amount

---

THE MENTAL STATUS EXAM[12] (CONTINUED)

4. Abstraction
   a. Proverbs
      i. Two heads are better than one. _____
      ii. People who live in glass houses shouldn't throw stones. _____
   b. Similarities
      i. Axe-saw: _____
      ii. Auto-bicycle: _____
5. Calculation and concentration
   a. $100 - 7$ (serially) _____
   b. $2 \times 3 =$ _____ $4 \times 3 \times 9 =$ _____

   $4 \times 12 =$ _____ $24 \times 3 =$ _____

   $8 \times 11 =$ _____ $96 \times 4 =$ _____

   $12 \times 13 =$ _____ $(8 \times 6) + 12 =$ _____

   c. If oranges cost 30¢ a dozen, how much do 18 oranges cost? _____
   d. A train leaves the station at 9:00 a.m. If its average speed is 50 m.p.h., at what time will it reach its destination 300 miles away? _____
   e. Reverse days of the week: _____
   f. Reverse months of the year: _____

   Remarks: _____
   _____

E. Insight
   1. Normal _____
   2. Impaired _____

F. Judgment
   1. Normal _____
   2. Impaired _____

(Formulated with the assistance of Jane Ryan, Associate Director of Nursing, Neuropsychiatric Hospital and Institute, University of California at Los Angeles)

---

of bleeding, bleeding between periods, emotional changes at time of period, difficulties with menopause, pregnancy

Musculoskeletal: Pain in joint or muscle, known illnesses or limitations

Neurological: Known illnesses, weakness, fainting, numbness, trembling, shaking

Endocrine: Known disease, temperature intolerance, changes in thirst, hunger

Hematological: Anemia, changes in bruising, bleeding[3]

Once the psychiatric and physical assessments of the client are completed, the nurse should have sufficient information about the client to begin to formulate a nursing diagnosis. The nurse may find, however, that there is a need for more information from the client, the family, or other sources (*e.g.,* laboratory tests). It is essential that

the nurse gather as much information as possible before completing the assessment phase of the nursing process.

The following Case Study shows how the assessment portion of the nursing process fits into the nursing care plan for a client. The assessment section includes the background information concerning the client, as well as a summary of the psychiatric history, the mental status examination, and the physical examination.

Case Study: The Nursing Process— Assessment

Background

Phil, a 20-year-old Caucasian college student, has just been admitted to a psychiatric unit. You have been asked to check his bag of belongings. You find a crumpled piece of paper with a poem on it, a pair of running shoes, and a small wallet with an expired driver's license. There is also a jacket, a small gold crucifix, some religious pamphlets, and an expired library card. Phil was brought to the unit by the police, who had found him in a shopping mall with a disheveled appearance, talking incoherently. He had refused to leave the mall, and seemed incapable of making decisions. There was no evidence of drug intoxication.

Later you assist the staff in going to each client's room to announce a special music program being offered on the unit. You find Phil in his room alone, dressed and lying on the bed. You introduce yourself and explain that the music program will start soon. Phil remains silent. He is motionless, and shows no expression. He does not seem anxious, although his expression indicates that he is preoccupied with his own thoughts and does not want to be disturbed. There is also some element of fear in his expression, although he does nothing to flee the situation. You describe typical music programs on the unit in a few sentences and encourage Phil to attend. You leave the room.

You discuss Phil with a member of the nursing staff. You find that the nurse has called the residence listed on the license in Phil's belongings. The telephone was answered by Ms. Andrews, the caretaker of a rooming house in which Phil rented a room.

Ms. Andrews stated that she had become increasingly concerned about Phil. He had enrolled in a nearby community college, but had stopped attending. He had become increasingly "nervous," according to Ms. Andrews, and seemed "scattered." He spent long hours in his room, and would occasionally fix himself meals. During this time, however, he seemed in a hurry and talked to no one, although he did not appear to have a hearing or speech problem. He did "move his lips at times, though, as if he was talking to someone, but he didn't say anything out loud." She noted that "his appearance was not very good at times."

According to Ms. Andrews, Phil had rented a room in the building for one year. Prior to that he lived with his parents, who helped Phil to move into the rented room but never returned. They occasionally called Phil, but he did not seem interested in what his parents had to say and even became "mad" on several occasions while talking with them. Ms. Andrews believed that Phil's parents helped him pay for his room and board. He has no job. His parents seem not to want to talk with Ms. Andrews when she answers the phone; they simply ask for Phil.

The staff on the unit continues to approach Phil and talk to him, but he does not respond. Phil paces the halls of the unit later in the evening, but he remains silent. He seems pensive and quiet. When he walks to the nurses' station to obtain his medication, he makes waving hand motions over the medication prior to taking it. He continues this behavior the next morning. The next morning he is called to the phone to accept a call from his landlady concerning his rented room, and he speaks a few words to her.

Assessment

Psychiatric History.
Identifying Data. Phil Robinson is a 20-year-old male Caucasian admitted to the psychiatric unit on December 1, 1988. Phil's personal belongings and his landlady have provided some information concerning Phil. The client has not spoken while in the hospital. The client is apparently single.

History. The client was brought to the hospital by the police, who found him disheveled in appearance and talking incoherently in a shopping mall. He refused to leave the mall. He showed no sense of judgment. He is considered gravely disabled.

Phil has been living in a rented room for one year. During that time he enrolled in college, but later did not attend. He became increasingly incapacitated during the past year. He would stay by himself in his room for long periods of time, and would speak to no one. He may have been experiencing hallucinations: his landlady reports that Phil talks to himself.

Phil's family did help him to move into the rented room, but have not visited Phil in the past year. Phil becomes agitated when talking with his parents on the phone. He has no known job or friends. He does have religious pamphlets and an expired library card as part of his possessions.

The client does not smoke and is slightly below his recommended weight. He has missed one meal during his day-and-a-half on the unit. He shows no violent tendencies.

While on the unit, Phil has not spoken to others on the unit and has attended no unit activities. He gives no response, verbal or nonverbal, to questions. He has been approached by assertive clients on the unit and seems quite skillful in disengaging from them. He did say a few words on the phone to his landlady.

Mental Status.
Appearance. Phil's dress and hygiene are unkept. Physically he appears to be his stated age, yet his sullen expression lacks the vibrance of a 20-year-old.

Behavior. He is withdrawn and silent. His posture is slightly stooped. His head is slightly bent as he continuously looks at the ground. His gait is slow yet steady. He is not hyperactive. He demonstrates the repetitive behaviors of pacing and hand gesturing over his medications just prior to taking the medication. The gesturing involves horizontal waving motions with both hands, one over the other. During the gesturing, his lips move as if he is saying something.

Affect. Phil's affect is flat and severely blunted. He shows no intense affective response to his surroundings.

Mood. He seems slightly frightened and severely withdrawn. He does not appear depressed, but seems vacant and lifeless.

Perception. He moves his lips at times as if talking to someone. He devotes attention to this private conversation and may be hallucinating.

RELEVANT RESEARCH

Six subjects on a mental health unit who had a medical (psychiatric) diagnosis of some type of depression were interviewed by one of three nurse researchers. After each interview the assessment material was summarized by the interviewers. The clients' charts were also reviewed to obtain the medical diagnoses and past psychiatric histories.

The three researchers then discussed the data gathered and identified nursing diagnoses. The researchers also identified the criteria they used in making the nursing diagnoses, and assessed whether the diagnoses would fit into other nursing and medical diagnostic schemes such as that developed by the North American Nursing Diagnosis Association (NANDA) or that developed by the American Psychiatric Association.

Results indicated that a total of twelve nursing diagnoses applied to the six clients. There was a lack of congruence between the nursing diagnoses and the medical diagnoses. Also, only three of the twelve diagnoses were similar to those in the NANDA classification. The lack of similarity pointed to how few nursing diagnoses there are in the NANDA classification that relate to psychiatric nursing, and the high level of abstraction in NANDA diagnoses. The latter judgment of the researchers points to the potential for care to be less individualized when based upon nursing diagnoses that are too general.

(Thomas M, Sanger E, Whitney J: Nursing diagnosis of depression. J Psychosoc Nurs Ment Health Serv 24:6, 1986)

Physical Assessment. Skin color is pale—appropriate for an individual who spends much time indoors. No vomiting noted. Pulse, blood pressure, and temperature are within normal limits, as are laboratory values for blood analyses. Neural reflexes are normal. There are no bruises. The client has eaten all but one meal while on the unit. The client cooperates minimally with the physical assessment and is slow to respond to verbal commands. Systems not mentioned are within normal limits on observation.

The Nursing Diagnosis

The assessment stage ends with the formulation of a nursing diagnosis. A nursing diagnosis is "a statement of a conclusion resulting from a recognition of a pattern derived from a nursing investigation of the client."[4] The recognition of the pattern is a complex process, guided by theories of human behavior. The nurse asks, "Based on theories of human behavior, what alterations from normal patterns are occurring?"

Research has provided some guidelines for selecting a pattern of behavior on which to focus nursing care. The *Relevant Research* describes the difficulty in arriving at meaningful nursing diagnoses (see box above).

Results of such research support the idea that nursing diagnoses are not simple derivatives of medical diagnoses. Nursing and medicine focus on different phenomena when working with clients. However, psychiatric nurses and psychiatrists must be aware of the diagnosis each places on a client so that all team members are informed of the concerns being dealt with in treatment.

In making the nursing diagnosis, the nurse looks for related facts that have been presented verbally and nonverbally by the client and the client's significant others. For example, the client may state that he goes for days without seeing anyone, and that the times when he was

happy in the past were the times when he had friends. The client may also state that he wishes he had friends today. A nonverbal clue could include a forlorn look as the client makes such statements. The nurse cognitively searches for the relationship among such facts presented by the client and then applies a label, or nursing diagnosis, to the group of facts.

Typically, a nursing diagnosis is not the same as a medical diagnosis. Gordon's definition helps to clarify the difference between the two:

> Nursing diagnoses, or clinical diagnoses made by professional nurses, describe actual or potential health problems which nurses by virtue of their education and experience are capable and licensed to treat.[6]

A nursing diagnosis tends to be more individualized than a medical (psychiatric) diagnosis. For example, in the case of the client mentioned above, the medical diagnosis may be "schizophrenia," while the nursing diagnosis could be "feelings of abandonment." While a medical diagnosis may focus on signs and symptoms, the nursing diagnosis focuses on a client's particular *response* to events.

A nursing diagnosis may change during the client's course of care. In the previous example, the nursing diagnosis could change from "feelings of abandonment" to "inadequate socialization skills" as the client's mood changes and the client begins to initiate interpersonal relationships. It is not unusual for a nurse to derive a diagnosis at the beginning of care and *change the diagnosis* as the care proceeds and the nurse establishes a more in-depth relationship with the client. A medical diagnosis, however, tends to remain the same.

Nursing diagnoses are central to care, and provide a way to summarize the variety of data about the client. Nursing diagnoses can be used to communicate the nature of the client's problems to nurses, the client, and the health care team. They also provide "index" words to use in reviewing the literature concerning the client's problems in order to determine typical etiological patterns of the diagnoses or recommended treatments. Nursing diagnoses also provide assistance in establishing goals for care. With a nursing diagnosis of "abandonment," the expectation is that at least one of the goals of treatment of the client will be a decrease in a sense of abandonment by formation of a relationship.

When health was viewed as only the absence of disease, the *medical* diagnosis was the only explicit basis for the direction of health care. However, because the well-being of the client involves more than pathology, the medical diagnosis clearly does not give enough direction to provision of mental health care.

For example, a client with a medical diagnosis of schizophrenia may be discharged and sent to a "board and care" home in the community. The home may be in a less desirable part of the community, and the client may be placed with other clients who have severe psychiatric/mental health care needs, and given an authoritarian type of daily supervision. Will the client be able to maintain a sense of well-being once discharged, or will the client deteriorate further and be readmitted to the mental health care system in an even more regressed state?

Because there is no medical diagnosis for "inadequate social skills," the client's interpersonal skills must be accounted for in a nursing diagnosis. Could the client benefit from working with the treatment team on a nursing diagnosis of "inadequate social skills?" Would achieving social competency help the client maintain a reasonable quality of life in the board and care home without regressing and having to be rehospitalized? Note that the client's sense of well-being and mental health status can depend equally on the nursing and the medical diagnoses.

Nursing and psychiatric diagnoses can complement each other. Medical diagnoses, for example, provide some direction for choice of medication, whereas nursing diagnoses provide reference points to use in determining whether the medications are beneficial because many nursing diagnoses describe particular behaviors.

In the research described above, the nursing diagnoses related to depression are not as general as are the medical diagnoses. For example, there are no psychiatric (medical) diagnoses for poor self-esteem, loneliness, or hallucinations. In most instances the nursing diagnosis is closer to the experience of the client. A client may not feel schizophrenic (a medical diagnosis), but may feel lonely (a nursing diagnosis). Carnevali mentioned that there is presently no rigid system for selecting a nursing diagnosis.[4]

In this text, those nursing diagnoses that best describe the encompassing client characteristics for a particular illness are used, including (1) the diagnoses in the *Psychiatric Nursing Diagnoses (Manual) I* developed by the American Nurses' Association,[1] and (2) the diagnoses developed at the Fourth and Fifth National Conferences on nursing diagnoses.[9] These can be found in the appendix of this text.

Some general principles for selecting psychiatric nursing diagnoses are suggested in the research of Thomas, Sanger, and Whitney:[17]

1. Use as few nursing diagnoses as possible. In the present health care system, many clients do not remain under treatment for an extended period of time. Hence, the nurse must be selective in the problems the nurse and the client focus upon. The researchers suggested use of two to four nursing diagnoses.

2. The diagnoses must be sufficiently specific to individualize care but sufficiently broad to capture, in one diagnostic label, a problematic pattern repeated by the client in many circumstances.

3. The diagnoses should be selected from those that are already identified in diagnostic schemes. This facilitates doing clinical research on the various diagnoses. This principle is not meant to limit the identification of patterns of behavior not previously identified. Psychiatric nursing, when compared with other disciplines such as psychiatry, is considered to be in the beginning stages of defining how it perceives human behavior in ways unique to psychiatric nursing. Giving premature closure to identifying patterns of behavior would be unfortunate.

4. The diagnosis must be stated in a nonjudgmental manner. The researchers tested whether the diagnosis met this criteria by asking themselves if they would share the diagnosis with the client.

5. The diagnoses should label patterns of behavior on which the nurse can work with the client. For example, for a client with the nursing diagnosis of "lack of interpersonal relationships," the nurse can help the client learn behaviors that are useful in making friendships. If the nursing diagnosis had been (inappropriately) "has no friends," the nurse would be expected, by the intent of this diagnosis, to provide friends for the client—an intervention that is impossible to perform because individuals select their own friends.

6. The diagnoses should focus on client problems, not nursing problems. In the case study presented in this chapter, an inappropriate nursing diagnosis would be "inability to gather interview data for assessment." The need to perform the assessment is the nurse's need, not the client's. One correct nursing diagnosis should be "mutism," since it focuses on the client's problem.

7. Nursing diagnoses are neutral. Terms that place negative connotations on the client, such as "irritating" or "repulsive," should not be used. Instead, the nurse should look for the internal mechanism within the client promoting behavior such as denial, fear, or conflict.

At the end of an assessment, the psychiatric nurse develops a summary of the assessment. MacKinnon and Michels[11] mention that the summary can contain a review of the major points of the psychiatric assessment as well as the internal psychological factors of the client that promote current problems. These internal psychological factors may include present difficult concerns or childhood events that triggered current concerns.

Returning to the Case Study introduced earlier in the

chapter, the summary statement and the diagnoses can now be added to the care plan.

Summary Statement

Phil is severely withdrawn and has not spoken to others while on the unit. He does respond to some verbal commands, and paces the halls or remains isolated. He is apparently hallucinating and has had periods of public displays of inappropriate behavior and disheveled appearance. He did say a few words to his landlady on the phone.

He has been isolated for a number of months. He did enter college, but became disorganized in his behavior and stopped attending. He has been agitated when on the phone to his parents while at his boarding house. He currently has little contact with his parents other than by means of the phone, and has no social ties.

Phil displays intelligence in his skill in avoiding interpersonal contact while on the unit. He is severely preoccupied with his internal processes and concerns, rather than merely being passive. He is sensitive, and has lost the interpersonal competency of engaging with others and asking for help. He has maintained his responsibilities in paying his rent, yet for the most part lives in his own world in a state of unreal aloneness.

Diagnosis

Nursing Diagnoses: Mutism
                     Withdrawn behavior

Deriving the Summary Statement

The statement summarizing the assessment data (including the nursing diagnosis) is not easy to derive. Typically, a nurse will meet with the client to do the assessment and later will write the summary and diagnosis section. After the assessment is written, the nurse may want to put it aside and ask the more difficult question, "Who *is* the client (Phil, in this case)?" Finding the answer requires that the nurse look at the whole of the client, not just one particular symptom, in order to determine the essence of the "whole" presented by the client. The nurse must focus on the overall image of the client and search for the nature of the intangible Self of the client. This can be difficult, because the many details of the psychiatric assessment can be seductive in giving the nurse a sense of control and knowledge. An example of the "essence" the nurse is looking for in Phil is a feeling of an unreal aloneness. This is the crux of his overall presentation, and the central component of his internal struggle.

Nursing diagnoses provide a means for the psychiatric nurse to give the behavior pattern a label that provides a summary of the central concern of the client—the concern that provides the greatest problem for the client in attaining a sense of well-being. The diagnosis is also a statement identifying behavior that the psychiatric nurse can assist the client in altering and improving. Once this pattern is identified, the nurse begins to develop the care plan.

Mutism and withdrawn behavior were selected as nursing diagnoses for Phil because they relate to competencies necessary for Phil's attainment of a sense of well-being: talking about his concerns facilitates his understanding of them, and as he understands his concerns he can test other behaviors that better serve his sense of comfort. To attain some understanding, Phil can work with others (clients and staff). Being with others means relating with others in a meaningful manner—the opposite of withdrawn behavior.

Planning

The planning phase of the nursing process determines the priorities of care. If a client is in acute psychological distress, for example, the nurse would focus on this event, provide care, and attend to other problems after the acute period has subsided. The planning phase includes the formation of a "nursing care plan."

The exact form of the nursing care plan depends on the setting in which the nurse works, and the individual preferences of the care providers. Typically, *the nursing care plan includes the nursing diagnosis, nursing interventions,* and *an evaluative and goals statement* to indicate what is expected at the conclusion of the nursing interventions. The development of the nursing care plan ends the planning phase of the nursing process.

Some care plans call for *long-term goals.*[14] Long-term goals pertain to expected client achievements in attaining or reestablishing emotional health and adaptation. Usually long-term goals are accomplished minimally in a matter of several weeks. These goals focus on such client achievements as:

1. Improvement of the client's condition ("The client will learn not to injure self but to talk with others about the client's concerns.")
2. Maintenance of the client's condition ("The client will keep clinic appointments.")
3. Slowing deterioration of the client's condition. ("The dying client will maintain communication with family.")

Short-term goals pertain to objectives that relate to the long-term goals but are written in measurable terms and contain an expected date of achievement (usually a matter of days). The short-term goals are definitive steps made by the client that indicate progress in meeting the long-term goals. In many cases there is more than one short-term goal for a particular long-term goal.

Examples of short-term goals are included in the "Evaluation Criteria" column of the nursing care plans in this text, especially in Part V.

A nursing care plan is more effective if it contains statements that are specific and tailored to the client. The evaluative statement(s) of the plan should include the exact behaviors the nurse would expect the client to demonstrate to indicate that a problem has been resolved.

The following Nursing Care Plan could be developed for Phil, the client discussed earlier in the Case Study.

NURSING CARE PLAN

The plan of care includes:

1. A long-term goal of satisfactory communal living
2. An immediate goal of talking with Phil's parents to gather information concerning Phil's history and present circumstances as well as data about the family relationships. Phil's college will also be contacted, with Phil's written permission, to obtain information about Phil.
3. The short-term goals of verbal behavior on Phil's part, and a willingness to relate to others. The lack of verbal communication will be considered in the following care plan.

ASSESSMENT	NURSING INTERVENTIONS	EVALUATION CRITERIA
NURSING DIAGNOSIS: Mutism		
SUBJECTIVE DATA Client has not verbalized.	1. Verbalize to client in daily therapeutic sessions. Pace with client if necessary. Provide orienting information. Make one statement to client at least every five minutes in session.	Within two days client will remain with staff during interview.
OBJECTIVE DATA Client has not responded when spoken to; is severely withdrawn, although paces.	2. Tell client what is expected of client. Say, "Use this time to talk about yourself," or "State in words what that gesture means."	Within three days client will respond verbally to statements made by staff or clients.

The evaluative criteria should be attainable by the client at the client's competency level. In the case of Phil, an evaluative criterion would *not* be, for example, "client converses in group therapy about his concerns." The client is not talking with anyone at this time. An expectation that the client would talk in group therapy would be unreasonable, because many individuals who are not mute find a group threatening at first.

Each care plan should be individualized. The plan should be written in pencil so that changes can be made as the client changes. Sensitivity on the part of the writer is helpful: the attempt to capture the essence of the problem and provide appropriate interventions brings a sense of reward to the clinician.

Intervention

Nursing interventions begin as soon as the nurse is within the visual range of the client. The client can learn much about the nurse, even if the nurse has said nothing. The client is also assessing how the client will be affected by the demeanor of the nurse. A nurse who sounds abrupt may promote a hesitant response from the client. It is useful to present an interested, listening perspective and adopt a demeanor of genuine caring.

Interventions are the actions the treatment team (or individual team members) perform with the client to promote a resolution of the problem described in the nursing diagnosis. Interventions are not a restatement of the nursing diagnosis. For example, if the nursing diagnosis is "poor self-esteem," the interventions would not include the phrase "promote self-esteem." Such promotion is assumed in labeling self-esteem as a problem.

Interventions are done in a purposeful manner. In the sample care plan included in this chapter, the nurse does not assume that the client will talk spontaneously if left alone. Rather, the nurse sits with the client and talks, even if the client does not respond. The nurse may comment on the daily schedule of activities of the unit, or on the need for the client to complete daily meal menus, or on other happenings in order to provide a "verbal environment" in which the client can participate.

Interventions are also "titrated," or adjusted to the needs of the client. The nurse will observe that, although professionals in the field diagnose, no client will *always* demonstrate behavior exactly exemplifying the diagnosis. *Even in one interview* the client can range from "psychotic" to more "normal."

In one instance, the client may be hallucinating (evidenced by the client's lips moving as if talking to someone, a preoccupied stare, and lack of response to communication). Five minutes later, the client may stop hallucinating and give an appropriate response to a question from the nurse. In one instance the nurse performs one type of intervention, and in the other instance another type. The process of titration is shown in Table 4-1.

The titration process takes concentration and diligence on the part of the nurse, and is the "work" the professional nurse does with psychiatric clients. Again, the psychiatric nurse does not do something *to* the client, but bases interventions on the needs of the client at the time.

Evaluation

While the processes of assessment, diagnosis, planning, and intervention are difficult, the evaluation of the effectiveness of nursing care is even harder, particularly in psychiatric/mental health nursing. Psychiatric/mental health nurses often become so involved in the complex care of the client that they find it difficult to be objective in reviewing their treatment to determine if their efforts with clients are working.

The "evaluation of nursing care is a feedback mechanism for judging quality and is designed to improve nursing care by comparing actual care given with standards for the care."[10] The evaluation portion of the nursing process in the Case Study of Phil includes those elements in the right-hand column of Phil's nursing care plan. For some clients, to remain with a staff person or therapeutic group for a period of time requires concerted effort. It is unclear whether Phil will be willing to remain with the nurse in a therapeutic session, or will leave the session.

The intervention most likely to be successful in prompting verbalization by Phil is to have others physically present with Phil and talking with him.

In respect to the second evaluation criterion of verbal responses made by Phil, it is thought that the intervention statements made by the nurse are so tailored to Phil's current needs and capabilities that Phil would verbalize as a result of the interventions. The evaluation stage transforms the nursing process into a continuing cycle. Does the client demonstrate the expected behaviors, after a stated period of time, to indicate that the client's problem or need has been resolved? If not, what aspects of the nursing care plan need to be revised? Was the nursing diagnosis correct? Did the interventions have sufficient impact with the correct frequency? Were the interventions given within the correct modality (individual, group, or family treatment)? Are the expected behaviors attainable? Many other pertinent questions could be asked to evaluate the effectiveness of the nursing process for a particular client.

For example, if Phil continues to be mute except when talking with Ms. Andrews, his landlady, could the team alter their plan and include Ms. Andrews in their approach? The team could add the intervention, "Call landlady and encourage her to visit Phil." This would be done after gaining Phil's written permission to do so. Phil may then verbalize more with the landlady and transfer this behavior to verbalizing with staff. The new evaluation criteria for this intervention would be, "Client verbalizes with others on unit within "X" days after landlady's visit."

Because the client's system is constantly changing and evolving through interactions with others and the en-

TABLE 4-1.
TITRATION OF NURSING BEHAVIORS TO MEET CLIENT NEEDS

CLIENT BEHAVIOR OR CIRCUMSTANCE	NURSE RESPONSE	RATIONALE FOR NURSE RESPONSE
Phil is a new client on the unit.	The student nurse goes to the client to introduce herself.	Approaching the client is a welcoming gesture. It also provides an opportunity to begin client assessment.
Phil is in his room.	The student says that there is an activity on the unit that Phil can attend.	Informing the client about an activity out of the client's room provides an opportunity to assess how the client will respond to others. Will the client welcome the opportunity of an activity, withdraw from it, or be ambivalent about it?
Phil remains silent. He seems preoccupied and apprehensive.	The student nurse describes the activity by saying, "The activity consists of various relaxation exercises done with different types of music . . ."	The client remains unresponsive after the student's initial remarks about the activity. Although the student titrated or adjusted her behavior according to client needs by going to Phil's room rather than expecting Phil to come to her, the description of the music activity here is more complex. With a less ill client the student might have had a rather effortless conversation about music activities on the unit.
		The student titrates comments to Phil's needs at the moment. Phil is apprehensive and appears to be hallucinating. The student did not know if she would be assigned to work closely with Phil, and she did not want to initiate an in-depth discussion with Phil if she would not be assigned to him. The priority at that time, then, was to remain focused on assisting Phil to accomplish the behavior that would best suit his needs, which was to begin to participate in the unit program as soon as possible.

RELEVANT RESEARCH

Perlman and others[15] studied the records of 404 psychiatric Medicaid clients from 35 free-standing psychiatric clinics in New York City. The results of the study indicated that basic information mandated by record-keeping standards was omitted from client records. The mental status and therapeutic plan sections of the Psychiatric Assessment were found to be less likely to comply with record-keeping standards. At the

hospitals there was a trend toward less thorough recording-keeping for Hispanic clients, when contrasted with that for black and white clients, probably due to language barriers between clinicians and clients. This study emphasizes the need for health care providers to be certain that all cultural aspects (including language) are considered when providing care.

(Perlman B, Schwartz A, Paris M et al: Psychiatric records: Variations based on discipline and patient characteristics, with implications for quality of care. Am J Psychiatry 139:1154, 1982)

vironment, it is essential that the steps of the nursing process continue to adapt to the changes in the client. Thus, in the evaluation process it is necessary to reassess the client's status, possibly formulate new nursing diagnoses, modify the existing care plan or develop a new one, and explore alternate interventions. The evaluation phase of the nursing process is cyclical in that the steps are repeated as frequently as is necessary. Figure 4-1 shows the constant flow of the nursing process through its repeated cycles for each client.

Cultural Concerns

In working with psychiatric/mental health clients, nurses are exposed to a variety of cultures, each of which has its own beliefs about health and illness. It is important that nurses be as aware as possible of the cultures of the clients with whom they work. However, given the diversity

of clients and cultures, it is impossible for nurses to be aware of all aspects of the culture of each client. In order to establish a strong nurse–client rapport, it is often better for the nurse to ask for the client's assistance in explaining cultural beliefs and practices.

The culture of the client has an impact on all aspects of the nursing process. For example, while performing a psychiatric assessment with a Native American client, the nurse might note that the client appears deferential because the client never makes direct eye contact with the nurse. The nurse's assessment would probably be incorrect, because some Native Americans consider direct eye contact a form of rude behavior.

Similarly, in planning, implementing, and evaluating nursing care, the nurse must be sensitive to the cultural backgrounds of clients. What may appear to be noncompliance on the part of the client may, in fact, be adherence to cultural or religious beliefs unknown to the nurse. The importance of culturally-sensitive care, particularly as it

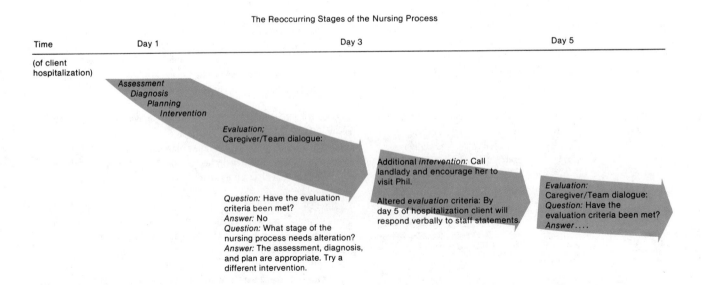

The Reoccurring Stages of the Nursing Process

Time   Day 1   Day 3   Day 5

(of client hospitalization)

Assessment
Diagnosis
Planning
Intervention

Evaluation;
Caregiver/Team dialogue:

Additional *intervention:* Call landlady and encourage her to visit Phil.

Altered *evaluation* criteria: By day 5 of hospitalization client will respond verbally to staff statements.

Question: Have the evaluation criteria been met?
Answer: No
Question: What stage of the nursing process needs alteration?
Answer: The assessment, diagnosis, and plan are appropriate. Try a different intervention.

Evaluation:
Caregiver/Team dialogue:
Question: Have the evaluation criteria been met?
Answer....

Figure 4-1. The evolving nature of the nursing process.

RELEVANT RESEARCH

In this study, 633 women employed in an academic setting responded to a set of questions to determine what effect certain factors have on the subject's mental health. Mental health was measured by the *General Well-Being Schedule.* The "system" factors thought to influence a person's sense of well-being were: physical health, religion, age, ethnicity, income, marital status, interpersonal relationships, educational level, and employment status.

The study used two perspectives on the client that are frequently found in nursing: a view of all aspects of the health–illness continuum, and a view of the client as a system. The focus of this study was the health component of the health–illness continuum. Variables other than psychological were examined, such as cultural (ethnicity), soci-

etal (interpersonal relationships), environmental (the number of people living with the respondent), and biological (physical health).

Findings of the study indicated that 66% of the subjects experienced a positive sense of well-being, 13% experienced severe distress, and 20% had moderate distress. A sense of greater well-being was associated with such factors as a higher income and Protestantism, whereas this positive feeling was not associated with marital status, age, ethnicity, educational level, and the number of hours worked each week.

The author concluded by stating that nurses are in a particularly advantageous position to study the factors that promote women's mental health. Many more studies are needed that document precisely the aspects of a woman's experience that promote mental health.

(O'Rourke M: The influence of social, demographic, employment, and health factors on the psychological well-being of employed women. Iss Ment Health Nurs 8:121, 1986)

relates to language, is described in the Relevant Research box above.

Prevention and the Nursing Process

The nursing process is implemented with clients who are at different degrees of *risk* of developing mental health problems. An assessment may not reveal acute problems, but the nurse should be aware of the potential for problems to develop later. At other times, treatment of the illness process is necessary so that a client can return to a peak level of functioning (*rehabilitation*). Different types of behavior are required of nurses as they attempt to *prevent* long-term effects of illness.

Primary prevention refers to the promotion of mental health and the prevention of illness.[8] An example of a nursing intervention at this level of prevention could include helping the parents of an ill child verbalize their feelings about their child's status. Primary prevention also refers to subtle attitudes on the part of the nurse, such as a sense of hope about the ability of a new mother to care for her infant or the patience of the nurse with a prediabetic client who is having difficulty grasping dietary concepts. Primary prevention involves using foresight, based on what is known about how illness develops, to intervene and offer guidance, assistance, or encouragement where it is needed.

Primary prevention also involves a focus on health. Some researchers have studied healthy behavior, or the "health" side of the health–illness continuum mentioned in the Introduction to this text. The following *Relevant Research* shows the relationship between system variables and mental health.

Secondary prevention refers to early case-finding and treatment of problems. An example of secondary prevention would be assessing a family for child abuse when certain cues are noted in family members. Early treatment includes providing quick and thorough crisis intervention for clients experiencing their first psychiatric hospitalization.

Tertiary prevention refers to rehabilitation or the return of clients to their peak level of functioning. While many clients may need weeks of treatment, special note should be made of the long-term (or chronic) psychiatric client. In many instances the psychiatric/mental health nurse is the only health care provider interacting professionally with such a person. Many gains can be made with these clients, but the nurse must understand that changes may be slow, or come in gradual steps. Nevertheless, the philosophy of nursing is that *change and growth can occur.*

Summary

1. The nursing process gives nurses a structure for providing professional care for clients.

2. The nursing process occurs within the context of the nurse's *therapeutic use of self.*

3. The nursing process includes the steps of assessment, diagnosis, planning, intervention, and evaluation.

4. The assessment phase of the nursing process includes examining all five components of the client as a system: the psychological, the physical, the societal, the cultural, and the environmental.

5. The nursing process includes the client as a co-participant in each step.

References

1. American Nurses' Association: Taxonomy for the Classification of Human Responses of Concern for Psychiatric/Mental Health Nursing. Kansas City, American Nurses' Association, 1986
2. American Psychiatric Association: Diagnostic and Statistical Manual of Mental Disorders-III-R. Washington, DC, American Psychiatric Association, 1987
3. Bates B, Hoekelman R: Interviewing and the Health History. In Bates B (ed): A Guide to Physical Examination. Philadelphia, JB Lippincott, 1987
4. Carnevali D: Nursing Care Planning: Diagnosis and Management. Philadelphia, JB Lippincott, 1983
5. American Nurses' Association: Standards of Psychiatric and Mental Health Nursing Practice. Kansas City, American Nurses' Association, 1982
6. Gordon M: Nursing diagnosis and the diagnostic process. Am J Nurs 76:1928, 1976
7. Hagerty B: Psychiatric/Mental Health Assessment. St Louis, CV Mosby, 1984
8. Hinsie L, Campbell R: Psychiatric Dictionary. New York, Oxford University Press, 1973
9. Kim M, McFarland G, McLane A: Classification of Nursing Diagnoses: Proceedings of the Fifth National Conference. St Louis, CV Mosby, 1984
10. Marriner A: The Nursing Process. St Louis, CV Mosby, 1986
11. MacKinnon R, Michels R: The Psychiatric Interview in Clinical Practice. St Louis, CV Mosby, 1971
12. Nursing Service, Ryan J: An Outline for a Psychiatric History. Los Angeles, University of California Neuropsychiatric Hospital and Institute, 1985
13. O'Rourke M: The influence of social, demographic, employment, and health factors on the psychological well-being of employed women. Iss Ment Health Nurs 8:121, 1986
14. Parsons P: Building better treatment plans. J Psychosoc Nurs Ment Health Serv 24:8, 1986
15. Perlman B, Schwartz A, Paris M et al: Psychiatric records: Variations based on discipline and patient characteristics, with implications for quality of care. Am J Psychiatry 139:1154, 1982
16. Popkess-Vawter S: Strength-Oriented Nursing Diagnoses. In Proceedings of Fifth National Conference: Classification of Nursing Diagnoses. St Louis, CV Mosby, 1984
17. Thomas M, Sanger E, Whitney J: Nursing diagnosis of depression. J Psychosoc Nurs Ment Health Serv, 24:13, 1986

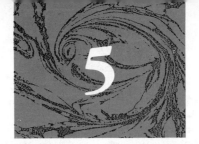

5

LORETTA M. BIRCKHEAD

IMPLEMENTATION OF THE NURSING PROCESS: THE THERAPEUTIC USE OF SELF

Learning Objectives

Upon completion of this chapter the student should be able to do the following:

1. Describe the Self/Other/Relationship conceptual framework as a guideline for understanding the psychological/social aspects of human nature.
2. Define the concepts of Self and Other, and describe their Relationship.
3. List appropriate nursing interventions for working with the Self, the Other, and the Relationship of Self and Other.
4. Describe two characteristics of the nurse therapist as a person.
5. Differentiate between empathy and sympathy.
6. List the stages of the nurse–client relationship and describe client behaviors in each stage.
7. List the steps of the learning process and interventions used by the nurse in each step.

8. Differentiate between the content of a psychotherapeutic interview and the process of the interview.
9. Differentiate among affect, mood, and emotion.
10. Describe the nurse's observations of clients demonstrating various levels of anxiety.
11. Explain nursing interventions for clients experiencing anxiety and panic.
12. Describe the influences of cultural differences on affect.
13. Discuss the manner in which nursing behavior facilitates client change.

Introduction

Developing a therapeutic working relationship with clients is the essence of psychiatric nursing. For that relationship to facilitate the client's psychological growth effectively, the nurse must integrate cognitive (intellectual) and affective (emotional) aspects of the self.

Effective mental health nurses are both intellectually astute and comfortable with emotions in themselves and others. Given appropriate cues, clients will describe a complex life, and nurses' cognitive skills will be used to understand and find meaning in the complexity. However, intellectual understanding and saying the "appropriate words" are not sufficient to bring about client change. Of equal importance is the affective (emotional) use of self, which involves two related processes. Nurses help clients to express and discuss their emotions, and they use their own emotional responses as a guide when asking clients about their emotions.

For clients to heal emotionally nurses must react emotionally, either verbally or nonverbally, to what is said. This does not mean that nurses become immobilized by a client's depression or that the nurse's emotional responses dominate the therapeutic work, but rather that clients can best attain a sense of well-being with nurses who are comfortable with emotions. As nurses refine and develop their emotional responses, clients become more comfortable with their own emotional lives.

The previous chapter described the psychiatric nursing process in detail. During the assessment stage of that process, psychological, societal, cultural, environmental, and biological aspects of the person are assessed. Nurses work at understanding clients' problems and the life circumstances that precipitated the problems. Nurses make lists of pertinent nursing diagnoses, plan care, intervene, and evaluate the effects of the interventions.

This chapter will focus primarily on the intervention aspect of the nursing process. The student will use the communication skills presented in Chapter 3 along with additional techniques presented here to interact effectively with clients. While using interventions to facilitate client growth, it is important that nurses remain open to new information about clients and adapt to clients' changes. The Self/Other/Relationship conceptual framework will be presented as the basis for the work of therapy and will serve as a guide for nurses in understanding psychological functioning.

The Importance of a Framework to Guide Practice

Many beginning nurses have difficulty knowing how to communicate with clients. Use of a framework, or a specific psychological theory, assists nurses by providing a guide for communication within the therapeutic relationship. The framework lists goals for treatment and techniques to use in promoting client change, and helps nurses to evaluate progress that is made. The framework also provides a consistent language for use with clients and other mental health practitioners. Therefore, use of a framework makes beginning nurses more comfortable in their new roles and facilitates communication with both clients and coworkers.

In addition, nurses who use a framework to guide practice are better equipped to deal with their own anxiety during the intervention process. Nurses who sense that maintenance of a useful focus on a client is not possible because of the nurse's personal preoccupation with emotion can continue to be effective with the client by relying on automatic technical (cognitive) responses consistent with the framework being used.

Because the framework establishes the clinician's approach to therapy, it has a significant impact on the client. If, for example, the client goes to a Freudian analyst for treatment, the clinician will focus on dreams and internal thoughts and feelings, as well as on developing insight into past and present behavior. However, if the same client goes to a professional who bases treatment on the interpersonal principles of Sullivan, the clinician will focus on the nature of previous interpersonal relationships and their effects on present relationships. Thus the client in Sullivanian therapy learns to think interpersonally, while the client in Freudian therapy becomes more intrapsychically oriented.

The Self/Other/Relationship Framework

Although many ideas used in psychiatric/mental health nursing may seem abstract and difficult to define, the work of therapy is guided by specific, concrete principles derived from the framework used by the nurse. The Self/Other/Relationship framework is presented here. It is based on the work of Harry Stack Sullivan (presented in greater detail in Chapter 6) and Hildegard Peplau, an expert in the use of interpersonal theory in psychiatric/mental health nursing practice.

Systems Theory: The Psychological and Societal Components of the Person

In the Self/Other/Relationship framework, the primary system components of the person are the psychological and the societal. Other components (environmental, biological, and cultural) are important, but the psychological component (Self) and the societal component (Other) are emphasized in the model.

The Self

The Self is *the* essential element, or the primary psychological dimension of the client with which the nurse works. The Self is probably best described as a *process*, just as running is a process. Running is not a physical object, and cannot be "held" or "treated" as physical matter, but it can be experienced. Similarly, the Self is a fluid process of awareness of experiences that include the Self, the Other, and the Relationship of the Self with Other(s).

The Self, Others, and Relationships With Others

The Self is the primary unit of concern in psychotherapeutic intervention because experiences that are dealt with are felt internally or within the individual. Although the "significant others" around the individual may foster a climate that produces certain emotions (as in the case of exhilaration at a sports rally), the emotion is nonetheless felt within the individual. These internal emotions can either promote or dissipate mental health.

The Self is also inseparable from Relationships with Others. As a result of this interrelatedness with other people, clients may be aware of any one of three experiences at a time: the Self, the Other, or the Relationship of Self and Other. These experiences, depicted in Figure 5-1, are viewed simultaneously from two different perspectives: the Self, as an entity unto itself, and the Self as inseparable from Relationships with Others. Relationships

have the capacity to promote or retard internal experiences (such as feelings) in the individual.

To be psychologically well-adjusted, the individual must view the Other as an entity with its own identity and description separate from the Self. To help the client achieve this understanding, our framework emphasizes the concept of *awareness*. As the client becomes more *aware,* the *Truth* or reality of the Other is understood by the Self. In other words, the Self views the Other objectively, *i.e.,* as the Other occurs, not as the Self distorts the Other or wishes the Other to be. The Self recognizes that the Other exists as a person outside the Relationship with the individual. Stated another way, the Other is viewed as a "person among people," *i.e.,* not only as a person in a significant Relationship with the Self. Failure to view the Other as a separate entity leads to various problems for the Self, such as the anxiety that the Self can experience when the Other (an important person in the life of the Self) engages in an activity without the Self. The Self feels rejected even when the Other clearly expresses caring for the Self. In this example, the Self is not perceiving the *Truth* of the Other. One of the greatest challenges of each person is to reconcile the separability of Self with the fact that the Self exists in Relationships with Others.

The separability/togetherness conflict is part of the contradictory character of the concept "Self." The Self is viewed as an entity unto itself, but at the same time the Self exists in a meaningful Relationship with Others. The Self is inseparable, yet distinct, from the Other. The unification of this contradictory idea is a primary goal for our framework for practice.

To summarize, the main psychological dimension of the person in psychotherapy is the Self. The Self is not a concrete, tangible quality, but rather an experience or feeling of awareness of the person. It is a fluid experience and may, at times, be clouded or unclear.

However, because people are fundamentally social beings, the Self cannot be defined as the only psychological experience. Indeed, the Self cannot be understood without also knowing who is significant to the client and what the relationship of the Self and Other is like. Psychological well-being comes, in large part, from a sense of awareness of Self and the Relationship of Self and Other.

Bonding and Attachment

Interpersonal relationships are based on "bonding" behavior among individuals. *Bonding* can be defined as an alliance of Self and Other in which the Self confirms the Truth of the Other. Bonding occurs on a continuum, from an absence of bonding to complete confirmation of the Other. Bonding is not possible unless the Self is aware of the True nature of the Other.

Bonding combined with *attachment* results in an experience of intimacy (love). Attachment is the Self's need to be with the Other to the extent that, when the Self is deprived of the Other, the well-being of the Self is decreased. Although the idea of "love" in contemporary culture is weighted with unrealistic expectations and

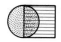

| The Self as an entity unto itself | The Other as known by the Self | The Relationship of Self and Others |

Figure 5-1. The three states of psychosocial experience.

even myths and fantasies, it can be surmised that bonding and attachment are together termed "love."

An example may help to clarify the meaning and interrelationship of these terms. A bond may exist between two clients on a unit. Each is cognizant of the Truth of the Other. Each Self sees the Other as that person actually is. Attachment is not present, however, in their relationship, because neither senses a need to be with the Other.

Each of these clients, however, has a significant Other, a spouse with whom the client experiences attachment (the need to be with the Other) *and* bonding (the cognizance of the Truth or the reality of the Other). Since both bonding and attachment exist, intimacy (love) is present between Self and this significant Other.

Nine different patterns of Self/Other/Relationship experiences can be observed at any one time in a client, as shown in Table 5-1. Problems can occur with a client in any of the possible patterns of Table 5-1. For example, the Self may express intimacy toward another, yet the Other express only bonding. Many other incongruities can occur among the various patterns. The nurse needs to assess the client to determine *which patterns are present.* Nursing interventions relevant to the difficulties in the patterns are shown in Table 5-2.

The Nurse Therapist as a Person

Self-Awareness

Effective nurse therapists need more than a theoretical understanding of clients. In order to deal with clients' emotional reactions (including grief, anger, aggressiveness, and depression), nurses must be able to look at themselves and examine their own feelings and reactions as people. Only when nurses understand and accept themselves will they be able to understand and accept clients' differences and uniqueness.

To become self-aware, nurses must analyze their thoughts, feelings, expectations, values, wishes, and needs, searching for compatibilities and incongruities. Are thoughts, feelings, and behavior congruent? Once the nurse becomes aware of incongruities, the process of integrating thought, feeling, and action can begin. Achieving self-awareness requires courage and the belief that nurses can tolerate self-knowledge and maintain a basic sense of well-being regardless of what is learned. The process can be painful as internal conflicts are identified; however, it is this pain that leads to emotional growth and the maturity necessary for nurses to guide clients through the process of psychotherapy.

Empathy

Empathy is the English translation of the German word "Einfuhling" coined by Theodor Lipps in 1885.[30] The literal meaning of the word is "feeling into;" it differs from sympathy, which means "feeling with." Empathy denotes an understanding of another for altruistic purposes, and this understanding must, in some verbal or nonverbal manner, be communicated to the other person. Empathic nurses use the skills of insight, compassion, identification, and understanding. The client's sense of the nurse's empathic attitude occurs on a continuum depending on how actively the nurse responds to the client.

Empathy describes a core process or an intervention through which the clinician works with the emotions or affects of the client. The ability to empathize has been described as the distinguishing characteristic of the committed nurse.[4] It adds a dimension of real understanding between client and therapist, and is one of the most important aspects of the helping relationship.

Differentiating Between Empathy and Sympathy

Sympathy can be defined as the existence of feelings identical to those of another person without accompany-

TABLE 5-1.
POSSIBLE *INTERACTION* PATTERNS OCCURRING IN THE EXPERIENCE OF SELF/OTHER/RELATIONSHIP

EXPERIENCES

1. *Self*—possible patterns include:	1. Bonding only (with the Other)
	2. Attachment only (with the Other)
	3. Bonding and attachment (intimacy) (with the Other)
2. *Other*—possible patterns include:	4. Bonding only (with the Self)
	5. Attachment only (with the Self)
	6. Bonding and attachment (intimacy) (with the Self)
3. *Relationship*—possible patterns include:	7. Bonding and attachment (intimacy) of the Self only (Other does not reciprocate)
	8. Bonding and attachment of Other only (Self does not reciprocate)
	9. Bonding and attachment of both Self and Other with each other

TABLE 5-2.
INTERVENTIONS FOR A LACK OF AWARENESS OF SELF/OTHER/RELATIONSHIP EXPERIENCES

EXPERIENCE	NURSING INTERVENTION
The Self	1. Explain the need for developing self-awareness. Explain the concepts of the Self/Other/Relationship framework to the extent that the client is capable of understanding. Use and define the words of the framework, *i.e.,* Truth, Awareness, Self/Other/Relationship, well-being.
	2. While listening to the client describe experiences, observe for the presence of anxiety and for unclear understanding of events. The presence of distortion (see explanation of distortion on pp. 87–88) indicates an awareness process that is restricted by anxiety.
	3. Examine the restriction of awareness. If you see a pattern in the type of restriction, determine the circumstance in which the pattern was learned.
The Other	1. Explain the importance of understanding the reality or Truth of significant others. Reiterate this throughout therapy, because anxiety concerning the Other will restrict awareness. The client will experience an increased sense of well-being as the process of awareness becomes more comfortable.
	2. Help the client define the nature of the Other, and the history and nature of the connection with the Other. Differentiate between bonding and attachment.
	3. Listen for a distortion of Truth about the Other. Help the client to compare the Other with any person in a similar situation. In what manner is the relevant Other distorted and how are similar Others not distorted?
	4. Determine the specific emotions aroused in connection with the Other that serve to foster restricted awareness. In what way can the Self manage such emotions in a different manner?
	5. Help the client define alternative ways of existing with the Other that will not arouse anxiety in the Self. The clinician and client may meet with the Other to gain awareness of the source of anxiety.
	6. Help the client determine what type of Relationship the client has with the clinician. Are bonding and/or attachment present?
The Relationship	1. Explain the nature of Self and Other and the importance of the Relationship as a potential cause for anxiety (and for positive feelings as well).
	2. Help the client describe the history and nature of the Relationship. Label patterns of interaction in which anxiety restricts awareness. Identify other emotions resulting from the anxiety.
	3. Observe and label the patterns identified above in a number of Relationships. Determine how the patterns were learned. Specify the nature of the bonding, attachment, and Relationship patterns.
	4. Help the client identify ways in which the Relationship would better suit the client's needs. When possible, help the client practice gaining awareness of the Relationship in the presence of the Other.
	5. Help the client determine if the relationship with the clinician is a bonding/attachment connection or a Relationship. Help the client maintain a sense of well-being while maintaining awareness of the Self, the Other, and the Relationship with the clinician.
The Self/Other/Relationship	Clients can shift from moment to moment among the various types of experience: the Self, the Other, and the Relationship. The clinician must listen for these shifts and change the focus of the therapeutic work accordingly.

ing behaviors of understanding the experience of the other. Forsyth[10] explained that empathy and sympathy are alike in that each is a conscious process and each occurs in the context of a relationship with another person. Yet, in the case of sympathy, the focus is on the content of an experience that is similar for both persons, not on the emotions of the other person. For example, a client may be grieving over the loss of a spouse. The nurse may have just experienced a similar loss. When the client denies any significance attached to the loss, a nurse who has not understood her own loss may say, "Yes, it's time to look toward the future," thus failing to understand and closing off the client's need to grieve.

Empathy in Psychotherapeutic Intervention

To Baumgartner,[4] the acquisition of empathy is an art in itself. She listed the following characteristic behaviors of nurses who have developed empathy to the highest possible degree:

1. The nurse accepts his or her own self.
2. The nurse consciously devotes energy to concentrating on the client's problems.
3. The nurse compares personal life events with the client's, temporarily experiences the feelings accompanying such situations (which are similar to the client's feelings), and through this process participates with the client in the client's emotional experience. The client then has the positive experience of having emotions shared, understood, and accepted by another person.
4. The nurse is able to tolerate the anxiety that the nurse feels as the emotions accompanying the client's experiences are felt. The nurse also tolerates the anxiety of having to wait until the client's emotions are understood. The nurse allows the client to "be who the client actually is" rather than forming premature conclusions about the client.
5. The nurse devotes effort to understanding the client intellectually.
6. The nurse does not place values on the client's feelings. The nurse accepts that the feelings stated by the client are, indeed, the client's feelings, and does not, by overlooking the client's true feelings, try to change the client into someone whom the nurse finds easier to deal with in therapy.
7. The nurse is fully aware of the client's entire emotional life, not just the aspects that are comfortable to the nurse.

The Stages of the Therapeutic Relationship

Peplau[24] described the stages of the nurse–client relationship as the orientation phase, the working phase, and termination. Each of these phases is described below.

Orientation Phase

In the orientation phase the nurse explains what will occur during the therapeutic process, including the following:

1. The name of the clinician who will be doing the interviewing
2. The purpose of the interview
3. The time when meetings will be held
4. The number and duration of meetings
5. The place where meetings will be held
6. The reason that the nurse will be taking notes, if that will be the case
7. Confidentiality

The purpose of the interview should be communicated in a manner that focuses on the client's concerns rather than on the nurse's concerns. The orienting information serves as a type of contract between the client and the nurse and forms a boundary for the client, *i.e.,* the client knows what to expect and can predict what will happen during the sessions with the nurse.

For example, a student nurse working on an inpatient unit could say, "Hello, Ms. Lopez, I'm Phyllis Jones, a nursing student. I would like to meet with you each day for an hour to discuss your current concerns. We can meet in interview room B. I will be taking notes during the interview to list dates and various topics that you mention. What you say to me will be held in confidence but I will share some of the information with my instructor. Also, if you say something about yourself that is important for the treatment team to know, I will share this information with them. However, I will tell you before talking with the team. One o'clock is a good time for me to meet with you—is that time all right for you?"

The Initial Interview

Peplau noted that certain client behaviors are often seen in initial orienting sessions. For example, clients may ask nurses to talk about themselves, or may try to enlist the sympathy of nurses, or may expect nurses to provide instant solutions to problems. If nurses observe such behavior, they should maintain the focus on the orienting information and clients' concerns.

As an attempt to avoid dialogue, clients may also ask nurses to go for a walk or accompany them to get coffee. The nurse can do these things with the client; however, if this happens often, it may shift the focus of the meeting away from client concerns. Behavior during the initial interview will set the tone for the sessions that follow. Typical nurse and client behaviors in an initial interview are found in Table 5-3.

The nurse should tell the client the amount of time left for the interview—usually when there are five minutes left. This provides for a natural closure to the session. Generally, sessions should not go past the time stated in the contract. Consistency provides a framework within which the client can learn limits and trust.

TABLE 5-3.
TYPICAL NURSE AND CLIENT BEHAVIORS IN THE INITIAL INTERVIEW

CLIENT	NURSE
Anxious because of psychosocial problems	Anxious because of interviewing a person who is anxious
Anxious because of talking with and getting to know a stranger (the nurse)	Anxious because of talking with and getting to know a stranger (the client)
Needs help	Needs to give assistance
Needs to be understood	Wants to understand
Wants an immediate solution to long-standing problems	Knows that problem clarification and resolution take time and effort
Wants to be free of psychological pain	Knows that psychological pain may not decrease immediately or may increase as problems are discussed. Knows that having a sense of hope fosters tolerance of the temporary pain
Wants a tangible remedy to problems	Knows that a sense of well-being is more how one takes care of things in everyday life. Knows that personal, internal change may be required
Wants Others to change	Knows that psychological health comes more from changes in Self than Other *and* the Relationship with Other

Establishing Rapport. The presence of rapport indicates a mutual connection between the interviewer and the client. Rapport indicates a sense of acceptance, the client of the nurse and vice versa. Each understands the typical behavior of the other and there are no surprises. The presence of rapport facilitates the demonstration of all components of the client's behavior. The client expresses thoughts and feelings more easily, and attempts to act on new coping patterns.

The nurse can establish rapport by acting in a manner that is respectful of the client. The nurse uses foresight to anticipate aspects of the therapeutic experience that may provoke anxiety in the client. The clinician then seeks to guide the client through such experiences. Providing clients with orienting information in order to reduce their anxiety is an example of this guidance. Rapport is also facilitated when the nurse is comfortable with the feelings expressed by the client and tactful in helping the client to understand them. There must be a feeling that the client and nurse can come to terms with difficult and painful experiences of the client with grace and courage. It is the rapport between client and nurse that creates this feeling.

Testing Behavior. Peplau[26] described *testing* as a characteristic of all interpersonal relationships. Friends test each other to determine where feelings and loyalties lie. For example, one may delay calling the other to determine if, indeed, the other will call instead, thereby denoting caring. In a similar manner, clients test nurses.

The establishment of trust between client and nurse is facilitated when the client tests the firmness with which the nurse holds to the contract established in the orientation phase of the therapeutic relationship.

Before making behavioral changes, the client tests the nurse to find out if the nurse is trustworthy. Old patterns of behavior, although ineffective, create a familiar sense of security, and the client will experience anxiety in changing them. This anxiety is more tolerable if the client can trust the competence and caring of the nurse.

Clients test nurses in a number of ways. Clients may attempt to establish a social relationship with the nurse, or request that the nurse tell the client how to live his or her life. Clients may test nurses by attempting to touch them. At times a client may appropriately use touch instead of words to communicate with a nurse; generally, however, psychotherapy consists of verbal exchanges.

Other testing behaviors include talking about irrelevant material to determine if the nurse will lose interest; shocking or surprising the nurse; talking about abstract or future-related topics; acting seductively; acting warmly toward the nurse in one meeting and coldly in the next; and praising the nurse in one meeting and berating her in the next.

Clients are frequently labeled with the pejorative term *manipulator* when they test the nurse; however, testing behavior is expected in all interpersonal relationships. The term manipulator is reserved for clients who attempt to have their own needs met at the expense of another person's well-being. For example, a client states that he does not have permission, yet, to leave the unit and wants the nurse to obtain a book for him. When the book is delivered and the client states that he no longer wants the book, he is manipulating. The nurse has been "used" only to give the client a sense of feeling good to the detriment of the other person.

Manipulation carries a heavier punitive label than testing. Manipulation is performed at the direct expense of someone else; it is not used in order to establish trust, as is testing behavior.

Working Phase

According to Peplau,[19] the orientation phase continues until clients understand the purposes and procedures of psychotherapy. When clients enter the working phase, they begin a more intense process of understanding themselves and the ways they need to change.

The client may demonstrate movement into the working phase in a number of ways:

1. The client may change in appearance. Appearance may either improve or worsen. When appearance worsens, the client may be beginning to face uncomfortable emotions. The energy of these emotions drains the client's available energy for maintaining a neat appearance. Rather than commenting on the client's appearance, the nurse should accept the current state of the client in the therapeutic process.

2. The client may deal with anxiety in a different manner. The client's anxiety may be directed more toward doing the work required by the interview. For example, if the client coped in the past by avoiding topics, the client may now be able to maintain a greater focus on a painful topic. The client may begin to examine life experiences after consistent encouragement from the nurse.

3. The client may begin to notice time during the session. For example, when the nurse states, "We have five minutes left in the interview," the client may say, "What? Only five minutes?" Other clients may arrive late for the interview when they previously always arrived on time. The client may make better use of the interview time and become more goal-oriented in the session. Rather than waiting to be asked for feelings about an incident, the client may voluntarily state feelings. This is a result of the nurse's consistent request for such information.

4. The client may recognize the nurse as a unique person. For example, the client may notice what time the nurse arrives on the unit.

5. The client may associate what is being discussed with what occurred in a previous session.

6. The client may use fewer testing maneuvers. The client may tell the nurse a secret, or describe some way in which the client used new coping abilities.

The Learning Process

The learning process, as described by Peplau,[23] facilitates the process of psychotherapy. As the nurse guides the client through the steps of the process, the client develops new behaviors to confront psychological concerns.

The seven steps of the learning process seen by Peplau are observation, description, analysis, formulation, validation, testing new behavior, and integration of new behaviors. They are described below.

Observation. The client who can *observe* notices what is happening by use of the senses. In order to assess whether a client can observe, the nurse can ask the following questions:

- "What do you see?"
- "What did you observe going on at the time of . . .?"
- "Who was with you at the time?"
- "Then what did you notice?"
- "What are you thinking now?"

Description. *Description* involves the ability to recall and recount the details of an experience or event.

In order to demonstrate competency of description, the client must be able to maintain a focus on the experience or event, verbalize its description, and relate the details of the experience or event. Beginning interviewers should avoid assuming the "rest of" the description or filling in data rather than asking the client for details.

A complete description provides the nurse with an idea of the following:

- *Who* was present during an experience or event
- *What* occurred (including the client's actions, thoughts, and feelings about the experience in both the past and the present)
- *Why* the event occurred
- *When* the event occurred
- *Where* the event took place
- The *meaning* of the event

Of course, the nurse asks the client to describe only significant events. During the description the nurse *listens for distortions* in the way the client describes the experiences or events. For example, the client who "had a problem with the family and left home" described the problem in this way:

> "Well, my Dad and I never got along. He was rough. I finally got a job to get away from home, but I lost it and had to go back. Then it started all over."

The goal is to have the client clearly describe experiences in detail and give realistic or valid meaning to such experiences. Naturally, the nurse needs much more information about this client, but from the statement the nurse can note at least two distortions of that process. The statement seems incomplete and vague, and perhaps has some other underlying meaning because of the following phrases:

1. "He was rough." This is an unusual way for a person to talk about a parent.

2. "It started all over." "It" is important because "it" is referred to as starting all over. This indicates that a particular family event has continued for some time, and that it was important enough that the client mentioned it as a part of the reason why the client came to the clinic.

Hearing these distortions, the nurse asked: "Describe the ways your father was 'rough,' as you stated." After considerable prompting the client stated that he had been abused as a child and an adolescent. If the nurse had not asked for clarification of "rough," the nurse might have simply recorded "family problems," and would not have known the true concern(s) of the client.

Statements the nurse may find useful in assisting the client through the description phase are:

- "Then what happened?"
- "Describe the . . . in detail."
- "Give me a detailed description of . . ."
- "What did you do (think, feel)?"
- "What did he say then?"
- "Who was present?"
- "Where was everyone standing?"

Analysis. *Analysis* is the ability to differentiate between relevant and irrelevant data. Analysis implies an understanding or scrutinization of information rather than a simple description. In the previous example, the client would demonstrate competency at analysis if he noted that the abuse he suffered was a very significant event in his life and/or if he noted the connection between being abused and leaving home.

Statements the nurse can make to help the client to work through the analysis steps are:

- "What is the meaning of . . .?"
- "In what way is . . . significant?"
- "What is the relation between . . . and . . .?"
- "What is similar in the two experiences?"

Formulation. *Formulation* is the ability to summarize the meaning of an event or experience. A conclusion is reached by connecting aspects of the experience described in analysis.

In the previous example, the client could state, "When I went back home after losing my job my father tried to push me around again. It made me remember all the times he had hurt me, and I got depressed."

Statements the nurse can use to help the client through formulation include:

- "How would you summarize why you came to the hospital?"
- "What is the reason that . . . happened?"
- "What is your pattern of behavior?"

Validation. To *validate* means to check one's own meaning of events or experiences with the meaning of others. Validation helps to clarify distortions.

In the example above, the nurse could state, "I understand that your father physically abused you. You left home when you found a job, but when you returned your father beat you again. This brought back memories of your past abuse and you became depressed." The client would indicate his ability to validate by agreeing with such statements or clarifying them as needed.

The nurse can assist the client through the validation step by using the following questions:

- "Do you mean that . . .?"
- "Is this the way it happened, that . . .?"
- "Am I correct in saying that . . .?"

Testing New Behavior. As a result of the previous steps, the client now decides to use different action to resolve the concern or problem. The client tests new behavior(s). In the example above, the client may decide to join a group of abused adults to see if discussing his problem with others decreases his depression.

Statements that can assist the client through the behavior testing step might include:

- "What has helped with your . . . in the past?"
- "Now that you understand the experience, what can you do differently?"
- "When this occurs again, what will you do?"

Integration of New Behaviors. After the client has tested new behaviors, the results are formulated (as in Formulation, above). If the new behaviors promote a sense of well-being in the client, the client is likely to adopt the new behaviors.

To guide the client through the integration step, the nurse could say:

- "Describe the result of trying your new behavior of. . . ."
- "What was the effect of the new behavior?"
- "As a result of the new behavior, how did you feel?"

Termination

Termination of the nurse–client relationship is a formal and necessary part of the relationship. If the nurse has had 12 to 15 interviews with the client, the entire last session usually concerns termination. Clients are reminded of termination prior to the final session(s), but usually it is discussed in more depth at the close of therapy. In general, termination issues are discussed after other problems have been resolved.

Peplau[25] stated that ideally termination occurs when both client and nurse believe it is appropriate. Termination occurs when the client has attained sufficient intellectual and interpersonal competencies to maintain a sense of well-being. When the client and nurse discuss termination, the client may demonstrate experiences of abandonment, loss, and anger.

Peplau presented a format for termination. The recommended steps of the termination process follow:

1. A summary by the client: the client is asked to summarize what has been accomplished in the therapeutic process.

2. A summary by the nurse and validation of the summary by the client: the therapist's summary includes the main themes of the therapeutic work, client strengths, problems examined, and outcomes of the therapeutic process. The tone is positive. The summary is based on the data presented by the client so that the client can understand what the clinician is saying. The nurse focuses on what the client has accomplished rather than on problems remaining.

   The nurse's summary follows the client's to avoid having the client repeat the nurse's summary. Also, after the nurse's summary the client is asked to validate whether or not the client agrees with the nurse's summary.

3. A consideration of the client's reaction to termination: the nurse may need to ask *repeatedly* about the client's feelings regarding termination, because the client may find it difficult to talk about such feelings.

4. Closing remarks: the nurse can say "goodbye" at the close of the last session. The clinician should not minimize the nature of the nurse–client interaction by closing with comments such as "See you around," or "Nice speaking with you."

Termination can provide a purposeful closure to what has been a meaningful relationship. The termination of the nurse–client relationship may be the first time the client has experienced an orderly separation from another person, and one in which the Other (the nurse) cared about the client's reaction to the loss of the relationship. Thus, a formal termination process can serve as a model of dealing with the experience of loss.

The Psychotherapeutic Interview

Overview

In psychotherapeutic interviewing, the nurse controls the purpose and procedure of the interview process. If the client attempts to ask the nurse personal questions, the nurse should redirect the client or review the meaning of the client's inquiries. The client, however, is responsible for the content of the interview.

The clinician uses interventions at one step above the current competency level of the client. *Competencies* are intellectual and interpersonal skills needed to maintain a sense of well-being. Thousands of competencies exist. A few examples of *intellectual* competencies include the ability to:

- Maintain a focus on a particular topic
- Compare two events
- Remember experiences
- Describe events

Examples of *interpersonal* competencies include the ability to:

- Share personal data with another person
- Tolerate feelings associated with the Other
- Engage in a Relationship with the Other
- Understand the Truth of the Other

In psychotherapeutic interviewing, the nurse presents a task for the client to respond to that is one step above the client's current competency level. For example, a nurse is working with Mr. Archer, a client who is not talking, makes seemingly random hand motions, and does not at present demonstrate the intellectual competency to describe experiences. (Description is an intellectual competency.) The nurse could say, "I see your hand moving, Mr. Archer. Tell me in words what you want to say." This intervention is aimed at the level of competency just above the client's current competency level. *In psychotherapeutic interviewing the focus is on client competency development.*

If the nurse had said, "You must have been upset last night because I understand that you didn't sleep," the nurse would *not* be intervening at one step above the current competency level of the client. The nurse's statement presumes that the client was upset and therefore didn't sleep, and that this is what the client wants to talk about. If the nurse addresses comments to the client's

hand motions and asks that the client place these actions into words so that the nurse can understand their meaning, the nurse is relating to the current behavior of the client (the hand motion). It is likely that the client will be able to progress into talking about the hand motion, since the client is currently involved with the hand motion (the client is "doing" the hand motion).

A skilled interviewer assists in the client's development by focusing on issues that are currently pertinent to the client. If the nurse pursues topics that are not relevant to the client, the client must then switch the focus. Irritation with the nurse would be a natural response in such a situation. The nurse's comments should be relevant to what the client is working on and capable of accomplishing.

Because the nurse–client interchange is primarily verbal, the nurse must use clear, precise statements. The nurse should allow the client time to respond, yet not allow lengthy silences when it does not seem that the client is trying to understand a thought or idea. The nurse should also ask one question or make one statement at a time; otherwise it may be difficult for the client to maintain the focus of the interview.

The psychotherapeutic interview does not involve a review of all that a client has experienced. Rather, in individual relationship interventions "samples of the problem experiences" are reviewed. The client's experiences are reviewed, not the nurse's. Generally, nurses should not discuss their own life experiences with clients. Birckhead[5] described clinical situations, however, in which the nurse's sharing of personal experiences may be appropriate. In one situation, a student nurse was the only professional person on an inpatient unit who shared a common cultural background with a client. The nurse shared past experiences of a family death with the client that Birckhead described as culturally appropriate in this particular situation. A full review of the appropriateness of such revelations by the nurse is not possible here. In general, a focus on the experiences of the *nurse* is inappropriate in psychotherapeutic work.

Statement of Purpose

The nurse's actual statement describing the purpose and activities of the interview to the client depends on the current mental status of the client. If the client is severely withdrawn and frightened, the statement of the purpose of the interview should be brief. For instance, the nurse could say, "Mr. Andrews, I would like to talk with you for 20 minutes about the reasons you are in the hospital." If the client is not severely ill and can comprehend what is being said, the nurse can use a more involved and less focused statement such as, "Mr. Banks, I am Pam Rahn, a student nurse on the unit, and I'll be here each week for three months. I would like to meet with you for 60 minutes each time I am on the unit to discuss your concerns."

The statement of purpose also depends on the goals of the interview in light of the total treatment of the client. If a nurse is leading group therapy on an inpatient unit for clients who are able to discuss what is occurring in their lives, the nurse need not state the purpose of the group therapy session at the beginning of each session. The nurse may talk about the purpose of the group individually with clients prior to admission to the group, but opening remarks at a session may deprive the group of the opportunity to "start" the group themselves.

A nurse who is involved in short-term therapy, however, may say, "Mr. Collins, I am Cheryl Lang, a nurse in the outpatient department. You and I will meet for 12 sessions to work on your concerns. Start by describing what brought you to the clinic." This statement of purpose assumes that the client has had some type of initial intake interview to determine that a short-term approach is needed. In the case of Mr. Collins, the treatment is expected to be short (12 sessions) and is expected to bring about important changes within the client. The approach is focused compared to other approaches, and for this reason it is likely that the purpose of each week's therapy will be stated at the beginning of each interview.

The client's understanding of the interview can also affect the nurse's statement of purpose. If the student and Mr. B have met for 30 minutes once a week for two weeks, and Mr. B understands his role in disclosing life experiences to the student and discussing them, the purpose of the interview need not be repeated. If, however, the nurse is working with a client who is not currently oriented to reality, she must repeat the purpose of the interview at the beginning of the interview in order to provide some sense of security for the client.

If a client is currently not in control of behavior, the nurse tells the client what to do. For example, if the client is hyperventilating, the nurse could tell the client to breathe deeply. In this example the nurse does not state the purpose of the interview, but focuses with the client on intervening. Even in this example, however, a brief statement of purpose could be given. The nurse could state, "Take deep breaths, Ms. C. You can breathe easier that way." In some situations, however, statements of purpose may confuse an anxious client and, indeed, take the focus off the suggested intervention.

The nurse's statement describing the purpose and activities of the interview depends on whether or not it is appropriate to state the expectation of a redirection of the client's life or internal experience as a result of the interview(s). The client has a right to know in what way psychological functioning will be affected by the therapeutic process. If a nurse is working with a client using short-term behavior therapy and the client is experiencing difficulties in controlling angry outbursts, the nurse could say, "Mr. DeLeon, I am Doris Richards, a nurse in the clinic. I will be working with you for eight weeks. The purpose of the work will be to decrease the incidence of your angry outbursts."

Stating the purpose of the interview is an important part of the interview process: it allows the client to know what is occurring and why, and it sets a formal, professional tone for the therapeutic process. Establishing the purpose forms a contract between the client and nurse so that both understand the focus of the interview. It is

professionally irresponsible not to inform the client about the purpose of the interview or to minimize the importance of the interview. The nurse can say, "Talk about what is important to you now," rather than saying, "I just want to talk with you a little bit about. . . ."

Occasionally, however, the purpose of the interview (in terms of changes the client can expect to experience) should not be stated. Examples of such cases include the client who is experiencing severe anxiety and is in a crisis state. In this instance it would be inappropriate to state, "Mr. Evans, as a result of discussion of your panic state you will come to understand the ways to decrease your anxiety and increase your coping skill." In instances of anxiety, the client is unable to understand the meaning of these words and needs direction to decrease the anxiety. The nurse could say, "Mr. Evans, come with me to the quiet room so you can calm down and become comfortable." The nurse may then say a few guiding phrases as she waits for the client to calm down.

Content and Process of the Interview

Psychotherapeutic work demands sensitivity and tact in discussions of issues that are not in the awareness of the client. Sensitivity is needed because some experiences of the client are so anxiety-provoking that they are not understood by the client and are kept out of the client's awareness.

The nurse understands what is not in the awareness of the client by using a conceptual framework in working with clients. For example, in the Self/Other/Relationship framework it is assumed that the Self has no meaning as an entity unto itself, but that it is interwoven with and affected by Others. A particular client may state that he has never had a friend and deny wanting or needing friends, but cry when saying this. The clinician could determine that there are problems in the bonding or attachment patterns of the Self with Other(s). The clinician would assume that this is true *because of the conceptual framework that provides a tool to understand the Self, not because the client states that he has problems in interpersonal relationships.*

The nurse must attend to two aspects of client behavior: the *content* (what has been said) and the *process* (what has not been said). The observable verbal and nonverbal behaviors of the client are the content of an interview. The client states that he has never had a friend and denies the need for a friend. This is the content of at least part of the interview. The tears of the client are also content, since they are observable.

The *process* of the interview is defined as the true meaning of an experience of a client that is not openly discussed. For example, the client is *not* stating: "I have never had a friend; I find it difficult to acknowledge that I need a friend; and I am crying because it saddens me to know that I have never had a friend." The client may not make such statements, because of fear of the nurse's reaction and confusion about his needs and feelings.

The nurse makes an interpretive leap here in stating

that the client has difficulties in Self/Other bonding or attachment. The nurse helps the client to understand by indicating where his difficulties lie (Self/Other/Bonding or Attachment concern, for example). The clinician then describes these concerns as problems requiring therapeutic work.

The nurse communicates problems to the client in a way that the client can accept. Therapeutic skill involves working with the client on problem areas that the client does not fully understand in a way that acknowledges the client's values and well-being.

Clients are likely to react negatively to authoritarian statements about what the nurse "sees as the real problem." Part of the skill in interviewing is to keep process comments within the range of the client's understanding. If authoritarian statements are made, the client will sense that the clinician is cold or distant and does not understand him or her.

The client and the nurse may disagree about the problem areas. For example, in defining problems for discussion in therapeutic work, the nurse may state that the client has difficulty establishing interpersonal relationships. The client may disagree. An appropriate response for the clinician would be, "I would like to keep in mind the possibility that interpersonal relationships are a concern." The client will usually agree to keeping interpersonal relationship concerns at least on a secondary problem list. The nurse can then explain how the conclusion was reached.

Language in the Interview

In psychotherapeutic interviewing the verbal exchanges have a primary importance. Peplau[20] considered words to be powerful instruments of change. "The language used by the therapist can have corrective impact on the language behavior of patients, which *then sets into motion subsequent changes in thought, actions, and feelings.*" The nurse's consistent use of language facilitates changes in the client's thoughts. The nurse needs to use language carefully, while continuing to listen to what the client is saying.

While there is no guarantee that using or avoiding specific words will bring about changes, the following list provides a few guidelines for the nurse's language use.

1. Present only one task for the client to consider at a time.

2. When using a yes/no question, be aware of whether you really want only a yes/no answer. A yes/no response is not conducive to further exploration and may seem to close discussion of the topic.

3. Be careful when using incorporative language (such as "we") with certain clients. If a client has problems with psychological boundaries, use the pronouns "you" and "I" to assist in differentiating the nurse from the client.

4. Avoid taking a position of authority with the client by ordering the client to do something, giving the cli-

ent permission to do something, or speaking for the client.

5. Be aware of "helpless" behavior of some clients. If a client says, for example, "I can't think of anything," the nurse should say, "Take your time and try."

6. Avoid the language of blame and criticism. This may be difficult when the nurse wants to agree that, for instance, the client's parents are "bad" people. Instead, look for the part that the client played in exchanges with the parents, and examine where change can occur.

Distortions of thoughts are evidenced by the language of the client. The goal in working with the client's language is to have the client use words that are easily understood by others. The following is a list of difficulties frequently found in the language of clients[21]:

Overgeneralization. The client may state, for example, "Everything happens to me." The nurse can reply: "Talk about one thing that has happened to you."

Erroneous Labeling. The client may state, "My boss is really stupid." This client may have come upon this label with inadequate data. The comment also exemplifies the client's tendency to label phenomena in the extreme: good or bad. The clinician, in this example, could say, "Describe an example."

Standardized Phrases. At times a client may use a word or phrase repeatedly, such as "That's fine." In this example the nurse could say, "What is fine?" or "You use the phrase 'That's fine.' When did you first start using it?" The client may not be able to remember when it was first used, but the nurse has opened a way for discussion of stereotyped phrasing. With such phrasing it is difficult to know the client's true response.

Focusing on the Nonactual. Peplau identified five subtypes of this category of client response.

1. Focusing on the future rather than discussing current concerns of the client. To assist the client in maintaining a focus on the present, the nurse could say, "Talk about one time that you were. . . ."

2. "If I were only. . . ." statements. The client talks about wishes rather than reality, as in the statement, "If only it was different." The nurse could ask, "In what way do you want it to be different?"

3. "Always or never" statements concerning the client's behavior. For example, the client may say, "I want to feel like I'm always in control." The nurse could say, "Talk about one time when you were not in control."

4. "Shoulds" or "oughts." When using these terms the client often uses self-blame or sets impossible goals. The nurse could say, "Who told you that you should do . . .?"

5. Doubts. The client may say, "I don't know" or "Maybe." The nurse could say, "Take your time and think about whether or not you. . . ."

Inadequate Cause–Effect Relations. The client may say, "My sister and the bulletin board over there." The nurse may not understand any relationship between the client's sister and the bulletin board. A problem arises when the client does not have the intellectual competency to tell the nurse the relationship between the sister and the bulletin board. However, the nurse can help the client to talk about what is probably a significant interpersonal relationship: the client's relationship with the sister.

Concreteness. When asked how she usually spends her time a client may say, "I don't spend it, I save it." The nurse could then say in a different way, "Talk about a typical day in your life."

Circumstantiality. The client does not talk directly about a concern. For example, a client may give many irrelevant details about an abusive parent. The nurse could say, "Before you go on, say some more about. . . ." The nurse can refocus the client's discussion onto more important aspects of a topic.

The Frequency and Setting

Frequency

The frequency of nurse–client interviews depends on a number of factors, including the following:

1. Whether or not the client is experiencing a crisis. If the client is in crisis, the sessions will be more frequent.
2. The period of time needed for the client to digest what occurs in the sessions. For example, some nurses in an outpatient setting prefer to see clients on a weekly basis to allow the client time to understand what has been discussed. A weekly schedule may be kept, however, simply because of routine.
3. The setting. On a locked inpatient unit the nurse may have a number of interviews with the client during the course of a day. On an open psychiatric unit the nurse ideally meets for an hour daily with each assigned client, during which time the nurse conducts individual relationship intervention with clients.

Regular nurse–client interviews have a long tradition in psychiatric/mental health nursing. However, scheduling interviews may be difficult because of inadequate staffing, use of large numbers of staff who are not nurses, and competing programs held on units. With personal motivation and team cooperation, however, this role of the nurse is preserved.

Related to the frequency of sessions is the continuity of the interviewer who conducts the sessions. Ideally, the nurse who assesses the client on admission should continue to work with the client throughout the hospital stay. It is impossible for the nurse to provide consistent interventions without spending repeated times with the client. By conducting repeated interviews, the nurse is able to understand the client's distortions of meaning that need clarification.

The client's daily interview with the psychiatric/mental health nurse should be one of the most important

parts of the client's day. Because the nurse observes the client actually living on the psychiatric unit, the nurse has valid information, gathered in current observation of the client, about the client's difficulties.

The Setting

It is important for the nurse to work with clients in settings that are conducive to psychotherapeutic dialogue. Noise should be minimized so that the interview can remain focused. The room in which the session is held should not distract the client from the psychotherapeutic focus. A medical examination room, because of its aura of sterility, may limit the ability of the client to express feelings.

Nurse–client interviews held in the room where the client sleeps may be adversely affected. Clients who use sexual connotations as a way of avoiding self-examination may be overly stimulated in a room with a bed. Other clients may take the opportunity to lie down, a posture which may not be conducive to client alertness and discussion.

Some clients become anxious when examining their lives and may need to leave the interview room temporarily. The nurse should not block the exit from the room.

When interview rooms are unavailable, a removed corner of a facility room can be used for the interview. It is the responsibility of the nurse to arrange for an appropriate meeting time and place. If there is not an ideal setting for the interview, the nurse makes use of the available facilities to promote the work with the client.

The Description of the Client's Life

In order for a nurse to understand fully an important event in a client's life, the client must first be asked to describe it. The client's detailed description of the event will enable the clinician to understand the client's difficulty in the situation. Without this description the nurse may erroneously attribute actions, thoughts, and feelings to the client, which can result in incorrect diagnoses, treatment plans, and staff attitudes toward the client. *Labels attributed to the client's behavior should be based on the client's description of that behavior.* Clinicians can facilitate client descriptions of actions, thoughts, and feelings by asking consistent questions over time.

The nurse's listening to a detailed description of the client's life is an important way for the nurse and client to get to know each other and to develop trust. The nurse and client participate in a learning process about the client's difficult life experiences. By asking for this information the nurse indicates (nonverbally) to the client, "I want to get to know you, and understand you, and I want you to see that you can trust me by the way I try to help."

The nurse should not badger the client for details nor should the nurse be interested only in obtaining the "facts." Of primary importance is how the client currently experiences the situation. Early in the therapeutic relationship some clients knowingly give incorrect information, but they will usually correct their statements as the relationship becomes more comfortable.

There are some clients who habitually lie to others, *e.g.,* those with an antisocial personality. Usually these clients are not treated in mental health care facilities because of their difficulty in interacting with other clients.

When the client is describing difficult experiences, positive and productive client interviews can be facilitated if the nurse guides the client first to describe actions, then to express thoughts about the experience, and finally to describe feelings about it.

When the description is sufficiently detailed the client can actually seem to relive the experience during the session. By reliving the experience with the client, the nurse can acknowledge that the thoughts and feelings of the client are appropriate to the circumstance. *Validation* is the process of acknowledging that the client's behavior is appropriate.

Many clients confuse thoughts and feelings. They mention no feeling, for example, when they describe a horrible situation. Without obtaining a detailed description of what actually happened, the nurse might easily validate that the situation was insignificant because the client does not express feelings about it. This would be a distortion on the part of the nurse due to inadequate data-gathering.

The opportunity for the client to experience emotions associated with significant experiences is a necessary part of the therapeutic relationship. Emotions are then "released," with a subsequent easing of tension. Typically, clients find it easier to identify emotions once they have described the situation in which the feelings occurred. The components of an adequate client description of an experience are found in the following box.

Interpretations

An interpretation is a summary statement, made by the clinician, of the meaning of the experiences of the client. The interpretation may pertain to one or more of the following phenomena:

1. *The meaning of the past as it relates to the present.* An example of an interpretive statement made to the client is: "In the past, Mr. Allison, you said that your relationship with your wife provided much security. Now that she is gone you wonder what the source of your security will be."
2. *The meaning of the present.* Example: "Mr. Allison, you seem to be avoiding sharing your feelings with the group."
3. *Inconsistencies in the components of behavior (actions, thoughts, and feelings).* Example: "Mr. Allison, you are describing a very sad time with the loss of your wife, yet you are laughing. Would you take a moment to examine your true experience?"
4. *The avoidance of one or more components of behavior (actions, thoughts, and feelings).* Example: "Mr.

COMPONENTS OF CLIENT'S DESCRIPTION OF AN EXPERIENCE

The client's description of an experience or event should include:

Who — Which individuals were present during the significant experience?

What — Exactly what was said by all parties? Obtain the client's best memory of the event. What was done by all of the individuals?

When — When did the experience happen?

Where — At what location did the experience occur?

Why — Although direct "why" questions can be challenging or threatening to the client, to what reasons can the client attribute the occurrence of the client's or other's behavior?

Effect — What was the effect (such as thoughts or feelings) of the experience on the client?

Result — What is the current status of Self and Others as a result of the experience? Are there unresolved thoughts or feelings as a result of the experience?

Allison, you have said that you cannot describe what happened the day your wife left. Please pause a moment and think about that day again. When did you usually wake up in the morning?" Here the avoidance of a description of an experience indicates at least an avoidance of a thought(s). Feelings may also be avoided, but this avoidance is difficult to validate without the description of the experience (actions) and the client's thoughts about the experience stated first.

The technique of interpretation has its roots in classical psychoanalysis,[17] in which interpretation is the process of making conscious the unconscious roots of the client's observable (surface) behavior. The use of an interpretation involves a loosening of the client's typical defenses. In the past the client has denied the true nature of the roots of current problems, and the use of an interpretation helps the client to get over the barriers of the defenses.

In classical, as well as more recent, theories of psychotherapeutic intervention, interpretation is widely used. The psychiatric/mental health nurse, operating within the appropriate context of individual relationship interventions, uses interpretations that can easily be understood by the client.

Timing is an important aspect of interpretation. If the client is not ready to hear the content of the interpretation, it may appear that the nurse is not paying attention to the state of the client. The nurse may seem to be pushing the client, and may appear to be nonempathic.

The interpretation must be succinct and accurate. If not, the nurse may appear to have "easy" or simplistic answers to the client's painful and important issues. To achieve high quality of interpretations, nurses should maintain their own personal growth in order to understand the nature of what clients present, discuss clients with peers, and remain students of human nature.

Barriers to the Interview Process

Client Behaviors and Nursing Interventions

Through the decades of working with clients, psychiatric/mental health nurses have identified and elaborated on certain client behaviors that facilitate or hinder the client's progression in psychotherapeutic work. Several of these concepts will now be reviewed, and interventions suggested.

Distortions of Meaning. Sullivan[29] wrote extensively about the development of distortions in the client's understanding of the meaning of events. Freud also developed a related concept of "transference." These will be discussed in more detail in Chapter 6.

Sullivan described distortions of meaning as a process wherein:

1. A situation occurs in which the client is a participant. For example, a wife is beaten by her husband.
2. The situation threatens the individual psychologically. The wife fears that her husband does not love her.
3. Because the client is threatened, the client becomes anxious.[22] The wife may say she is nervous.
4. Anxiety prevents the client from understanding the meaning of what is occurring in the situation. The client attributes a *distorted* understanding to the event. If a person is jogging and attempts to read a sign, the sign will appear blurred. The sign will also be blurred in the jogger's memory. Similarly, as the client attempts to remember the nature (or the meaning) of a past traumatic event, the meaning will be blurred because of the anxiety experienced during the event. The wife, for example, may search for a cause of her beating and believe erroneously that she deserved the beating.
5. Because of anxious feeling and distorted thoughts, the client behaves in ways that do not support well-being. A wife, for example, remains with her husband although he beats her.
6. If a situation in the present is similar to a traumatic event in the past, clients tend to repeat previous ineffective behavior. One reason clients seek help is to overcome this behavioral pattern. The battered wife will continue to remain with her husband despite the fact that he beats her.

Nursing Interventions.

1. Ask the client to give a detailed description of the situation. In addition to providing the nurse with the necessary information, describing an event may help the client take a more objective view of its significance.
2. Listen for distortion of meaning by applying the Self/Other/Relationship framework.
3. Assist the client to clarify the meaning of the event. With a client who claims to have no feelings about the departure of his spouse, despite being admitted to the hospital for suicidal behavior, the nurse might use the following approach: "Mr. Malone, you have described a situation in which your wife of 20 years, whom you loved very much, suddenly left home. How do you think any individual would feel in this situation?" This approach attempts to "place" the client outside his own circumstance so that he can take an objective view of the situation.
4. Label new meanings for the client when necessary. In the example above, if the client had not been able to identify his feeling the nurse could have said, "Mr. Malone, I wonder if you were depressed after you found out that your wife left." In this example, the nurse could have chosen the label "angry" if she had sensed that the client's primary response was anger. By labeling, the nurse can assist the client to regain the ability to identify feelings about past experiences.
5. Discuss repeating patterns of distortion with the client. The nurse can clearly view the development and nature of current experiences in the client's life by personal observation. When there is good rapport between client and nurse, the client may participate in a useful, but perhaps painful, review of distortions occurring in the present.

Severe Distortions of Meaning by the Client. The nurse intervenes in severe distortions of meaning by using an interviewing technique called *decoding*. Decoding is a psychotherapeutic technique whereby the nurse states an understanding of a client's distorted words or actions in terms that can be understood by both nurse and client.

For example, a client may say frequently, "I am the king of the world." The nurse can first state, "I do not understand. What do you mean when you say that you are the king of the world?" The client may not respond with a message that can be understood, however. The nurse can then make an interpretation of what the client is talking about. The nurse might say, "I want to understand what you are talking about. Are you saying that you would feel better about yourself if you were the king of the world?" or "Do you think your statement about being the king of the world relates to your poor sense of self-esteem?" The nurse would then wait for a response.

In decoding it is important to remember that the first intervention is to have the client edit the speech so that it becomes understandable to others. If the client cannot do this, the nurse then makes a statement about a possible meaning of the distorted language. An interpretation that is too far removed from the obvious, however, may make the client believe that the nurse is distancing herself or himself from the client, and does not care about the client. If an interpretation is too far removed, clients may respond with greater confusion.

Distortions of Meaning by the Nurse. Distortions of meaning can occur within psychiatric/mental health nurses, just as they do within clients. Nurses' distortions are responses to clients in the form of thoughts and feelings that reflect nurses' own experiences rather than the Truth of the clients. The development of distortions of meaning within nurses occurs in the same way that it does within clients. Distortions can prevent nurses from becoming aware of the Truth of the Other of clients.

For nurses to grow, they must be able to identify their own distortions of meaning and act to clarify them. Because nurses understand the process of identifying and resolving distortions, this process should take place within a short period of time, usually during the meeting with the client. If the nurse cannot clarify the distortion during the session with the client, the clarification should take place before the next session or the nurse should discuss the interview with a professional peer in order to attain clarity.

Distortions on the part of the nurse are not unusual or wrong. The important element is that the nurse is aware of the experience of the distortion; clarifies the distortion; uses the clarification to aid in understanding the client; and then relates differently to the client. The following example demonstrates the process of the nurse using his own distortions to help promote the well-being of the client.

The nurse sees Mr. Stevens in daily hour-long sessions while the client is hospitalized on an inpatient psychiatric unit. During the second session, Mr. Stevens leaves the interview room and does not return. The nurse, Jeff Howard, sits for a few minutes, thinks that Mr. Stevens is inadequate and a coward for leaving, and himself leaves the interview room. Jeff ignores Mr. Stevens for the rest of the day.

After the nurse leaves the hospital and goes home, he thinks about Mr. Stevens. He also dreams about the client. The dream consists of a large, menacing figure telling Jeff that he is inadequate and ineffective.

When the nurse awakes he thinks about the dream. He also associates his feeling of inadequacy in the dream with how he felt after Mr. Stevens walked out of the session. He also thinks about the feeling of loss he had when the client left the session. The nurse knows that he is competent because he has received positive feedback from his peers and other clients.

Jeff then realizes that the client's exit from the session reminded him of an experience he had when he failed at doing something that he wanted to do effectively. He now understands that everyone fails at times, and everyone feels ineffective at times. Also, everyone has experienced the loss of someone who was important to them, as in the sense of abandonment when Mr. Stevens left the session.

The nurse understood that the client was important

to him as a person and was worthy of his respect, and Jeff genuinely wanted to help Mr. Stevens. The nurse knew that he did not have to think of Mr. Stevens as someone who was abandoning him because Jeff did something wrong. This is the distortion on the part of the nurse.

The nurse approached Mr. Stevens the next day to begin the session. He started by asking the client to describe what had been going on that prompted the client to leave the session. Jeff did this with the attitude of wanting to understand, and to support the development of the client, not to tell Mr. Stevens that he was wrong for leaving the session or to express his anger.

Jeff also explained that it is important for Mr. Stevens to attend the session so that the client can use that time to clarify what is occurring. Mr. Stevens cast doubt on the nurse's statement, saying, "No one cares what anyone else says." The nurse and client then discussed the client's experiences of not having others who care about him. After this session the rapport between the nurse and client improved, and the client shared his concerns.

In this example, *the client shared his true concerns because the nurse understood his own behavior (his thoughts that he was ineffective and his feelings of being inadequate).* In this example, the nurse did not ignore his feelings, but rather *used his feelings to understand what was occurring with the client.* The nurse asked about the client's avoidance of the session because he had a thinking and feeling response to the client. Because the nurse asked, the client talked about his true concern: not having others who care about him.

Resistance. *Resistance* is the process wherein the client avoids the Truth about Self or Other, or the Relationship of Self or Other. Resistance can take many forms, such as

Not coming for a scheduled psychotherapeutic interview with the nurse
Silence
Statements to the effect that the nurse is the "one with the problem"
Talking about unimportant topics
Forgetting to follow some part of the mutually agreed upon treatment plan
Seductive behavior toward the nurse

Resistance occurs because the awareness of Truth may be painful. It may be very uncomfortable for a client to acknowledge, for example, that his wife has permanently left him. Human beings cannot simply withstand all painful events. Human beings show enormous strength to withstand struggle *and* a vulnerability at times to pain. There are no simple methods to determine when the client is ready to assume increasing "amounts" of Truth.

Resistance may also occur because of inertia, in which the client adheres to old familiar patterns of behavior. This can occur even when the old patterns are dysfunctional. Some individuals do not understand the process of change, wherein they can take control of their lives and subsequently increase the sense of well-being.

Others do not know the experience of joy in living and expect a life of depression. Resistance can also occur because clients do not have the necessary skills for increasing their sense of well-being.

Resistance may be more common when the client experiences anxiety in the interview with the nurse. The client may fear the reaction of the nurse to the Truth of the client, and may then resist because of the experience of anxiety. The nurse can assist the client to understand this anxiety.

Nursing Interventions.

1. Facilitate a trusting relationship. When the client trusts the therapist there is less need for resistance.
2. Discuss the client's pattern of resistance. The client can provide the nurse with answers to questions that will help to clarify the reasons for resistance, e.g., When does it occur? What is the client experiencing at the time? What does the client feel might happen if the resistance behaviors aren't used? Is the nurse somehow encouraging the resistance? What behaviors could the client use other than resistance?

It may take repeated reviews with the client before the nurse perceives any change in the resistance pattern.

Cultural Impact on the Therapeutic Process

Culture can be defined as the values, customs, ideas, and habits of a group of people. There is virtually no area of the psychotherapeutic process that is not affected by the cultural background of the client and nurse. If the cultural norms of nurse and client are substantially different, they will have difficulty achieving an empathic relationship. On the other hand, if the client and nurse have a very similar cultural background, the therapeutic experience may be based on too narrow a perspective; the client may not learn to deal with issues that lie outside their shared cultural norm.

Nurses must be conscious of their own potential for distorting client experiences that lie outside their cultural backgrounds. Brantley[7] described a process of anti-black racism that can occur in the psychotherapeutic process. Brantley described this racism as the formation of decisions, policies, and behavior on considerations of race for the purpose of maintaining power over a particular group. Racism may be overt or covert, conscious or unconscious, and committed by an individual or by a group.

In the psychotherapeutic process racism can occur through the nurse's inability to empathize with or relate to the experiences of a client with a different ethnic background, or through the nurse's inability to discuss racism toward the client occurring inside the nurse. The results of such racism may include the client's termination from treatment, a decreased sense of hope in the client, and a sense in the client that personal destiny cannot be controlled.

Brantley[7] suggested the following interventions to use in cases in which racism occurs:

1. Assist the client to explore coping mechanisms and to develop more productive ways of dealing with the anxiety triggered by racism.
2. Encourage the client to voice frustrations experienced as a result of racism.
3. Do not minimize racial issues in therapy, but explore these topics in terms of the impact on the client's psychological functioning.

The *meaning* attributed to psychological complaints is another important area of the relationship between culture and therapy. In a study of Caucasian American and Hong Kong Chinese students at the University of Hawaii, White[33] examined the meaning attributed to illness by these two groups. White asked 15 students in each group to read a list of psychosocial problems and then to describe "what it would be like to have the problem" and "what might cause such a problem." The problem list included phenomena such as "crying for no apparent reason" and "feeling guilty." The research found that the American students inferred a psychological reason for complaints, while the Chinese students more often described situational pressures or academic concerns as causes of problems.

These explanations are described by White as "culturally-specific."[33] The Americans in the study were individual-centered; the Chinese were situation-centered. Such cultural contrasts in the interpretation of complaints raise important problems for the diagnosis and treatment of psychological concerns in Chinese individuals. The Chinese minimization of what is psychological (emotions, for instance) would be seen in Western psychotherapeutic thinking as denial. Yet, because of the common Chinese explanation of complaints as nonpsychological, the inference of denial may be "unnecessary, untestable, or both."[33]

Activity versus passivity on the part of the nurse is another area in which cultural differences between client and clinician are demonstrated. Uzoka[32] studied the differences between active and passive therapists in individual therapy with Nigerian clients. Most clinicians in the study were trained in the West, where inactivity on the part of the clinician is encouraged.

In the study, 28 Nigerian students and staff members were assigned to work in therapy with either an active therapist (highly verbal and directive) or a passive therapist (minimally verbal or directive). Results indicated that subjects in a group in which the therapist was active demonstrated greater verbalization, attended more therapy sessions, and demonstrated greater self-disclosure than did subjects working with a passive therapist.

In traditional African therapy the therapist (the native doctor) does most of the verbalization. It is thought that subjects in the study who worked with an active clinician demonstrated greater self-disclosure (as well as other behaviors) because the active Western clinician more closely resembled the African therapist. Typical *passive* clinicians would have to change their techniques (and become more active) in order to treat effectively at least some African clients. This study demonstrated the need to adapt one's behavior at times to meet the needs of the client.

Understanding Behavior

Behavior is composed of thoughts, emotions (feelings), and actions (including speech). All psychotherapeutic intervention deals with one or more of these aspects of behavior. The American Nurses' Association has classified the range of human emotional responses, as shown in the list below.

Thoughts are internal cognitions that cannot be directly observed but are inferred from what the client says.

Emotions (feelings) consist of affect and mood. *Affect* is the outward display of internal emotion, such as a facial expression. *Mood* is the internal, felt aspect of emotion. For example, a frown may be the outward display of the internal mood of irritation.

Mood cannot be observed, but it can be identified by asking clients how they feel. Clients may say, for example, that they are depressed or elated. Mood can also be assessed from clients' actions. For example, while partici-

pating with others in a game, a client taps one hand on the table and glares at someone who is delaying the game. The client's eyes widen and the body stiffens. The nurse can surmise that the mood of the client is anger.

Some clients cannot differentiate between thoughts and feelings. If asked, "What did you think about your wife leaving you?" a client may respond, "She just did it." This response does not answer the nurse's question, and indicates that the client cannot communicate what he thinks about his wife leaving him. A more appropriate response to the question would have been, "I think she should have stayed at least long enough to discuss the problems."

Feelings are internal sensations of emotion such as joy, happiness, sadness, anger, lust, frustration, irritation, and loneliness. Clients commonly label a thought when they are asked to label a feeling. For example, when asked to state his feelings about his wife's leaving, the client said, "She's a traitor." The client stated his perception of the meaning of the wife's departure rather than his feelings. A more appropriate reply would have been, "I felt enraged."

Biological Aspects of Emotion

The neuropsychology of emotion has been studied in recent years. Investigators have sought to understand the link between the central nervous system and affect. Rime and Giovannini[27] reported on the physiological patterns of reported emotional states. They asked 689 adults in seven European countries to describe four emotional experiences and the physical sensations present during the experiences.

Most subjects reported the presence of some physiological sensation during an affective experience. The reported sensations included: change in temperature, perspiration, increased blood pressure, chest or breathing symptoms, stomach troubles, and muscular reactions. Increased blood pressure and muscular changes were the symptoms most frequently reported. Symptoms associated with positive emotions, such as joy, included a pleasant feeling of arousal, warm temperature, and increased blood pressure.

Other authors have described the relationship of cognition and affect as they occur in the central nervous system. Izard[14] stated one possible description of the relationship between affect and cognition as follows: individuals have values that they hold as important; when they find themselves in particular situations they compare their expectations of what should occur in a situation with their cultural values. For example, most southern Europeans (such as Italians) expect a more active or obvious expression of emotional joy in their peers than do most northern Europeans (such as those from Great Britain).

Individuals experience certain physiological responses depending on their values. The physiological responses are mediated by the autonomic nervous system. Individuals perceive physiological reactions and label

---

EMOTIONAL HUMAN RESPONSE PATTERNS IDENTIFIED BY THE AMERICAN NURSES' ASSOCIATION

30.01   Impaired emotional experience
   30.01.01   Anger/rage
   30.01.02   Anxiety
   30.01.03   Disgust/contempt
   30.01.04   Distress/anguish
   30.01.05   Envy/jealousy
   30.01.06   Fear
   30.01.07   Grief
   30.01.08   Guilt
   30.01.09   Helplessness
   30.01.10   Hopelessness
   30.01.11   Joy/elation/happiness
   30.01.12   Loneliness
   30.01.13   Sadness
   30.01.14   Shame/humiliation
   30.01.15   Surprise/startle

American Nurses' Association: Taxonomy for the Classification of Human Responses of Concern for Psychiatric/Mental Health Nursing Practice (Working Draft). Kansas City, American Nurses' Association, 1986

them as certain types of emotion (joy, anger, sadness, or fear). People vary in their thresholds for visceral perception, which may account for pathological development of affective responses. Also, differences in sympathetic–parasympathetic balance may be a source of differences in temperament among individuals.

Heilman and Satz[13] summarized much of the work done in the field of the neurological relationship to emotion. Their assumption was that all emotional behavior is influenced by neurological processes. Without critical neurological mechanisms, emotions would not occur.

Heilman and Satz stated that emotions have three components: a subjective feeling, observable behaviors (for example, the facial expression that accompanies the sensation of a feeling), and physiological changes. The authors focused on physiological changes. Their findings came from different types of studies. Some concerned brain lesions that alter behavior, using brain-injured clients as subjects. Other studies considered the findings from experimental animal research and from research with "normal" human subjects.

In studies[14] of normal subjects, stimuli were shown first to the subjects' left visual field and then to the right visual field. Neurologists then determined which brain hemisphere processed certain types of stimuli. It was found that emotional stimuli were perceived more accurately when presented to the right brain hemisphere. The right hemisphere has a special and dominant influence on the reception and expression of emotions. People with right-hemisphere brain damage cannot understand emotional expressions of others. They also have problems making emotional faces and have decreased emotional arousal responses.

Further evidence linking particular neurological patterns with specific emotional responses is seen in clients with basal ganglia disorders. Some clients with these disorders have emotional changes, such as depression, that are thought to be related to neurotransmitter disturbances such as monoamine metabolism difficulties.

Theories of Affect

According to Green,[11] Freud viewed affect as a biological phenomenon related to memories and ideas rather than to feelings. He emphasized the negative consequences of affect on thought processes, and believed that we must master affects by thoughts, and confront affects with facts. The following are some of Freud's ideas on affect:

1. Affect is a quantity of energy that accompanies life events. It is similar to the electrical charge of a nervous impulse.

2. When a person's ego is threatened by an extreme amount of negative affect, the person acts to moderate the excess of affect.

3. The ego acts to discharge excess affect by taking some action such as working out in an exercise center. The quantity of affect is divided rather than being entirely attached to traumatic experiences in the cli-

ent's life. For example, a client experiencing extreme anger when abandoned as a child might handle the large amount of energy attached to the anger by shifting some of it to visions of people who look or talk like the child's parents.

Brierly (as described by Green) was the first major writer to recognize affect.[11] She described affect as the ideas an individual has about significant others. The affective development of an individual precedes the individual's recognition of separateness from the mother. Brierly emphasized the relationship between thought and affect, and stated that the astute clinician is capable of both intellectual insight and affective understanding.

Carl Rogers[16,28] wrote extensively about the importance of affect and mood in a client's psychological experience. Rogers advocated a counseling relationship that includes warmth and responsiveness on the part of the therapist, a permissive climate in which the client can easily express feelings, and freedom from coercion and pressure by the therapist. Clinicians using Rogers's approach respond to the client's affect. The clinician is then required to "get behind the words of the client and into his feeling world to obtain an accurate empathic understanding."[28]

Tomkins,[31] whose work began in the 1950s, was the first contemporary psychologist to view emotions as a person's primary motivational system. From studies of the expression of emotion, Tomkins derived nine primary affect types: interest, enjoyment, surprise, fear, anger, distress, shame, contempt, and disgust.

Aylwin[3] also described a "cognitive" view of affect. She saw cognitions (or thinking) from the standpoint of "representations" that are used in the thought process. The different types of representations are *inner speech* or verbal representations, *visual imagery* or mental pictures, and *imagery* or an imagined role play.

Aylwin elaborated that each type of representation or cognitive style is associated with particular affects. Individuals have a unique preference for a cognitive style(s) and associated affects. For example, an individual who has a cognitive style of imagined role play may experience the affects of fear, anxiety, and joy, because these affects are found in conjunction with *action* (which occurs in the imagined role playing).

The Definition of Affect: A Synthesis

The various views of affect have been discussed, but the search continues for a succinct definition. Denzin[8] has written one of the best reviews of the major writers on affect. He quotes Stanislavski's definition of affect (termed "emotion" in Stanislavski's work): Emotion is a lived, believed-in, temporary body experience that permeates a person's consciousness. In the process of being experienced, the emotion plunges the person into a new reality—the reality changed by the emotional experience. Because emotion is also a unique world solely contained within itself, it is a *self-feeling*.

The components of this definition worth emphasizing are:

1. Emotion is sensed or felt by the individual experiencing the emotion.
2. The individual believes in the presence of the emotion. It is understood to be present even if the individual is not able to state the nature of the emotion.
3. The emotion is temporary. For psychiatric clients, however, there is more to be said about the temporary nature of emotions or affect. Schizophrenic clients may have experienced the negative emotional effects of criticism and intrusiveness (overinvolvement) from family members long before actually demonstrating the signs and symptoms of the disorder. The clients *repeatedly* experienced negative emotions within themselves; the emotions were not temporary. The individuals then adjusted to repeated negative internal emotions by closing themselves off emotionally, developing angry, negative personality styles, or adopting other patterns of living that perpetuated this isolation.
4. Emotions are accompanied by a physiological reaction. Individuals may sense their stomachs "turning into knots," for example. These reactions can serve as a signal that emotion is present although, as stated by Aylwin, many individuals are not astute enough to define the experienced emotion.
5. The affect of an individual influences others around the individual. This idea is also in keeping with the systems perspective of this text. The Self of the client as well as the Others around the client (the *social* component) are influenced by affect. For example, an anxious mother may precipitate anxiety in the infant.
6. In addition to having an influence on others, the emotion is also a "self-feeling"; it refers back to the individual feeling it. Denzin echoes the conceptual framework for psychiatric/mental health nursing discussed in this text, particularly the dual nature of part of psychological reality: *both* the self *and* the self's relationships with others constitute the emotional nature of the person.

Clients often exhibit a variety of behaviors in response to their emotions. Behaviors frequently seen in nurse–client interviews are summarized in the following box.

Anxiety: The Core Affect

Anxiety is one of the core phenomena with which the psychiatric nurse works. The Fifth National Conference on Nursing Diagnoses added anxiety to the list of nursing diagnoses.[34] It also strongly recommended that further study be made of the differentiation of anxiety from other emotions, such as fear. The highlighting of anxiety by the conference members follows a rich tradition in the men-

---

COMMON CLIENT BEHAVIORS RESULTING FROM EXPERIENCING EMOTIONS IN NURSE–CLIENT INTERVIEWS

1. Fear of not being accepted
2. Guilt or shame for having feelings
3. Withdrawal
4. Fear of being exposed
5. Fear of a loss of control
6. Fear that once emotions are released, nothing will be left
7. Uncertainty about the result of sharing feelings
8. A positive feeling of unburdening
9. A positive feeling that the client can experience caring from another person (the nurse) when expressing emotions

---

tal health sciences of the study of anxiety. The psychiatric nursing classification scheme of the American Nurses' Association[1] (ANA) lists anxiety as a nursing diagnosis.

Kerr[15] summarized Freud's work in anxiety. Although Freud described the experience of anxiety only minimally, he formulated two theories of anxiety. According to his later theory, anxiety occurs when the ego senses real or potential danger related to the threatened release of one's impulses or separation from significant others. To Freud, anxiety has a physiological rather than a psychological nature.

Sullivan[29] also considered the phenomenon of anxiety through much of his work. He defined anxiety as virtually all basic types of emotional suffering. Anxiety includes anxiousness, guilt, shame, dread, feelings of personal worthlessness, "eerie loathing," and other less definable but still painful feelings.

Although Sullivan's definition is not concise, it points to the diffuse nature of anxiety. To a great extent anxiety is empathized from others in the context of interpersonal relationships. Anxiety is extremely unpleasant, and the individual organizes behavior to avoid anxiety and to maintain a sense of security.

Anxiety is difficult to work with because it does not have an obvious cause. Because of its nonspecific character, anxiety cannot be "willed" away. High levels of anxiety prompt a disorganization within the individual; the person becomes incapable of meeting personal needs and resolving the anxiety-promoting situation.

Yocom[34] compared fear with anxiety. Fear and anxiety are affects and cannot be avoided in life. In fear, the affect of apprehension has a *tangible* quality to it, because the source of the fear is identifiable. An example of the affect of fear would be the emotion experienced when riding a steep roller coaster. Once the threat promoting the fear is removed, the affect of fear disappears.

"The diffuse and undifferentiated quality of anxiety refers to the level in the personality at which the threat is experienced."[34] With anxiety, it is the *core* or *essence* of the individual that has been threatened. Fear does not strike at this core.

As the nurse observes an anxious person, the individual may be restless, unable to sleep, trembling, and preoccupied with self. The person may shuffle the feet, have poor eye contact, or demonstrate extraneous movements, facial tension, a quivering voice, and increased perspiration.

The intensity and duration of anxiety are determined by the individual's perception of the event and coping skills. Many cultural differences in response to anxiety can be noted.

Hallam[12] reported that Mahorney described anxiety from the standpoints of learning theory and biological theory. Learning theory describes a situation in which a stimulus associated with punishment evokes anxiety. When the punishment is removed, the stimulus continues to evoke the anxiety response.

Biological theories of anxiety include the finding that lactate infusion will produce panic attacks in clients who are prone to such attacks, but rarely in those who are not. Also, anxiety attacks can be blocked by monoamine oxidase inhibitors or tricyclic antidepressants, two groups of drugs used in the treatment of mental illness. These drugs are thought to exert their effects through the activity of biogenic amines, especially norepinephrine.

Benzodiazepines are the most popular of the agents used in the treatment of anxiety. These drugs are thought to exert their effects by facilitating the activity of another neurotransmitter, aminobutyric acid. Neurons have specific receptor sites for the benzodiazepines. Because of the difference in responsiveness of the receptor sites, scientists may find biological evidence to suggest a distinction between the various anxiety-related conditions.

Hallam's[12] work on anxiety is notable for its discussion of panic (anxiety) attacks. However, Hallam also made the point that anxiety can be a symbol for the *effects* of interpersonal actions *and* physiological responses. According to Hallam, when clients state that they are anxious, they may be referring to their beliefs, identity, or any number of other aspects of their lives. In keeping with the systems perspective, Hallam described the causes of anxiety as biological, psychological, and sociological.

Hallam also described research findings on the prevalence of anxiety complaints. Anxiety is the fifth most common diagnosis made by general practitioners. Between 4% and 5% of the population is treated for anxiety complaints each year. Complaints of generalized anxiety are the most common, followed by phobias and panic. Only about one fourth of these subjects received mental health care within the previous year. Women are several times more likely than men to complain of anxiety or receive a diagnosis of anxiety. In 1981, one in five British women received prescriptions for the benzodiazepine class of tranquilizers during the course of a year.

In *The Diagnostic and Statistical Manual, III-R (DSM-III-R)*, the American Psychiatric Association[2] lists various disorders related to anxiety. Listed under Anxiety Disorders are Agoraphobia, Social Phobia, Simple Phobia, Panic Disorder, Generalized Anxiety Disorder, Obsessive Compulsive Disorder, and Posttraumatic Stress Disorder. The diagnostic criteria for these disorders are included in Table 5-4.

Nursing Care of Anxiety

Peplau[18] wrote classic works in psychiatric/mental health nursing on the topic of anxiety. She stated that anxiety is an energy that is related to cultural or social needs. Since it is an energy, it cannot be studied directly; it "must be studied through its transformation into effects on behaviors." By observing clients the nurse can note both the presence of anxiety and the intensity of the anxiety.

Peplau wrote primarily for the nurse working directly with clients using a verbal approach. She focused on clients experiencing momentary anxiety *not* necessarily of the nature of a formal Anxiety Disorder as defined in the DSM-III-R. Because anxiety is experienced by many psychiatric/mental health clients regardless of medical diagnosis, this focus is appropriate. Peplau delineated the degrees of anxiety as follows:

1. *Mild Anxiety.* The person is alert and the use of senses is increased. Motor behavior is enlivened and the person is more interested in what is going on.

2. *Moderate Anxiety.* At this level of anxiety the perceptual field is reduced. Other effects may be present, such as muscular tension. The person sees and hears less. As at the mild level of anxiety, the motor behavior of the person is more active. At both mild and moderate levels of anxiety the person is still in control, and is capable of learning.

3. *Severe Anxiety.* With severe anxiety the perceptual field is reduced to a very small proportion; whole perceptual events are not noticed. Peplau reports that in some instances the focus may be on scattered details. While there is a heightened awareness, it is ineffective because it is focused on only a small portion of the perceptual field. Connections between details may be distorted.

   Motor behavior is less organized in the person with severe anxiety than it is at the previous two levels. The client may, for example, exhibit restless motor behavior that lacks purpose.

4. *Panic.* Panic is seen in many psychiatric clients, not only in those with the medical diagnosis of a Panic Disorder. In experiences of panic the individual perceives only the smallest detail and loses control. The person senses terror and may magnify a detail (such as an insignificant object in the room) beyond proportion in order to sense some control. As with severe anxiety, the connections of meaning between details is distorted. It is an intensely uncomfortable experience; some clients describe it as if their very selves were disintegrating.

Peplau delineated the steps in the development of anxiety as follows:

(Text continues on p. 96.)

TABLE 5-4.
ANXIETY DISORDERS (PSYCHIATRIC)

DIAGNOSTIC CRITERIA FOR PANIC DISORDER

A. At some time during the disturbance, one or more panic attacks (discrete periods of intense fear or discomfort) have occurred that were (1) unexpected, *i.e.*, did not occur immediately before or on exposure to a situation that almost always caused anxiety, and (2) not triggered by situations in which the person was the focus of others' attention.

B. Either four attacks, as defined in criterion A, have occurred within a four-week period, or one or more attacks have been followed by a period of at least a month of persistent fear of having another attack.

C. At least four of the following symptoms developed during at least one of the attacks:
    1. Shortness of breath (dyspnea) or smothering sensations
    2. Dizziness, unsteady feelings, or faintness
    3. Palpitations or accelerated heart rate (tachycardia)
    4. Trembling or shaking
    5. Sweating
    6. Choking
    7. Nausea or abdominal distress
    8. Depersonalization or derealization
    9. Numbness or tingling sensations (paresthesias)
    10. Flushes (hot flashes) or chills
    11. Chest pain or discomfort
    12. Fear of dying
    13. Fear of going crazy or of doing something uncontrolled
    Note: Attacks involving four or more symptoms are panic attacks; attacks involving fewer than four symptoms are limited-symptom attacks.

D. During at least some of the attacks, at least four of C symptoms developed suddenly and increased in intensity within ten minutes of the beginning of the first C symptom noticed in the attack.

E. It cannot be established that an organic factor initiated and maintained the disturbance, *e.g.*, Amphetamine or Caffeine Intoxication, hyperthyroidism.
    Note: Mitral valve prolapse may be an associated condition, but does not preclude a diagnosis of Panic Disorder.

DIAGNOSTIC CRITERIA FOR 300.21 PANIC DISORDER WITH AGORAPHOBIA

A. Meets the criteria for Panic Disorder

B. *Agoraphobia:* Fear of being in places or situations from which escape might be difficult (or embarrassing) or in which help might not be available in the event of a panic attack. (Include cases in which persistent avoidance behavior originated during an active phase of Panic Disorder, even if the person does not attribute the avoidance behavior to fear of having a panic attack.) As a result of this fear, the person either restricts travel or needs a companion when away from home, or else endures agoraphobic situations despite intense anxiety. Common agoraphobic situations include being outside the home alone, being in a crowd or standing in a line, being on a bridge, and traveling in a bus, train, or car.
    Specify current severity of agoraphobic avoidance:
    Mild: Some avoidance (or endurance with distress), but relatively normal lifestyle, *e.g.*, travels unaccompanied when necessary, such as to work or to shop; otherwise avoids traveling alone.
    Moderate: Avoidance results in constricted lifestyle, *e.g.*, the person is able to leave the house alone, but not to go more than a few miles unaccompanied.
    Severe: Avoidance results in being nearly or completely housebound or unable to leave the house unaccompanied.
    In Partial Remission: No current agoraphobic avoidance, but some Agoraphobic avoidance during the past six months.
    In Full Remission: No current agoraphobic avoidance and none during the past six months.
    Specify current severity of panic attacks:
    Mild: During the past month, either all attacks have been limited-symptom attacks (*i.e.*, fewer than four symptoms), or there has been no more than one panic attack.
    Moderate: During the past month, attacks have been intermediate, between "mild" and "severe."
    Severe: During the past month, there have been at least eight panic attacks.
    In Partial Remission: The condition has been intermediate, between "In Full Remission" and "Mild."
    In Full Remission: During the past six months, there have been no panic or limited-symptom attacks.

DIAGNOSTIC CRITERIA FOR 300.23 SOCIAL PHOBIA

A. A persistent fear of one or more situations (the social phobic situations) in which the person is exposed to possible scrutiny by others and fears that he or she may do something or act in a way that will be humiliating or embarrassing. Examples include: being unable to continue talking while speaking in public, choking on food when eating in front of others, being unable to urinate in a public lavatory, hand-trembling when writing in the presence of others, and saying foolish things or not being able to answer questions in social situations.

B. If another disorder is present, the fear in A is unrelated to it, *e.g.*, the fear is not of having a panic attack (Panic Disorder), stuttering (Stuttering), trembling (Parkinson's disease), or exhibiting abnormal eating behavior (Anorexia Nervosa or Bulimia Nervosa).

C. During some phase of the disturbance, exposure to the specific phobic stimulus (or stimuli) almost invariably provokes an immediate anxiety response.

(Continued)

TABLE 5-4. (CONTINUED)

DIAGNOSTIC CRITERIA FOR 300.23 SOCIAL PHOBIA

D. The phobic situation(s) is avoided, or is endured with intense anxiety.
E. The avoidant behavior interferes with occupational functioning or with usual social activities or relationships with others, or there is marked distress about having the fear.
F. The person recognizes that his or her fear is excessive or unreasonable.
G. If the person is under 18, the disturbance does not meet the criteria for Avoidant Disorder of Childhood or Adolescence.
   Specify generalized type if the phobic situation includes most social situations, and also consider the additional diagnosis of Avoidant Personality Disorder.

DIAGNOSTIC CRITERIA FOR 300.29 SIMPLE PHOBIA

A. A persistent fear of a circumscribed stimulus (object or situation) other than fear of having a panic attack (as in Panic Disorder) or of humiliation or embarrassment in certain social situations (as in Social Phobia).
   Note: Do not include fears that are part of Panic Disorder with Agoraphobia or Agoraphobia Without History of Panic Disorder.
B. During some phase of the disturbance, exposure to the specific phobic stimulus (or stimuli) almost invariably provokes an immediate anxiety response.
C. The object or situation is avoided, or endured with intense anxiety.
D. The fear or the avoidant behavior significantly interferes with the person's normal routine or with usual social activities or relationships with others, or there is marked distress about having the fear.
E. The person recognizes that his or her fear is excessive or unreasonable.
F. The phobic stimulus is unrelated to the content of the obsessions of Obsessive Compulsive Disorder or the trauma of Posttraumatic Stress Disorder.

DIAGNOSTIC CRITERIA FOR 300.30 OBSESSIVE COMPULSIVE DISORDER

A. Either obsessions or compulsions:
   1. *Obsessions:*
      a. Recurrent and persistent ideas, thoughts, impulses, or images that are experienced, at least initially, as intrusive and senseless, *e.g.,* a parent's having repeated impulses to kill a loved child, a religious person's having recurrent blasphemous thoughts
      b. The person attempts to ignore or suppress such thoughts or impulses or to neutralize them with some other thought or action.
      c. The person recognizes that the obsessions are the product of his or her own mind, not imposed from without (as in thought insertion).
      d. If another Axis I disorder is present, the content of the obsession is unrelated to it *e.g.,* the ideas, thoughts, impulses, or images are not about food in the presence of an Eating Disorder, about drugs in the presence of a Psychoactive Substance Use Disorder, or guilty thoughts in the presence of a Major Depression.
   2. *Compulsions:*
      a. Repetitive, purposeful, and intentional behaviors that are performed in response to an obsession, or according to certain rules or in a stereotyped fashion
      b. The behavior is designed to neutralize or to prevent discomfort or some dreaded event or situation; however, either the activity is not connected in a realistic way with what it is designed to neutralize or prevent, or it is clearly excessive.
      c. The person recognizes that his or her behavior is excessive or unreasonable (this may not be true for young children; it may no longer be true for people whose obsessions have evolved into overvalued ideas).
B. The obsessions or compulsions cause marked distress, are time-consuming (take more than an hour a day), or significantly interfere with the person's normal routine, occupational functioning, or usual social activities or relationships with others.

DIAGNOSTIC CRITERIA FOR 309.89 POSTTRAUMATIC STRESS DISORDER

A. The person has experienced an event that is outside the range of usual human experience and that would be markedly distressing to almost anyone, *e.g.,* serious threat to one's life or physical integrity; serious threat or harm to one's children, spouse, or other close relatives and friends; sudden destruction of one's home or community; or seeing another person who has recently been, or is being, seriously injured or killed as the result of an accident of physical violence.
B. The traumatic event is persistently reexperienced in at least one of the following ways:
   1. Recurrent and intrusive distressing recollections of the event (in young children, repetitive play in which themes or aspects of the trauma are expressed)
   2. Recurrent distressing dreams of the event
   3. Sudden acting or feeling as if the traumatic event were recurring (includes a sense of reliving the experience, illusions, hallucinations, and dissociative [flashback] episodes, even those that occur upon awakening or when intoxicated)
   4. Intense psychological distress at exposure to events that symbolize or resemble an aspect of the traumatic event, including anniversaries of the trauma
C. Persistent avoidance of stimuli associated with the trauma or numbing of general responsiveness (not present before the trauma), as indicated by at least three of the following:
   1. Efforts to avoid thoughts or feelings associated with the trauma
   2. Efforts to avoid activities or situations that arouse recollections of the trauma
   3. Inability to recall an important aspect of the trauma (psychogenic amnesia)

(Continued)

TABLE 5-4. (CONTINUED)

DIAGNOSTIC CRITERIA FOR 309.89 POSTTRAUMATIC STRESS DISORDER

    4. Markedly diminished interest in significant activities (in young children, loss of recently acquired developmental skills such as toilet training or language skills)

    5. Feeling of detachment or estrangement from others

    6. Restricted range of affect, *e.g.,* unable to have loving feelings

    7. Sense of a foreshortened future, *e.g.,* does not expect to have a career, marriage, or children, or a long life

D. Persistent symptoms of increased arousal (not present before the trauma), as indicated by at least two of the following:

    1. Difficulty falling or staying asleep

    2. Irritability or outbursts of anger

    3. Difficulty concentrating

    4. Hypervigilance

    5. Exaggerated startle response

    6. Physiological reactivity upon exposure to events that symbolize or resemble an aspect of the traumatic event (*e.g.,* a woman who was raped in an elevator breaks out in a sweat when entering any elevator)

E. Duration of the disturbance (symptoms in B, C, and D) of at least one month
    Specify delayed onset if the onset of symptoms was at least six months after the trauma.

DIAGNOSTIC CRITERIA FOR 300.02 GENERALIZED ANXIETY DISORDER

A. Unrealistic or excessive anxiety and worry (apprehensive expectation) about two or more life circumstances, *e.g.,* worry about possible misfortune to one's child (who is in no danger) and worry about finances (for no good reason), for a period of six months or longer, during which the person has been bothered more days than not by these concerns. In children and adolescents, this may take the form of anxiety and worry about academic, athletic, and social performance.

B. If another Axis I disorder is present, the focus of the anxiety and worry in A is unrelated to it, *e.g.,* the anxiety or worry is not about having a panic attack (as in Panic Disorder), being embarrassed in public (as in Social Phobia), being contaminated (as in Obsessive Compulsive Disorder), or gaining weight (as in Anorexia Nervosa)

C. The disturbance does not occur only during the course of a Mood Disorder or a psychotic disorder.

D. At least 6 of the following 18 symptoms are often present when anxious (do not include symptoms present only during panic attacks):

    1. Motor tension

        1. Trembling, twitching, or feeling shaky

        2. Muscle tension, aches, or soreness

        3. Restlessness

        4. Easy fatigability

    2. Autonomic hyperactivity

        5. Shortness of breath or smothering sensations

        6. Palpitations or accelerated heart rate (tachycardia)

        7. Sweating or cold clammy hands

        8. Dry mouth

        9. Dizziness or lightheadedness

       10. Nausea, diarrhea, or other abdominal distress

       11. Flushes (hot flashes) or chills

       12. Frequent urination

       13. Trouble swallowing or "lump in throat"

    3. Vigilance and scanning

       14. Feeling keyed up or on edge

       15. Exaggerated startle response

       16. Difficulty concentrating or "mind going blank" because of anxiety

       17. Trouble falling or staying asleep

       18. Irritability

E. It cannot be established that an organic factor initiated and maintained the disturbance, *e.g.,* hyperthyroidism, Caffeine Intoxication.

---

1. The individual has an expectation in mind. For example, a client on a psychiatric unit may expect that his wife will visit or he may expect imagined voices to carry out hallucinated threats. Everyone has expectations, and some people's are more active than others'.

2. For some reason the expectation is not met. The expectation may have been unreasonable, or others who were a part of the expectation may not have carried out their obligation to the client. For example, the spouse of the client mentioned previously may not have visited the hospital.

3. The client feels the discomfort and powerlessness of anxiety.

4. The feeling of anxiety is not resolved, and the energy of this feeling is transformed into behavior. This transformation may be automatic, because the transformation assists in reducing the anxiety. It would be useful if the behavior consisted of talking with a psychiatric/mental health nurse about the feelings accompanying the unmet expectations. However, the client may discharge the energy of the anxiety in behaviors that are not productive. A client may state that another client does not "do her job right and makes me angry." According to Peplau, if the client could state the situation more accurately, he would say, "I expected my wife to visit me. She did not. I became anxious. I changed my anxiety to anger and I directed it toward the other client to blame her."

Nursing Interventions. Peplau[18] reported that the steps for intervention in anxiety do not occur in the same order as the steps in the development of the client's anxiety. The nurse does not discuss the client's justification for the behavior, because the dialogue will have no conclusion or may develop into a "power struggle" between the nurse and client about the justification. The client in such a power struggle may feel defensive and sense that the nurse is an antagonist rather than an ally. The nurse begins by observing transformations in the anxiety and the relief behavior. The following steps are taken:

1. Name the affect anxiety. The nurse could ask, "What are you feeling now?" The client has to *name* the feeling. Because many clients have lost the intellectual competency to label their feelings, the nurse would then ask, "Are you anxious now?" Although the nurse is guessing the client's affect at the time, if the client does not have the competency to label the feelings, the client *can* begin to regain or learn this competency by using the nurse's language. Also, the nurse uses knowledge of the various emotions to conclude that anxiety is the emotion being experienced.

   The client may deny feeling anxious, ignore the nurse's statement, admit to feeling a "little anxious," or admit to feeling anxious. If the client does not acknowledge the presence of anxiety, the nurse will need to repeat attempts to assist the client in labeling emotions. The client will successfully name emotions *with the nurse's repeated, consistent approach.* It may help if the nurse points out observations. The nurse could say, "Are you anxious now? I notice you are moving around in your chair."

2. Connect the named affect (anxiety) with the relief behavior. Once the client acknowledges the presence of anxiety, the nurse connects the name of the emotion (anxiety) with the relief behavior. The nurse could ask, "What are you doing to decrease the feeling of anxiety?" There are many possible relief behaviors. In the previous case, the client became angry at another client.

Having the client make this connection accomplishes a number of things. The client is assisted in learning or relearning the connection between the events that result in anxiety. Because of the overwhelming and pervasive nature of affect, the client may not have felt in control of the affect; understanding the connections provides a sense of security in knowing that control may be possible. Also, the nurse avoids giving the impression of reading the client's mind. The nurse talks with the client about the *observable* behaviors demonstrated by the client that indicate what was occurring within the client. The nurse and client would label "getting angry" at another client as the observable relief behavior. Labeling decreases the mystery of the forces that operate in the client's illness and promotes the client's sense of security.

3. Label the expectation, need, or want that the client had that was disappointed. The nurse could ask, "What occurred before you became angry?" The client could respond, "I expected my wife to visit."

4. Label the disappointment in the client's expectation. The nurse could ask: "What happened instead?" The client could respond, "She didn't show." The nurse and client would then review the entire sequence in the development of the relief behavior as a transformation of anxiety. They would then develop new behaviors that could be used to handle the anxiety-provoking behavior more appropriately.

It is important to note that, as the nurse guides the client through these steps, the client may become anxious with the nurse. This anxiety is generally mild to moderate, so the nurse should continue working with the client. The client is not, to use Peplau's terminology, a fragile piece of china that will break.

The nurse can work with the client experiencing anxiety. The nurse can ask the client to name the present emotion. The client would then go through the intervention steps mentioned above. The nurse could also elect to titrate the responses to the client in order to promote the client's ability to maintain a focus on the topic and not discuss the presently felt anxiety. Titrating means to finely adjust one's remarks according to the ability of the client to use the nurse's statements effectively.

The nurse, for example, may sense the client's anxiety rising to a disorganizing level (but not to the severe or panic level) when the client labels the expectation that was disappointed. This may be difficult for many clients because of a sense of self-respect and pride, and difficulty in admitting that another person has hurt them. The nurse could say, "Take your time" or "Take a deep breath. This is difficult work." These interventions help the client control anxiety while the psychotherapeutic work continues.

The nurse would elect to titrate responses when sensing that the benefit to the client from talking about a topic other than anxiety is greater than the benefit from changing the focus to the client's present experience of anxiety. Selection of the focus (a topic other than the client's anxiety, or the experience of the present anxiety) is a matter of judgment and art on the part of the nurse.

Panic Disorders

Hallam[12] reviewed a number of studies concerning married women who experience panic attacks. The symptoms emerge or are exacerbated as part of a *couple's* attempt to adjust to one another and to the constraints, demands, and conflicts of marriage. Women with panic attacks have many of the characteristics fostered in a social system in which women are taught to take a passive role. Clients are unassertive, lack social skills, and are overdependent on others. They tend to attribute distress to external sources, which is in keeping with the tendency to avoid interpersonal conflict. In general, women with a panic disorder are more dissatisfied with their role in life than are their partners. The clients are not to blame; being told that one is not a capable and worthy individual would lead to dissatisfaction.

Hallam described the development of a Panic Disorder as follows:

1. There is ongoing conflict within the client. This cannot be resolved because of fears of loneliness and lack of independence.
2. Chronic anxiety and depression occur.
3. The client experiences a series of panic attacks. The client has inadequate skills to deal with stress or with interpersonal issues.
4. The client finds the internal experience of symptoms of panic (such as a wave of heat felt going through the body) uncomfortable. The symptoms become unconditioned stimuli that elicit the anxiety response. These symptoms are considered aversive by the individual because they signal the presence of other aversive consequences, such as loss of control and even illness or death.

    Agoraphobics do not typically report a fear of supermarkets, open spaces, buses, or other such situations, but rather a fear of experiencing panic in these situations. Given the symptoms (listed under Panic Disorder in DSM-III-R)[2] that can trigger a panic attack, one can understand the "generalized and irrational nature of the anxiety complaints."[12] Such symptoms occur as a subtle part of everyone's experience at one time or another, and the client may not be aware of the complex sequence of events through which the anxiety response is learned.
5. Clients become obsessed with the symptoms of anxiety and become fearful of loss of control, illness, or even death.
6. The client adjusts to the panic disorder by increasingly limiting interpersonal experiences.

Treatment

Treatment for panic disorders consists primarily of behavioral therapy, such as gradual exposure to anxiety-provoking stimuli and relaxation techniques. Hallam also re-

ported that drug therapy with imipramine can be effective in some cases.

Nursing Care of the Client in Panic

The psychiatric/mental health nurse must be familiar with panic levels of anxiety. Peplau[22] stated that "in panic there is immediate, extraordinary, extreme discomfort." Panic mobilizes a large quantity of energy within the person that must be used: the client must do *something*. Peplau described work with many types of clients experiencing panic, not simply those with the medical diagnosis of Panic Disorder.

Clients may engage in random movements, repetitive actions, crying, or other behaviors. Some clients can maintain sufficient control to try to understand their current state with the assistance of a professional. Peplau mentioned that the behaviors clients demonstrate in instances of panic depend on previous patterns of coping with anxiety and current interpersonal circumstances, such as whether or not nurses are available to assist the client in coping.

Peplau[22] listed six basic nursing interventions for panic:

1. *Nurses must control their own anxiety.* Nurses can accomplish this by having no expectations of the client. If the nurse expects an "ideal client" and the client does not behave in this manner, the nurse will experience anxiety. The nurse's thinking will become disorganized and, following Sullivan's theory, the nurse will empathize personal anxiety to the client. The client must then deal not only with the client's own anxiety, but also with the nurse's. This places an unfair burden on the client.
2. *Remain with the client.* The feeling of panic includes sensations of terror and horror. "These feelings should not have to be experienced alone, without the presence of another person who is concerned and competent in this particular experience." The "presence of another person provides a tangible reference point . . . through which an outward reality-based pull (or) an external focal point is provided for the (client)." When a client has no such reference point, the only focus for the client is the panic. The client's awareness of panic will produce more panic.
3. *Do not touch the client.* At times the nurse may feel a need to touch the client. This may be because the nurse is at a loss for other useful interventions or because the nurse wants to "control" the client. The client in panic may misinterpret such gestures. Children experiencing a temper tantrum may be an exception to this rule.
4. *"Use no content type of input."* Because of the overwhelming emotion, the client can neither engage in the learning process nor concentrate on verbal input or problem-solving.
5. *"Inputs that are given should be clear, direct, simple, (with) the fewest number of words per sentence possible."* The nurse's tone of voice should be calm, not challenging or burdensome. Only a few words

can be understood by the client because of the intellectual disorganization present in panic. The few words that the nurse speaks are used to provide the sense that there is a competent, professional person present with the client; to engage what little ability the client in panic does have to attend to reality; and to begin to direct the energy of the panic toward a productive channel. The nurse could say, for example, *"Stop that." "Sit." "Say it in words."*

6. *Administer fluids.* The client in panic may not notice thirst, and water should be offered.

All clients do not need to be isolated. For some clients this will increase the panic. In other instances the remaining clients on the unit may need to have the client distanced to some degree, at least at one end of the corridor of a unit, for example, in order not to become overly anxious themselves.

It is preferable that nursing interventions begin before the client reaches the panic level of anxiety. However, this is not always possible. Staff members should not be blamed if a client experiences panic. The staff and client need to be aware of what promotes panic and how to cope with it. Awareness involves understanding, not blame or criticism.

Posttraumatic Stress Disorder

Posttraumatic Stress Disorder (PTSD) is another anxiety disorder. Birckhead[6] stated that PTSD is a severe emotional reaction to experienced trauma. The trauma is usually so severe that it would be difficult for anyone to adjust to it. Reactions to the trauma may occur shortly after the traumatic event(s) or years after the event(s). Examples of experienced trauma include war, incest, a concentration camp experience, and a natural disaster. Clients' reactions may include reliving or reexperiencing the traumatic event, hyperalertness, a lack of concentration, and others. Treatment of PTSD can include counseling and use of the behavioral techniques mentioned above. The psychiatric nurse can play an important role in such counseling, using techniques described in Part IV of this text.

Well-Being

In the last decade, *positive* emotions have become more of a focus for study in the mental health sciences. Previously, concern centered on negative emotions. A focus on positive emotions serves a number of purposes. It promotes understanding of the goal of mental health care (not just the absence of mental illness, but the presence of a positive state). Understanding the "health" end of the health–illness continuum also provides a clearer picture of the illness aspect by enabling the two parts to be contrasted. Also, a focus on the health aspect of well-being allows the client a sense of determination and perseverance, even in the midst of the client's pain of mental illness. Positive emotions are possible; there is hope, and there is an existence other than emotional pain.

Well-being is defined in various ways. In one view it is subjective—it is a person's own belief about what constitutes happiness. Other definitions of well-being refer to some external criteria, such as success. A third definition views well-being as a preponderance of positive affects over negative affects.

Influences on a Sense of Well-Being

A number of factors are associated with increases or decreases in a sense of well-being. Thoreau wrote that well-being comes from activity; others have emphasized a detachment from the routines of everyday life.

The question of what promotes a sense of well-being is important to the mental health sciences. Interventions can attempt to correct pathology and/or promote health. For example, a depressed individual may take medication to decrease pathology or may become involved in a social club to increase social support, thereby promoting well-being. Some clients who do not respond to interventions that decrease pathology may benefit from measures that promote well-being. Focusing strictly on factors that decrease pathology leaves out a whole realm of interventions that promote health.

Factors Associated with a Sense of Well-Being

Subjective States. A sense of well-being is closely linked with self-esteem, and is more likely to exist in those who have a sense of internality, *i.e.,* a feeling that outcomes are attributable to one's self rather than to outside sources.

Income. Even when varying levels of education are taken into account, as income level increases so does a higher sense of well-being. Imbalances in income are also important. Mental illness increases in periods of economic downturn, but this effect is greatest in communities where there is an unequal distribution of income. In such communities economic troubles do not touch everyone in the same manner. Although two communities may have the same amount of overall income, in a community where there is unequal income distribution, feelings of injustice and deprivation relative to others can actually decrease a sense of well-being among the disadvantaged in that community.[9]

Social Interaction. Extroverted individuals tend to be happier than introverts. People who are active socially generally have an improved sense of well-being even if they are not in good health or are from lower-income groups. Several researchers have found that having a love relationship is a significant predictor of life satisfaction, and that love is the most important resource for happiness.[9]

Additional Demographic Factors.

1. Health has been found to affect the sense of well-being because of its impact on how people feel physically and how active they are able to be.

2. Black individuals, even those who are well-educated and have high incomes, generally have a lower sense of well-being than whites.

3. Unemployed men and women have a lower sense of well-being than those who are employed. However, women working inside the home as homemakers are generally as happy as those who go outside to work.

4. Educational level seems to have little effect on well-being.

5. Religious participation appears to have a positive effect on well-being.

6. Sleep disturbances and lack of exercise are associated with a low sense of well-being.

Level of Prevention

Primary prevention refers to the promotion of mental health. At this level of prevention much can be accomplished if the nurse is aware of all aspects (positive and negative) of the client's life. The nurse's attitude can show that the challenges of life can be faced with strength.

At the *secondary level* of prevention (or early case findings), the nurse uses the systems perspective to make a complete assessment and confronts most problems quickly. An advantage of using the systems perspective in working with clients is that the nurse assesses and intervenes where necessary in any component (psychological, physical, societal, cultural, or environmental) of the person in which there is a need or problem.

In *tertiary prevention* the nurse assists the client with rehabilitation. A great deal of psychiatric/mental health nursing is concerned with interventions used with clients who are attempting to reverse some illness condition. At this level of prevention, a conceptual framework can help the nurse to formulate a perspective with which to understand the client.

Facilitating Client Change

The term *therapeutic use of self* means that the psychiatric/mental health nurse's behavior is an instrument for client change. As discussed earlier in this chapter, behavior consists of thoughts, feelings, and actions.

Impact of the Nurse's Behavior on the Client

Thoughts. The nurse expends mental effort or energy to understand the Truth of the experiences of the client. Given the very complex behavior of clients at times, this is a major contribution on the part of the nurse.

Feelings. The nurse reacts on an emotional level with the client (within the limits of a professional relationship) in order to understand the Truth of the client. In this way the nurse serves as a role model for clients as they learn to become comfortable with their own emotions.

Actions. The nurse acts in ways that promote the well-being of the client. Such actions include using words to reorient the client to a room or pacing with a mute client.

Some specific *nursing behaviors* are associated with client change:

1. An ability to identify emotional pain

2. A willingness to allow clients to progress in therapy at their own pace. Some clients move through the various stages quickly, while others will not benefit unless they go through each step slowly.

3. An ability to tolerate the client's emotions. Typically, health care providers unconsciously moderate their own behavior in order to obtain a level of emotional release from the client that they can tolerate.

4. Use of interventions that assist the client to release emotions, *e.g.,* a soft voice or a comforting gesture. Prompting responses or at times even silence is useful. The appropriate approach is determined from client cues. The following box identifies nursing behaviors that encourage a client to share emotions.

5. An ability to empathize and identify client emotions

Specific *client factors* also tend to facilitate change:

1. The presence of emotional pain serving as a motivating factor for change

2. The belief that clients must change themselves rather than others

---

APPROPRIATE NURSE BEHAVIORS WHEN CLIENTS EXPERIENCE AND SHARE EMOTIONS

1. Acceptance
2. Verbal and nonverbal messages to the client indicating that experiencing and sharing emotions is appropriate (such as nodding in acknowledgment of what has been said, reflecting back to the client what has been said, and using a voice tone of concern)
3. Returning for scheduled interviews with the client to demonstrate an ability to work with, and accept, the client's emotions
4. Verbal responses to the client indicating that the nurse understands what the client is thinking and feeling. These responses provide some sense of structure when the client deals with previously unexpressed emotions.

3. A desire to change specific behavior and an understanding of why that behavior exists
4. A willingness to work with a therapist to guide the change process
5. The ability to trust the therapist
6. Sharing with the therapist the emotions that are tied to traumatic life events
7. Gaining insight into problematic behavior and the reasons it occurs
8. Releasing emotions as necessary

Focusing on the Client's Strengths

People have an inherent ability to change in both constructive and destructive directions. All clients have the potential to grow, no matter where they are on the health–illness continuum. Keeping this in mind can help the nurse to continue working with a client even when early interventions do not appear to effect change. Wanting to abandon the client is a natural response when the nurse is faced with extremely inappropriate client behavior. However, a consistent intervention approach can eventually work with the client, even if changes occur very slowly.

The nurse must remember that the psychiatric/mental health client is a person with actual and potential strengths. The nurse can find strengths in the client regardless of the depth of illness. These strengths may occur in any component of the client system. Looking for these strengths and building on them help to build the client's sense of well-being. Some examples of client strengths include: consideration of other people (a societal component of the client) or demonstration by a young client of deep respect for older people as part of the individual's cultural heritage (a societal component of the client); the ability to overcome a fear, as evidenced by remaining in group therapy even when it is difficult for the client to do so (the psychological component); maintaining a proper diet and rest (the biological component); the ability to provide shelter for oneself (the environmental component).

Summary

1. The Self/Other/Relationship conceptual framework provides a guideline with which to understand psychological functioning.
2. Sympathy is different from empathy. The focus of sympathy is on the content of an experience that is familiar to both the client and the nurse, not on the emotions of the other person. The focus of empathy is on the client's emotions; the client experiences the nurse's altruistic attempt to understand the client.
3. The psychotherapeutic interventions include the phases of orientation, working, and termination.

Each phase is marked by typical client behaviors and useful nurse responses.
4. The learning process is a clearly defined set of principles for use in conducting a psychotherapeutic interview.
5. Common client behaviors have been identified that serve to block client change; these may include resistance and distortions. Testing behavior on the part of the client is expected.
6. Nurses typically experience their own personal distortions, which can affect their clinical work. These must be examined carefully and resolved.
7. Psychotherapeutic work includes a willingness on the part of the nurse to work with emotions—both the client's and the nurse's.
8. Anxiety can block the client's ability to learn in the psychotherapeutic interaction.

References

1. American Nurses' Association: Taxonomy for the Classification of Human Responses of Concern for Psychiatric/Mental Health Nursing Practice (Working Draft). Kansas City, American Nurses' Association, 1986
2. American Psychiatric Association: Diagnostic and Statistical Manual of Mental Disorders, DSM-III-R. Washington, DC, American Psychiatric Association, 1987
3. Aylwin S: Structure in Thought and Feeling. London, Methuen, 1985
4. Baumgartner M: Empathy. In Carlson C (ed): Behavioral Concepts and Nursing Intervention. Philadelphia, JB Lippincott, 1970
5. Birckhead L: Identification as an Appropriate Component of Therapeutic Growth and Development. Issues in Mental Health Nursing 6:73, 1984
6. Birckhead L: Intervening with Middle-Aged Families and Post-traumatic Stress Disorder. In Wright L, Leahey M (eds): Family Nursing Series. Springhouse, PA, Springhouse Publishers, 1987
7. Brantley T: Racism and Its Impact on Psychotherapy. Am J Psychiatry 140:1605, 1983
8. Denzin N: On Understanding Emotion. San Francisco, Jossey-Bass, 1984
9. Diener E: Subjective Well-Being. Psychol Bull 95:542, 1984
10. Forsyth G: Exploration of Empathy in Nurse–Client Interaction. Advances in Nursing Science 2:53, 1979
11. Green A: Conceptions of Affect. Int J Psychoanal 58:129, 1977
12. Hallam R: Anxiety: Psychological Perspectives on Panic and Agoraphobia. New York, Academic Press, 1985
13. Heilman K, Satz P: Neuropsychology of Human Emotion. New York, Guilford Press, 1983
14. Izard C: Approaches to Developmental Research on Emotion–Cognition Relationships. In Bearison D, Zimiles H (eds): Thought and Emotion: Developmental Perspectives. London, Lawrence Erlbaum Associates, 1986
15. Kerr N: Anxiety: Theoretical Considerations. Perspect Psychiatr Care 16:36, 1978
16. Meador B, Rogers C: Person-Centered Therapy. In Corsini R (ed): Current Psychotherapies. Itasca, IL, Peacock, 1984
17. Nemiah J: Classical Psychoanalysis. In Arieti S (ed): American Handbook of Psychiatry. New York, Basic Books, 1975
18. Peplau H: Anxiety Development: Panic. In Field W (ed): The

Psychotherapy of Hildegard E. Peplau. New Braunfels, TX, PSF Productions, 1979

19. Peplau H: Criteria for a Working Relationship. In Field W (ed): The Psychotherapy of Hildegard E. Peplau. New Braunfels, TX, PSF Productions, 1979

20. Peplau H: Interviewing as a Language Competence Development. In Field W (ed): The Psychotherapy of Hildegard E. Peplau. New Braunfels, TX, PSF Productions, 1979

21. Peplau H: Language and Its Relation to Thought Disorder. In Field W (ed): The Psychotherapy of Hildegard E. Peplau. New Braunfels, TX, PSF Productions, 1979

22. Peplau H: Manifestations of Anxiety and Intervention. In Field W (ed): The Psychotherapy of Hildegard E. Peplau. New Braunfels, TX, PSF Productions, 1979

23. Peplau H: The Process and Concept of Learning. In Burd S, Marshall M (eds): Some Clinical Approaches to Psychiatric Nursing. New York, Macmillan, 1963

24. Peplau H: A Concept of Psychotherapy. In Field W (ed): The Psychotherapy of Hildegard E. Peplau. New Braunfels, TX, PSF Productions, 1979

25. Peplau H: Termination and the Use of Summary. In Field W (ed): The Psychotherapy of Hildegard E. Peplau. New Braunfels, TX, PSF Productions, 1979

26. Peplau H: Testing Maneuvers and Interpretations. In Field W (ed): The Psychotherapy of Hildegard E. Peplau. New Braunfels, TX, PSF Productions, 1979

27. Rime B, Giovannini D: The Physiological Patterns of Reported Emotional States. In Scherer K, Wallbott H, Summerfield A (eds): Experiencing Emotion: A Cross-Cultural Study. London, Cambridge University Press, 1986

28. Rogers C: The Necessary and Sufficient Conditions of Therapeutic Personality Change. J Consult Psychol 21:95, 1957

29. Sullivan H: The Interpersonal Theory of Psychiatry. New York, WW Norton, 1953

30. Szalita A: The Use and Misuse of Empathy in Psychoanalysis and Psychotherapy. Psychoanal Rev 68:3, 1981

31. Tomkins S: The Quest for Primary Motives: Biography and Autobiography of an Idea. J Pers Soc Psychol 41:306, 1981

32. Uzoka A: Active Versus Passive Therapist Role in Didactic Psychotherapy with Nigerian Clients. Soc Psychiatry 18:1, 1983

33. White G: The Role of Cultural Explanations in "Somatization" and "Psychologization." Soc Sci Med 16:1519, 1982

34. Yocom C: The Differentiation of Fear and Anxiety. In Kim M, McFarland G, McLane A (eds): Classification of Nursing Diagnoses: Proceedings of the Fifth National Conference. St Louis, CV Mosby, 1984

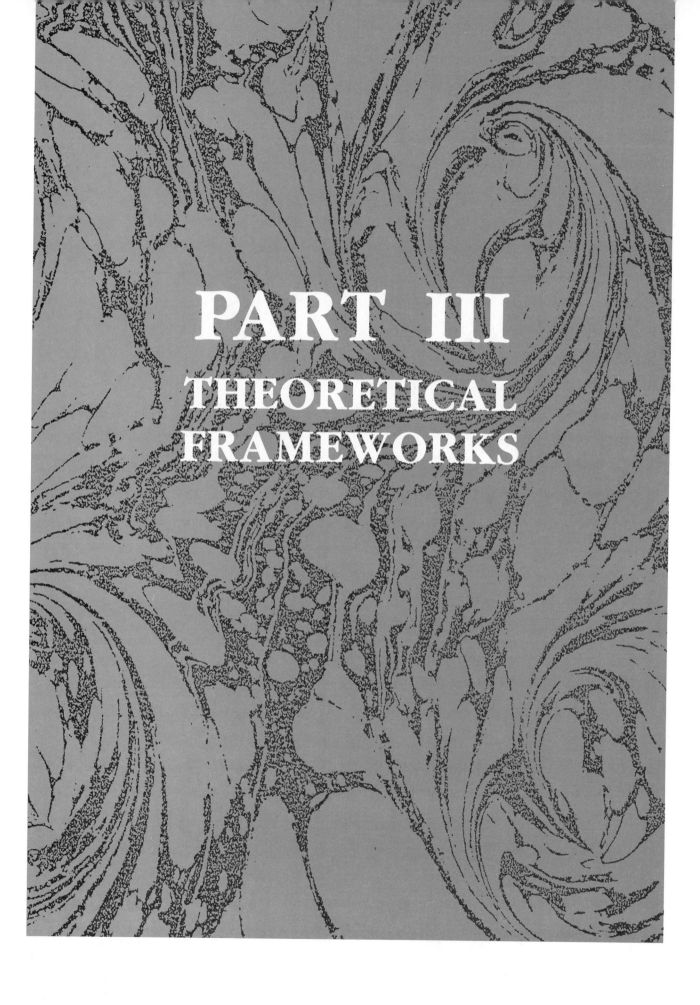

PART III
THEORETICAL FRAMEWORKS

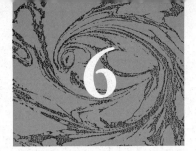

JOY DAN GRAVES AND RONDA MINTZ

DEVELOPMENTAL THEORIES

Learning Objectives

Upon completion of this chapter the student should be able to do the following:

1. Define the term "developmental."
2. Identify the major tenets of the medical model.
3. Differentiate among the id, the ego, and the superego.
4. Define the relationship of instincts to the id, the ego, and the superego.
5. Describe the role of the unconscious in mental health problems.
6. Define each defense mechanism identified in the psychoanalytic approach.
7. Identify the emphases of ego psychology and object-relations theory that are different from emphases of the psychoanalytic perspective.
8. Identify the points of focus of the interpersonal theory of psychiatry.
9. Describe the nature of the client-centered therapist's approach.
10. Differentiate between stimulus–response learning and observational learning.
11. List ways in which each developmental theory is useful to nursing.

Introduction

Psychiatric/mental health nursing theory incorporates theories from the social sciences, relating them to the unique relationships between nurses and clients in the mental health care setting. To understand fully the vast scope and richness of psychiatric nursing today, it is essential to understand the evolution and expansion of theoretical frameworks embracing the field of nursing since the turn of the century.

From a developmental standpoint, three classical theorists continue to remain prominent in the literature today: Sigmund Freud, Erik Erikson, and Jean Piaget are most often cited for their landmark effects on psychiatry and the social sciences. The work of these three theorists can be called "developmental," because they seek to define internal and/or external forces or events that shape the person's path of increasing psychological maturity or specialization. The authors also consider what might inhibit development. Chapter 7 discusses in detail the work of these three theorists and their impact on current conceptualizations of infant and child development. Rather than focusing on specific theorists, this chapter will describe the historical evolution of several of the most prominent models shared by the disciplines involved in the treatment of psychiatric clients. A time line showing the dates of significant developmental theoretical models is included, in Figure 6-1.

The Medical Model

Blaney[6] described the medical model as composed of four characteristics. First, the medical model assumes an organic cause of illness. Second, the model proposes that some underlying condition leads to the observed symptoms. Third, the model includes the concept that individuals have no responsibility for their behavior—mental illness is similar to physical illness in that there is a cause of the illness that is outside the control of the individual. The fourth characteristic includes the concept that various symptoms can be ordered into syndromes; hence the development of classification schemes such as the *Diagnostic and Statistical Manual of Mental Disorders-III-Revised.*[2]

At the end of the 19th century, researchers and physicians struggled to assess and describe mental disorders in order to develop a systematic organizational scheme. They felt that, if a classification system could be developed, disease processes could be identified and cures researched and tested. Emil Kraepelin first distinguished mental disorders in a categorical way. In 1899, he delineated two classifications: *dementia praecox,* a degenerative process occurring in an individual; and *manic-de-*

pression, a nondegenerative process. In both categories the disorders were seen as organic, with the disease process occurring in the central nervous system. Once these diagnostic categories were established, research moved toward identification of the cause as either *external* (such as an ingested poison or foreign substance) or *internal* (a biochemical reaction causing abnormal and inappropriate behavior in individuals). Viewing a mental disorder as having psychological, rather than biochemical, origins was regarded as outrageous and inconceivable by the medical model activists.

In 1938, electroconvulsive therapy (ECT) was introduced as the treatment of choice for depressed persons, enhancing the medical model of mental disease. Although controversial, and deemed barbaric and primitive by some, shock therapy (using electrodes attached to specific points at the patient's hairline) proved highly successful as a somatic treatment modality. In the 50 years since then, extensive improvements have occurred in the application of ECT, and positive effects of the treatment continue today with selected clients.

In the 1950s, the medical model was enhanced by the introduction of chlorpromazine (Thorazine). Originally prescribed as an antihistamine, chlorpromazine effectively reduced the symptoms of psychotic clients. Within a few years, Thorazine became widely used as the treatment of choice for schizophrenic persons, who had previously been labeled untreatable and chronically insane. Other antipsychotic medications followed, and imipramine (Tofranil), the first antidepressant medication, was accidentally discovered. In the late 1960s the

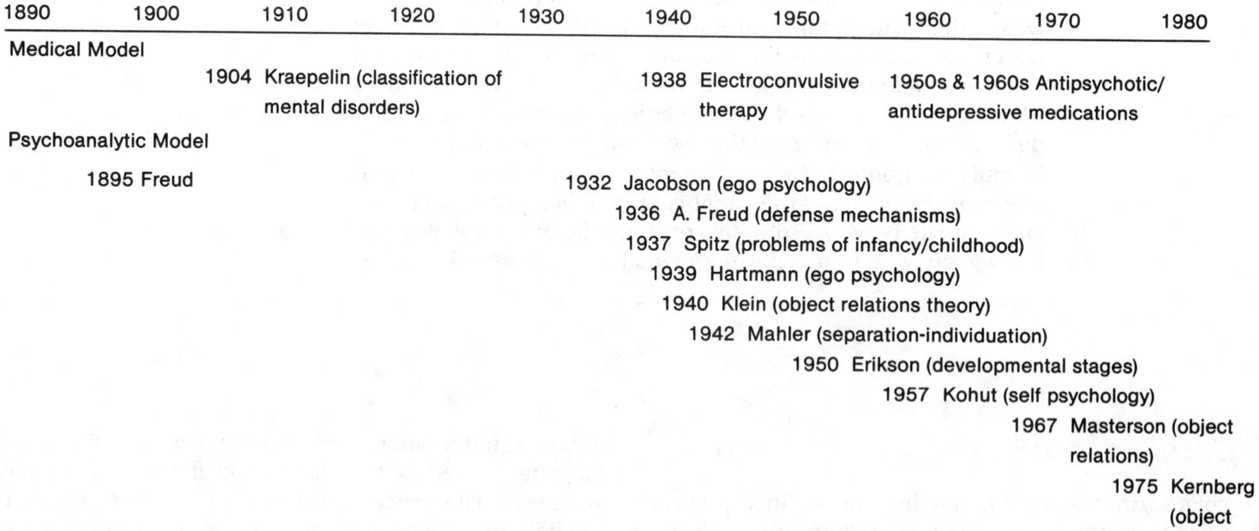

1890	1900	1910	1920	1930	1940	1950	1960	1970	1980

Medical Model

1904 Kraepelin (classification of mental disorders)

1938 Electroconvulsive therapy

1950s & 1960s Antipsychotic/antidepressive medications

Psychoanalytic Model

1895 Freud

1932 Jacobson (ego psychology)

1936 A. Freud (defense mechanisms)

1937 Spitz (problems of infancy/childhood)

1939 Hartmann (ego psychology)

1940 Klein (object relations theory)

1942 Mahler (separation-individuation)

1950 Erikson (developmental stages)

1957 Kohut (self psychology)

1967 Masterson (object relations)

1975 Kernberg (object relations)

Interpersonal Model

1938 Sullivan (interpersonal theory)

Humanistic Model

1960 Rogers (client-centered psychotherapy)

Figure 6-1. The development of theoretical models.

biochemical implications of manic-depressive disorders became known when lithium carbonate, a salt, became the treatment of choice for clients who cycled between states of euphoria and dysphoria.[19]

Significance to Nurses

Inpatient and outpatient psychiatric treatment of mental disorders today includes the use of medications and, in extreme cases, ECT. Medications may be used as an adjunct to psychotherapy and/or to a behavioral treatment program. Nurses need a thorough understanding of the different medications used for psychiatric disorders, because the dosages vary and side-effects are quite common and can be debilitating. Accurate and quick diagnosis of side-effects is a key contribution of nurses working in interdisciplinary teams using the medical model. Nurses also provide client education concerning the usefulness of medications, appropriate dosages, and side-effects.

The medical model receives much emphasis in psychiatry. This emphasis is demonstrated in research and treatment priorities concerning the organic basis of mental illness. Nursing accepts a broader view of mental illness, in that "mental" concerns are seen as having not only physical implications for causation and treatment, but also environmental, psychological, societal, and cultural implications.

The Psychoanalytic Model

In the 18th century, Franz Mesmer's work (1734–1815) in the field of hypnosis was the origin of psychoanalytic technique. Mesmer gazed into a highly disturbed patient's eyes to quiet the person. He would touch people's hands or make movements over them to calm them. Although his techniques were quite popular and attracted numerous clients, Mesmer was a very controversial figure and a commission was appointed to investigate his methods. The commission dismissed Mesmer as a fraud and labeled his technique, mesmerism, simply the result of suggestibility. Nevertheless, the concept of hypnosis as a treatment for psychopathology in patients was enhanced.

Interest in hypnosis remained at a relatively low level, however, until Jean Martin Charcot (1825–1893), a French neurologist, equated susceptibility to hypnosis with pathological states, especially hysterical neurosis. Other scientists in France equated hypnosis with normal behavior and labeled it suggestibility.

Hypnosis was first used on hysterical patients by Joseph Breuer. He called this *talking therapy,* or *cathartic therapy.* He found that under hypnosis patients could recall traumatic events they were normally unable to remember. Many times their symptoms disappeared after one session. He was interested in relief of symptoms and in why certain events were lost to a person's memory. As he became more successful, he became frightened be-cause many of his patients began to have sexual fantasies regarding him.

After studying with Charcot, Sigmund Freud also began to use hypnosis with his clients in Vienna. As did Breuer, he found that his clients had sexual fantasies about him. Freud's clients fascinated him, and he recognized the sexual fantasies as a process of the unconscious mind. In a scientific manner Freud began to classify and document his findings. From this work he concluded that the unconscious mind plays an important role in determining behavior. Thus, the unconscious mind became the foundation on which Freud's psychoanalytic theory was formulated. Freud abandoned the use of hypnosis and spent the bulk of his theory development on conversations (in one-to-one sessions) with his clients. At the same time, Breuer was experimenting with similar techniques. In 1895, Freud and Breuer together published *Studies in Hysteria,* a landmark piece of work delineating Freud's theory of the unconscious. Freud and Breuer later parted when Freud's work led him to pursue the sexual component of mental disorders and hysteria, which ultimately evolved into Freud's psychosexual theory and the noted Oedipal complex theory (discussed in Chapter 7).

The Theory of the Unconscious

Freud's theory of the unconscious mind developed when he postulated that nervous peoples' symptoms and behaviors have meaning—that they are derived from unconscious desires and instincts that have been repressed. To organize the concepts of the conscious and unconscious, he constructed a topographical theory of personality. He also constructed a structural theory, in which the structure of personality consists of the id, the ego, and the superego.[8,9,10]

Freud focused on instincts. A *psychological instinct* is ". . . the psychical representative of the stimuli originating from within the organism and reaching the mind. . . ."[17] There are four principal characteristics of an instinct: the aim, the object, the source, and the impetus. The *aim* of an instinct is satisfaction. The *object* is the person or thing through which the instinct is able to achieve its aim. The *source* is the somatic process that occurs in an organ or part of the body, the stimulus of which is represented in mental life by an instinct. The *impetus* refers to force or energy created by the instinctual stimulus. Freud's belief that all instinctual energy rests in the id is called the *dynamic theory of personality.*

The id is the reservoir of the instinctual and unconscious drives. It furnishes all the energy for the operation of the other two systems. It cannot tolerate increases in energy, which are experienced as uncomfortable states of tension.

The ego is the part of the personality that establishes a relationship with the environment through conscious perceptions, feelings, and actions. The ego serves to control impulses from the id and the superego, and has an established pattern of ego defenses designed to protect the ego from overwhelming anxiety.

The superego is the last to develop, and is an internalized moral arbitrator. Its main function is to strive for perfection, inhibit the impulses of the id, and persuade the ego to substitute moralistic goals for realistic ones.[10,11,12]

Defense Mechanisms

As stated previously, the ego assists in the distinction of reality from unreality, as well as protecting the organism from pain or discomfort experienced as a result of aggressive or sexual expression.[8] Therefore, with pressure exerted by the id, the ego inhibits or alters inappropriate urges or statements into more meaningful and appropriate behavior. With a protective stance, the ego calls on defense mechanisms to cope with desires that are socially inappropriate. Freud's primary focus was on the defense mechanism of *repression,* which he noted in his clients when they apparently had no recollection of early childhood memories yet could recall these events while in a hypnotic trance. This unconscious forgetting of events, affects, ideas, and/or impulses is the underlying basis for all defense mechanisms. It is activated to prevent the disruption of the ego, and hence of the self-concept of the individual. Defense mechanisms also have in common the following: they always function at the unconscious level; and they alter, deny, and/or distort reality to avoid the experience of anxiety. Anna Freud[8,9] expanded on her father's theory of the unconscious and added to his list of existing defense mechanisms, all of which are still considered useful.

Table 6-1 presents the defense mechanisms currently seen in psychiatric nursing and psychiatry. The list includes eleven unconscious mechanisms and one conscious mechanism, suppression, which is considered by many to be both the conscious counterpart to repression and a defense mechanism. Descriptions of each mechanism, and case examples, are also given. Psychiatric Nursing Diagnoses I (PNDI)[1] uses these mechanisms as nursing diagnoses listed under "Defensive Human Response Patterns." Table 6-2 lists the components of nursing diagnoses applicable to defense mechanisms.

TABLE 6-1.
DEFENSE MECHANISMS

NAME	DESCRIPTION	EXAMPLE
Repression	The unconscious elimination of unacceptable ideas, affects, events, and/or impulses from conscious awareness	An adult who was physically abused as a child has no memory recall of her childhood.
Denial	Refusal to accept and process any thought, wish, need, or event that is perceived as threatening and anxiety-producing	A child believes her father will live at home again, although her parents were just divorced.
Projection	Emotional rejection of unacceptable feelings or thoughts through the process of attributing them to or seeing them in others	A hospitalized male adolescent from a verbally abusive home views a confronting statement made by a staff member as hostile and negative.
Identification	To pattern oneself after another person, (usually in a position of authority) in order to relieve feelings of helplessness and unimportance	A newly admitted, shy, 10-year-old begins to wear makeup and dress like her primary nurse.
Introjection	The incorporation of another person's values and attitudes, even if they are in contrast to the individual's existing beliefs and values	A usually unmotivated student begins to excel in school after bonding with his nurse therapist in treatment.
Displacement	The transferring of an emotion from its original source to a less threatening, more acceptable person or object	A neglected and emotionally deprived child stops feeding his goldfish.
Intellectualization	To distance oneself from the emotional experience of a painful event by focusing solely on the cognitive and rationale aspects	An adult who tragically lost his wife in a plane crash provides specific details of the pilot's errors and the traffic controller's response, without any tears or expressions of pain or loss.
Rationalization	To justify or make tolerable through motives, behaviors, and emotions what is really intolerable to the individual	When a teenager is not invited to a party, she tells herself that she really needs to study that night and wouldn't have been able to go anyway.
Sublimation	Diverting unacceptable instinctual urges or drives into socially acceptable channels that serve society	A man with a very strong sex drive becomes a screen writer of R-rated love stories.
Reaction formation	The adoption of attitudes and behaviors that are the opposite of impulses or urges felt, but disowned	An adult who harbors anger toward her parents for being abusive during childhood becomes an advocate for the improvement of nursing care homes for the elderly.
Undoing	To attempt to counteract the effects of doing something perceived as unacceptable by repetitiously performing the reverse action or behavior	A disturbed male adolescent engages in repeated hand-washing after thinking sexual thoughts about his mother.
Suppression	The *conscious* removal of unacceptable thoughts or feelings from the awareness	A female adolescent on a diet refuses to acknowledge her hunger in order to continue to lose weight.

TABLE 6-2.
PSYCHIATRIC NURSING DIAGNOSIS I: *DEFENSIVE HUMAN RESPONSE PATTERN*

Excess of or deficit in defenses
  Impaired functioning of defenses
    Denial
    Displacement
    Fixation
    Introjection/identification
    Isolation
    Projection
    Rationalization
    Reaction formation
    Regression
    Repression
    Sublimation
    Turning against the self
    Undoing
  Impaired appropriateness of defenses
  Impaired focus of defenses
  Impaired range of defenses
  Excess of or deficit in defenses

(American Nurses' Association: Taxonomy for the Classification of Human Responses of Concern for Psychiatric/Mental Health Nursing Practice. Kansas City, American Nurses' Association, 1986)

Freudian Concepts

Freudian analysis is still practiced in its strictest form. The major components of Freud's analytic treatment are also used in modified form today. While many theorists have expanded Freud's original constructs in a movement away from id-centered analysis, even with modifications Freud remains the father of psychoanalysis and the originator of what is now considered intensive personality reconstruction, or psychoanalysis.[14]

The major focus of treatment is the understanding and "reliving" of the client's past life in the therapeutic encounter. The psychoanalyst, being objective, quiet, nonintrusive, and attentive, stirs up old feelings and conflicts from the client's childhood. These feelings and patterns of communicating become activated with the psychoanalyst as a means of displacement from past significant others onto this present relationship with the therapist. This unconscious process of repetition of past attitudes, emotions, and fantasies is called *transference*.[26] The tranferential process of bringing forth from the past painful experiences and then analyzing their significance results in freeing the self from the tension of the painful experiences. Hence, transference is the crux of psychoanalytic work. With freeing from the past come growth and a healthier development that can then lay the path for a happier and more satisfying way of life.

A second, yet related, Freudian concept is the use of *interpretation* as a treatment technique. In a Freudian interpretation, a present problem is seen as being related to a past conflict.[10] Most likely, an issue that arises in the relationship with the psychoanalyst is interpreted as similar to a situation occurring with the client's mother or father. For example, if a client cancels a therapy appointment because she scheduled another important appointment at the same time, Freudian analyst might look at this as a client's need to avoid closeness or intimacy with the analyst, or the need to place other people above the relationship with the analyst, perhaps in the same way that the client's father always cancelled family events at the last minute due to business complications. This comparison of past and present is a psychoanalytic interpretation, and is essential in analyzing the transference placed onto the psychoanalyst and the therapeutic relationship.

The third essential ingredient is the reaction of the psychoanalyst to *countertransference,* a conflict or dynamic with the client. Freud incompletely addressed this concept in 1910, and again in 1915, leaving post-Freudians open to their own interpretations and conclusions as to what Freud really meant. Freud did suggest that it was essential for practicing psychoanalysts to undergo their own analysis in order to resolve their own past conflicts and dynamics, thereby reducing the possibility of a countertransferential error with a client. Countertransference can include: an aggressive feeling, such as anger or competition with the client; loving and positive feelings, such as taking pride in a client's accomplishments or thinking about the client above and beyond other clients; or sexual feelings, with erotic thoughts and dreams of seducing the client—to name only a few forms. Post-Freudians have continued to investigate and expound on types of, and meanings behind, countertransference. At present they tend to agree that countertransference is not necessarily bad or a flaw, as long as it is recognized, identified, and worked through. Most often this is done in a psychoanalyst's own analysis or in clinical supervision meetings.[13]

Ego Psychology and Object-Relations Theory

During the 1940s there were many theoretical expansions of Freud's psychoanalytic concepts. Led by Anna Freud, theorists began to focus on the ego construct as the process of psychic organization, in contrast to Freud's emphasis on the id and impulses as the driving force of human behavior. Ego psychology, the psychoanalytic movement of the 1940s, was born, and was perpetuated by numerous post-Freudian theorists including Hartmann,[16] Kris,[25] and Jacobson.[18] It was extended many years later with the work of Mahler,[28] and Blanck and Blanck.[4,5] Anna Freud's major contribution was her delineation of defense mechanisms that serve to protect the ego. Hartmann's work, alone and in collaboration with the theorists listed above, delineated how the psyche is formed, the roots of aggression, and the role of the ego in relation to superego formation.

Ego psychologists believe that the ego is present from the beginning of life. The theory states that, because the ego has its own set of instincts and its own energy supply, development proceeds from a primitive, undifferentiated ego that exists at birth to an independent and separate ego. This proposition differs substantially from Freud's original hypothesis, in which he suggested that the ego derives all of its psychic energy from the id. The concept of development, from birth through the life cycle, is central to ego psychology; development is thought to be continuous, and composed of crucial landmarks. Pathology is considered a consequence of malformation that occurred somewhere along the developmental continuum. In order for there to be a logical development, there needs to be an organizing principle that encourages and directs the evolution of the ego and strengthens its functioning.

In 1968, Mahler[27] delineated *the separation–individuation process* as the specific organizing process whereby major aspects of behavioral and intrapsychic life are formed. In her theory, *separation* is defined as the point at which the child achieves a sense of differentiation from the mother, and hence, from the world at large. *Individuation* is considered to be the evolution of ego functions such as autonomy, memory, and cognition, which help to create a sense of being with self-contained boundaries.[29] Mahler's theory looks at human growth and development as representing changes in the way a person differentiates between experiences relating to the "self" (the person) and experiences relating to an "other," (another person, *i.e.,* the mother). The "other" is considered an object in the growing child's world. Therefore, the mother–child dyad is the primary, most important, love relationship that a newborn is exposed to. It is theorized that the experiences of this relationship have a major influence on a growing child's future attachments to significant others, thought of as *object relationships.*

Mahler formulated a theory of *human symbiosis* as a developmental framework for children and adolescents. The theory originally derived from observations of psychotic children interacting with their mothers in comparison to nonpsychotic children interacting with their mothers. Mahler's central theme was that all psychological life can be traced back to the universal symbiotic conditions in infancy that make physical life possible among humans. It is the unique psychobiological rapport between mother and infant that allows for physical survival of the child who is totally dependent on the external environment for need gratification.[29] With only a primitive, unintegrated ego, the infant easily conforms to the harmony of the mother's verbal and nonverbal behaviors, whether she serves as a healthy or a pathological object.[28]

Three separate, but overlapping, phases of psychological development are delineated in Mahler's complex separation–individuation process. The third phase is divided into four subphases, as listed in Table 6-3. *Symbiosis,* the phase before separation–individuation, is described as an *interdependent oneness* in which both mother and child believe that, without each other, the other will perish. The infant behaves and functions as if the dyad were indestructable, with one common boundary of togetherness. As the child enters Phase III, *separa-*

tion–individuation, Mahler describes the process whereby the mother, in her role as a buffer for her curious, exploring child, gradually encourages the differentiation of the child's inner and outer worlds. By 18 months of age, concomitant with mastery and consistent use of running and physically separating repeatedly from the mother, the child experiences a major conflict, most noticeable during the *rapprochement* subphase. Should the child satisfy the inner curiosity for exploration and adventure away from the mother (suggesting independence), or should the child remain close and within proximity of the mother (maintaining the dependent need for the mother's protection)?[28] Adaptive resolution of this major conflict requires that the toddler feel that the attachment to the parent is safe, regardless of the increase in physical distance from the mother.

The parents play a significant role in the toddler's success at this critical subphase. If the mother is unable to separate her needs from her child's, a symbiotic relationship remains, preventing the child from being able to separate inner needs from the mother's. In this example, a major disturbance follows, in which these children are unable to define themselves as separate or distinct from their parents.[29] If, on the other hand, the mother withdraws her support too suddenly for her child's dependency needs to be fulfilled, allowing for a sense of security, the child's movement toward greater independence will be stifled as autonomy becomes equated with rejection, and thus danger. The child is then caught between engulfment of symbiosis, if moving toward the mother, or the devastating experience of abandonment, if moving away. If either extreme occurs, future separation–individuation experiences will also be experienced maladaptively and resolved ineffectively, based on this first attempt in the child's first four years.

To many psychoanalysts, object-relations theory is seen as a subset of ego psychology, with Mahler's work seen as a part of both psychological constructs. Today, ego psychology appears to focus more on the delineation and assessment of ego function, while object-relations theory focuses more on the intricacies of self–other differentiation from a developmental perspective. That trend was led by Melanie Klein[21,22,23] who in the 1940s looked at the structural and dynamic relationships between the child's self-representation and the object-, or other-, representation.

Object-relations theory has been described as an examination of the structural and dynamic relationships between self-representation and object-representation.* The object refers to the primary mothering person who is the *object* representation, and the infant who is the *self* representation. The infant expects to be fed, protected, and nurtured. This is the average expectable environment within the mother–child dyad.[33]

Within the previously described theoretical framework, the theme of developing levels of object relations can be examined. In the developmental mode, infants move through *primary narcissism* (involvement with self), *need gratification* (obtaining what is necessary to

* References 15, 16, 20, 22, 28

TABLE 6-3.
MAHLER'S SEPARATION–INDIVIDUATION PROCESS

PHASE 1: NORMAL INFANTILE AUTISM (first month of life)
A state of hallucinatory disorientation in which the infant exists in a half awake–half sleep state. The infant is unaware of a distinction between inner and outer stimuli, or the existence of a separate external reality.

PHASE 2: SYMBIOSIS (one through five months)
The infant behaves and functions as if the mother–infant dyad were omnipotent with one common boundary of togetherness. According to the youngster, mother and child are one and mother can anticipate and know the child's every need and want, thus fulfilling them instantaneously.

PHASE 3: SEPARATION–INDIVIDUATION

SUBPHASE A: *Differentiation* (five through nine months)
This subphase is denoted by a decrease in total bodily dependence on the mother with the beginning of walking. This locomotion enacts the first physical separateness from the mother; pulling away from the mother, and visual and tactile exploration of the total environment begins as well.

SUBPHASE B: *Practicing* (nine through fourteen months)
Mastery of walking is the goal in this subphase. The child can now actively move from and return to the mother. The child's awareness of separation and individuation is evident with the growth and functioning of the child's self-awareness and emerging personality. The child is also aware of a special bond with the mother, and strives to make the mother proud and confident.

SUBPHASE C: *Rapprochement* (14 through 24 months)
This is a chaotic period of rediscovery and acknowledgement of the mother as a separate individual. As separateness grows, there develops an increasing need to share every new skill and experience, concomitant with a great need for the mother's devoted love. Feelings of anger and rage toward the mother surface when it becomes apparent that the mother can't predict and understand every need and wish the child has.

SUBPHASE D: *Consolidation of Individuality and Beginnings of Emotional Constancy* (third year)
This is an extremely important intrapsychic period, in the course of which a stable sense of entity is attained. This phase includes the establishment of a measure of self-constancy, along with external person (object) constancy. A transition occurs in which the more primitive ambivalent love relationship with the mother changes into a more mutually satisfying love relationship. An image of a constant and nurturing mother becomes internalized in the establishment of emotional and feeling components of the personality.

---

survive), and *object constancy*. For example, when infants are born, the primary concern is for self. The need for initial survival in a strange environment does not allow infants to consider anyone but self (narcissism). Meeting infants' needs for food, shelter, and love is called *need gratification*. As these needs are met by a constant object (mother), infants develop a sense of knowing someone will be there to feed, clothe, and love them. Thus, they develop a sense of object constancy.[17,22,28] This theoretical framework provides the basis for a holistic view of humans.

Introjection (taking in) of the object begins in the first few months of life when infants split the whole object (mother) into parts—the good object (good mother) and the bad object (bad mother). For example, the good mother feeds the infant when it is hungry, and the bad mother does not. Survival is the basic postulate behind infants' need to do this, because infants are dependent on their mothers for life. Infants fear annihilation when their aggressive impulses come to the foreground, and they must *split* the good from the bad in order to survive. If there is no splitting, the loss of the good object, if only temporary, is felt by the infant as anguish, and is intensely mourned for. The loss of the good object is felt with such sorrow and desolation by every infant until the good ob-

jects are secured within themselves that Klein calls this state of anxiety the *depressive position*.[22,23] Infants must first split the good object (good mother) from the bad object (bad mother), and then integrate them into a whole object (a mother who has both good and bad qualities). The process of achieving this is an important part of development. Figure 6-2 depicts the internal process of the infant as the infant first splits the good and bad aspects of the mother, and later integrates the two.

Present-day object-relations theorists include Masterson,[30] whose concepts are presented in Chapter 19, Personality Disorders, and Kernberg.[20] Kohut,[24] who had a background in object-relations, ventured into a separate subset of psychological theory with his focus on the self as an integral part of treatment. He began a new construct, the field of *self psychology*.

In the psychoanalytic institutes and conferences today, much deliberation about and validation of the differing theories still occurs, serving to provide psychotherapists and their clients with varying and at times controversial viewpoints as to the optimal course of treatment. Many of the leading psychoanalysts favor one theorist, yet are also able to integrate other theorists' constructs and ideology into their conceptualizations of their clients' treatment. Keeping in mind their differing psy-

Object Relations

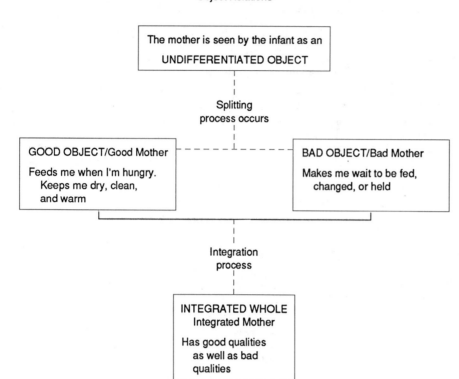

Figure 6-2. Object relations theory is demonstrated in an infant's view of its mother, first as an undifferentiated object. The infant then splits the view, seeing the mother as entirely good or entirely bad at any specific time. Finally, integration takes place, whereby the infant is able to see both good and bad qualities in the mother.

chological frameworks, ego psychologists and object-relation theorists would most likely agree that (1) treatment is provided on an individualized basis, centered on the dynamics and conflicts of the particular client, and (2) the need to work through and resolve past familial experiences requires intensive treatment, encompassing two to five weekly sessions over a period of many years.

Significance to Nurses

Having a foundation in psychoanalytic theory is essential for psychiatric nurses because: it encourages nurses to see clients in the present as well as in the past; it provides a strong theoretical basis for many of the later psychological theories; psychiatric nurses will work with psychiatrists and their clients who are in psychoanalysis; it is important to understand the tenets of this field; much of the current literature that looks at personality disorders focuses on a psychoanalytic framework to understand the origins of these complex diagnoses; most of the common psychiatric terms are rooted in Freudian concepts, such as transference and countertransference; psychiatric nurses often experience a heightened transference from psychiatric clients due to the milieu structure and the amount of time nurses spend with the clients, and therefore it is important for nurses to understand, in depth, the complexities of transference; psychiatric nurses often experience heightened countertransference with their clients, also due to the structure of the milieu and the issues that clients stir up in nurses.

The Interpersonal Theory of Psychiatry

Harry Stack Sullivan developed the interpersonal theory of psychiatry, and is well known for his work with schizophrenic patients. In 1922 he was one of two psychiatrists in the United States who believed that individuals with schizophrenia were curable or treatable. Although he was influenced by Freud and went through a brief classical analysis period, he abandoned Freud's pleasure principle and theories of psychosexual development. Like Freud, Sullivan believed a person's past history enters into present behavior, and he looked for arrested development. He felt that the interpersonal relationships in the home, school, or environment influenced an individual's development. In 1938 he began developing his theory, in which he proposed four generic factors that influence interpersonal development:[35,36]

1. Biological potentiality
2. The level of maturation
3. The results of previous experiences
4. Foresight

He felt that personality developed over a period of 20 or more years, in contrast to Freud's belief that development took place in the first five years. He proposed that personality developed as a result of a person's social relationships, and he felt that these could be greatly modified by favorable or unfavorable conditions.

Sullivan treated schizophrenics as individuals, rather

than as cases, in order to assist clients to build self-esteem. He set up a special ward for male schizophrenics at Sheppard and Enoch Pratt Hospital in Maryland, and trained the health care workers in using his concepts.[34,35,36]

The core of Sullivan's theory is maximizing satisfaction (*euphoria*) and minimizing insecurity (*tension*). Basic to maximizing satisfaction is meeting the biological needs for food, air, water, sex, and elimination. In addition, needs that are both biological and psychological are the needs for power and physical closeness.[35,36] Tension results when a bodily need is not met, and tension continues to rise until satisfaction is gained. In the same manner, tension results when interpersonal security is threatened if a significant person offers disapproval. This can be real or imagined disapproval. With his focus on infancy, Sullivan explored how anxiety within the mother was transferred to her infant.[35] This transferring process was originally termed *empathy* in his early writings. In the interpersonal relationship with the mother, the growing child formulates a self-system, a means of organizing events in the environment to defend and minimize anxiety while searching for, and securing, satisfaction. Sullivan coined the *good-me, bad-me,* and *not-me* components of the self-system that a child learns through experiences in childhood. Positive and approved-of behaviors are the good-me. Negative behaviors are the bad-me. Behaviors that generate heightened levels of anxiety, thus forcing the child to deny participating in the behavior, are termed not-me.

Infancy is the stage of development in which individuals are essentially helpless. The mothering person becomes the focus of the infants, and in the early stages of infancy they are unable to differentiate themselves from their mothers. When all of their needs, biological and psychological, are met, they experience a state of euphoria or complete satisfaction. Tension arises when the needs are unmet, and continues to rise until the needs are met. Sullivan believed tensions in the mothering person are also felt by the infant. Toward the end of infancy, development of language allows the infant to perceive the good mother and the bad mother, which are precursors of the good-me, bad-me, and not-me.

Childhood is the stage of development when individuals begin to learn the essentials of their culture. Language is a primary developmental task for children, and their parents remain their primary interpersonal relations. If the children do not experience too many disappointments in having their needs met, they will learn to sublimate their impulses into socially acceptable channels. If there is too much tension, children may not be able to respond in a positive way to affection from other people. This anxiety may result in a lack of self-confidence and self-esteem.

The *juvenile era* is the stage of development when individuals need peers. It is a time for becoming social, gaining scholastic skills, learning to compete, and learning to cooperate. Children learn that they must adjust to the outside world because they are no longer the center of attraction. They learn about group identification and what it means to be outside the group. During this period, children learn to use *selective inattention:* whatever occurs that they don't understand is ignored. Excessive use of this defense can lead to problems in establishing healthy interpersonal relationships. During this period children also learn to postpone gratification, and learn to think in a more mature, logical fashion that allows foresight.

Preadolescence is the stage of development when there is a need for an intimate relationship with a peer of the same sex. This friendship, when fully developed, is always a reciprocal relationship. This is the precursor to learning to love another person. If there have been too many traumas in the earlier stages of development, intimate relationships may be impaired, and loneliness can become a way of life.

Early adolescence is the time when intimacy with the same sex begins to take second place to interest in the opposite sex. Daydreaming and fantasies abound, and chums may discuss the best way to win favors from the opposite sex. This is the stage when sexual patterns develop. The adolescent has a need for personal security, intimacy, and sexual genital satisfaction.

Late adolescence and maturity is the stage of development when the individual who has attained a pattern of sexual intimacy moves into a pattern of mature interpersonal relationships. During early and late adolescence, the task is to come to terms with lust. If these experiences are not fraught with opposition, a more mature person, who is capable of genuine intimacy with another person, emerges. If too many tensions are experienced, regression to the earlier juvenile era occurs, and the person becomes an egocentric (self-centered) person.[35]

Significance to Nurses

Sullivan's theory is important for psychiatric nurses because psychiatric nursing is about interpersonal relationships. Sullivan encourages empathy development and the ability to listen in a positive and genuine way. Peplau's theory of nursing is strongly influenced by Sullivan's work. To use Peplau's framework effectively, nurses should also be familiar with the tenets of Sullivan's work, because psychiatrists and their clients are involved in Sullivanian psychotherapy, and understanding the treatment approach of the psychotherapist can benefit the client and the interdisciplinary treatment team. Because Sullivan influenced other contemporary theorists, to understand current psychotherapeutic debates, a knowledge of Sullivanian treatment is strongly recommended.

Client-Centered Psychotherapy

Carl Rogers, an American psychologist, was born into a close-knit farming family. Rogers stated that his early teachers encouraged his ability to be original and unique in his thinking. He later spent two years in a theological seminary that was committed to a freedom of philosophical thought, and that respected honest attempts to resolve problems.

Rogers studied clinical psychology, including Freudian theory and behavioral psychology. Rogers also studied the ideas of Rank, who felt that individuals have self-directing capacities that emerge through psychotherapeutic intervention. Rank's ideas complimented Roger's beliefs about the dignity of individuals, as well as his extensive experience with clients.[31]

In the 1940s, Roger's methods of therapy became well known. At this time two major influences dominated the field of psychotherapy in the United States: psychoanalysis and directive counseling. *Directive counseling* involved the concept that therapists are *experts* who diagnose their subjects and select the direction clients take in therapy. These clinicians act with little regard for what clients think about themselves. Rogers wrote that his "disillusionment with these techniques inevitably occurred as therapists discovered that, even though they *knew* what was wrong with a client and *what* the client should do to change, neither of these aspects of the therapists's knowledge promoted the client's changing his/her behavior."[32]

Rogers proposed a counseling relationship that includes warmth and responsiveness from the therapist, a permissive climate in which the client's feelings can be expressed easily, and freedom from pressure and coercion on the part of the therapist. Roger's approach is called *client-centered,* to focus on the growth-producing factors in the client. Rogers viewed the client as one whose self-concept had developed in an incomplete manner. Clinicians using Roger's approach *respond to the client's affect.* The clinician is then required to "get behind the words of the client and into his feeling world (to obtain an) accurate empathic understanding."[32]

If a therapist firmly demonstrates an attitude of respect for, and confidence in, the client's capacity to live a healthy and positive life, Rogers believed that the client would then experience an increase in self-respect and self-confidence. With a climate of unconditional acceptance and positive regard, Rogers contended that the client would realize the unconscious material, and with this knowledge present behavior and feelings would change.

Significance to Nurses

One of the most essential ingredients required by a psychiatric nurse using the client-centered model, is the ability to exude warmth and respect for the client, regardless of degree of pathology, socioeconomic lifestyle, or occupation. Roger's theory clearly emphasizes the need for the listener to respect and warmly accept the client as a person first. Second, nurses must encourage development of self-respect and self-confidence. Rogers addresses how these aspects of the client can be developed in the context of the relationship. Third, with a stronger emphasis on the "here and now," Rogers presents a realistic theoretical construct that can be used in the psychiatric hospital milieu with fast-paced, changing clients having multiple diagnoses and levels of psychopathology.

Learning Theories

Recently, learning theorists recognized that people learn better if they are told what is happening and what to expect. They learn from watching others perform modeling behavior, which is rewarded or punished.

Stimulus–response learning and observational learning theory are complex areas that have generated numerous hypotheses and many research studies.

Stimulus–Response Learning

John Dollard and Neal Miller[7] adapted learning theory to encompass the sociological behavior of the human being. Specifically, Miller and Dollard stated that human behavior is learned, and expanded learning theory to include the social conditions under which learning takes place. *Social learning theory,* therefore, is firmly based on learning theory, in which all important social behaviors are understandable through familiar psychological principles of learning.[7] This theory was a milestone in stimulus–response psychology because it demonstrated that social analysis can be combined with experimental methods—for example, social research can be done using objective data and objective analysis of the data.

Observational Learning

Bandura and Walter's[3] work on learning by imitation is classic, and is known today as *modeling.* The three major forms of learning that can be attributed to learning through the observation of a model include:

1. Learning new patterns of behavior
2. Learning to increase or decrease the intensity of a previously learned inhibition (to repress, or control a feeling or behavior)
3. Learning to imitate the behavior of others without acquiring new patterns of behavior

Observational learning involves four basic processes:

1. Attention to the model
2. Retention of relevant model cues
3. Reproduction of the model's performance
4. Motivation incentive to perform, known as reinforcement

Developmentally, a child learns new patterns of behavior, learns to increase or decrease behavior, and learns to imitate parents or other significant people in the environment through observational learning.

Significance to Nurses

Learning theory is important in psychiatric nursing because much of the therapeutic work done includes teaching new, more adaptive methods of coping. To be sure that clients are in an optimal state to receive this knowledge suggests that nurses must have a good foundation in learning theory. Second, many of clients' maladaptive behaviors have been learned, and thus can be altered and relearned if clients are provided with the right combination of learning material and comfort. Third, most child and adolescent psychiatric units utilize a behavioral, and/or social learning, organization to work with the clients. To be able to work effectively with the clients in these units, mastery of learning theory is suggested.

Summary

1. Personality development occurs as a result of both physiological and psychological processes.
2. Consistent patterns of development do occur, and can be predicted.
3. Important psychic structures in the psychoanalytic model include the id, ego, and superego.
4. Defense mechanisms develop to protect the ego from overwhelming anxiety.
5. Mahler's theory encompasses the use of separation-individuation as the major organizing principle of human development.
6. Sullivan's interpersonal theory emphasizes the importance of interpersonal interaction and one's development and sense of well-being.
7. Rogers's client-centered theory encourages self-respect and self-confidence.
8. Learning theorists are concerned with the physical readiness of the individual to develop cognitive skills.
9. Bandura and Walters's work on learning by imitation (modeling) is an important contribution to developmental theory.

References

1. American Nurses' Association: Taxonomy for the Classification of Human Responses of Concern for Psychiatric/Mental Health Nursing Practice. Kansas City, American Nurses' Association, 1986
2. American Psychiatric Association: Diagnostic and Statistical Manual-III-Revised. Washington, DC, American Psychiatric Association, 1987
3. Bandura A, Walters R: Social Learning and Personality Development. New York, Holt, Rinehart & Winston, 1963
4. Blanck G, Blanck G: Ego Psychology: Theory and Practice. New York, Columbia University Press, 1974
5. Blanck G, Blanck G: Ego Psychology II: Psychoanalytic Developmental Psychology. New York, Columbia University Press, 1979
6. Blaney P: Implications of the Medical Model and Its Alternatives. Am J Psychiatry 1332:9, 1975
7. Dollard J, Miller N: Learned Drive and Learned Reinforcement. In Dalbir, Stewart J (eds): Motivation. Baltimore, Penguin Books, 1973
8. Freud A: Psychoanalytic Psychology of Normal Development. In The Basic Writings of Anna Freud, Vol VIII, 1970–1980. New York, International Universities Press, 1969
9. Freud A: The Ego and the Mechanisms of Defense. New York, International Universities Press, 1966
10. Freud S: The Basic Writings of Sigmund Freud. Brill A (ed). New York, The Modern Library, 1938
11. Freud S: The Ego and the Id. New York, WW Norton, 1960
12. Freud S: New Introductory Lectures on Psychoanalysis: New York, WW Norton, 1965
13. Gorkin M: The Uses of Countertransference. New York, Jason Aronson, 1987
14. Graves J: Psychoanalytic theory—a critique. Perspect Psychiatr Care 11:69, 1973
15. Guntrip H: Schizoid Phenomena, Object Relations, and the Self. New York, International Universities Press, 1969
16. Hartmann H: Ego Psychology and the Problem of Adaptation. New York, International Universities Press, 1958
17. Horner A: Object Relations and the Developing Ego in Therapy. New York, Jason Aronson, 1979
18. Jacobson E: The Self and the Object World. New York, International Universities Press, 1964
19. Kaplan H, Sudock B: Modern Synopsis of Comprehensive Textbook of Psychiatry. Baltimore, Williams & Wilkins, 1966
20. Kernberg O: Object Relations Theory and Clinical Psychoanalysis. New York, Jason Aronson, 1976
21. Klein M: Some Theoretical Conclusions Regarding the Emotional Life of the Infant. In Riviere J (ed): Developments in Psycho-Analysis. London, Hogarth, 1952
22. Klein M: Notes on Some Schizoid Mechanisms. In Envy and Gratitude. New York, Basic Books, 1957
23. Klein M: Envy and Gratitude and Other Works, 1946–1963, Vol III. New York, Free Press, 1975
24. Kohut H: The Restoration of the Self. New York, International Universities Press, 1977
25. Kris E: On some vicissitudes of insight in psychoanalysis. Int J Psychoanal 37:445, 1956
26. Maddi S: Personality Theories: A Comparative Analysis. Homewood, IL, Dorsey Press, 1973
27. Mahler M: On Human Symbiosis and the Vicissitudes of Individuation. New York, International Universities Press, 1968
28. Mahler M, Pine F, Bergman A: The Psychological Birth of the Human Infant. New York, Basic Books, 1975
29. Mahler M: Selected Papers of Margaret M. Mahler, M.D., Vols I and II. New York, Jason Aronson, 1979
30. Masterson J: Treatment of the Borderline Adolescent: A Developmental Approach. New York, John Wiley & Sons, 1972
31. Meador B, Rogers C: Person-Centered Therapy. In Corsini R (ed): Current Psychotherapies. Itasca, IL, Peacock, 1984
32. Rogers C: The necessary and sufficient conditions of therapeutic personality change. J Consult Psychol 21:95, 1957
33. Segal H: Introduction to the Work of Melanie Klein. New York, Basic Books, 1973
34. Sullivan H: Schizophrenia as a Human Process. New York, Putnam, 1962
35. Sullivan H: The Interpersonal Theory of Psychiatry. New York, WW Norton, 1953
36. Sullivan H: The Psychiatric Interview. New York, WW Norton, 1970

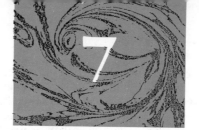

MARGARET L. FRANKS AND DIANA E. OLSON

GROWTH AND DEVELOPMENT ACROSS THE LIFE SPAN: A SYSTEMS PERSPECTIVE

Learning Objectives

Upon completion of this chapter the student should be able to do the following:

1. List Erikson's eight stages of man and the tasks associated with each stage.
2. List each developmental period and the appropriate age range according to Freud's psychosexual developmental theory.
3. Describe how Piaget's stages of development apply to client behavior.
4. Discuss the implications of the various theories for your client's developmental stage, assessing for physical and emotional problems.
5. List Kübler-Ross's five stages of dying, and give examples of behaviors within each stage.

Introduction

Although the process of human development is complex, nurses need to be aware of the various psychological, sociocultural, and biological factors present. Change, growth, and adaptation are the main themes of development. It is important for nurses to understand the process of growth and development in order to be able to assess whether clients are progressing above or below normal parameters. An understanding of growth and develop-

ment also allows nurses to appreciate the individuality of each client as clients progress through the various stages. Determining whether a lack of progress in selected areas is indicative of an illness process facilitates early case-finding (primary prevention) when expected levels of growth and development are not achieved.

Biological changes are accompanied by psychological and sociocultural tasks in each stage of development. The rate of growth varies in each stage because individuals vary in their rates of development. In this chapter, the concepts of biological, psychological, and sociocultural development and environmental effects are integrated into each developmental stage in the life cycle.

Growth is defined as the physiological progress through which the person "assimilates or transforms essential, nonliving nutrients into living protoplasm." Cell size increase is an example of growth. *Development* includes those physiological processes whereby an "individual progresses from an undifferentiated state to a highly organized and functional capacity." Cell specialization is an example of development. Development implies an "increase in skill and in complexity of function."[7] Increased psychological specialization accompanies physiological growth and development.

As mentioned in the Introduction, systems theory is a perspective that psychiatric/mental health nurses use to understand the client. The client is viewed as a unique human being who is a "system" of parts. These parts of the system are the psychological, cultural, biological, societal, and environmental components. In this chapter, systems theory will be explained, using the work of Putt as a reference.[29]

General Systems Theory

Many scientists (including nursing scientists) have found it useful in their practice to look at nature as a system. The word system implies a collective. Hence, nature is seen as a collective of parts. Both the parts and the collective of parts have their own definition and characteristics.

Systems theory (or general systems theory) was developed by Ludwig von Bertalanffy, who attempted to formulate principles common to diverse systems encountered in a wide variety of scientific disciplines. Many disciplines, including nursing, use systems theory.

A *system* can be defined as a set of relationships between objects and their properties or attributes.[29] Relationships tie the system together, making it a functional unit. In the field of chemistry, one such relationship is a chemical bond. In the field of psychiatric/mental health nursing, an important relationship is the interpersonal bond between the Self and Others.

Around every individual is an *environment*. This environment affects the system and may cause changes in the system. In Figure 7-1, the "environment" is presented as an element of the person because the environment affects the person, as in the example of an individual's neighborhood. Other system elements that influence the person are societal, psychological, biological, and cultural factors.

The nurse uses systems theory by keeping the following systems theory principles in mind:

1. Every system has a *structure,* or an arrangement of parts. For example, a Self has a particular type of arrangement, such as a bond or attachment with significant Others. Systems theory directs us to look at the structure or arrangement of parts of the system. Other conceptual frameworks, such as the concep-

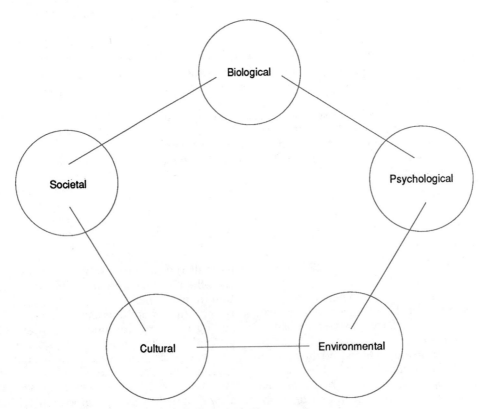

Figure 7-1. The interdependent units of systems analysis.

RELEVANT RESEARCH

The purpose of this study was to determine nurses' degree of awareness of the impact of parental alcoholism on children. A random sample of 500 nurses was drawn from a Board of Nursing list of all nurses registered to practice in a Midwestern state. These nurses were sent questionnaires designed by the authors to measure knowledge of the impact of parental alcoholism on children with alcoholic parents, as well as selected characteristics of the respondents. A total of 265 nurses completed the questionnaires.

Content validity of the questionnaire concerning the impact of alcoholism on children was established by two nationally recognized individuals who work with the children of alcoholics. Reliability of the tool was assessed by administering the tool to 30 nurses. Internal consistency of the tool using Cronbach's Alpha was r = .76.

Two thirds of the respondents reported having contact with alco-

holics in the clinical setting, while 40% stated that they had similar contact with children of alcoholics. The majority of the sample were staff nurses, and 48% worked full-time. Forty-two percent of the respondents worked in medical-surgical nursing, while 10% worked in psychiatric nursing.

The subjects were generally knowledgeable about the effects of parental alcoholism on children. These items in the questionnaire included references to the children's feelings of powerlessness. The nurses were less knowledgeable about the long-term effects on the children. Most subjects did not know that children of alcoholics are more likely to become chronically depressed or suicidal; to become alcoholics or marry alcoholics; or to minimize their feelings. Only 11% of the nurses remembered hearing specifically about the children of alcoholics in their nursing education program.

Arneson S, Schultz M, Triplett J: Nurses' knowledge of the impact of parental alcoholism on children. Arch Psychiatr Nurs 1:251, 1987

tual framework of Self and Others presented in Chapter 5, that come from outside systems theory are needed to describe further the structure of *parts* of the system.

Each discipline will have its own conceptual framework to further define each of these principles listed for describing a system.

2. Each system has a characteristic *process* or way of functioning. Within each system (and between the system and the environment), matter, energy, or information is processed.

3. Each system is part of a *hierarchy of order*. For example, a family system is part of a *suprasystem* of a particular culture, and within this same family system are subsystems, *e.g.,* each particular family member. The aspect of interest to the nurse at a particular time is referred to as the system or the "unit of analysis." The focus or "unit of analysis" may change as client needs change.

An example of the need for the nurse to change the clinical focus or unit of analysis is described in

a study by Arneson, Schultz, and Triplett[1] (see the above Relevant Research box). The authors found that, although nurses were knowledgeable about adult alcoholism, few understood the long-term effects on the children of alcoholics. This indicates a difficulty in shifting the nurse's unit of analysis from the identified client, the alcoholic, to others affected by the disease (the children). Figure 7-2 demonstrates the need to shift focus.

4. Within a system there is an *interdependence* of parts. One part or subsystem can affect an entire system. However, the degree of this effect occurs on a continuum.

5. Systems can be either *closed* or *open,* depending on what the system lets out into the environment or what the system allows in from the environment.

6. Healthy systems maintain a *steady state,* or a state of relative adaptation. A system in a state of equilibrium may be a rigid one that is vulnerable to environmental changes.

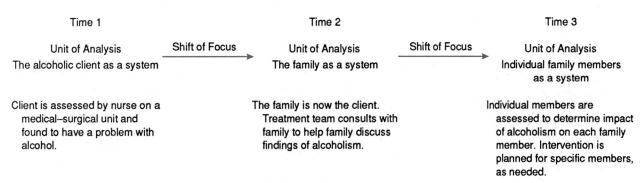

Figure 7-2. The shift of focus or unit of analysis by a medical-surgical nurse.

7. Systems can self-correct by using *feedback*. Feedback is a process whereby a portion of the output of matter, energy, or information from the system to the environment is returned from the environment to the system as *input*. Through the use of this input, the system can adjust itself. For example, a system (the family) has just moved to a new location. Family members extend greetings to their neighbors (output). The neighbors return the greeting (input back to the system). The family then adjusts its processing in response to this input to extend greetings on a permanent basis.

8. A closed system tends to become random in its organization and to dissipate its energy. This tendency is termed *entropy*. The final effect of entropy is death. The evolution of a system toward higher complexity is termed *negentropy*.

9. A system contains parts that have particular roles. As one family member will be a *controller* of decision-making, another will be a *trigger* to signal the presence of anxiety in the system, and so on.

10. A system is a *whole*. A system as a whole is more than the simple addition of its parts; it has a character of its own. For example, a particular group therapy collection of people has a "group feeling" to itself that is much more than looking at individual personalities within the group.

The following sections will emphasize the importance of particular system (person) parts—on the growth, development, and well-being of the system (see Fig. 7-1).

Childhood

Childhood is the first 12 years of the life cycle. It is divided into four main stages: prenatal, infancy, early childhood, and late childhood. Change and adaptation dominate the life of a child from the moment of conception through the last year of childhood. Physical changes are the fastest and most dramatic of the entire life cycle during the prenatal and early years. Accompanying the physical changes are important psychological and social changes and adaptations. Studies in developmental psychology have demonstrated that patterns of growth and change exist in all stages of life, starting with childhood. The patterns are thought to be due to powerful inner forces or pressures for growth interacting with stimulation from the environment. Although development proceeds according to a predictable sequence, individuals develop at different rates. One baby will walk at 9 months, whereas another one will walk at 16 months of age. Individuals have their own styles of development. Some progress cautiously and slowly, while others take periodic big leaps.

Prenatal Development

At conception, millions of sperm are released by the male and move forward, approaching and surrounding the ovum. Only one sperm enters the membrane to fertilize the ovum or form a fertilized cell. The sperm, completely submerged in the ovum, dissolves, and its genetic material is set free. The genes of the two parents combine to form a new individual. At seven weeks of gestation, the developing embryo is about 1¼ inches long, and already beginning to differentiate into the systems and body parts that make up a human being. By the eleventh week, the unborn baby, now called a fetus, is about three inches long and weighs one ounce. The fetus can kick and turn its head; it has fingernails, toenails, eyelids, vocal cords, lips, and nose, and its sex can be identified. By the end of four months, the fetus is about 6 inches long and weighs 7 ounces. All of the organs have been formed, and the remainder of its life *in utero* is spent in continued growth and refinement of structures.

Environmental factors affect the life of the fetus in the uterus. Good maternal nutrition is an absolute requirement. During pregnancy a mother needs about 20% more calories than usual and approximately twice as much protein. Her daily intake should include fresh fruits, vegetables, and grains for adequate fiber. In countries with severe food shortages, the rate of stillbirths and premature births increases sharply.

Cultural factors also affect the life of the fetus. A pregnant black woman may engage in the practice of "geophagy," or eating clay and dirt. This practice was common in Africa. It was believed to be beneficial to the mother and unborn child. The clay was in fact rich in iron. When clay was not available in the U.S., Argo starch was substituted. This practice can lead to anemia, because the starch gives the feeling of fullness. The more starch that is eaten, the greater the anemia, and the more the person craves the clay or starch.[36]

A woman's cultural background plays a dominant role in how she cares for herself during pregnancy. For example, there is the belief in some cultures that certain foods and medicines have an inherent "hot" quality and can therefore cause diaper rash in newborn infants; as a result, the expectant mothers avoid these foods during pregnancy. The concept of balance is important in many cultures. The hot–cold theory is an example from some Hispanic cultures.[18] The hot–cold theory designations do not depend on the temperature of the food or medicine, but rather on the presumed effects in the body. The Chinese believe in the opposing but complementary forces of Yin and Yang. Yin is all that is negative and female. Yin is dark, wet, and cold. Yang is positive and masculine. It is bright, sunny, and warm.[6] Commitment to cultural beliefs varies among individuals depending on their age, education, social class, and degree of acculturation. The nurse must assess the acculturation of clients to surmise which beliefs and health practices they may ascribe to.

Biological Factors

Illness in the mother, especially during the first trimester, can affect the unborn child. During the 1960s an epidemic of rubella, or German measles, affected many mothers early in their pregnancies. Their babies had defects such as deafness, cataracts, and heart disease. The connection between rubella and birth defects has been implied by clinical research.[32] Thalidomide, a mild tranquilizer, was used to treat morning nausea. Thalidomide caused deformities in hundreds of children. Diseases and drugs can cause damage at any stage of prenatal development. Pregnant women have been advised not to use common drugs, such as alcohol, caffeine, nicotine, and mild tranquilizers.

Maternal stress can cause spontaneous abortion. Thus, psychological factors can affect the fetus and have been thought to cause an increased incidence of malformation in babies. An increased number of anomalies were noted during and after World War II in children of mothers who experienced severe stressors unrelated to nutritional deprivation.[32]

Infancy

Biological Development

A baby is born weak and helpless but ready for growth, change, and adaptation in the life ahead. At birth the nervous system and the muscular system are very immature, and the brain is only one fourth of its adult size. Due to this lack of maturity, the movements of the newborn appear to be uncoordinated and weak. *Reflexes* are the basic mechanisms of response. Some of the major reflexes in the newborn are: the *Moro* or *"startle" reflex,* which may occur in response to any sudden internal or external stimulus, such as a loud noise; the *rooting reflex,* in which babies, when hungry, turn their mouths in the direction of the cheek that is touched;[32] the *palmar grasp reflex,* in which newborns curl their fingers tightly around a small object placed in the palm of the hand; the spontaneous *stepping reflex,* which takes place when the soles of the baby's feet touch an object or surface and the baby makes walking motions; and the *flexor withdrawal reflex,* which protects the newborn by withdrawal of a limb from a source of pain.[4] Blinking the eyes in response to a touch on the eyelid or bright lights, and turning the head to the side to protect the airway if the infant is placed in a facedown position, are other examples of protective reflexes. Most of these reflexes are lost within the first months of life, but sensory development continues.

It is important for the nurse to be aware of infant reflexes, because some clients revert to these reflexes when they experience emotional pain as adults. When these behaviors occur, the nurse should note the behavior and the topic the client is discussing at the time.[38]

Recent research indicates that the newborn is able to see objects by the second day of life, and later becomes able to fixate or to stare at an object. The newborn has a preference for the human face, particularly the mother's face. Providing reciprocity of interaction is very important in infancy. Bowlby found that infants directed four behaviors toward caretakers: following, smiling, clinging, and crying.[3] When these attachment behaviors were unrewarded, severe psychological and physiological responses occurred. The infants did not attempt to communicate, and became stiff and unresponsive.

The newborn has an aversion to bright lights, but sharply contrasting colors and moderately bright, lighted objects will elicit a prolonged fixation behavior.[13] By the third month, binocular coordination is demonstrated when an object is moved about in front of the infant's face.[30] Newborns respond to noises from pans, cans, bells, and whistles, and some respond to human voices by the tenth day. The sense of smell is rather poorly developed in the newborn, as is the sense of taste. The tactile sense of skin is not well developed in the newborn, but by the end of the first year the infant is capable of locating a source of irritation or pressure.

Psychosexual Development

Freud, the founder of the psychoanalytical school of development, believed the prime motivator of human behavior was *libido,* or sexual energy. He called his theory "the psychosexual stages of development."

At birth the infant seeks pleasure, and immediate gratification of all needs. The primary area of gratification is the mouth and lips. Freud called this the *oral stage,* which lasts from birth to age 15 months. The objects of gratification are the breast, bottle, and thumb. Energies of the infant are directed toward nursing and the relationship to the parenting figure. The infant takes in stimuli from the environment, and is particularly sensitive to tactile stimuli. These stimuli are important for later cognitive and emotional development. A continued relationship to the mother's body is important for achieving this tactile stimulation and laying the groundwork for the stages to come.[7]

Cognitive Development

Piaget, a Swiss philosopher trained in zoology, was interested in developmental psychology.[29] Piaget's investigations into the nature of thought and language were mostly clinical. He observed children and their behavior, formulated hypotheses, and then altered the circumstances to test the hypotheses. Piaget's stages of development focus on the child's cognitive or intellectual processes. His first stage is the *sensorimotor,* which lasts from birth to 24 months. Intellectual development proceeds sequentially, as does physical development. As infants grow, their perceptions become finer. Almost from birth, infants prefer to look at a human face. They recognize their parents or primary care-givers, and reserve the most winning smiles and pleasant gurgling sounds for them. Infants also discover ways to affect the world. If they push a ball, it rolls away; if they cry, somebody comes to them. Infants absorb information through the senses and explore the world through physical (motor) activity. The concept of *object permanency* is an important intellectual development. By the age of six months, most infants realize that an object exists even if it can not be seen. Infants will start to look for things or objects. More important, they realize that if the mother leaves the room she will return, that is, she still exists.[28]

One of the infant's most basic needs is for *attachment,* which refers to the bonding or closeness between

TABLE 7-1.
A COMPARISON OF THREE THEORISTS' STAGES OF DEVELOPMENT

AGE	FREUD PSYCHOSEXUAL STAGES	ERIKSON SOCIOCULTURAL STAGES	PIAGET COGNITIVE STAGES
Birth to one year	*Oral stage* Erotic area centered in the mouth. Child sucks and bites, gains pleasure from the mouth. Mother figure needs to provide consistent feeding and nurturing.	*Task:* Trust vs. mistrust Child needs to feel cared for, to have more satisfying experiences than frustrating ones. Child needs to be fed and feel secure. Trust is a confidence in sameness.	*Sensorimotor stage* Baby uses only reflex behavior. Does not have words or symbols for thinking. Parents need to provide stimulation.
One to three years	*Anal stage* Pleasure is centered in the anus. Child enjoys examining bowel movements, and begins to gain control over them. Withholding or giving are traits established during this stage.	*Task:* Autonomy vs. shame and doubt Control of bowel and bladder gives toddler a sense of autonomy. Muscular coordination improves. Toddler has lots of energy and asserts independence by saying "No." A feeling of badness or shame arises from parental punishment. If toddler is never allowed independence, will doubt abilities	*Preoperational thought:* ages two to seven years Child has language and can begin to use symbols for objects. Child has no logical thinking, but generalizes. Child needs independent learning. Intuitive thought leads to faulty conclusions. Child uses assimilation to gain information.
Three to six years	*Oedipal stage* Child loves the parent of the opposite sex. Wants to have that parent all to self. Resolution comes when child decides to grow up to be like the same-sex parent and marry someone like the mother or father. Discovers genitals, and infantile masterbation begins.	*Task:* Initiative vs. guilt Child begins to initiate own actions, no longer merely imitates. Children, if not allowed to explore, may feel guilty about their questions and curiosities.	
Six to twelve years	*Latent stage* No psychic energy is invested in sexual desires. Energy is diverted into cultural mastery and intellectual activities of school.	*Task:* Industry vs. inferiority Children want to do things well. They get rewards at home and at school for doing well. School is the work of children, and they develop habits there that will affect them in later life. These are relatively calm years. If children fall behind at school or do not interact well with peers, they feel inferior.	*Concrete operations:* ages seven to twelve years Children develop ability to use some abstract thought and to discover concrete solutions to everyday problems. Accommodation (the ability to modify ideas to fit reality) increases.
12 to 18 years	*Genital stage* Freud's last stage of growth and development Individual reaches sexual maturity. Earlier conflicts regarding sex reemerge at this time. It isn't an easy time for most people. Sexual feelings return to the mature genitals, and any sexual behavior not involving the genitals is immature behavior.	*Task:* Identity vs. role confusion Adolescents must bring together everything they have learned about themselves and what kind of people they are. They struggle for independence from parents, take on new ideas, reject old ideas, and choose vocations and standards of life. If they are not able to make these decisions about their lives, confusion results.	*Formal operations* Adolescents become able to make use of hypothetical reasoning. They learn to experiment, and can look at reality and use abstract thinking. This level of thinking is the highest level a person can reach. The person is now able to live in the present, the past, and the future.
18 to 35 years		*Task:* Intimacy vs. isolation People commit themselves to affiliations, partnerships, and marriage. There is an emotional intimacy with friends, and a sexual intimacy with a mate. The person who allows intimacy has the capacity to maintain individuality without losing relationships. Avoidance of close relationships is indicative of a failure to gain a sense of intimacy, and results in isolation.	

(Continued)

TABLE 7-1. (CONTINUED)

AGE	FREUD PSYCHOSEXUAL STAGES	ERIKSON SOCIOCULTURAL STAGES	PIAGET COGNITIVE STAGES
35 to 65 years		*Task:* Generativity vs. stagnation. Adults actively participate in establishing or teaching the next generation. The theme is one of caring and concern for others, as well as productivity and creativity. The failure of the above results in stagnation and being minimally involved with others.	
65 years to death		*Task:* Ego integrity vs. despair. Older adults, when looking back over their lives, should view them as acceptable and orderly, and as having purpose; they are satisfied with the way their lives have evolved, and would not change things. The opposite of this is a feeling of despair that one's life has been a failure; the person is full of regrets.	

the child and the mother or primary care-giver. Attachment in infancy is necessary for emotional, social, and intellectual development.

When the child is 12 to 14 months old, the beginning of language occurs. By this age, the child can understand a great deal of what is being said. Thus, it is possible for the parent to give a command or send a warning message. The child starts to speak in words or phrases. This is a breakthrough for the child, since the emotional and intellectual gains and rewards are great.

Sociocultural Development

Erikson, a lay psychoanalyst who studied under Freud, identified eight stages of humans, attempting to explain human development according to clearly identifiable periods during which the foundations for certain behaviors were established.[10] Erikson differed from Freud in that he viewed humans as *social* beings rather than beings controlled by psychosexual motives. Erikson's stages all require the accomplishment of a task to successfully pass through the stage. The task for infancy, birth to one year, is *trust.* Trust is the infant's sense of the world as a satisfying, warm[10] place where care and love are given and protection is offered. The significant relationships that occur during this phase influence all future ones. If trust is not established, the infant could have difficulty establishing close relationships in later stages of development. Table 7-1 summarizes the developmental stages of Freud, Piaget, and Erikson for each age group.

Cultural considerations related to infancy include the finding that some Hispanic cultures believe that a person can look at a child in an admiring way and put the evil eye or *mal ojo* on the child. If you touch the child while looking at it, you break the spell. The *mal ojo* will cause the child to cry and become sick. Rubbing the child all over with an egg and saying prayers will help cure this problem. In Vietnamese culture it is very bad to touch the child on the head. It is believed that this interferes with the child's spirit. It is the nurse's responsibility to assess the cultural beliefs of the family when caring for a young

child. The nurse must decide how cultural practices can be included in treatment plans. To ignore such cultural beliefs may limit the nurse's effectiveness.

Early Childhood

Early childhood, ages two to five years, is a period in which the child grows and matures, and assumes greater physical activity and knowledge of the world. Children separate themselves from their parents and engage in closer relationships with peers.

Biological Development

Significant growth occurs between ages two and five years. Body proportions begin to resemble those of an adult. Fat tissue decreases, while muscle tissue increases. The skeleton becomes harder and larger, making the child more sturdy. The nervous system develops; the brain has grown to about 90% of its adult weight, and the nerve fibers are almost mature. The five-year-old child is now ready to deal with greater intellectual challenges. The child can run, jump, climb, throw, and catch a ball. Fine motor skills develop, including the ability to tie shoes or print letters.

Psychosexual Development

In Freud's second stage of psychosexual development, the libidinal energy moves to the anus. The *anal stage* is 15 months to 3 years of age. The toddler begins to experience some control of bowel and bladder functions at this time. The child experiences pleasure from the act of defecating. In this period, the child is asked for the first time to delay gratification over bodily functions. Toilet training sets up a situation in which the child can receive either approval or disapproval from the parents, depending on the child's willingness to delay gratification or have immediate pleasure. The child may love to play with feces, which parents usually have difficulty tolerating. The use of clay, finger paints, and sand help satisfy this instinctual need in a more acceptable way.

Freud's third stage, the *phallic,* involves a shift of the sexual energy to the genitals. This is also called the Oedipal stage for males. In it, the male directs his energies toward the mother in competition with the father. In the female, this is referred to as the Electra complex. The male child imitates the way the father gives affection to the mother. The male fears retaliation by the father in the form of castration. The child resolves this conflict of wanting the mother and fearing the father by deciding to grow up to be like the father. The child uses the defense mechanism of repression to resolve this conflict unconsciously. Identification with the adult of the same sex allows successful completion of this stage by the three- to six-year-old child.

Cognitive Development

Piaget defined the cognitive development period as the *preoperational stage,* meaning that the child cannot perform a mental operation requiring flexibility or an expanded view. Although children's language is similar to that of adults, their thinking processes and capabilities are not the same as in adults. Two- to four-year-old children cannot categorize objects in more than one dimension—for example, an object cannot be both round and red. The thinking of children is egocentric. Children believe that theirs are the only viewpoints. Children cannot see or understand another's feelings. They are surprised when you do not see things their way.[28] Children gain knowledge and practice problem-solving through play. Preschool children, like infants, are rooted in the sensory world and learn by concrete experiences. They are able to think symbolically, using symbols to represent ideas. Learning is through imitation without understanding of cause-and-effect relationships. Concept formation is beginning for preschoolers, however. They become aware of objects as concrete and separate from the environment. Language is used to get attention, to gain information, and to promote and maintain relationships.

Four- to seven-year-old children are able to integrate concepts on more than one dimension. They can conceive of groups, or classes, as having a relationship. This is the beginning of the system that continues to develop as they mature.

A nurse can find examples of clients' behavior illustrating Piaget's principles. A particular hospitalized client, Ann, believed that the television commentator was talking to her when he said the word "and." This behavior indicates the preoperational characteristics of egocentrism and the inability to see other's perceptions, focusing rather on a detail.

Sociocultural Development

Erikson sees the developmental task to be accomplished in early childhood as *autonomy vs. shame and doubt.* One- to three-year-olds need to become independent of parents and seek out new experiences. Supportive parents can help children develop their own skills and abilities and make some decisions for themselves. If parents are too restrictive or continually put down the child's efforts, feelings of self-doubt can arise and the child may become timid and passive.

Autonomy is also gained with a sense of control over bowel and bladder functions. Shame and doubt can be instilled by parents by rigidity in bowel training and demands for perfection that the child cannot reach. Toilet training also serves as a socializing mechanism for children. They learn that the act of elimination, regardless of where they are, is socially unacceptable. The desire to please others is present at the age of two, so they try to make their care-taker happy by doing what that person desires. Children also learn that others enjoy them more when they are dry and clean.[32]

The next stage, from three to six years, is when young children begin to develop their own identities. Erikson describes the task for this period as *initiative vs. guilt.* Children are developing consciences, internalizing the values of their parents. If they do something wrong or even think about doing something wrong, they may feel guilty. If the parents provide support, help, and understanding, children will continue to try to do the right behaviors.

Play is an important mode of learning and expressing, as well as a source of pleasure to children. Children deal with their experiences and make sense of the world through play. "Imaginative play" is a mechanism for dealing with feelings. "Doctoring" or "nursing" can help children deal with the powerful emotions that arise when visiting the doctor or hospital. Children progress from solitary play to cooperating with other children in a group. They need to explore, discover, and experiment to use this initiative. They also have curiosity about their own bodies. They may be found exploring their bodies and playing with their genitals. Guilt may arise from parental overreaction to this behavior. The parents' matter-of-fact attitude about the children's play, and the use of distraction, will help to resolve this stage successfully. Children also learn social roles and responsibilities and modes of coping to reduce anxieties as greater awareness of the feelings of love, hate, anger, and tension develops.

Later Childhood

The years between ages 6 and 12 are known as *later childhood.* Dramatic changes occur during this span. Six-year-olds start school, eager to learn to read and write, while children of age 12 years are physically and emotionally on the verge of adolescence.

Biological Development

The nervous system develops rapidly. Neurological maturity is reached by about age eight years, and rapid expansion of cognitive and body competencies occurs. Prolonged physical exercise can be tolerated. Basic motor skills improve steadily from ages 6 to 12 years. Fine motor skills continue to develop and improve. For example, a child learns to write, and the handwriting improves steadily.

Psychosexual Development

Freud's *latency stage* of six- to twelve-year-olds is a relatively calm period. Freud was unable to discern any sexual energy focus—thus the term *latency* for the stage. Children develop more intellectually at this time. Behaviors include same-sex groupings. Boys' clubs, Girl Scouts, or clique activities are important. Sex is rejected, as is the opposite sex. This is the time of the true homosexual period; the affinities of children are with those of their own sex. Children begin to move out of the family system and are exposed to the values and attitudes of others through school, peers, and church.

Cognitive Development

School-age children must adapt themselves to the complexities of the school situation. Piaget calls this the *concrete operations period,* encompassing seven to eleven years of age. This period involves using reasoning through real or imaginary situations. Cause-and-effect relationships begin to be recognized. Classification skills, or the ability of children to differentiate and coordinate two crucial properties of a class, develop. Children can also begin grouping, which means they can do a series of operations, such as forming combinations and rearranging them.[28] For example, they may group objects, such as balls, in one pile. They then classify the balls by color, *e.g.,* all red balls in one spot and all yellow balls in another.

When children perform concrete operations, they use the skill of conservation. *Conservation,* one of Piaget's concepts, involves the ability to see that a quantity does not change even if the form does. Children realize that the amount of water does not change even when poured from a short glass into a tall thin one. This ability leads to the beginning of abstraction and early problem-solving.[29]

Sociocultural Development

The task Erikson describes for this stage is *industry vs. inferiority.* The work of the child is school. Children who excel at school, who relate well with peers, and who have feelings of self-worth are setting the tone for later experiences in life. Children become part of a group. School has its own rules, regulations, objectives, goals, and definition of excellence. Some children may have their sense of industry weakened at school and need to have it built up at home or by special assistance in school. Some of these children may accept the verdict that they are inferior, and will want to withdraw in despair. Others will compensate to overcome feelings of inferiority by excelling in different areas. For example, the child who is unsuccessful as an athlete may strive to excel in mathematics or science.

Children in this stage are able to see a need for reciprocity and equality between individuals. A belief in the sacredness of human life is developed. A school-age child usually has a predominant partner or chum of the same sex. There is a decreasing dependency on the family, with more self-direction becoming evident, although the school-age child continues to imitate the behaviors of adults. Additional developmental tasks in this stage include developing positive attitudes toward other social, racial, and economic groups, and giving and receiving affection from family members and friends without expecting immediate return from the other person.

Bilingual and bicultural educational programs are needed for children who speak little or no English. Thus, ethnic minorities can share with the existing culture and in turn enrich their own cultures. Oral language is the primary or "true" language. Writing and reading are dependent on the child's competency in oral language. Teachers and care-givers may need to be reminded of this fact in language development.

Mental Health in Childhood

The presence or absence of mental health in a child is difficult to determine. In assessing the mental health of a child, the setting or background in which the child is living and developing should be considered. The relationships among members of the family are important—for example, the relationship between the parents, parents and child, and child and siblings. Child-rearing practices and warmth and affection within the family group influence the mental health of the child.

When a young child is hospitalized for an emotional problem, it is imperative that the nurse assess the child's family situation. The interdependence of the family members is significant, as the child frequently mirrors problems of a dysfunctional family. The family system is one of the few systems the child knows, and thus it is important to the emotional growth of the child.

In children, dysfunctional behaviors such as feeding problems, sleep disturbances, or speech impairments (lisping or stuttering, or mutism) may be signs of mental health problems. Childhood schizophrenia, early infantile autism, and hysteria are examples of severe mental health problems.[37]

Adolescence

Change and growth are highly visible components of adolescence, the period of life between ages 12 and 19 years. Because of the rapid and startling changes that occur, some authors refer to this period as a rebirth—a renaissance of body and mind. The individual finally abandons childhood and begins the struggle toward adulthood. Adolescence is, for some individuals, the most difficult and significant period of their lives.

Some cultures have tried to assist adolescents in the

journey to adulthood through various rites, rituals, and ceremonies called the *rites of passage.* For example, among the Delaware Indian tribe of North America, a girl who started her first menstrual period had to depart from the tribe and live in a special hut. Her head was wrapped for 12 days so that she could see nobody. She had to submit to fasts and vomiting, and did no labor while she was in this unclean state. After the period, she was washed and clothed anew but kept in solitary confinement for two months. Then she was brought out and declared eligible for marriage.[15] In contemporary Western society, many adolescents have only vague notions of the guidelines for reaching adulthood.

Biological Development

The most dramatic characteristics of adolescence are the onset of puberty and the physical growth that brings the body to sexual maturity.

Girls usually begin to mature between ages 10 and 13 years, earlier than boys. The ovaries and genitals develop. At about 12 years of age, girls menstruate for the first time. The menstrual cycle is initiated at puberty as two hormones, estrogen and progesterone, are produced by the ovaries. The female pelvis increases in width to accommodate the passage of an infant during the birth process. Protective layers of fat develop under the skin, giving the girl a softer, more rounded appearance. The secondary sex characteristics also emerge. The breasts enlarge and develop, and body hair appears.[39]

Males also experience six years of physical and sexual growth. The genitals and testes mature, and the testes begin to produce sperm and testosterone, the primary male sex hormone. Between the age of 13 and 15, boys may experience a sudden growth in height. Their bodies grow larger and stronger than do girls' bodies due to increased skeletal muscle mass. Secondary sex characteristics appear, including growth of the beard and axillary and pubic hair. The texture of the skin changes and there is increased oil production, which can cause acne. The deepening of the voice results from the growth of the larynx.[39]

When adolescents have reached sexual maturity, the sexual desires are often repressed or delayed, causing confusion and frustration. Adults generally want adolescents to delay sexual gratification until a later date, which may correspond to college, college graduation, finding a real job in the adult world, or some other index of emotional maturity.

As adolescents discover their growing bodies, their biological self-concept becomes extremely important. They spend increased time in front of mirrors studying themselves. Typically, they fear that they may be abnormal or not developing correctly. Boys want to look like other boys and fear that they may be too short or not muscular enough. Girls want to look like other girls; they worry that their breasts are not developing rapidly enough or that their bodies look too boyish and straight. Adolescents are self-conscious about their physical appearance, and can be easily hurt when criticisms or even suggestions about their appearance are made.

Psychosexual Development

Freud's last stage of development is the *genital stage,* when the individual has reached sexual maturity. The sexual drive is now located in the genitals. The adolescent has heightened sexual drives, often expressed in physical ways. This stage marks the culmination of the previous stages. Freud saw the goals for this stage as establishment of heterosexual relationships, separation from libidinal attachment to parents, and increased independence from parents.

According to Freud, individuals who successfully complete this stage will be able to participate freely in both love and work in creative and gratifying ways. Unsuccessful resolution results in individuals who do not progress developmentally and who do not have a well-defined sense of self.

Cognitive Development

In Piaget's learning theory, the stage of *formal operations* begins at about 11 years of age and develops through the teens and adulthood. Piaget and other learning theorists agree that capability in learning depends on the forms of thinking that one is cognitively capable of performing. There are several characteristics of the stage of formal operations. Adolescents can understand metaphors and can perform experiments, as in the chemistry laboratory. They are able to conceptualize a plan based on hypothetical events, consider more than one variable, and identify appropriate strategies of action. Individuals are capable of making self-appraisals. Adolescents are capable of directing thoughts and emotions toward abstract ideals or institutions, such as systems of government or political beliefs. They need guidance and frequent contact with adults, such as teachers and parents, to remain aware of the realities of life. Many adolescents believe that they are unique, which can lead to magical thinking. This means that they believe that they are not subject to the same rules or regulations as other people. A girl may believe that she cannot get pregnant, or a boy may think that he cannot be injured or killed in a car or motorcycle accident. Egocentric, magical thinking may lead to disasters for teenagers and their families; it explains the reasoning that allows some adolescents to risk their futures or their very lives. By the end of adolescence, egocentric feelings and thoughts decrease and individuals realize that, although they are unique, universal rules also apply to them and they share a great deal with other people.

Moral Development

Adolescents make major advances in wisdom and the ability to exercise judgment. Kohlberg's research on moral development reveals that the vast majority of adolescents advance to a stage of moral development that is characterized by respect for law and order and a smoothly functioning society. Some adolescents advance to the highest stage of morality, characterized by the belief in, and respect for, the ideals of human equality and the sanctity of life. Although moral development occurs in previous growth and development stages, the adolescent period marks a "transition from a morality based on laws made by others to a more mature morality based on one's own judgment and convictions."[21]

Sociocultural Development

Erikson sees the task for the adolescent as *identity vs. role confusion*. In this search for personal identity, adolescents gradually come to see themselves as distinct people, separate from their parents and deciding on the kind of person they are in terms of attitudes, beliefs, interests, likes, dislikes, and values. Adolescence is a time of confusion and inner turmoil. The physical, intellectual, and moral developments demand a new self-concept.[11]

The task of identity formation, according to Erikson, is a dynamic process that evolves throughout the life cycle. The components of identity formation are the construction of what the person is and the ability to maintain an acceptable balance between the individual's self-concept and the expectations of society as a whole. The result is a continuing adaptation in search of a "good fit" between the changing self and the changing society. If adolescents are to continue to develop in self-actualizing ways, they need to accomplish successfully the tasks of developing a sense of basic trust, a sense of autonomy, a sense of initiative, and, finally, a sense of industry. These are necessary for the mastery of the skills needed in the adult work world.[25] This identity depends on the synthesis of all the accrued and unique experiences of the individual's life. Young people need their own cognitive skills and aid from older, more experienced people—some who have already achieved a sense of their own identity—in order to achieve a degree of balance between social roles and social demands.

Failure to achieve this identity task results in confusion about every fact of life, such as sex, love, future work, and personal philosophy. One way adolescents work through this confusion is to try different roles on a temporary basis. One individual may try dancing, another may try acting, and still another may try law or politics. In this way, young people get some idea of the tasks assigned to the role and the lifestyle associated with the role before committing themselves to the role on a permanent basis.

Affiliation: Best Friends and Peer Group Influences.

A best friend is an individual with whom one can explore the world, the self, the other's ideals, and fantasies. The best friend is very important to the adolescent. Adolescents spend hours on the telephone with friends, sharing the happenings of the day and exploring their thoughts. Parents and other family members are often excluded from these conversations. This relationship helps the teenager to see through the eyes of another.[24]

The peer group, a collection of individuals who share common age, ideas, and goals, also has a great influence on the adolescent. The group bolsters self-esteem by making distinctions between their own characteristics and those of the other "out" groups. Often these characteristics are shown by a distinctive way of dressing, by

taking drugs, or by resisting authority. These activities unite the group against outsiders. The group behaviors can also be viewed as a necessary measure designed to protect the teenagers against loss of identity. Social and peer groups provide a sense of security and self-esteem, while the individuals withdraw from emotional dependence on their families and begin to set their own goals and values.

By the end of adolescence, young people have adjusted to the physical changes in their bodies and have awakened to love and to loneliness. Usually they have a desire for adult privileges, yet an apprehension about adult responsibilities.

During young adulthood, the period beyond the teen years, many men and women make serious inroads into the adult world in terms of job selection, lifestyle, and long-term emotional commitment. At the other end of the continuum are the "dropouts" or delayed adolescents who remain uncommitted and unconcerned. These people may take several more years to evolve an identity or make career decisions. During youth, some people may try to reject the society, its culture, and its values. They may turn to other lifestyles or exotic ways of living. They may be attracted to religious "cults," which give them rules to live by and thus prolong the time when they do not have to make their own decisions about life.

At the end of adolescence and during young adulthood, the individuals are ready to begin the next stage; leaving home and beginning their own families.

Mental Health in Adolescence

Adolescence, with its turmoil, depressions, longings, and loneliness, may produce severe emotional problems. Some adolescents rebel against parental and societal values. They reject the behaviors that society considers normal. They may begin abusing alcohol or other drugs. They may become truant from school or drop out. They may suffer depression to the point of attempted or actual suicide. They may "act out" in antisocial behavior, causing conflicts at home, at school, and with the law. Eating disorders are common among adolescent females. For some adolescents, the stresses and changes of this stage are so severe that they retreat into fantasy or delusions accompanying schizophrenia.

The adolescent is beginning to move out of the family system to become a participant in other systems: peer groups, work groups, school, and community. If the family system has clear boundaries and roles, the adolescent will usually feel free to move into the other larger systems. Dysfunctional family systems increase the confusion and stress of adolescence. The family system should be neither too dependent, causing inefficiency in roles, nor too independent, causing premature disengagement of the adolescent.

Adulthood

Adulthood spans the years from ages 20 to 65 and over. Young adulthood covers ages 20 to 40. Middle adulthood is called "middlesence" and covers the ages of 40 to 65 years. "Senescense" or old age begins at age 65, and includes the 70s and beyond. All stages of adulthood are characterized by change and adaptation as the various assigned developmental tasks, sometimes accompanied by the corresponding "crises," are resolved and completed.

Young Adulthood

In the first phase of young adulthood, individuals must "pull up roots" and separate from their parents, develop personal value systems, and achieve independence. College, the army, the Peace Corps, and similar institutions offer ways of trying different roles without making long-term commitments. Major changes in attitudes usually occur during this period. Exposure to different people and values helps individuals become more flexible in their thinking and point of view. The second phase of young adulthood is termed *The Trying Twenties* by Sheehy.[32] Young people usually enjoy independence but feel some pressure from parents and peers to settle down. The third phase of young adulthood takes place in the decade of the 30s, with the *Age Thirty Transition.* This is followed by the *Settling Down Period.*[33]

Biological Development

Biological development is at its peak, and cognitive skills attain their highest levels, in young adulthood. The skeletal system completes its growth by age 25, but retains the ability to form new bone at any time. This ability is necessary for the healing of fractures. Muscular efficiency is at its highest during the 20s. Muscular strength starts to decline in the 30s. This explains why professional athletes frequently retire by 35 years of age. In the late 20s, the skin begins to lose moisture and becomes dry, and lines around the eyes and mouth begin to show. Adequate fluids and a well-balanced diet help to maintain appearance and health. Gray hair and baldness may appear in the late 20s, sometimes to the chagrin of the individual.

Cholesterol levels in the blood increase after age 21. High levels are correlated with fatty deposits in the blood vessels, which can lead to circulatory problems, particularly of the heart. Young men are more likely to have elevated cholesterol levels than are young women. In a study by Johnson, race, gender, and weight are known to influence hypertension in young adults.[20] This research found that black females have the highest incidence of hypertension, followed by black males, white males, and white females. Obesity was found to increase blood pressure. There are no specific changes in the respiratory system during this period. It is important for an individual to participate regularly in physical exercise to develop and maintain the capability of the heart and lungs for maximal oxygen uptake.

The digestive system decreases production of ptyalin (an enzyme that digests starches) after age 20. Other than that, the digestive system remains the same during young adulthood. Young people may have ulcerative colitis, an inflammatory condition of the colon and rectum. This is classified as a psychophysiological disease. "Wisdom teeth," or third molars, erupt at around age 20 or 21. Frequently, third molars cause problems and have to be extracted.

The major changes in the perceptual system are in the eyes. The lenses begin aging in infancy. Because the lenses grow without shedding the older cells, they become thicker, less elastic, and more opaque. The change is gradual, and the young person usually will not notice any change in visual acuity until after age 35 years. Hearing levels peak at age 20 and then gradually decline. About age 32, some people complain of a hearing loss, although most people are not bothered by appreciable hearing loss in young adulthood. Taste, touch, and smell function normally during young adulthood. Sensory deprivation does occur, and can cause behavior changes in an individual. These include changes in the ability to think and reason, disorientation, anxiety, fear, depression, hallucinations, and delusions.[34]

The kidneys play a dominant role in facilitating physiological homeostasis by excreting metabolic waste products and regulating water content, salts, and acid–base balance. The genitals have reached adult size, and are maintained at that size and functioning level throughout the 20s and 30s. Sexual responses and functioning remain at a high level throughout this period.

Cognitive Development

Cognitive development in the young adult years has not been studied sufficiently. Intelligence may be divided into two functions, fluid intelligence and crystallized intelligence. *Fluid intelligence* is involved in organizing and reorganizing information in the process of solving problems. Some of the broad measures of fluid intelligence include working with geometric figures and matrices, and inductive reasoning. Fluid intelligence decreases throughout adulthood because it depends on speed of thinking, dexterity, and short-term memory.

Crystallized intelligence represents an accumulation of knowledge gained from experience, and includes the necessary tasks defined by the culture. Fluid intelligence plays a role in the development of crystallized intelligence, that is, the ability to solve problems and reorganize information is necessary in order to learn through experience. The ability to learn through experience increases with age. Young adults are busy increasing crystallized intelligence throughout this stage of the life cycle.[32]

Piaget discusses intellectual development in terms of quantitative vs. qualitative changes. *Quantitative intelligence* refers to the amount of knowledge or information an individual has at his or her disposal at any given time; *qualitative intelligence* refers to major changes in thought processes. Qualitative changes usually stop when the young adult has reached the stage of formal operations, while quantitative changes continue. Piaget notes that a major change in the cognitive development of the young adult is the loss of adolescent egocentrism.[39]

Between the ages of 21 and 30, 65% of adults in advanced countries reach Piaget's stage of formal operations.[21]

It is interesting to note that about one third of the young adult population apparently use preoperational or concrete operational reasoning to meet the challenges of living in a highly technical society. The general effect of the above on the self-actualization process may be detrimental.

Sociocultural Development

The developmental task of young adulthood, according to Erikson, is *intimacy*. This task includes the need for real sharing. As adolescence is phased out, intimacy is phased in. In the United States, intimacy is never achieved by some people. Our culture places much less attention on this phase of development than on the earlier stages. The result is isolation. The successful young person is able to establish independence from parents, establish an intimate relationship with another person, learn to express love responsibly with more than sexual contacts, become established in a vocation or profession, join a congenial social group, and, finally, become an involved citizen of the community. Inadequate resolution of the task may lead to disturbances in sex role performance. For example, the person may withdraw from encounters with others. Inability to achieve a sense of intimacy may be reflected in the rising divorce rate in our society, although the divorce rate is also influenced by many other factors.[38]

Because many choices and decisions are made in the early and mid-20s, often under pressures exerted by parents or peers, it is inevitable that some of the choices or decisions will prove to be less than satisfactory to the individual. For these persons, a developmental crisis occurs, which Sheehy calls "*Catch 30.*"[33] This crisis develops between the ages of 28 and 32 years. Individuals may decide to change their situations or the direction of their lives by altering goals. For example, a man who has been busy developing his career and enjoying his independence may decide that he is not fulfilled. He may decide to initiate an intimate relationship with a woman for the purpose of exploring the possibilities of love, marriage, and parenting. Another young man may decide to end an unsatisfying marriage relationship, while a third young man may choose to change jobs or professions. Women may make the same decisions about the nonsatisfying situations in which they find themselves. For some, "Catch 30" means breaking with their pasts and restructuring their lives by making radical changes. After the crisis of "Catch 30," the middle and late 30s are years of consolidation and gradual growth. Men and women seek long-term goals and deeper, more lasting friendships and relationships. They feel more at ease; life becomes more understandable and more predictable. Sheehy describes this phase as "a time of rooting and extending." Individuals put down new roots by marrying, relocating, buying houses, establishing themselves in new jobs, or deciding to have children. A new seriousness and dedication to goals are characteristic of this phase.[33]

Young Adulthood and Stress

Stress reactions, which include physiological changes, are the result of intolerable levels of anxiety that occur at any time during the early adult years. A big examination in college, a wedding or divorce, a first child, a new job, or physical injuries due to accidents are all common stimuli or precipitants of stress. Environmental chronic stress experiences, such as driving in city traffic, listening to screaming children or barking dogs, or four years of graduate school, can produce ulcers or weight problems if the individual cannot develop strong coping mechanisms. Suicide is the third leading cause of death, and many times is related directly or indirectly to the experience of stress. Alcohol or drug abuse is a common problem during this stage of development.

Accidents in this age group reach a peak at about 21 years of age, and 50% of disabling accidents occur before 35 years of age. Males are involved in accidents more often than females. Accidents may result from aggressive behavior—for example, fighting, reckless use of motor vehicles, or misuse of dangerous power tools. Accidents are more likely to occur when an individual is under pressure or duress; it follows that this age group experiences accidents. All of these experiences can and do have an effect on the mental health of the individual. Various diagnoses of mental illnesses, such as anxiety reactions, depression, and adjustment reactions, are common.

Young adults are actively involved in setting up their own family systems. The ease with which they are able to do this depends on the role of their own family system and other support systems. This transition period is difficult, and young adults feel stress in establishing new roles as wage earners, child rearers and intimate partners. Some react to these stresses by withdrawal and stay with their original family system, while others integrate successfully.

Middle Adulthood–Middlescence

The years from age 40 to age 65 are usually considered middle age, or *middlescence*. Important physical and psychological changes occur. There are also changes in the roles assigned to individuals, such as reversal of parent–child roles, work roles, and social roles.

Biological Development

Due to the sociocultural emphasis on youth and youthful appearance, an individual may be inclined to ignore, deny, or hide the physical signs of aging. In spite of the attempts to deny it, each person ages and proceeds toward senescence.

From age 40 until the end of middle age, bone mass decreases. Calcium loss from bone tissue occurs and, in some people, osteoporosis occurs. There may be a loss in height, particularly in women. Changes in the joints, such as the hip joint, are also due to the loss of elasticity of cartilage, and hardening or thickening of collagen fibers. Some middlescent adults become more sedentary, and the muscles slowly begin to decrease in mass, structure, and strength. Muscle loss is also caused by the changes in collagen fibers; the loss of elasticity causes sagging or drooping of abdominal, breast, and facial muscles. The middle section of the body enlarges, and people have to buy clothes designed for middlescence.[25]

The integument usually remains intact until about age 50, if the person is in good health and eating a well-balanced diet. At about 50 years of age wrinkles, the result of many factors, begin to appear. The first step is the aging of collagen fibers. Body water content begins to decrease, and fat content begins to increase. As the skin loses water, it becomes thinner, drier, and more easily damaged. Due to weakening of the underlying muscle and fibrous tissue, the subcutaneous tissue pushes through, causing the skin to balloon or "bag" under the eyes. In our youth-oriented culture, plastic surgery can repair this age-related process, if the individual feels that it is necessary. The hair does not grow as quickly, it thins out, and it may become gray. The function of the central nervous system is maintained in early middlescence or in the 40s.

People in their 50s may experience slowing of the reflexes, decreased muscular activity, decreased memory, and slower responses to environmental stimuli. Thus, middlescent people are more prone to trauma, accidents, and injuries. Some losses in the special senses, hearing and smell, may be noticed at about age 50. Visual losses are more pronounced in early middlescence—primarily farsightedness or hyperopia, which can be helped by glasses or contact lens.[12]

Heart function is maintained in the early middlescent years by activity, both at work and in recreational activities. After age 45, as the individual becomes more sedentary, heart muscles begin to lose their tone; rate and rhythm changes occur. Hypertrophy of the left ventricle occurs in some people and may be associated with atherosclerosis or arteriosclerosis. Degenerating cardiovascular tissues can lead to death in middlescence.

The gastrointestinal system is less affected by aging than is the cardiovascular system. There is a known gradual decrease in the normal gastric juices, acids, and enzymes necessary for normal digestion. By age 60, middlescents may have eliminated certain foods from the diet because the foods don't "agree" with them, or they may complain about intestinal disorders, such as constipation.

The efficiency of respiratory functioning in the middle years may be related to smoking. Smoking increases the likelihood of respiratory disease and decreases respiratory efficiency. By age 60, however, the lung tissues become thicker and less elastic, causing a decrease in breath capacity.

The normal function of the renal system is maintained in early middle age. With aging, however, there is a gradual loss of nephrons, the functional units of the kidney. Therefore, there is a decrease in renal functioning. Also, diseases of the kidney, such as cancer, glomerulonephritis, or stone formation, contribute to a decrease in kidney function.[39]

In women, menopause is a characteristic sign of middle age. Menopause usually occurs between 45 and 55 years of age. The reproductive function ceases, and the body's production of estrogen and progesterone drops off sharply. Hormone (estrogen) replacement therapy is used to treat menopausal symptoms, particularly "hot flashes."

With men, there is no abrupt cessation of reproductive ability. There is, however, a gradual decrease in the production of the male hormone testosterone. A small percentage of men may also experience symptoms associated with the transition period between middle age and older age. Symptoms include "mood swings, insomnia, lassitude, decreased sexual potency, and vasomotor instability." Most men report that these symptoms disappear in two to three years.[26]

In the middle years, men tend to become more concerned about their general health. Men appear to be somewhat more satisfied with their bodies than are women. Physical appearance, then, may be more important for women than for men. Cosmetic surgery, spas, weight control centers, make-up, hair conditioners and dyes, skin creams and ointments, and vitamin therapy have become big business as middlescents try to appear younger. Because American society is "youth-oriented," the middlescents try to remain youthful.

Cognitive Development

Individuals in their 40s can function at a high level intellectually. Experience and maturity give them an advantage over younger adults when organizational ability or decision-making is required. In their 50s, some individuals experience a gradual loss in mental function due to changes in hormones and enzymes, as well as loss in motor and sensory functions.

Recent research, based on longitudinal methods (in which the same individuals are tested as they grow older), reveals slight decreases in cognitive ability in the 50s. The aging of central nervous system tissues is also responsible for the decline in performance or fluid intelligence. Crystallized intelligence remains stable throughout the middle years. The combination of crystallized and fluid intelligence into one measure called *omnibus intelligence* shows an average that remains at the same level throughout the life cycle. Education, health, activity, and stimulation are more important factors than is aging in maintaining cognitive functioning.[32]

Individual creativity remains very high throughout the middle years. Creative works depend on both crystallized intelligence and knowledge of human experiences through the humanities and social sciences. The production of creative works reaches a peak in the 30s, and continues to increase until the 60s.[9] The motivation to be creative and to learn is very great in many individuals in this age group. Many continue their education, complete degree programs, and obtain professional credentials.

Mid-Life Crisis or Transition

The *mid-life crisis* generally occurs at about ages 40 to 45, and seems to give rise in many individuals to creative impulses and work. This fact has been documented by many well-known writers and artists. The crisis is apparently precipitated by the individual's assessment that "youth" is fleeting and that old age is approaching and becoming a reality. For some individuals, it is painful to realize that their aspirations since adolescence and young adulthood may never be realized. "What is it that I really want for myself and others?" becomes the issue in this crisis. Choices must be made and priorities set. A new life structure will be formed on the basis of the choices and new priorities. The aspirations of youth may be changed or lowered to fit into the new life structure, or for some the aspirations may be raised to a higher level of attainment, such as actively seeking a higher educational degree. The character of family relationships may change considerably, for better or for worse; the nature of the work life may deteriorate, or it may improve. Some people face an isolated middle adulthood for the late 40s, 50s, and early 60s, while others become more successful at work, feel more fulfilled in family and social roles, and actually enjoy middlescence.[24]

Sexuality, Culture, and Middlescence

In our culture, the relationship between a woman's youth and beauty and a man's strength and virility is taken for granted. Therefore, many men and women in the middle years begin to question their abilities or adequacies in sexual performance. Old wives' tales about the effect of menopause on a woman's sexual desires and ability are well known and are believed by many people, even today. Actually, many women report that relationships with their significant others improve, and that sexual relations become more important and more enjoyable. A man may perceive changes in health, strength, and sexual drive, which can alter his self-concept and therefore his sexuality. The loss of sexual responsiveness is more likely to be caused by psychological factors than caused by physiological factors. Other factors that can also have a negative effect on a male's sexual responsiveness are career preoccupation, economic pursuits, fatigue, alcohol, or "fear of failure." With adequate rest, relaxation, and healthful habits, a man is likely to maintain sexual interest and activity throughout middlescence.

Social Development

The developmental issue during middlescence, according to Erikson, is *generativity vs. stagnation*. During this stage, the human qualities of caring, loving, guiding, and teaching are extended from the family and close friends to nonrelatives or strangers, especially younger people. *Generativity* is the concern for, and active participation in, the nurturing of the next generation, expanding parental love to brotherly love. Many roles of the middle years permit people to function well and fulfill this task. Teachers, doctors, nurses, and psychologists are examples of professional roles in which generativity can be accomplished. If generativity is not accomplished, the negative resolution is self-absorption, which can result in a sense of *stagnation*[25] or lack of growth.

A woman who has had the nurturing role as a wife and mother for many years may not feel the need to seek actively more of the same tasks. She may find other fulfillments: developing a career, or some other creative endeavor.

Middle-aged adults may become parents to two generations. They may have their children to "parent" even when the children are "out of the nest." This may include financial aid, emotional support, or babysitting. In addition, they may find themselves "parenting" their own parents and children by economic support or personal care, which may extend to having the aging parents (or children) living in their home with them. The reversal of parent/child roles can present problems, not only to the middle-aged children, who report anxiety, guilt, and depression, but also to the aging parents.[25]

Today more parents are becoming grandparents during the middle years. A majority of middlescent grandparents report emotional fulfillment in the role of grandparent. Depending on the person, the meaning attached to being a grandparent differs as will the style of relating to the grandchildren. Being a grandparent can mean being a teacher, a mentor, or a playmate. It can also involve giving money and gifts to the grandchildren, as well as emotional support. Through all of these activities, many grandparents feel that they contribute to the welfare of their grandchildren. Some grandparents report feeling psychological distance from their grandchildren, possibly because they are too busy with their own lives or because they do not approve of their children's lifestyles.

Other tasks assigned to this period are accepting and adjusting to physical changes; developing "new" satisfactions as a mate; making an art of friendship; and using leisure time with satisfaction, progressing toward retirement, or actually adjusting or adapting to retirement.

Middlescence and Illness

The morbidity and mortality rates for coronary artery disease are high in middlescence. Surgery offers hope to some people who suffer from this disease, while others are treated by medication, diet, and controlled exercise programs. Other chronic health problems include cancer, pulmonary disease, and diabetes.

Mental health problems can occur in people who have had no previous history of mental illness. Most middle-aged adults cope effectively with the stressors of role change, role reversal, and loss. When they are unable to cope, they may experience depression, or abuse alcohol or drugs. *Involutional melancholia* occurs during the involutional period, a time of diminishing bodily vigor and energy, and is a fairly common psychiatric diagnosis. The main symptom of involutional melancholia is depression and sometimes paranoia. In women, it may occur between ages 40 and 55, while in men it may be later, ages 50 to 65.

Senescence

Aging is a natural phenomenon. It refers to the changes that occur throughout the life cycle, accounting for the differences in structure and function between youthful and elderly persons. The population of the elderly in the United States has increased rapidly. Old age, or *senescence,* is thought to begin at age 65, and continues throughout the 70s and beyond. The number of people over 65 years of age was 3.1 million in 1900, 9.0 million in 1940, 23 million in 1976, and 27 million in 1982, which meant that one out of every eleven individuals in the U.S. was in the aged group. It is projected that in 2030 the number of aged persons will be 66.6 million, or approximately 21% of the population will be over age 65 years.[16,38] (See Figure 7-3.) The over-85 group will have grown from the present 2.2 million to 13 million.[17] This dramatic increase in the number of elderly people has future implications for social planning and economic distribution. Health and medical care, housing, and adequate nutrition will probably continue to be problems for the aged. Most elderly persons live on fixed incomes derived from Social Security or private retirement plans. Many elderly persons now work at part-time jobs to increase their meager incomes. This practice will probably continue beyond the year 2000. The mandatory retirement age has been raised by law to 70 to increase the working years allotted to individuals. Seeking employment is a serious problem for older workers, simply because their skills may be obsolete. Employers are hesitant to employ older workers because they may need to be ''retrained'' and the number of years remaining in their work lives is limited.

Changes in individuals' interpersonal functioning occur in old age. The parents of the elderly are dying or dead, their children have matured and have their own homes and families, and grandchildren are born and a new role of grandparent opens. After retirement from work, they may lose contact with their peer group of workers. Spouses may be ill and die; close friends die; and new friends and companions are needed to fill the void created by the long list of losses. New roles need to be developed and accepted by older people if they are to have a meaningful life. The decrease in income at retirement may make it difficult to pursue new interests and to develop new roles.

The Study of Aging

Gerontology, the study of aging, includes components of biology, psychology, and sociology, along with culture and subcultures. *Geriatrics* refers to the field of medicine that deals with the health problems of the aged. Preventive and palliative aspects of health are also included in geriatrics. The aging process is further divided into the following categories:

1. *Social aging* refers to the social roles and habits of individuals. As aging progresses, people experience a loss in meaningful social interaction due to the loss of spouses and close friends.

2. *Biological aging* refers to the physical changes in the body systems and cells during the latter decades of the life cycle. Biological changes occur at different rates in different individuals. One woman may show advanced aging processes at age 60 years and be quite dependent, while another woman may continue in the middle-age roles, appear much younger than her 70 years, and still be employed.

3. *Cognitive aging* refers to the altered or reduced capacity of an individual to learn new information and new behaviors.

4. *Affective aging* is the reduced capacity of a person to adapt to an altered environment. For example, el-

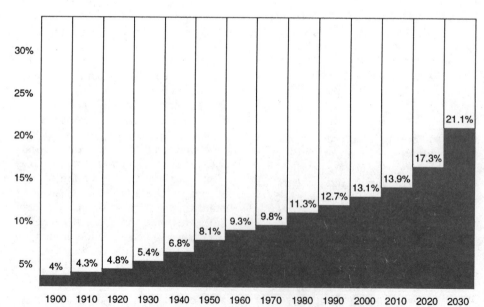

Figure 7-3. Percentage increase in the aged (over 65 years of age) population of the United States (1900–2030).

derly persons frequently have difficulty in orienting themselves when they are moved to a hospital or nursing home.

Biological Development

All the body systems are affected by the aging process; organ reserves are diminished, and the repair process occurs at a much slower rate than when individuals were younger. Biological theories of aging stress both genetic and environmental or extrinsic factors in the aging process.

Changes in Physical Appearance. The appearance of the integument, or skin, changes a great deal. Both the secretory and the excretory glands of the skin decrease in function, and the skin becomes dry, wrinkled, less elastic, and withered-looking (Fig. 7-4). Overexposure to the sun is known to accelerate these changes, and also causes an increase in the number of pigmented areas as well as potentially cancerous skin lesions. The skin retains its function of protecting the body in aging. The layer of fatty tissue beneath the skin tends to disappear, and the roundness of the extremities and trunk is lost. The hair becomes thinner and turns white.

Skeletal Changes. The tissues of the joints stiffen, causing a decrease in the range of movement in the joints. The older person may complain of pain and stiffness in the joints. Demineralization of bone tissue occurs, and the bones become brittle. The aged person may

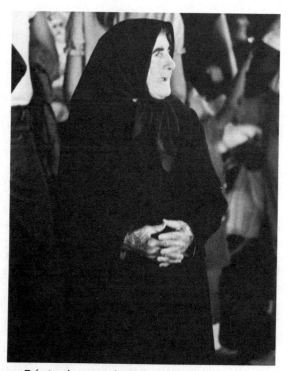

Figure 7-4. Aged woman dressed in traditional widow's clothing waiting at an airport in Portugal. (Photograph by Richard Hannen)

suffer fractures of the bones with very little or even no trauma. Common areas for fractures are the hip and vertebrae. Osteoporosis causes an actual loss of bone tissue. The mobility of the older person decreases, and movement becomes slower. Loss in number and bulk of muscle fibers also occurs.

Cardiovascular Changes. The cardiovascular system is subjected to great stresses, and probably suffers its greatest degenerative changes in old age. Generally, the output volume of the heart is reduced and the amount of oxygen-carrying blood in all body parts is subsequently reduced. The linings of the blood vessels are changed by the degenerative process. *Atheromas,* or fatty plaques, are deposited in the innermost lining, which, when coupled with the growth of fibrous tissue in the middle lining of the blood vessels, causes the increased rigidity of arteriosclerosis or "hardening of the arteries."[31]

Respiratory Changes. The mechanical efficiency of the lungs is decreased because of the aging process. Additional respiratory effort is needed to obtain the necessary amount of oxygen. Respiratory movements of the chest are reduced as a result of the increase in fibrous tissue in the chest wall and lungs. Inspiratory and expiratory volumes are decreased. Lower respiratory tract diseases and infections occur more often in the aged person, while upper respiratory tract infections are more common in younger individuals.[31]

Nutritive Changes. The enjoyable social function of eating may become more difficult for the aged individual due to loss of teeth, periodontal disease, and changes in the structure of the jawbone. Chewing may become so difficult that a modification in the diet may be necessary. Atrophy of the taste buds and a decreased sense of smell further diminish the pleasure of eating. In general, the digestive system maintains its function quite well in the aged, although diminished production of digestive juices and loss of muscle tone and activity throughout the gastrointestinal tract give rise to the common complaints of indigestion and constipation. Antacids and laxatives are purchased very often by elderly people. Protein foods, fresh vegetables, and fruits are more expensive than carbohydrate foods, so the elderly eat more crackers, breads, and cereals. They can develop anemia and vitamin deficiencies, and become prone to infections. "Meals on Wheels" and meals at senior citizen centers help this group obtain better nutrition.

Sensory and Neurological Changes. Due to a decreased blood supply, the nervous system suffers a generalized impairment. In senescence, the brain gets only 90% of the blood that it received in the early middle years of life. The neurons, or nerve cells, are replaced by nonfunctional connective tissues, which results in forgetfulness, irritability, and lack of adaptive abilities. In the eye, cataracts develop and color perception is diminished. The ciliary muscle loses its elasticity and functions less well in accommodating to light level changes. Driving a car or crossing a busy street becomes more hazardous for the elderly person. Hearing losses are more pronounced and vestibular functions decrease, so that the older person is more prone to falls and accidents.

Changes in the Genitourinary System. Kidney function is reduced, and there is also a loss of control in urine elimination. Loss of elasticity and diminished muscle tone in the ureters, bladder, and urethra contribute to urinary incontinence. Training for urine control, if successful, can improve the morale and sociability of the aged person. Sexual ability may continue into the 80s and beyond. The lack of a suitable partner or the fear of failure are known causes of a diminished sexual desire or activity. If general health is fairly good, the elderly person can continue to enjoy sexual activities throughout most of the life cycle.

Psychological Development

Behaviors that are learned and repeated over many years may become overlearned or done automatically. Overlearned behaviors are the most difficult behaviors to change. Also, individuals who have lived and coped with life's frustrations and problems for 75 years probably have behaviors and opinions that are fixed, and are resistant to change. It is traumatic to old people when they are forced to learn new ways of living: when they are restricted by a new diet, or forced to move from their own home to a child's home or a nursing home. Old behaviors, habits, and opinions must be altered to fit into a new environment.

Perception is the process of interpreting or attaching meaning to sensory input. Aged people have a constant background of neural noise that makes it more difficult for them to sort out and perceive complex sensory input. Memories from the past have had more time to consolidate and are stronger. Newer memories are the first to fade and last to return, compared to old memories.[12]

Acquisition of new knowledge is more difficult for older people than for younger students. However, given the opportunity for learning at an appropriate pace, aged people can master new material quite well. Education and continued stimulation appear to be important in maintaining intellectual capacity in old age. Adult education programs should be continued to meet the needs of the elderly.

In Maslow's hierarchy of needs, once the basic biological needs have been met, the person is able to seek gratification of the higher needs. These include, for example, security needs, social needs, and ego needs. Finally, the person may attain a state of self-actualization. Many older people live in a state of severe poverty and are unable to obtain food and decent housing. Social Security payments, old age assistance, and private pensions or resources provide some of the aged with a measure of financial security. These individuals may move to a higher level.[12] The elderly have the same need to love and be loved as do younger people; however, they may not have the opportunities to meet these needs. They may be separated from families, friends, and work associates, and it becomes more difficult to enter new groups. Adaptation to new groups is difficult. The ego needs for self-esteem and respect from others remain the same as in earlier stages. Older people need to have a goal or a purpose to satisfy the ego needs. The tasks at the highest level—being creative and altruistic—are important in order to get attention and approval from others and to compensate for the loss of loved ones and the loss of physical attractiveness.[12]

Sociocultural Development

The last stage of development, according to Erikson, is the stage of *ego integrity vs. despair.* In this stage, there is a new challenge or final opportunity to relive again what was and rethink what might have been. If the individual can look back on life's experiences, accomplishments, and both achieved and unachieved goals with a feeling of satisfaction, a sense of ego integrity develops. The negative side of the task is anxiety and despair. A person may try to make up for the past by "good deeds." If the sense of ego integrity outweighs the sense of despair, a final strength, *wisdom,* will result. Wisdom can be used and passed on to the following generations. Wisdom also gives meaning to life's experiences.[25]

For most people, success in aging is related to their ability to make a place for themselves in society where they can grow older and achieve fulfillment through strategic participation for as long as possible.[27] In a cross-cultural study of the aged, Simmons concluded that there are five wishes shared by older people everywhere: to live as long as possible, to hoard waning energies, to continue sharing in the affairs of life, to safeguard seniority rights, and to have an easy and honorable release from life.[35]

Women tend to outlive men by about seven years in the United States. After age 65, there are one third more women than men. This gives rise to a new group of disadvantaged: older, single women, who may be excluded from social gatherings.[5] The nonworking wife loses an important role of homemaker and companion when her mate dies. Depression and suicide may follow the loss of the spouse. Older men and working women face a crisis point as a result of a role loss at retirement. Retirement is defined as the separation of an older worker from a job that was performed for pay. It is socially approved unemployment, usually beginning between 65 and 70 years of age. Although all of us expect to retire, very few make plans for retirement or go to counseling programs.[2] Postretirement seminars and counseling can help retirees to adjust to a new status and to role changes in society. Many men experience severe depression, and suicide may result.

Senescence and Stress

Stress is a universal experience in life. Adaptation to stressful events requires energy. Aged individuals have had a great deal of stress placed on their bodies during their lifetime. After prolonged exposure to stressors, the resistance breaks down and exhaustion becomes inevitable. The older person has less energy available for adaptation and is therefore more vulnerable. Reserves of energy for adaptation cannot be entirely replaced, and each stressful event leaves the individual with a diminished supply. How aged individuals adapt to stress is determined by how well they adapted to stress in earlier years.[12]

Mental Health in Senescence

Mental illnesses in senescence cover a full range, from minor problems to psychoneuroses to psychoses. These are often associated with poverty, physical impairments, and chronic illnesses. These people may need long-term protective care. Damage to the brain caused by deterioration or neurological disease can result in the inability to think clearly and effectively.

Two degenerative disorders are Alzheimer's disease and Pick's disease. Alzheimer's disease results in the impairment of memory for recent events and a loss of orientation for time and place. This may be accompanied by an inability to speak (aphasia). A person with Pick's disease experiences difficulty in concentration and learning and an inability to react on an emotional level that is appropriate to the stimulus. For example, a man who has just been told of his wife's death may respond, "That's all right."[11] Depression related to the many losses at this stage of life can be fairly common, and should be assessed carefully to differentiate it from degenerative intellectual functioning.

In the final analysis, how well people adapt to old age is, in part, determined by how well they adapted to changes in other phases of life. If they experienced a crisis each time a new adjustment or adaptation was necessary, then they will probably experience difficulty in adjusting to old age.

Dying and Death

Dying and death are the last task, the final crisis, and the final adaptation for an individual. Thus, death becomes a part of each person's life cycle; it is the inevitable outcome for all of us. Often an awareness of death influences our quality of living, possibly starting in the middle years when mortality becomes a recognized reality. During the older adult years, a person is asked to adjust to physical impairments, slowing mobility, loss of financial income after retirement, possible illness and death of spouse or significant other, and some loss of meaningful interactions. Now a person is asked to adjust to the last great loss, the loss of self with all the meaning that is attached to the self. Of course, death can occur at any age, and it has different meanings to a person at different stages in the life span. From age three to five years, the child does not recognize death as a final event. From age five to nine years, the child personifies death as a ghost or "death personage" who takes people away. At about 10 years of age,

the child finally recognizes death as a terminal event, an inevitable outcome. The adolescent focuses on a sense of being and not on longevity. The quality of life is important, not the quantity. This fact may help to explain why suicide ranks very high as a cause of death for adolescents. Thoughts about dying and death bring about a sense of frustration, disappointment, and anger for the young adult who may now be on the threshold of "becoming." In the middle years, the individual is deeply involved with others: spouse, children, grandchildren, friends, neighbors, and peers at work. Death is feared because it represents a threat to all these very meaningful relationships. Increased reflection about one's life and the meaning attached to it comes with aging. Butler[4] considers that the life review is a natural and universal process in old age. Old people may go over and over their lives, questioning the sense and worth of it all. Coping with dying involves making peace with themselves and possibly making restitution for some of their failures in life.

Kübler-Ross[22,23] spent many years working with dying patients, and has summarized her observations of a person's needs and behaviors in the five stages of dying.

The first stage is *denial and isolation*. The initial response and defense mechanism is "No, not me" or "The test label got mixed up." This gives the client a little time to understand what is happening, that is, that death is approaching.

The second stage is *anger*. "Yes, I am going to die, but why must it be me? I lived a good life and worked hard; it is just not fair." The nurses, doctors, and family members may become targets for the anger. After some of the anger is resolved, the person moves on to the next stage.

The third stage of dying is the *bargaining* stage. In this stage the client searches for a means of prolonging life. Frequently, bargains are made with God. For example, a client may decide to give all of his estate to the care and welfare of the indigent or to give his body for scientific study after his death, if he can have an extra three years of life and happiness with the people he loves.

Depression is the fourth stage of dying. The main cause for depression is loss. Real loss is associated with health loss, hospitalization, separation from familiar surroundings and loved ones, and, finally, the impending loss of life itself. Clients need time to work through this stage before they can move on to the last stage.

Acceptance is the fifth and last stage of dying. This is not necessarily a happy stage or a happy acceptance. The client finally accepts the fact of the inevitable, death itself, and becomes more calm, not depressed or angry. It is important to the dying person that a close, "significant other" sit quietly nearby and share the last days and hours. In the stage of acceptance, the family often needs understanding and support. Some family members become upset when the client "gives up" and is ready to die.[21]

The care of the dying client in a hospital is very important. The quality of the care is influenced by the attitudes of the professionals and nonprofessionals who provide care.[16] Sometimes, due to family wishes, clients are deceived or shielded from the truth. Denial of the client's poor prognosis may also be a reflection of the professional staff's need to deny their own mortality. The dying lose their right "to set their house in order" if the truth is denied. Also, they may not be permitted to verbalize feelings or emotions about this painful experience.[13]

A client may speak of impending death in symbolic language. The nurse is obliged to stay with the language of the metaphor. For example, if a man talks about driving a truck down a long, dark road, the nurse should not say, "I don't believe you are talking about driving a truck. I think you are talking about dying." A better response might be "Tell me more about driving the truck and the long, dark road."[14]

Many times an optimal response for a care-giver is just being there with the patient, holding the patient's hand, and perhaps talking a little, following the patient's cues. Many dying clients have stated that they do not want to be alone or "anesthetized" by drugs. They would like pain medication as needed, but they want to have an awareness of the last total experience, death.[13]

Summary

1. A person may be viewed as a system with many components or parts.

2. The system of the person includes psychological, biological, and social components along with cultural and environmental aspects.

3. An understanding of theories of growth and development assists the nurse in evaluating an individual's functioning.

4. The psychosexual stages of development developed by Freud revolve around the individual's need to cope with instinctual drives.

5. Piaget formulated a model of growth and development founded on the child's cognitive or intellectual processes.

6. Erikson viewed the person as a social being and expressed the stages of growth and development as containing tasks specific for each stage.

7. Differences in behavioral expectations for specific growth and development stages occur across varying cultures.

8. The childhood period of growth and development includes the period of the most dramatic physical changes and adaptation demands—the first 12 years of life—and necessitates a supportive environment.

9. Adolescence includes the period between 12 and 19 years. It is marked by dependent/independent attitudes on the part of the adolescent.

10. Adulthood spans the years from 20 to 65. During this time individual identity is formed, as are intimate relationships in which one's life is shared with significant others. The individual initiates and develops a work role.

11. Senescence is the period after 65 years of age. This stage is marked by a need to develop new roles that facilitate a sense of meaning in life and that replace lost roles, such as worker or parent.

12. Dying and death is the last task of an individual. Some individuals go through five stages of dying, including: denial, anger, bargaining, depression, and acceptance.

References

1. Arneson S, Schultz M, Triplett J: Nurses' knowledge of the impact of parental alcoholism on children. Arch Psychiatr Nurs 1: 251, 1987

2. Atchley R: Social Forces and Aging: An Introduction to Social Gerontology. Belmont, CA, Wadsworth, 1985

3. Bowlby J: Attachment and Loss, Vol I, II. New York, Basic Books, 1969

4. Brazelton TB: Neonatal behavioral assessment scale. In Clin Dev Med 50:1973

5. Butler R, Lewis M: Aging and Mental Health. St Louis, CV Mosby, 1983

6. Chung H: Understanding the Oriental maternity patient. Nurs Clin North Am 112:67, 1977

7. Cratty B: Perceptual and Motor Development in Infants and Children. Englewood Cliffs, NJ, Prentice-Hall, 1979

8. Deledsi J: Principles of Growth and Development. In Hill P, Humphrey P (eds): Human Growth and Development Throughout Life: A Nursing Perspective. New York, John Wiley & Sons, 1982

9. Dennis W: Creative Productivity Between Ages Twenty and Eighty Years. J Gerontol 21:1, 1966

10. Erikson E: Identity: Youth and Crisis. New York, WW Norton, 1968

11. Erikson E: Childhood and Society. New York, WW Norton, 1950

12. Franks M, Graves J: Old Age. In Lugo J, Hershey G: Human Development. New York, Macmillan, 1979

13. Frantz R: Visual Perception from Birth as Shown by Pattern Selectivity. In Stone L, Smith H, Murphy B (eds): The Competent Infant: Research and Commentary. New York, Basic Books, 1973

14. Garfield C: The Human Side of Death and Dying. Symposium at University of California at Irvine, 1976

15. Gaster T: The New Golden Bough (abridged work of Sir James Frazer). New York, New American Library, 1975

16. Gelman D, Hager M, Gonzalez D et al: The Family. Newsweek, May 6, 1985

17. Graves J, Franks M: Dying and Death. In Lugo J, Hershey G: Human Development. New York, Macmillan, 1979

18. Harwood A: The Hot–Cold Theory of Disease: Implications for Treatment of Puerto Rican Patients. JAMA 216:1153, 1971

19. Humphrey P: The Adolescent. In Hill P, Humphrey P (eds): Human Growth and Development Throughout Life: A Nursing Perspective. New York, John Wiley & Sons, 1782

20. Johnson A: Evans County, Georgia, Cardiovascular Study: Race, Sex, and Weight Influences of the Young Adult. Am J Cardiol 35:523, 1975

21. Kohlberg L, Gilligan C: The Adolescent as a Philosopher. Daedalus 100:1051, 1971

22. Kübler-Ross E: Death: The Final Stage of Growth. Englewood Cliffs, NJ, Prentice-Hall, 1975

23. Kübler-Ross E: On Death and Dying. New York, Macmillan, 1971

24. Levinson D: The Seasons of a Man's Life. New York, Knopf, 1978

25. Lugo J, Hershey G: Human Development. New York, Macmillan, 1979

26. Modigh A: The Young Older Adult. In Hill P, Humphrey P (eds): Human Growth and Development Throughout Life: A Nursing Perspective. New York, John Wiley & Sons, 1982

27. Myerhoff B, Simic A: Life's Career—Aging: Cultural Variations on Growing Old. Beverly Hills, Sage Publications, 1978

28. Phillips J: The Origins of Intellect: Piaget's Theory. San Francisco, WH Freeman, 1975

29. Piaget J: The Origins of Intelligence in Children. New York, WW Norton, 1966

30. Putt A: General Systems Theory Applied to Nursing. Boston, Little, Brown and Co, 1978

31. Roberts S: Cardiopulmonary Abnormalities in Aging. In Burnside I (ed): Nursing and the Aged. New York, McGraw-Hill, 1981

32. Schuster C, Ashburn S: The Process of Human Development. Boston, Little, Brown and Co, 1985

33. Sheehy G: Passages. New York, EP Dutton, 1974

34. Shelly J: Sensory Deprivation. Image 10:49, 1978

35. Simmons L: Aging in Preindustrial Societies. In Tibbets C (ed): Handbook of Social Gerontology. Chicago, University of Chicago Press, 1960

36. Spector R: Cultural Diversity in Health and Illness. New York, Appleton-Century-Crofts, 1985

37. Topalis M, Aguilera D: Psychiatric Nursing. St Louis, CV Mosby, 1986

38. U.S. Department of Commerce, Bureau of the Census: Statistical Abstract of the United States. Washington, DC, U.S. Department of Commerce, 1984

39. Vander A, Sherman J: Human Physiology. New York, McGraw-Hill, 1985

40. Vasta R: The Unconscious Lie in Psychoanalysis. Unpublished doctoral dissertation, California Graduate Institute, 1985

41. Wadsworth B: Piaget's Theory of Cognitive Development. New York, McKay, 1971

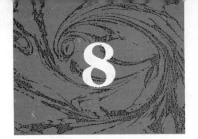

LORETTA M. BIRCKHEAD

STRESS AND STRESS MANAGEMENT

Learning Objectives

Upon completion of this chapter the student should be able to do the following:

1. Explain the concept that stress is a part of everyday life.
2. Describe the therapeutic use of self in working with clients' stress at any particular level of prevention.
3. Explain how a positive experience in life can also be a stressor.
4. List diseases that can result from uncontrolled stress.
5. Describe a client in the latter stages of the General Adaptation Syndrome.
6. Describe one stress management technique.

Introduction

Stress is an everyday fact of life. You can't avoid it.[7]

Stress *is* present in life. Indeed, stress is such an ever-present part of life that it is frequently overlooked. When stress occurs and a person must adapt, the stress may be beyond the individual's adaptive ability. Physical and emotional changes then occur and, if the person is vulnerable or if the changes are intense or chronic in nature, disease may result.

One of the purposes of this chapter is to help the clinician appreciate the pervasiveness of stress in our lives and the implications of long-term stress for health and illness. The effects of stress can be lessened with life-style changes. Modifications in lifestyle are significant challenges, and usually require professional assistance to be successful.

The Biological Perspective

Cannon, a physiologist, was the first person to describe the body's reaction to stress. When he studied stress in the early years of the 20th century, he identified the *fight-or-flight* response to stress. In this response, when confronted with a threat, the body either prepares to combat the threat or retreats from the threat.[8]

Selye, a physician, also studied responses to stress. He defined stress as the state manifested by a particular syndrome that consists of all the nonspecifically-induced changes within a biological system. Selye developed the idea of a *General Adaptation Syndrome* (GAS). Selye wrote:

> I call this syndrome "general" because it is produced only by agents which have a general effect upon large portions of the body. I call it "adaptive" because it stimulates defense and thereby helps the acquisition and maintenance of a stage of inurement. I call it a "syndrome" because its individual manifestations are coordinated and even partly dependent upon each other.[22]

According to Seyle, a GAS occurs in three stages, as follows.

1. *The alarm reaction* is the initial response. In this stage, the stressor (that which produces stress) is first felt and the body expresses a generalized call to arms of defensive forces within the body to repel the stressor. The stressor may cause death instantly (as in a car crash), even in stage one. In another example, a female executive identifies heavy job pressures as a stressor. She and her nurse practitioner discuss her weight gain and increased cholesterol level, and consider how these factors may be a result of stressors in the client's life.

2. *The stage of resistance* is one of adaptation or resistance to the stressor. In this second stage, the individual remains exposed to the stressor that was not repelled in stage one. Selye noticed a number of physiological differences between stages one and two. For example, in stage one the cells of the adrenal cortex discharge its hormone. In stage two, however, the gland stores a reserve of the hormone. In the case of the female executive, job stressors remain, she takes no stress management actions, and physiological changes continue to occur. She experiences arm pain.

3. In *the stage of exhaustion,* after continued exposure to the stressor, the adaptation facility is lost, signaling the start of the stage of exhaustion. As all adaptive energy is lost, the individual dies. *Thus, unremitting stress eventually breaks the body's protective mechanisms.* Selye believed that we are continuously exposed to potentially pathogenic microbes, yet they cause no disease until we are exposed to stress. In

most instances, disease is not due to a germ as such, but to the *inadequacy of our reactions against the germ.*[22] In the above example, the executive has a heart attack.

Selye was concerned that the term *stress* was used loosely. The lack of clarity about the meaning of stress added to the confusion about the concept. Therefore, he also described what stress is *NOT:*

1. Stress is not nervous tension. Selye explained the body's physiological stress reaction as an automatic one that can be considered without use of the psychological terms of anxiety or feelings of stress. Selye stated that stress can be produced in cell cultures grown outside the body.

2. Stress is not the result of trauma. Normal activities, such as a good laugh, can produce considerable stress without producing conspicuous damage. In reality, stress cannot be avoided, because during every moment of our lives some demand for life-maintaining energy exists. Complete freedom from stress is death.

3. Stress is not a deviation from a homeostatic or steady state of the organism. Any biological function (such as the movement of a finger) causes deviations from a resting state of the organism.

4. The pattern of the *reaction* to stress is not random. It affects certain organs in a selective manner. While certain organs are affected in a particular manner, the stressor itself is nonspecific in its operation. Only diseases in development of which the effects of a *nonspecific* stressor play a major role are called diseases of stress or adaptation. Furthermore, no disease is due to stress alone, because the cause of nonspecific responses to the stressor will always be modified by various "conditioning factors" (such as an individual's genetic predisposition) that alter disease *proneness.*

There is little justification to call the instantaneous death from a traumatic injury to the spinal cord, for example, a disease of adaptation. The damage is inflicted so rapidly that there is no time for any adaptive process. In diseases of adaptation, however, there are insufficient or faulty *reactions* to stressors. For example, a person undergoing a divorce frequently feels nervous. If the individual does nothing to moderate the stress response, ulcers may develop. This example highlights the importance of an individual's lifestyle in dealing with stress. For example, does an individual's lifestyle include being alert to a prolonged stress response, and knowing stress relief techniques?

In describing the biological operation of the General Adaptation Syndrome (GAS), Selye[21] stated that the exact nature of the body's alarm signals that first relay the stress message has not been identified. These signals may be metabolic by-products released during activity or damage, or they may be caused by the lack of a vital substance consumed whenever any demand is made on an organ. However, because there are only two systems that connect all parts of the body with each other—the nervous system and the vascular system—the alarm signals use one or both of these pathways.

Although the exact nature of the first signals of stress is unknown, the existence of these signals is known by their effects. These effects include the discharge of ACTH (adrenocorticotropic hormone), involution of the lymphatic organs, enlargement of the adrenal glands, changes in the corticoid hormone content of the blood, fatigue, and many other signs. Eventually the stressor, through the operation of the alarm signals, excites the hypothalamus, which acts as a bridge between the brain and the endocrine system.

The effects of a stressor will depend on the individual's general health level, which determines the body's reaction to the stressor. Although all stressors have specific effects, they do not elicit exactly the same responses in all organs. The same stressor acts differently in different individuals, depending on the factors that determine the reactivity of the person to the stressor. For example, a person without social supports may have a more difficult time adjusting to the loss of a spouse than will someone with many social supports.

In Figure 8-1, certain cells of the hypothalamus release a chemical messenger to the pituitary, causing a discharge of ACTH into the circulatory system. After reaching the adrenal cortex, ACTH triggers the secretion of corticoids (mainly glucocorticoids), such as cortisol or corticosterone. These corticoids provide energy for the adaptive reactions necessary to meet the demands of the stressor. Also, the corticoids facilitate other enzyme responses and suppress immune reactions, along with inflammation, to help the body coexist with pathogens.

There are a number of feedback loops in the chain of biophysiological events involved in a stress response. For example, if there is a surplus of ACTH, a feedback channel returns some of the ACTH to the hypothalamus–pituitary axis, which shuts off further ACTH production. Also, a high blood level of corticoids similarly prevents too much ACTH secretion.

Another important pathway helps to mediate the stress response: stress hormones, such as the catecholamines, are freed to activate general adaptation mechanisms. Adrenaline is secreted to make energy available, to increase the pulse rate, to elevate the blood pressure and the rate of blood circulation in the muscles, and to stimulate the central nervous system. Also, the blood coagulation mechanism is enhanced as a protection against excessive bleeding if injuries are sustained in the encounter with the stressor. Many other biological changes result from the occurrence of stress.

Selye stated that emotional arousal is one of the most frequent activators of the GAS. However, it is not the only factor, since stress reactions can develop in clients exposed to trauma while under anesthesia. Because of the variety of stressors, scientists frequently use the terms "neurogenic stress" or "psychogenic stress" when talking about stress reactions stemming from biological or psychological sources, respectively.

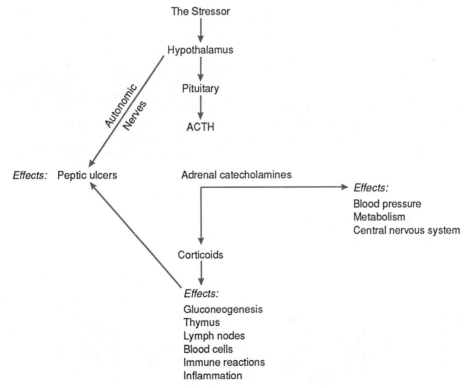

Figure 8-1. The pathway of stressor effects.

(Adapted from Selye H: The Stress Concept Today. In Kutash I, Schlesinger L (eds): Handbook on Stress and Anxiety. San Francisco, Jossey-Bass, 1980.)

While the GAS is characteristic of many organisms and of both sexes, differences between the sexes begin to appear when the degree to which a person can withstand stress, or the types of changes within the environment that cause stress, are examined.[15] Sex differences in response to stress are shown in Table 8-1.

Under normal conditions, women have higher levels of circulating estrogens than do men, while men have higher levels of circulating androgens. Estrogen may be a factor in the lower incidence of vascular and hypertensive diseases in women because they have greater levels of circulating lipoprotein, which removes cholesterol from the vascular system. In contrast, men have increased amounts of another type of lipoprotein that carries cholesterol into the arterial wall (which may be associated with increased cardiovascular illness).

During exercise, men produce a greater working capacity than women because their bodies supply more oxygen to the skeletal muscles during stress. Also, women generally have lower lung capacities than men, probably as a result of differences in body size. Men have greater hemoglobin capacities and greater oxygen capacities than women.

Studies have shown that females are less likely than men to respond to emotionally-arousing stimuli (stress) by a release of epinephrine. This is true whether the situation requires a passive or an active response. Males respond to stress in a more aggressive manner than females, which may be due to larger amounts of circulating androgens. Women are more prone to depression and introversion than men. Whether these behaviors are learned or hormonally-mediated is still controversial.

Many of the physiological mechanisms involved in stress responses are not fully understood. Although differences between the sexes in stress response exist, each time an individual (male or female) is exposed to a stressor there is a tendency to learn the nature and degree of activity needed to resolve the experience, and the individual develops greater ease in handling the demands of the stress. Thus, there remains the bio-psycho-social interrelationship of factors that work together for more efficient stress management.

The Psychological Perspective

Freud discussed emotional trauma and hypothesized that traumas occur when an excessive influx of stimulation overexcites the psychic apparatus (the psychological make-up or consciousness).[10] He accounted for differences in the response of individuals to the same *external* stress event by proposing that there are variations in "stimulus barriers" among individuals. This barrier to stimulation regulates the entry of perceptions from external events into the consciousness of the person. Freud proposed that, when an external stressor is anticipated or actually perceived, anxiety is activated. As anxiety increases, the stimulus barrier is increased. The person erects a protective internal barrier to the painful feeling of anxiety. The result is reduced stressful input, and the individual feels better.

According to Freud, the barrier to *internal* stimulation consists of defense mechanisms, such as repression or projection. However, the pressure to express the emotions aroused by traumatic events remains long after the original trauma.

Freud noted that there is often a lag period between the traumatic event and the appearance of symptoms. Once symptoms appear, however, they have a tendency to persist for a long time after the stressful event. There is also a bland acceptance of the symptoms: individuals tend to overlook their own symptoms.

Freud believed that memories of childhood trauma are not always true memories, but a fantasy elaboration of childhood situations. Thus the traumatic events, which were so stressful, did not always represent only an external stress, but could also involve internal components. As mentioned earlier, events have *meanings* that are unique to a particular individual. It is easy to understand that meanings of events can be distorted in situations of intense stress responses and anxiety. The nurse can help clients clarify such distortions. Once the psychological barriers to stress are erected, it can be a formidable challenge to dismantle them so that new meaning related to traumatic events can enter.

Freud also mentioned that a traumatic event, or the

TABLE 8-1.
SEX DIFFERENCES AND STRESS

CONDITION	WOMEN	MEN
Normal	Higher level of circulating estrogens	Higher level of circulating androgens
	Circulating lipoprotein removes cholesterol.	Circulating lipoprotein carries cholesterol into arterial wall.
Exercise	↓ Physical working capacity	↑ Physical working capacity
	↓ Lung capacity	↑ Hemoglobin capacity
	↓ Blood volume	↑ Energy expenditure
Stress-producing	↓ Epinephrine release	↑ Epinephrine release
	↑ Behavioral inhibition	↓ Behavioral inhibition

(Adapted from Martinson I, Anderson S: Male and Female Response to Stress. In Kjervik K, Martinson I (eds): Women in Stress: A Nursing Perspective. New York, Appleton-Century-Crofts, 1979)

stressor, may produce a variety of symptoms. However, after the traumatic event there is a tendency to repeat some aspect of the experience. This repetition can take the form of behavioral or biological responses, such as heart palpitations, in situations that are symbolic representations of the original trauma.

An example of a behavioral repetition is seen in a client who was repeatedly blamed by her parents for not "doing things right." In working with the nurse, the client learned that what her parents called "right" was actually *their* view of appropriate behavior, rather than an intrinsically correct view. As an adult, however, the client reacted to others by attempting to be correct. She often labeled herself as "incorrect" and wrong when there was, in reality, no evidence that she was incorrect. The client often reported feeling a lack of self-worth. She was obese and had cardiac problems. She was repeating a behavior pattern learned as a child. In working with such a client, the nurse uses the nursing principles of obtaining (1) a thorough description of the client's definition of Self (which is distorted in some way), and (2) a realistic definition of Self.

Freud's ideas about the individual's control of consciousness are explained in the box below.

It should be mentioned, however, that even the steps leading to inadequate coping behaviors can serve a purpose. It is unrealistic to expect that people can cope with all experiences in life. Victims of natural disasters, for example, may need to deny (distort) that the disaster had any effect on their life. Likewise, psychiatric clients may need to minimize or repress their memories of harmful childhood experiences. Defenses such as denial and minimization serve the purpose of curbing the painful experience of anxiety associated with events. At a later time, the implications of events can be seen more clearly and their "danger" to the sense of well-being can be decreased. When continued and extensive use of defenses begins to limit functioning or relations with others, the value of the defenses diminishes.

Another area of development in the history of the study of stress is viewed from a "cognitive" perspective. One reason for the variation in individual responses to stressful events is that people differ in the registration and interpretation of stress events, as well as in styles and capacities of responding to stress.

Lazarus, an experimentalist in psychology, studied the cognitive processes of appraisal used in coping with threat. Lazarus and Coyne[12] considered emotions as responses to cognitions (thoughts). The degree of threat appraised and reappraised by the individual leads to variations in emotions, such as anger, sadness, and elation.[11]

The individual perceives an event, which is appraised as a threat or a nonthreat. The individual does a primary appraisal of the threat, and then calls up responding resources. The primary appraisal may result in an automatic coping response or in positive emotions. The primary appraisal may also result in a secondary appraisal, which involves a comparison of the threat with coping resources. Actually, several (secondary) reappraisals of the threat are made to determine if the threat exceeds the individual's coping capacity. The discrepancy between the degree of threat and available coping capacities accounts for the emotions or actions activated. An individual may respond to a perceived threat with anger, which may then be reduced when a "safe" signal is received after reappraising the threat and coping resources through cognitive processing.[7] The following box depicts how cognitive processes affect emotion.

THE MANAGEMENT OF EVENTS IN AN INDIVIDUAL'S CONSCIOUSNESS

Step 1.   Stressor occurs.
Step 2.   Meaning is attached to the stressor.
Step 3.   No anxiety is provoked.
Step 4.   No defenses are created; the individual copes with the stressor.

or

Step 3.   The meaning provokes anxiety.
Step 4.   Defenses are created to deal with the anxiety

and

the meaning of the stressor is distorted.
Step 5.   The individual repetitively copes inappropriately with the stressor.

(Adapted from Horowitz M: Stress Response Syndromes. New York, Jason Aronson, 1976)

THE EFFECT OF COGNITIVE PROCESSES ON EMOTION

Primary appraisal of threat results in:
1.   Automatic coping (attack or avoid)

or

2.   Positive emotion (such as elation)

or

3.   Secondary appraisal (comparison of threat and coping resources)
↓
   a.   Emotion reduction (through an appropriate discharge of emotions or through defenses)

or

   a.   Direct action and/or emotional arousal (attack, avoidance, inaction, or listlessness)

(Data from Lazarus R, Coyne R: Cognitive Style, Stress Perception, and Coping. In Katash I, Schlesinger L (eds): Handbook on Stress and Anxiety. San Francisco, Jossey-Bass, 1980)

The Sociological-Cultural Perspective

Levine and Scotch[13] bring to the study of stress their expertise in the areas of sociology, anthropology, and epidemiology. They report that various broad sociocultural phenomena can serve as sources of stress. These sources include the following:

1. Differences between the structure of particular families and those that predominate in their social environment. An example of this stressor could be a black family living in a predominantly white neighborhood.
2. Different aspects of the life cycle of families. Stressors in this category are the stages of marriage, the "empty nest" syndrome when children leave the home, retirement, and the death of a spouse.
3. Role conflict. Stressors in this category might include the conflict between the need of parents to work and their need to participate fully in child care.
4. Stressors related to work. Job dissatisfaction, job responsibilities, or organizational stress among levels of management and the workers are typical stressors.
5. Social isolation. Rural community living serves as a stressor for some individuals.
6. Socioeconomic class and race. Conditions are more stressful for those at lower socioeconomic levels of a society than for those near the top. An individual's racial makeup can determine such characteristics as place and type of residence, friendships, leisure time activities, educational opportunities, and socialization resources in the environment.

Current Perspectives

The psychiatric nursing diagnoses of the American Nurses' Association (PNDI)[1] do not include "stress response." In the mental health sciences the term "anxiety" is frequently used to label an uncomfortable internal experience or feeling, rather than "stress" or "stress response." PNDI does include many internal experiences (such as distress, anguish, disgust) that indicate an underlying anxiety.

The *Diagnostic and Statistical Manual-III-R* of the American Psychiatric Association[2] has one stress-related diagnosis, Posttraumatic Stress Disorder. This disorder involves the development of characteristic symptoms following a psychologically traumatic event that is generally outside the range of usual human experience. Examples of stressors promoting such a response are combat, natural disasters, rape, and incest. As with PNDI, the psychiatric manual of mental disorders typically focuses on the term "anxiety" to refer to the symptom-producing feeling, not "stress." This is the tradition of the mental health sciences.

Current ideas involved in the study of stress include descriptions of the manner in which stress enters our lives and affects us. Trygstad,[25] for example, studied stress and coping in psychiatric nursing. One of her findings indicated that working relations among staff were more frequently a stressor for psychiatric nurses than were the clients.

Future advances in the study of stress and its effects will include an increased awareness within individuals of the reality of stress, its effects, and stress management. For many people, stress is not a personal concern. For example, individuals may continue to smoke or drink excessively or to maintain excess weight although these behaviors constitute stressors on biophysiological function. A person may be affected biologically by smoking, but not affected by the knowledge of the effect of smoke (the stressor) on the individual's health. This is complicated by the fact that smoking may reduce stress in the short run.

Once the individual personalizes the stress, making it relevant to the individual, the person must then choose to change and adopt a lifestyle of continued stress awareness and management. Changing and adopting a new lifestyle is challenging, and this change may itself be stressful.

The Effects of Stress

Smith and Selye[24] report that stress-related diseases are increasing. Between 50% and 80% of all disease phenomena are associated with stress. Peptic ulcers, bronchial asthma, arthritis, heart attacks, alcoholism, cancer, and mental disorders are all examples of diseases thought to be associated with stress.

Health depends on the adaptive energies of the individual in meeting the effect of stressors. Table 8-2 details various diseases associated with stress. Specific increases or decreases in hormones triggered by the occurrence of stress are listed. Diseases or symptoms frequently associated with these hormonal changes are also presented. The diseases listed are only a few of the possible responses to stress.

Morse and Furst[17] also describe symptoms related to stress. They describe the fight-or-flight response as being triggered by the autonomic nervous system, especially the catecholamines. Table 8-3 lists the symptoms and diseases caused by catecholamine overproduction.

The information gained by studying stress helps nurses understand the occurrence of stress. In Table 8-3, for example, one result of catecholamine production is muscular contraction, which causes headaches, neck pain, and other muscular difficulties. The clinician identifies these symptoms and the client's need for stress management and lifestyle changes. Other common signals seen frequently by nurses include impaired breathing, increased excitability, sweating, and altered perceptions.

Beck[4] notes that reactions to stressors are found in all cultures and that these reactions activate survival

TABLE 8-2.
THE RELATIONSHIP OF HORMONAL OR PHYSIOLOGICAL ACTIVITY AND SOME SYMPTOMS OR DISEASE STATES

CHANGES IN HORMONAL OR PHYSIOLOGICAL ACTIVITY	DISEASE OR SYMPTOMS
↑ Gluconeogenesis	Diabetes mellitus
↓ Gluconeogenesis	Hypoglycemia
↑ Protein breakdown	Muscle wasting, delayed healing
↓ Excretion of K+	Cardiac arrhythmias
↑ Vasoconstriction	Hypertension
↓ Blood to kidney	Kidney disease
↑ Antiinflammatory response	Respiratory infectious diseases
↓ Immunity	Cancer
↑ Proinflammatory response	Allergies
	Gastrointestinal disturbances
↑ Blood clotting	Coronary thrombosis
↑ Metabolism	Hyperthyroidism

(Adapted from Smith M, Selye H: Reducing the Negative Effects of Stress. Am J Nurs 79:1955, 1979)

mechanisms. For example, one response to threat is sweaty palms, which assist in cooling the body and promoting muscular activity. However, another response is nausea. Although nausea and vomiting may have assisted primitive people to discharge the contents of the stomach and to prepare peripheral circulation for flight, this response is not considered adaptive in most people to-day. There are many biological responses to threat that are not adaptive and that promote disease.

Beck's ideas of the origin of responses to threat *assist in removing self-blame from those who experience stress and stress-related illnesses.* Individuals today have much to learn in developing adaptive responses to stress, rather than expecting physiological mechanisms to carry the burden of stress adaptation. Clients may participate more readily in stress management programs if they perceive that having a stress-related illness is not wrong. Clients can be taught that their bodies are reacting in "primitive ways," and that these physiological reactions can result in disease, if not checked in proportion or degree. Stress management practices can help clients to use mental and physical energy to overcome the effects of diseases resulting from extreme or prolonged stress.

The Nature of Stressors Associated With the Stress Response

General Categories of Stressors: A Systems Perspective

Howard and Scott[11] state that the initial stressor causing problems in the organism can be categorized by the location of the stressor or the meaning of the stressor to the person (see Table 8-4). The table also includes the five

TABLE 8-3.
POTENTIAL SYMPTOMS AND DISEASES CAUSED BY CATECHOLAMINE OVERPRODUCTION DURING STRESS

SITE	ACTION	POTENTIAL SYMPTOM OR DISEASE
Skin	Vasoconstriction	Pallor
Liver	Excess glucose	Diabetes
Lungs	Excessive dilation	Impaired breathing
Lungs	Increased breathing rate	Hyperventilation
Stomach, intestines	Lining irritated	Ulcers
Blood vessels	Increased tendency to clot	Heart attack or stroke
Blood vessels	Increased blood pressure	Hypertension
Heart	Muscle damage	Heart damage or death
Motor nerves	Increased excitability	Muscle tremors
Muscles	Partial contraction	Headache, backache, jaw ache, shoulder pain, neck pain
Palms and soles	Increased sweating	Malodor
Eyes	Increased visual perception	"Beady" eyes
Mouth	Decreased saliva	Xerostomia (dry mouth)
Blood lactate	Waste product	Acid–base imbalance
Uric acid	Waste product	Gout
Cholesterol and fatty acids	Energy	Heart attack or stroke

(Morse D, Furst M: Stress for Success, p 68. New York, Van Nostrand Reinhold, 1979)

TABLE 8-4.
DIMENSIONS OF STRESSORS

MEANING OF THE STRESSOR	LOCATION OF THE STRESSOR		
	INSIDE THE PERSON	BETWEEN THE PERSON AND THE ENVIRONMENT	OUTSIDE THE PERSON
"Symbolic" meaning of the stressor (subjective)	The psychological	The societal (interpersonal)	The cultural
"Nonsymbolic" meaning of the stressor (objective)	The biological	The biological-environmental exchange	The environmental

(Adapted from Howard A, Scott R: A Proposed Framework for the Analysis of Stress in the Human Organism. Behav Sci 10: 146, 1965)

foci of analysis of a human system mentioned in the Introduction to this book (the environmental, societal, cultural, psychological, and physical), wherein the stressor originates its effect.

Psychological Components of Stress

To function, human beings need to maintain some degree of psychological health; to maintain health, individuals must have a satisfactory interpretation of a stressor. In this sense a stressor is "symbolic," because the individual thinks and evaluates the stressor by using highly individualized and personal interpretations. A client with cardiac disease may label a problem a "minor hassle," while a nurse may call the problem a stressor that could result in cardiac damage.

Social and Cultural Components of Stress

Social and cultural components are related to stressors that arise from living among and with others. For example, if a couple finds out that their child has a terminal illness, considerable stress is placed on the family group.

Some authors have considered job-related stressors, specifically those experienced by nurses.[19] Birckhead[5] developed a scale to indicate the degree to which nurses sense that they receive support from one another in their job setting. The focus of this scale is on *groups* of nurses. Birckhead views group support among nurses as essential for effective coping with stress in the work environment, and as essential for effective client care. One item on the scale is as follows:

> On my unit there is a joy that comes from our having pride and confidence in the way in which we strive to improve patient care.

> Strongly Agree   Agree   Undecided   Disagree   Strongly Disagree

This question is an obvious reference to the positive gains, such as personal joy, that can come from a support-

ive group. Nurses can respond to this scale as a point of departure for a discussion about their supportive relationships with each other.

Trygstad also studied the work environment, focusing on stressors for psychiatric nurses. This research is summarized in the Relevant Research box on p. 147.

Biological Stress

Changes in the body's internal organic system can upset the body's balance, creating problems. For example, during pregnancy biological changes cause "morning sickness," a problem or challenge to be reviewed and solved or ameliorated. Biological changes involve a physical (objective) alteration that is more easily known (nonsymbolic) than are subjective (symbolic) aspects of stress.

Environmental Stress

External stimuli can also create problems. Examples might include air pollution or the temperature of the atmosphere. Pollution can cause serious breathing problems for those with respiratory illness. Also, for older adults with few financial resources, not having money to pay a fuel bill can be a major stressor.

The Symbolic Meaning of Stress

The emphasis on the symbolic aspects of stressors is important. Stressors can be symbolized either as "challenges" or as "problems." It is possible to work with challenges because they are within the potential range of control of the person, even if only in the way the person symbolizes or thinks about the stressor. Problems denote barriers and difficulties rather than potentials. Nurses must question their own views of stressors. Do nurses view stressors as "challenges" or "problems" for the clients? Do clients become more involved in life-style changes when nurses perceive the stressors as challenges rather than problems?

RELEVANT RESEARCH

The purpose of Trygstad's study was to identify individual staff nurse stressors in psychiatric nursing. The sample consisted of 22 registered staff nurses working on nine psychiatric units at private or federal hospitals. All participants were female and had worked in an acute psychiatric setting for from one to six years. Twenty-seven percent of the sample held an associate degree, 46% held a baccalaureate degree, and 9% held a master's degree.

Data were collected through interviews of staff nurses by a researcher. Participants were asked to describe stressful experiences.

The researcher found that staff relationships on the units accounted for one third of all stressors identified, and included working relationships among RNs, LVNs, nursing assistants, and psychiatric technicians. Specific problems included ineffective communication, fighting among staff, and unresolved friction among staff members.

Seventeen percent of the stressors involved problems with head nurses and supervisory practices. Physicians were responsible for 9% of the stressors identified. Physicians were identified as stressors when they ignored nursing input and did not fulfill their responsibilities.

Resource shortages (such as a lack of personal space) accounted for 10% of stressors identified. Client-related problems accounted for 13% of all stressors. The stressor described most often in relation to clients was chronicity.

The Self was perceived as a stressor 13% of the time. Self stressors included self-doubt and the perception that the nurse was not performing well. Organization practices, such as devaluation of the nurse, were identified as stressors 6% of the time.

This study increases understanding of the work and stress of the psychiatric nurse. The work role and setting can then be examined to determine where changes can be made in order to decrease job stress.

(Trygstad L: Stress and coping in psychiatric nursing. J Psychosoc Nurs Ment Health Serv 24:23, 1986)

It should be noted, however, that a certain amount of stress is essential to a sense of well-being. This type of stress is called *eustress*. Selye[20] stated that there is a great deal of confusion about what stress actually is and how to deal with it. Stress is the body's nonspecific response to any demand placed on it, whether or not the demand is pleasant. Changing a flat tire and changing sleeping habits are both stressful, and both produce similar biological responses. It is not clear why positive stress, or eustress, places far less demand on the body than does "bad" stress, or distress.

Because stress cannot be totally eliminated, individuals should aim to understand typical lifestyle patterns and stress responses and then try to adjust their lives for effective functioning. One person's style of living may be to work long hours at a fast pace, while another may function at a slower pace with few complexities. Selye remarked that the difficulty arises when an individual attempts to force the self beyond normal stress tolerances.

The Nature of Stressors

A number of authors have attempted to determine the nature of stressors affecting individuals. Holmes and Rahe[9] developed a scale of stressors or stressful events. Individuals of varying backgrounds were asked to rank the amount of adjustment needed to cope with each life event. The resulting list is called the Social Readjustment Rating Scale (see Table 8-5). The numerical ratings were assigned by 394 individuals, who originally ranked the items after being told that marriage was equivalent to 50 units (Life Change Units, or LCU). The individuals in the study were from varying backgrounds, ages, and economic classes.

In developing the scale, Holmes and Rahe thought that, if stress results in disease, people experiencing a high degree of stress should report more illness than people reporting only a little stress. Their theory was supported when they found that people who scored between 150 and 199 LCUs in 1 year had a 37% chance of experiencing disease the following year. Those scoring between 200 and 299 had a 51% chance, and those scoring over 300, had a 79% chance.

Life Experience Stressors

Marks[14] developed a Life Events Survey, designed to assess the number and impact of ongoing episodic life events specific to individuals in college. The list of events in the survey was developed by combining a number of commonly-used life event lists, and included work or school, finances, health, romantic relationships, home, friends and family life, and personal events, such as being robbed. Individual scores on this survey can be compared with scores from other students. Marks' research is an example of attempts to help individuals in particular groups, such as college students, to find stressors specific to their current life experiences through the use of a scale tailored to their potential stressors.

Developmental Age Stressors

Simmons's[23] work presented a description of stress in the midlife years, and is an example of work being done on stressors associated with specific age periods. For example, the developmental period of the midlife years extends from ages 20 to 60 years. In the first part of this stage (20 to 28 years), individuals question the nature of the

TABLE 8-5.
SOCIAL READJUSTMENT RATING SCALE

EVENTS	SCALE OF IMPACT
Death of spouse	100
Divorce	73
Marital separation	65
Jail term	63
Death of close family member	63
Personal injury or illness	53
Marriage	50
Fired at work	47
Marital reconciliation	45
Retirement	45
Change in health of family member	44
Pregnancy	40
Sex difficulties	39
Gain of new family member	39
Business readjustment	39
Change in financial state	38
Death of close friend	37
Change to different line of work	36
Change in number of arguments with spouse	35
Mortgage over $10,000	31
Foreclosure of mortgage or loan	30
Change in responsibilities at work	29
Son or daughter leaving home	29
Trouble with in-laws	29
Outstanding personal achievement	28
Wife begins or stops work	26
Beginning or ending of school	26
Change in living conditions	25
Revision of personal habits	24
Trouble with boss	23
Change in work hours or conditions	20
Change in residence	20
Change in schools	20
Change in recreation	19
Change in church activities	19
Change in social activities	18
Mortgage or loan less than $10,000	17
Change in sleeping habits	16
Change in number of family get-togethers	15
Change in eating habits	15
Vacation	13
Christmas	12
Minor violations of the law	11

(Holmes T, Rahe R: The Social Readjustment Rating Scale. Psychosom Res 11: 214, 1967)

world and their place in it. Existing relationships with previously important individuals, groups, and institutions are modified or terminated. The person examines and modifies the self that was formed in the preadult world. The possibilities of the adult world are examined, and the individuals imagine themselves as a part of it. An initial adult identity is consolidated. The first part of the midlife period includes a juggling between exploring alternatives and creating a stable life structure.

Although it is necessary for health care providers to be aware of stressors associated with specific populations (such as members of a certain age group), each change experienced by individuals can serve as a type of loosening from a previous phase. Within this loosening change, improvement and learning take place, so that the individual is at an even *higher* level of actualization and well-being than before the change. Changes (including losses) can be viewed as problems or challenges within which to grow.

Coping Skills for Adjusting to Stress

For many individuals, disease is the end result of a stress process. However, individual persons can be aware of the subtle clues to distress. For example, people can notice that when they search for, and crave, altered emotional states they take a drink of alcohol. This signal of searching for, and craving, alcohol is a clue to the loss of control over alcohol. The individuals can be aware of their personal responses (psychological and biological) and use this information to do something different, such as learn stress management.

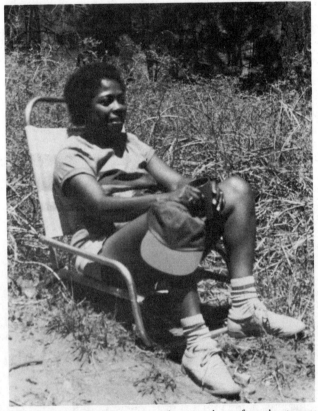

Figure 8-2. Periodic times spent relaxing and away from the stresses of day-to-day life assist in maintaining one's physical and emotional health.

Stress management gives some sense of personal power to individuals. Personal styles of coping with stress afford a sense of mastery as well as a sense of well-being.

The Therapeutic Use of Self and Levels of Prevention

Stress management can be done with clients at the primary, secondary, or tertiary prevention level. An advantage of stress management at the primary level of prevention is that it works well with clients who are not ill, and who can benefit from learning ways to promote wellness. Health promotion is accomplished by reducing stress through the use of stress management.

In primary prevention, the nurse can demonstrate the therapeutic use of self in finding the pattern of stressors in the client's life. The nurse can help the client to identify typical stress responses and can develop, with the client, a style of stress management that fits the client's patterns of living (Fig. 8-2). In making use of the therapeutic use of self the nurse gets to know the complexities of the client's *unique* style of living. The nurse also provides a sense of hope and belief in the individual by showing that the client can effect a change in stress response.

Much of the work in psychiatric/mental health nursing emphasizes the therapeutic use of self with ill clients. This work falls within the categories of secondary and tertiary prevention. For example, school nurses can perform early case-finding (secondary prevention), by reviewing cases of adolescents with marked changes in behavior (such as belligerence and truancy). By demonstrating in-

LIFESTYLE AND HEALTH QUESTIONNAIRE

Directions: Circle the numbers that best depict you and your life during the last year.

	ALMOST NEVER	SELDOM	OFTEN	ALMOST ALWAYS
Psychological:				
1. I have one regular activity which allows me to express myself (*i.e.,* at work and/or at home).	1	2	3	4
2. I feel comfortable with how my life is going right now.	1	2	3	4
3. I know what feelings I experience when I am stressed.	1	2	3	4
Interpersonal:				
1. My family relationships are good.	1	2	3	4
2. I maintain two close friendships.	1	2	3	4
3. My life includes opportunities for me to touch others, be touched by others.	1	2	3	4
4. I am involved in one close relationship.	1	2	3	4
5. My relationships fulfill my needs.	1	2	3	4
Biophysical:				
1. My personal health care practices are good (teeth, eyes, etc.).	1	2	3	4
2. I am content with my sexuality.	1	2	3	4
3. I avoid overuse of drugs, alcohol, tobacco.	1	2	3	4
4. I am aware of certain measures that tell how my body is coping with stress (*e.g.,* blood cholesterol level, blood pressure, resting pulse, pulse on exertion).	1	2	3	4
Sociocultural:				
1. My present job is fulfilling.	1	2	3	4
2. I allow time in my life to work on my spirituality.	1	2	3	4
3. I am involved in one community resource group.	1	2	3	4
Environmental:				
1. My environment at home is comfortable to me.	1	2	3	4
2. My environment is relatively free from pollutants/allergens/noise.	1	2	3	4
3. I exercise sufficient precaution in promoting my physical safety in my environment.	1	2	3	4

(Adapted from Baldi S, Costell S, Hill L et al: For Your Health: A Model for Self-Care. South Laguna, California, Nurses Model Health, 1980)

PHYSICAL AND EMOTIONAL SIGNS OF STRESS

Mark the following as they apply to your life during the last year:

	Often	Sometimes	Never
Tired feelings	____	____	____
Gaining and/or losing weight	____	____	____
Colds	____	____	____
Backaches	____	____	____
Headaches	____	____	____
Stomach troubles	____	____	____
Sadness	____	____	____
Trouble concentrating	____	____	____
Trouble falling asleep	____	____	____
Anxiety	____	____	____
Alcohol/drug use	____	____	____
Bowel problems	____	____	____
Menstrual cramps	____	____	____
Confusion	____	____	____

How many times did you mark "often" or "sometimes" in this section?

What other physical or emotional signs or messages has your body given you during this last year?

Do you see a connection between events in your life in the past year and your bodily reactions?

(Adapted from Baldi S, Costell S, Hill L et al: For Your Health: A Model of Self-Care. South Laguna, California, Nurses Model Health, 1980)

---

terest in the client and by using expert interviewing skills, the nurse can gain the trust of the adolescent while trying to determine if particular stressors are affecting the student. Cases of child abuse/neglect can be found in this manner, as well as other problems.

Tertiary prevention is demonstrated by nurses who help ill clients perform deep breathing exercises, role play difficult interactions for the clients, and so on. These techniques help clients control stressful experiences.

Stress Management

Nurses are in a position to observe stress situations in clients, to assess stress responses (using the rating scales of events, biological measures, and behavioral observations), and to help clients adopt lifestyles that include stress management.

The first step in stress management is to assess the client's present lifestyle and level of health. Baldi et al[3] developed a workbook for this assessment. They believe that improvements in exercise, relaxation, nutrition, and play can help people stay healthy and handle everyday stresses. They also emphasize that individuals are responsible for getting and staying healthy. This idea of responsibility revolves around the concept of self-care defined by Orem. Baldi defines self-care, using Orem's ideas, as the practice of activities that individuals initiate and perform on their own behalf to maintain life, health, and a sense of well-being.

To adopt a healthy lifestyle, the person has to make important decisions and take risks. Behavioral changes can be accomplished at any age or state of health. A supportive environment helps facilitate these changes, as does the attitude that change may take time, and that mistakes are understandable if long-term changes are expected.

The questionnaire on the previous page helps to assess a client's overall lifestyle and health. This questionnaire does not have right or wrong answers, but helps the individual to begin thinking about areas in need of change. Scores for each section can be added, as can the total score. If the score is under 36, the respondent may want to examine several life areas to determine if changes are needed in order to live a more comfortable life.

The box at the left lists physical and emotional signs of stress, and is used in stress response assessment. When completing the questionnaire, individuals are also asked to list other physical or emotional signs or messages they have received in the last year.

Baldi lists certain ways that individuals cope (see Table 8-6). The list includes some coping responses that are harmful for individuals, and others that are healthy. *The techniques are tailored to the individual* in keeping with the nurse's therapeutic use of self.

Baldi describes the use of "contracting" as a technique for making lifestyle changes. A contract is a client's agreement with self or with another person to accomplish a specific goal in a set period of time. The Stress Management Self-Contract Form shown in Figure 8-3 is an example.

There are a number of ways to facilitate the effectiveness of the self-contract. It is important to set only one goal at a time, and to allow a realistic amount of time to reach the goal. A baseline should first be determined: persons completing the contract should determine how they are doing now in the particular area before deciding what needs to be changed.

It is useful to allow a free day, two or three times per week, during which the individual does not have to follow the contract strictly. The contractor must also be aware of behaviors or acts that help or hinder reaching the goal. Finally, if the contract is to be taken seriously, the rewards and costs section must be completed. If the person fails to complete the contract, the person should view this as an effort made to change, and should try again.

TABLE 8-6.
TECHNIQUES OF STRESS MANAGEMENT

Which of the following methods of managing stress do you usually use? Do you consider them "healthy" for you or "harmful" for you?

Complete the following worksheet:

TECHNIQUE	HEALTHY FOR ME	HARMFUL FOR ME	TECHNIQUE (continued)	HEALTHY FOR ME	HARMFUL FOR ME
Listening to music			Listening to self-improvement tapes		
Physical activity			Overworking		
Having sex			Self-pity		
Smoking cigarettes			Having a temper tantrum		
Overeating			Going for a ride		
Drinking liquor			Praying		
Knitting/sewing			Chewing gum		
Cooking			Spending money		
Taking drugs (street or prescribed)			Writing poetry		
Trying to ignore the problem			Daydreaming		
Pretending it doesn't bother you			Biting fingernails		
Thinking things over			Playing an instrument		
Going to a movie or watching TV			Moping, isolating yourself, doing nothing		
Talking with friends			Talking to a therapist		
Leaving town			Talking to a spiritual guide		
Throwing things			Reading spiritual literature		
Cleaning the house			Add your other ways here:		

(Adpated from Baldi S, Costell S, Hill L et al: For Your Health: A Model for Self-Care. South Laguna, California, Nurses Model Health, 1980)

Cognitive Style and Coping

The *cognitive model* of coping abilities also emphasizes how people appraise what is being experienced and use this information to shape the course of events.[12] A "cognitive appraisal" is an individual's judgment about demands and constraints during continuing transactions with the environment and resources, as well as options for managing the transactions. These evaluative processes determine the person's stress reactions, the emotions experienced, and the outcomes of the adaptations. Cognitive appraisal processes are selective and sometimes idiosyncratic. Each person has his or her own view of experience.

The emphasis on cognition and coping is not as simple as determining the accuracy of one's reality-testing.

My Goals of Stress Management are

Short-term—by the end of six weeks I will   *have attended 6 aerobic dance classes*

Long-term—by the end of six months I will   *have attended aerobic dancing twice weekly*

Planning (all the steps I will take to reach my goal):

    1.   Schedule a baby sitter
    2.   Find a leotard
    3.   Call to obtain a class schedule
    4.   Arrange meals so I do not eat just prior to class

Thoughts About My Reaching My Goal

Helpful thoughts: *I will feel better*
                      I will enjoy the music

Nonhelpful thoughts: *I'll quit*
                        Others will be better than I

My Reward (if I meet my goal):   *a new dress*

The Cost (if I fail to meet my goal):   *wax my car*

Evaluation Date: *2/25/89*

I agree to help in reviewing this contract.   I agree to strive towards this goal.

Jack Thompson   *1/12/89*   *Jill London*   *1/12/89*
(Support person)   (Date)   (Your signature)   (Date)

Figure 8-3. Stress management self-contract form.

(Adapted from Baldi S, Costell S, Hill L et al: For Your Health: A Model for Self-Care. South Laguna, California, Nurses Model Health, 1980.)

Indeed, defensive functioning can be advantageous to the individual. A client with a recent spinal injury may deny the poor prognosis so that the sense of loss is not overwhelming and does not interfere with rehabilitative efforts. The client who denies the prognosis may be more ready, during the rehabilitative period, to devote energy to rehabilitative efforts than will someone who focuses on life with a loss of function.

In line with the importance of cognition in coping with stress, it may be useful for individuals to examine their needs and wants, particularly when making difficult decisions or comparing the potential negative implications of making certain choices. These examinations are useful in situations in which people cannot move toward or away from something, and are caught in agonizing decisions. Energy is directed toward indecision rather than no growth.

Figure 8-4 describes a method for charting needs and wants, and determining the possible negative implications for making a particular choice.

The Relaxation Response

There are numerous methods available to manage stress. Books on stress management techniques are available and include techniques such as assertiveness training, transcendental meditation, the use of affirmations, and other practices. Some clinicians who work with clients experiencing stress advocate relaxation techniques to assist in adjusting to stress. Morris[16] uses a relaxation technique involving alternatively tensing and relaxing seven groups of muscles. Research indicates that this is one of the most useful techniques for producing a sense of total relaxation. In many instances relaxation can be achieved on the first attempt to use the method.

In *Progressive Relaxation,* the client is instructed to tense each group of muscles for 10 seconds and then relax them for 60 seconds, progressing from the arms and hands to the legs and feet. The client must be willing to participate in this relaxation technique and must have no physical injury that contraindicates it. Music and soft lighting can potentiate the effects of the technique.

Paul[18] describes common misunderstandings and misuses of the relaxation technique proposed by Morris. These misunderstandings, and their corrections, include the following:

1. *Misunderstanding:* Relaxation is regarded as an "extra" that may be of some help when added to an existing therapeutic program.
   Correction: Relaxation training is most effective when it is an *integral* part of a program; it is often the central therapeutic procedure of a program.
2. *Misuse:* Relaxation is used routinely without regard for the time and manner of its introduction.

Correction: Each client is an individual, and the technique of relaxation training should be introduced and used with the client as indicated by the treatment needs of the client. *It is inappropriate simply to hand a client a cassette tape containing relaxation technique instructions, with no explanation.* The client and the technique are then set for failure. The explanation should include a statement of the purpose of relaxation training and generally what the client will hear on the audio tape.

3. *Misunderstanding:* Clients do not need to understand the nature of relaxation training and how it works.

    Correction: It is important for clients to understand the nature of stress, its physiological and psychological components, and the changes that relaxation can bring. Clients have varying reactions to relaxation techniques, and these need to be explored in counseling sessions.

4. *Misunderstanding:* Clients do not need to be motivated or assisted to practice regularly.

    Correction: Some clients attain benefit from relaxation training only after weeks of practice.

5. *Misuse:* There is failure to facilitate transfer of the training to real life situations.

    Correction: Techniques of relaxation are more effective if they are presented as a remedy for specific problems.

Paul's work can be generalized to the nurse's role in coping with stress. Individuals can improve their ability to adjust to stress. The goal is not to remove stress, but to adopt stress management skills that promote self-care. The nurse can serve in a key role in the client's stress management. The nurse can assess the client's stress responses, help the client examine daily life experiences to ascertain the nature of the stressors, and guide the client to adopt improved means of stress management.

The Instant Calming Response

In working with a client learning stress management, the nurse must emphasize a disciplined approach to stress management, including regular use of stress management techniques such as meditation or progressive relaxation. However, clients can also be taught more *immediate* stress management techniques. These can be used when the person has no time to prepare to use the techniques.

In learning the *Instant Calming Response,* the client explores with the nurse the immediate behaviors that promote a sense of calm. These actions may include deep breathing, counting to five, assuming a body position that evokes a sense of calm (such as holding one palm against the other), stretching, and others. The client can practice these behaviors in a calm period and report on their use during periods of stress.

Other Stress Management Techniques

Stress management techniques are increasingly being used in nursing practice. Brallier,[6] a nurse whose practice focuses on stress management, details many stress management techniques. She uses a systems approach, as described in the Introduction to this book, in working with clients. She focuses on typical stressors and stress responses, nutrition, exercise, societal (group and family) experiences, cultural experiences, spirituality, and how the environment affects the person's stress level. Several stress management techniques described by Brallier include:

1. *Biofeedback:* the use of instruments to assess the body's biological stress response (by measuring muscle tension)
2. *Autogenics:* concentration on positive, relaxing phrases to decrease stress (such as repeating to one's self, "My mind is calm and quiet.")
3. *Imagery:* the creation of a perception to invoke a sense of relaxation. For example, one could image a quietly running stream.
4. *Meditation:* the practice of spending quiet times in which one attempts to experience peace and an absence of thoughts about daily living
5. *Body movement:* movements such as those in Yoga and Tai Chi
6. *Hands-on methods:* approaches such as massage and acupressure

Additional techniques include listening to music, exercise, problem-solving, and talking with a friend or a professional counselor.

The Therapeutic Use of Self: A Summary

As stated in the Introduction to this book, students come to the therapeutic interchange with their own unique backgrounds and knowledge. Using these, students focus on the uniqueness of the clients. Students respond to clients using interventions directed toward pertinent client needs.

The use of the nursing process implies that, in working with clients and their stress experiences, nurses will understand the nature of stress and how it can affect health. Nurses then use their own selves—their own talents in establishing positive, healing relationships with clients—to understand stress in clients' lives.

In order to discover the details about the client's management (or lack thereof) of stress, the nurse must demonstrate a belief that stress needs attention. Also, the nurse must value the importance of changes in the client's lifestyle to cope better with stress.

At each step in the nurse's work with the client (as-

ASSESSMENT FORM

Needs and Wants (with an example)

Question: *Where should I live during college?*	Alternatives (Each alternative is assigned a measure of 1 to 10, with 10 being the highest in terms of the particular alternative best fulfilling the need)		
	1	2	3
Needs (Must have. Each has a value of 10):	*With parents*	*Dormitory*	*Own apartment*
1. *Quiet* =10	10 × 10 = 100	10 × 5 = 50	10 × 9 = 90
2. *Privacy* =10	10 × 6 = 60	10 × 7 = 70	10 × 10 = 100
3. *Time with friends* =10	10 × 6 = 60	10 × 10 = 100	10 × 8 = 80
4. *Convenience* =10	10 × 9 = 90	10 × 10 = 100	10 × 9 = 90
Others: _____			
	Total 310	Total 320	Total 360
Wants (Not a "must" but do have some importance. Each is assigned a value from 1 to 10, with 10 indicating the highest value.)	(Each alternative listed above is assigned a measure of 1 to 10, with 10 being the highest in terms of the particular alternative best fulfilling the want.)		
1. *Private phone* =4	4 × 5 = 20	4 × 0 = 0	4 × 10 = 40
2. *Meals accessible* =5	5 × 10 = 50	5 × 10 = 50	5 × 3 = 15
3. *Easy parking* =2	2 × 10 = 20	2 × 2 = 4	2 × 4 = 8
4. *Safety* =2	2 × 10 = 20	2 × 10 = 20	2 × 9 = 18
Others: _____			
Totals from Needs and Wants columns:	Total 110	Total 74	Total 81
	Total 420	Total 394	Total 441

Figure 8-4. (*Facing page*) An assessment form for determining needs and wants. (*This page*) Weighing the possible negative implications of choice.

sessment of stress effects, lifestyle change planning and implementation, and evaluation of the effectiveness of lifestyle changes), nurses use many of their abilities. Nurses respond with clients to change patterns of daily living that have been part of clients' experience for years. When nurses employ the Therapeutic Use of Self, clients can most effectively be assisted to make the changes required for stress management.

Summary

1. Stress is a natural, unavoidable aspect of life.
2. Disease can result from excessive stress over a prolonged period.
3. Patterns of physiological reaction to stress have been identified. For example, the discharge of adrenocor-

ASSESSMENT FORM (Continued)

Potential Negative Implications
of Choice with the Highest Number of Points

Things that could go wrong if the choice is that alternative receiving the highest number of points:

Things that could go wrong with choice of: *living in an apartment*

	Probability (1 to 10)	Severity (1 to 10)	Product (Probability × Severity)
1. *Roommate doesn't pay rent*	1	1	1
2. *Burglary*	3	5	15
3. *Can't be with friends*	1	10	10
4. *Noisy neighborhood*	4	8	32
5. *Time involved in fixing apt.*	1	1	1
6.			
7.			

Note: Generally, anything with a 50+ score may need to be eliminated or modified as an alternative. Score of 170–180+ indicates that there are serious reasons to eliminate the alternative.

Total 59

ticotropic hormone (ACTH) is one of the first signals of stress.

4. Stress management techniques can minimize the harmful effects of stress.

5. To be effective, stress management techniques must be tailored to the client's needs and attributes.

6. The nurse employs the Therapeutic Use of Self to establish and maintain a professional relationship through which the stress management plan is implemented with the client.

References

1. American Nurses' Association: Taxonomy for the Classification of Human Responses of Concern for Psychiatric/Mental Health Nursing Practice. Kansas City, American Nurses' Association, 1986
2. American Psychiatric Association: Diagnostic and Statistical Manual-III-R. Washington, DC, American Psychiatric Association, 1987
3. Baldi S, Costell S, Hill L et al: For Your Health: A Model for Self-Care. South Laguna, California, Nurses Model Health, 1980
4. Beck A: New Directions Cognitive Therapy. Programs for Mental Health Professionals, University of California at Irvine, Winter, 1984
5. Birckhead L: The Effect of the Nurse Support System on Patient Teaching. Unpublished doctoral dissertation, Boston University, Boston, Massachusetts, 1978
6. Brallier L: Successfully Managing Stress. Los Altos, California, National Nursing Review, 1982
7. Davis M, Eshelman ER, McKay M: The Relaxation and Stress Reduction Workbook, 2nd ed. Oakland, California, New Harbinger Publications, 1982
8. Greenberg J: Comprehensive Stress Management, Dubuque, Iowa, William C. Brown, 1983
9. Holmes T, Rahe R: The social readjustment rating scale. Psychosom Res 11:214, 1967
10. Horowitz M: Stress Response Syndromes. New York, Jason Aronson, 1976
11. Howard A, Scott R: A proposed framework for the analysis of stress in the human organism. Behav Sci 10:145, 1965
12. Lazarus R, Coyne J: Cognitive Style, Stress Perception, and Coping. In Kutash I, Schlesinger L (eds): Handbook on Stress and Anxiety. San Francisco, Jossey-Bass, 1980
13. Levine S, Scotch N: Social Stress. Chicago, Aldine, 1970
14. Marks T: Self-Schemata and Vulnerability to Depression. Unpublished dissertation, University of California at Los Angeles, 1982
15. Martinson I, Anderson S: Male and Female Response to Stress.

In Kjervik K, Martinson I (eds): Women in Stress: A Nursing Perspective. New York, Appleton-Century-Crofts, 1979

16. Morris C: Relaxation therapy in a clinic. Am J Nurs 79:1958, 1979

17. Morse D, Furst M: Stress for Success. New York, Van Nostrand Reinhold, 1979

18. Paul B: Relaxation Training—The Misunderstood and Misused Therapy. In McGuigan E, Lime W, Wallace J (eds): Stress and Tension Control. New York, Plenum Press, 1979

19. Scully R: Stress in the nurse. Am J Nurs 80:912, 1980

20. Selye H: On the real benefits of eustress. Psychol Today: 60, 1978

21. Selye H: The Stress Concept Today. In Kutash I, Schlesinger L (eds): Handbook on Stress and Anxiety. San Francisco, Jossey-Bass, 1980

22. Selye H: The Stress of Life, p 32. New York, McGraw-Hill, 1956

23. Simmons S: Stress During the Mid-Life Years. In National League for Nursing: Responding to Stress: Community Mental Health in the 80s. New York, National League for Nursing, 1981

24. Smith M, Selye H: Reducing the negative effects of stress. Am J Nurs 79:1953, 1979

25. Trygstad L: Stress and coping in psychiatric nursing. J Psychosoc Nurs Ment Health Serv 24:23, 1986

ELIZABETH OJALA

BEHAVIORAL RESPONSES TO ILLNESS

Learning Objectives

Upon completion of this chapter the student should be able to do the following:

1. Describe four areas of societal expectations of sick role behavior.
2. Describe how people suffering from chronic or emotional illness may have difficulty meeting societal sick role expectations.
3. Understand the implications of noncompliance with societal sick role expectations.
4. Understand how each of the five universal family features may influence familial behavioral response to illness.
5. Understand the importance of looking at the behavioral response to illness of individuals or families from their point of view.
6. Describe how cultural beliefs and practices may influence behavioral response to illness.
7. Identify areas of information regarding cultural beliefs and practices that would assist in making an accurate nursing assessment.
8. Understand how clients' unique perception of their illness influences their behavioral responses to illness.
9. Describe behaviors clients may exhibit in attempting to manage their responses to illness.
10. Provide a rationale for supporting clients' efforts to manage their responses to illness.

Introduction

Nursing practice encompasses many roles. Nurses help to prevent illness; promote and maintain health in the well; care for the sick; promote recovery; or help clients to die with a sense of dignity. Nursing practice covers the entire health–illness continuum, from optimal health at one end to death at the other. To fulfill nursing's many roles, nurses must understand all facets of illness, including what causes it, how to prevent it, the effects it produces, and what promotes recovery from illness. Another area pertinent to the understanding of illness is the client's behavioral response to illness.

Many nurses are frustrated by behavior of clients, such as the client who plans to return to work only two days after admission to intensive care units following a myocardial infarction, or the newly-admitted adolescent who refuses to get into a hospital gown, or the client with cancer of the larynx who refuses to have a laryngectomy, even when death will result if surgery is not performed. These clients exhibit behaviors in response to their illnesses, rather than symptoms of the illnesses themselves. However, many nurses find it rewarding to work with clients with recently diagnosed diabetes who actively seek information about regulating the disease, or with clients who eagerly push themselves to walk a little further each day after suffering a stroke. These clients also exhibit behavioral responses to their disease states. As the client examples illustrate, clients' behavioral responses to illness can promote or hinder recovery. Because it is nursing's role to promote recovery, nurses should understand the dynamics underlying clients' behavioral responses to illness. This chapter examines the factors that influence these responses.

Societal Sick Role Expectations

Society has certain expectations regarding appropriate sick role behavior that influence the behavior of those who are ill. Parsons[7] determined that those societal expectations fall into four areas. When people are ill they are expected to: (1) stop functioning in all or part of their usual social roles; (2) accept help from others; (3) want to get well; and (4) seek competent help. Each of the societal sick role expectations will be discussed here in relation to behavioral responses to illness.

First, *people who are ill are expected to stop functioning in all or part of their social roles.* Social roles include activities such as going to work, attending social events, caring for children, and performing household duties, as well as performing community service. How many and which social roles are not fulfilled during illness is, of course, dependent on the stage and severity of the disease. For example, although it is considered appropriate to cancel a dinner engagement when a person is coming down with the "flu," that is not generally considered an adequate reason for not going to work. Once a person is recognized as ill with the flu, it is appropriate

not to go to work, and the person may be relieved of all or part of other responsibilities as well. On the other hand, an ill person is expected to stop engaging in recreational activities immediately. Most employers find it unacceptable for employees not to come to work but to keep dinner engagements.

When illness is chronic, role function is affected over long periods of time. If the illness is also severe, the person's social role functioning may become severely restricted, leading to an impoverishment of role function. For example, in order to recover from the disease, a person suffering from Guillain-Barré syndrome may be forced to cease all motor activities for several months. Inability to perform motor activities affects the performance of many social roles. A severely arthritic person may be forced to give up more and more activities as the arthritis becomes more severe. If a person is forced to give up driving a car, becomes unable to ride a bus without assistance, and cannot walk for long distances, social role functioning outside of the home becomes quite restricted. A person who is chronically depressed may lose the ability to function adequately at work or at home. In addition, the inability to relate to others in a warm, friendly manner may drive away old friends and prevent the formation of new relationships. Over time, emotional illness, as well as physical illness, can lead to social role restriction.

In the case of emotional illness, societal expectations regarding fulfillment of social roles during illness may not be as clear as they are for physical illness. When people have the flu, others perceive them as ill and support their staying in bed and not performing usual social role functions. When individuals are depressed, others may not perceive them as ill because the difficulties are of an emotional and cognitive nature, and are not as obvious as physical incapacitation. Others may perceive the emotionally ill as aloof (because they are withdrawn), hard to get along with (because they are irritable), or rigid (because they are afraid), rather than ill. As a result of these perceptions, others may not see a need for emotionally ill people to be relieved of social role function. Perhaps it is only when emotionally ill people become completely unable to fulfill their social role functions that others recognize them as ill.

Thus, when people are ill, they are expected to stop functioning in all or part of their usual social roles. Which roles and how many they cease to carry out are dependent on the stage, length, and severity of the illness. Emotional illness, as opposed to physical illness, may not be as readily perceived as illness. Therefore, relief from social role functioning may not be seen as necessary.

The second societal expectation of ill people is that *they accept help from others.* How much and what type of help is accepted is relative to how ill the people are perceived to be. For example, if people are unable to get out of bed, they are expected to accept help with meals and household chores. If individuals are able to care for themselves at home but unable to go to work, they may be expected to accept the help of co-workers on a project. Chronic illness may require help from others on a long-term basis, creating an image of chronically ill people as helpless and dependent. That image may be difficult for the chronically ill person to accept. In the case of emotional illness, it may not be clear when a person needs help or what kind of help can be given. An emotionally ill person may be able to work and take care of household responsibilities, yet be preoccupied and easily upset, causing the quality of work and interpersonal relationships to suffer. Others may perceive that something is wrong and want to help, but not know what to do. Others may offer what they think is help, and have it rejected as not helpful. It is difficult for an emotionally ill person to accept help if it is not offered, or if the assistance that others offer is not perceived as help.

Thus, an ill person is expected to accept help from others. How much and what type of help is expected to be accepted is dependent upon how ill the person is perceived to be. In the case of chronic illness, the need for help on a long-term basis can lead to an undesirable image as a dependent person. In the case of emotional illness, a person may have difficulty accepting help because it may not be offered, or what is offered may not be seen as helpful.

The third societal expectation of ill people is that *they should want to get well.* Sick people are sent get-well cards and wishes for a speedy recovery. Remaining in the sick role beyond the time expected for an illness is viewed negatively. People who stay in bed and let others wait on them long after they are capable of getting up and returning to usual functioning are seen as shirking responsibility. People are expected to want to return to usual role functioning and, as soon as they are capable of assuming usual functioning, they are expected to do so.

In the case of chronic illness, societal expectations complicate the individuals' situation. It may be that, as much as they may want to, they can't "get well"—they can only strive to resume as many of their pre-illness capabilities as possible. This inability to resume all prior functioning within a certain period of time can create feelings of guilt and shame in chronically ill people. They may feel that others see them as lazy, or may view themselves as worthless.

In an emotional illness, the societal expectation that the person wants to recover is also complicated. What the emotionally ill person does to get well may appear to be very different from what a physically ill person does to get well. When a person is physically ill, it usually promotes recovery to avoid strenuous activity and to rest and relax. However, strenuous activity may aid in recovery from depression, and rest and relaxation may create social isolation when the person needs companionship and communication with others. Because the behavior of emotionally ill people may not be perceived as health-seeking behavior, it may not appear that they want to get well.

People suffering from a chronic emotional illness are in an even more complicated position with regard to societal expectations. It is not likely that they will recover completely from their illness. Therefore, they will continue to need assistance in carrying out social role func-

tioning. At the same time, they may be viewed by others as not wanting to get well or, worse yet, as not ill. The person's continued dependency on society may be viewed negatively.

The fourth societal expectation of ill people is that *they are expected to seek competent help.* When people are ill, they are expected to be seen by competent professionals, and to comply with the prescribed treatment. Generally, in our society a health professional is viewed as competent. However, in some cultural groups the assistance of a lay helper, such as a "curandero" or medicine man, may be sought. Regardless of the society, the ill person is expected to seek competent help.

In chronic illness, the need for competent help diminishes as the ability to affect the client's condition decreases. Therefore, at some point, contacting the health professional may be discouraged while self-care and independence are encouraged. This transition can create confusion in the societal expectation that, when a person is ill, competent help should be sought. However, some chronically ill clients may no longer benefit from professional help.

There are difficulties when emotionally ill people seek competent help. There is still a stigma attached to emotional illness. Those who find that they have a mental illness may wonder if others will remain friends. This question represents an underlying fear that they might not be as acceptable if they are emotionally ill. The same reaction seldom occurs with physical illnesses. Emotionally ill people are thought of as lacking willpower and being irresponsible, filled with sin, or even dangerous. A person experiencing an emotional illness may believe or fear that these negative connotations are true. Therefore, even acknowledging emotional illness may produce anxiety in an emotionally ill person. If people do not acknowledge illness, they will not seek competent help. Sometimes emotionally ill people acknowledge that they suffer from emotional illness, yet may not see the need for professional assistance. They may feel that family and friends can help, and spend hours discussing problems with them. In addition, obtaining professional help may be threatening for emotionally ill people because it may signify weakness or, worse yet, that they are "losing their minds."

Once people admit that they need professional help, it is usually a new experience to obtain help. Most people have been to medical doctors and have been cared for by nurses at some point in their lifetime, whereas people seeking psychological help are usually doing it for the first time. Who is sought: A psychiatrist, psychiatric nurse, social worker, psychologist, family counselor, or clergyman? The variety of professionals who work with emotional problems may confuse the emotionally ill person. The belief that a professional cannot help them anyway may complicate the search for help. The emotionally ill person, in order to seek competent help, must overcome some or all of these barriers. When a person is emotionally unstable, these barriers may seem insurmountable; therefore, emotionally ill people may not seek competent help in a timely manner.

People suffering from chronic or emotional illness may have more difficulties in meeting societal expectations. These difficulties affect the behavioral responses exhibited by people who are emotionally ill, and especially of those who are chronically emotionally ill. If societal expectations are not met, society disapproves. This disapproval may be translated into "It's not okay to be emotionally ill," or "You're not okay because you're emotionally ill." As a result, people suffering from emotional illness are caught in a situation in which they are ill and are expected to conform to "proper" sick role behavior and yet, due to the chronic or emotional nature of their illness, may not be able to conform. Social disapproval, real or imagined, can lead to guilt feelings and embarrassment or shame. How these feelings of guilt, embarrassment, or shame may be manifested in behavior will be discussed in the section on individual behavioral response.

Familial Behavioral Response to Illness

Aside from rare instances of institutionalization, most people are born into, and raised in, families. Within the family unit children are socialized and taught the values, beliefs, and practices that influence their behavior throughout their lives. Just as society has expectations regarding sick role behavior, families have expectations regarding how family members should behave and be treated when they are ill. These expectations influence the family's behavioral response to the illness of a family member. In order to understand families' behavioral responses to illness, it is important to realize that all families are unique and, at the same time, share certain features with all other families. An examination of the features that all families share can help in understanding familial behavioral response to illness.

Spradley[8] identified the following as the most important universal family features:

1. Every family is a small social system.
2. Every family has its own cultural values and rules.
3. Every family has structure.
4. Every family has certain basic functions.
5. Every family moves through stages in its life cycle.

Each universal family feature will be discussed in relation to behavioral response to illness.

The Family as a Social System

A family is a small social system. As a system, the members of the unit are interdependent and strive to maintain balance. The illness of a family member upsets the balance of the family unit, causing the members to compensate for the imbalance. Therefore, what affects one member of the family unit affects them all. For example, if the youngest son in the Adams family is hospitalized with an asthma attack, the mother and father may spend long periods of time with him at the hospital. As a result, the teenage daughter may assume responsibility for making the family's dinner and doing the laundry, as well as supervising her 10-year-old brother after school each day. The 10-year-old brother may assume responsibility for taking out the trash. The father may assume responsibility for cleaning the house and grocery-shopping while the mother is at the hospital. In this way, the family compensates for the imbalance created by the mother's and father's absence from the home during the son's hospitalization.

In some situations, the family may not be able to compensate for the imbalance in the family system, or may find that secondary problems are created by their efforts to compensate. For example, if the illness of a family member is severe or life-threatening, the family may become so anxious about the illness that they are unable to perform their routine responsibilities, much less shift roles and responsibilities. As a result, the family system may become severely imbalanced, resulting in a chaotic and nonnurturing situation. Or, as a result of their efforts to compensate, secondary problems may be created. In order to compensate for her mother's absence during an illness, a teenage daughter may have to give up her extracurricular activities in order to babysit her brother. As a result, she may feel anger and resentment, and be irritable and unkind toward her brother. He, in turn, may feel hurt and unloved, and respond by aggressive behavior at home and at school. Secondary problems have erupted as a result of the family's efforts to compensate for the original problem, the illness of the mother.

Illness of a parent may create worry and anxiety in the children. If they are asked to assume additional responsibilities while a parent is ill, they may find it difficult to make the adaptation back to their previous roles and responsibilities. For example, a community health nurse received a referral from a school nurse regarding an eight-year-old girl who was missing school because of complaints of stomach pains. The child was examined by a physician and found to be healthy. During a visit to the home, the mother reported to the nurse that her daughter complained every morning of a stomach ache and begged not to go to school. The mother allowed her to stay at home, although she did not feel that her daughter was physically ill. When questioned about recent family events, the mother shared that her husband had suffered a heart attack a month previously. He had been home for two weeks and was due to start back to work that week. An interview with the child revealed that the child was worried about her mother and did not want to leave her at home alone while she was at school. The child felt that her mother needed her at home. In fact, when her father had been hospitalized, the daughter had been allowed to stay home with her mother and "help out" for a few days. The child, unable to make the transition back to her previous role, continued to see herself as her mother's caretaker.

As a social system, families have boundaries. The family unit forms a bond that separates it from the rest of the world. Nursing recognizes that bond when stipulating that only family members may visit a patient. The strength of the family bond differs from family to family. However, when outside forces threaten the family unit, that bond may become very strong. Illness in a family member may cause outside forces to threaten the family. For example, if school authorities judge that one child in a family needs psychological help, the family may feel threatened. As a result, the family may deny that there is anything wrong with that child and refuse to have any involvement with school authorities or mental health professionals. Nurses must remember that their well-meaning interventions may be viewed as threats to the family unit. As a result, the family may shut professionals out or resist help.

Families are not closed systems, since they allow interaction between family members and external social systems such as school, church, and other community organizations. A job outside the home is also an interaction between family and external systems. As a result, there is a give-and-take between the community and the family unit. In the event of illness, a family may draw on outside social systems for assistance and support. At the same time, the family may need to withdraw some or part of their involvement in outside social systems. Some families routinely draw on outside social system support yet give little back. Other families routinely give more than they receive. A family that is used to giving may find it difficult to accept assistance when it is needed. They may struggle to preserve the family's independence as a matter of honor. It is important for nurses to assess how a particular family usually interacts with outside social systems to understand how the family may react to outside assistance when a family member is ill.

Another characteristic of families as social systems is that they have goals. According to Spradley, the overall purpose of families is "to establish and maintain an environment that promotes the development of their members."[8] How each family meets that purpose is unique. For example, one family may see provision of a stable environment as important to the development of its members, and therefore turn down an offer of promotion for the father that would involve relocation to another state. Another family may see provision of a variety of environments as important to the development of its members, and therefore seek job opportunities that allow them to live in foreign countries. How a family carries out its overall purpose and goals affects how it responds to the illness of a family member. For example, if the need arises for a family member to be hospitalized in another city, the first family in the example above will probably find it more stressful than the second family.

Families are small social systems composed of interrelated parts. Therefore, what affects one family member affects the whole unit. Families have boundaries that set them apart from other social systems, and they also interact with other social systems. Families work toward a common purpose of fostering the development of their members. How each family meets that purpose is unique. To understand the behavior of families, nurses should view them as social systems.

Cultural Values and Rules of the Family

Families share broad cultural values that are passed on from generation to generation, as well as values that are derived from current society, religion, and other social influences. Families develop their own special values and ways of operating that can be called their "family culture." These cultural values are translated into beliefs about health and illness. The family's health beliefs strongly influence how they behave in response to illness of a family member. For example, if a family has a present value orientation and believes there is no point in worrying about tomorrow, they may show a lack of interest in discharge planning for a family member until the day of discharge. On the other hand, a family that has a future value orientation may request information regarding discharge plans before that information is even available.

Behaviors that may seem illogical or detrimental to a client's health may be very logical when understood in relation to the family's point of view. If a family believes that illness is caused by factors external to the person, it is illogical to them that introspection can assist in recovery from an emotional illness. As a result, the family may refuse to allow a member to participate in psychotherapy, but instead may seek a treatment to drive the evil spirits out. If a family that believes that all problems are to be discussed and solved within the family is forced to seek outside help for an ill member, they may view the need for external help as a family failure. As a result, the family may have difficulty providing information regarding what they consider private family matters. If a family reveres the elderly, they will probably scorn the idea of placing a grandmother in a nursing home and care for her at home, even if it places considerable strain on the family. If a family believes that individuals should not disagree with authority figures, they may agree to the plan of nursing care even though they have no intention of following through on the care as planned. To prevent misunderstandings, client noncompliance, management problems, and, consequently, poor care, nurses should assess the family's health values, beliefs, and ways of operating prior to planning nursing care.

Each family has prescribed roles and responsibilities. The roles and responsibilities of each member, and how they will carry them out, are determined by the family. In a single-parent family, the one parent may be responsible for disciplining the children. In another family, the financial support of the family may be shared among the mother, father, and eldest son. In the event of illness, roles and responsibilities are usually disrupted. The amount of disruption depends on the flexibility of the family, and the roles and responsibilities that are affected. A flexible family is able to shift roles and responsibilities as the need arises. For example, the father is able to assume responsibility for the mother's household tasks when she is ill. A family that is not as flexible may become paralyzed when the mother becomes ill and the father is unwilling to do "women's work." If the ill family member assumes a role that cannot be filled by another family member, more disruption will occur. For example, if the father is the sole financial support of the family and the mother has never worked outside the home and has three young children at home, the father's illness may be devastating to the family. It is important, then, for nurses to determine what roles and responsibilities the ill family member usually fulfills within the family, as well as how those roles and responsibilities are being fulfilled during the illness.

Family members usually have several roles to play. For example, a mother is a daughter, may be a wife, and may be a sister. The responsibilities of the different roles may, at times, be difficult to fulfill. In one instance, a mother sought assistance from a community mental health nurse when her nine-year-old son began wetting his bed, something he had not done since he was four years old. In discussing recent events in the family, the mother mentioned that her 21-year-old sister had just been diagnosed with acute lupus erythematosus. She cried, and expressed the fear that her sister would die. She said that she had always functioned as her "little" sister's care-taker, and now felt helpless to do anything for her. In addition, as the eldest child in her family, she had always been the member who organized the family in times of crisis. However, in this case she felt unable to do anything to support her parents and sister. She described herself as anxious and sad, and appeared preoccupied and overwhelmed by her situation. The nurse felt that she was probably not attending to her son's needs in the usual manner. As a result, he reacted to his mother's anxiety and preoccupation by regressing to an earlier behavior of bed-wetting. In this example, the mother had difficulty fulfilling all of her various roles. As a result, a behavioral problem erupted in her son. It is important to be aware of all of the various roles a person usually fulfills and to understand that trying to fulfill all those roles may, at times, be difficult.

The concentration of power within a family is also part of a family's culture. In one family the power may be concentrated in one individual (or parent) who makes all the decisions and exerts control over the other family members. In another family the power may be distributed more evenly between both parents. In yet another family the power may even be shared somewhat by the children, who are allowed to participate in family decision-making. The concentration of power within a family affects how the family behaves when a family member is ill. Most likely, if the concentration of power is with one person, that person will decide if a family member is ill, and when and from whom the family member will seek treatment. Therefore, it is important for nurses to determine which family member has the authority to make decisions regarding treatment. If a family power figure becomes ill, the person may continue to exert that power from the sick bed. As a result, the nurse may find that the client, although hospitalized, is not resting but rather is on the telephone and having visitors most of the time. If the client becomes too ill to continue to exert power, the family may ignore the illness because they may be unable

to see the person in a dependent and powerless role. In this case the family may have difficulty continuing to function effectively because family members are unaccustomed to making decisions and exerting control. In a family in which the power is distributed more evenly, the illness of one member, even a parent, may be adjusted to with little difficulty because the other family members are accustomed to making decisions and exerting control.

If a family member who has always assumed a powerless and dependent role within the family becomes ill, the family may readily accept the dependent role that the illness may demand. In this case, however, the family may have difficulty letting the family member recover, and may foster the person's dependency long after the person has recovered from the illness. If, as may be the case in emotional illness, a family member has been unable to function mentally for a period of time, the family may have difficulty trusting the individual to make sound decisions and exert control over his or her own or other family members' lives after recovery. This lack of trust may undermine the confidence of the family member who is trying to get well. An examination of the concentration of power within a family can provide the nurse with information that is vital to good care-planning. Therefore, efforts should be made to determine where the power lies within a family.

Knowledge of the family "culture," including values, beliefs, practices, roles and responsibilities of each member, and how the power is distributed, provides necessary background information for assessing how the illness of a family member may affect the family unit. Behaviors exhibited in response to the illness of a family member that may seem illogical without an understanding of the family culture become logical when they are looked at from the family's point of view. An examination of the family culture helps the nursing professional become aware of the family's point of view.

Family Structure

All families have structure. That structure may consist of the traditional nuclear family of father, mother, and children; blended families of divorced parents and their children; a single-parent family of mother or father and children; an extended family of grandparents, mother, father, and children; or a kinship network of several generations living in close proximity and sharing goods and services as well as roles and responsibilities. In the time of illness, the family structure affects how roles and responsibilities are adjusted and how family functions are carried out. When the mother of a single-parent family becomes ill, it may be devastating for the children because they have no other adult to provide for their physical needs. On the other hand, when one member of a kinship network becomes ill, the other members can more easily take over the ill member's roles and responsibilities. Nurses should determine the family structure in order to be able to predict how devastating the illness of a family member may be for family functioning.

Family Functions

Families have functions that they must carry out. Spradley identified six functions typical of the American family today.[8] Those functions include provision of affection, security, identity, affiliation, socialization, and controls. A family provides *affection* for its members by showing each other that they are loved and supporting each other emotionally. A family provides *security* for its members by meeting their physical needs and being a safe place within which they can develop. A family provides its members with an *identity* by providing guidance and feedback about themselves in relation to family expectations. A family provides *affiliation* for its members by providing an automatic group membership. A family *socializes* its members by transmitting their attitudes, values, goals, and expected behaviors to its members. A family *controls* its members by exerting control over their conduct, assigning roles and responsibilities, and regulating how resources are to be used. Looking at families from the perspective of the functions they fulfill, it should be evident how important individuals' families are to them.

During an illness of a family member, the family's ability to function may be affected. An ill family member may not be able to fulfill the usual roles and responsibilities. Therefore, the other family members may not be provided the usual affection, feedback, controls, and so on. On the other hand, the family's ability to provide its usual functions for the family member may be limited when the member is ill. When a family member must be removed from the home due to illness, it may be especially difficult for the family to provide its usual functions. Once the family member is removed from the home, the family is able to exert little, if any, control over the welfare of the individual. For example, if a young boy is hospitalized and the parents are unable to stay with him and provide his care, the ability of the family to provide affection and control is diminished. The family is expected to trust the ability of the hospital staff to provide physical security and a safe environment for their young boy. The child loses his identity as the youngest son in the Jones family, and becomes the male patient with pneumonia in Room 233. Further affecting his identity may be the fact that he is expected to behave differently as a patient in the hospital than he does at home. If the child remains hospitalized for a long period of time, the family's ability to socialize their young member may be affected as well.

In the case of the hospitalization of a parent, the removal of the parent from the home affects the ability to provide the usual affection, security, socialization, and control for the spouse and children. Small children may be restricted from visiting the parent. Visits with other children and spouses may be hampered by a lack of privacy and hospital regulations such as "Don't sit on the bed." The family may, at the same time, be very concerned over the welfare of the hospitalized parent and feel frustrated and saddened about their inability to provide for the parent in their usual ways.

When a family's ability to provide the usual functions is threatened or lost, the family reacts to that event. Feelings of loss of control over the situation and an inability to help the ill member may, in turn, create feelings of frustration, anger, and sadness. The family may show these feelings by angry, demanding behavior or sarcastic, complaining behavior toward the health professionals providing care for their family member. It may be difficult for nurses to deal with this behavior and to understand why the family behaves in this manner.

Exploring the feelings motivating the family's behavior may help the nurse understand the behavior and, in turn, be better able to deal with it in a constructive way. For example, when a young child is hospitalized and the mother is not allowed to (or cannot) remain with her child in the hospital, the mother may fear for the child's safety and security and grieve over her inability to provide the ill child with affection. Although the mother may want the nurses to care for her child in a nurturing manner, she may also resent their ability to provide for her child when she cannot. Rather than being happy when the nurses tell her how good the child was when bathed that day, she may respond with irritation. In another example, a husband is hospitalized and the wife feels overburdened at home and anxious about her husband's welfare. The wife may need affection from her husband. The lack of privacy in the hospital allows for little physical intimacy, and may limit verbal intimacies as well. As the wife sits forlornly beside her husband's bed, feeling this need, a nurse walks in with a friendly smile. The nurse comments that the client must be feeling better for he has been able to keep the nurses laughing all morning. Rather than being happy that her husband is feeling better, the wife responds with a sarcastic remark to the nurse and leaves the hospital early. In these examples, the behavior of the mother and the wife may seem inexplicable to the nursing staff. Only by understanding the feelings underlying the behavior do the nurses make sense of the behavior.

Complaints by the family about the care that is given to their family member are often irritating to nurses. However, when the complaints are viewed within the framework of usual family functions, they make sense. Families usually provide for the safety, nutrition, hygiene, and appearance of their family members. Therefore, it is logical that they are concerned about the quality of the food the client is being fed, the way the client looks, and whether the side rails are up on the bed. Seemingly small things, such as combing a client's hair, washing his or her face, cleaning glasses, or changing a soiled pillow case may be very important to a family because they usually have control over these patient-care areas. In dealing with family complaints, it is useful to find out exactly what the family expects and wants for its member. If the family expectations are unrealistic or seem unreasonable, explore with the family why they feel it is necessary for the client to have that care. This is done to discover the feelings underlying the family's desires. Assume that there is a logic underlying the family's desires and that they are reasonable people. A little time and understanding helps the family deal with the difficulties of having a member hospitalized. As a result, any problems that exist due to family complaints can be resolved more easily.

In the case of an emotionally ill family member who is hospitalized, all previous discussions apply. In addition, it is likely that the family's functioning has been disrupted before the hospitalization because of the family member's behavior. For example, if a parent is experiencing depression, the ability of that parent to provide affection had probably diminished before hospitalization. In the case of alcoholism or drug abuse, the member's aggressive or unpredictable behavior may have already caused other family members to feel insecure and unsafe. Aggressive behavior of a child may have caused the family to feel that they are unable to exert control over that member. Antisocial behavior of an adolescent may create guilt in parents who feel they have failed to socialize that member. The senile behavior of an elderly grandmother may have caused the family to feel that they are unable to provide a safe environment for her. If the hospitalization is preceded by an acute episode of abnormal behavior, such as a suicide attempt, an attempt to harm another person, a manic buying spree, or a psychotic break with reality, the family will probably have experienced strong emotions, ranging from shock and fear to rage. Hospitalization may be viewed as a relief, an injustice, an outrage, or a last resort. Strong reactions to the hospitalization of an emotionally ill family member should be anticipated by the nurse.

Further complicating the hospitalization of an emotionally ill family member may be other factors, such as the member's being placed in a locked unit, the necessity for physical restraint, the bizarre behavior of other clients on the unit, or angry, threatening behavior the family member directed toward other family members. The family may react in numerous ways. They may withdraw and leave as quickly as possible. They may be apologetic and embarrassed by their member's behavior. They may be angry, demanding, and nonsupportive of the hospital staff's efforts. They may express guilt and sorrow over their perceived inability to bring their child up "right." Or they may act as if the hospitalization is a routine event and seem unaffected by it. It is important for the nurse to observe, and seek to understand, the family behavior. Information regarding what behaviors, if any, precipitated the hospitalization and what the hospitalization of the family member means to the family should be sought in order to assess the family situation. The family should be encouraged to express feelings regarding the hospitalization. Efforts should be made to help the family avoid any further family disruption.

The fact that all families carry out certain functions is an important universal feature in relation to helping nurses understand why families behave as they do in the face of illness. No other universal family feature points out so clearly how important the family is to an individual. During illness, nursing care provides for individuals some or all of the functions usually provided by the family. It is important to remember that the family provided those functions before the client's illness, and will do so again.

Family Life Cycles

The last family universal feature concerns what Duvall described as the *family life cycle*.[4] Duvall described families as going through a series of developmental stages, from a newly married state through the rearing, raising, and letting go of children, into retirement and being a couple again, and finally to the death of both spouses. She described families as continuing to carry out their basic functions throughout the life cycle. In addition, she identified certain tasks specific to each developmental stage that were to be accomplished by the family. Not all families go through their life cycles in the same way as the typical nuclear family described by Duvall. Other family structures, such as the single-parent family, are common today, and those structures cause the developmental tasks to vary. However, regardless of their structure, the family goes through a family life cycle.

The effect of the illness of a family member during different stages of the family life cycle will vary in relation to what is occurring during that stage. Therefore, the response of family members to illness during different stages of the life cycle will also vary. For example, if a wife becomes severely depressed during the first year of a childless couple's marriage the illness may affect the couple's establishment of a mutually satisfying relationship. However, the husband may react to the wife's illness with patience and understanding, feeling that the illness may help them to get to know each other better. If, however, the wife becomes severely depressed after the birth of the couple's first child, the couple's adjustment to their infant and the infant's development may be affected. In this case, the husband may not be as patient and understanding with his wife, for he may see the effect that his wife's illness is having on their new baby and, as a result, react with resentment and anger.

In another situation, the reaction of the family to aggressive, uncontrollable behavior of their five-year-old child may be one of tolerance. However, aggressive, uncontrollable behavior exhibited by that same child during adolescence will probably not be tolerated, and may be feared. Illness may cause a family to return to a previous developmental stage, such as when a child suffers a schizophrenic episode during college years, resulting in the child's returning to live with the parents. The parents' reactions in this situation may include resentment at having to resume their former care-taking functions, or relief at having regained their child. The diagnosis of a chronic illness after retirement will probably be met with a different response than it would have been during a family's working years. Alcoholism and drug abuse will probably be met with a different family response if in an elderly family member than if in a young family member. A wife will probably react differently to being told that her husband has a terminal illness when he is 90 years old than she would have when she and her husband were young. The effect of illness on the family differs according to the developmental stage of the family. As a result, the behavioral response to the illness of a family member differs. It is important for nurses to take into consideration the stage of the family cycle when planning care for the family.

As each of the five universal family features was examined in this section, it was pointed out that the family, as a unit, is a strong determinant of the behavior of its members and that the illness of a family member causes a behavioral response in the family unit. Overall, an examination of the universal family features revealed that, in order to understand the behavioral response of families and their members, nurses must look at the illness situation from the family's point of view. An assessment of the factors involved in each of the universal family features can help nurses become aware of the family's point of view. The box below provides a list of general family assessment areas.

Cultural Influences on Behavioral Response to Illness

An old Navajo man refuses to have a colostomy, although he understands that without it he will die from cancer of the stomach. When asked why, he says, "Because right now I'm known as Hostine Yassie, and if you operate on me, I'm going to be known as 'The Old-Man-Who-Shits-Through-His-Stomach.' I'm not going to do it."[3]

A Mexican-American father storms into the Head

Start Clinic where his son had received a smallpox vaccination three days earlier. He is very upset with the nurse who gave the vaccination, and shows her the reddened, swollen area where the vaccination was given. He feels that the site is infected and his child will become ill. He says that he did not give permission for this to be done to his child.[5]

A school nurse sees a 13-year-old Mexican-American girl who was referred by a teacher. The girl complains of sleeplessness and loss of appetite, and appears anxious. The nurse contacts the girl's parents and recommends that she be seen by the community mental health nurse at the neighborhood health center. Follow-up of the referral reveals that the family did not take her to the health center but called in a "curandera" to treat her.[5]

A 15-year-old boy from a rural mountain town is hospitalized for observation and testing after he ceases talking following a traffic accident. After a week of hospitalization during which no physical cause is found, several relatives arrive for a visit. The boy speaks to his relatives with no apparent difficulty.[5]

A Hawaiian family visits their 21-year-old son who has been hospitalized in an inpatient psychiatric unit. The family stays all day and evening, praying, talking, and listening to each other. When asked to leave they refuse, saying they were doing "ho'oponopono."[6]

What do these seemingly unrelated examples of behavior have in common? These are examples of behavior that occurred as a result of cultural values and beliefs. Tripp-Reimer describes culture in the following way:

> Culture is the total lifeways of a human group. It consists of learned patterns of values, beliefs, customs, and behaviors that are shared by a group of interacting individuals. More than material objects, culture is a set of rules or standards for behavior.[2]

A group's culture pervades all areas of life, from how they speak to how they decide who is ill and how they are to be treated. Therefore, culture is a strong determinant of behavior. In the previous examples, culture was a determinant of behavioral response to illness. The old Navajo determined that life was not worth living if it meant having a colostomy. His behavior was consistent with the Navajo belief in the quality of life.[3]

The Mexican-American father was acting from the point of view that only he, not the child's mother, had the authority to determine whether or not his son received a vaccination. His behavior was consistent with the Mexican-American paternalistic culture. In addition, the father believed that when his son was injected with the agent that causes smallpox it would give him the disease, rather than promote immunity.[5]

The Mexican-American family was operating from the point of view that their daughter was suffering from "susto pasado," and that the person to treat her was a curandera.[5]

In the case of the rural mountain boy, the staff attempted to derive an elaborate psychological explanation for the sudden return of the boy's speech. However, when they mentioned their theory to the boy's family, the boy's brother said, "Wouldn't, not couldn't. Doesn't like

FAMILY ASSESSMENT QUESTIONS

1. How has illness upset the equilibrium of the family?
2. What compensatory actions has the family taken?
3. Has family equilibrium been restored?
4. Have secondary problems erupted as a result of a compensatory action?
5. What are the family's beliefs about the illness?
6. How does the family think the illness should be treated?
7. What roles and responsibilities does the ill member have, and how are they being fulfilled during the member's illness?
8. Where is the concentration of power within the family?
9. What is the family structure?
10. How are the physical and safety needs of members provided for?
11. How is guidance and feedback given to family members?
12. How strong is the bond among family members?
13. Are any socialization behaviors apparent?
14. How is control exerted over family members?
15. What stage of the family developmental cycle is the family experiencing?
16. Is the family having any difficulty completing their developmental tasks?

strangers." And the boy's father said, "Should have asked the boy."[5] The boy's response was consistent with the verbal style of his rural mountain culture.

The Hawaiian family was carrying out the Hawaiian practice of "ho'oponopono," in which they believe the family unites their emotional and spiritual forces to enable the ill member to receive help. During the ho'oponopono, faults are identified and released and forgiveness is sought and received. Thus, both the wrongdoer and the wronged are released from each other. The practice of ho'oponopono is consistent with the Hawaiian belief that conflicts within humans are the direct cause of illness.[6] For the nurse to understand fully a client's behavioral response to illness, the behavior must be interpreted in relation to the cultural values and beliefs underlying it.

Working in cross-cultural health programs or in "any program in which some of the staff are of a culture different than some of the patients," nurses could probably recount numerous examples of misunderstandings between health care professionals and clients that have occurred as a result of cultural differences.[3] It is when cultural differences cause misunderstandings that cultural influences on behavior become most apparent. Such misunderstandings result in client noncompliance and, consequently, poor health care. Therefore, nurses should assess client's cultural values, beliefs, and practices prior to planning nursing care.

It is important to remember that all people have a cultural heritage, and that nurses' own cultural values and beliefs influence their behavior in working with clients. Nurses cannot free themselves completely from their own evaluative system. However, they can adopt a "culturally relativistic" perspective from which they attempt to understand the client's behavior in the context of the client's own culture (evaluative system).[2]

It is not practical to expect that nurses will have a thorough knowledge of the cultural beliefs and health practices of all the different groups of people that they may encounter. Also, it is important to treat clients as individuals, rather than assuming that they have certain beliefs and practices as a result of being members of a particular group of people. Each client's beliefs and practices must be thoroughly assessed to ensure that nursing care is based on mutually satisfactory goals and a realistic treatment plan. Information regarding clients' health beliefs and practices that will assist in making adequate assessments is presented in the box on this page.

In obtaining information about a group's cultural values and beliefs, it is important to remember that observation, listening, and indirect questioning may be more useful than attempts to question people directly about their cultural practices. Nurses should keep in mind that all people have a cultural heritage, and that their cultural heritages influence the ways they provide care. It is important to use the nursing process to provide care that is appropriate to a particular cultural group.

CULTURAL ASSESSMENT QUESTIONS

1. What value does good health have for the client? Is it a high or a low priority?
2. What is a state of illness considered to be? Within the family, who determines when a member is ill?
3. What conditions and behaviors are considered abnormal?
4. Is a difference between physical and mental illness recognized? What is considered physical and what mental?
5. What do the client and family believe causes illness? What do they believe caused this illness?
6. How are common illnesses usually treated?
7. How are ill people expected to behave?
8. Are people other than health professionals used to treat the illness?
9. What role does the family assume in caring for an ill family member?
10. What are typical attitudes toward mental illness and the mentally ill?
11. Do differences exist between the client's and the family's interpretation of the illness situation?
12. What are the client's and the family's goals in relation to the illness situation?

The Individual's Behavioral Response to Illness

Individual behavioral responses to illness are based on several factors: basic societal expectations for sick role behavior, and how those expectations affect behavioral response; universal family features that all families share, and how the family responds to illness in light of the universal features; and cultural values and beliefs about illness that help to determine individual behavioral response. These perspectives provide a background for understanding the responses of the person facing illness, an important part of psychiatric/mental health nursing.

The individual facing the prospect, or experiencing the actuality, of illness faces a change in existence. Illness brings many possibilities: pain, suffering, and/or death; loss of mental and physical function; inability to fulfill roles and carry out responsibilities; and a need for reliance on others. Illness endangers the physical, psychological, and social self. As such, illness poses a threat to the integrity of the individual. The exact nature of that threat differs from one individual to another, however, and depends on how each individual perceives the illness situation.

Each person perceives illness in a unique way. Therefore, patients who seem to be facing similar illness situations will have different points of view about their situations. For example, two 50-year-old men who have just sustained myocardial infarctions are lying side-by-side in the intensive care unit and thinking different thoughts. Mr. Warren is thinking, "Well, I guess it all finally caught up with me. I knew I should have taken the doctor's advice and slowed down a little. I should have lost a few pounds and quit smoking, too. Now I'm going to be laid up here in the hospital, and will miss out on the negotiations for the TCA deal. I wonder who they'll get to handle it?" Mr. Samuels is thinking, "I can't believe this. Yesterday I was down at the beach riding my bike, and today I'm lying here in the hospital with a heart attack. I took care of myself all these years. I don't smoke or drink. I watch what I eat and work out every day, and look what happens to me. How could this happen to me? Is this it? Am I going to die?"

Both men perceive the myocardial infarction as a threat to themselves. However, Mr. Warren's perception is focused on the threat his illness poses to his ability to work, while Mr. Samuels sees his illness as a threat to his existence. Furthermore, Mr. Warren sees his illness as having occurred as a result of his failure to take care of himself. As a result of the two men's unique perceptions of their illness situation, a similiar situation provokes two very different threats.

Fear and anxiety are common responses to the threat of illness. Specific fears that the individual may have include fear of financial ruin, fear of being unattractive to others, fear of becoming a burden to one's family, fear of getting old, fear of losing one's status at work, fear of dying, fear of pain and suffering, fear of specific medical and nursing procedures, fear of losing part of one's body, and fear that one will not receive care. In the case of emotional illness, individuals may fear being labeled as mentally ill, loss of control of cognitive functions, not being able to be helped by others, being abandoned by family and friends, becoming suicidal, becoming aggressive and hurting someone else, being seen as less than competent, and being dependent on someone else. Other emotional responses that may be provoked in response to the threat of illness include guilt, anger, shame, embarrassment, sadness, disgust, frustration, and despair. For instance, a person may feel guilt about nonfulfillment of customary responsibilities; anger about an inability to function independently; shame about loss of control of body functions, such as elimination or cognition; embarrassment about changes in appearance as a result of illness; sadness about the family's concern, disgust about not being able to walk, frustration about the slow recovery process, or despair about the recurrence of a previous illness.

In some cases, rather than provoking fear, anxiety, or other unpleasant emotions, illness provides relief from them. For example, if a man has been existing in a very stressful environment for a period of time and then becomes ill, it may be a relief to be able to give up the usual social role functioning and assume the helpless, dependent behaviors of the sick role. Being ill may be the only acceptable way for the individual to cease trying to deal with an overwhelmingly stressful environment. Knowing that he is "ill" may then put his mind at ease. Some individuals take the situation one step further and not only feel relief over being ill but enjoy it, because of the attention it provides them or because preexisting dependency needs can now be met. In these individuals, anxiety may be aroused as a result of having to give up being ill and the "secondary gain" that illness provides them. Rather than provoking unpleasant emotions in an individual, illness may at times provide relief from such emotions. However, in most cases illness is perceived as a threat, and unpleasant emotions are aroused.

As a result of the threat that illness presents and the accompanying emotional arousal, an individual faced with illness feels a need to take some sort of action to manage the threat and decrease the emotional arousal. The behaviors that each person exhibits in an attempt to do this are, of course, unique to the individual. For example, Mr. Warren may attempt to decrease his frustration over not being able to fulfill his usual work role by demanding that a telephone be installed at his bedside and insisting that he be allowed to have visits from his coworkers. He may attempt to decrease his guilt over not having taken care of himself by talking about his lifestyle and asking the nurses to provide him with information on quitting smoking and losing weight. Mr. Samuels, in order to deal with his bewilderment over having had a heart attack, may ask the nurses repeatedly how he could have had a heart attack when he was so healthy. He may attempt to deal with his fear that he might die by lying rigidly in his bed and praying. Both men are attempting to decrease their emotional response and deal with the threat of their illness. However, the behaviors they use in their attempts to manage their response to their myocardial infarctions differ greatly.

Other examples of behaviors that individuals may exhibit in attempting to manage their responses to illness are the following:

An 80-year-old woman with a fractured hip fears becoming a burden to her daughter. She seeks out a social worker, and actively plans her transfer from the extended care unit to a nursing home. In order to deal with her fear of losing her memory, she makes lists of everything she wants to remember.

A 16-year-old boy with recently diagnosed diabetes is angry because he must alter his lifestyle and be different from his friends. He ignores his diabetic diet and refuses to take insulin.

A 21-year-old athlete who has sustained severe injuries in an auto accident fears that he may never walk again. He talks about his rehabilitation process as a challenge and sets daily goals for his rehabilitation program.

A 14-year-old girl who has been admitted to an inpatient psychiatric unit fears being exposed to her peers as "mentally ill." She makes her parents promise not to tell her friends where she is, and calls her best friend to tell her she is home in bed with "strep" throat.

These examples of behavior demonstrate individuals' conscious attempts to manage the threat of their illnesses and decrease their emotional responses. Another way individuals may react to their illnesses is by using unconscious mental maneuvers, or defense mechanisms, to protect themselves from experiencing the threat of their illness and the unpleasant feelings that may be aroused. Through the use of defense mechanisms, unpleasant feelings are minimized or eliminated completely.[1] There are numerous defense mechanisms that may be employed in managing the threat of illness (see Chap. 7). However, two defense mechanisms that are of particular interest are avoidance and denial.

Denial has been described as a "mechanism that the ego uses to shut out external reality that is too frightening or threatening to tolerate. The person sees, hears, or perceives the event through any of the senses but refuses to recognize it consciously."[1] Denial occurs in situations in which the perceived threat is too overwhelming for the person to deal with. By keeping the perceived threat from being consciously recognized, denial serves to protect the person's emotional equilibrium. Examples of denial behaviors include the following:

A 38-year-old woman, whose mother died of breast cancer, is told during her physical exam that she has a lump in her breast that must be checked for cancer. During lunch that day she tells a friend that the doctor gave her a clean bill of health.

An 84-year-old woman who lives alone is reported by her daughter to have a drinking problem and is treated by her physician for a broken finger. When the physician asks her how she sustained the fracture, the woman gives a detailed explanation of how she twisted her finger getting out of her rocking chair. She denies having fallen or drinking alcohol.

A 35-year-old man whose mental state has been deteriorating due to a highly stressful work environment is confronted by his boss with evidence that he has become significantly less effective at work. He denies that his performance has changed.

A 13-year-old girl is treated in the emergency room for a series of self-inflicted superficial lacerations on her wrists. When asked why she has tried to hurt herself she replies, "I wasn't trying to hurt myself. I just wondered how it would feel."

The defense mechanism of *denial* keeps the individual from ever experiencing the perceived threat of the illness. Consequently, the unpleasant emotional response that would have been aroused is prevented from occurring.

Avoidance is a defense mechanism similar to denial. However, rather than being an unconscious refusal to *recognize* a traumatic reality, it is an unconscious refusal to *encounter* a traumatic reality because it would provoke an unpleasant and undesired emotional response.[2] Examples of avoidance behaviors include the following:

A 45-year-old man who previously has had an allergic reaction to the dye used during an angiogram is scheduled for a heart catheterization the next day. When the nurses attempt to inform him about the preparation for, and procedures of, the catheterization, he changes the subject to other aspects of his care, such as his salt-free diet and medications.

A 70-year-old man with arthritis is admitted for a hip replacement, and is told by his physician that he cannot continue to live independently and must be transferred to a facility where he can receive some assistance. The man argues with his physician about this, and says that he will not go. When the nurses attempt to discuss his feelings regarding the transfer to a supervised facility, the man changes the subject to a discussion of the progress he has made in physical therapy. When the social worker comes to see him at a prearranged time, he is not in his room.

A 16-year-old boy who has been admitted to an inpatient psychiatric unit fears that he may lose his girlfriend as a result of his emotional illness. He receives a message that his girlfriend has called and wants him to call her back. He does not return the call.

A 60-year-old man who has been treated for a leg ulcer for the past three months fears that the community health nurse will no longer take care of him once his ulcer heals. The ulcer is almost healed, and the nurse judges that the client is capable of caring for his leg himself. When the nurse attempts to praise the man for his independence and discuss termination of her visits, the man repeatedly asks her questions about some aspect of his wound care.

The defense mechanism of avoidance keeps individuals from experiencing unpleasant emotional responses by causing them to avoid the threatening situations. If the traumatic realities are never encountered, they are not experienced as threatening and the emotional responses are not aroused.

Individuals deal with the perceived threat of their illness and the accompanying emotional arousal by attempting to decrease the threat and the emotional arousal. Individuals may attempt to manage their responses to illnesses through conscious efforts to do something about them or through the use of unconscious mental maneuvers that allow them to minimize or completely eliminate their emotional responses to the threat of their illness.

The behaviors manifested as a result of individuals' attempts to manage their responses to illness may range from enthusiastic participation in the care to complete denial of the illness. At times the behaviors exhibited may seem illogical, nonfunctional, or even detrimental to individuals' health or recovery from illness. Before judging the behaviors as needing to be eliminated or changed, nurses need to remember the following:

1. The behaviors may be quite logical when looked at from the client's point of view.
2. The behaviors function, in most cases, to reduce the emotional impact of the threat of the illness, and thereby help clients maintain emotional equilibrium.
3. The behaviors represent clients' best efforts at exerting some control over their present situation.

If nurses fail to understand the logic underlying clients' behaviors and seek to disrupt, discourage, or eliminate the behaviors, they may take away from clients that which they are able to do to protect themselves from the threat of their illness. Nurses can undermine clients' ability to exert some control over their situation. Furthermore, the idea that clients are defenseless in the face of their illness and must rely on care-givers for relief and protection is reinforced. Therefore, rather than emphasizing changing clients' behaviors, nurses should first seek to understand how clients perceive their illness situations, what the illnesses are, and what they are trying to do to deal with their emotional responses to their illnesses. Based on this information, nurses should plan interventions that provide support for behaviors that help clients maintain their emotional equilibrium. The following clinical examples exemplify what occurs when clients' behaviors are not recognized and understood, as well as how nurses can support clients' behaviors.

The Therapeutic Use of Self

As mentioned in the Introduction to this text, nurses make use of their selves in nurse–client relationships to assist clients to grow and change. Part of this use of the self is the response of nurses to clients' *needs,* rather than just to clients' symptoms of illness. In the case discussed

earlier in the chapter about the client with a leg ulcer, the nurse relates to the client about the healing of the ulcer, as well as to the client's thoughts and feelings about the termination of the professional relationship with the nurse.

To employ the therapeutic use of self effectively, nurses must assess clients' behavioral responses to illness, as well as symptoms of the illnesses. Because symptoms of illnesses are usually obvious, they are easier to assess than behavioral responses, which can be overlooked, particularly when clients use denial or avoidance. Nurses must also be aware of their own reactions to clients, which might prevent them from focusing on the clients' responses to the illnesses.

The nature of the therapeutic use of self involves assisting clients to work on their problems and concerns, not those of the nurses or other health care professionals. Clues to the nature of the essence of clients' responses to illness come directly from clients. In this way, clients are treated individually, and are thoroughly and objectively assessed for their responses to illness and the appropriateness of those responses.

Several points should be noted regarding effective therapeutic use of self with clients' responses to illness:

CLINICAL EXAMPLES

A student nurse was assigned to care for Ms. Falk, a 52-year-old retired army captain. When first encountered, Ms. Falk had just been diagnosed with severe heart disease and scheduled for open heart surgery. As the primary nurse, the student was to prepare Ms. Falk for surgery as well as attend to her other needs. On the first day, the student walked into the client's room prepared to give her pre- and postoperative information and instructions. However, when the subject of surgery was brought up, Ms. Falk began discussing how her arthritis had been acting up again. Subsequent attempts to discuss the surgery resulted in Ms. Falk's ignoring the topic and discussing something else. Eventually the student left the client's room, feeling frustrated at not having accomplished her purpose.

The next morning the student nurse gave Ms. Falk written information regarding the surgery. She asked the client to read it, and said she would return later to discuss it and answer any questions. Ms. Falk thanked the student and said she would read the information. When the student delivered Ms. Falk's lunch tray, she asked if Ms. Falk had read the information. The client said she had not. The information was nowhere in sight. Ms. Falk then began discussing a trip she had planned to the Orient. She talked at length about all the places she had visited while in the army, and said it made her feel good to think of being in those places again. When the student left that day, Ms. Falk smiled and thanked her for listening. The student felt good about being thanked, but continued to feel she was failing to prepare her client for surgery.

The day before Ms. Falk's surgery, the student was determined to accomplish her goal. She walked into Ms. Falk's room and said, "Ms. Falk, you are having open heart surgery tomorrow. It is important that you understand what is going to be happening to you before, during,

and after surgery. I am here to give you that information." Ms. Falk turned to the student and angrily replied, "Don't you think I know I'm having surgery? Don't you think I think about it? What are you going to tell me about it that I don't already know? Leave me alone!" The student left the room feeling upset and confused over what had happened. She knew she had hurt Ms. Falk in some way, but did not know what she had done. A short time later she went by the client's room and found Ms. Falk lying in bed sobbing. The student said she'd like to help if Ms. Falk could tell her what was wrong. Through her sobs Ms. Falk managed to tell the student that she was terrified of having the surgery, because her father had died during surgery and she feared she would do the same. She said she didn't want to have the surgery but knew she must, and felt powerless to do anything about her situation. Ms. Falk went on to say that she had been dealing with her feelings by trying not to think of the surgery. It helped her to pretend that it wasn't going to happen. She said she just wanted to ignore the surgery until it was over and she could begin her process of recovery.

The student then understood why the client had behaved as she did. Ms. Falk was using avoidance to deal with her fear of dying during surgery. As a result of the student's repeated attempts to inform the client about the surgery, Ms. Falk was not able to continue to use avoidance. Consequently, she experienced anger, fear, and sadness in response to the threat of her illness. The student knew then how to prepare Ms. Falk for her surgery. She supported Ms. Falk's expression of emotions that day. However, when the client began ignoring her surgery again, the student supported that behavior too. The student was with Ms. Falk the next morning when she was wheeled into the operating room. They talked about snorkeling in crystal clear cerulean waters.

CLINICAL EXAMPLE

Mr. Post was a 45-year-old man with amyotrophic lateral sclerosis, a disease that causes rapidly progressive muscular atrophy and eventually results in death. Mr. Post was paralyzed from the waist down, and required assistance with all of his basic daily activities. He was described by the nurses as a difficult patient because his care was very time-consuming. He was very particular about his care and "impossible to please."

One day Mr. Post was assigned to a new graduate nurse. He entered the client's room with some anxiety because he had been told that Mr. Post was a difficult client. Mr. Post greeted the nurse by saying, "Well, I see you're a new one. I guess I'll have to tell you all about my routine and how I like things done." The nurse told Mr. Post that his plan of care had been explained to him and that, although he was new, he would do his best. As the nurse began to gather equipment for the client's bath, Mr. Post stopped him and told him he always used the toilet first. As the nurse proceeded to set up a Hoyer lift to transfer Mr. Post, the client stopped him and gave detailed instructions as to how to lay the straps under him and carry out the transfer. Before long, the nurse realized that Mr. Post had detailed instructions for him regarding every small step of his care. It was as if the client didn't trust him. Each time the nurse tried to anticipate the next step, Mr. Post stopped him and told him how to do it. Any deviation from what Mr. Post described as his "ritual," caused him to become irritated with the nurse. In turn, the nurse was becoming irritated with the client.

It was almost lunchtime and they had barely started Mr. Post's A.M. care. The nurse was fatigued from trying to anticipate Mr. Post's desires, so began waiting for Mr. Post to tell him what to do next and how to do it. Suddenly, things began to go more smoothly and the nurse felt himself relaxing and enjoying caring for Mr. Post. Mr. Post became more amiable and forgiving of any small errors the nurse made. As a result, the A.M. care was finished on time, and Mr. Post complimented the nurse on his abilities. The rest of the day progressed smoothly, with both Mr. Post and the nurse feeling happy and satisfied.

The other nurses were surprised to hear that things had gone so well between the nurse and Mr. Post. They were curious to know what he had done. What the nurse had done was to allow the client to tell him what to do and how to do it. By doing this he had supported Mr. Post's need to have his care performed in a ritualistic manner, and had thereby allowed him to exert control over his life in one of the few ways left to him. In addition, the nurse had freed himself from the impossible task of trying to do things perfectly and please the client.

Mr. Post's behavior was his way of dealing with the threat of his illness. He never disclosed what threatened him about his illness. It is likely that he feared the progressive and inevitable loss of control over his body, and eventual death. He did tell the nurse he was trying to get all his legal papers in order before he lost the use of his arms, and spent each afternoon filing the stacks of legal documents surrounding his bed. (Mr. Post was a lawyer, who had held a position of some prominence prior to his illness.)

1. Do not assume that responses observed in the client are part of the client's personality. The responses may be "new" to the client, and may represent the client's response to illness.
2. The nurse can determine the presence of responses to illness by first working with the client on the obvious problem or circumstance. In the case of the 60-year-old man with the healing leg ulcer, the nurse first discussed the leg ulcer and the fact that it was healing, and that the nurse would no longer be visiting. The client then demonstrated his response to the illness—the defense of *avoidance*. He repeatedly asked questions about his wound care rather than move ahead to act on his ability to perform his own care.
3. Once clients have described their illnesses, ask them to also describe what they think and feel about having the illness. In this manner the client and nurse can label the pattern or the response to the illness. The client may need to approach this labeling gradually, and the nurse may be most effective in assisting with the labeling by having the client talk about how the illness has changed the client's life, the client's initial reaction to the illness, and so on.
4. Labeling the response to the illness may be the extent to which client and nurse discuss the response.

For example, clients going to open heart surgery may not want to talk about having the surgery because it arouses high anxiety. Clients may prefer to talk about other topics, but they *do want the nurse to be near them for support and comfort.*

5. The nurse and client may determine that the client's response to the illness may constitute a nursing diagnosis. The client may be experiencing a stress response to the illness, and nurse and client can work on stress-reducing interventions. Clients who use avoidance and denial may need consistent interviews with the nurse in order to establish a trusting relationship in which the client may begin to examine the illness experience and the accompanying denial and avoidance.

Summary

1. Providing optimal nursing care includes applying the nursing process not only to the stated illness of the client but also to the family's and the client's behavioral responses to illness.
2. When illness is perceived as a threat, unpleasant emotions such as fear, anger, denial, and others may be provoked in the client and the client's family.

3. Clients respond to illness in their own unique ways. Clients must be assessed to determine if there are responses to illness that need consideration by the nurse and client.

4. Individuals may attempt to manage their illness through unconscious mental maneuvers. Denial and avoidance allow people to minimize the emotional impact of the presence of illness.

5. Regardless of the types of behavior that clients demonstrate, the behaviors are the clients' best efforts to manage their responses to illness.

6. The nurse's role is to determine what the client is doing to deal with the response to illness and to provide support for client behaviors that help the client maintain emotional well-being.

References

1. Barry P: Psychosocial Nursing Assessment and Intervention. Philadelphia, JB Lippincott, 1984
2. Bellack J, Bamford P: Nursing Assessment: A Multidimensional Approach. Belmont, California, Wadsworth, 1984
3. Brownlee A: Community, Culture, and Care. St Louis, CV Mosby, 1978
4. Duvall E, Miller B: Marriage and Family Development, 6th ed. New York, Harper & Row, 1985
5. Hymovich D, Barnard M: Family Health Care. New York, McGraw-Hill, 1973
6. Paglinowan L: Ho'oponopono. Alu Like Hawaii Center handout, 1984
7. Parsons T: The Social System. New York, The Free Press, 1964
8. Spradley B: Community Health Nursing Concepts and Practice, 2nd ed. Boston, Little, Brown and Co, 1985

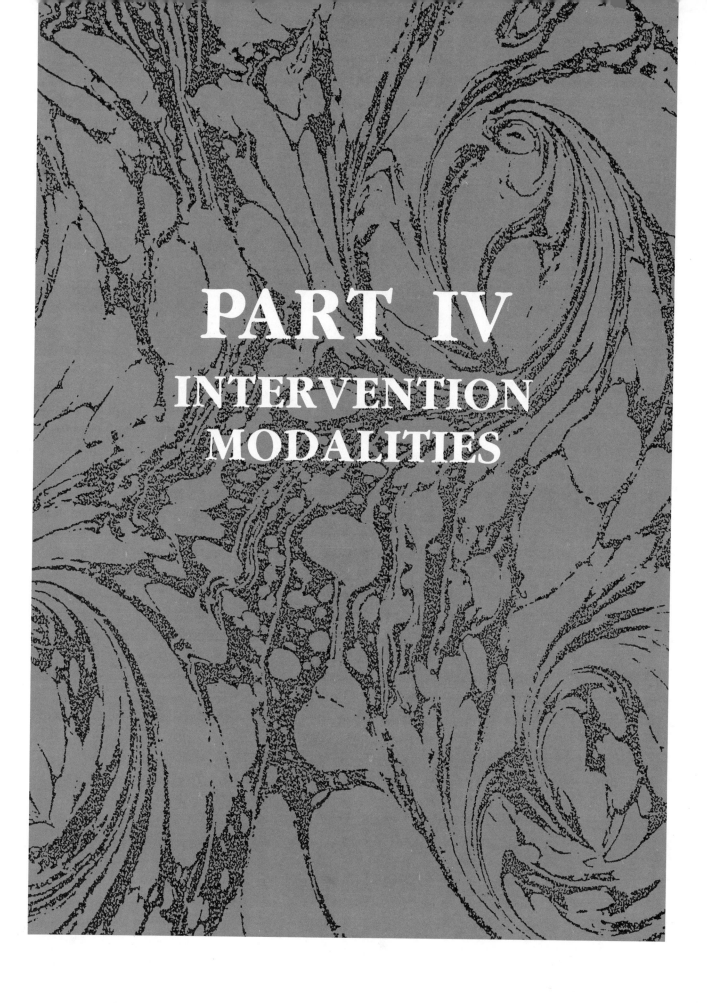

PART IV
INTERVENTION MODALITIES

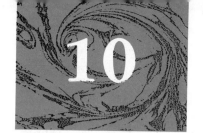

LORETTA M. BIRCKHEAD

INDIVIDUAL RELATIONSHIP INTERVENTION

Learning Objectives

Upon completion of this chapter the student should be able to do the following:

1. Describe the history of intervening with clients using individual relationships.
2. Differentiate among the functions of the psychotherapists, counselors, and nurses using individual relationship interventions.
3. Describe the stages of the client change process in psychotherapeutic intervention.
4. Describe the meaning of "resistance to change."
5. Identify commonalities among various psychotherapeutic interventions.
6. Differentiate among the various short-term therapy approaches.
7. Describe the applicability of short-term approaches to nursing.
8. Identify clients who are suitable for particular short-term approaches.
9. Discuss ethical issues found in psychiatric/mental health nursing practice.

Introduction

When psychotherapists talk with each other about the field of psychotherapy, there is generally an overall framework within which their discussions take place. This framework includes the concepts of:

The site of the psychotherapy, *e.g.,* outpatient, inpatient, day-care, homecare

The diagnosis of the client

The intervention "modality" in which the client is seen: is the client interviewed individually, in a group, or with the family (or only the spouse) present?

The theory used in working with the client

The severity of illness

The stage of the relationship with the client (the beginning, the middle, or the termination phase)

The outcome of the work

This chapter will focus on only one modality of treatment: interventions performed in the context of the *individual* relationship between the clinician and the client. Numerous individually-oriented psychotherapies have been used in the past, and new models of care are being formulated today. In addition to reviewing these various models of care, this chapter will also explore commonly held goals for, and methods of, individual relationship intervention.

The chapter will examine *short-term therapy.* Short-term therapy is currently used more often because of the lack of financial assistance available for long-term treatment and because of recent findings demonstrating the effectiveness of short-term treatment in many cases.

For centuries, individuals have sought help for their maladies. Both the nature of the problems and the treatments accepted for them are culturally defined. To the Hopi Indian, for example, symptoms are due to witchcraft, and therapy consists of magic. Historical writings refer to healings performed by priests, shamans, and other physicians of previous time periods. Regardless of the culture, the healing process depends on an agreed-upon diagnosis that is verified by a person with training in the healing process.[11]

Because of the varieties of disorders and clinicians who treat them in different cultures, it is difficult to define psychotherapy. Many definitions are too broad, and specify neither the disorder nor the remedy. In practice, psychotherapy is defined more by the nature of *the clinician* who treats the problem than by the disorder or what is done in treatment. This is the case in medical treatment. For instance, closing a wound is still "closing a wound," whether it is done by a doctor, a dentist, or a nurse, yet the doctor, dentist, or nurse brings to the wound-closing the perspective specific to their discipline. In mental health care, talking with a client about feelings occurring as a result of an individual's divorce may appear the same, regardless of whether it is done by a psychiatrist, psychiatric nurse, social worker, or psychologist. Each clinician brings, however, a different perspective to the work.

Psychotherapy can be defined as a method of alleviating specific intrapsychic and/or interpersonal difficulties through the use of specific therapeutic procedures, practiced by skilled professionals.[11] This definition highlights the fact that the practice of psychotherapy is based on scientific principles. Clinicians are not random in their approaches, but use a process (such as the nursing process) to define the problem, plan, and intervene according to established principles of what can be expected to be effective in particular circumstances. The word "skilled" in the definition points to the fact that true psychotherapy is done by professionals who have been educated in the field of psychotherapy. Psychotherapy performed by trained professionals began at the end of the 19th century.[11]

Do nurses practice psychotherapy with clients? Typically this skill is learned at the master's degree level of nursing education. Nurses practicing in the field of psychiatric/mental health nursing with baccalaureate degrees typically practice "relationship interventions." Looking at brief interactions of relationship intervention and psychotherapy, an observer may see no difference. Differences do appear, however, over a longer period of observation.

Relationship intervention is a useful title for the methods used by psychiatric nurses in working with clients because change is fostered through the client's relationship with the nurse and others. *Individual relationship intervention* is defined as the nurse–client clarification of the client's interpersonal relationships. The following points elaborate on this definition:

1. Clarification occurs through the use of the nursing process.
2. The therapeutic use of self (the Self of the nurse) is the channel through which the nurse exerts an effect on the client.
3. Individual relationship intervention assists the client to change by means of the clarification of the nurse–client Relationship, the Relationship of the client with Others in the client's current life, and the Relationship of the client with Others in the client's past.
4. While the process of change occurs by clarifying the client's *Relationships,* the client also grows in the areas of intellectual and interpersonal competencies. Hence, in the work with the psychiatric nurse, the client grows both internally and in Relationships with Others.

    The nurse and client may consider the client's personal thoughts, feelings, or actions, or the client's Relationships with Others. These considerations are described in Chapter 5.
5. The word "clarification" implies the presence of some distortion of meaning held by the client. These distortions are one primary reason clients seek mental health care. The nature of distortions is described in Chapter 5.

This chapter is entitled *Individual Relationship Intervention* to capture the essence of the nursing skills that have become a part of the traditional role of the psychiatric/mental health nurse. Concepts of individual relationship intervention are found in the literature of psychotherapy and counseling, as well as in the roles of psychiatric/mental health nurses developed during the latter part of this century. Material from psychotherapy and counseling will be discussed in terms of the aspects that pertain to the nurse's role and because the psychiatric/mental health nurse must be aware of the fields of counseling and psychotherapy in order to understand the work of other mental health professionals.

The Origins of Individual Psychotherapy

Freud is credited for making psychological treatment a \specific therapy. Initially he used hypnosis to assist in the recall and clarification of repressed, unconscious material. Freud later abandoned hypnosis and began using the technique of *free association* to uncover the unconscious thoughts of clients. In using free association, the clients are asked to say spontaneously whatever comes to mind, without editing the expressions.

Hence, free association was one of the first specific *therapeutic procedures* used in psychotherapy. Freud provided a wealth of specific techniques for problems, and gave us much of the initial body of knowledge used today in practicing the skills of psychotherapy.

Freud also developed the idea that mental illness begins in the client's childhood. As he used the free association technique, many clients talked spontaneously about traumas experienced in their childhoods. Through Freud's insistence on the childhood etiology of mental illness, he distinguished psychoanalysis from faith healing. This distinction created a new discipline of psychotherapy.

Mental Health Care Professionals

Orne[11] stated that within the early psychoanalytic movement the technical aspects of the therapeutic method were not directly related to other forms of medical practice. Orne also noted that medical education, with its orientation to (objective) physical pathology, could even impede the clinician's grasp of the *subtle* behavioral factors that are so important in the psychotherapeutic process.

Note the tendency here to separate the physical processes from the psychological. Nursing seeks to minimize this split by viewing the client as a whole (system), composed of interrelated parts.

By placing the psychotherapeutic method *outside* medical practice, it was also noted that many capable *nonmedical* personnel were able to do psychotherapy. In Europe, in the early years of practice, psychoanalysis was taught in universities and did not depend on medicine (for referrals). Over time, however, that changed. In the 1940s the European influence on American psychotherapeutic practice placed it within the confines of medicine, where it remained for many years.

A number of factors opened the field of psychotherapeutic practice to clinicians other than psychiatrists (physicians), including the following:[11]

1. There were not enough psychiatrists.
2. Nonmedical psychotherapists, who function well in treating children, became popular.
3. School guidance counselors increased in number.
4. The work of Carl Rogers, whose psychotherapeutic practice was much different from that of traditional psychotherapy, became popular. Rogers formulated the *person-centered approach*. This approach is humanistic, and seeks to provide the client with positive self-regard so that the growth potential of the client can be maximized. Rogerian therapists do not use psychiatric diagnoses, and do not assume any medical responsibilities.

    These few comments demonstrate some of the differences between the Rogerian model of practice and the traditional psychotherapeutic approach. Rogerian psychotherapists began to see many clients who once would have been seen only by a psychiatrist.
5. After World War II the clinical psychologist movement grew. These psychologists were academicians who scientifically tested many of the clinical phenomena espoused by traditional psychotherapists. Psychologists were also interested in the clinical application of their knowledge base. They developed numerous psychological tests to assess psychological function objectively, and began their own clinical practices.
6. After World War II other disciplines demonstrated the capability of doing psychotherapy. In 1956, clinical specialists in psychiatric/mental health nursing were first graduated. Today clinical nurse specialists assume many roles in psychotherapeutic practice, including private practice. Similarly, psychiatric social workers perform many roles once performed only by psychiatrists.[12]
7. *Behavior therapy* was seen as an alternative to traditional psychotherapeutic practice. According to behavior therapists, symptoms are learned responses that must be "unlearned" and replaced by other, more adaptive behaviors. This theory was an extreme change from the traditional medical psychotherapeutic model that viewed symptoms as external manifestations of internal processes.

Therapeutic Processes and Their Differences Among Clinicians

Up to this point, various terms have been used to refer to the therapeutic process or procedural approaches. In this section the terms psychotherapy, counseling, and individual relationship intervention will be differentiated and discussed in the light of eight variables. Cochrane[4] differentiated between psychotherapy and counseling according to the following eight variables: goals of treatment, focus of treatment, methods, role of the client, role of the therapist, timetable of the process, level of preparation of the clinician, and length of treatment.

The clinical specialist in psychiatric/mental health nursing typically practices psychotherapy and has a master's degree in psychiatric/mental health nursing. Individual relationship intervention includes responsibilities suitable for baccalaureate level-prepared nurses, but it must be emphasized that the baccalaureate nurse is *not* a psychotherapist. Baccalaureate nurses can promote profound change in (with) clients. However, the title *psychotherapist* is usually reserved for clinicians who have attained skills through additional educational and clinical practice. Although baccalaureate nurses may demonstrate the skills of master's-level clinicians, they cannot be considered psychotherapists because they do not have the necessary educational and clinical preparation. Psychotherapists typically have a master's degree in an area related to the practice of psychotherapy, plus one or two years of supervised clinical practice. Psychotherapists usually take an exam after their master's degree to demonstrate their ability in the field of psychotherapy. Master's-prepared clinical specialists in psychiatric/mental health nursing may take the Certification exam offered by the American Nurses' Association. Certification is the ANA's recognition of the completion of preparation as a clinical nurse specialist.

Distinctions among the psychotherapist, the counselor, and the nurse using individual relationship intervention are described below and summarized in Table 10-1.

1. The goals of treatment
   a. *Psychotherapists* consider ways in which clients can accept themselves as they are, and how they can attain a sense of wholeness.
   b. *Counselors* consider how clients need to change in order to adjust to various role demands and expectations of themselves and others (*e.g.,* how to engage with others in social conversation).
   c. *Nurses* using individual relationship intervention consider ways in which clients can attain a sense of well-being as they evolve within their societal, psychological, cultural, environmental, and physical circumstances.
2. The focus of treatment
   a. *Psychotherapists* assist clients with the clarification of internal realities, such as conscious and unconscious memories. The clients' pasts are typically of concern because past traumas are thought to dictate current problems.
   b. *Counselors* assist clients to focus on reality concerns of the present, such as academic decisions.
   c. *Nurses* using individual relationship interven-

TABLE 10-1.
DISTINCTIONS AMONG TYPES OF THERAPISTS

DISTINGUISHING CHARACTERISTICS	TYPE OF THERAPIST		
	PSYCHOTHERAPISTS	COUNSELORS	NURSES USING INDIVIDUAL RELATIONSHIP INTERVENTION
Goals of treatment	Self-acceptance, wholeness	Adjustment	Sense of well-being as one grows as a system
Focus of treatment	Clarification of conscious and unconscious experience, past traumas	Present reality concerns	Removal of barriers to a sense of well-being, through examination of conscious memories of the past as they relate to the present
The method of therapy	Helping client to find answers through interpretation and discussion of what blocks understanding	Guidance in choice selection	Use of the nursing process through the therapeutic use of self
Client's role	Explorer in understanding	Learner of better coping skills	Learner about the self and interaction with others
Therapist's role	Promoting client's uncovering and examination	Warm, permissive attitude, influencing voluntary behavior change	Facilitating clarification of distortions and fulfillment of client's competencies
Therapist's view of the client	An individual who is troubled by the past and resists changing	An individual who cannot problem-solve effectively	An individual viewed as a system not attaining a competency level due to anxiety
Level of preparation of the clinician	A Master's degree, with supervised clinical work	A baccalaureate degree and certificate, or a master's degree; supervised clinical work	A baccalaureate degree with supervised clinical work
Length of treatment	Several months (for short-term therapy) or several years	Months	Less than a year

tion assist clients in removing or decreasing internal or external barriers to a sense of well-being. For example, if a client on an inpatient psychiatric unit is angry after a family visit, the nurse might talk with the client in order to understand this feeling. The nurse and client might consider the past, but only as it relates to the present, and only in terms of conscious memories.

3. The method of therapy
   a. *Psychotherapists* promote a form of internal examination in which clients are helped to derive an interpretation and understanding of internal conflicts and drives. Psychotherapists may use dream analysis, analysis of clients' resistance to treatment, or interpretations explaining clients' experience (such as reactions to the therapist).
   b. *Counselors* use a form of guidance in which clients make choices or adjustments that are needed.
   c. *Nurses* emphasize the use of the nursing process in working with clients. One way of intervening with clients is by employing the therapeutic use of self, described in a later section of this chapter. Many nurses also emphasize, as an example of the therapeutic use of self, the *learning process* whereby clients develop understanding (learning) about the barrier(s) to well-being.

4. The role of the client
   a. To *psychotherapists,* clients are participants with the clinician in the study of the client. Clients may have any degree of severity of illness.
   b. To *counselors,* clients are those who develop more effective behaviors in order to cope with the environment. Clients are not considered to be severely ill.
   c. To *nurses* using individual relationship intervention, clients have definite strengths and are worthy of respect and intervention to attain higher goals, regardless of the level of mental health. The natural growth processes of clients unfold as they work with nurses on selected problems. The relationship is similar to that of the conductor and the skilled musician. Clients are experts in their own lives (the instruments). Nurses assist with the refinement of the internal tone of the instruments (the psychological and physical aspects of the client systems) and the interaction of those instruments with others (the environmental, societal, and cultural aspects). Clients may have any severity of illness.

5. The role of the therapist
   a. *Psychotherapists* are facilitative and encouraging companions who assist in the focus on clients' lives. Clients are viewed as individuals who have the answers within themselves and who do the exploratory work.
   b. *Counselors* are seen as warm and permissive people who influence voluntary behavior changes on the part of clients.
   c. *Nurses* using individual relationship interven-

tion are facilitators or guides who assist clients in removing barriers to understanding by:
   i. Clarifying distortions of meaning in selected problem areas, and
   ii. Assisting clients to attain interpersonal or intellectual competencies (see Chap. 5 for a discussion of distortions and competencies)

6. The conceptualization of clients by therapists
   a. *Psychotherapists* view clients according to a variety of models of human development. Frequently the models include the ideas that the client's past needs review to release the tension of memories of the past, and that clients will resist change even if they are coming to therapy to change.
   b. *Counselors* view clients as individuals who cannot problem-solve effectively.
   c. *Nurses* using individual relationship intervention *intervene* with clients according to a particular theory or model of care. The model is broad and includes the *system elements* of psychological, physical, environmental, cultural, and societal variables and how these variables promote or retard clients' sense of well-being.

7. The level of preparation of the clinician
   a. The *psychotherapist's* minimum educational preparation is a master's degree (1½–2 years in length), with supervised clinical experience during and after the program.
   b. The *counselor's* educational preparation is varied, and includes a baccalaureate degree, a master's degree, or certificate training and some supervised clinical work.
   c. *Nurses* practicing relationship interventions have a baccalaureate degree in nursing and supervised clinical work (in a college or university program) with clients needing psychological intervention. Nurses continue to obtain professional supervision of their work, by professional peers, after graduation.

8. The length of treatment
   a. *Psychotherapists* conduct an in-depth exploration of the individual. The in-depth exploration may take several months (for some short-term forms of therapy) or a number of years.
   b. *Counselors,* in contrast to psychotherapists or nurses, provide more direct and goal-oriented therapy. It can last many months, as in the case of clients who are learning what may seem like simple activities of daily living.
   c. *Nurses* using individual relationship intervention generally engage in the therapeutic process for less than a year. In individual relationship intervention, the base from which areas of focus are selected is very broad, because the client is seen as a system. Once the assessment is done, the nurse uses a model of care to help the growth of the client in selected priority problem areas.

In summary, *psychotherapists* explore the internal mechanisms of the self of clients in order to help clients attain an integration of their psyches. The past is explored for thoughts and feelings that have been troublesome or denied. *Counselors* use a particular model of intervention and help clients adapt to external demands placed on them. Discussions with the client are more superficial and supportive. The approach is task-oriented, and definite problems are solved. *Nurses* view clients as systems and help clients to attain a sense of well-being. Through the nursing process, the nurse guides the client in reviewing conscious thoughts and feelings in order to regain or develop interpersonal and intellectual competencies.

The Therapeutic Use of Self

As discussed in the Introduction to this book, nurses establish certain contexts in their work with clients. These contexts are professional relationships with clients. In these relationships, nurses provide for the "therapeutic use of self" (the nurse's Self) in their therapeutic endeavors with clients.

In individual relationship intervention, the therapeutic use of self takes on broader dimensions (although these aspects can be found in the nurse's use of Self in other types of treatment as well). These points include:

1. Nurses have their own unique sets of cultural beliefs, motivations, skills, and patterns of reacting and behaving. Nurses must be aware of how they present themselves to clients. They must be able to describe themselves as if they are observing themselves.

2. In the therapeutic use of self, nurses assist clients by creating positive, healing relationships with clients. They form professional alliances with clients.

3. Nurses make use of their cognitive and affective responses to clients in order to understand better what within the clients produces such responses. Nurse responses to clients are not "good" or "bad"—they simply occur. Nurses must be aware of these responses, however, so that they can use their own responses to understand clients better. Responses to clients may also be referred to as "countertransference" (see Chap. 6).

4. In the therapeutic use of self, nurses follow the lead of clients in the therapeutic work. To the extent possible, nurses respond and work with the content or problems initiated by the clients.

Nurses doing individual relationship intervention can be thought of as experts in human nature. The idea of human nature involves understanding the "true" present-moment concerns of the clients' systems from a wide knowledge base (the psychological, societal, cultural, physical, and environmental aspects). The goal of clients and nurses is a full and free expression of the human nature of the client. This nature is growth-oriented, and worthy of respect. When barriers to the expression of the human nature of clients are removed, clients experience a sense of well-being.

Working with clients' *true* concerns (mentioned above) involves as much art as science on the part of the nurse. The therapeutic use of self involves providing an atmosphere for clients in which the nature of the clients (including heartfelt concerns) can unfold. Then nurses "see the Self" of the clients which, prior to working with the nurse, was hidden by any of a variety of defenses, enabling the client to feel safe.

The Basic Tenets of Psychotherapy

There are many types of psychotherapy that share the same basic principles.[11] Qualification of these tenets, with respect to the work of nurses, is given in the listing below when necessary.

1. Clients are not fully aware of the nature of the reasons for their behavior. Typically, nurses work only with what is conscious or what is easily made conscious.

2. The actual causes of behavior seen in severe mental illness are multiple and complex. The causes can be determined, at least partially, through long periods of work with clients. Because nurses generally work with one client for less than a year, problems are usually more easily definable in terms of both the nature of the problem and what promotes the occurrence of the problem.

3. Symptoms are expressions of psychological needs and motives.

4. Symptoms are expressions of underlying difficulties. Clinicians treat not the symptoms but the underlying problems.

5. Clinicians assist clients in becoming aware of the needs and motives that play a part in their difficulties. In this way, psychological growth occurs and specific symptoms are eliminated.

6. Clients must express their thoughts and feelings to the clinician, regardless of how difficult the expression may be.

7. The psychotherapist's role is to assist the client to understand, not to tell the client what to do. Clinicians assist clients in becoming aware of what they really want and bringing suppressed motives and feelings into awareness.

8. Specific techniques used by clinicians include:
    a. The encouragement of free expression
    b. The interpretation of dreams (Nurses typically work only with what is conscious or easily made conscious.)
    c. Inquiry into specific thoughts and feelings associated with events
    d. An analysis of distortions in the meaning of events and experiences

9. Clients are not passive recipients of care, but are active participants in the therapeutic process.

10. Clients will often experience uncomfortable feelings in the therapeutic sessions.

In addition to these basic, shared beliefs about the nature of treatment, there are also several shared beliefs about the nature of psychological difficulties. To most psychotherapists, psychological problems can best be understood developmentally: problems in the client's developmental past are now causing conflict. Clients can obtain a "cure" for this conflict by undergoing psychological treatment.

The Change Process in Psychotherapeutic Intervention

Although mental health care professionals cannot promise a "cure" for problems, client changes *do* occur as a result of psychotherapeutic intervention. In this section some of the commonalities of change, as it occurs in psychotherapy, will be discussed. Specific topics include the nature of the expected changes and some generalities about the ways in which changes occur. Specific interventions used by psychiatric/mental health nurses with clients are discussed in Chapter 5 on the therapeutic use of self.

When thinking about change, imagine a small stream beginning on top of a mountain. The stream joins other streams, and together they form a river. The river empties into a bay or the ocean. The psychological life of an individual is represented by this network of water channels. The psychological life is composed of various traits, feelings, thoughts, memories, and fantasies similar to the streams mentioned above.

These various components are derived from a common ground that gives rise to the streams. This common ground is similar to the social group in which individuals are born and live. The common ground has its own culture (or group of beliefs) and values; it also provides an environment for the person that, hopefully, is rich in the proper nutrients for the development of the well-being of the person.

To take this analogy further, the water contains certain physical characteristics. The hydrogen and oxygen molecules have their own physical description. These physical properties help define the nature of the substance. Similarly, people have physical properties. These properties set certain requirements for other components of the person as a system. For instance, the physical property of the system needs others to provide food when the person is an infant. This sets requirements for the social components of the infant's life. The care-taker, for example, must come to feed the infant.

The psychological life of the person is comparable to that of a stream system. Changes in some part of the stream system can be made by affecting the ground around the spring, the stream, the river, or the entrance of the river into the bay or ocean. Comparing this water system to the psychological life of the individual, one can say that:

1. The ground around the spring and the spring are the prenatal, infancy, and childhood growth and development stages of the individual. Many theorists (such as Freud) believe that personality is formed at an early age and that, in order to bring about change, the clinician and client must consider the difficulties that occurred during these periods and what conflicts and defenses against these difficulties were (and are) experienced by the client.

   In order for clients to consider these growth and development stages, they must feel comfortable doing so and must recall memories of these stages. This takes time, and therefore years of therapy may be required in order to understand these growth and development eras. This type of therapy is termed *psychoanalysis,*[5] and requires extensive training after a master's or doctoral degree.

2. The feeder streams can be compared to factors in the life of a client that promote a sense of well-being. These factors include the individual's characteristic responses to interpersonal situations. Some theorists believe that these characteristic responses are affected by present circumstances. For example, individuals may continue to select anger in interpersonal situations, despite the fact that there are other ways to respond, or the substance abuser may continue to include other substance abusers in his or her social group.

   Theorists believe that individuals can be helped by working with the characteristic patterns of behavior that the individual is currently using, without having the client extensively review the occurrences of infancy and childhood. This type of treatment is termed *psychoanalytic psychotherapy,* and is practiced by those with extensive training after a master's or doctoral degree. The psychoanalytic psychotherapist does not deal extensively with the entire developmental foundation of the person, but works with a select few feeder streams that are central to the illness process. This type of therapist also works with feeder streams that may be hidden from view among rocks and bushes (the unconscious). This type of therapist helps clients to determine the nature of meanings that are important to them, but that are emotionally painful and therefore not in their conscious awareness.

3. The river is the "derivative" of the feeder streams, and can be compared to the psychological Self of the individual. The river is obvious. Similarly, the psychological Self is not hidden, as are some feeder streams, mentioned above. The psychological Self is in the present consciousness or awareness of the client. For some clients (such as those with schizophrenia), the ability to verbalize about reality in a way that can be understood by others may be lost temporarily. In such cases, nurses still have the goal of conversing with the client about present reality, and use certain

techniques to maintain this focus on reality with the client.

Individual relationship intervention is the work with the client's psychological content, of which the client is aware or can easily be helped to awareness. In this approach, the client and nurse may discuss a few historical causes of the client's present psychological situation, but this description is clearly related to present difficulties.

Nurses will also take into account the other components (cultural, environmental, physical, and social) of the client as a system, particularly as these variables affect the client's psychological state. Again, discussions with the client concerning these variables are stated in a manner clearly understood by the client and the nurse. To use the example of the stream system, the focus of the nurse is on the river and the individual streams that affect the river in an obvious fashion. Nurses do not deal with infancy and childhood growth and development, as is done in psychoanalysis. Also, nurses do not deal extensively with hidden meanings affecting the psychological reality of the client (the hidden streams dealt with by the psychoanalytic psychotherapist). Nurses help clients to produce change by working with aspects of the client system that are different from those focused on by other mental health professionals.

Steps of the Change Process

Janet A. Rodgers[13] reviewed Kurt Lewin's writings on the three-step procedure of change. These steps include: *unfreezing, moving,* and *refreezing.*

1. *Unfreezing* means stopping old habits. It is possible that unfreezing occurs only when there is a threat to the self-system and anxiety is present in the client. The client may only thrust forward into new territories of behavior, so to speak, when the client's discomfort in relation to the problem(s) has become so great that the shell of old patterns cracks.

    During this period of unfreezing, some form of psychological safety must be available to support the client; hence the importance of the clinician's ability to be empathic, as mentioned previously.
2. The client begins *moving.* The client experiences a slight decrease in discomfort. The propensity and motivation for growth occur. Clients look for words of encouragement or for cues as to a direction to take. They see that a difference is possible, or that an alternative movement can be made. Clients think differently, either about their new selves or about the mechanisms of change itself. Perhaps clients think about how others will respond or are responding to them differently.
3. When the new behaviors (thoughts, feelings, and actions) become comfortable to the client and are reinforced by the client or by others, a *refreezing* of the *new* behavior occurs. Some degree of permanency of the behavior is acquired.

Clinician-Related Variables That Facilitate Change

Research indicates that clinicians who use the psychoanalytic technique of the "neutral mirror" (exemplified by answering a client's question with a question to the client) seem to do *less* well with their clients than those who relate more warmly, actively, and empathically.[10] If clinicians cannot expect the mere silent presence of another human being to effect change, what clinician-related variables facilitate change? The following traits of clinicians appear to help:

Warmth
The ability to be empathic while remaining objective
Appearance
Sophistication
Values
Genuineness of interest
The ability to be nonjudgmental
Respect for the client
Maturity
Tact
A firm belief in the clinician's ability to help
Flexibility

Clinician Techniques That Facilitate Change

Several approaches used by clinicians appear to facilitate change in clients, whereas others do not. Horvath[7] studied one specific approach: the *demands* presented to clients by clinicians that they alter their self-concepts. Horvath studied 87 unassertive individuals who were placed randomly in four types of imaginary role-playing situations. One group was asked to display characteristics of people with healthy self-concepts. The other groups were presented with tasks not related to the demand to display characteristics of healthy self-concepts.

Horvath found that only the group presented with the demand to demonstrate a good self-concept increased significantly in assertiveness and self-esteem, while decreasing in social discomfort. According to Horvath, the results of the study support the idea that general therapeutic factors involve *the need for the therapist to demand that clients* improve their self-concept. While there are problems with the study (such as the fact that the study did not use actual clients or clinicians), it points the way to possible understanding of some of the commonalities of effective therapies. Some of these factors include the clinician's providing for:

1. Insight or cognitive awareness, by interpreting for the client what has occurred in the experience of the client
2. The release of the client's emotions
3. A discussion of the nature of the relationship of the client and the clinician
4. An emotionally accepting and objective response to the client

5. Explicit or implicit approval or disapproval cues for the client as to what is appropriate
6. Implicit suggestions and persuasion for the client
7. Identification of the clinician as a role model for the client
8. Encouragement of communication and honest self-scrutiny
9. Inspiration of the client's hope for help
10. A sense of mastery on the part of the client
11. The establishment of a termination date at the beginning of therapy

Resistance to Change

Certain client variables related to change are important in considering what client traits are likely to promote client change. According to Marmor, the client characteristics that foster change are:[10]

1. expectancies for treatment
2. motivation to change
3. the capacity to relate to others

However, these characteristics do not apply to some clients with whom nurses work. In particular, clients who are severely depressed or schizophrenic may be unable to relate (they may be mute), or may not have expectations for treatment because past interpersonal interactions have meant disparagement.

Nursing's mandate is the rehabilitation of *all* individuals regardless of "social or economic status, personal attributes, or the nature of health problems."[1] Nursing believes that each person has "an inherent capacity for change." These beliefs ensure that nurses will not abandon clients who do not have the characteristics often considered to be prerequisites for effective psychotherapeutic intervention. For many difficult clients, nurses must first reach out, over a period of time, in order to establish even a beginning relationship. Typically, if nurses do not reach out to clients, the clients do not relate to the nurses and are not motivated to change. In many instances, if nurses do not reach out to clients no one does, and clients maintain a poor quality of life. When nurses attempt to establish professional, goal-oriented relationships with ill clients, the growth potential of the clients is tapped and progress begins, even if only in small steps.

Rodgers[13] described *resistance to change* as another commonality of clients in therapy. Most people find it difficult to change. *Resistance* means that change is blocked by various client behaviors. "Because *no one* can change all his beliefs and still retain his sanity, people frequently prefer problems that are familiar to solutions that are not."[13] In a society in which so much is changing, it is not surprising to find many individuals hanging on to past ways of behaving rather than welcoming change. Some of the causes of resistance include:

1. The threat of facing reality
2. Fears of the reactions of others if clients disclose information
3. Fears of abandonment by others if clients alter their behavior

4. Clinicians' fears of changes in clients (*e.g.,* can clinicians tolerate the release of emotion if clients face certain concerns? Can clinicians who, as do most human beings, like stability, accept new, different "people" in the clients?)
5. The clients' lack of experiences in which changes were constructive rather than destructive
6. The clients' lack of experience in knowing the liberating effects of change
7. Insufficient information about the nature of the changes that are expected
8. Insufficient information about the nature of the steps needed to effect change
9. The internal or external experience of pressure to change, whether from the clients or from others. This occurs particularly when clients are given no decision-making power in the change process.

The behaviors demonstrated by clients resisting change may include:

1. Silence
2. Avoidance of a topic or changing the subject
3. Attempts to infer that the clinician has "the problem"
4. Anger
5. Talk about irrelevant topics
6. Avoiding or coming late to interviews
7. Minimizing the importance of the therapy or the clinician as a person
8. Hopelessness

Behaviors Indicating the Occurrence of Change

When has change taken place in clients? This depends on how clinicians (and clients) define mental health. The following list contains several typical changes expected of clients by clinicians:[10]

1. Decreased symptoms
2. Increased sense of well-being
3. Self-actualization
4. The ability to adapt to circumstances
5. Greater emotional maturity
6. The ability to love unselfishly
7. The ability to have satisfying sexual relationships
8. The ability to work effectively
9. Social responsibility
10. Productivity
11. Insight into the nature and source of the presenting problems

Short-Term Therapy

Currently there is growing research, practice, and interest in *short-term therapy*. The purpose of short-term therapy is to offer psychotherapeutic intervention to clients within a brief period of time, usually in less than 12 hours of psychotherapeutic intervention. The interest in brief therapy has arisen for a number of reasons, including:

1. Lack interest in therapy of longer duration on the part of many clients
2. The unsuitability of many clients for longer-term therapy because of inappropriate cognitive or emotional characteristics (to be explained later in this section)
3. Clinicians' need to be accountable for clearly stated objectives and treatment plans. This focused approach lends itself to short-term therapy.
4. The decline of the willingness of health care insurance providers to pay for long-term treatment, thus necessitating a short-term approach
5. Ethical questions regarding the legitimacy of lengthy treatment when shorter treatment may be just as effective

The study of short-term approaches to therapy is important for nursing. Clinical specialists in psychiatric/mental health nursing, prepared at the master's degree level, may elect to do short-term psychotherapy exclusively in their practice or in conjunction with the use of a longer-term approach with other clients. Baccalaureate-prepared psychiatric nurses do not do long-term psychotherapy, but can find the focus, and some techniques, of short-term therapy very suitable for their practices.

Thompson[18] described the usefulness of Peplau's principles of psychiatric/mental health nursing in short-term individual therapy. In particular, Thompson found Peplau's ideas concerning the various roles required of the nurse in working with clients, interventions for anxiety, and phases of the nurse–client interaction useful in doing short-term therapy.

Commonalities Among Short-Term Approaches

There are many different types of short-term therapy. There are, however, certain features that are common to most short-term interventions, including:[3]

1. All short-term approaches limit the number of sessions.
2. All short-term approaches necessitate the rapid development of a relationship between the clinician and the client. Rapport must be established quickly.
3. Problems must be defined quickly.
4. Goals are focused, and few in number.
5. The clinicians are verbally active.
6. At times, the clinicians make rapid decisions based on incomplete data.

Types of Short-Term Therapy

According to Clarkin and Frances,[3] providing categories for the various short-term therapies is difficult, in part be-

cause each approach shares commonalities with others. The authors defined one classification system based on clinical usefulness composed of five types of short-term therapy: crisis intervention, and psychodynamic, behavioral, problem-solving, and family therapy. Definitions of each of these forms of therapy will follow later in the chapter.

Research continues into the effectiveness of each of the above-mentioned approaches. Clarkin and Frances[3] have reviewed some preliminary results, such as:

1. In a study comparing brief, dynamically-oriented therapy vs. behavior therapy, researchers found no difference in the client outcome ratings, although behavior therapy clients rated themselves as more improved. Another researcher found improvement in clients receiving brief psychodynamic therapy (behavior therapy) compared to clients receiving no therapy (the control group), who did not improve.
2. Behavioral techniques have been found to be more useful than other forms of treatment in specific cases, such as phobias, social difficulties, and sexual dysfunction.
3. Couples therapy has been found to be superior to individual treatment for marital discord.
4. Family crisis intervention has been found to be more effective than traditional, inpatient psychiatric care.
5. Studies comparing traditional, long-term therapy with short-term therapy *have failed to demonstrate* the superiority of long-term treatment.

Now that a classification of short-term therapies and a limited examination of the research in the field have been provided, the nature of several of the types of short-term therapy will be discussed. Part of the task of the clinician is to determine which type of therapy is best suited for specific clients.

Crisis Intervention

While crisis intervention is examined in detail in Chapter 13, it is discussed briefly in this chapter to provide a comparison with other short-term therapies.

Clarkin and Frances[3] stated that crisis intervention involves treatment usually lasting less than one month. It is an *intensive,* goal-directed approach, used to resolve a recent crisis of major proportions. The client is assisted in restoring a pre-crisis (or higher) level of functioning. The treatment may involve daily, prolonged sessions and admission to a short-term, inpatient psychiatric unit. Family members may be asked to provide support; the client may receive medications.

Because of the client's symptoms and distress, immediate treatment is necessary. The client may, for example, be suicidal. Typically, the stress that produces the symptoms provides a clear focus for treatment: the client, for example, may have just lost a job and have symptoms of recent origin.

Clients who benefit most from crisis intervention are those who are willing to participate in treatment and to take medications. The social system of the client should support the client.

The goals of crisis intervention are the relief of symptoms and the prevention of a more severe illness. Another goal is the development or recall of coping skills that can be used by the client to meet and cope with the crisis.

Alternatives to Crisis Intervention.

If crisis intervention is not suitable for the client, the clinician must decide which other form of short-term therapy is appropriate or if long-term therapy is suitable. Overall, indications for short-term therapy include:[3]

1. A specific stressful event caused the client's symptoms.
2. A goal is defined for what the client and clinician will accomplish in a brief amount of time.
3. The client is willing to participate in treatment.
4. The client can make use of personal resources for adaptation (or use those of his or her social group in conjunction with the client's own resources) after treatment.
5. The client can take care of his/herself.
6. The client does not require crisis intervention or hospitalization.
7. The client cannot pay for longer-term treatment.

The client is *not* considered suitable for short-term treatment if:

1. The client has pervasive psychiatric problems (such as schizophrenia or persistent, impulsive behavior).
2. The client's problems are sufficiently complex that they cannot be clearly defined in a limited amount of time.
3. The client is not motivated for brief work. Long-term treatment may assist in the development of more of a motivation for change.
4. The client needs prolonged contact with a clinician because of pervasive anxiety or the need to resolve interpersonal issues that can be recreated and resolved with the clinician.

Once it is determined that the client is suitable for short-term treatment other than crisis intervention, the clinician must then decide which short-term approach is best. Four other short-term therapies are described below:

Brief Psychodynamic Therapy

Brief psychodynamic therapy is generally the same as long-term psychodynamic psychotherapy, but takes place in a condensed period of time. This technique is differentiated from other approaches by the fact that it makes use of the clarification of "unconscious wishes, fears, and defenses"[3] in order to resolve a conflict that is limited in complexity. Brief psychodynamic therapy seeks personality change in the focused conflict area (problem) as well as relief of symptoms.

Several major theorists propose using brief psychodynamic therapy. While these theorists will not be re-viewed here, it should be mentioned that these clinicians typically select only clients whose psychological trauma occurred at an early age, or clients experiencing problems with separation from others.

Most clinicians who use brief psychodynamic therapy also examine the nature of the client's reaction to the clinician. It is thought that the way the client reacts to the clinician is a reflection of the ways the client learned, at an early age, to react to others who were part of the perceived psychological trauma. Hence, if the client can correct the defenses built up against childhood traumas (which are repeated with the clinician), improvement will be seen. This process is termed *transference,* and is described in greater detail in Chapter 6, Developmental Theories.

Clients best suited for brief psychodynamic therapy are those whose problems are psychological conflicts stemming from trauma experienced early in life. These clients have also had successful interpersonal relationships in the past, are expressive, and relate to the clinicians. The clients must be able to define the problems with the clinician. The clients are motivated to change their behavior, and are relatively sophisticated in being able to review clearly what has happened in their lives. The clients understand the reality of what is expected in treatment. There is a willingness to tolerate the painful feelings that are explored, and clients can state potentially threatening feelings about the clinician openly to the clinician. The clients must have achieved certain productive levels in life, evidenced by work, education, or interpersonal behaviors. Typically the clients are intelligent.

Clarkin and Frances[3] mentioned that there are several contraindications to the use of brief psychodynamic therapy, including: psychosis, substance abuse, a serious suicide attempt, extreme impulsive behavior, and the inability to focus on one problem in therapy.

Brief Problem-Solving Therapy

The central aspect of *brief problem-solving therapy* is the focus on a description and resolution of a specific problem in the client's life. Some of the techniques used in this approach include: discussing with the client the various courses for resolving the problem, giving advice, role-playing, emotional reassurance, and changes in the living conditions of the client.

The goals of brief problem-solving therapy are a decrease in distressing symptoms, improved adaptation of the client to the problem, the use of new or previously forgotten skills to resolve the troublesome situation, and an improvement in the client's self-esteem. The goals of treatment do *not* include clarification of the unconscious, as does brief psychodynamic therapy. Brief problem-solving therapy also does not produce personality change. In many cases, this type of therapy is used when the client has functioned well prior to the onset of the problem.

Clients who do best in this type of treatment cooperate with the clinician's suggestions and interventions, and are willing to make changes. Clients who are *not* suited for brief psychodynamic therapy are also not suited for brief problem-solving therapy.

Brief Marital or Family Therapy

Brief marital or *family therapy* is based on the idea that clients' problems arise because of what is occurring in their interpersonal relationships. Improvements can take place by intervening with the family group.

Clients who can benefit from brief marital or family therapy have recognizable family issues or concerns (*e.g.,* problems involving negotiating the roles and responsibilities of various family members), or there are obvious ways in which the family group is involved in the problem. There are also cases in which a pressing concern in the family group needs resolution (*e.g.,* a divorce).

Family groups suitable for this type of intervention can discuss interpersonal behaviors without intense negative feelings, can agree with the therapist on a treatment plan, and are interested in changing the way family members relate to one another.

Clarkin and Frances[3] list several important factors that might preclude family therapy: the insistence of one or more family members on concealing personal information, the need of a family member to focus on developing a personal sense of identity rather than a "family identity," and the presence of complex problems requiring longer treatment (*e.g.,* extensive psychological pathology of one or more family members).

Brief Behavior Therapy

A variety of behavior therapy techniques have been developed to treat *specific* clinical problems, including:

1. *Systematic desensitization:* A graded series of anxiety-provoking stimuli are presented to the client at the same time that a response (such as relaxation) is elicited.
2. *Implosion:* Learned fears (such as memories of war combat) are extinguished by their repeated presentation to the client. Strong emotional responses are elicited at first, but the intensity of the responses decreases with repeated exposure to the feared stimuli.
3. *Cognitive approaches:* Techniques are used that emphasize the importance of one's thoughts in producing behavior change. Clinicians help clients obtain a more rational understanding of events in order to change nonproductive thought patterns. This approach is based on the idea that irrational beliefs keep people from enjoying life, reaching their potential, and obtaining optimum health.[14]
4. *Operant techniques:* The techniques used are based on the idea that behavior is a result of the environmental consequences of the behavior. Treatment techniques are based on rearranging environmental consequences of events by reinforcing (through a reward) the behavior that is desired.

These techniques can be done in individual, group, or family settings. They can be used with clients exhibiting anxiety, panic attacks, hyperventilation, social phobias, depression, social skills deficits, and compulsive rituals.

Research Concerning the Effectiveness of Short-Term Therapy

Husby[8] studied the changes reported by 33 clients who had received short-term psychodynamic therapy, two and five years after treatment. All but four clients reported *positive* changes such as relief of symptoms, improved self-understanding, increased self-esteem, and improved interpersonal functioning. Husby reported that all of these changes could not have been attributed to spontaneous remission. Although this study did not use a control group, a needed element in the research, most clients reported at the two-year follow-up that they felt that the therapy was still working for them. The four clients who did not report changes were more severely ill at the start of the study, so a deteriorating effect of the therapy for these clients was probable.

Strupp[16] reported on an intensive exploratory study of two clients who were part of a larger study, the Vanderbilt Psychotherapy Research Project. He compared the effects of the brief therapy done with two clients by a lay counselor (a college professor who agreed to do counseling). One of the clients improved and the other did not, but both clients were able to enter into an initial positive relationship with the counselor, which was facilitated by the counselor's accepting and respectful attitude.

The client who improved made use of the counselor's accepting attitude. The other client's defenses forced him to sidetrack the counselor's interventions and, later, to develop a hostile attitude and become disillusioned with the counselor.

Thus, the diverse treatment outcomes were a result of the differences in the clients' personality structures and in the lay counselor's limitations in dealing with them. In the case of the client who did not improve, the provision of "empathy, warmth, and unconditional positive regard is not a sufficient condition for therapeutic change."

Specifically, the lay counselor lacked the professional's ability to:

1. Develop themes presented by the clients in a therapeutic fashion.
2. Maintain an objective view of the clients' psychological difficulties.
3. Label hidden themes presented by the clients.
4. Label the barriers clients use to avoid gaining an awareness of what they are doing in their lives.
5. Compare the clients' reaction to the clinician with the nature of the clients' difficulties with others.

Hill and Hoch[6] reported on their successful work as nurse therapists at an outpatient clinic in Winnipeg, Canada, where they did short-term therapy. They found that client problems best suited for short-term therapy included: treatment involving a theme of independence or dependence (*e.g.,* clients having difficulty separating from their families), low self-esteem, and unresolved grief.

Ethical Concerns in Individual Relationship Intervention

Whether the clinician is doing long-term or short-term therapy, psychoanalysis, or individual relationship intervention, ethical concerns are always present in the therapeutic experience. A question here is whether or not the clinician choses to consider ethical issues. At one point in the history of mental health care, the professionals were "in charge." Today the mentally ill and their families "maintain the right to make choices and determine the course of treatment."[15]

Related to ethical concerns, Karasu states that society is now experiencing an "Age of Ethical Crisis" compared to our previous "Age of Anxiety."[9] This age of ethical crisis has a number of components, including:

1. A progressive loss of faith in traditional institutions
2. Mistrust of authority
3. A renewed concern for human rights
4. A disappointment with mental health care sciences and their inability to solve the problems of society
5. Anti-elitism (the professionals' misuse of power to maintain the unequal distribution of resources in society)

Questions related to psychotherapeutic intervention include: whether traditional mental health care institutions meet the needs of the population; whether professionals, entrusted with responsibility for providing care, have the interests of clients in mind; and whether the rights of clients are protected in mental health care.

These questions should be expected. Traditionally, the treatment of the mentally ill has evoked an image of "controller" and "vulnerable victim" who cannot provide consent for treatment because of illness. Also, both psychiatry and philosophy (traditionally the field in which ethical matters are extensively studied) have discussed ethical concerns in their fields in highly abstract terms and principles. The pressing every-day concerns of clients seem removed from these abstract discussions.

Clinicians in psychotherapeutic practice were once removed and left undisturbed in the confines of their offices. Now clinicians are questioned by other clinicians about their methods, ideas of mental illness, and other topics. This is not surprising since there are more than 250 models of psychotherapeutic methods, with the proponents of each claiming that theirs is the correct method of treatment. Clinicians are also questioned by clients themselves, who are confused about methods of therapy as well as about the power of the therapist. Increasingly,

clients expect (and have the right to) treatment that is understandable. They demand that clinicians be held accountable. Clients expect to have a part in planning and evaluating their treatment with the clinician. Therapists can no longer expect blind reverence.

Professionals in mental health care cannot ignore ethical questions. Historically, professionals have been relatively blind to ethical concerns.[2] Ethical issues are often overlooked because they are not apparent. Clinicians may ignore ethical topics because they, like all human beings, have internal forces that motivate people toward *both* right and wrong.

Ethics Defined

Ethics is a code of morality of a person or group of people, such as a professional group. *Morality* is the distinction between right and wrong conduct. The mental health sciences, on the other hand, are concerned with the establishment of facts and knowledge. From one point of view, ethics and psychiatric/mental health nursing, are two separate areas of study and are almost opposite in focus. Psychiatric/mental health nursing is concerned with describing human nature and validating its ideas about what "is true" about human nature. Ethics is concerned with prescribing actions, and forming judgments, based on what "ought to be."[9]

Yet, "the lines become less sharply drawn when the complexities of social reality are considered, as when the therapist is obliged to act as a 'double agent' to accommodate conflicts of interest."[9] Conflicts of interest occur between the client and therapist, as well as between third parties to whom the therapist has some allegiance. For example, a conflict of interest would exist between a client and a clinician if the clinician gave a disturbed client an injection of medication to calm the client, regardless of the wishes of the client. An example of a conflict involving a third party would be seen in the termination of inpatient treatment for a client because of the end of insurance reimbursement, despite the fact that the client remains mentally ill.

Examples of Ethical Dilemmas

Extensive discussion of the variety and number of ethical dilemmas that occur in psychiatric/mental health nursing is beyond the scope of this text. However, several issues commonly faced by psychiatric/mental nurses are discussed below.

There is a *tendency of some clinicians to favor certain social or client types over other individuals.* An example of this judgment is seen in the idea of some clinicians that women who are battered by their spouses are masochistic. This judgment by clinicians favors individuals who are *naturally* assertive. If clinicians understood the effects of socialization on battered women, who believe that there is no other life for them outside of their marriages, the clinicians would judge these women differently. These women would not be thought of as "masochistic," but rather as the unfortunate victims of society's conditioning.

Clinicians' own values can influence their judgments. At one time it was thought that the psychotherapeutic process was value-free. This idea is now considered a fallacy. Clinicians are not "neutral." Because the clinicians mentioned in the example above select to talk about masochism, and not about how the clients have been socialized, the clinicians' values are shown. The fact that most clients are responsive to the direction of clinicians is evidence of the power and influence that clinicians can have over clients. At the present time, psychotherapeutic science cannot determine when "reality" (for clients) is being considered in the therapy sessions and when the content is predicated on clinicians' values. The values of clinicians may not coincide with clients' reality.

The question of the influence of the clinician's own values is one of the most pervasive and unexplored ethical dilemmas of the psychotherapeutic process. One apparent question is whether or not *clients* really know what they want. If clients are caught in a conflict or are experiencing high levels of anxiety, can clinician silence simply be a matter of "allowing clients to make their own decisions"? Clinician values are always present.

An example of an ethical dilemma occurred in a crisis team in a mental health clinic. A severely delusional individual was brought in after having been found walking on the runway of a major airport. Should the client's right to freedom dictate that the client not be hospitalized, or should the priority be the protection of others who may be harmed by the client's presence on the runway? This dilemma is confronted by clinicians (if they are aware of the dilemma) in a multitude of less dramatic examples.

Another dilemma occurs in relation to the issue of *whether to encourage clients to adapt to social reality or to encourage rebellion of clients against social reality.* This dilemma is exemplified by a client who is uncertain about his or her sexual preference. Should the client be subtly encouraged to adapt to social reality and "pass" for being a heterosexual, or should the client be encouraged to stand up for his or her homosexual or lesbian rights and rebel against the dictates of society. What promotes comfort for the client? When does clinician bias enter the treatment?

Do clients have the freedom to change or to not change? Related to this dilemma is the question of whether clients should be placed in psychiatric hospitals against their will.

Should individual clients be hospitalized against their will rather than treating the social system? In many cases, if a social group is in conflict, an individual client may be less able to withstand the tension of the conflict. For example, if the parents in a family are having a conflict, the adolescent child may be most affected and require hospitalization. Should this *individual* pay the price (hospitalization and the stigma of being labeled a "psychiatric patient") simply because the mental health care professionals and institutions do not know how to treat the system as a whole (the family in this example)? Knowing the nature of the system may demonstrate that the client is behaving in a *reasonable* fashion within an *un*reasonable environment.

Should a therapeutic technique be selected without the permission of the client? An example of this dilemma would be admitting a client to a unit that functions by using behavior modification (the rewarding and/or punishment of selected behaviors), without allowing the client the choice of the treatment technique. In such a situation, should the client be told about the lack of focus on self-awareness in behavior modification, and that the client will not select the behaviors that are reinforced?

Confidentiality is an ethical dilemma discussed in Chapter 34 on the law and psychiatric/mental health nursing. An example of this issue is the decision of whom to talk to about the condition of a client. If a mute, and seemingly severely ill, client is admitted to a mental health unit, can (or should) the staff call the family for information concerning the client? Would making such an inquiry violate the rights of the client?

Another example of an ethical dilemma concerns *whether clinicians should decide ethical dilemmas according to patient needs, physician needs, or hospital (institution) needs.* Swider, McElmurry and Yarling[17] reported on their study concerning decisions about an ethical dilemma made by baccalaureate nursing students. They found that students more frequently made decisions based on institutional needs, than on client or physician needs (see Relevant Research box).

Guidelines for Working With Ethical Dilemmas

The study of ethics involves judgments. Judgments are different from clinical decisions based on scientific research. Because psychiatric/mental health nursing is a science it seeks to further define its scientific base. At the same time the profession must examine its art, part of which includes ethical *judgments*. Because of the nature of judgments, ethical questions will not be resolved in a short amount of time. The following guidelines offer some direction for working with ethical concerns.

1. Clinicians should constantly be aware of, and alert to, the input of their values into clinical situations. This awareness can be facilitated with a clinician peer who can offer an outside perspective on the nature of the part the clinician adds to the treatment.

2. Clinicians should accept, as a career objective, the constant need to understand ethical concerns. In what may seem like small steps, the disparity in ethical judgments can become the knowledge of science by means of research. Such a career objective also decreases the tendency to deny ethics-related questions and to make hasty judgments concerning questions of right and wrong.

RELEVANT RESEARCH

This study examined the solutions to an ethical dilemma given by 775 senior baccalaureate nursing students (from 20 randomly-selected schools). The ethical dilemma was presented to discussion groups of students in the form of a case concerning a 34-year-old mother who was administered an overdose of an IV anti-cancer medication after a mastectomy. The client subsequently died. The nursing staff felt that the physician who administered the drug was only marginally competent. The physician told the family only that the client had suffered a severe reaction to the drug. When the nurse on the unit expressed strong reservations about what the family had been told, the attending staff requested that she not complicate the situation and said that it was an honest mistake. The nurse checked the chart where the physician had written the medication order, and found that the dose ordered was ten times the normal dose. Students in the discussion groups were then asked what the nurse should do.

The students reviewed the case with a faculty member. The groups' decision about the nurse's action in the ethical dilemma were categorized as (1) client-centered (reflecting nursing responsibilities to the client/family), (2) physician-centered (reflecting nursing responsibilities to physician needs), or (3) bureaucratic (hospital)-centered (reflecting nursing responsibilities to the employer). Examples of client-centered responses included informing the family of what had happened and letting the family choose their course of action. Physi-cian-centered responses included taking the incident before a board of the physician's peers. Bureaucratic-related responses included responses such as filing an incident report.

Of the 1,163 decisions mentioned by the students, 9% were client-centered, 19% were physician-centered, and 60% were bureaucratic-centered. Other responses, which could not be categorized, accounted for 12% of the responses. Group responses did not differ significantly by education, clinical experience, or previous experience with ethical dilemmas. When asked to list the first decision to be made, none of the decisions were client-centered. Eighty-nine percent were bureaucratic-centered, and 8% were physician-centered.

Subjects in this study began with the hospital system in resolving the dilemma. In response to the question of when the nurse should stop pursuing the matter and resolve the ethical dilemma, the student responses indicated no consensus. There was no agreement as to when the nurse had fulfilled her responsibilities in this case.

The researchers concluded that nurses are pulled in many directions in their decision-making, and that some confusion exists among nurses about their ultimate ethical responsibility. The researchers advocated peer support to facilitate discussion of the meaning of one's choices, developing an awareness of the implications of decisions concerning ethical dilemmas, and discussion of the nurse's autonomy within the hospital system.

(Swider S, McElmurry B, Yarling R: Ethical Decision-Making in a Bureaucratic Context by Senior Nursing Students. Nurs Res 34:108, 1985)

3. Clients and clinicians should openly state their views of what each believes is occurring at each step of the therapeutic process. Do both label the same phenomena as the problem? Do both agree to the nature of treatment needed? Do both agree that this method of treatment is the best method for the problem? The establishment of a mutual contract limits the power of the clinician over the client and safeguards the rights of the client.

Although psychiatric nursing bases its practice on interventions that have received theoretical and research support, the ethical issues found in practice have received much less attention. Clinicians have an obligation to recognize ethical issues and resolve them, taking into account the needs and rights of clients.

Summary

1. Individual relationship intervention by nurses can be contrasted with the work of a psychotherapist or counselor according to the focus and goals of treatment, the length of the nurse–client relationship, and the techniques that are used.

References

1. American Nurses' Association: Statement on Psychiatric and Mental Health Nursing Practice. Kansas City, American Nurses' Association, 1976
2. Bloch S, Chodoff P (eds): Psychiatric Ethics. Oxford, Oxford University Press, 1984

3. Clarkin J, Frances A: Selection criteria for the brief psychotherapies. Am J Psychother 36:166, 1982

4. Cochrane C: Toward a distinction between counseling and psychotherapy. Georgia Psychol 6:13, 1984

5. Dewald P: The process of change in psychoanalytic psychotherapy. Arch Gen Psychiatry 35:535, 1978

6. Hill S, Hoch M: 12-hour psychotherapy. Can Nurse 72:30, 1976

7. Horvath P: Demand characteristics and inferential processes in psychotherapeutic change. Consult Clin Psychol 52:616, 1984

8. Husby R: Short-term dynamic psychotherapy. Psychother Psychosom 43:23, 1985

9. Karasu T: Ethical Aspects of Psychotherapy. In Bloch S, Chodoff P (eds): Psychiatric Ethics. Oxford, Oxford University Press, 1984

10. Marmor J: Change in psychoanalytic treatment. J Am Acad Psychoanal 7:345, 1979

11. Orne M: Psychotherapy in Contemporary America: Its Development and Context. In Arieti S (ed): American Handbook of Psychiatry, 2nd ed. New York, Basic Books, 1975

12. Peplau H: Psychiatric nursing: Past, present, and future. Paper presented at the Neuropsychiatric Institute, University of California at Los Angeles, November 1, 1982

13. Rodgers J: Theoretical considerations involved in the process of change. Nurs Forum 12:160, 1973

14. Sideleau B: Irrational beliefs and intervention. J Psychiatr Nurs 25:18, 1987

15. Smoyak S: Ethical perspectives. J Psychiatr Nurs 24:7, 1986

16. Strupp H: Success and failure in time-limited psychotherapy. Arch Gen Psychiatry 37:831, 1980

17. Swider S, McElmurry B, Yarling R: Ethical decision-making in a bureaucratic context by senior nursing students. Nurs Res 34:108, 1985

18. Thompson L: Peplau's theory: An application to short-term individual therapy. J Psychiatr Nurs 24:26, 1986

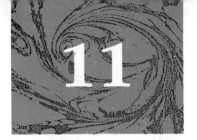

GWEN MARRAM VAN SERVELLEN
AND LORETTA M. BIRCKHEAD

GROUP THERAPY

Learning Objectives

Upon completion of this chapter the student should be able to do the following:

1. Identify the types of group approaches used with client problems and differentiate among them.
2. Discuss the nature of group functioning that guides nursing practice in group work.
3. Identify the basic leadership functions and interventions used in group work.
4. Describe the implications of client or clinician cultural variables for group therapy.
5. Summarize the role of the nurse in enhancing the benefits of group membership for clients.
6. Summarize the role of the nurse in assisting the group to attain its goals.

Introduction

The use of groups in psychiatric clinical practice and in mental health is a promising development with broad impact on the prevention, treatment, and restoration to health of many individuals. The increasing use of group therapeutic modalities is, in part, the direct result of the acknowledgement that groups exist, that group dynamics (as in a peer group) must be considered to account adequately for human behavior, and that desirable conse-

quences for individuals in groups can be enhanced deliberately.[12]

Groups offer a number of benefits to members. These include support, education, increased problem-solving ability, increased understanding of interpersonal relationships, and, for the psychiatric client, improved reality testing.

As Marram[12] stated: "No better opportunity exists than in a group experience for individuals to learn how they are uniquely different, yet, at the same time, like others." Groups can be a comforting experience to those who have experienced a difficult environment.

Nurse group leaders use the unique and common aspects of individuals to encourage others to reveal their problems and get help from the group. At the same time, nurse group leaders become increasingly aware of how their own backgrounds and experiences with groups determine their current reactions to the group including their fears and desires.

Historical Development of Group Interventions

The first accounts of the benefits of group therapy began with Joseph Hersey Pratt, in 1905. Dr. Pratt, an internist, developed the home sanatorium treatment. He gathered tuberculosis patients together in small groups at Johns Hopkins Hospital. Designed for poor patients who were unable to afford inpatient treatment, his program organized outpatients into groups of approximately 20 people. His didactic (lecture) groups were organized as weekly classes that considered the physical and emotional aspects of tuberculosis.[20] He lectured to group members about strict hygiene, diet, and rest. He offered support, hope, and encouragement to his patients, which was very meaningful to patients whose lengthy illness was discouraging. By 1930, Pratt had established the first clinic in which a group method was the primary therapeutic effort. His writings span a period of 50 years and help to document the impact of the group process on individual members. He understood the importance of mutual support created by the common bond among patients with the same disease. Pratt was the first practitioner of modern group psychotherapy in the United States.

In 1921, E. W. Lazell published the first literature concerning the treatment of psychiatric patients in groups.[18] He used the group method to treat war veterans with diagnoses of psychotic schizophrenia. Like Pratt, Lazell used a lecture method. Again, the emphasis was to encourage, inspire, and bring hope to these patients. At the same time, the groups focused on education about every-day living problems.

It was not until World War II that group techniques played a major role in psychiatric treatment. Just prior to WWII, group methods turned toward social group formation and used theatrical production to assist members. In Great Britain, Joshua Bierer formed social clubs for the treatment of the mentally ill. Like Lazell, Bierer attempted to help members through use of problem-solving techniques and by focusing on daily living. He also sought to make members' attitudes toward life more positive. His methods included entertainment, painting, writing, and group discussions.

Shortly after Bierer's work with the mentally ill, Jacob Moreno introduced a more formal approach to group psychotherapy. In an historical sense, Moreno's group method is the oldest model because it can be traced back to 1910. This approach later became known as *psychodrama,* and is still used today in many psychiatric settings for the treatment of the mentally ill, as well as in the training of psychiatric/mental health professionals. Psychodrama is a form of group treatment that uses drama and theatrics to reproduce members' problems while acting out conflicts and feelings in a safe environment. Only two or three members are "on stage" at any one time, but the total group benefits vicariously from watching the dynamics of interpersonal relationships acted out in the group meetings. Moreno, who coined the term "group psychotherapy," is credited with founding the first professional journal dealing with group work and starting the first professional organization for clinicians interested in group work.

Other early developments in group work include the advances of several psychoanalytic group psychotherapists in the late 1920s and early 1930s. Many psychotherapists believe that group psychotherapy began with Freud's observations in 1919, in which he saw the dynamics of the interplay among individuals in a group setting. He believed that there was a definite pattern of interaction among members that facilitated the therapeutic process. Three additional psychoanalytic psychotherapists had an impact on the development of group work, including Alfred Adler, Alexander Wolf, and Samuel Slauson.

Most well-known were Adler, who used group psychotherapy in child guidance work, and Wolf, a psychiatrist and psychoanalyst who applied psychoanalytic principles to the treatment of individuals within group settings. Wolf, instead of treating the whole group through encouragement, persuasion, and education, analyzed individuals' interactions with other members. This was psychoanalytic treatment of the individual in a group context. Topics of focus were conflicts and patterns of interaction recalled from the individual's past. The group setting was similar to the family group. By 1947, Wolf had started to hold seminars in psychoanalytic group therapy at the New York Medical College. Slauson, also using psychoanalytic techniques, was best known for the development of activity groups for children. He began his work with children and adolescents at the Jewish Board of Guardians during the late 1930s. He eventually called his approach "activity group therapy." It emphasized the expression of children's conflicts and inner feelings through sports, games, art, and crafts.

During World War II, group psychotherapy became more widespread because it made possible the treatment of large numbers of individuals with few clinicians. In the mid-1960s, the age of groups began. Therapy groups, encounter groups, leaderless groups, marathon groups, task groups, and psychodrama were becoming commonplace in U.S. psychiatry. To this day, the group approach is recognized for its ability to treat large numbers of people by relatively few psychotherapists.

Many types of group psychotherapy emerged after World War II. Among these was the *Tavistock method,* a group dynamics approach to group psychotherapy. The author of the Tavistock method, Wilfred Bion, adopted, along with his colleagues Foulkes and Ezriel, an approach to psychoanalytic group therapy that encouraged the analyst to give careful attention to forces in the group that provided greater or lesser cohesion.[18] His theory of groups attempted to establish universal laws of group behavior and group development, whether or not the groups were therapeutic. True to its psychoanalytic tradition, the Tavistock model treated the group like a single person. The leader's interpretations were always directed to the group as a whole. Individual patients in psychoanalysis would be encouraged to examine their own feelings and behaviors carefully during the sessions in order to better understand their underlying feelings.

Another growing influence was the importance attributed to intensive group experiences. Among those interested in the possibilities of this model was Carl Rogers. Rogers's intensive group experiences focused on helping a person find genuine authenticity in relationships with others. From this came the *encounter group method,* through which a variety of specific techniques, including psychodrama and guided fantasy, enabled the members to discover their true selves, hidden beneath social and professional facades. By the early 1960s, Rogers referred to the intensive group experience as the *basic encounter group,* and William Schutz had developed his own variation of the encounter group at the Esalen Institute in California.

In encounter groups, leaders became freer to express themselves, and participants were allowed to dramatize their problems rather than just state them. Group therapy methods were applied to "normal" individuals as well as to those with psychiatric problems.

Today, specialized group methods are used in a broad range of educational, health, and welfare settings. These include child guidance clinics, schools, delinquency programs, mental hospitals, correctional institutions, and general hospital settings.

Types of Group Work

For nurses, the practice of group work with clients is diverse, and occurs within the framework of illness prevention and treatment as well as that of health restoration. The following sections identify some of the forms of group work that psychiatric/mental health nurses may use in their professional practices.

The major contribution of groups to the experiences of members are social, cultural, and psychological. Group norms are formulated and values emerge, based on the social and cultural dimensions of the group. These norms and values influence members' concepts of self and their sense of self-esteem. Perceptions of individuals that they are like others in the group influence the formulation of shared values.

Traditional Forms of Group Psychotherapy

Group psychotherapy (or a psychotherapy group), in contrast to "therapeutic group work" and "self-actualization groups," is the branch of psychiatry and psychotherapy concerned with the use of group process, and other methods, to treat psychopathology. *Psychopathology* means disturbances in mood, thought, or character that originate in the complex interplay among cultural, physical, psychological, environmental, and social aspects of a person's existence.

Since its beginnings in the early decades of the 20th century, group psychotherapy has undergone extensive expansion. It is now practiced by people from a variety of backgrounds, including psychology, nursing, social work, and psychiatry. The types of groups may vary in nature from analytic group psychotherapy, based on a psychoanalytic approach to unconscious content, to group psychotherapy, based on communication and interpersonal interpretations of here-and-now events.

In the past, group psychotherapy was used as a transition phase for patients terminating individual therapy and to prepare for community life and then help clients discharged from hospitals. More recently, however, apparent benefits of group psychotherapy have included (1) maintaining individuals in the community without hospitalization, and (2) treating clients exclusively with group psychotherapy.

Most patients undergoing (or who have undergone) psychiatric treatment have experienced a breakdown in interpersonal relationships. This experience often leads to feelings of rejection, unworthiness, isolation, and inadequacy. Group psychotherapy has been effective in helping individuals to establish more successful relationships by encouraging them to relate to other people in the group, and to resolve some of their former problems and conflicts. An important by-product of this process is that the clients usually experience support from the group, with increased feelings of self-worth as well as increased awareness of the reasons for their troubles. Individuals are expected to identify with the group's goals for health, and are encouraged to test new and more effective patterns of adapting to the stress they experience. Clients also experience increased self-esteem from the cohesiveness of the group, providing feelings of belonging and opportunities for members to assist one another.

The methods used in group psychotherapy to help individuals resolve problems in relating to others, and to help them assume more successful patterns of adapting, may differ from group to group. Types of group psychotherapy, for the most part, can be distinguished by their emphasis on (1) personality reconstruction, (2) insight without reconstruction, (3) remotivation, (4) problem-solving, (5) reeducation, or (6) support. Psychotherapy groups can include inpatient, outpatient, or clinic groups with one or more of the above emphases. The subtypes of group psychotherapy groups are discussed below.

Within the realm of inpatient and outpatient services, psychotherapy groups vary in intensity and are distinguishable in their aims. The aims and intensity of these groups depend on the philosophy and treatment practices of the ward and staff, as well as on the capacities of the clients and the nature of their illnesses. The aim or emphasis of these groups ranges from personality reconstruction to offering support.

Personality reconstruction groups take an intensive analytical view of individuals in groups. These groups may employ dream analysis, free association, and transference reactions as content of the group discussions. Each individual is analyzed within a group context, which is presumed to be a replay of each client's primary family group.

Insight without reconstruction groups are a less intense form of group treatment that may be analytical in nature but focus more on the here-and-now of interpersonal relationships in the group. The emphasis is on the hows and whys of interpersonal relationships in the group, but the focus relies more on the current communication processes of group members. Changes in members' behavior are expected, but are believed to be achieved through insight into current relationships rather than knowledge of past deep-seated phenomena.

Birckhead[2,3] has described the need for insight-oriented group work on inpatient psychiatric units with severely ill clients. The author described the role of the nurse as the group leader, and suggested specific interventions for establishing and maintaining these groups.

Remotivation groups use a variety of strategies to encourage clients to communicate and interact with one another, and to demonstrate behaviors believed to be linked with decreases in symptoms. These groups encourage appropriate social and interactional responses. Often, the nurse teaches the norm, or the accepted social response, by informing about and reinforcing certain behaviors. Clients who have undergone long-term institutionalization or who have suffered chronic or regressive psychiatric illness or human interactional neglect often are not familiar with appropriate and acceptable behaviors, and are good candidates for this type of group experience.

Problem-solving groups, like remotivation and reeducation groups, concentrate less on insight and much more on knowledge of specific concerns and alternatives, as well as on the process of resolving present conflicts and making here-and-now decisions. Problem-solving groups in inpatient settings may relate to issues of orientation and discharge, for example. Other groups, used quite frequently on wards and in communities, strive to remotivate and/or reeducate clients.

Reeducation groups are useful for withdrawn, institutionalized clients. These groups encourage, for example, appropriate social responses. The techniques used by the leader of reeducation groups are information-giving, role-playing, and reinforcing appropriate behaviors. Clients who have suffered long psychiatric illnesses and are socially inept are good candidates for this type of group experience.

Support is an ingredient of many types of group psychotherapy. When it becomes the distinguishing feature of the group, it forms a subtype of group work. Support groups do not seek to achieve psychological insight or personality reconstruction, but help members maintain a functional or semifunctional adaptation to their environment, given the existing illness of the client and the resources available. The nurse does not threaten the client's defense structure (*e.g.,* the client's use of denial or resistance) in these groups, but reinforces and supports the client in the basic tasks of communicating or giving and receiving information. In an inpatient setting, common problems of ward living are typical areas of discussion. In outpatient settings, problems of daily living are often discussed, including how to get along with members of one's family, making financial ends meet, and adapting to the prescribed treatment and/or medication regimen.

Variations of Group Psychotherapy in Psychiatric Services

In addition to the inpatient and outpatient groups described above, there are a number of special modifications in group psychotherapy for psychiatric clients with whom nurses work. For the purpose of this discussion, they will be referred to as: (1) inpatient milieu groups, (2) special problem groups, and (3) multiple-family and married couples' psychotherapy groups.

It must be recognized that within various psychiatric/mental health settings there are always overlapping and interacting group influences that can affect clients. Not only are clients exposed to formal group psychotherapy, but they also interact with staff in less structured community, or milieu, groups.

The recognition that clients' therapeutic experiences are not strictly the result of organized and insulated group efforts has done much to alter conceptions of what happens in the minute-to-minute interactions among clients and staff. Prior to this recognition, such "informal" interaction was viewed as less significant and somewhat less valid than were formal group meetings. Nor was this interaction appreciated for its capacity to affect clients' behavior. Nurses, perhaps because of their continual exposure to these interactions, were probably the only group aware of the diagnostic and therapeutic potential of informal interactions.

Psychiatric wards that are viewed as continuously functioning therapeutic milieus are *therapeutic communities.* The therapeutic community, based on group principles, represents as much a philosophy of treatment as it does a type of approach. The idea of a therapeutic community increased in the orientation of psychiatric wards after World War II. It began in Western Europe, where there was a shortage of therapists and a great sense of community responsibility.[9]

There are several operational components of the therapeutic community approach. These include extensive use of occupational, recreational, and industrial therapy programs; vocational rehabilitation; development of patient government; psychotherapy groups; and group work.

Nurses in a therapeutic community are responsible for helping to create and maintain a culture that can foster healthy personalities. They are expected to support and encourage clients in every phase of treatment and, in

RELEVANT RESEARCH

This study was based on the idea that self-help groups are effective in promoting recovery and rehabilitation of people who share a common problem. The two factors thought to have an impact on recovery are leadership by a nonprofessional who has recovered from the problem, and acceleration of group identification due to the shared problem. In this study, the sample consisted of 28 clients on a psychiatric unit with a primary diagnosis of reactive depression. Each client had, within six to twelve months prior to psychiatric hospital admission, experienced the loss of an important person, the loss of a job, or other personal losses, triggering a reactive depression. The subjects were randomly assigned to one of two self-help groups or to one of two control groups.

Each experimental group consisted of clients, the investigator, and a lay leader. The lay leader was an ex-client who had been hospitalized four years previously with a depression due to a loss. Control group members returned to their usual activity which was "free time."

A total of four group meetings were held, one each on consecutive days, for all groups.

Data were analyzed using mean proportions calculated for each group on the pretest and posttest. The influence of the self-help group treatment was determined by using a one-tailed Difference of Proportions test. There was a significant difference between the groups on the Beck Hopelessness Scale, with the experimental group showing significantly less hopelessness than the control group. There was also a significant difference between the groups on the Thorton Learned Helplessness Index, supporting the idea that members of the support group would experience a decrease in feelings of helplessness because of the self-help group. The importance of this exploratory study lies in its ability to document changes in individuals with reactive depression who experience short-term support groups that have nonprofessional group leaders who share a common experience with all group members.

(Rothlis J: The effect of a self-help group on feelings of hopelessness and helplessness. *West J Nurs Res* 6:155, 1984)

their minute-to-minute interaction with clients, to convey appropriate responses and behavior. These norms, transmitted to clients by nurses, are part of a total therapeutic community culture, and in some instances are norms the client will be obliged to abide by outside the hospital community.

The range of therapy groups that focus on *special client problems,* rather than on global issues of daily living, is impressive. These groups can be found in both inpatient and outpatient facilities, and increasingly in agencies such as centers for special problems.

These therapy groups address a specific problem of concern to all the clients in the group. Homogeneity in these groups is a powerful influence on the problems, and creates a climate of acceptance while encouraging clients to discuss seriously their fears and concerns. Examples of these groups include special problem groups for substance abuse, eating disorders, and the physically and sexually abused. Research on addiction and alcoholism problems seems to indicate that homogeneous groups of people with these problems are far more successful than mixing them in heterogeneous therapy groups. In many instances, special problem groups deal with socially inappropriate behaviors. When patients or clients who exhibit socially disapproved-of behaviors are put together in a group, they experience a greater feeling of understanding and acceptance, whereas in heterogeneous groups they anticipate discrimination and social isolation—reactions that may, in fact, occur.

Multiple-family and married couples' psychotherapy groups (both inpatient and outpatient) are another special type of group psychotherapy. *Multiple-family group therapy* draws on aspects of group and family therapy. Family therapy uses a systems theory approach, and treats all family members together in sessions. The client with symptoms is the *identified patient,* but the entire family system is believed to be dysfunctional, causing the individual's problems. The combined multiple-family group approach is a variation of traditional family therapy in which the group process and input of other family groups have an impact on change in the individual family. The leaders use social pressure and group norms to elicit change in each family and, at the same time, offer support to the family system through feedback from other families who have suffered the same problems. Multiple-family therapy groups consist of a number of families (usually not more than four, depending upon the size of the families). The *identified patients* of each individual family system are included in the group. The families may be confronting similar problems (*e.g.,* substance abuse, anorexia, or psychiatric illness) exhibited in the identified patient.

Other variations in family group therapy are the *married couples' or significant others' groups.* These groups include the spouse or live-in mate of the identified patient. The goals are similar to those of multiple family group therapy, namely, to increase the couples' insights into their interactional and communication problems, to provide a training ground for experimenting with change, and to achieve change through mutual support from people who have had similar experiences.

Therapeutic Groups

There is a second major type of group work with which nurses should be acquainted, because they are frequently asked to be group leaders. For the purposes of this discussion this type of group will be referred to as *"therapeutic groups for nonpsychiatric clients."*

Formerly, group processes and methods were largely confined to the treatment of psychiatric clients. However, the use of group work with the nonpsychiatric population is now widespread. Group methods are currently used with a large number of client populations to promote mental health and prevent mental illness due to psychophysiological stress.

Group psychotherapeutic techniques are used to support physically ill or recovering clients, the aged, youth with psychosocial developmental stress, and even socially-displaced members of the community. Although the distinction between therapeutic groups and group therapy may seem to be arbitrary, some important differences exist.

Therapeutic groups and group therapy may be differentiated by (1) how big a role emotional stress has played in the individual's current level of health (or illness), and (2) the primary objective of the group experience. In group psychotherapy, the members' complex emotional problems are of primary concern; the central objective is the treatment of the emotional disturbance manifested in members' thoughts, feelings, and actions. In therapeutic groups, longstanding and complex emotional problems are secondary to physical illness, normal growth and developmental crisis, or social maladjustment. In this case, the primary objective of the group experience is not treatment of extensive emotional problems but prevention, education, and treatment of focused emotional problems occurring in the client's recent history.

Therapeutic groups, unlike psychotherapy groups per se, have developed from the efforts of a variety of disciplines, including social work, psychology, and nursing, as well as psychiatry. Pratt first introduced therapeutic groups in 1905 when he organized tuberculosis patients together in small groups for a therapeutic purpose. Therapeutic groups in medical hospital settings were used in the 1940s in the training and practice of psychiatric social workers. After that, groups led by psychologists and social workers began to appear more frequently in general hospitals, in the community with families, in clinics and rehabilitation centers, and in detention homes for delinquent children. Much of this work was referred to as "group counseling."[13]

The use of therapeutic groups in nursing practice is the result of at least three important factors: (1) nurses' involvement with social workers in groups, (2) the growing attention of nurses to the psychosocial factors in illness, as well as in growth and development, and (3) the increased interest of mental health nursing in group work with a variety of nonpsychiatric client populations. The coexistence of social workers and nurses in health and welfare agencies has frequently led to collegial relationships.

These relationships have encouraged the use of nurses as co-leaders in groups led by social workers, and eventually the leadership of groups by nurses themselves. At the same time there has been an increasing interest and concern among nurses (in schools, in community health, and on medical–surgical wards) for the psychosocial ramifications of growth and development and of illness. Nurses have been particularly concerned when the illness originates from a psychological problem or when illness and hospitalization create secondary psychological stress. Paralleling this concern has been the interest of mental health nurses in nonpsychiatric clients. Currently nurses are exploring the various uses of therapeutic groups for a number of types of clients. For example, groups are being formed with patients on medical–surgical units (such as kidney transplant, preoperative cardiac, stroke, cancer, or ulcer patients), with high school and primary school children requiring guidance and counseling, with the aged in nursing homes and convalescent hospitals, and with clients in the community, such as unwed mothers and delinquent youths.

Meetings held for clients with premenstrual syndrome (PMS) are an example of support groups run in outpatient medical settings. Levitt[10] and others reported on groups held during visits to a hospital-based PMS program. Many women are hesitant to talk about PMS symptoms and feelings with friends. They fear that others will consider them mentally ill. In the PMS group, women experience peer support, increased self-esteem, and a decreased sense of aloneness or uniqueness because of their illness.

The focus of therapeutic groups differs from that of psychotherapy groups. Therapeutic groups work with "normal," or basically healthy, individuals. The individuals may, however, be undergoing some form of situational or normal growth and development crisis. Situational crises may result from illness, disease, accidents, or any combination of these. Growth and development crises arise from inadequate or borderline adaptation to the requirements of a current psychosocial stage of development. With either type of crisis, certain emotional reactions occur that may be painful and distressing to the individual. Generally, if the individual is supported and counseled during the crisis period, there should not be a progression to severe emotional disorder.

Because this process deals with preserving mental health rather than treating mental illness, it is appropriate to describe it as an educative and preventive measure rather than as a treatment measure. Therapeutic groups are concerned with preventing further psychological deterioration and with educating individuals so that normal adjustment to situational and developmental crises will occur.

Therapeutic groups are used with a variety of general hospital clients, including some who are physically disabled, infectious, preoperative, or postoperative, and those for whom hospitalization is a regulative measure. Group work with the chronically physically ill (stroke patients, aphasiacs, the blind, multiple sclerosis victims, epileptics, and diabetics) is described in the literature. Group work with preoperative clients—for elective abdominal surgery, for example—has been found successful in uncovering concerns and instructing clients. Group work with tuberculosis clients has been a long-time use of therapeutic groups with people who have medical problems.

Leaders of therapeutic groups with medical–surgical clients have held two different perspectives about the purpose of these groups. Some leaders focus on modifying disruptive behavior of these clients on the unit; others focus on alleviating stress due to hospitalization and illness. The former approach strives to modify what is assumed to be preexisting psychological illness exacerbated by the presence of physical illness or disability. The latter approach does not attempt to correct preexisting psychological illness, nor does it assume that there is a preexisting illness inherent in the patient's current adaptation. This approach characteristically strives for a change in perception and a decrease in disabling anxiety and frustration. It is also expected that the members' potentials and capacities for effective coping and interaction with those around them will improve. This approach may also incorporate family members in the group along with clients, primarily because family members are often involved in clients' concerns, indirectly and directly, and often affect clients' ability to cope.

Although these two approaches vary, they share a number of common features. Both approaches emphasize the need to help clients work through present stress situations rather than the need for long-term analysis of clients' psychological problems. Both approaches recognize the difficulty that staff on units have in coping with emotional problems of patients, and seek to alleviate disruptive behavior either directly, using the former approach, or indirectly, using the latter. Both approaches stress a renewed or increased capacity to cope effectively with a change in role or altered lifestyle. The difference in these approaches lies in how each would implement these objectives for clients. The former approach modifies the client's behavior; the latter approach alleviates anxiety and frustration that accompany illness and hospitalization.

Group work with the aged in nursing homes and convalescent hospitals is another example of therapeutic group work with nonpsychiatric clients. The most important goal of these groups has been remotivation, to stimulate interaction among the aged clients and to help group members renew their sense of independence. These groups address the problems of social disengagement that often accompany growing dependence on others, as well as the loss of significant others in the clients' lives. A predominant philosophy regarding the aging process is that social disengagement by the elderly can be normal and natural. It is not healthy for all, however. For some clients, it is a process that may lead to severe patterns of withdrawal, increased dependency, and severe depression. For depressed clients, social disengagement should be discouraged. Improved social relations among aged persons are felt to be quite helpful, regardless of the fact that a member's social disengagement is more normal than abnormal. Improved social relations are believed to give more meaning and satisfaction to the aged. Characteristically, the aged are faced with losses that may foster increased apprehension or resignation, or both. They may experience the loss of a spouse, close friends, memory and mental acuity, economic security, dignity, independence, familial surroundings, work, and feelings of usefulness.[4] In addition, they face changes in their body image and certain physical crises. Each of these experiences is traumatic; considered together, they are heavy burdens to bear at an age at which an individual's will or energy to confront problems directly has slackened.

The benefits to individuals in these groups are many and varied, from improving attitudes about themselves to facilitating communication and alleviating the effects of social isolation. Frequently, the health and welfare problems of members, as well as their feelings about loss of loved ones, are discussed in these groups. Burnside,[4] in weekly group meetings with regressed, long-hospitalized convalescent clients, devised various ways of decreasing the sensory impoverishment of members. Group discussion stimulates members' thinking processes and widens their viewpoints. Shere,[19] who worked with a group of mentally fit elderly people of ages 85 and over, noted the following benefits: (1) increased self-respect, (2) diminished feelings of loneliness and depression, (3) reactivated desires for social exchange, (4) reawakening of intellectual pursuits, and (5) development of capabilities for resuming community life.

Therapeutic groups with individuals facing developmental crises (e.g., learning problems experienced by school-aged children or the mid-life crisis faced by adults) are other examples of the use of therapeutic groups with nonpsychiatric clients. Understanding the crises, an awareness of the available choices, and the consequences of one response or another are frequently the foci of these groups. The assumption underlying this approach is that through group discussion members will be guided to choose more mature actions that will, in turn, be socially acceptable to others.

In summary, a number of group therapy formats are available to nurses. In choosing the type of group appropriate for clients, it is important to know the alternatives that exist and the potential benefits of each group format. Table 11-1 presents a list of the various types of group work, with aims and suitable clients listed for each type.

The baccalaureate-prepared psychiatric/mental health nurse can function effectively as a group leader in problem-solving groups, support groups, inpatient milieu-setting groups, special problem groups (such as substance abuse groups), multiple family and married couples' groups that focus on a special problem (such as coping with a dying family member), and therapeutic groups. The following discussion addresses the various theoretical notions underlying nurses' intervention in groups.

Theoretical Frameworks in Group Work

While many psychiatric theories have guided group leaders' decisions to use one or more interventions, the fol-

TABLE 11-1.
TYPOLOGY OF GROUP WORK

TYPES OF FORMATS	MAJOR AIMS	TYPES OF CLIENTS
GROUP PSYCHOTHERAPY Inpatient and outpatient groups Therapeutic milieu Special problems groups Multiple family and couples' groups	1. Personality reconstruction 2. Insight without reconstruction 3. Problem-solving 4. Remotivation and reeducation 5. Support	Psychiatric clients and/or their families
THERAPEUTIC GROUP WORK Groups with clients who suffer acute or chronic physiological disturbances Groups with the aged Groups with developmental or situational crises	1. Problem-solving 2. Education 3. Support	Nonpsychiatric clients and/or their families

lowing frameworks are useful in helping beginning practitioners to intervene in small group therapy or therapeutic groups. The frameworks to be considered here are interpersonal, communication, and group process theories.

From a general systems theory viewpoint, groups are organizational structures with different subparts or subsystems. The members are one subsystem; the leader is another. The nurse's interventions affect the members and, hopefully, influence them toward more adaptive functioning of each member in the subsystem.

The significance of the interpersonal framework, according to Sullivan,[21] is that the leaders have direct impact on the members, as well as the members having impact on one another. The following brief summary shows how group interaction, when viewed as an interpersonal process, affects the members.

The Interpersonal Framework

The Origin of Emotional Behavior in Interpersonal Interactions

Sullivan believed that all behavior (thoughts, feelings, and actions) is attributed to interpersonal interaction, not innate drives or instincts within individuals. Sullivan focused heavily on the mother–child relationship, but also on the patterns of interaction throughout the individual's development. For example, sequential interactions in a group can be viewed as a cause-and-effect process, a result of the immediate social and interpersonal context. In this case, the feelings and behaviors of one member could be analyzed as a direct result of the behavior of one or more group members and/or the group leaders.

The Basic Need for Interpersonal Security

Sullivan believed that each individual has an inherent need for interpersonal security, and that the basic deter-

rent to security is anxiety. Anxiety is viewed as the chief disruptive force in interpersonal relationships.

In group interactions, anxiety may appear at varying levels. Anxiety arises from an individual's insecurity in relating to others, and can be allayed if there is a basis of trust. In a group, the nurse should secure trust, reduce anxiety, and build interpersonal security. This role is discussed in the next section devoted to nursing interventions in group work.

Correcting Distortions About Others With Feedback

Another interpersonal concept that directly influences group members' behavior is feedback from others. Feedback corrects the distortions people have about their current interactions. Sullivan believed that individuals have a capacity to *inattend selectively* (or to be inattentive to what promotes anxiety) and to distort certain aspects of their interactions with others. They may think that other people don't like them or are displeased with them when others do not have those feelings. The ability of individuals to seek validation from one another is important in treating mental illness and promoting health. In groups, nurses use various sources of feedback (members and the leaders themselves) to correct distortions that develop, and teach that validation is a necessary step in formulating conclusions about oneself and others.

The following example shows how feedback can be used to clarify distortions. The group took place in a day treatment program, and met three times a week. One member, Mr. Lee, made the following statements at various times during the group:

"I lost my job a month ago, but it doesn't bother me."
"Did I tell you about the last job I had? It involved. . . ."
"My boss laid me off, but it doesn't matter."
"On my last job I got to run the big machine all by my-self."

Group members pointed out, with the nurse's assistance, that Mr. Lee did indeed seem to care about losing his job, but that he had difficulty sharing his feelings. At first Mr. Lee denied this feedback, but with continued supportive feedback he began to clarify the distortion of his dismissal and feelings toward his boss and the loss of his job.

The Communication Framework

It is important for nurses to understand communication when working with groups. A great deal of the communication that takes place in groups is nonverbal—facial expressions, body position in relationship to others, gestures, and behavior *do* communicate. While individuals communicate verbally in groups, nonverbal communications are *as important* as verbal exchanges, and should be a focus of the nurse group leader. Frequently the nurses' role is to acknowledge messages (even nonverbal ones) and to validate their meaning.

Along these lines, communicating occurs on multiple levels. Watzlawick[22] indicated that there is both a *manifest content,* or apparent level, in messages, and another part of the transmitted message that reveals how the sender perceives the relationship with others, usually a more *latent* or covert aspect of the message.

An example of a group with manifest and latent content is seen in a group led by a nurse on an inpatient psychiatric unit in which clients were learning to identify and express feelings. One group member, Max, superficially described his feelings about being hospitalized. When the nurse encouraged other group members to describe their feelings, Max sighed, looked irritated, stood up, and went to the opposite end of the room. These behaviors demonstrated Max's manifest, or observable, message.

The nurse hypothesized that Max's latent content included his present irritation with the nurse, a reaction to the nurse's attempt to assist Max out of his resistive stance. The nurse understood this latent content as a statement of how Max viewed his relationship with the nurse: he was irritated with her. In this example, the nurse stated, "Max, I noticed that you moved away from me when I asked other group members to describe their feelings. What were you feeling toward me at the time?" With group support, Max defined how he didn't want to talk because he had nothing in common with anyone in the group and looked on the nurse as a "jailor." The group members praised Max's strength for attending the group and honestly describing his thoughts. Eventually Max became more comfortable in the group.

The *exchange model* of communication is another important communication model used to examine group behavior.[7] In this model, group members learn about themselves from others. In the interchanges among group members, one individual may acquire another's words and may live in another person's world. Real change occurs in individuals when there is a very personal and intimate exchange of people with each other.

Homans, Thibaut, Kelly, and Leavy all emphasize the social exchange nature of interactions among people.[7]

The Group Process Framework

Closely related to the idea of manifest and latent content is the phenomenon of *group process.* Yalom[23] refers to group process as *what is really going on* in the group, but about which no one is talking. In practice, the word "process" is used in a variety of ways, including:

1. What is really going on in the group, but not talked about
2. The running commentary used to describe the various verbal and nonverbal events in the group. Clinicians use this meaning to describe what went on in a group.
3. The cause of events that took place in the group

In Yalom's definition, the process is important because it is the present-moment reality and an example of how group members live their lives. When examples of distortions and problematic behavior are displayed, as in the case of a client who says he is not angry while shouting profanity at another person, they become the content for group discussion.

In working with the process of a group, nurses can state what is observed in a group member's behavior and ask what the behavior means. This must be done with tact and respect, because random or casual requests for clients to interpret their behavior can be threatening and alienating.

In group interactions, members frequently give and receive confusing messages or communications. Because clear communication is an important social skill, and nurses are interested in fostering it, they will frequently interpret messages that are sent and received, and teach members about the subtleties of communicating.

The Interpretation of Messages

In addition to the complexities of communication, the nurse will also teach the group that messages are not always sent the way they are intended. Messages connote and denote different things to different people. The specific culture, ethnic group, sex, and age of group members can affect the interpretation of messages.

In a group situation in which several members are sending and receiving multiple messages, at various levels, both covert and overt, it is possible for misunderstandings and distortions to occur. It is important for members to understand that in the group, as in society, the messages they send may not be same as the messages that are received. Members frequently learn the complexity of communication by becoming aware of the incongruency of others' perceptions of the messages they send. In the group setting, social skills and knowledge are enhanced by the nurse's awareness of these basic principles.

In a client group in a home for older adults, for example, the nurse found that it was frequently necessary to ask clients to repeat or clarify what they had said in order to increase the frequency of clear communication. These clarifications took time from the group, but were interventions that enabled each group member to understand exactly what was being said in the group.

Groups in Flux

Groups can be viewed as a gathering of individuals who interact in response to tensions felt in the group. The occurrences within a group are members' attempts to reduce the tensions in the group. Although these tensions are believed to arise from the interactions of members, they must also be modified by the group in order for the group to remain intact. Nurses should be aware that the content, decisions, and interaction in the group are a factor of the group's experience of, and need to reduce, tension. They need to know what these tensions are, and how they manifest themselves in individuals' behavior. The group's need to get direction, advice, and information from the nurse, for example, may be a reaction to their fears of being independent and taking more responsibility for directing the group themselves.

In an example from a four-bed inpatient psychiatric intensive care unit, the nurse working on the unit admitted a new client. The three other clients became restless and more verbal. Two clients began to make demands for such things as extra snacks and extended T.V. time. The nurse viewed this behavior as a result of tensions arising from a change. The change was the addition of a new client to a group in which the members had become accustomed to one another. The nurse responded to demands from the clients by restating the limits established on the unit in a tactful, but firm, tone. She introduced the new client, and then guided the other three clients to an activity room, accompanied by another staff member, to decide on a group activity. The nurse then completed the admission of the client.

Group Phases

Because groups are in a constant state of fluctuation, it is necessary to understand the various stages and phases that groups can be expected to experience. Several group process theorists have attempted to isolate the exact stages through which groups pass. The theory by Bennis and Shepard[1] about phases of group development is considered one of the classic theories.

Bennis and Shepard, in describing phases of group development, identify dependence and interdependence as the major issues of internal uncertainty that are common to, and important in, all groups. *Dependence* refers to the group's handling and distribution of power; *interdependence* is the members' feelings about closeness with others in the group. Bennis and Shepard describe the group as it moves from phase I, dependence, through phase II, interdependence.

In another analysis of group phases and stages of development, Schutz[17] related phases of group develop-

ment to the establishment and maintenance of relations among members in reference to certain interpersonal needs, such as intimacy and control. He explained that to function effectively the group must find a comfortable balance of (1) the amount of contact members have with each other, (2) control and influence, and (3) personal closeness. He conceptualized three issues of group development, usually assumed by the group in the following sequence: *inclusion, control,* and *affection.* In the initial sessions, Schutz maintained, members need to feel included and to include others. Fulfillment of these needs usually constitutes the beginning activity of the group. Members also need to influence others, and to be influenced, if the group is to make decisions. Without this influence, no decision-making system can be effective. During the working phase of the group, members must be preoccupied with the issue of who will control or direct the group, and to what extent others will share in the control. Finally, members need to express and receive affection. Not only is it necessary for individuals to relate to each other with sufficient warmth and closeness for group processes to proceed, but at certain points expression of warmth and affection is appropriate. At termination, for example, members are usually evaluating the growth of the group and are occupied with warmth and close feelings toward the group as a whole and toward certain members in particular.

The quality of group movement, or the degree to which group process becomes either functional or nonfunctional, is another important consideration for the nurse. For example, according to Schutz's theory, if the group achieves a viable level of closeness and a process of control over its members so that effective interaction occurs, the group is *adaptive* or *functional.* If, on the other hand, the group has not met members' needs for inclusion, is too controlling, and does not permit a level of interpersonal intimacy, a *maladaptive* or *dysfunctional* state exists.

The nurse must assess how adaptive the group is. If the group is dysfunctional, the nurse must assess the degree and causes of the dysfunction. Providing for members' needs for inclusion, control, and affection—for the expression and reception of these interpersonal processes—is one way the nurse can intervene to move the group toward a more functional state.

Other theorists have proposed frameworks for psychiatric group work practice that emphasize using group conditions to change individuals. One such theory is that proposed by Sarri and Galinsky,[15] who focus on the regularities and consistencies of group development that can be ascertained. They emphasize that this theory is based on a number of assumptions, including: (1) the group can be used as an efficient vehicle for individual change, (2) the group is not an end in itself—the purpose is not to create an enduring system but to maximize the potential of the group for individual change, (3) group development can be directed and controlled by the clinician's actions, and (4) there is no one, optimal way in which groups develop.

According to these authors, group development can

be divided into seven discreet stages, based upon the events that characterize these stages. The *origin phase* refers to the events leading to the composition of the group. Occurrences in this phase influence later group development. For example, the initial orientation of members to the group has a significant impact on later social organization. Major variables believed to affect further group development are the size of the group, members' characteristics, initial orientation, and environmental location of the group. Phase two is the *formative phase,* and is characterized by the initial activity of group members in seeking similarity and mutuality of interests. Initial commitments to group purpose, emerging interpersonal ties, and a quasi-structure can be observed at this phase. *Intermediate phase I* is the third phase in the group's development. It is characterized by a moderate level of group involvement and group cohesion, clarification of purposes, and involvement of members in goal-directed activities. The fourth phase, called the *revision phase,* is characterized by a challenge by group members to the existing group structure, and is accompanied by modification of group purposes and operating procedures. *Intermediate phase II* is the fifth step in group activity. It is characterized by a higher level of integration and stability than that in intermediate phase I. The sixth phase is called the *maturation phase,* and is characterized by stabilization of group structure, purposes, and operating and governing procedures, expansion of the culture of the group, and the existence of effective responses to internal and external stresses. The last, or seventh, phase is referred to as the *termination phase.* Dissolution of the group can occur for a variety of reasons: goal attainment is complete, maladaptation has occurred, there is lack of integration, or a predetermined time to terminate the group arrives.

Other, less linear, concepts of group development are proposed by systems theorists. Sampson and Marthas,[14] Durkin,[5] and others use systems theory to explain group development.

The living systems concept, applied to group dynamics, proposes that a group is composed of interrelated elements that function together and engage in an exchange relationship with its environment, *e.g.,* the agency in which the group is housed. To understand the group in relation to any dimension at any one time, we must first understand its location and function within an equilibrium-maintaining system. One of the major properties of all systems, and all groups, is their tendency to seek some point of balance or equilibrium. Systems restore homeostasis whenever events disturb the organizing state of balance.

In summary, various theories assist nurses to analyze group behavior and the behavior of individuals in a group setting. These theories help practitioners understand aspects of group functioning and group intervention.

The last section of this chapter describes the role of the nurse in group development. The discussion is based on a framework of common nursing leadership functions and interventions in a group therapy or therapeutic group setting.

Leadership Functions and Interventions

The idea of group leadership functions is not new. Many of the basic group psychotherapy texts suggest various functions of the leader or group therapist. Yalom,[23] Sampson and Marthas,[14] and Marram[12] have all detailed the functions of group leaders. In addition, Schurman[16] enumerated five functions that are especially appropriate for the nurse group therapist. These functions include (1) orienting individuals to the group, (2) helping members clarify their thoughts and feelings, (3) redirecting questions so that they are answered by members, (4) helping all members to participate, and (5) acting as a resource person.

Leadership is a basic requirement for an effective group experience. It fosters constructive norms and values, based upon functional interpersonal relationships. It contributes to the attainment of group goals, and hence the viability of the group for its members and leaders.

The three basic functions that assist the nurse to intervene appropriately and effectively include: (1) facilitating the natural benefits of group membership (such as increased understanding of interpersonal behavior), (2) maintaining a viable group atmosphere so that these benefits can occur, and (3) supervising group growth by using interventions that are specific to the stage or phase of group development at the present time.

Certain natural benefits have been ascribed to interpersonal relationships. Broadly speaking, these are need satisfaction and security. In the context of groups, this also means a sense of belonging and feelings of companionship.

Yalom[23] explained that group therapy sets in motion a set of curative features that are not possible in other forms of therapy. These include:

1. *Acceptance*—by group members
2. *Universalization* or *universality*—realizing the common quality of one's problem(s)
3. *Reality-testing*—the opportunity to check out old distortions about how others feel and think about the individual
4. *Altruism*—the opportunity to care and share with others in the group
5. *Ventilation* or *expression*—of problems and fears
6. *Interpersonal interaction*—with other group members and leader(s)
7. *Information-gathering*—imparting and receiving information
8. *Group cohesiveness*—a feeling of belonging and unity

The group leader, by establishing and maintaining a group, facilitates the members' abilities to benefit from group interaction.

Nurses must realize the benefits of group membership and encourage clients to join and participate. Positive attitudes on the nurses' part will help clients overcome their initial resistances and fears, as is shown in the following relevant research.

RELEVANT RESEARCH

This study was based on the idea that self-disclosure is an important variable in group psychotherapy with chronic schizophrenic clients. Eighteen open- and closed-ward male clients from a large psychiatric hospital participated in the group psychotherapy program. The clients were assigned to one of three therapy groups. It was believed that the more clients perceived therapists to be facilitative, the greater would be the clients' degree of self-disclosure. Based on comparisons of mean scores among the groups, the findings suggested that clients who viewed the therapist as more approachable made significantly more self-revelations than those who viewed the therapist as less approachable. The study reinforced previous evidence that greater perceived therapist interpersonal facilitativeness yields higher self-revelation in members.

(Strassberg D, Roback H, Anchor K, et al: Self-Disclosure in Group Therapy with Schizophrenics. In Roback H, Abramowitz S, Strassberg D (eds): Group Psychotherapy Research: Commentaries and Selected Readings. New York, Krieger, 1979)

Nurses can safeguard the achievement of benefits to clients throughout the life of the group. Viability of the group rises when the members understand that they are free to talk about their concerns, free to experiment with new behaviors in the group, and safe in remaining in the group. Nurses can best assist clients by demonstrating unconditional, positive regard for all members, by supporting clients, and by encouraging members to validate their perceptions of other members.

As a group leader, the nurse is responsible for supervising the growth of the group. In this capacity, the nurse assists the group in identifying its goals, rising above its tensions, and evaluating its progress toward meeting its goals.

The essential functions of the nurse as a group leader suggest a number of interventions. Specific interventions will be addressed here in light of various stages or phases of the therapeutic group experience. Several specific interventions are listed in Table 11-2.

Group Phases and Stages[12]

Stage 1: Psychosocial Environments Conducive to Self-Expression

In the beginning stages or phases of group work, deciding on the direction of the group (its goals and its purposes) is most important. Without objectives and purposes, group functions are arbitrary and confused.

Contracting with members for change is an important step in conveying to the membership that the group has control over, and responsibility for, the change it will make in its individual participants. *Contracting* is the process through which the leader formulates an agreement regarding the focus of the group and the expected outcomes. Before members can fully commit themselves to the group, they must understand the purpose of the group, how the purpose will be achieved, what they can expect from the leader and the other members, and what is expected of them as individuals.

The nurse should recognize that finalizing the objectives of the group may encourage self-disclosure by some members but does not ensure interaction. It promotes members' sharing of thoughts and feelings, but the nurse's skill in creating interpersonal safety is needed on an ongoing basis.

Jourard[8] stressed that self-disclosure leads to knowledge of self, and is an important goal of the therapeutic process. Self-disclosure is enhanced by the attitudes of acceptance, understanding, and positive regard communicated by the nurse.

These attitudes must be delivered in a framework of appropriate *norm-setting*. Norms that foster group safety and support are negotiated early in the group. The nurse might state, "It is important that everyone participate" and "Members can respect the statements of others by not interrupting." These conditions become the groundrules for member interaction, and assist the group in reaching a situation in which it is safe to disclose and get help with problems in the group.

Stage 2: Responsibility for Change

Once members have a basic sense of trust and confidence in the group and in the group's leader(s), real work on problems can begin. Usually, four to eight sessions into the life of the group (if the membership has been rather constant), the nurse will note that members have a clearer notion about how they can be helped by the group and how they might help others. Members will have a better understanding about what behaviors are appropriate and will begin to give feedback to one another about their behavior.

This stage marks the beginning of members' ability to face specific problems and to take responsibility for making changes. Members will, for example, accept the idea that they have trouble communicating clearly or have difficulty handling their anger appropriately, and

TABLE 11-2.
INTERVIEWING SKILLS

LEADER(S)' INTERVIEWING TECHNIQUE	GROUP MEMBER RESPONSE	OUTCOME
1. *Giving information:* "My purpose in offering this group experience is. . . ."	Further validates assumptions: "How is this going to happen?"	Leader(s) and members enter into a dialogue in which members get more information to make decisions and build trust in group experience.
2. *Seeking clarification:* "Did you say you were upset with John because he said that?"	May try to restate thoughts or feelings: "Yes, I guess I was upset."	Members become aware when they are not clear, and learn to identify thoughts and feelings more precisely, at the same time taking responsibility for them.
3. *Encouraging description and exploring* (delving further into communication or experiences): "How did you feel when Joann said that to you?"	Elaborates on the message: "I didn't like it very much."	Members deal in greater depth with an experience in the group—again, taking responsibility for their reactions. (This example also places events in time or sequence, lending further perspective to group events.)
4. *Presenting reality:* "Would other group members think Joann was unstable if they interviewed her for a job? You don't appear shaky to me."	Listens and considers other possibilities	Members compare perceptions of self with other's perceptions of them.
5. *Seeking consensual validation* (seeking mutual understanding of what is being communicated): "Did I understand you to say that you feel better now than you did last week?"	Offers further clarification: "Well, yes, I'm better than last week but not as good as I'd like to be."	Group and leader(s) learn how members view their progress, while improving their own self-evaluation skills.
6. *Focusing* (identifying a single topic for discussion: "Maybe we could identify one problem you have and talk more about that."	Channels thinking: members may think of the most puzzling problem they have.	Group and leader(s) identify specific topics they can resolve before the meeting ends. They increase their understanding of one problem before jumping to others.
7. *Encouraging comparison* (asking members to compare and contrast their experiences with others in the group): "How did the rest of the group handle this problem"?	Group members share their experiences as they relate to the topic.	Leader(s) and members gain greater insight into their commonalities and differences, and learn from one another alternate ways of responding to problems.
8. *Making observations:* "You look more comfortable now, John, than you did at the beginning of the meeting." *or* "The group has been silent for the last five minutes."	Group members have something to respond to: "I feel more at ease now." *or* "I think we are quiet because we are bored."	Group members and leader(s) place attention on significant events and can elaborate on their meaning.
9. *Giving recognition or acknowledging:* "John, you are new to the group."	Feels acknowledged and included: "Yes, I'm John, and I came here because. . . ."	Members view specific instances as important, and leader(s) reinforce the behavior or event they choose to notice; in this case, the desire to come to group.
10. *Accepting* (not necessarily agreeing with the communication, but receiving it with openness): "Yes, I hear you say that you don't know if you want to be in the group or not."	Feels heard and understood without fear of attack	Members learn that even *unacceptable* attitudes can be talked about, and perhaps any thought is not so horrible that they cannot share it.
11. *Encouraging evaluation* (asking the group as a whole, or individual members, to judge their experience): "When Marilyn gives you support, do you feel better?" *or* "How did we do in helping Joann with her problem"?	Members reflect on progress made: "Not exactly, because I don't know if I can trust her to be honest." *or* "It was hard. I'd like to know from her."	The criteria for success become clearer to members, and new directions may be formulated as a result of the discussion.
12. Summarizing (condensing, in a few sentences, what has occurred): "The group discussed several issues and problems today; they were: . . ."	Members recall significant points and close off consideration of new or extraneous topics.	Members and leader(s) place events in perspective, identifying salient points of a group session. Such a summary can lead to a better understanding of group process.

(Marram G: The Group Approach in Nursing Practice. St Louis, CV Mosby, 1978)

will begin to ask the group for help. They may try out new behaviors within and outside of the group, and ask others to give their opinions about the changes. At this stage, members can usually accept feedback because they have a certain basis of trust in the group: the group knows them and will not respond in a harmful manner.

At this stage, too, members are better able to clarify distortions about their relationships with other people. Members realize that they must validate their perceptions of other people, their families, spouses, and parents, the staff, and/or their bosses at work.

However, the nurse should not be surprised when the apparent ease of the group in discussing and resolving members' problems is periodically mixed with resistance. Not all growth in groups is free of pain. Sometimes feedback from others is difficult to accept, no matter how true it may be. Also, changing old patterns of response in interactions with others is difficult, and takes time. When members begin to be impatient with one another and hostile confrontation ensues, they may be resisting awareness of their own Selves.

According to Johari's Window (in Luft)[11] there are four aspects of the self, of with which we may or may not be aware. These quadrants are: (1) the part of the self of which we are aware and of which others are equally aware, (2) the self that we are aware of and of which others are not, (3) the self of which we are not aware, and others are aware, and (4) the self that neither we nor others are aware of. These aspects of the self are depicted in Figure 11-1.

In the first phase of the group, the members deal with material that is nonthreatening, *e.g.,* material that the clients can acknowledge about themselves in front of themselves and others. During the middle phase of the group, there is a greater probability that members may be confronted with what they were not aware of, but is discernible by the group. Through feedback from others, members gain knowledge and information about themselves.

It is likely that the group will be more lenient in judging members than the members are of themselves. In some cases, members may acknowledge that they have the same problem, the same fear, or the same undesirable habit as another member. This process supports members who may be sharing important self-revelations for the first time.

Therapeutic problem-solving can best be achieved in the working phase of the group. There is a tendency for relevant material to arise in the group, and the group is able to offer support. Real and fantasized problems that

Awareness of Actions, Feeling, and Motivations

Client is aware, others are not aware	Client is aware, others are aware
Others are aware, client is not aware	Others are not aware, client is not aware

(Luft J: Group Processes: An Introduction to Group Dynamics. Palo Alto, California, National Press Books, 1963.)

Figure 11-1. Johari's window.

concern clients may be identified. The need for change may be realized from others' feedback. Alternatives can be discussed. The group has a commitment to bettering the experience of its members.

When a group member attempts a change, success is assigned to the individual but felt by the group. The group may feel as much pride as the individual who has achieved the change. Likewise, the group's ability to help one member has individual meaning for each and every member. Being part of the group that helped someone get better reinforces the members' sense of self-worth and dignity.

The leader serves an important function in group success by reinforcing individuals' attempts to change. Inviting a group member to attempt a change inside the group, encouraging the group to report on the change they see, and showing interest in how the change has worked outside the group will reinforce members' sense of responsibility and control over their lives.

Stage 3: The Perspective on Self and Others Through Change

From the perspective of the group leader, the task of the third stage of the group is to bring a termination to the group. In assisting this process, the nurse focuses on the impact the group has had on each member, and helps the group confront the experience of loss due to termination of the group.

Like termination of a significant one-to-one relationship, the ending of group relationships can arouse feelings of anxiety and loss that lead to temporary episodes of regression to old, problematic behaviors in some members. The leader should provide sufficient opportunity for members to express their feelings and gain perspective about their separation from the group, the leader, and individual members. The leader is obliged to bring up the subject of group termination at least two to three sessions in advance of the last session, depending on how long the group has met, how frequently the group met, and how intense the group experience has been. Nurses may stimulate self-disclosure of feelings about termination through various means, including communicating their own feelings about the group's terminating and what the group has meant to them.

Termination is a time to assess the group's progress and to evaluate the experience. When group work is one modality in a sequence of subsequent treatment programs, the nurse should help the members evaluate the progress they have made in the group and the problems needing attention in other aspects of the program, or in the future.

The leader must be aware that, because separation and loss generate painful feelings in many members, the group, individuals within the group, and the leader may resist dealing with the termination issue. The group may cope by avoiding discussions about termination, denying that they have feelings, and denying the importance of the group and leader to them. The leader may feel anx-

RELEVANT RESEARCH

The authors, both children of Holocaust survivors, discussed their reactions and experiences in leading nine short-term awareness groups designed for other children of Holocaust survivors. They evaluated their role as leaders, and examined countertransference, personal motivation, and the establishment of goals in the group. Many of the conclusions resembled the leaders' experiences in other professional support groups with individuals who had undergone a trauma or had had to cope with a common social predicament. The authors cautioned about leaders' tendencies to "rescue" members. The group members had undergone painful experiences that had to be relived in order to work through them. This involved the leaders' eliciting details of the atrocities that needed to be confronted if members, and the group as a whole, were to grow.

The authors noted that they had had to strive to:

1. Not become overly sympathetic about the depression and losses of the parents of group members, as described by the group members. If the group leaders became too sympathetic, they attempted to have group members understand the experiences of *their* parents rather than to help clients to deal with their own sources of pain. Fogelman and Savran reported that work on *clients' feelings* is especially important because of the tendency of survivors' children to be overprotective and to feel guilty about their parents, who have suffered so much. If the members' feelings are not the focus, the guilt feelings will block members' ability to express their deep reactions as children of Holocaust survivors.

2. Become comfortable with hearing about the horror of the Holocaust. If the leaders are not comfortable, they are unlikely to do meaningful work with children of survivors.

3. Become familiar with the Jewish experience prior to, during, and following the Holocaust. By studying these experiences, the clinicians can better understand the clients. Hence there is no dictate against working with clients of a different sociocultural group, but the clinicians should learn about the history of the particular group, how members respond in a group situation, beliefs about mental health, and so on.

The authors described how *group work in particular* benefited these clients by:

1. Assisting members to achieve a sense of identity. Many felt alienated from others because of their cultural uniqueness.

2. Assisting members to learn about the details of their cultural group in an atmosphere of acceptance. (Many children of Holocaust survivors are not informed about the Holocaust because the parents fear that they will scar their children's lives with awareness of such horror.)

3. Assisting members to learn from others how to deal with their feelings toward their parents (such as anger felt toward parents— a reaction normal for all children).

(Fogelman E, Savran B: Brief group therapy with offspring of Holocaust survivors: Leaders' reactions. Am J Orthopsychiatry 50:96, 1980)

ious about discussing separation, may feel pangs of guilt (if the group did not accomplish all of its goals), or may disengage emotionally from the group. Individual members may act out their resistance by regressing, terminating their attendance prematurely, changing the subject inside the group, or insisting that the group continue. A group that has had many positive emotional experiences may collaborate to continue group meetings past the designated termination date, although without the group leader.

Sociocultural Variables in Group Work

A number of particular situations occur in group work as a result of the sociocultural backgrounds of group members, the leader, or both. Some of these situations include:

1. If the leader is from a different sociocultural group than are some or all of the group members, will group members from the same sociocultural group

as the leader attempt to form a clique with the leader, to the exclusion of other group members?

2. If one group member is the only representative from a particular sociocultural group, will this group member be isolated from the rest of the group?

3. If group members and the leader share a particular sociocultural origin, will the group generally be as effective as a group in which members and/or leader are from mixed sociocultural backgrounds?

Fogelman and Savran[6] describe a case study of the last culture-related group phenomenon listed above. The authors are children of Nazi Holocaust survivors, and have described their experiences in leading nine different awareness groups designed for children of Holocaust survivors. Hence, in these groups the leader and members shared a cultural heritage.

Summary

1. Different group approaches exist that can be selected for use according to member characteristics and leadership style preferences.

2. A number of theoretical frameworks describe group functioning. The models include a focus on interpersonal interaction, the group's communication patterns, and the group process.

3. Leadership functions serve to promote the group's attainment of group goals while facilitating members' productive work in the group.

4. Cultural differences among group members (and the leader) must be taken into account to provide a group atmosphere in which group members can feel accepted and free to express themselves.

5. Nurses function as group leaders and co-leaders in a variety of groups at each level of prevention.

6. Group leadership techniques, such as seeking clarification and promoting member comparison of experiences, foster group development.

References

1. Bennis W, Shepard H: A theory of group development. Hum Rel 9:415, 1956
2. Birckhead L: Techniques for group psychotherapy on inpatient units. Issues Ment Health Nurs 6:127, 1984
3. Birckhead L: The nurse as leader: Group psychotherapy with psychotic patients. J Psychosoc Nurs 22:24, 1984
4. Burnside I: Working With the Elderly: Group Process and Techniques. Boston, Jones & Bartlett, 1984
5. Durkin J (ed): Living Groups: Group Psychotherapy and General Systems Theory. New York, Brunner/Mazel, 1981
6. Fogelman E, Savran B: Brief group therapy with offspring of Holocaust survivors. Am J Orthopsychiatry 50:96, 1980
7. Greenberg R: The Nurturance Phenomenon: Roots of Group Psychotherapy. Norwalk, Connecticut, Appleton-Lange, 1986
8. Jourard S: Healthy Personality. New York, Macmillan, 1974
9. Kalkman M, Davis A: New Dimensions in Mental Health/Psychiatric Nursing. New York, McGraw-Hill, 1980
10. Levitt D, Freeman E, Sondheimer S et al: Group support in the treatment of PMS. J Psychiatr Nurs 26:23, 1986
11. Luft J: Group Processes—An Introduction to Group Dynamics. Palo Alto, California, National Press Books, 1963
12. Marram G: The Group Approach in Nursing Practice. St Louis, CV Mosby, 1978
13. Marram-Van Servellen G: Group and Family Therapy. St Louis, CV Mosby, 1984
14. Sampson E, Marthas M: Group Process for the Health Professions. New York, John Wiley & Sons, 1977
15. Sarri R, Galinsky M: A Conceptual Framework for Group Development. In Glasser B, Sarri R, Vinter R: Individual Change Through Small Groups. New York, Free Press, 1974
16. Schurman M: Five functions of the group therapist. Am J Nurs 64:108, 1964
17. Schutz W: The Ego, FIRO Theory, and The Leader as Completer. New York, Holt, Rinehart & Winston, 1968
18. Shaffer J, Galinsky D: Historical Introduction and Overview. In Shaffer and Galinsky (eds): Models of Group Therapy and Sensitivity Training. Englewood Cliffs, New Jersey, Prentice-Hall, 1974
19. Shere E: Group Work with the Very Old. In Kastenbaum R (ed): New Thoughts on Old Age. New York, Springer, 1964
20. Spotnitz H: The Couch and the Circle. New York, Knopf, 1961
21. Sullivan H: The Interpersonal Theory of Psychiatry, New York, WN Norton, 1953
22. Watzlawick P: An Anthology of Human Communication. Palo Alto, California, Science and Behavior Books, 1963
23. Yalom I: The Theory and Practice of Group Psychotherapy. New York, Basic Books, 1975

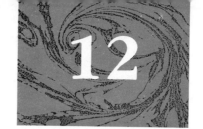

12

JILL IONE LOMAX AND GWEN MARRAM VAN SERVELLEN

FAMILY THERAPY

Learning Objectives

Upon completion of this chapter the student should be able to do the following:

1. Describe the characteristics of functional and dysfunctional family systems.
2. Make basic assessments of family dynamics.
3. Describe different types of family therapy.
4. Identify the three phases of family therapy.
5. Identify appropriate goals of family therapy.
6. Plan appropriate interventions for basic problems in family systems.
7. Identify families at risk for family violence.
8. Appreciate the basis of family resistance to therapy.
9. Identify his or her impact, real or potential, on the family system.

Introduction

Most, if not all, clients are part of an active family system. For clients who have frequent contact with family members, hospitalization disrupts their normal routine for better or worse. How family relationships will be maintained during hospitalization, or altered as a result, is a concern for staff as well as clients and their families. If nurses are to understand clients holistically and be effective members of the treatment team, they must appreciate the importance of family dynamics and the interactions between the family system and the hospital system.

Although student roles in hospital settings are restricted, students become an inescapable and important part of the milieu, including that part in which the family and hospital systems interact. This chapter focuses primarily on those family dynamics and therapeutic interventions that students are likely to observe or be a part of in medical–surgical as well as psychiatric hospital settings. The importance of the interplay among nurse, client, and family will be addressed.

Family therapy is a branch of psychotherapy that applies knowledge about family process to the diagnosis and treatment of the psychopathology of the individual family member as well as of the family as a unit. There are several theories of family therapy that guide assessment, diagnosis, goal selection, and the choice of interventions. These theories overlap and are continuing to evolve. This chapter presents an eclectic theoretical approach appropriate to the basic student. More advanced students are referred to the chapter references for an in-depth study of specialized approaches.

The Historical Development of Family Therapy

Some historians believe that the roots of family therapy can be traced back to the early work of Freud. In 1909 Freud resolved the phobia of a five-year-old boy by treating the boy's father.[10] Nevertheless, Freud did not pursue this approach but continued to see patients apart from their families. Although he regarded early family life as the background for current symptomatic behavior, he believed it confused the therapeutic process to include the family in therapy sessions.

In the early 1940s the therapeutic focus continued to be psychoanalytic in nature and very narrow in scope. A few therapists, however, began to see the benefits of including family members in their treatment of individuals. The child guidance movement, which began in the 1940s, influenced therapists to involve the family. Usually, however, the child was seen by a psychiatrist, and the rest of the family was seen by a social worker. The benefits of working with the child and family together were generally unrecognized.

Prior to World War II most psychotherapists were bound by their theoretical orientation to the practice of one-to-one therapy. After the war the sudden reuniting of families brought a number of interpersonal, social, and cultural problems, and the public turned to mental health professionals for solutions. Therapists found themselves working with problems involving divorce, marital discord, emotional breakdowns in family members, delinquency in children, and many other circumstances affecting the family as a whole. Although the traditional, psychoanalytic framework was inadequate to help with these problems, a large number of professionals continued to confine their treatment to the family member with the emotional symptoms and ignore the dysfunction within the family unit.

According to Goldenberg and Goldenberg,[12] 15 behavioral sciences and professional disciplines directed their attention to analyzing the family. In the late 1940s and early 1950s five scientific and clinical developments merged to form what is now referred to as "the family movement" in mental health.[12] These developments included:

1. The extension of psychoanalytic treatment for a wide range of emotional problems, including work with whole families
2. The introduction of systems theory, with its emphasis on exploring relationships among parts that make up an interrelated whole
3. The investigation of the family's role in the development of schizophrenia in one of its members
4. The development of the fields of child guidance and marital counseling
5. The increased interest in group therapy and milieu therapy as alternatives to individual therapy

In the early 1950s more therapists began to experiment with family therapy, but they rarely talked or wrote about it. Those who saw families, somewhat clandestinely, feared the rejection of their peers. Attempts were made to avoid alienating the psychiatric establishment, which viewed families as irrelevant in the treatment of psychopathology. Consequently, much of this early work went unrecognized.

By the late 1950s family therapy was practiced more frequently and more openly. More and more clinicians and researchers were publishing their views and findings. Today there are multiple theoretical approaches to the treatment of families. Among these are structural family therapy (Minuchin and Montalvo), strategic approaches (Bateson, Erickson, Haley, Jackson, Weakland), and communication therapy (Satir).

Family therapy is thought by some to be a form of group therapy in which the nuclear family is the unit of analysis. However, the majority of family therapists view the family as a behavioral system with unique properties. Emotional disturbances of individual members are regarded as the consequences of conflicts among family members. For example, the behavior of a seven-year-old boy wetting his pants in public may be a demonstration of family conflict, and would be resolved by focusing on the family as a unit rather than only on the young boy. In traditional family therapy the entire family is treated as a unit. The goal is to resolve or reduce significantly the pathological conflicts and anxieties within the unit.

The Family Approach to Therapy With Individuals

A growing body of research demonstrates that families can play crucial roles in the etiology of family members' problems and in their treatment and recovery as well.*

* References 4, 11, 13–15, 18, 26, 30

RELEVANT RESEARCH

The authors point out that a body of recent research has demonstrated a strong relationship between mental illness and marital disharmony and dissatisfaction. They studied the marital relationships between two groups of couples to determine whether the number and kind of marital problems differed between groups. One set of couples had a spouse with a physical illness, and the other set had a spouse with a chronic psychiatric condition.

Twelve depressed patients and their spouses attending an outpatient psychiatric department were compared with 12 patients with rheumatoid arthritis and their spouses and 12 cardiac patients and their spouses. The results of the study suggested that depression had a much greater impact on marital life (from both the patients' and the spouses' viewpoints) than did rheumatoid arthritis or cardiac illness—two common chronic physical illnesses. Depressed patients and their spouses ranked highest in marital dissatisfaction, followed by arthritic patients and spouses, and then followed by cardiac patients and their spouses. Depressed patients and their spouses had the most marital and sexual problems, and they were the most dissatisfied with their work and social activities. The authors concluded that depression may have a greater impact on marital life than does chronic physical illness.

(Vanger N, Bridges P: Marital problems in chronically depressed and physically ill patients and their spouses. Compr Psychiatry 27:127, 1986)

Specifically, the involvement of family members in the treatment process may significantly improve the client's prognosis, shorten hospitalization, decrease the recidivism rate, and increase or maintain health. In addition, the individual's problems often create or exacerbate problems for other family members. By the time of hospitalization, the entire family may be stressed and frustrated and in need of therapeutic attention.

In the past, whole families occasionally were hospitalized for the treatment of psychiatric problems.[1] Today, however, it is only the most impaired member of the family, or the person identified as such, who is hospitalized. Treatment approaches may be based on *monadic* (biological or intrapsychic) models or *dyadic* (interpersonal/systems) models. The behavior and intrapsychic life of the individual can be changed by both approaches. Although the monadic approach may be the more practical in cases in which family participation is impossible, the behavioral and intrapsychic changes that occur in the individual as a result of altering the family's transactional patterns are thought to be more quickly achieved and longer-lasting.

Families can play a crucial role in clients' adherence to medical treatment. Some people are easily persuaded by their families to adhere to or reject prescribed medication and dietary programs and other medical recommendations. Nurses can help to improve a client's prognosis by assessing family relationships and including the appropriate family members in treatment planning. For example, if a client is instructed to take medication after discharge, it may be as important to teach the family about the medication as it is to teach the client. Families who have misconceptions or apprehensions about medications may be reassured and become less apt to sabotage the individual's health care. If a client is required to follow a special diet, it is particularly important to educate and enlist the support of those who shop for groceries and prepare the meals.

Well-functioning families may benefit from therapeutic family intervention during times of crisis. Crisis periods may result from normal life events such as pregnancy, birth, children leaving home, retirement, illness, and death. In these cases the goal of therapy is to preserve the family's strengths rather than to correct any particular dysfunction. Interventions are designed to help people understand and tolerate their reactions to change, and the problems presented by that change, and to provide sources of support for all members. Some or all members may need guidance in identifying options, weighing pros and cons, and selecting an acceptable response to change. An example is the family members of the client with Alzheimer's disease who are grieving and confused about what they can and should do for their loved one. These individuals need assistance in coping with an uncertain situation.

A Multidisciplinary Approach to Family Therapy

The formal and disciplined practice of family therapy has been developing since the 1950s. Pioneers with diverse educational backgrounds have made significant contributions. Currently, social workers, psychologists, psychiatrists, nurses, and clergy provide therapy to families. Mental health clinicians come from educational programs that place varying degrees of emphasis on theoretical and experiential training in family therapy. The mental health system is in the process of charting the specific training a family therapist should have to be most effective. State laws and institutional policies regarding the right to practice continue to vary. Concerns about territorial boundaries and power relationships, as well as concerns about proper educational preparation, influence who does and does not practice family therapy in any given setting.

Historically, social workers have been the most active in advocating and providing family therapy. Nurses, in spite of the frequency with which they interact with families, are least likely to act as family therapists. Recently, however, nurses with a master's or doctoral degree in psychiatric/mental health nursing are joining the ranks of autonomous family therapists. These advanced-practice nurses usually have certification in psychiatric/mental health nursing from their state licensing board or the American Nurses' Association. Nurses with less training may function as co-therapists along with psychiatric social workers, psychologists, or psychiatrists.

Family therapy can be conducted by one or two therapists. One of the therapists is often, but not necessarily, the client's primary therapist. Co-therapists usually complement each other by being of different sexes or coming from different disciplines. The co-therapy relationship is very special and needs care and attention as does any relationship. The co-therapists must establish a complementary working relationship in order to be effective. Time must be spent together before and after sessions to compare observations about the family, establish compatible goals and the means to reach those goals, and evaluate the work that is done. Overall, they must maintain productive lines of communication and foster the optimal atmosphere for cohesive therapeutic interventions with family members.

Regardless of who is designated to do the formal therapy, many different staff members interact with the family. These interactions may be brief or extensive. They may take place during formal meetings or during informal contact when the family phones or visits in search of information and progress reports. If these interactions are random, uncoordinated, disorganized, and lacking in clear goals (which is too often the case), the client, family, and staff can all suffer. An individualized plan for working with each family needs to be developed so that clear goals are established, and there is a clear understanding of who does what to achieve those goals. Coordinated plans can be implemented if staff members work together cooperatively rather than independently or competitively.

The Role of Supervision in Family Therapy

Family therapists need to learn more than just information about functional and dysfunctional family process and techniques for interventions. They also need to learn about themselves and their roles in the therapeutic process. This learning can best be accomplished with frequent and long-term supervision by experts.

Particular attention is given to the relationship that is established between the family and the nurse. When the family and the nurse form a therapeutic alliance, a new system is created—the therapeutic system. The nurse's professional values and knowledge influence the formation of this alliance. The nurse's personal dynamics also affect, and are affected by, the family. In addition, nurses' experience in their own families of origin and current families injects an unavoidable subjectivity into their work. This subjectivity may help or hinder the formation of a therapeutic alliance and the ability of the newly-formed system to establish and achieve appropriate goals. The ideal relationship involves empathy toward each family member. On occasion, however, the therapist may side with one member for personal reasons. In these instances therapeutic goals are exchanged for personal ones. For these reasons, supervision is invaluable.

Inevitably therapists make mistakes. These mistakes are more easily corrected when supervision is available. Experienced family therapist Braulio Montalvo believes that "any family can absorb and orient the therapist and direct him away from his function as a change agent; that any therapist can be caught behaving with the family in ways that will reinforce the very patterns that brought them to therapy."[22] Supervision can be a vital source of advice and guidance for the therapist and, subsequently, provide opportunities to learn and grow.

Supervision can be done live (*e.g.,* when the supervisor is present in the room or behind a two-way mirror), from audio/video tapes, or from self-reports. Supervision can occur on a one-to-one basis or in a group setting. There are proponents for the benefits of each supervisory format, and nurses might benefit most by experiencing each one. A common form of supervision for beginning students occurs in a co-therapy relationship with a senior clinician. In this way the beginner observes first-hand how and when to intervene by watching the senior therapist. Analysis of the dynamics of the interactions with the family occur spontaneously in pre- and postsession meetings between the co-therapists.

A Broad Definition of Family

Although it might appear that everyone knows what a family is, attempts to reach a consensus on a definition have yet to succeed. Conceptions about the appropriate membership in and functions of the family and the roles of its members are changing as our society changes. For example, legal battles currently are being fought about the acceptability of marriage between homosexuals and the adoption of children by single heterosexual and homosexual men and women.

A liberal definition of family is: any group of people who have formed an enduring interconnected network of relationships. Such a definition does not require that the people involved live together or have legal or genetic ties. A more specific definition identifies the family as the basic social group to which people belong. This primary system of socialization exerts the greatest influence on both the development and the continuation of a person's behavior. As such, the family provides the essential function for society of transmitting cultural values and traditions through the generations. In this definition, too, biological and legal connections, while common, are neither sufficient nor necessary determinants of family membership.

United States society consists of many different cultures and lifestyles that contribute to the formation of various types of families. Generally speaking, the *nuclear family* consists of a married man and woman and their offspring. The *step-family* contains one or more children who are related biologically to one parent but not to the other. The *extended family* includes members from three generations or aunts, uncles, cousins, or other relatives. In addition, there are *single-parent families. Adoptive families, family-care homes,* and *foster families* care for children who are not able to be with their biological parents. Other arrangements exist as well, such as grandparents raising grandchildren, children raised by orphanage personnel, and so forth. All adults come from a *family of origin,* which may be any of the aforementioned families. Also, there are married or cohabiting couples (heterosexual or homosexual) without children.

It is important to know who the client does and does not consider to be a family member. Assessment can begin with the simple question: "Who is in your family?" It is significant to note who is not mentioned as well as who is mentioned. If the people omitted live with the client or are closely related genetically or legally, then an understanding of their exclusion is important. The clinician's personal identification of a client's family is relevant to the extent that it disagrees with the client's definition. Problems arise when staff seek to exclude from consideration people whom clients include in their family system and vice versa. The prudent and sensitive nurse respectfully accepts the client's identification of family members.

Deciding who should be involved in family therapy sessions can be difficult. It may be important, but not practical, to include a family member who plays a valuable role in the developmental life of the family but lives in a distant town. Patients may want to include people who refuse to participate or may not wish to involve others who seek involvement. The therapist's decision on whom to invite or exclude is a major therapeutic intervention in itself. Family therapy sessions have included lovers, friends, landlords, and care-takers in addition to parents, siblings, spouses, and children.

The Family as a System

According to systems theory, a system consists of parts that have two things in common: (1) the parts are interconnected and interdependent, and (2) each part is related to the other in a stable manner over time.[28] The individual human organism is a system, the family unit is a system, but people riding on a public bus are not. If a system has a continuous flow of elements or information entering and leaving, then it is an *open system.* If there is no such flow, it is a *closed system.*[28]

Families are open systems in transformation. They go through natural developmental stages and phases of change brought on by the processes of birth, childhood, adolescence, leaving one's family of origin, coupling, beginning the process of family development over again with one's own children, later adult life, decline, and death. Each stage requires structural modifications in the family's membership and organization. How the family deals with these life changes offers clues about the strengths and weaknesses of the family system.

Families also consist of special functional *subsystems.* These include the marital subsystem (parents), the sibling subsystem (children), and the individual parent–child subsystem. Developmental tasks accompany the formation of each subsystem.

In order to form the foundation of a developing family, the two individuals forming a couple must separate from their families of origin and any previous couple system. Old relationships change and new ones develop with the friends and family of the new partner. Another task for the couple is to develop a mutually satisfying lifestyle together. Many decisions must be made, such as how money will be earned and spent, who will shop, how they will share a bedroom, who will do the housework, and so forth. A major decision, in fact, is how the couple will go about making decisions.

Before or after the problems of coupling have been successfully solved, the two-person system may become a three-person system. The process of child-bearing and child-rearing brings new stress to the system. New subsystems emerge (mother–child, father–child, perhaps grandparent–child), and changes occur in existing relationships. If and when a second child is born, the sibling subsystem emerges; once again, reorganization of roles and relationships takes place. Who takes care of the baby, who washes dishes, how will money be spent now? What disciplinary measures are taken, and by whom? Who gets whose attention, and when, and how?

As members of the sibling subsystem and parent–child subsystem, children begin to prepare for the variety of relationships they will encounter for the rest of their lives. As children enter and leave adolescence, the process of change and adaptation continues.

The Functional Family

Repeated exposure to dysfunctional families sometimes leads clinicians to have a jaundiced view of all families and to lose sight of the existing strengths and adaptive features of family systems and individual personalities. Life is a problematic process filled with normal developmental stresses. A functional family is not free of stress, but it is able to cope without compromising healthy functioning for any significant length of time.

All families go through developmental stages, although not all families go through the same stages in the same order. The healthy family system proceeds relatively smoothly through its developmental stages. It is able to complete the appropriate tasks in each stage and modify roles, rules, and patterns of interaction as it adjusts to the demands of each succeeding stage.

Table 12-1 lists the ideal characteristics of a healthy family. Although few families can be expected to exhibit all of these traits, a healthy family strives to behave in the following ways, and in many instances it succeeds.

Clinicians base their practice on the following assumptions about families and their functioning:

TABLE 12-1.
IDEAL CHARACTERISTICS OF A HEALTHY FAMILY

1. Parents are each well-differentiated, having developed a sense of self before separating from their families of origin
2. Clear separation of generational boundaries within the family. The children should be free of the role of saving a parent or the parental marriage
3. Realistic perceptions and expectations by parents of each other and of their children
4. Loyalty to the family of procreation is greater than that to the family of origin
5. Spouses put themselves and each other before anyone else, including the children; the marriage, however, is not a symbiotic one that excludes the children. The children ought not to feel that to be close to one parent means they are alienating the other
6. Encouragement of identity development and autonomy for all family members. Successful development in the children will mean that they will leave home at some point to start families of their own
7. Nonpossessive warmth and affection expressed between parents, between parents and children, and among the siblings
8. The capacity to have open, honest, and clear communication and to deal with issues with each other
9. A realistic, adult-to-adult, caring relationship between each parent and his/her parents and siblings
10. An open family in the sense of involvement with others outside the family, including extended family and friends. Outsiders are allowed inside the family.

(Reprinted with permission from Framo JL: The Integration of Marital Therapy With Sessions With Family of Origin. In Gurman AS, Kniskern DP (eds): Handbook of Family Therapy, p 139. New York, Brunner/Mazel, 1981)

1. The family is the basic social group to which members of society belong.
2. The family is the primary socializing agent for individuals, and it exerts the greatest influence on both the development and the continuation of a person's behavior.
3. The family serves the essential function for society of transmitting cultural values and traditions through the generations.
4. The family system evolves through developmental stages.
5. Family members proceed through developmental stages within the family.
6. Current family membership changes due to events such as birth, death, divorce, and separation.
7. Families have internal strengths and resources.
8. Family systems are changeable.
9. Changes in the dynamics of the family system lead to changes in all members.
10. Changes in the psychodynamics of individuals within the family affect all other family members.
11. Family therapy facilitates changes in the family system.
12. Family therapists must be skilled at assessment, goal formation, interventions, and evaluation in order to facilitate healthy changes in the family system.

The Dysfunctional Family

It is possible to identify a dysfunctional family system by contrasting it with the well-functioning family. Sedgwick[25] points out that the mental health of a family is, in part, interchangeable with family "effectiveness"; that is, a family is deemed healthy if it successfully executes activities to meet family and individual needs and, at the same time, satisfies societal expectations. Sedgwick identifies the role of the family as follows:

1. To gather information
2. To make and implement decisions
3. To resolve conflict and provide for individual growth and development
4. To create an emotional context fostering self-disclosure, trust, cooperation, and acceptance
5. To engage in productive and adaptive activities with regard to internal needs and external societal expectations[25]

These activities may be viewed as essential for effective family function and, thus, as criteria for the health of the family. However, one must remember that even these roles, although apparently universal criteria, are not without bias.

Although authors differ in the specificity of their ideas of family mental health, most believe that it is the outcome of many factors interacting together. It is the result of the interactions among family members, between the family unit and the larger social system, and between sociocultural subsystems and individual family members. It is important, therefore, to judge the health of a family in the context of this multifaceted framework.

The DSM-III-R identifies three categories in which family dysfunction is treated distinctly from the problems of individuals. These categories are diagnostic of system problems, that is, problems in the interactions of members of the family system. They are:

V61.10 Marital Problem
V61.20 Parent–Child Problem
V61.80 Other Specified Family Circumstances[3]

Some agencies use these categories. Others prefer to diagnose problems in terms of the individual's pathology and focus only secondarily on how the individual's problems affect, and are affected by, the family system.

Nursing diagnoses are being developed and will be more widely used within the profession in the next decade. The following list from the Seventh National Conference of the North American Nursing Diagnosis Association (NANDA) contains those diagnoses that apply to the family as a whole:

3.2.2 Family processes, altered
5.1.2.1.1 Coping, ineffective family: Disabled
5.1.2.1.2 Coping, ineffective family: Compromised
5.1.2.2 Coping, family: Potential for growth[20]

In addition, the following diagnoses can be used to identify relationship difficulties within the family:

3.2.1.1.1 Parenting, altered: Actual
3.2.1.1.2 Parenting, altered: Potential
9.2.3 Violence, potential for: Self-directed or directed at others[20]

The taxonomy of nursing diagnoses by the American Nurses' Association includes the following diagnoses that can be used in family assessment:

21.02 Aggression/violence toward others
   21.02.01 Abuse—physical
   21.02.02 Abuse—sexual
   21.02.03 Abuse—verbal
   21.02.04 Assaultive
   21.02.05 Homicidal
   21.02.06 Temper tantrums
23.01 Impaired family role
   23.01.01 Dependence deficit
   23.01.02 Dependence excess
   23.01.03 Enmeshment
   23.01.04 Role loss/disengagement
   23.01.05 Role reversal[2]

A wealth of literature focuses on the family and its dysfunctional process. The following discussion is a summary of the specific theories regarding family pathology.

Inside a family group basic interpersonal needs are expressed, negotiated, and met. When needs are not fulfilled, the family is stressed; stress in turn can result in dysfunction, but dysfunction also breeds stress. In this way the process of stress and dysfunction is circular, and it is often the role of the nurse to break the chain of events by dealing with stress and dysfunction simultaneously.

The concept of family dysfunction is addressed by Bowen.[6] Bowen does not apply a medical model to families, but perceives families as functional and dysfunctional. Families may channel their struggles through individual family members. These family members, in turn, are identified in "sick" roles, but it is incorrect to apply a diagnostic label to the individual. Most family therapists,

as previously noted, do not view symptoms as the exclusive possession of an individual identified patient but, instead, believe they are caused by the dysfunction of the family as a whole.

Jackson and Satir[17] and Haley[16] share with Bowen a nonmedical-model view of family and individual pathology. They address dysfunction in terms of communication. Although Satir[24] attributes the symptom of dysfunctional communication to the individual within the family, she believes that the dysfunctional communicator resides in an environment that provokes or maintains the dysfunction.

If the presence of communication dysfunction in individuals is examined, it is possible to clarify the nature of the total family's dysfunction. For Satir, the dysfunctional communicator has unfulfilled needs for self-esteem and self-worth within the family unit; this problem is symptomatic of a dysfunctional family. A functional family is one in which individual attainment and preservation of self-esteem take place.

An alternate view of family group pathology is the structural theory presented by Minuchin.[21] Unlike Satir, Minuchin focuses on dysfunction from a broader perspective by looking not only at the members' communications but also at the inherent structure of the family system. Minuchin is a systems theorist, and he views the internal working of the family in relation to systems and subsystems. This larger view of the family and its pathology centers around the following conceptual framework.

According to Minuchin, a family must master various developmental tasks from origination to expansion to dissolution. These tasks require modification of the family structure, which is accomplished through boundary negotiation and modification. If boundaries are so rigid that they do not allow negotiation, dysfunction will result. *Boundaries* are the specific rules of a subsystem that determine expectations about who is to participate and how. Minuchin identifies three basic characteristics of boundaries. They may be *enmeshed,* in which case boundaries are diffuse, making relationships too close. They may be *disengaged,* in which case they are too rigid, and, therefore, relationships are too distant. Or they may be *clear,* in which case rules are negotiable, and members' needs for individual growth and supportive affiliation are met. For Minuchin, the presence of enmeshed or disengaged relationships is not in itself symptomatic of family dysfunction. He explains that the degree and persistence of these characteristics are the clues to dysfunction.

Minuchin's concept of boundaries is illustrated in the typical case of a couple who have a child. The nature of the mother–child relationship for the first several months is naturally enmeshed; at the same time, the husband–wife relationship may become disengaged. These occurrences in the family subsystems are expected in Western culture. However, if these conditions continue into early childhood, the family probably would exhibit a great deal of stress, discernible in the behavior of family members as well as in the quality of interpersonal communication.

How well the family copes with stress determines its level of function or dysfunction at any moment (Fig. 12-1). One type of stress identified by Minuchin is *transitional stress,* which occurs during the addition and loss of family members. Marriage, the birth of a child, the death of a spouse, and so forth, all call for basic structural changes within the family. Another type of stress on the family is what Minuchin refers to as *idiosyncratic problems.* These problems are unique to each family, and require adjustment and adaptation. They can include, for example, the presence of genetic disease in a child.

Stressful contact between the family and forces outside the family is a third source of stress. An example is the difficult blending of the family's cultural practices and values with those of the neighborhood and the larger society. One final stress identified by Minuchin is the stressful contact of one member with forces outside the family. One member's deviation from societal expectations, for example, affects the family as a whole. A parent's arrest for driving while intoxicated causes family stress and may require special changes in the behavior of the various subsystems in the family.

Principles of Family Functioning

Family Homeostasis

Systems theory guides our understanding of family dynamics as well as our understanding of the family as an entity. Applying this theory, the family is seen as a unit of interdependent parts and processes. Each family member's behavior influences and is influenced by the behavior of every other member. A circular causality exists, and it is difficult, if not impossible, to determine just which behavior occurs first.

Stresses and strains affect all living systems, and like any living organism a family attempts to achieve and maintain a state of equilibrium or *homeostasis.* The family

system is delicately balanced, and it struggles to maintain that balance as it undergoes change. The family must balance opposing forces if it is to maintain its integrity. For example, a son may desire to choose autonomously a profession that conflicts with his parents' expectations for him and their desire to influence him. How this conflict is resolved will be critical to the ability of the family to prevent estrangement and remain functionally intact.

The family's homeostasis is threatened when one member deviates from behavioral norms established by the system. Seeking to maintain homeostasis, the family may deny the deviation, rationalize its existence, pressure the individual to conform, or assume the individual's normal responsibilities by shifting roles and power relationships. For example, the family may ignore a member's sudden nonsensical communication. An older sibling may assume the care of a younger sibling when their mother becomes disabled. After a man who usually makes major family decisions becomes ill, his wife may assume his responsibilities.

Once the system achieves a new equilibrium of interrelationships, the renewed health of the individual may be just as disrupting and difficult to accommodate as was the initial illness. If the aforementioned husband becomes well and tries to resume his leadership role in the family, he may find his wife unwilling to resume a subordinate role and his children reluctant to consult him as they had previously.

Intact families are not necessarily healthy families. It is important to note that equilibrium for some families may protect pathology as well as health. Sometimes the pathology of an individual serves a homeostatic function for the family. It is not unusual in such cases for a second family member to become ill when the first becomes healthy. It is important, therefore, to look for how the client's pathology might fit into the family system as a whole. The following Clinical Example serves as an example.

When this so-called homeostatic mechanism is not flexible, the improved health of any one individual family member may be short-lived as a result of the system's nat-

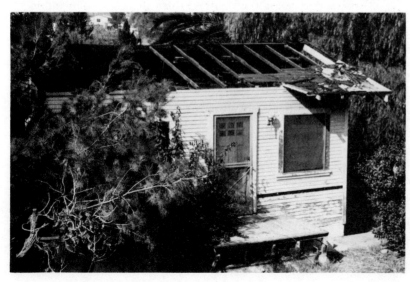

Figure 12-1. The damaged house symbolizes the problems many families have faced in attempting to cope with the stresses of living with others.

CLINICAL EXAMPLE

The Smith family knew that their son George was frequently truant from high school and performed poorly academically and socially when he did attend. Periodically the school authorities complained of George's smoking, petty theft, and vandalism in the form of graffiti; he was suspended from school for these actions. His parents were worried and fought with each other about how to handle their son, but they showed no inclination to seek professional help until he was arrested for setting a fire on campus. George finally received individual therapy at the age of 15; the parents refused family sessions. During his last two months in individual therapy, he remained in school and no longer set fires, stole, or seriously acted out in any way. Up to this time George's

17-year-old sister, Bess, had been the "model child," giving her parents and school officials no cause for concern. At the time of George's reformation, Bess exhibited truant behavior for the first time and was suspended for drinking on campus. Although George had changed, the family system with its need for one "good" child and one "bad" child remained intact.

If conjoint family therapy could have been done with all four members of this family, the goal would have been to adjust their system so that homeostasis was reset to accommodate and maintain health and a high level of functioning for all members.

ural attempt to regain its accustomed equilibrium. The well-functioning family is able to adjust its homeostatic set point and incorporate positive changes. The impaired family is not.

Family Rules

The family system, like any system, is governed by rules that help maintain homeostasis. Family *rules* are organized and repetitive behavioral patterns that are established and maintained by family members. Family rules direct members to behave in predictable ways. Rules govern the patterns of interaction, roles, and divisions of labor and power within the family. In other words, rules determine much of who does what, how, and when.

Some rules are overt and openly acknowledged and discussed, such as "Never raise your voice at the dinner table" or "Mom balances the checkbook, Dad mows the lawn, and brother and sister take turns doing the dishes." Other rules are covert, understood but not openly discussed, such as "Mother is much more likely than Dad to give permission to stay out late (so ask Mom)" or "Our son isn't serious about things and can always be counted on to be lighthearted."

When family rules are broken, temporary or long-term chaos and instability result, depending on the family's ability to correct the rule-breaker or its flexibility to accommodate change. In the examples about not raising voices at the dinner table and the son's expected lightheartedness, a family might know how to handle the son's momentary verbal tantrum during dinner, but they would be disoriented and paralyzed if he brandished a knife. Other families, of course, might have a high tolerance for verbal and physical fighting, including knife play. Their tolerance might be sustained by beliefs such as "All families fight," "You only hurt the ones you love," "No one is really going to get hurt," or other beliefs about each other that provide an acceptable place for this behavior within the system.

It is usually only when a person's behavior persistently and noticeably breaks a significant and rigid rule,

and with sufficient magnitude, that outside help is sought to restore order and stability. Some families might enter therapy because of their inability to tolerate normal expressions of anger by one member, while other families might wait until the family member has been repeatedly assaultive. Clinicians can help families identify and examine the rules of their systems so they can modify those rules that are excessively rigid or loose, unrealistic, or conflicting. Ideally, the rules operating in healthy families enable members to coordinate internal changes with external or contextual changes, and maintain healthy functioning for everyone.

Family Myths

Some family rules enter the realm of family myths. *Myths* are beliefs shared by all family members about each other that are not altered despite evidence of their falsehood. The reality distortions function as homeostatic mechanisms by dictating how members should behave in certain situations—for instance; "Mother will have a nervous breakdown if she hears bad news" (so never tell her what is really going on); "Father doesn't drink, and if he does it is not a problem" (so don't worry and don't talk about it); "Everyone in our family gets along; no one really gets angry" (so don't acknowledge being angry and don't show it).

These families do not know how to act intimately and to express their feelings openly with each other. Members act as if they do not trust each other's ability to handle stress, conflict, and disappointment. Their protective actions effectively reduce their level of intimacy with each other.

When someone challenges a family myth and behaves contradictorily to the myth's injunctions, the family becomes fearful that chaos may ensue. In order to prevent this fear and chaos, the family system exerts subtle pressure on insiders and outsiders to accept and support the myths. Clinicians, as well as family members, are subject to this pressure and may be just as susceptible to its power. When these attacks are subtle, even experienced therapists can be blinded and seduced into supporting the myths. Some families will punish clinicians for challenging their myths by attacking their professional credentials, intelligence, integrity, and even sanity. If therapists have the same myths operating in their families, they may be even more inclined to overlook certain truths. For example, clinicians who have never acknowledged and understood their own alcoholic or abusive family systems are likely to believe a family's denials about drinking or accept statements that the victim of battering "provoked the incident."

Family myths may be revealed when members make blanket statements about each other—for example: "Billy is just like his father—athletic and stupid," "Johnny is nothing but trouble," and "Mary never has any problems." These myths are dangerous because they restrict role flexibility, retard growth, and impair self-esteem. Myths prevent the full expression of family members' individuality and complexity. Thus, Billy may never fulfill his potential as a student, Johnny's strengths may be suppressed, and Mary's problems may be overlooked to the detriment of her health.

Myths such as "If it weren't for Johnny, we would be a happy family" support the family's identification of one of their members as the client, the one whom the clinician should "fix." Although a therapist may superficially accept this myth as a means of gaining entry into the family system, the skilled clinician will engage everyone in the process of change. The myth then gives way to the reality that indeed everyone is responsible for the healthy functioning of the family, and that the power for happiness or unhappiness does not lie with one person.

Another myth is that family members have an inherent knowledge about each other that is similar to ESP. Perceived boundaries between self and other are blurred such that one member simply "knows" what another is silently thinking or feeling, as if that person were oneself—for instance: "Johnny knows what is expected of him (without being told)," and "Mary knows I love her (without my saying so)." When miscommunication occurs, the message sender may believe the receiver simply is being perverse. Subsequently, the sender may become frustrated and angry.

To improve communication, a therapist asks family members to state clearly to each other what they think and feel. Resistance to this intervention is common, however. The notion that family members really might be strangers to one another threatens their sense of security and perceived intimacy. They frequently will deny their estrangement. Not only might the message sender insist that "Martha knows what I mean; I don't have to spell it out," but Martha may be just as eager to act as if she understands. She, too, does not want to believe that she does not understand. At this point the therapist can reassure the family, in a style acceptable to them, that miscommunication happens in the closest and most loving families, and that all families need to take the time to explain and reexplain a lot of things to each other if they are to remain close.

To complicate matters, of course, some family members really want and like their distance from each other.

Vague and incomplete messages are deliberate. The clinician's efforts to have them speak clearly and directly to one another will be resisted, lest their indecipherable messages be understood and unwanted intimacy occur. In this case, it would be important to understand the reasons underlying the lack of desire for intimacy.

Family Roles

A *role* is a complex set of behaviors derived from cultural influences, family rules, and personal proclivities. Roles are assigned by the family system and accepted by the individual. They can be broad or narrow in scope. Examples of roles are breadwinner, care-taker, peacemaker, decision-maker, disciplinarian, and so forth. Each family member can have several roles, both in and outside of the family. Conflict results when these multiple roles are not compatible with each other. Conflict also results when members do not agree on who assumes which role.

The common myth that one member of a family is responsible for the family's ills leads to the establishment of a set of roles that structures the *scapegoating* process. The dynamics of scapegoating involve three players—persecutor, victim, and rescuer. The persecutor is usually a parent, the victim is often a child, and the rescuer (the person who tries to protect the scapegoat from the persecutor) may be the other parent or another member of the family.

Sometimes the clinician, who enters into the family system, becomes caught up in the process and becomes the rescuer or another persecutor, or displaces the old victim and becomes the new scapegoat for the entire family. When the family members band together and blame the therapist for their problems, they may appear unified in a healthy way and elect to leave therapy at this point. However, this newly-found cooperation will be short-lived as long as the family needs a scapegoat. Once therapy is terminated, the unchanged system will require that one of their members again assume the role of scapegoat. The solution to their destructive process is to increase each individual's sense of responsibility for self and to create a jointly-owned sense of responsibility for family life.

Role relations should allow for changes in individuals and accommodate the developmental stages of the family. The parent–child complementary roles of the nurturer and the nurtured must evolve and change for the children to learn to care for themselves and achieve autonomy. The family system must adjust roles when the usually healthy breadwinner becomes disabled. Clinicians can assist families to clarify and agree on roles through the processes of communication and negotiation.

Cultural Influences on the Family

Just as a person's behavior can be better understood in the context of his or her family life, so can the family be

CLINICAL EXAMPLE

A mother brings her anorexic 17-year-old daughter to a psychiatric hospital. The mother is unpacking the daughter's suitcases and arranging her things in the room while the daughter wraps her arms around herself and watches from a corner. The following verbal exchange takes place after this nonverbal interaction.

Daughter (grumbling): "Oh, Mom, what are you doing?"
Mother (breezily): "I'm just unpacking your things. I don't think they have enough hangers here for you."

The mother and daughter are obviously sending messages to each other beyond the literal meaning of their behaviors. These messages exist even when neither participant is aware of delivering or receiving them. The mother's behavior could be saying, "I need to be needed by you.

If you do this and other things for yourself, then you might find that you don't need me, and I want to prevent that from happening." Or, perhaps she means, "I'm feeling guilty for your being here, and I'm trying to do something for you to make amends, and this is all I can think of to do."

The meaning of the daughter's behavior could be, "I want to do this for myself, and I don't know how to stop you from doing it for me," or "I'm really glad you're doing this for me, because if I start doing more things for myself I may become so independent that I lose you (or make mistakes and feel inadequate). But I'm embarrassed to admit this, so I'll pretend that I'm upset—but not so upset that you'll really stop." The exchange between the mother and daughter also could be demonstrating the possibility that it is the mother's wish, much more than the daughter's, that the daughter be hospitalized.

---

better understood by appreciating its social and cultural contexts. Cultural values affect the rules, roles, and myths in any family. In his introduction to *Ethnicity and Family Therapy* by McGoldrick, Pearce, and Giordano, Irving Levine observed that "ethnocultural factors are more powerfully played out in family relations than in any other arena."[19]

Routine assessments of families should include information about their ethnic background and country of origin, how long they have been in the United States, their fears and hopes about migration, and the language they speak most fluently. Of particular importance is the presence of family members in other countries, the level of contact with these members, whether or not they are expected to come to the United States, and so forth.

It is not reasonable to expect that a family will quickly or easily assimilate the set of values and manners of mainstream U.S.A. Families that migrate to the United States may feel the pressures of conflicting values.[27] For example, the Latino family that values interdependence may suffer initial adaptation difficulties as well as later intergenerational conflicts after their migration into a predominantly Anglo society that values independence.[5]

The cultural values of both the family and the therapist influence the relationship between them. Clinicians must be aware of the impact of their own cultural values on their assessments of the family's strengths and weaknesses. For example, interdependence in Latino families may appear to other Latinos to be normal, but it may appear to the nonLatino observer to be pathological fusion.[5] There is no need to eradicate cultural differences, but there is a need to acknowledge these differences and to learn strategies for coexistence.

Family Communication

A family's patterns of communication are indicative of its functioning. All behavior in a social context is communi-cation, whether the behavior is verbal or nonverbal, conscious or unconscious. As the saying goes, "One cannot not communicate." Nonverbal behavior, in the form of facial movements, body postures, gestures, silence, grooming, and choice of clothing, reveals as much about ourselves as the rate, rhythm, tone, inflection, timing, and word selection in our speech.

There are two aspects to any communication. The *denotative* aspect is the literal message or the content. The *metacommunicative* aspect is the meaning behind the literal message or, in other words, the message of the message. Metacommunication says a great deal about the relationship between sender and receiver. The denotative aspect is usually clear and obvious. The metacommunicative aspect can be hidden and quite difficult to understand.

One example involves the husband who, while reading the newspaper, remarks to his wife as she enters the room, "The baby is crying." The denotative information about their child is obvious, but it is only part of what the husband is communicating to his wife. The metacommunication is veiled and depends on the relationship between husband and wife and on the context in which the statement is made. Hence, the husband could be saying: "Stop what you are about to do and attend to the baby," or "I'm going to be irritable right now (because I usually am when the baby cries), so be forewarned," or "Don't say anything, because I'm listening to the baby to see if I should go to her," or something else entirely.

The above Clinical Example is another example of how metacommunication takes place and might be encountered by the nurse.

Cultures, groups, families, and individuals develop their own rules for coding information and for deciding what, when, and how that information should be communicated. A universal set of rules does not exist. Although family members attempt to impose the same set of rules on each other, mutual compliance does not necessarily develop. When it does not, misunderstanding and conflict can occur. Miscommunication and conflict also occur between patients and therapists. It is important for therapists to remember that not all behavior means the same thing to all people. Clinicians should not assume that they know what patients are "really" saying. Without validation from the sender, the receiver can validate only the message that was received, not the message that was intended.

Problems also result when restrictions are imposed on communication. Children whose parents literally insist that they be "seen and not heard" may resort to the use of destructive nonverbal communication to meet their need to communicate. When thwarted, the child's communication will be transformed but will not disappear.

Another communication problem develops when a person gives two conflicting messages. One example is a father who demands that his child not defy him, yet complains that the child does not act independently. Another example is a mother who stiffens when hugged, yet complains when her child does not approach her affectionately. The parents in these examples are conflicted about what they want, and, therefore, they put the children in a bind. A potential solution exists when open discussion is permitted, and the child can comment on the bind and ask, "Did you mean this or that? What do you really want me to do?"

However, if the parent denies the mixed messages and conditions the child not to question the dilemma, the child must accept the parent's conflicting messages in all their impossibility. This inability to comment on the bind is referred to as being "in a double bind." A *double bind*, therefore, is an interaction in which one person demands a response to a message containing mutually contradictory signals while the other person is unable either to comment on the incongruity or to escape from the situation.

Repeatedly being in a "damned-if-you-do and damned-if-you-don't" bind produces bewilderment, anger, and ultimately withdrawal. Being hopelessly caught in repeated double binds, however, could possibly lead to psychosis. Double-bind situations have been found to occur repeatedly in families of schizophrenics.[4]

We communicate information about ourselves both consciously and unconsciously. Likewise, information about others is received both consciously and unconsciously. It is a common experience to learn something consciously for the "first" time, and then realize that we knew it all along.

It is generally accepted that what we communicate unconsciously is truth, whereas the information we consciously communicate may or may not be the truth. However, even when we lie or withhold information, we are communicating something about ourselves. The boy who breaks a window and then says "I didn't do it" is sending the message, "I don't want to be punished," or perhaps, "I feel terrible about myself for doing this, and I don't want to feel this way." The boy's mother may or may not receive the hidden message. She may believe him, or she may know he is lying but misinterpret the message behind his lie.

People desire to understand and be understood. The most desired communication, however, is the sending and receiving of information that increases self-esteem. When this communication is thwarted, anxiety occurs. For instance, the boy who broke the window ultimately wants to feel good about himself. If telling the truth threatens his self-esteem more than telling a lie does, then he probably will lie. If he feels better lying, then he will be anxious when his lies are not believed. Whether or not a person wishes to communicate a truth or a falsehood, the goal of that communication is usually to help the person feel good.

Fears of rejection and criticism are likely to activate dysfunctional communication. The dysfunctional communicator, guided by threats to self-esteem, will do the following:

1. Overgeneralize
2. Send incongruent messages
3. Act as if a message was sent when, in fact, one was not
4. Send incomplete messages but act as if the messages were complete
5. Act as if he or she is not responsible for the message that is sent by using vague pronouns ("one believes" or "you feel" rather than "I think" or "I feel")

Conversely, the functional communicator is able to:

1. Differentiate objectivity (descriptions of a person, place, thing, or event) from subjectivity (thoughts and feelings about the person, thing, or event)
2. Speak directly to the person for whom the message is intended
3. Be relevant
4. Say what is meant and mean what is said
5. Deliver congruent messages (messages in which verbal and nonverbal behaviors communicate the same information)
6. Avoid being too vague or too specific. (The person who supplies endless details, qualifications, and explanations is as dysfunctional as the person who omits necessary pieces of information and whole connections.)
7. Hear what others say
8. Accept responsibility for one's own communication

Family therapy expert Virginia Satir views the psychological problems of individuals in terms of poor self-esteem and poor communication skills.[24] The individual's environment is believed to provoke, or at least sustain, the dysfunction. Responsibility for good communication belongs to all involved. High self-esteem and good communication skills enable family members to be more assertive and negotiate openly with each other for what they want. Low self-esteem and poor communication skills induce passivity or aggression.

Because high self-esteem and clear, honest, and direct communication are interconnected, nursing interventions are designed to develop both. Treating all family members with a positive regard and teaching and role-modeling functional communication are basic interventions for achieving these goals.

RELEVANT RESEARCH

This study was based on the premise that many families are most vulnerable when one of their members is about to be discharged from the psychiatric hospital. Major concerns for families are: (1) a lack of understanding of mental illness, (2) alienation from professionals, (3) coping with their emotional reactions, and (4) meeting their own needs. An exploratory descriptive research design was used to determine how a support group for families of psychiatric clients could help them deal with their concerns. Seven people volunteered for the study group that met six times. Individual unstructured interviews were held before and after each group session.

The themes of each group session were categorized as either man-

agement issues or emotional issues. Management issues were defined as problems for which families sought specific solutions. These included: (1) their relationship with the health care system, (2) their relationship with the client, and (3) their need to take care of themselves. Emotional issues included worry and frustration resulting from an unclear understanding of emotional illness, bitterness and confusion about the lack of help they had received, sadness related to pessimism about the client's future, and worry about the right way to respond.

The group sessions appeared to help the families improve their coping skills. The authors concluded that family group interventions can be a powerful and effective method for assisting families.

(Rose L, Finestone K, Bass J: Group support for the families of psychiatric patients. J Psychosoc Nurs Ment Health Serv 23(12):24, 1985)

In addition, the nurse can encourage families to clarify and take responsibility for their messages by pointing out vague, incomplete, and mixed messages. Helping family members reveal their hidden messages and decipher the messages of others, so that problems can be dealt with more easily, takes skill and sensitivity. These interventions should be designed to resolve conflict while maintaining self-esteem. This can be done by accentuating the positive aspects of the problematic messages and turning them to their best advantage. For example, a mother who needs to be needed and her daughter who needs to be independent can be helped to identify the things the mother can do for the daughter that do not interfere with the daughter's process of maturation. This approach praises the motivations of both mother and daughter and permits both to be "right" without either one having to lose or feel guilty. Interventions that induce guilt rarely help. Criticizing the mother for interfering with her daughter's development and chastising the daughter for not being mature may threaten their self-esteem and provoke their defensiveness. Defensiveness protects the status quo and prevents change.

Family Reactions to Hospitalization

A variety of reactions accompany the hospitalization of a family member.[26] They include any or all of the following: relief, fear, sadness, grief, anxiety, guilt, confusion, anger, and happiness. Family members can be happy to receive help, yet be apprehensive about what that help will entail. A typical comment heard by nursing staff is, "We're so pleased George is finally in the hospital getting help; how soon can he leave?" Another common mixed reaction is, "Martha is so much better! What do you mean she's being discharged Tuesday?"

Hospitalization may provide an immediate reduction

in family tension. If family members believe the client is the source of their problems, or if the client believes the cause of distress lies with the family, then hospitalization can be perceived as a welcomed vacation from one another. However, relief may quickly be followed by hurt and anger in the person being hospitalized and by guilt in the family back home.

Sometimes the problems at home have exhausted everyone to the extent that they are no longer helping themselves or one another. A family member's physiological impairment, depression, psychosis, or destructiveness toward self or others may be so severe that only a hospital can provide a safe and therapeutic environment. In these cases, hospitalization can reduce the family's sense of helplessness and assist the family to restore its equilibrium.

Hospitalization also can increase chaos in the family system. Although the presenting problems have disrupted normal routines, hospitalization can disrupt them even further. A single mother in the manic phase of a bipolar illness may be functioning poorly at home, but family life may be in complete disarray while she is away. Hospitalization can induce fears of abandonment in those left at home as well as in the one left in the hospital. Sometimes separation anxiety helps motivate people to try very hard to resolve the problems that separated them. When too intense, however, this anxiety can provoke premature discharge and flight from therapy. On the other hand, some families may try to use hospitalization as a way of avoiding their problems.

Families turn to outside help usually under duress and with mixed feelings about accepting that help. Up to the time of hospitalization the family may have denied or tolerated the problems. Denial does not necessarily disappear once a decision is made to seek help. Reassurance that nothing is wrong, or that whatever is wrong will be corrected quickly and painlessly, may be the type of help that is really sought. Many families expect the client to regain normal functioning immediately as a result of hospitalization. They may expect the client to take part in household chores, to work at a job, and to remember to do important things.

Psychiatric problems are not easily remedied. Compounding the problem is the stigma placed on people with psychiatric problems. Hospitalization, therefore, can bring a loss of self-esteem to the client or the whole family. Some families are affected by cultural beliefs that families should deal privately with their problems, no matter how severe. These families reluctantly turn to outside help, much to their embarrassment or shame, only when they have exhausted all available remedies. They do not share information easily with outsiders about their history, thoughts, and feelings. Subsequently, therapy becomes a painful process.

Family members frequently wonder, not always aloud, what their part is in the etiology and treatment of the client's problems. An inability to tolerate fears about culpability or responsibility may contribute to their denying the client's problems or withdrawing from the client. By supporting and reassuring the family, the nurse can facilitate effective engagement or reengagement in the therapeutic process.

Family Resistance to Therapy

Resistance to effective family therapy can come from the client, the client's family, the clinical staff, or the hospital administration. Some staff may feel solely responsible for client care. They may believe that family involvement is an intrusive and complicating factor and, therefore, something to be discouraged. Many families feel intruded upon by staff and the whole therapy process. They may feel threatened by potential changes in the client or themselves.

Power struggles can develop between families and staff when their concepts of treatment differ. These power struggles are defensive maneuvers motivated by anxiety in both parties. Staff become anxious when they believe they are responsible for developing a healthier family system, and, despite their best efforts, the family does not behave as they "should." Likewise, families become anxious when they cannot influence staff to do what they want, especially when what they want is to be left alone and not be pressured to change.

Change is a stressful process even when the change is positive and in the direction that people desire. The family that has adapted to problems has reached an equilibrium that it will fight to maintain, consciously or unconsciously. When one family member changes, the whole family is challenged to (or threatened with) change. Sometimes one member of a dysfunctional family becomes healthier and serves as a catalyst to improve the health of others in the system. Sometimes, however, a client becomes healthier within the hospital system or outpatient therapeutic environment, only to be pressured by the family system to resume the unhealthy behaviors at home because they help maintain the family's homeostasis.

This is not to say that family members truly wish to sabotage improvements in themselves and each other. Sometimes they simply do not know how to endure the pain of change. While clinicians may believe that "the pain has to get worse before it gets better," they should not be surprised when families are put off by pain altogether. Exposing and exploring distressing conflicts is not a normal instinct.

A variety of defenses are employed by families to avoid the stress of change. They include attacks on the staff's credentials ("Who are you to suggest we change?"), blaming the identified client ("He's the problem; change him, not us"), anger at the identified patient ("If it weren't for you, we wouldn't be in this mess"), and withdrawal from therapy ("Therapy isn't helping" or "We'd like to continue but the car broke down"). A sensitive nurse understands the pain that is inherent in change and respects the family's need to retain as much autonomy in and responsibility for deciding what their problems are and what they are going to do about them as possible.[30]

Characteristic Family Behaviors During Therapy

There are four basic types of family involvement in the care of the ailing family member. The entire family or individual members can be overinvolved, uninvolved, pseudoinvolved, or therapeutically involved. Nurses can help maximize therapeutic involvement by understanding the different types of involvement, identifying and working with the family's strengths, empathizing with the family's fears, and minimizing their own power struggles with families.

The Overinvolved Family

The overinvolved family essentially is enmeshed with the client. Boundaries between individuals are blurred, and members feel overly responsible for each other's behavior and for the fulfillment of each other's needs. They feel personally responsible for the care that the staff provides for the client, and they can be quite vigilant in overseeing that care. Separation anxiety is provoked by the hospitalization and the staff's restrictions on contact with the client. They may show their anxiety by challenging visiting-hour restrictions, demanding special favors, and criticizing staff's care of the patient. Staff who feel competitive with the family are prime candidates for engaging in power struggles with the family over who is in charge of deciding and implementing client care.

The overinvolved family's expectations that they can be all things at all times to the client are unrealistic and can become quite burdensome. When these families become overwhelmed, they generally endeavor to bring the staff into their enmeshed system and transfer their burden of responsibility onto the staff. The family's sense of responsibility toward the client is fulfilled if they can persuade staff to provide the constant attention and gratification that they cannot. Staff who allow themselves to be pressured into assuming this role eventually find themselves feeling frustrated with their own limitations and then angry with the family for its unrealistic expectations.

It is important to work with the overinvolved family collaboratively, rather than competitively, and not succumb to a "winner-take-all" approach to client care. Collaboration can be achieved by directing the family's attempts to help toward tasks at which they can succeed. Effective directing requires tact and ingenuity. When successful, it reassures the family that their contributions are important and will not be rejected. The following is an example. Martha's anxious mother begins to dominate the family meeting by interrupting the nurse and by speaking for Martha, who can and should be speaking for herself. A collaborative response by the nurse could be, "Let me hear first from Martha, and when she is finished I want you to add what you know to be important information so I don't miss anything." This response helps structure the interview so the nurse can ask necessary questions. This response conveys to the mother that her contribution is valued, and it also enables Martha to assume more responsibility for her own thoughts and feelings. This type of intervention will need to be repeated, and it does not magically end the problems of enmeshment between mother and daughter. However, it does allow mother and daughter to practice behaviors that help them delineate healthier boundaries and still work together as a team.

The Uninvolved Family

In contrast, the uninvolved family may never visit or call the client or meet with the staff. When they do, however, their anxiety about their role in client care is as apparent as that of the overinvolved family. They may feel quite helpless and, therefore, want to shift all responsibility for the client's well-being onto the staff. Hospitalization can bring relief to these families. They feel threatened by their sense of inadequacy when the staff or the client seek their involvement. These families may withdraw, go on vacation, or be "too busy" to participate in family sessions. Their disengaged relationship with the client may be longstanding or may be a temporary maneuver to decrease their anxiety. Home visits for the client and impending discharge can increase the family's anxiety when they feel ill-equipped to deal with the client or the client's illness.

Eliciting support from the uninvolved family is difficult because access to them is so limited. Relentless pursuit, in the form of phone calls or letters or cornering them during their rare visits to the client, can be counterproductive. The most successful overtures are likely to be those that carefully structure and limit their participation to clear and manageable tasks. Asking them to attend a meeting in which the agenda is open-ended and vague generally increases their anxiety. An effective opening statement to enlist a husband's assistance in discharge planning might be, "I will meet with you and your wife if you would like to know what your wife's limitations are likely to be when she returns home. I can talk with you about what you both can do to make things as easy as possible in spite of her limitations." This approach might engage the husband's nondefensive interest and elicit a limited, but workable, commitment to meet and discuss discharge plans.

The Therapeutically Involved Family

The therapeutically involved family is a well-functioning family that works collaboratively with staff to maximize the health of all its members. They are realistic about their strengths and weaknesses and are open to interventions that offer improvements. This does not mean that they assume a submissive role and unquestioningly accept all recommendations. Collaboration involves negotiation between the family and staff on a treatment plan that is suited to the needs of that family.

Types of Family Therapy

Intervention can be done with families in an informal setting on a limited basis. Family visits to a member in the hospital or calls to staff for information provide staff with opportunities for assessment and teaching that may greatly benefit client care. Formal family therapy, however, refers to a scheduled series of sessions in which family functioning is the focus. These sessions may last several weeks to several years if conducted on an outpatient basis (Fig. 12-2). The nurse is frequently a co-therapist in either family therapy or multiple-family group therapy.

Multiple-family group therapy benefits several families simultaneously through the application of group therapy techniques and principles. The multiple-family group may or may not include the hospitalized family members. The group leader facilitates discussions around specific issues or themes—for example, the impact of psychiatric problems and hospitalization on the family system, alcoholism, sexual or physical abuse, single-parent families, parents of teenagers, families with members who have schizophrenia or Alzheimer's disease, and so forth.

Common anxieties and questions are discussed in an effort to identify, understand, and resolve problems. Participants are helped to compare and contrast themselves with each other, offer and receive observations about each other, and develop greater objectivity about themselves. By experiencing peer group identification and support, families feel less isolated and embarrassed about problems, become more willing to acknowledge and discuss their experiences, and become more receptive to change. Families often share successful coping

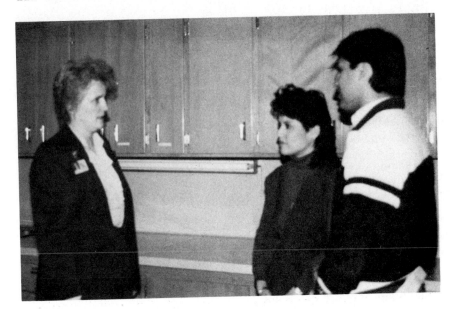

Figure 12-2. A psychiatric nurse (left) assessing a couple in their home.

skills or reinforce to each other what therapists have said to them. As knowledge and receptivity to change increase, tension usually decreases.

The Process of Family Therapy

Family therapy, like other types of therapy, occurs through a process. There are three phases in this process: the initial or *engagement phase,* the *working phase,* and the *termination phase.* There are no clear boundaries between these phases, and no specific time periods are spent in each phase. The working and termination phases may begin at the same time as the engagement phase. Although the divisions are somewhat arbitrary, they help delineate the different tasks in therapy.

There are certain expected outcomes of the family therapy process. These outcomes are outlined in the following manner:

1. Problems are clearly identified and resolved to the greatest extent possible.
2. Communication skills are improved. Messages become clearer and more honest, and are delivered directly to the person for whom they are intended.
3. Family members are better able to identify and disclose their thoughts and feelings to one another.
5. Techniques for problem-solving and conflict resolution are improved.
6. The healthy functioning and autonomy of the identified client are increased.
7. The family receives information about relevant health issues and appropriate community resources.
8. The family is able to identify signals that problems are recurring and has a plan of action for handling any recurrence.

The Engagement Phase

The engagement phase produces the cornerstone of therapy. It may last a few minutes or several months, and it may recur as often as necessary during the entire course of therapy. The primary tasks in this phase are to develop a therapeutic alliance, identify the problems in the family, and establish the goals for treatment. These tasks form the basis of contract negotiation between the family and the therapist.

Developing a Therapeutic Alliance

In family therapy the entire family system is considered to be the client. The identified client often is seen as the symptom-bearer or representative of problems within the family system. The development and maintenance of a therapeutic alliance between the hospital and family systems enable everyone to join forces and work together on problems. Although all participants have responsibility for creating and sustaining this alliance, the nurse has special responsibilities that accompany the professional role.

Nurses are in a special position to facilitate the family's entry into the hospital system because they are often the first staff with whom the family has significant contact. Nurses have a vital role in helping family members feel that they are a welcome and essential part of the treatment team and in eliciting the family's commitment to therapy. Families can be alienated by staff who treat them as outsiders or trespassers.

The style and pace of aligning with the family are determined individually. Skilled nurses accommodate to the family's style of interaction rather than expect the family to accommodate to theirs. This blending with the family does not necessitate becoming a chameleon and acting exactly as the family acts, but it does involve adapting one's style to the family's in a complementary fashion. The appropriate opening exchange may involve a social conversation or the immediate discussion of a problem to be solved. Whichever occurs, the demeanor of the nurse conveys support for the family's involvement in treatment and a willingness to understand their situation.

During the initial contact the family is likely to be stressed, functioning less than optimally. Although the context in which they meet is familiar to the nurse, it is likely to be strange and uncomfortable for the family. The family is in strange surroundings in the hospital and is trying very hard to maintain its integrity under adverse conditions. In these circumstances families initially may be confused and fearful, which can lead them to be hostile or withdrawn. Few families can be expected to understand the hospital system, let alone enjoy their presence in it.

The initial interview with a staff member may be the first time the family has openly discussed their problems together. They may have many questions, fears, and hopes that are difficult for them to express. They may be worried about being blamed by the staff and, therefore, may be reluctant to acknowledge and explore certain difficulties. Because there is no consensus regarding the etiology of most psychiatric problems, it is usually best to convey a neutral attitude regarding causality. Staff can redirect a family's tendency to blame one another by emphasizing the family's potential to help one another and by providing a positive and nonjudgmental environment in which the entire family can join in the therapeutic process.

It is essential to identify and work collaboratively with the family member or members who influence and make the major decisions regarding therapeutic issues. This information can be elicited by asking who decided that the client enter the hospital, who decided that the family enter therapy, and so forth. Eliciting information about how the family makes major decisions may uncover the existence of unhealthy power imbalances in the system.

Reorganization of power relationships may be helpful to the family. This change, however, usually can be made and sustained only in long-term outpatient therapy. Therefore, the task of the nurse in the short-term hospital is not to shift the family's balance of power but to work with the family system as it exists. Nevertheless, it is helpful to engage the non-power brokers because they, too, have important contributions to make and may be affected by the problem that brought the client to the hospital.

Identifying Problems and Goals

The first step in solving a problem is to identify the problem in terms of behaviors that can be changed. A major source of conflict can be disagreement among family members about what the problem is. By asking each member to discuss the problem from his or her viewpoint, this conflict can be addressed openly. In addition,

by valuing each member's viewpoint, the clinician engages everyone in the therapeutic endeavor.

The family may need the clinician's help in identifying problems in behavioral and quantifiable terms. Consider the example of a husband who complains that his wife is "depressed and sometimes acts crazy" and that they "don't get along." His wife responds, "I just don't feel like doing anything." To understand and resolve their problems it is necessary to identify the sequence of behaviors occurring between the two of them. The following questions can elicit this information: What are the things your wife normally does that she doesn't do now? Who's doing those things now? What is she doing when you say she acts "crazy"? What do you do when she acts this way? What responsibilities does she presently carry out although she is depressed? What do you expect your wife to do that she doesn't do now? Answers to the same or related questions should be elicited from the wife in order to compare perceptions and expectations. It is important to keep in mind that the answers from the person who is questioned first may influence the answers from the person who is questioned next. It should also be noted that "what" questions usually elicit the most practical information. "Why" questions tend to intimidate people because they often are unanswerable and, therefore, should be avoided when possible.

This couple's history and list of complaints may reveal a shifting in roles and a set of unfulfilled expectations about each other's behavior. Regardless of whether it is believed that the wife's depression is induced biologically or psychologically, this couple needs to decide how they are going to interact, who is going to do what, when it is going to be done, and so forth.

Because families tend to label their problems as belonging solely to one member (the scapegoat or the identified client), the next step is to redefine the problem as everyone's problem: one that affects everyone and is affected by everyone. Expanding the problem so that everyone is included may meet with resistance. It may take a great deal of skill and finesse to help the family accept that "you are all in this together, and the solution lies in what each of you can do to help the others." This approach places the responsibility for success onto the family system as a whole and not just onto one member of the system (the identified client) or someone outside the system (the therapist).

Each family member is asked to describe the successful and unsuccessful ways in which each has already tried to solve or cope with the problem. The clinician emphasizes that the family is now in a position to try new behaviors. At this point the therapist negotiates the goals of therapy and contracts with the family for small changes.

Contract negotiation concludes the engagement phase of therapy and begins the working phase. The contract identifies the participants in therapy, the problems that will be addressed, the expected outcomes, the frequency and length of sessions, and the length of time that therapy is expected to last. The contract may or may not include the methods by which changes will occur. Successful therapy focuses on changes that are realistic and attainable in a reasonable period of time. Families and therapists can make the mistake of attempting overly-ambitious changes and thus doom themselves to frustration and disappointment.

Assessment Tool for Family Interview

The order in which information about the family is gathered will be flexible and depend on the natural flow of the therapeutic interaction. It is not always possible to gather all of the following information in the initial interview, nor are the items mentioned intended to include everything that a clinician might need to know about a family. Skilled interviewers not only elicit the information that they believe is relevant but also encourage clients to reveal the information they believe is significant.

An interviewing style that selectively blends tact, empathy, neutrality, matter-of-factness, and firmness enables the clinician to gather all important data, including that which clients might find intrusive, threatening, or irrelevant. Data from the assessment interview should include:

A. Data about the client and each family member:
  1. Name and relationship to client
  2. Sex
  3. Age
  4. Who lives with whom, where, and for how long, and whether anyone desires or expects a change in the living arrangements
  5. Education (highest grade completed, major, history of learning disabilities)
  6. Employment history
  7. Source of economic support
  8. Significant physical health problems (past and present)
  9. History of psychiatric services (when, how long, modality, problems addressed, outcome, reason for termination)
  10. Other available support systems (church, friends, group memberships)
  11. Religious background and relevant religious beliefs (for example, "Illness is a sin," "devils" are responsible for the problem, "Prayer is the answer")
  12. History of drug and alcohol use
  13. History of being physically or sexually abused or abusive
  14. Other relevant developmental, family, and social history (for example, divorce, separations, deaths, pregnancies not resulting in live births, recent move, economic problems)
B. The interactional style of the family (who initiates or disrupts conversation on what topics, who talks to whom, who talks for whom)
C. Perception of the problem according to (1) the client, (2) each family member, and (3) the clinician
D. Goals of treatment desired by (1) the client, (2) each family member, and (3) the clinician
E. Contract with client and family and their reactions to it (treatment modalities, frequency and length of sessions, goals, expected length of therapy)

The Working Phase

During the working phase new behaviors are promoted and tested. This phase begins when the family's resistance gives way to the therapist's skills at facilitating risk-taking. It is important for the therapist to promote a sense of competence in all family members as they begin to express themselves more clearly and experiment with new behaviors.

The trend today is toward shorter hospital stays. The shorter the stay, the less time there is to spend in the working phase. Therefore, there is limited opportunity to attempt fundamental changes in the family's style of communication, role relationships, and functional organization. Long-term outpatient therapy is more appropriate for attempting to achieve these goals.

The aim of inpatient interventions is symptom reduction, education, development of coping strategies, and assessment for outpatient referrals. This crisis-oriented approach emphasizes the present, the here-and-now, and deemphasizes the past. The major tasks are to decrease anxiety and to help the family decide what they are going to do *now*, given their current circumstances.

The overall goal of family therapy is improved family functioning. This general goal may involve large and complex changes that become manageable and attainable only when broken down into smaller and more specific steps. This breakdown is what is meant by contracting for small changes.

Sometimes families fear that their problems are being trivialized when the focus is placed on one example of their problems. However, when one episode of miscommunication is explored in depth or time is spent resolving one apparently small conflict, the family, in fact, is learning and practicing the process of effective communication or conflict resolution. Later, then, they can apply their newly-learned skills to other, similar problems. It is not necessary to resolve all problems in therapy, but it is important to learn the process by which problems are resolved.

The Termination Phase

The main tasks in the termination phase are to solidify achievements, evaluate progress toward the stated goals, plan how to handle possible recurrence of the original problems, and establish appropriate follow-up care, if necessary. Sometimes the presenting problems are resolved during the working phase only to recur later, often during the termination phase. Rather than feeling discouraged, the family can be reassured that this set-back is a normal and temporary part of the stress of termination. If learning has taken place, the family will recognize the signals of a relapse and will know what to do when they occur.

Not all families, of course, remain in therapy through the planned termination phase. Some families withdraw from therapy before engagement takes place, or during the working phase, or abruptly upon completion of the working phase. Some families do not see the importance of the termination phase, just as some individuals do not see the importance of completing a prescribed series of medication once their symptoms go away. Also, some families do not tolerate the ritual of saying goodbye.

Each therapy session also has a termination phase. The session is summarized and decisions are made about the next step. Details are clarified about the next session, and the family knows whom to call between sessions for information and in case of an emergency. The structure provided for the periods between sessions helps decrease anxiety and chaos and eases the family's sense of abandonment and helplessness.

Table 12-2 outlines the phases of family therapy. Specific instructions are included for the therapist to use as a guide for conducting formal family therapy sessions. This guide is not meant to include everything the clinician would do, nor are the tasks necessarily to be performed in the order given.

Special Problems With Violent Families

Family violence has received increased attention in the last two decades. Popular media, clinical journals, and textbooks have made it clear that Americans have serious concerns about child abuse and neglect, the battering of wives and husbands by each other, and the battering of the elderly by their adult children.

What is family violence? To a great extent this term implies value judgments. Some people believe corporal punishment of any kind is cruel and unnecessary, whether or not physical injury occurs. Other people believe it is the parents' duty to correct their children through necessary spankings. Some people believe it is a man's right to discipline his wife and children by any means he sees fit.

Odum defines family violence as "those behaviors of family members that are intended to result in the physical or psychological trauma or pain of another member, or in that member's failure in normal growth and development."[23] Odum states that violence is a deliberate, aggressive set of actions, whereas abuse may be passive, like acts of omission that lead to a child's failure to thrive. Violence and abuse often occur together. An important distinguishing feature of violence is that it is almost always believed to be explosive and life-threatening, and, therefore, it creates disabling fear in the victim. Spousal rape and incest are two forms of family violence. *Incest* is defined as "any physical contact between parent and child that has to be kept secret."[7]

Theories of violence come from the fields of biology, neurophysiology, psychology, sociology, and anthropology, but the causes are not fully understood. Social learning, cultural attitudes, hormonal levels, brain disorders, heredity, and alcohol abuse all may predispose an individual to violence.[8] Therefore, an assessment of these factors is important in the identification of families at risk for violence. It is important to remember, however, that no single factor is always associated with violence. For instance, although there are striking relationships between the abuse of alcohol and homicidal and suicidal behavior, not all alcoholics become violent after drinking.

The following typical characteristics have been identified in families at risk for domestic violence.[23] The same factors also make the family unlikely to seek counseling or other health care:

- Poor self-esteem in one or more members
- Resistance to the external environment and lack of spontaneity in social or interpersonal activities
- Belief in corporal punishment or strict disciplinary habits
- Excessive expectations beyond innate capacities of family members
- Patriarchal family structure and rigid role prescriptions
- Inadequate social supports
- Denial of any problems

Also, families in which abuse is an intergenerational phenomenon are more likely to exhibit patterns of family violence.[29]

Levels of Prevention in Family Violence

The role of the nurse in the assessment and treatment of family violence is important. Nurses, as noted earlier, work with families in a variety of settings. The role of the nurse can be viewed from a broad context to include primary, secondary, and tertiary prevention.

Primary prevention deals with assessing families prone to family violence. Nurses working in home health care, outpatient clinics, and public health programs see families over a prolonged period of time. They can observe the extent to which the families fit the profile of families prone to violence. Assessments can be made with answers to the following questions: Are members of the family acting in self-deprecatory ways? Do they lack certain interpersonal or social skills? Is corporal punishment a pattern used in the family? Do the parents or spouses hold unrealistic expectations for their family members? Are roles rigidly assigned and enforced? Is the family patriarchal in nature? Does the family lack the necessary social supports for functioning in the community? Do the adults in the family fail to recognize their problems and have poor coping skills?

Nurses may be the first to identify a violence-prone family. In this capacity they will document the evidence and seek or provide early supports for the family. Referrals can be made to include family members in educational support programs in schools and childcare settings. Educational support groups for parents and home health care assistance also may be available.

Secondary prevention deals with the early detection and adequate treatment of actual cases of abuse. Bruises, cuts, lacerations, broken bones, and burns are signs of abuse and can be detected in the emergency room, out-

TABLE 12-2.
PHASES OF FAMILY THERAPY

I. Engagement Phase
  A. Develop a therapeutic alliance.
    1. Identify relevant family members.
    2. Negotiate the date, time, place, and group composition of the initial meeting.
    3. Prepare to receive the family (chairs, ashtrays, tissues, audio/visual equipment, privacy).
    4. Introduce yourself (name, discipline, role in health care system).
    5. Negotiate the setting (rearrangement of furniture, acceptance or nonacceptance of smoking and audio/visual recording).
    6. Explain the reason for meeting.
    7. Engage all members.
    8. Accommodate to the family's style and language.
    9. Facilitate empathic exchange among all present.
    10. Judiciously disclose information about yourself that facilitates a therapeutic alliance.
    11. Listen without judgment; accept, and attempt to understand, the beliefs and values of all members.
    12. Search for strengths.
  B. Identify problems and goals.
    1. Ask each person to identify the problem.
    2. Ask what changes each person desires.
    3. Ask what each person expects to happen as a result of therapy.
    4. Elicit relevant history.
    5. Answer questions clearly and directly.
    6. Avoid offering premature advice and solutions.
    7. Negotiate the initial contract (who will attend sessions, how often, expected length of therapy, initial goals).
    8. Summarize the meeting and clarify agreements about the next session.
    9. Formulate the initial hypothesis and treatment plan.

II. Working Phase
  A. Maintain existing strengths.
    1. Assist the family to identify their strengths as individuals and as a unit.
    2. Review the contract as often as necessary.
  B. Facilitate new behaviors.
    1. Structure sessions to achieve goals.
    2. Provide a nonthreatening environment.
    3. Build self-esteem.
    4. Redefine problems in interactional terms.
    5. Teach and facilitate clear and direct communication among members.
      a. Interrupt repetitive, ineffective, and dysfunctional communication.
      b. Point out discrepancies.
      c. Spell out double messages.
      d. Spell out nonverbal messages.
    6. Prescribe tasks to be done during or between sessions (new roles, chores, or other behaviors).
    7. Summarize each session and contract for the next session.
    8. Modify the hypothesis and treatment plan when necessary.

III. Termination Phase
  A. Evaluate progress towards goals from the viewpoint of the therapist and each family member.
  B. Discuss everyone's feelings about termination and expectations for the future.
  C. Recognize the limits of change.
  D. Discuss the possibility of relapse and what the family should do if it occurs.
  E. Agree on an appropriate plan for follow-up care.

---

patient clinic, physician's office, and inpatient setting. Victims may hint at the trouble by making references to having secrets or wanting to talk about something but not knowing where to begin.

The cycle of family violence may be more easily broken at times of crisis. When the family's homeostasis is shaken and the family is thrown off balance, they may be more receptive to support and counseling and better able to change what seem to be rigid patterns of interaction. When the victim or perpetrator is hospitalized, some form of family therapy is always advisable, both during confinement and immediately afterwards. The aim of treatment is to make the best use of available resources when the family system is in a state of disequilibrium.

Therapeutic communication is an essential nursing skill in working with an abusive family. Therapeutic communication includes rapport-building, active listening, maintaining a nonjudgmental attitude, and minimal advice-giving in the early stages of the relationship. The family must establish a sense of trust with the nurse. All prob-

lems presented by the family should receive attention. Active listening includes observing nonverbal and verbal patterns of interaction.

The nurse will contribute significantly by identifying stressors that precipitate or intensify violence as a pattern of interaction. Nurses can identify repetitive interactions in the family that escalate anger, hostility, and aggression. When these interactions occur, the nurse can divert the attention of the family to healthier ways of responding. Role-modeling and teaching nondefensive listening can assist the family, but sustained learning of new patterns may not be possible in the early stages of intervention.

Nursing interventions that help all family members build self-esteem and positive self-images will make a significant contribution to the efforts of the treatment team. During secondary prevention the treatment team assesses the need to report findings to the authorities. State laws outline the circumstances in which health care professionals are mandated to report suspected abuse.

Tertiary prevention includes effective planning of

care to prevent future episodes of family violence. In the case of child abuse, sexual abuse, and wife-battering, sometimes the only solution is to separate the victims from the perpetrators. Imprisonment of perpetrators, foster-home placement of severely abused children, and nursing-home placement of abused elderly persons are sometimes the only ways to provide safety. Other measures include shelters, which provide a temporary haven for victims. These remedies usually are employed only when there is no real possibility of maintaining a safe environment at home. Nurses may be able to assist families with placement. They should assess the kind of care that is needed, the programs that exist to assist the family, and the wishes of the family. The ideal solution eliminates or eases the problem while producing a minimal amount of social, psychological, and economic hardship on the family. Although the ideal solution may be to keep the family intact, this is not always possible or advisable. The nurse needs to appreciate the fact that separation of family members can create a great deal of shame, guilt, and anxiety. At this time the supportive rapport the nurse has established with the family can assist them in coping with the hardships of dissolution.

In summary, family violence is prevalent and appears to have increased over the last two decades. It is a special problem that requires a wide-range approach. Nurses can make significant contributions in the early diagnosis and referral of cases, the treatment of victims and perpetrators, and the supportive maintenance of the family in the aftercare phase of treatment. Nurses at the graduate level are prepared to provide private counseling services. These services may include couple and family therapy, rape counseling, and group therapy for perpetrators.

Summary

1. Family intervention, like other forms of therapeutic intervention, is an art as well as a skill.

2. Although it is very important to have a theoretical framework that guides the nursing assessment and choice of goals and interventions, there are no rigid rules that can be followed in the course of family work. The blending of the nurse's personality with the personalities of the family members also contributes to the nurse's choice of words and gestures and provides an authentic use of self in the therapeutic exchange.

3. Effective nurses monitor their own motivations and goals as they seek to achieve the therapeutic goals established with the families.

4. The basic role of the beginning nurse clinician is to be an effective participant-observer and a supportive, therapeutic change agent. In this role the nurse strives to:

   a. Foster a positive emotional atmosphere of acceptance and warmth.

   b. Promote the natural benefits of family membership.

   c. Engage the family in the treatment process.

   d. Facilitate productive contact among family members.

   e. Promote self-esteem in all family members.

   f. Teach and facilitate clear and assertive communication among members.

   g. Facilitate role clarity and the establishment of healthy roles in the family system.

   h. Assist the family to establish boundaries between members that preserve individual differences, thereby providing for normal growth and development of the family system and all its members.

   i. Assist the family to develop more effective coping and problem-solving strategies.

5. By involving the family in therapy, the natural benefits of family membership can be maintained, induced, restored, or enhanced.

6. Family violence is a special problem in the treatment of families and requires a broad range of interventions.

7. Family work can be rich and rewarding for all participants and should be undertaken with the knowledge that there are many methods by which families can be assisted to learn, grow, and adapt to life's stresses.

References

1. Abroms G, Fellner C, Whitaker C: Admissions of whole families. Am J Psychiatry 127:1363, 1971

2. American Nurses' Association: Taxonomy for the Classification of Human Responses of Concern for Psychiatric/Mental Health Nursing Practice (working draft). Kansas City, Missouri, American Nurses' Association, 1986

3. American Psychiatric Association: Diagnostic and Statistical Manual of Mental Disorders-III-R. Washington, DC, American Psychiatric Association, 1987

4. Bateson G, Jackson D, Haley J et al: Towards a theory of schizophrenia. Behav Sci 1:251, 1956

5. Bernal G, Flores-Ortiz Y: Latino families in therapy: Engagement and evaluation. J Mar Fam Ther 8:357, 1982

6. Bowen M: The Use of Family Therapy in Clinical Practice. In Haley J (ed): Changing Families. New York, Grune & Stratton, 1971

7. Burgess AW: The Sexual Victimization of Adolescents. Rockville, Maryland, National Institute of Mental Health, 1985

8. Campbell J: Theories of Violence. In Campbell J, Humphreys J (eds): Nursing Care of Victims of Family Violence. Reston, Virginia, Reston Publishing, 1984

9. Framo JL: The Integration of Marital Therapy With Sessions With Family of Origin. In Gurman AS, Kniskern DP (eds): Handbook of Family Therapy. New York, Brunner/Mazel, 1981

10. Freud S: Analysis of a Phobia in a Five-Year-Old Boy (1909). In Complete Works of Sigmund Freud, vol 10. London, Hogarth Press, 1955

11. Glick ID, Clarkin JF: The Effects of Family Presence and Brief Family Intervention for Hospitalized Schizophrenic Patients: A Review. In Harbin HT (ed): The Psychiatric Hospital and the Family. New York, Spectrum, 1982

12. Goldenberg I, Goldenberg H: Family Therapy: An Overview. Monterey, California, Brooks/Cole, 1980

13. Greenley JR: The Patient's Family and Length of Psychiatric Hospitalization. In Harbin HT (ed): The Psychiatric Hospital and the Family. New York, Spectrum, 1982

14. Gurman AS, Kniskern DP: Research on Marital and Family Therapy: Progress, Perspective, and Prospect. In Garfield SL, Bergin AE (eds): Handbook of Psychotherapy and Behavioral Change: An Empirical Analysis, 2nd ed. New York, John Wiley & Sons, 1978

15. Gurman AS, Kniskern DP: Family Therapy Outcome Research: Knowns and Unknowns. In Gurman AS, Kniskern DP (eds): Handbook of Family Therapy. New York, Brunner/Mazel, 1981

16. Haley J: Family Therapy: A Radical Change. In Haley J (ed): Changing Families. New York, Grune & Stratton, 1971

17. Jackson D, Satir V: A Review of Psychiatric Development in Family Diagnosis and Family Therapy. In Ackerman N, Beatman F, Sherman S (eds): Exploring the Basis for Family Therapy. New York, Family Service Association, 1961

18. Johnson A: Mutual expectations: How family members view the social role of the mental health center client. J Psychosoc Nurs Ment Health Serv 24:35, 1986

19. Levine IM: Introduction. In McGoldrick M, Pearce JK, Giordano J (eds): Ethnicity and Family Therapy. New York, Guilford Press, 1982

20. McLane AM (ed): Classification of Nursing Diagnoses: Proceedings of the Seventh Conference of the North American Nursing Diagnosis Association. St Louis, CV Mosby, 1987

21. Minuchin S: Families and Family Therapy. Cambridge, Massachusetts, Harvard University Press, 1974

22. Montalvo B: Aspects of live supervision. Fam Process 12:343, 1978

23. Odum R: Family Violence. In Logan BB, Dawkins CE (eds): Family-Centered Nursing in the Community. Menlo Park, California, Addison-Wesley, 1986

24. Satir V: Conjoint Family Therapy, 3rd ed. Palo Alto, California, Science and Behavior Books, 1983

25. Sedgwick R: Family Mental Health: Theory and Practice. St Louis, CV Mosby, 1980

26. Spitzer SP, Weinstein RM, Nelson HL: Family Reactions and the Career of the Psychiatric Patient: A Long-Term Follow-Up Study. In Harbin HT (ed): The Psychiatric Hospital and the Family. New York, Spectrum, 1982

27. Szapocznik J, Scopetta MA, Arnalde M et al: Cuban value structure: Treatment implications. J Consult Clin Psychol 46:961, 1978

28. von Bertalanffy L: General Systems Theory: Foundations, Development, Applications. New York, George Braziller, 1968

29. Walker L: The Battered Woman. New York, Harper & Row, 1979

30. Withersty DJ, Kidwell ER: Measuring the Effects of Family Involvement on a Psychiatric Inpatient Unit. In Harbin HT (ed): The Psychiatric Hospital and the Family. New York, Spectrum, 1982

DONNA AGUILERA

CRISIS INTERVENTION

Learning Objectives

Upon completion of this chapter the student should be able to do the following:

1. Describe a historical trend fostering occurrences of crises.
2. Identify the differences between crisis intervention methodology and traditional methods of psychotherapy.
3. Differentiate between maturational and situational crises.
4. Identify the balancing factors that determine whether or not individuals will go into crisis when they are in hazardous situations.
5. Describe examples of the nurse's role in crisis intervention.
6. Identify specific life experiences that have the potential to precipitate a crisis.
7. Identify a person in crisis from reported and directly observed behavioral clues.
8. Describe how cultural differences among people affect the crisis intervention process.
9. List three major areas of focus to include in the assessment of an individual in a crisis situation.
10. Plan and implement interventions, appropriate to the skills learned, for an individual in crisis.
11. Describe characteristics of the nurse's therapeutic use of self in crisis intervention.
12. Recognize the intrinsic limitations of crisis intervention methodology and its potential in nursing situations.

Introduction

As stated in previous chapters, human beings are viewed as biopsychosocial entities and, as such, are unique. In crisis intervention, nurse therapists seek to return clients to a high level of wellness. The goal is to restore clients to their previous state of equilibrium, or to homeostasis. The therapist reinforces individuals' strengths and minimizes their weaknesses while they are in a state of crisis. The objective is to move clients from a passive, dependent state to an active, independent state in a short period of time.

As defined by Caplan,[12] crisis may occur when the individual faces a problem that cannot be solved. Inner tension, signs of anxiety, and difficulty in functioning all increase during extended periods of emotional upset. Typically, the individual functions at a relatively even level but experiences cognitive and emotional disorganization during the crisis period. Although crisis theory is not used extensively when describing individuals with a long history of severe mental illness, these individuals can experience rises and falls in their level of functioning. Typically, crisis theory focuses on relatively healthy persons who are experiencing temporary, overwhelming obstacles to their sense of well-being.

A person in crisis is at a turning point. The individual faces a problem that cannot readily be solved using the coping mechanisms that worked before the crisis. As a result, tension and anxiety increase, and the individual becomes less able to find a solution. A person in this situation feels helpless, caught in a state of great emotional upset and unable to take independent action to solve the problem. Crisis intervention can offer the immediate help that a person in crisis needs in order to reestablish equilibrium.

Increasing awareness of sociocultural factors that can precipitate crisis situations has led to the rapid evolution of crisis intervention methodology. This chapter presents the nursing process within a crisis theory model, focusing specifically on the problem-solving approach to crisis intervention.

The Historical Development of Crisis Intervention

Today we hear talk of the changes in our lives that have been made by "urbanization" and "technology." A closer study of these changes will show the impact they have had on families and individuals.

Before the industrial and technological revolutions, most people lived on farms or in small rural communities. Most were self-employed, either on farms or in small, associated businesses. When sons and daughters married, they were likely to remain near their parents, working in the same occupations. In this way, trades and occupations became links between generations. Families tended to be large and, because family members lived and worked together and relied chiefly on each other for

social interaction, they developed strong loyalties and a sense of responsibility for one another.

Contemporary urban life, however, does not encourage or allow this kind of sheltered, close-knit family relationship. People who live in cities are likely to be employed by a company and paid a wage. They work with business associates and live within a neighborhood rather than with just their immediate families. Because of housing conditions and the necessity of living on a wage, families in cities usually consist of parents and unmarried children.

The differences between rural and urban life have important repercussions for individual security and stability. The rural, extended family offered a large and relatively constant group of associates. Family size meant that there was always someone to talk to, even about a problem involving two family members. But urban life is highly mobile and there is often a rapid turnover in business associates and neighbors. There is also no certainty that these relative strangers will share the same values, beliefs, and interests. All of these factors make it difficult for people to develop trust and interdependence outside the immediate family. In addition, urban life often requires that people meet each other superficially, in specific roles, and in limited relationships, rather than as total personalities.

All of these factors taken together mean that people in cities are more isolated than ever before from the emotional support provided by the family and close familiar peers. As a result, there are few role models to follow, the demands of urban life are constantly changing, and coping behavior that was appropriate and successful in previous times may be hopelessly ineffective today. This creates a favorable environment for the development of a crisis. Table 13-1 summarizes the historical development of crisis theory and intervention.

Historically, the diagnostic manual of the American Psychiatric Association does not focus on crisis-related behavior. The Adjustment Disorder category, however, does relate to responses to a relatively recent identifiable stressor, which is similar to the description given to crisis events. The box on page 232 includes a list of psychiatric diagnostic criteria for an Adjustment Disorder.[3]

Theoretical Frameworks

The crisis approach to therapeutic intervention has been developed only within the past few decades and is based on a broad range of theories of human behavior, including those of Freud, Hartmann, Rado, Erickson, Lindemann, and Caplan. Its current acceptance as a recognized form of treatment cannot be directly related to any single theory of behavior; all have contributed to some degree.

An overview of the theoretical development of crisis intervention creates an awareness of the broad knowledge base incorporated into present practice. Although not all theories of human behavior are necessarily dependent on Freudian concepts, and only a selected few are presented here, the overview begins with the psychoana-

TABLE 13-1.
THE HISTORICAL DEVELOPMENT OF CRISIS THEORY AND INTERVENTION

DATE	EVENT
Pre-urbanization	Family members lived close to one another, developed family loyalties, and assisted each other in crisis periods.
Circa 300 B.C.	Hippocrates, a medical doctor, stated that a crisis is a sudden cessation of a state that gravely endangers life.
Urbanization	People became more mobile; family members were not necessarily available during a period of crisis.
Early 20th century	Concerned groups formed suicide centers, such as the National Save-a-Life League in New York City.
1930s and 1940s	Research in crisis theory began with the work of Quierdo, Lindemann, Caplan, and Erickson.
	Quierdo began an emergency first-aid service similar to the approach used during World War II and the Korean and Vietnam Wars. Combat troops who suffered from temporary personality disorganization were evacuated quickly to a treatment location near the combat zone rather than to the rear area. The individual regained equilibrium and could return to the front line with more ease.
	Lindemann conducted studies that made significant contributions to crisis theory, especially in the area of bereavement reactions.
	Caplan provided a detailed definition and description of crises. Caplan also addressed the concept of crisis intervention in terms of helping crisis victims avoid long-term and severely debilitating mental illness. He labeled three types of preventive measures: primary, secondary, and tertiary prevention.
	Erickson's research provided the concept of two types of crises, maturational-developmental and accidental-situational.
1946	Congress passed the National Mental Health Act to provide a method for financing mental health research and training and to establish community mental health centers in which individuals (including those in crisis) could receive treatment.
1950s	The Joint Commission on Mental Illness and Health studied the nation's mental health problems. In response, President John Kennedy helped with the passage of the Community Mental Health Center Act of 1963. Financial grants were available to states to develop public mental health centers.
1960s	Telephone crisis hotlines were developed, using both professional and paraprofessional volunteers to assist crisis victims on a 24-hour basis. Examples of hotlines include those for suicide and for drug abusers.
1970s	Nurses began development of theory in crisis intervention. Nurses worked on special crisis inpatient units with clients needing intensive crisis intervention.
Present	Crisis theory development continues in the areas of spouse abuse, AIDS, child abuse and neglect, elder abuse, stress and burnout, and disaster assistance. Criminal justice agents (police) are the primary crisis interveners of our society because they are usually the first agents on the scene.

(Adapted from Hendricks J: Crisis Intervention: Contemporary Issues for On-Site Interveners. Springfield, Illinois, Charles C Thomas, 1985)

lytic theories of Freud because these are a major basis for further investigation of normal and abnormal human behavior. The fundamental procedures of crisis intervention and brief psychotherapy are derived from hypotheses based on studies of the reasons for normal, as well as abnormal, human behavior.

General Theories Supporting the Concept of Crisis

Psychoanalytic Theory (Freud)

Sigmund Freud was the first theorist to demonstrate and apply the principle of *causality* as it relates to psychic determinism.[6] Simply put, this principle states that every act of human behavior has its cause, or source, in the history and experience of the individual. It follows that some cause is operating, whether or not the individual is aware of the reason for the behavior. Present behavior is caused or determined by one's past experience. This psychic determinism is the theoretical foundation of psychotherapy and psychoanalysis.

Since the end of the 19th century, the concept of determinism and the scientific bases from which Freud formulated his ideas have undergone many changes. Although the ego-analytic theorists have subscribed to much in the Freudian position, there are several respects in which they differ. These seem to be extensions of Freudian theory rather than direct contradictions. As a group, these theorists conclude that Freud neglected the direct study of normal, healthy behavior.

Ego-Analytic Theory (Hartmann)

Heinz Hartmann, an early ego analyst, was profoundly versed in Freud's theoretical contributions.[37] He postulated that Freud's psychoanalytic theories could prove valid for normal, as well as for pathological, behavior. Hartmann began with the study of ego functions and distinguished between two groups: those that develop from conflict, and the others that are "conflict-free," such as memory, thinking, and language, which he labeled "primary autonomous functions of the ego." He considered these important in the adaptation of the individual to the environment. Hartmann emphasized that an individual's adaptation in early childhood, as well as the ability to continue adapting to the environment in later life, had to be considered. Hartmann's conception of *the ego as an organ of adaptation* required further study of the concept of reality. He also described the search for an envi-

DIAGNOSTIC CRITERIA FOR ADJUSTMENT DISORDER

A. A reaction to an identifiable psychosocial stressor (or multiple stressors) that occurs within three months of onset of the stressor(s)

B. The maladaptive nature of the reaction is indicated by either of the following:
   1. Impairment in occupational (including school) functioning or in usual social activities or relationships with others
   2. Symptoms that are in excess of a normal and expectable reaction to the stressor(s)

C. The disturbance is not merely one instance of a pattern of overreaction to stress or an exacerbation of one of the mental disorders previously described.

D. The maladaptive reaction has persisted for no longer than six months.

E. The disturbance does not meet the criteria for any specific mental disorder and does not represent Uncomplicated Bereavement.

(American Psychiatric Association: Diagnostic and Statistical Manual of Mental Disorders-III-R. Washington, DC, American Psychiatric Association, 1987)

---

ronment as another form of adaptation—the fitting-together of the individual and the society. He believed that, although the behavior of the individual is strongly influenced by culture, a part of the personality remains relatively free of this influence.

Adaptational Psychodynamics (Rado)

Sandor Rado developed the concept of *adaptational psychodynamics,* providing a new approach to the unconscious, as well as new goals and techniques of therapy.[54] Rado saw human behavior as being based on the dynamic principle of *motivation and adaptation.* An individual achieves adaptation through interaction with its culture. Behavior is viewed in terms of its effects on the welfare of the individual, not just in terms of cause and effect. The organism's patterns of interaction improve through adaptation, with the goal of increasing the possibilities for survival. Freud's classic psychoanalytic technique emphasized the developmental past and the uncovering of unconscious memories, and less importance was attached to the reality of the present. Rado's adaptational psychotherapy, however, emphasizes *the immediate present* without neglecting the influence of the developmental past. Primary concern is with failures in adaptation "today," what caused them, and what the client must do to learn to overcome them. Interpretations always begin and end with the present; preoccupation with the past is discouraged. As quickly as insight is achieved, it is used repeatedly as a beginning to encourage the client to enter into the present, real-life situation. Through practice, the client instinctively reacts with new patterns of healthy behavior. According to Rado, this automatic reaction, not insight, is ultimately the curative process. He believed that it takes place not passively, in the doctor's office, but actively, in the reality of daily living.[47]

Epigenetic Development (Erickson)

Erik Erickson further developed the theories of ego psychology, complementing those of Freud, Hartmann, and Rado, by focusing on the *epigenesis of the ego.*[51] Epigenetic development is characterized by an orderly se-quence of development at particular stages, each depending on the previous stages for successful completion. Erickson perceived eight stages of psychosocial development, spanning the entire life cycle of the individual and involving specific developmental tasks that must be solved in each phase. The solution that is achieved in each previous phase is applied in subsequent phases. Erickson's theory is important because it offers an explanation of the individual's social development as a result of encounters with the social environment. See Chapter 7 for a further discussion.

Crisis Theories

Lindemann

Lindemann's[36] initial concern was in developing approaches that might contribute to the maintenance of good mental health and the prevention of emotional disorganization on a community-wide level. He chose to study bereavement reactions in his search for social events or situations that *predictably* would be followed by emotional disturbances in a considerable portion of the population. In his study of bereavement reactions among the survivors of those killed in the Coconut Grove nightclub fire, he described both brief and abnormally prolonged reactions occurring in different individuals as a result of a loss of a significant person in their lives.

In his experiences in working with grief reactions, Lindemann concluded that it might be profitable for investigation, and useful for the development of preventive efforts, to construct a conceptual frame of reference around the concept of an emotional crisis, as exemplified by bereavement reactions. Certain *inevitable events* in the course of the life cycle of every individual can be described as perilous situations—for example, bereavement, the birth of a child, and marriage. He postulated that in each of these situations emotional strain is generated, stress is experienced, and a series of adaptive mechanisms occur that can lead either to mastery of the new situation, or to failure with more or less lasting impairment to function. Although these situations create stress for all people who are exposed to them, they become crises for individuals who (by personality, previous experience, or other factors in the present situation) are especially vulnerable to this stress and whose emotional resources are taxed beyond their usual adaptive resources.

Lindemann's theoretical frame of reference led to the development of crisis intervention techniques, and in 1946 he and Caplan established a community-wide program of mental health in the Harvard area, called the Wellesley Project.

Caplan

According to Caplan,[12] the most important aspects of mental health are the state of the ego, meaning the stage of its maturity, and the quality of its structure. Assessment of its state is based on three additional areas: (1) the capacity of the person to withstand stress and anxiety, and to maintain ego equilibrium, (2) the degree of reality recognized and faced in solving problems, and (3) the repertoire of effective coping mechanisms employable by the person to maintain a biopsychosocial balance.

Caplan believed that all the elements that compose the total emotional milieu of the person must be assessed in an approach to preventive mental health. The material, physical, and social demands of reality, as well as the needs, instincts, and impulses of the individual, must all be considered as important behavioral determinants of crisis intervention.

As a result of his work in Israel (1948) and his later experiences in Massachusetts with Lindemann and with the Community Mental Health Program at Harvard University, Caplan evolved the concept of the importance of crisis periods in individual and group development.[11]

Crisis occurs "when a person faces an obstacle to important life goals that is, for a time, insurmountable through the utilization of customary methods of problem-solving. A period of disorganization ensues, a period of upset, during which many abortive attempts at a solution are made."[12]

In essence, the individual is viewed as living in a state of emotional *equilibrium, with a goal of always returning to, or maintaining, that state.* When customary problem-solving techniques cannot be used to meet the daily problems of living, the balance, or equilibrium is upset. The individual must either solve the problem or adapt to the lack of a solution. In either case, a new state of equilibrium will develop, sometimes better and sometimes worse for positive mental health. There is a rise in inner tension, signs of anxiety, and disorganization of function, resulting in a protracted period of emotional upset. Caplan refers to this as "crisis."

Types of Crises

A significant feature of Erickson's theory is the elaboration of particular types of crises. He dealt, in particular, with the problem of adolescence and saw this period as a *normative crisis,* that is, a normal maturational phase of increased conflicts, with apparent fluctuations in ego

strength. His theories provided a basis for the work of others who further developed the concept of types of crises.[22] The types of crises are mentioned below.

Maturational crises are those in which the individual is going through a particular growth and development stage and undergoes the conflicts normally associated with these stages. In adolescence the independence/dependency conflict with parents and others, and the physiological changes associated with adolescence, can cause a feeling of disorganization and crisis. Another example is retirement, in which individuals who have developed much of their life activity in the context of their job, suddenly find themselves with no focus for their activity. Their life may seem hollow, and their life transition may necessitate pervasive role changes in their family. The retired individual may need to develop new levels of intimacy with a spouse or risk marital conflict as well as the conflicts involved in the career change.[22]

Situational crises are associated with accidental events such as natural disasters, rape, or the sudden death of a significant other. These crises are not expected and involve some loss perceived by the individual as devastating.[22]

Developmental Phases of Crisis

According to Caplan,[13] there are four developmental phases in a crisis:

1. There is an initial rise in tension as habitual problem-solving techniques are tried.
2. There is a lack of success in coping as the stimulus continues and more discomfort is felt.
3. A further increase in tension acts as a powerful internal stimulus, and mobilizes internal and external resources. In this stage, emergency problem-solving mechanisms are tried. The problem may be redefined, or there may be resignation and the giving-up of certain aspects of the goal as unattainable.
4. If the problem continues and can neither be solved nor avoided, tension increases and a major disorganization occurs.

Some events may cause a strong emotional response in one person, yet leave another apparently unaffected. Much of this difference is determined by the presence or absence of factors that can effect a return to equilibrium.

Balancing Factors Affecting Equilibrium[1]

In the time between the perceived effects of a stressful situation and the resolution of the problem, there are three recognized balancing factors that may determine the state of equilibrium. Strengths or weaknesses in any one of the balancing factors can be directly related to the onset of crisis or to its resolution. These balancing factors are perception of the event, available situational supports, and coping mechanisms, as shown in Figure 13-1.

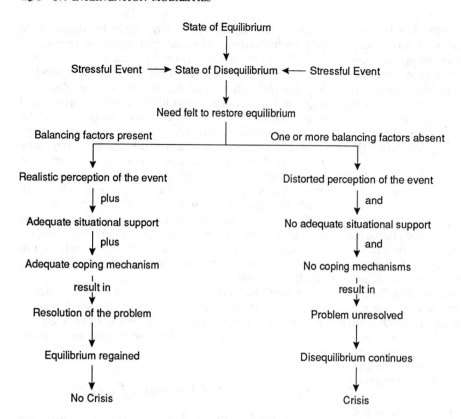

Figure 13-1. Paradigm: The effect of balancing factors in a stressful event. (Aguilera DC, Messick JM: Crisis Intervention: Theory and Methodology, 6th ed, p 69. St Louis, CV Mosby, 1986.)

The upper portion of the paradigm in Figure 13-1 illustrates the "normal" initial reaction of the individual to a stressful event. In the left column, the balancing factors are operating and crisis is avoided. In the right column, however, the absence of one or more of these balancing factors may block resolution of the problem, thus increasing disequilibrium and precipitating crisis.

Fig. 13-2 demonstrates the use of the paradigm for presentation of subsequent case studies. Its purpose is to serve as a guideline to focus the reader on the problem areas. An example of its applicability is presented in the cases of two people affected by the same stressful event. One resolved the problem and avoided crisis; the other did not.

Why do some people go into crisis when others do not? Figure 13-2 illustrates the cases of two students, Sue and Mary. Both fail a final examination. Sue is upset but does not go into crisis. Mary goes into crisis. Why does Sue react one way, and Mary differently, to the same stressful event? What "things" in their present lives make the difference?

Perception of the Event

Cognition, or the individual's understanding of a stressful event, plays a major role in determining both the nature and the degree of coping behaviors. Differences in cognition, in terms of the event's perceived threat to an important life goal or value, account for large differences in coping behaviors. The concept of cognitive style proposed by Cropley and Field[18] suggests a certain uniqueness in the way people take in, process, and use information from the environment.

Cognitive styles, or a person's characteristic modes of organizing perceptual and intellectual activities, play an important role in determining an individual's coping responses to daily life stresses. According to Inkeles,[25] cognitive style helps to set limits on information-seeking in stress situations. It also strongly influences perceptions of others, interpersonal relationships, and responses to various types of psychiatric treatment.

For example, under stressful situations a person whose cognitive style is identified as *field-dependent* relies heavily on external "objects" (such as familiar people) in the environment for orientation to reality. This type of individual uses coping mechanisms such as repression and denial. In contrast, the *field-independent* person prefers intellectualization as a defense mode.

If the event is perceived realistically, the relationship between the event and feelings of stress will be recognized. Problem-solving can be appropriately oriented toward reduction of tension, and it is more likely that the stressful situation will be resolved.

Lazarus[33,34] focused on the importance of *appraisal,* the mediating cognitive process, to determine the various coping methods used by individuals. This recognizes that coping behaviors always represent an interaction between the individual and the environment; and that environmental demands of each unique situation will initiate, form, and limit coping activities that may be required in the interaction. As a result, people engage in diverse behavioral and intrapsychic activities to meet actual or anticipated threats. Appraisal, in this context, is an ongoing

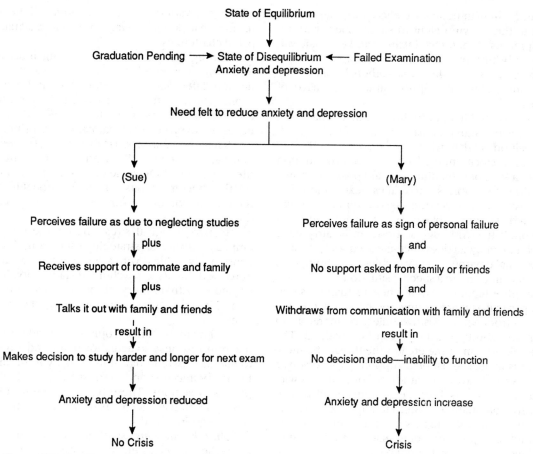

State of Equilibrium

Graduation Pending ⟶ State of Disequilibrium ⟵ Failed Examination
Anxiety and depression

Need felt to reduce anxiety and depression

(Sue)

Perceives failure as due to neglecting studies
plus
Receives support of roommate and family
plus
Talks it out with family and friends
result in
Makes decision to study harder and longer for next exam

Anxiety and depression reduced

No Crisis

(Mary)

Perceives failure as sign of personal failure
and
No support asked from family or friends
and
Withdraws from communication with family and friends
result in
No decision made—inability to function

Anxiety and depression increase

Crisis

Figure 13-2. Paradigm applied to case study. (Aguilera DC, Messick JM: Crisis Intervention: Theory and Methodology, 5th ed, p 71. St Louis, CV Mosby, 1986.)

perceptual process by which a potentially harmful event is distinguished from a potentially beneficial or irrelevant event in one's life.

When a threatening situation exists, a *primary appraisal* is made to judge the perceived effect of the event on one's future goals and values. This is followed by a *secondary appraisal,* in which an individual perceives the range of coping alternatives available, either to master the threat or to achieve a beneficial outcome. As coping activities are selected and initiated, feedback cues from changing internal and external environments lead to ongoing *reappraisals* or to changes in the original perception.

As a result of the appraisal process, coping behaviors are never static. They change constantly in both quality and degree as new information and cues are received during reappraisal activities. New coping responses may occur whenever new significance is attached to a situation.

If, in the appraisal process, the outcome is judged to be too overwhelming or too difficult to be dealt with using available coping skills, an individual is likely to resort to the use of intrapsychic defensive mechanisms, such as denial, to repress or distort the reality of the situation. An appraisal of a potentially successful outcome, however,

is likely to lead to the use of direct action modes of coping such as attack, flight, or compromise.

If the perception of the event is distorted, there may be no recognition of a relationship between the event and feelings of stress. Thus, attempts to solve the problem will be ineffective, and tension will not be reduced.

In other words, what does the event mean to the individual? How is it going to affect the future? Can the individual look at it realistically, or is its meaning distorted? In the example, Sue sees failing the examination as the result of not studying enough, or of concentrating on the wrong material, and decides it will not happen again. On the other hand, Mary thinks that failing the examination makes her a failure; she feels threatened and believes she will never graduate from college.

Situational Supports

Situational supports are people who are available and can be depended on to help solve the client's problem. Situational supports strengthen the individual against feelings of insecurity and reinforce feelings of ego integrity.

By nature, human beings are social, and dependent on others in their environment to supply them with reflected appraisals of their own intrinsic and extrinsic values. In establishing life patterns, certain appraisals are more significant to individuals than others because they tend to reinforce the perception individuals have of themselves.

Loss, threatened loss, or feelings of inadequacy in a supportive relationship may leave the individual in a vulnerable position, so that, when the person is confronted with a stressful situation, the lack of situational support may lead to a state of disequilibrium and possible crisis.

Appraisal of self varies across ages, sexes, and roles. The belief system that forms the basis of self-concept and self-esteem develops out of experiences with significant others in one's life. Although self-esteem is fairly static within a certain range, it does fluctuate according to internal and external environmental variables that impinge on it at a specific time and in a specific situation.

When self-esteem is low, or when a situation is perceived as particularly threatening, the person needs and seeks others from whom positive inflective appraisals of self-worth and ability to achieve can be obtained. The lower the self-esteem or the greater the threat, the more need there is to seek situational supports. Conversely, a person will strive to avoid or withdraw from contacts with individuals perceived as threats, real or imagined, to self-esteem. Any potentially stressful situation can provoke questions of self-doubt as to how one is perceived by others, the kind of impression being made, and the real or imagined inadequacies that might be disclosed.[41]

Success or failure of a coping behavior is always strongly influenced by the social context in which it occurs. The environmental variable most centrally identified is the individual's significant others. It is from them that individuals learn to seek advice and support in solving daily problems. Confidence in being liked and respected by peers is based on past testing and reaffirmations of their expected supportive responses.

Any perceived failure to obtain adequate support to meet psychosocial needs may provoke, or compound, a stressful situation. The receipt of negative support is equally detrimental to an individual's self-esteem.

Sue (see Fig. 13-2) talked to her roommate about her feelings about failing the exam; she even cried on her shoulder. She also called home for reassurance from her family. In effect, she found someone to support her during this stressful event.

Mary did not feel close enough to her roommate to talk about the problem. She had no close friends whom she trusted. Fearing their reaction, she did not call home to tell her family about failing. Mary did not have anyone to turn to for help; she felt overwhelmed and alone.

Coping Mechanisms

Over the years the term *coping* has been used interchangeably with similar concepts, such as adaptation, defense, mastery, and adjustive reactions. Coping activities take a wide variety of forms, including all the diverse behaviors that people engage in to meet actual or anticipated challenges.

Through the process of daily living, individuals learn to use many methods to cope with anxiety and reduce tension. Lifestyles are developed around patterns of response which, in turn, are established to cope with stressful situations. These lifestyles are individual, and quite necessary to protect and maintain equilibrium.

Some theorists propose that coping (as well as other) behaviors are acquired or learned through the course of life experiences. Once the behaviors are found to be useful, they become habits that are functional if they lead to the elimination of the stimulus or tension that activated them.

In psychological stress theory, the term "coping" emphasizes various strategies used, consciously or unconsciously, to deal with stress and tension arising from perceived threats to psychological integrity. It is not synonymous with mastery of problematic life situations; rather, it is the process of attempting to solve the problems.[33]

Coleman[16] defined coping as an adjustive reaction made in response to actual or perceived stress in order to maintain psychological integrity. Within this concept, human beings respond to stress by attack, flight, or compromise reactions. These become complicated by various ego-defense mechanisms whenever the stress becomes ego-involved.

Attack reactions usually attempt to remove or overcome the obstacles perceived as causing stress in life situations. These reactions may be primarily constructive or destructive in nature. *Flight, withdrawal,* or *fear reactions* may be as simple as physically removing the threat from the environment (such as putting out a fire) or removing oneself from the threatening situation (running away from the fire area). They may also involve much more complex psychological maneuvering, depending on the perceived extent of the threat and the possibilities for escape.

The early work of Cannon in 1929[10] provided a basis for later systematic research on the effects of stress on the human organism. According to Cannon's "fight or flight" theory, reactions of acute anxiety, similar to those of fear, are vital to readying the individual physiologically to meet any real or imagined threat to self. From his studies of homeostasis, Cannon described the mechanisms whereby human and other animal life systems maintain steady life states, with the goal always to return to such states whenever conditions force a temporary departure.

Compromise or *substitution reactions* occur when either attack on or flight from the threatening situation is perceived as impossible. This method is most commonly used to deal with problem-solving, and includes the accepting of substitute goals or changing internalized values and standards.

Masserman[40] demonstrated that, under situations of extended frustration, individuals find it increasingly possible to compromise for substitute goals. This often involves the use of rationalization, a defense mechanism whereby "half a loaf" soon appears to be "better than none."

Tension-reducing mechanisms can be overt or covert, and can be consciously or unconsciously activated. They are generally classified into behavioral responses such as aggression, regression, withdrawal, and repression. The selection of a response is based on tension-reducing actions that have successfully relieved anxiety and reduced tension in similar situations in the past. Through repetition, the response may pass from conscious awareness during its learning phase to a habitual level of reaction as a learned behavior. In many instances individuals may not be aware of how or why they react to stress in given situations. Except for vague feelings of discomfort, the rise and consequent reduction in tension may pass almost unnoticed. When a novel stress-producing event arises and learned coping mechanisms are ineffective, discomfort is felt on a conscious level. The need to "do something" about the stress becomes the focus of activity, narrowing perception of all other activities.

Normally, *defense mechanisms* are used constructively in the process of coping. This is particularly evident whenever there is danger of becoming psychologically overwhelmed. All such mechanisms are seen as important for survival. None is equated with a pathologic condition unless it interferes with the process of coping. An example of the latter are destructive defenses used to deny, to falsify, or to distort the perception of reality.

According to Bandura,[5] the strength of the individual's conviction of his or her own effectiveness in overcoming or mastering a problematic situation determines whether coping behavior will even be attempted. People fear and avoid stressful, threatening situations that they believe exceed their ability to cope. They behave with assurance in situations in which they judge themselves able to manage and expect success eventually. The perceived ability to master problem situations can influence the choice of coping behaviors, as well as the persistence used once a behavior is chosen.

People usually rely on available coping mechanisms when they have a problem. Some people sit down and try to think about the problem, or discuss it with a friend. Some "cry it out" or try to get rid of their feelings of anger and hostility by swearing, kicking a chair, or slamming doors. Others may argue with friends, or react by temporarily withdrawing from the situation in order to reassess the problem. These are just a few of the many coping methods people use to relieve their tension and anxiety when faced with a problem. Each method may have been used at some time in the developmental past of the individual, been found effective to maintain emotional stability, and become part of the individual's lifestyle in meeting and dealing with the stresses of daily life.

Sue discussed her problem with her roommate; this reduced her tension and anxiety. She was able to solve the problem, and decided that for the next exam she would study more. Her tension and anxiety were reduced, equilibrium was restored, and she did not have a crisis.

Mary withdrew. She was unable to use, or did not have access to, coping skills, so her tension and anxiety increased. Unable to resolve the problem and unable to function, she went into a crisis.

The Therapists in Crisis Intervention

The Nurse

The need to work effectively in crisis situations is intrinsic to the nursing profession. Crises happen in all areas of nursing practice, in the context of psychiatric emergencies, or in premature births, or in emergency rooms. Wright[58] expressed the experiences of nurses with crises:

> For us, in the front line of illness, accidents, and emergencies, crisis assumes much more personal meaning. We may be faced with the patient, his family, and friends feeling totally overwhelmed and impotent, and being disturbed by some very powerful feelings. This more individual application of the word brings it closer to our own experience and makes 'crisis' more disturbing.

This quote is not meant to emphasize the disturbing nature of crises to the nurse, although such a reaction can occur in the nurse, but to emphasize the frequency with which nurses find themselves working with clients in crisis. Indeed, in health care institutions such as medical or psychiatric hospitals, the nurse is typically the first professional person in "the front line" of care to deal with the crisis.

The preparation of the nurse for crisis work includes education in the meaning of crisis; understanding how and why the crisis event affects the client; and training in crisis intervention techniques. The nurse also receives clinical experience in crisis work during student rotations in the emergency unit, in psychiatric hospitals, and in community health nursing. The box on page 238 describes various locations and roles of nurses who practice crisis intervention.

Hollenkamp and Attala[23] described the use of nurses in the Women's Crisis Shelter for battered women in Belleville, Illinois. This shelter initiated a health program in 1982, out of a recognition of the health needs of women in the shelter. Traditionally, there had been a lack of medical care for the clients who did not have access to a physician. A health program was started at the shelter itself in which a small group of nurses began delivering health care to the women and children as they entered the shelter. "The women and children are screened for acute and chronic illnesses and injuries through an inquiry into health history and current complaints, and a physical assessment."[23]

The functions performed by the nurses include crisis intervention, physical assessment, health teaching, team-building with other staff in the shelter and in the community, and management of health problems, including psychological concerns.

NURSING SETTINGS FOR CRISIS INTERVENTION

1. The psychiatric setting
   Examples: A crisis unit
   An observation unit
   With suicidal/homicidal clients
   With clients who have just gained some difficult emotional insight
   With staff who meet with a psychiatric nurse to discuss staff burnout as a result of working in a crisis environment
2. The medical setting
   Examples: The emergency unit
   Medical/surgical units where clients are informed of diagnoses or prognoses
   Medical/surgical units where clients experience side-effects of drugs or the worsening of a condition
   With staff who meet with a psychiatric liaison nurse to discuss staff burnout as a result of working in a crisis environment
3. Labor and delivery
   Examples: With the pregnant woman who is afraid of delivery
   With the mother and father following the delivery of a child with a birth defect
4. The community
   Examples: The psychiatric nurse doing home care (see Chap. 30) or working in a community mental health center
   The community health nurse who also is visiting clients in the home, although not for identified psychiatric problems of clients
   Community disaster teams
   The nurse serving as liaison to the police department
   The nurse serving as co-worker/trainer of crisis hotline staff

---

The use of crisis intervention skills is important for the nurses working in such a shelter. The clients have left abusive situations at home; frequently they have no personal effects, money, transportation, or employment; they may have physical injuries; few or no support systems may be available to them; and they may have one or more children who are dependent on them for care. These clients exemplify individuals in crisis who have multiple concerns that are temporarily overwhelming and who need the skills of a nurse. Pothier[49] reports that the nurse is underutilized in such community work, but can serve at the "leading edge" of practice by offering services to individuals with needs such as those of the women in the Women's Crisis Center.

Further examples of psychiatric nurses on the "leading edge" of practice include:

1. *Student* nurses studying crisis intervention who work in the community with policemen to formulate crisis teams for working with family disturbance calls[55]
2. Psychiatric nurses who coordinate the placement of individuals in homes of families who assist clients in coping with a crisis over a three- to five-day period.[9]

Paraprofessionals

Rusk[53] reported an increased trend toward the use of paraprofessionals in functions once considered only within the domain of the highly-skilled professional. Leaders in community mental health were keenly aware of the many dangers inherent in random, unplanned deprofessionalization of major mental health functions. Concern was voiced about the lack of definitive, established criteria for the different levels of educational preparation and experience required of those who conduct various "therapies." Increasing numbers of paraprofessionals are now being provided with additional education and training to function as consultants or "therapists" in mental health centers.

As new roles and careers have been created, some are being formed within well-structured, formal educational and training programs. Others, however, have evolved gradually and informally, often in response to specific needs of innovative programs.

A prototype of the model for new careers in mental health was established by Lincoln Hospital Mental Health Services in New York City. According to Collins,[17] in a report on this program, local residents were trained to serve as mental health aides in neighborhood mental health service centers. Rather than functioning as extensions of the professional, the aides serve as liaisons to help bridge the social and experimental gap separating the middle-class professionals and the lower-class clients.

Non-Mental Health Professionals

Other resources for manpower that have been recruited into liaison activities with community programs are *non-mental health professionals.* These are professional individuals who serve primarily other functions within their communities. Common to all is their traditional role of helping people who are in trouble. Included in this group are the medical professionals, teachers, lawyers, clergy, policemen, firemen, social and welfare workers, and so on. In the course of their daily work activities, these highly-skilled individuals can be found functioning in what could be called the front lines of preventive mental health care. They are frequently in contact with individuals and groups who are in potential crisis situations because of a loss, or the threat of a loss, in their lives. Most often these professionals become the initial contact made by a person in crisis. Many new programs have been developed to include them as active participants on treatment teams.

Nonprofessional Volunteers

Nonprofessional volunteers are another human resource being recruited by mental health centers. Not only are they used in the traditional volunteer roles, but they are also seeking training to develop skills to meet their human needs to be creative, to help others, to be recognized, to learn new skills, and to become meaningful members of treatment teams.

Crisis hot lines, initially established by professionals and community leaders, rely heavily on nonprofessional volunteers for their 24-hour-a-day, 7-day-a-week services. According to Clark and Jaffe,[14] these hot lines seem to have originated in both the traditional mental health care institutions and in groups of private citizens. Nonprofessionals were carefully selected, intensively trained, and closely supervised in these original psychiatric emergency centers.

Team Approach to Crisis

A recent development has been the increasing use of the team approach to crisis intervention. Crisis team members are selected, on the basis of their expertise, to meet the specific needs of each client in crisis. Crisis team members vary with the structure and requirements of individual mental health centers, as well as with the geographic and socioeconomic needs of the community. The unique skills of each member are used from the time of initial contact until the crisis is resolved and follow-up support is no longer believed to be necessary.

Team membership is open-ended, expanding and contracting within highly flexible boundaries. Leadership of each team depends on the member who has the skills and expertise most appropriate to help the individual resolve the crisis. This is not to say, however, that ultimate professional responsibility is removed from the physician. Rather, there is a broader delegation of authority to make decisions in treatment planning.

Nurses, psychiatrists, psychologists, and social workers may work as a team in a crisis intervention unit in a psychiatric hospital. The client in crisis is hospitalized for from one to five days, and intensive work is done to help the client resolve the crisis. Team members rapidly enlist the support of significant others in the client's environment, and quickly involve the client in individual, group, and family counseling.

Local mental health centers often have an emergency plan for a crisis team mobilization in the event of a disaster in the community, such as the flooding of homes. In such an event, the team works to first attend to acute medical and psychiatric needs of the victims. In the first hours after the crisis event, "all activities must be directed at developing useful procedures that will be of immediate value to the victims."[15]

As mental health professionals, psychiatric nurses serve to provide mental health care to crisis victims. A family, for example, who lost their home in a flood had a wife who was angry and hostile and a husband who experienced alcohol withdrawal. Cohen[15] reported that in this family the mental health professional was able to elicit a story of marital difficulties between the couple prior to the disaster. "There existed a strong, dependent need to control the other's behavior."[15] Both spouses agreed to a transfer to a local hospital. The mental health care professional called the hospital during the transfer of the couple, and prepared it for the couple's arrival. The crisis team member also shared with the hospital staff the nature of the couple's behavior within the crisis context of the disaster.

Crisis team members working with victims of disasters also maintain close communication with each other. This is encouraged by a team leader who regularly keeps members informed of the activities of the total team.

After the immediate crisis period and for up to six months after the disaster period, a psychiatric nurse and other mental health professionals plan with victims how their life can be restructured after the devastating effects of the disaster. Victims, for example, need help in relocating or obtaining disaster relief. They also may need help to maintain the relationships within the family unit if the unit was conflict-laden prior to the disaster.

The Therapeutic Use of Self

According to Caplan,[13] human beings are constantly faced with a need to solve problems in order to maintain equilibrium. When they are confronted with an imbalance between the difficulty (as they perceive it) of a problem and their available repertoire of coping skills, a crisis may be precipitated. If alternatives cannot be found, or if solving the problem requires more time and energy than is usual, disequilibrium occurs. Tension rises and discomfort is felt, with associated feelings of anxiety, fear, guilt, shame, and helplessness.

One purpose of the crisis approach is to provide the consultation services of a therapist, such as a nurse skilled in problem-solving techniques. This does not mean that the nurse will have an answer to every problem. However, the nurse will be expected to have a ready and informed competency in problem-solving, guiding, and supporting the client toward crisis resolution. The therapeutic goal for the individual seeking help is the establishment of a level of emotional equilibrium equal to, or better than, the pre-crisis level.

Crisis intervention involves "exploring and examining the present situation with the client and/or the client's family. This is not an intellectual exercise but must involve the feelings of the client, and this is undertaken by helping the client to feel safe with the nurse."[58] There are a number of occurrences that may increase the difficulty in enabling the client to feel safe with the nurse. The nurse may be in a uniform, which can seem impersonal. There may be confusion at the scene, diverting the

Relevant Research

This report presents a description of a crisis-oriented residential treatment program and a cost-effectiveness analysis of the crisis-oriented center. The center described is one of 13 similar programs in the state of California.

The center (called La Posada) was developed as an alternative to hospital treatment. It combines two separate treatment modalities: the crisis intervention model, and the halfway house or social rehabilitation model. The program offers one to two weeks of intensive crisis intervention therapy in a home environment for acutely psychotic and suicidal clients whose degree of control over their behavior does not require a locked hospital unit.

Upon measuring the characteristics of clients at La Posada, the author found that 33% of the clients admitted to the program over a 1½-year period were "decompensating clients who do not yet require hospitalization." Such admissions are examples of *secondary prevention,* which includes early case-finding and treatment. In the case of La Posada, the treatment focuses on functioning of the client in the environment in order to increase independence; individual, group, and family therapy; and continuing socialization that resembles community living. To account for the remaining percentages of admissions to the program, the author found that 30% were direct admissions to La Po-

sada; 28% were admissions of individuals who had stayed a few days on a locked psychiatric hospital unit; and the remaining individuals voluntarily decided to be treated at La Posada rather than face involuntary psychiatric hospital admission.

Eight to ten residents usually live at La Posada at any one time. The program is staffed by various professionals at all times. Approximately 270 clients are admitted to the program each year. Over a 20-month period, 71% of admissions were "acutely psychotic and severely depressed clients." Most clients were "chronic patients" with a norm of four psychiatric hospitalizations prior to admission to La Posada.

Entering La Posada means "becoming part of a familylike community, which in turn imparts certain behavioral expectations in a powerful yet noncoercive manner." These expectations are *greater than expectations typically found* in other traditional psychiatric hospital units, according to the researcher.

Symptoms decrease within two to three days of the client's entering the program. Discharge typically occurs within nine days of admission, and at discharge clients are involved in outpatient therapy. "The cost per day per crisis treatment at La Posada is one third of the cost per day of hospitalization."

(Weisman G: Crisis-oriented residential treatment as an alternative to hospitalization. Hosp Community Psychiatry 36:1302, 1985)

client's attention. There may be a number of individuals who could use the nurse's assistance, and the client may not want to take the nurse's time. It is hoped that the nurse's "empathy and individuality will help the nurse to understand the client's difficulties and feelings."[58]

According to Wright, the nurses first offer their sense of humanity. The nurse is concerned with the "pain, distress, and difficulty"[58] of the client. The nurse expresses this empathically to the client. Importantly, the nurse evaluates whether or not the client understands that the nurse is empathic. For example, the client may sigh deeply after the nurse has expressed an understanding of the client's distress, and seem unburdened. Clients who do not seem to receive caring from another individual, such as the nurse, can be told verbally that the nurse is concerned. The nurse could say, "I can imagine that what you lost was very important to you. That must hurt you deeply." Some clients, in times of crisis, are oriented only to themselves and simply will not hear empathic messages from the nurse. With these clients, the nurse can listen and encourage the client to talk about the crisis experience.

Morley and others[43] recommended seven attitudes that are important adjuncts to the specific crisis intervention techniques. In essence, these constitute the general philosophical orientation necessary for the full effectiveness of the nurse-therapist.

1. It is essential that the therapist view the work being done not as a "second-best" approach but as the treatment of choice with clients in crisis.

2. Accurate assessment of the presenting problem, not a thorough diagnostic evaluation, is essential to an effective intervention.
3. Both the therapist and the client should keep in mind throughout the contacts that the treatment time is limited, and should persistently direct their energies toward resolution of the presenting problem.
4. Dealing with problems not directly related to the crisis is not appropriate in this kind of intervention.
5. The therapist must be willing to take an active, and sometimes directive, role in the intervention. The relatively slow-paced approach of more traditional treatment is inappropriate in this type of therapy.
6. Maximum flexibility of approach is encouraged. Diverse techniques, such as serving as a resource person or information-giver and taking an active role in establishing a liaison with other helping resources, are often appropriate in specific situations.
7. The therapist's goal is explicit. Energy is directed entirely toward returning the individual to at least the pre-crisis level of functioning.

When faced with clients in crisis, it is common for nurses to experience stressful emotions such as fear, anxiety, confusion, or nervousness. It is crucial, however, that nurses be extremely careful not to transmit their emotions to the client. If this happens, clients have to deal with their own crisis as well as the secondary burden of the nurses' emotions. A client in crisis is frightened and vulnerable, with feelings of being out of control. Extra emotions at this time, caused by the nurse, could force clients into aggressive or potentially lethal outbursts of emotion.

Rather than displacing their emotions onto the clients, a better and healthier alternative for nurses is to talk about their feelings with supervisors or experienced crisis intervention nurse-therapists. Many new nurses find it helpful to role-play a crisis intervention situation with other staff nurses or professionals in order to allay their anxiety and fear before finding themselves in a crisis situation. Therapeutic use of self tools are role-modeled and shared to give the new nurse a feeling of security and know-how for impending situations.

Levels of Prevention

Hendricks[22] reported that some "individuals are crisis-prone due to specific circumstances in their lives that help them be more susceptible to crises." Crisis-prone people may demonstrate one or more of the characteristics in the following box. A nurse functioning at the primary level of prevention who cares for clients demonstrating such characteristics can talk with the client to clarify the meaning of the characteristics to the client and to discuss possible behavioral changes. Such a dialogue may decrease the likelihood of the development of a crisis.

If the first interaction that a nurse has with a client utilizes crisis intervention techniques detailed in this chapter, then *tertiary prevention* is being implemented as the nurse strives to bring the client back to a previous level of functioning. It would be safe to say, therefore, that both primary and secondary prevention techniques had been ineffective if the client had been in contact with health care professionals preceding the crisis. However, in the majority of situations, the client did not come to the attention of a health care professional until the crisis was impending. Most often, the client turns to nonprofessionals first—a spouse, a friend, or another family member who is not equipped to intervene with the magnitude of emotions at hand. The best intervention for the untrained person is to refer the client to crisis intervention professionals immediately, in hope of avoiding the crisis stage—therefore intervening on a *secondary prevention* level, described in other chapters in this text.

Cultural Considerations

All of the ethnic, racial, occupational, and age groups who live at the socially-, culturally-, and economically-deprived margins of society are usually categorized by some as "lower-class." Much of the tone of literature about them has had a negative quality. Socioeconomic programs have always seemed to be more interested in what could be done *for* them, rather than what could be done *with* them. Recently there has been an emphasis on a new theme, that of recognizing the strengths of these groups, rather than just their weaknesses, and of going into their communities and working in a cooperative effort *with them* to make the changes that the deprived groups feel are most necessary.

Nurses are well aware that the attitudes of society toward mental illness are a keystone in the development of any treatment program. These attitudes should be determinants of the goals of the services that are offered. To be effective, a program should be meaningful to, and seen as needed by, the community groups it is meant to reach.

Crisis intervention is not restricted to people at lower sociocultural or economic levels. However, because of a variety of factors, it is thought that crisis intervention techniques are more effective for those at this level than are other types of therapy.

Jacobson[26] stated that motivating forces have universal elements that precede cultural differences. Typically, people are wary of strangers, and need time to assess new situations and strangers in the environment. Under stressful circumstances they are usually guarded in their speech and controlled in their actions. In emergency situations such as fires, earthquakes, and other catastrophes, individuals work together freely; barriers to communications are lowered, and sociocultural levels are disregarded. This also occurs when a person is in a crisis and comes for help. The element of strangeness is quickly overcome as the client and the nurse concentrate on relieving the symptoms of stress, although they may be from different sociocultural backgrounds.

The time-limiting factor of crisis intervention is a distinct advantage with individuals in lower sociocultural and economic groups who focus on the present and want relief of their symptoms as soon as possible. Crisis inter-

---

CHARACTERISTICS OF CRISIS-PRONE INDIVIDUALS

1. Unemployment, underemployment, or dissatisfaction with their present occupation or position
2. Drug abuse (including alcohol)
3. Difficulty coping with minor problems, *i.e.,* problems encountered by the general population on an everyday basis
4. Low self-esteem, persistent feelings of insecurity
5. History of unresolved crises or emotional disorders
6. Underutilization of support systems or minimal access to support systems (personal, family, social)
7. Few permanent relationships (personal, employment, homes)
8. Feelings of alienation from others (family, friends, society)
9. Demonstrates impulsiveness and an uncaring attitude
10. History of frequent personal injuries and/or frequent involvement in property damage incidents

(Hendricks J: Crisis Intervention: Contemporary Issues for On-Site Interveners. Springfield, Illinois, Charles C Thomas, 1985)

vention is directed toward helping individuals solve specific problems. In crisis intervention, changes in personality traits and behavioral changes are not expected, nor are they the focus of therapy sessions. This lessens the threat to clients, because individuals do not have to expose a complete pattern of living, that may be different from those of the therapists.

Community mental health centers serve individuals from different sociocultural levels. Psychotherapy for an extended period of time may be too expensive for an average middle-class family or person, and it may not be needed if a crisis situation exists. Those who may now be considered middle-class may have originally come from a lower sociocultural background, and may retain misconceptions about psychotherapy and mental illness.

Referrals to community mental health centers come from many sources. Family physicians may decide that individuals need help with emotional problems and refer them for assistance; attorneys, juvenile authorities, clergy, family-service agencies, and others may also make referrals. The community itself is usually aware, through publicity (radio, television, newspapers, word-of-mouth, and liaison personnel), of a mental health center's function and the services available. Because of this publicity and the center's location in the community, it may serve many "walk-in" clients.

Conversely, referrals *from* a community mental health center are also diversified and are usually highly-individualized. Individuals may be referred directly for hospitalization if they are dangerously suicidal or homicidal; for longer-term therapy after crisis intervention for chronic problems; to a family service agency, if needed; or to a rehabilitation center.

The attitudes about mental illness in our society continue to be less than favorable. An aura of fear and anxiety still surrounds overt mental disturbance. Much of this is the result of the distorted ideas about what happens when a person "goes crazy" or "insane"—ideas that have been reinforced by the mass media.[56] Many movies, television programs, and works of fiction about mental illness include elements of fear, loss of control, and questionable "recovery." Some of these are believable, yet are grossly exaggerated for impact and saleability.

Lower sociocultural and economic groups, in particular, generally fear mental illness.[45,46,52] Often, they fail to admit the presence of a mental illness until there are overt psychotic behaviors. Frequently, they ask for outside help only when individuals become a danger to themselves or to others. Frequently, the first "help" that people in these groups receive is from the police, who are called in to protect the family and others from the mentally-ill person. Too often, the family still tries to keep the disturbed member at home, until it is too late and the individual becomes unmanageable.

Many cultural reasons exist for this. Many people still consider mental illness an inherited trait, passed on from generation to generation. To admit that there is a history of mental illness "in the family" could destroy plans for pending marriages or business associations, and, most certainly, the family's status in the community.

Those from lower socioeconomic groupings fear mental illness for good reason. Hollingshead and Redlich's study[24] showed that individuals in lower socioeconomic groups constituted the largest population in state hospitals, and received more custodial care. Individuals from lower socioeconomic levels saw mental illness as *craziness,* not as illness. They saw institutionalization as the only answer. Fearing this end, they avoided seeking help, even when it was obviously needed.

Other factors have been recognized as pertinent, basic needs of sociocultural and economic groups that must be met in treatment programs.* Generally, people in these groupings are here-and-now oriented because they cannot afford to wait for tomorrow and later. Too often theirs is a day-to-day existence. They have no reason to save for a rainy day because for them it rains every day.

Crisis intervention is appealing because of its cost. If day laborers have to choose between keeping clinical appointments and getting a few hours of work, they will have to have concrete proof that they will get help if they keep the appointment, and will expect immediate feelings of relief from their symptoms.

Socioculturally- and economically-depressed families have had long experience with help from outsiders; the past history of social intervention from outsiders has not done much to build their trust. Many have learned to mistrust the well-intentioned social welfare agencies that saw fit to move the aged or infirm away from their homes and into institutions "for their own good." They are familiar with situations in which children have been taken from "unfit" parents and placed in foster homes or similar child care agencies. Too often their families have been measured against middle-class norms and found lacking in stability. Ineffective outside action has led only to further instability. How can they be expected to trust the mental health profession? Historically, the mental health profession has taken adverse actions against them or neglected them completely.

Even more concretely, until they have proof that conversation or "talking treatment" crisis intervention will help them, their basic needs for survival will outweigh any appeals to them to help identify their emotional needs. Not knowing what to expect or value from psychiatry, they cannot be expected to express their needs immediately.

The Therapeutic Process in Crisis Intervention

Differences Among Therapeutic Modalities

While the therapeutic process in crisis intervention has some elements in common with other therapeutic mo-

---

* References 8, 21, 38, 52, 59, 23, 39.

dalities, there are distinct differences. Specifically, crisis intervention differs from psychoanalysis and brief psychotherapy in its goal, focus of treatment, and duration, and in the behavior of the therapist. The differences between crisis intervention and psychoanalysis and brief psychotherapy are outlined in Table 13-2.

Psychoanalysis

In *psychoanalysis,* the goal of therapy is to restructure the personality; the focus of treatment is on past traumatic experiences and the freeing of the unconscious. Psychoanalytic psychotherapeutic procedures are usually divided into two functional categories: the *supportive* (suppressive) and the *uncovering* (exploratory or expressive) procedures. The therapist's role is nondirective, exploratory, and that of a passive observer. This type of therapy is indicated for individuals with neurotic personality patterns. The length of therapy is indefinite, and depends on the individual and the therapist.

Brief Psychotherapy

Brief psychotherapy aims to remove specific symptoms and to prevent the development of deeper neurotic or psychotic symptoms. Its focus is on: the past, as it relates to the present situation; repression of the unconscious; and the restraining of drives. The role of the therapist is indirect, and that of a participant observer. The basic tools used are psychodynamic intervention coupled with medications or environmental types of interventions. Indications for brief psychotherapy are acutely disruptive emotional pain, severely disruptive circumstances, and situations endangering the life of the individual or others. It is also indicated for those who have problems that do not require psychoanalytic intervention. Another indication involves the life circumstances of the individual: if the person cannot participate in long-term therapy, which implies a stable residence, job, and so forth, brief therapy is advocated to alleviate disruptive symptoms. The average length of treatment is from one to twenty sessions. Some dynamic brief psychotherapy approaches condense the longer-term psychoanalytic work into a brief time period, but not all clinicians practice according to this model.

It is imperative that the patient feel relief as rapidly as possible, even during the first therapeutic session. The span of treatment can be any reasonable, limited number of sessions, but is usually more than six and fewer than twenty. Circumstances associated with disrupted functioning are more easily accessible if they are recent. Generally, only active conflicts are amenable to brief psychotherapy. Disequilibrated states are more easily resolved before they have crystallized, acquired secondary gain features, or developed into highly maladaptive behavior patterns.

Crisis Intervention

The goal of *crisis intervention* is the resolution of an immediate crisis. The therapist's role is direct, suppressive (in seeking to aid the client attain emotional control), and that of an active participant. Techniques vary, and are

TABLE 13-2.
MAJOR DIFFERENCES BETWEEN PSYCHOANALYSIS, BRIEF PSYCHOTHERAPY, AND CRISIS INTERVENTION METHODOLOGY

	PSYCHOANALYSIS	BRIEF PSYCHOTHERAPY	CRISIS INTERVENTION
GOAL OF THERAPY	Restructuring the personality	Removal of specific symptoms	Resolution of immediate crisis
FOCUS OF TREATMENT	1. Genetic past 2. Freeing the unconscious	1. Genetic past as it relates to present situation 2. Repression of unconscious and restraining of drives	1. Genetic present 2. Restoration to level of functioning prior to crisis
USUAL ACTIVITY OF THERAPIST	1. Exploration 2. Passive observer 3. Nondirective	1. Suppressive 2. Participant observer 3. Indirect	1. Suppressive 2. Active participant 3. Directive
INDICATIONS	Neurotic personality patterns	Acutely disruptive emotional pain and severely disruptive circumstances	Sudden loss of ability to cope with a life situation
AVERAGE LENGTH OF TREATMENT	Indefinite	One to twenty sessions	One to six sessions

(Aguilera DC, Messick JM: Crisis Intervention: Theory and Methodology, 5th ed, p 27. St Louis, CV Mosby, 1986)

limited only by the flexibility and creativity of the therapist. Some of these techniques include: helping the individual to gain an intellectual understanding of the crisis; assisting the individual to bring feelings into the open; exploring past and present coping mechanisms; finding and using situational supports; and anticipatory planning with the individual, to reduce the possibility of future crises. The indications for this type of therapy are an individual's (or family's) sudden loss of ability to cope with a life situation. The average length of treatment is from one to six sessions.

Crisis intervention extends logically from brief psychotherapy. The minimum therapeutic goal of crisis intervention is psychological resolution of the individual's immediate crisis and restoration to *at least the level of functioning that existed before the crisis period.* A maximum goal is improvement in functioning above the pre-crisis level.

Caplan emphasizes that crisis is characteristically *self-limiting,* and lasts from four to six weeks. The crisis is a transitional period, representing both the danger of increased psychological vulnerability and an opportunity for personality growth. In any particular situation the outcome may depend, to a significant degree, on the ready availability of appropriate help. On the basis, the length of time for intervention is from four to six weeks, with the median being four weeks.[26]

Because time is limited, a therapeutic climate is generated that commands the *concentrated attention* of both therapist and patient. A goal-oriented sense of commitment develops, in sharp contrast to the more modest pace of traditional treatment modes.

Approaches to Crisis Intervention

Jacobson and associates[27,28] state that crisis intervention may be divided into two major categories: generic and individual. These two approaches are complementary.

Generic Approach

A leading proposition of the *generic approach* is that there are certain recognized *patterns of response* in most crises. Many studies have substantiated this thesis. For example, Lindemann's[35] studies of bereavement found that there is a well-defined process that a person goes through in adjusting to the death of a relative. He referred to these sequential phases as *grief work,* and found that failure of a person to grieve appropriately, or to complete the process of bereavement, can lead to future emotional illness.

Subsequent studies of generic patterns of response in stressful situations have been reported. Kaplan and Mason[31] and Caplan[13] studied the effects on the mother of the birth of a premature baby, and identified four phases or tasks that she must work through to ensure healthy adaptation to the experience. Janis[29] suggested several hypotheses concerning the psychological stress of impending surgery and the patterns of emotional response that follow a diagnosis of chronic illness. Rapoport[50] de-

fined three subphases of marriage, during which unusual stress can precipitate crises. These are only a few of the broad research studies that have been done in this field.

The generic approach focuses on the *characteristic course of the particular kind of crisis* rather than on the psychodynamics of each individual in crisis. Specific intervention measures are designed to be effective for all members of a given group rather than for the unique differences of one individual. Recognition of these behavioral patterns is an important aspect of preventive mental health.

Tyhurst[57] suggested that knowledge of patterned behaviors in transitional states, occurring during intense or sudden change from one life situation to another, might provide an empirical basis for the *management* of these states and the prevention of subsequent mental illness. He cites as examples the studies of individual responses to community disaster, migration, and retirement of pensioners.

Jacobson and associates[28] stated that generic approaches to crisis intervention include "direct encouragement of adaptive behavior, general support, environmental manipulation, and anticipatory guidance. . . . In brief, the generic approach emphasizes (1) specific situational and maturational events occurring to significant population groups, (2) intervention oriented to crisis that is related to these specific events, and (3) intervention carried out by non-mental health professionals."[28]

This approach is a feasible intervention mode that can be learned and implemented by nonpsychiatric physicians, nurses, social workers, and others. It does not require a mastery of knowledge of the intrapsychic and interpersonal processes of an individual in crisis.

Individual Approach

The *individual approach* differs from the generic in its emphasis on assessment, by a professional, of the interpersonal and intrapsychic processes of the person in crisis. It is used in selected cases, usually those that do not respond to the generic approach. Intervention is planned to meet the unique needs of the individual in crisis and to reach a solution for the particular situation and circumstances that precipitated the crisis. This differs from the generic approach, which focuses on the characteristic course of a particular kind of crisis.

Unlike extended psychotherapy, there is relatively little concern with the developmental past of the individual. Information from this source is seen as relevant only for the clues that may result in a better understanding of the present crisis situation. Emphasis is placed on the immediate causes of disturbed equilibrium and on the processes necessary for regaining a pre-crisis or higher level of functioning. Jacobson cited the inclusion of family members or other important people in the process of the individual's crisis resolution as another area of differentiation from most individual psychotherapy. In comparison with the generic approach, he viewed the individual approach as emphasizing the need for greater depth of understanding of the individual's biopsychosocial process, with interventions oriented to the individual's unique situation, and carried out only by mental health professionals.

Change: The Problem-Solving Approach In Crisis Intervention

Another approach in crisis intervention considers the *sequence of reasoning* that must be done for an individual to resolve a crisis and change. Problem-solving requires that a logical sequence of reasoning be applied to a situation in which an answer is required for a question and in which there is no immediate source of reliable information.[7] This process may take place either consciously or unconsciously. Usually the need to find an answer or solution is felt more strongly when such a resolution is most difficult.

The problem-solving process follows a structured, logical order of steps, each depending on the preceding step. In the routine decision-making required in daily living, this process is rarely necessary. Most people are unaware that they may follow a defined, logical sequence of reasoning in making decisions. Often they only realize that some solutions seem to have been reached more easily than others. Finding out the time, or deciding which shoe to put on first, rarely calls for long, involved reasoning; usually the question arises and the answer is found without any conscious effort.

Factors Affecting the Problem-Solving Process.

Depending on past experiences related to the immediate problem, some people are more adept at finding solutions than are others. Both internal and external factors affect the process at any given time, although initially there may be only a temporary lack of concrete information. For example, when a driver finds himself lost because of a missing road sign, how much finding the right directions means to him in terms of his physical, psychological, and social well-being could affect the ease with which he finds an answer to the problem. Anxiety increases in proportion to the value he places on finding a solution. If he is only out driving for pleasure, for example, he may feel casually concerned; if he is under stress to be somewhere on time, his anxiety may increase according to the importance of his reaching his goal.

When anxiety is kept within tolerable limits, it can be an effective stimulant to action. It is a normal response to an unknown danger. It is experienced as discomfort, and helps the individual to mobilize resources to meet the problem. But as anxiety increases there is a narrowing of perceptual awareness, and all perceptions are focused on the difficulty. When problem-solving skills are available, the individual is able to use this narrowing of perceptions to concentrate on the problem at hand.

If a solution is not found, anxiety may become more severe. Feelings of discomfort become intensified, and perceptions are narrowed to a crippling degree. The ability to understand what is happening and to make use of past experiences gives way to concentration on the discomfort itself. Individuals become unable to recognize their own feelings, the problem, the facts, the evidence, and the situation in which they find themselves.[48]

Although problem-solving involves a logical sequence of reasoning, it is not always a series of well-defined steps. According to Meyer and Heidgerken,[44] it usually begins with a feeling that something has to be done. The problem area is generalized, rather than made specific and well-defined. Next, there is a search of the memory in an attempt to come up with ideas or solutions from previous similar problems. March and Simon[39] refer to this as "reproductive problem-solving," and its value is greatly dependent on past successes in finding solutions.

When no similar past experiences are available, individuals may next turn to "productive problem-solving." Here they are faced with the need to construct new ideas from more or less raw data. They have to go to sources other than themselves to get facts. For example, the driver looking for the road sign may find someone nearby who can give him the needed new data—directions to the right road. If there is no one nearby, he will have to find some other source of information. He may resort to trial and error, and with luck and patience find the way himself. Finding a solution in this way may meet a present need, but the information gained may not always be applicable to solving a similar problem in the future.

Problem-Solving in Crisis Intervention.

Dewey[19] proposed the classic steps or stages of problem-solving: (1) a difficulty is felt, (2) the difficulty is located and defined, (3) possible solutions are suggested, (4) consequences are considered, and (5) a solution is accepted. With minor modifications, these steps in problem-solving have been persistent over the years. Johnson[30] simplified problem-solving by reducing the number of steps to three: preparation, production, and judgment.

In 1962, Merrifield and others[42] conducted extensive research on the role of intellectual factors in problem-solving. They advocated return to a five-stage model: preparation, analysis, production, verification, and reapplication. The fifth stage was included in recognition of the fact that the problem-solver often returns to earlier stages of the five-stage model in a kind of revolving fashion.

According to Guilford,[20] the general problem-solving model involves the following processes: (1) input (from environment and soma), (2) filtering (attention aroused and directed), (3) cognition (problem sensed and structured), (4) production (answers generated), (5) cognition (new information obtained), (6) production (new answers generated), (7) evaluation (input and cognition tested, answers tested, new tests of problem structure, new answers tested).

Steps in Crisis Intervention: The Nursing Process

There are certain specific steps involved in the technique of crisis intervention.[43] Although each step cannot be placed in a clearly-defined category, typical intervention would pass through the following sequence of phases:

Assessment

The first phase is the assessment of the individual and the problem. This requires the use of active focusing techniques on the part of the therapist to obtain an accurate assessment of the precipitating event and the resulting crisis that brought the individual to seek professional help. The therapist may have to judge whether the person seeking help presents a high suicidal or homicidal risk. If clients are thought to be dangerous to themselves or to others, referral is made to a psychiatrist for consideration of hospitalization. In the event that hospitalization is not deemed necessary, the intervention proceeds. The initial hour may be spent entirely on assessing the circumstances directly related to the immediate crisis situation.

It is important that both the therapist and the client be able to define a situation clearly before taking any action to change it. Questions are asked such as, "What do I need to know"? and "What must be done"? The more specifically the problem can be defined, the more likely it is that the "correct" answer will be sought.

Clues are investigated to point out and explore the problem or what is happening. The therapist asks questions and uses observation skills to obtain factual knowledge about the problem. It is important to know what has happened within the immediate situation. How the individual has coped in past situations may affect present behavior. Observations are made to determine the client's level of anxiety, expressive movements, emotional tone, verbal responses, and attitudinal changes. The client may cry, look exhausted, ask the same question repeatedly, or look disheveled.[4]

It is important to remember that the therapist's task is to focus on the immediate problem. There is not enough time and no need to explore the patient's past history in depth.

One of the therapist's first questions is usually, "Why did you come for help today?" It is important to emphasize the word *today*. Sometimes individuals try to avoid stating why they came by saying, "I've been planning to come for some time." The therapist's usual reply is, "Yes, but what happened that made you come in *today?*" Other questions to ask are, "What happened in your life that is different? When did it happen?"

In a crisis, the precipitating event has usually occurred within 10 to 14 days before the individual seeks help. Frequently it is something that happened the day before or the night before, and could include: threat of divorce, discovery of a spouse's extramarital relations, finding out that a son or daughter is using drugs, loss of a boyfriend or a girlfriend, loss of a job or status, an unwanted pregnancy, and others.

The next area on which to focus is the individual's perception of the event: What does the event mean to the client? How does the individual see its effect on the future? Does the client see the event realistically, or is its meaning distorted?

The client is then questioned about available situational supports: What person in the environment can the therapist find to support the client? With whom does the client live? Who is the client's best friend? Whom does the client trust? Is there a member of the family to whom the client feels particularly close? Crisis intervention is sharply time-limited, and the more people involved in helping the person, the better. Also, when therapy is terminated, if others are involved and familiar with the problem they can continue to give support.

The next area of focus is to ascertain what the person usually does when a problem arises that cannot be solved: What coping skills are used? The client is asked the following questions: "Has anything like this ever happened to you before? How do you usually abate tension, anxiety, or depression? Have you tried the same method this time? If not, why not, if it usually works for you?" If the client's usual method was tried and it did not work, the therapist asks why. The therapist also asks the client for suggestions of ways to reduce symptoms of stress. Something is usually suggested; coping skills are very individual. Methods of coping with anxiety that have not been used in years may be remembered. One man recalled that he used to "work off tensions" by playing the piano for a few hours, and it was suggested that he try this method again. Since he did not have a piano, he rented one; by the next session his anxiety had reduced enough to enable him to begin problem-solving.

One of the most important parts of the assessment is to find out whether the individual is suicidal or homicidal. The questions must be very direct and specific: "Are you planning to kill yourself or someone else? How? When?" The therapist must find out and assess the seriousness of the threat. Is the individual merely thinking about it, or has a method been selected? Is it a lethal method—a loaded gun? Has a tall building or a bridge been picked out? Can the client tell you when he or she plans to do it—for example, after the children are asleep? If the threat does not seem too imminent, the individual is accepted for crisis therapy. If the intent is carefully planned and details are specific, hospitalization and psychiatric evaluation are arranged in order to protect the client or others in the community.

Diagnosis

As noted earlier in this chapter, a crisis event precipitates emotional strain and stress.[36] This strain shows itself in a multitude of potential symptoms. Some individuals withdraw when experiencing a crisis. Others do not withdraw, but become ineffective in their various roles.

The classifications of nursing diagnoses describe several diagnostic categories related to crisis responses. These include:

21. Alterations in Conduct/Impulse Control (includes 21.06, Disorganized Behavior)[2]
23. Alterations in Role Performance (includes 23.01.04, Role Loss/Disengagement, and 23.02.01, Withdrawal)[2]

Coping, ineffective family: Compromised[32]
Coping, ineffective family: Disabling[32]
Coping, ineffective individual[32]
Grieving, dysfunctional[32]

Planning Therapeutic Intervention

After an accurate assessment is made of the precipitating event(s) and the crisis, intervention is planned. This is not designed to bring about major changes in the personality structure, but to restore the person to at least the precrisis level of equilibrium. Information is also sought to determine what strengths the individual has, what coping skills may have been used successfully in the past and are not being used presently, and what other people might be used as supports for the individual. Alternative coping methods, not presently being used, are sought. This step is essentially a thinking process in which alternatives are considered and evaluated against past experience and knowledge, as well as in the context of the present situation.

In the planning phase, goals are established. In an example of parents who feel their premature baby may die and are therefore in crisis, short-term goals state that the parents will understand the exact status of their child's health, and that they will express feelings they are suppressing. Long-term goals include making the parents understand why they are in crisis, testing new ways of coping, and restoring family functioning.

Intervention

The nature of intervention techniques is highly dependent on the skills, creativity, and flexibility of the therapist. Morley[43] suggested that therapists can intervene with patients by:

1. Helping the individual gain an intellectual understanding of the crisis. Often the individual sees no relationship between a hazardous situation occurring in life and the extreme discomfort of disequilibrium that is being experienced. The therapist can use a direct approach, describing the relationship between crisis and the event in the client's life.

2. Helping the individual discuss present feelings that may not be easily accessible (Fig. 13-3). Frequently the person has suppressed some very real feeling,

such as anger or other inadmissible emotions toward someone that should be loved or honored. The feelings involved may be denial of grief, feelings of guilt, or incompletion of the mourning process following bereavement. An immediate goal of intervention is the reduction of tension by providing a means for the individual to recognize these feelings and bring them into the open. It is sometimes necessary to produce emotional catharsis (such as crying or verbalizing anger) and to reduce immobilizing tension.

3. Exploring coping mechanisms. This approach requires assisting the person to examine alternative ways of coping. If, for some reason, the behaviors the patient used successfully in the past to reduce anxiety have not been tried, the possibility of their use in the present situation is explored. New coping methods are sought; frequently, the person devises some highly original methods that have never been tried before.

4. Reopening the social world. If the crisis was precipitated by loss of someone significant to the person, the possibility of introducing new people to fill the void can be highly effective. It is particularly effective if supports and gratification previously provided by the "lost" person can be achieved to a similar degree from new relationships.

In addition to the points mentioned above, specific directions may be given for what should be tried as tentative solutions. This enables the individual to leave the first session with some positive guidelines for going out and testing alternative solutions. At the next session the individual and therapist evaluate the results and, if none of these solutions has been effective, they work toward finding others.

In summary, the therapist identifies: (1) the crisis-precipitating event, (2) symptoms that the crisis has produced in the individual, (3) the degree of disruption evident in the individual's life, and (4) the plan for intervention. Planned intervention may include one technique or a combination of several techniques. The individual may be helped to gain an intellectual understanding of the crisis, or helped to explore and ventilate

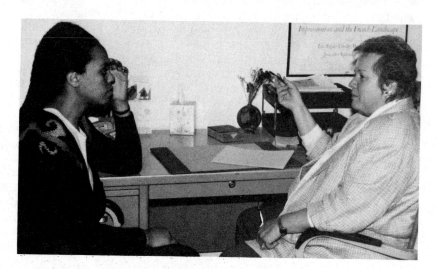

Figure 13-3. A psychiatric nurse works with a client in crisis.

feelings. Other techniques may be to help the individual find new and more effective coping mechanisms or use other people as situational supports. Finally, a plan is presented for helping the client to establish realistic goals for the future.

Evaluation

An *evaluation* is made to determine whether or not the planned action has produced the expected results and goals attained. Appraisal must be objective and impartial in order to be valid. Has the individual returned to the usual or a higher level of equilibrium in functioning? The problem-solving process is continued as the therapist and the individual work toward resolution of the crisis.

In this last phase of the nursing process, the therapist reinforces the adaptive coping mechanisms that the individual has used successfully to reduce tension and anxiety. As coping abilities increase and positive changes occur, they may be summarized to allow the client to reexperience and reconfirm the progress that has been made. Assistance is given, as needed, in making realistic plans for the future, and there is a discussion of ways in which the present experience may help in coping with future crises.

Case Study

The following case study illustrates how a therapist worked effectively in crisis intervention with a married couple whose sociocultural background was different from her own.

Tony and Marta, a young married couple with four small children, came to a crisis intervention center and requested help. They had originally gone to their parish priest for advice, and he recommended that they seek professional help at a nearby community center. Tony, an unskilled laborer, worked as a maintenance man for an airline. He had finished the eighth grade in school. Marta had finished nine years of school and had worked in a garment factory until just before the birth of their first child. They lived in a poor section of town, in a house owned by Tony's mother. Their only recreation was watching television. Tony usually worked six or seven days each week.

Tony was very angry and suspicious at the beginning of the session; Marta appeared frightened and was reluctant to talk. When asked by the therapist "why they had come to the center today," Tony replied that he thought his wife was "crazy"; he then began to explain her behavior. The afternoon before, Marta had caught their oldest son (Joe, nine years old) playing with matches behind the house. She had flown into a rage, pulled him into the house, and burned his arm by holding it over the flame of the kitchen stove. Tony's mother had walked in while Joe was screaming. The grandmother, having learned what had happened, grabbed Marta and forced her arm over the flame so she "could see how it felt." When the therapist asked Marta if this was true, she nodded her

head and began to cry. The therapist asked to see Marta's arm. Together they removed the bandage from the large, second-degree burn. Marta said she had put a patented burn medicine and a dressing on it. The therapist told Marta that she would like a doctor to see her arm to possibly give her an antibiotic prescription and some medicine to help relax. A medical consultation was arranged. While Marta saw the physician, the therapist met with Tony.

(Therapist's note: This maneuver served two purposes: first, it showed Marta and Tony that the therapist wanted to provide immediate help; and second, by a nonjudgmental attitude and acceptance of their behavior, the therapist established a basis for rapport.)

When Tony was alone with the therapist, he dropped his defensive attitude and showed his true concern for Marta's irrational behavior. When questioned about Marta's usual manner of coping with problems, he stated that he really did not know; usually she just "blew up" at him; since it did not bother him, he ignored it. He stated that he loved his wife and children and he believed that she loved him and the children, too. When asked what he and Marta usually did together, and with the children, for pleasure, he said, "Are you kidding? I work six or seven days a week—hard! I come home and I'm tired; I have a few beers, eat, and usually fall asleep in front of the T.V." When asked what Marta usually did, he stated that she "takes care of the house and the kids."

When Marta returned from the medical consultation, the therapist repeated what Tony had said. Marta replied, "That's true—that's all I do: take care of his mother's crummy house and the kids!" Tony burst out immediately, "You have never gotten along with my mother—you hate her!" Marta said that she did not hate her; she just did not like her "always butting into our business, and you always taking her side against me and the kids! I've told you I don't like living in *her* house, where she can walk in and out anytime she wants to. I want a place I can call my own. We pay her rent; we can pay rent someplace else—and get a better house too!"

Tony said, "You never told me you didn't want to live in Mother's house." Marta replied, "I have, but you never listen!"

When asked about the possibility of moving, since Marta was unhappy with the living arrangements, Tony said his mother would "not understand," but, he continued, "Marta and the kids mean more to me than anything."

The therapist thought at this time that she should refocus on the problem that had brought them into the center. She asked Marta about burning Joe's arm. Marta said, "I was tired and upset. All I ever hear are the kids yelling and Tony's mother butting in and telling me everything I'm doing wrong with the kids and the house. Tony never tries to help or even listen to me. I just felt like I was cracking up!"

Tony was asked if there was any way he could help Marta. The therapist explained that taking care of four small children every day without a few hours "off" can be very exhausting. The therapist went on to tell Tony that his work kept him in contact with people all day, whereas

Marta had no contact with anyone except his mother (who was an added irritant) and the children. Marta said that if only she could look forward to talking with him when she was upset, or even if she could go over to a friend's house for a few hours once or twice a week—"anything to get away for a few hours!"—she knew she would be all right.

Tony, very reluctantly, said that he would put the kids to bed one night for Marta so she could go to a friend's house. The therapist said that it sounded like a wonderful idea, and that it would be good for both of them to get out for a few hours together to talk things over. Their reaction was a cautious silence.

When Tony and Marta came for their next session, it was very obvious that they had had a good week. They were talking together quite animatedly when the therapist came into the waiting room to get them for their appointment. She remarked how well and happy they looked. Marta started talking about their week: Tony had put the kids to bed one night, as he had said he would, and she had gone to a friend's house to visit. She said it was really great to be out for a few hours. When Tony was asked how he had managed with the children, he looked embarrassed and said, "It was a mess! I don't know how she ever manages them all—no wonder she gets so tired!" It seemed that Tony could not get the children to go to sleep, or even stay in bed, without Marta there to control them. Finally, he had brought them all into the living room to watch television. When they had fallen asleep he had carried them to bed, one by one. The highlight of the week had come when Tony told his mother not to come to the house and bother Marta. He had said that if she did, he and Marta would find another house and move. This had made Marta feel so much better that she had backed down a bit and told her mother-in-law that she could visit them, but that she ought to call in advance to say that she was coming. The therapist told them how well they were doing in working toward solving their problem, but cautioned them that there would be good weeks and bad weeks. If they began to talk *with* each other when problems arose, rather than *at* each other, they could work out solutions more easily.

At the next session Marta had apparently returned to her pre-crisis state, and Tony and she were relaxed and comfortable with each other and the therapist. Tony began by saying that they both really felt that they were capable of handling their problems now and did not want to return for more visits. He said that he now could really understand Marta's feelings of being "hemmed in" and "trapped" when she was with the children constantly—all day, every day. He said a friend at work had invited them over for dinner the Saturday before and, instead of refusing as he usually did, he had accepted. He had asked his mother to stay with the children, and he and Marta had gone to dinner. He said that as he had watched Marta laughing and talking he had realized how much he had missed their being together, alone, "like before we were married. I watched her and realized how pretty and young she really is and how much I love her. I'm going to do everything I can to help her with the kids—I know we can make it now!" The therapist agreed and wished

them luck, and told them if they needed help again to feel free to return to the center.

Summary of Case Study

The therapist in this situation, although from a middle-class background, was aware of the sociocultural background of her clients, and this knowledge was invaluable in her approach toward working with them. Her attitude was nonjudgmental, concentrated on getting some immediate "help" (the medical consultation), and focused on assisting them with their problem. She worked on the "here-and-now," and was very directive. Although she offered suggestions, no attempt was made at major changes in behavior. The terminology was kept at a concrete level. She attempted to give them the feeling that she was there to help them and that she would be there in the future, if necessary.

Summary

1. Crisis intervention can fulfill needs for immediate problem-solving.
2. Crisis intervention is direct, is short-term, and seeks to assist the client to return to the level of functioning (or a higher level) that existed prior to the crisis event.
3. The types of crises include (a) maturational, those crises normally associated with particular developmental stages, and (b) situational, those accidental events that can precipitate a crisis in coping.
4. Balancing factors determine whether an individual will experience a crisis. They include: how the individual perceives the crisis event, the availability of supports (resources) to use in coping with the crisis, and personal coping skills.
5. The nurses' therapeutic use of self includes the ability to establish trust quickly with the clients, to assist clients to deal with their emotions. At the same time nurses must effectively cope with their own emotions, and remain flexible in therapeutic approaches.
6. Nurses can identify with clients certain characteristics that may indicate a tendency or proneness toward experiencing crises.
7. Nurses use the problem-solving approach of the nursing process to label clients' problems rapidly and work with the clients to resolve the crises.

References

1. Aguilera D, Messick J: Crisis Intervention: Theory and Methodology. St Louis, CV Mosby, 1986
2. American Nurses' Association: Taxonomy for the Classification of Human Responses of Concern for Psychiatric/Mental Health Nursing Practice (working draft). Kansas City, American Nurses' Association, 1986
3. American Psychiatric Association: Diagnostic and Statistical Manual of Mental Disorders-III-R. Washington, DC, American Psychiatric Association, 1987

4. Baird S: Helping the family through a crisis. Nurs 87 17:66, 1987
5. Bandura A, Adams N, Beyer J: Cognitive processes mediating behavioral change. J Pers Soc Psychol 35:125, 1977
6. Bellak L, Small L: Emergency Psychotherapy and Brief Psychotherapy. New York, Grune & Stratton, 1965
7. Black M: Critical Thinking: An Introduction to Logic and Scientific Method. Englewood Cliffs, New Jersey, Prentice-Hall, 1946
8. Bloch H: An open-ended crisis-oriented group for the poor who are sick. Arch Gen Psychiatry 18:178, 1968
9. Britton J, Mattson-Melcher: The crisis home: Sheltering patients in emotional crisis. J Psychosoc Nurs Ment Health Serv 23:18, 1985
10. Cannon W: Bodily Changes in Pain, Hunger, Fear, and Rage. New York, Appleton, 1929
11. Caplan G: A public health approach to child psychiatry. Ment Health 35:235, 1951
12. Caplan G: An Approach to Community Mental Health. New York, Grune & Stratton, 1961
13. Caplan G: Principles of Preventive Psychiatry. New York, Basic Books, 1964
14. Clark T, Jaffe D: Change within youth crisis centers. Am J Orthopsychiatry 42:675, 1972
15. Cohen R: Crisis Counseling Principles and Services. In Lystad M (ed): Innovations in Mental Health Services to Disaster Victims. Rockville, Maryland, National Institute of Mental Health, 1985
16. Coleman J: Abnormal Psychology and Modern Life. Chicago, Scott-Foresman, 1950
17. Collins J: The paraprofessional: I. Manpower issues in the mental health field. Hosp Comm Psychiatry 22:362, 1971
18. Cropley A, Field T: Achievement in science and intellectual style. J Appl Psychol 53:132, 1969
19. Dewey J: How We Think. Boston, Boston Health Co, 1910
20. Guilford J: The Nature of Human Intelligence. New York, McGraw-Hill, 1967
21. Hartog J: The mental health problems of poverty's youth. Ment Hyg 51:85, 1967
22. Hendricks J: Crisis Intervention: Contemporary Issues for On-Site Interveners. Springfield, Illinois, Charles C Thomas, 1985
23. Hollenkamp M, Attala J: Meeting health needs in a crisis shelter: A challenge to nurses in the community. J Comm Health Nurs 3:201, 1986
24. Hollingshead A, Redlich F: Social Class and Mental Illness. New York, John Wiley & Sons, 1958
25. Inkeles A: Social structure and the socialization of competence. Harv Ed Rev 36: 1966
26. Jacobson G: Crisis theory and treatment strategy: Some sociocultural and psychodynamic considerations. J Nerv Ment Dis 141:209, 1965
27. Jacobson G: Crisis theory. New Dir Ment Health Serv 6:1, 1980
28. Jacobson G, Strickler M, Morley W: Generic and individual approaches to crisis intervention. Am J Pub Health 58:339, 1968
29. Janis I: Psychological Stress: Psychoanalytical and Behavioral Studies of Surgical Patients. New York, John Wiley & Sons, 1958
30. Johnson D: The Psychology of Thought and Judgment. New York, Harper & Row, 1955
31. Kaplan D, Mason: Maternal reactions to premature birth viewed as an acute emotional disorder. Am J Orthopsychiatry 30:539, 1960
32. Kim M, McFarland G, McLane A: Classification of Nursing Diagnoses: Proceedings of the Fifth National Conference. St Louis, CV Mosby, 1984
33. Lazarus R: Psychological Stress and the Coping Process. New York, McGraw-Hill, 1966
34. Lazarus R: The Psychology of Coping: Issues in Research and Assessment. In Coelho D, Hamburg D, Adams J (eds): Coping and Adaptation. New York, Basic Books, 1974
35. Lindemann E: Symptomatology and management of acute grief. Am J Psychiatry 101:101, 1944
36. Lindemann E: The meaning of crisis in individual and family. Teachers Coll Rec 57:310, 1956
37. Lowenstein R: Psychology of the Ego. In Alexander F, Eisenstein S, Grotjahn M (eds): Psychoanalytic Pioneers. New York, Basic Books, 1966
38. McMahon J: The Working Class Psychiatric Patient: A Clinical View. In Riessman F, Cohen J, Pearl A (eds): Mental Health of the Poor. New York, Free Press, 1964
39. March J, Simon H: Organizations. New York, John Wiley & Sons, 1963
40. Masserman J: Principles of Dynamic Psychology. Philadelphia, WB Saunders, 1946
41. Mechanic D: Social Structure and Personal Adaptation: Some Neglected Dimensions. In Coelho D, Hamburg D, Adams J (eds): Coping and Adaptation. New York, Basic Books, 1974
42. Merrifield P: The Role of Intellectual Factors in Problem-Solving. Psychol Monogr 76:10, 1962
43. Morley W, Messick J, Aguilera D: Crisis: Paradigms of Intervention. J Psychiatr Nurs 5:538, 1967
44. Meyer B, Heidgerken L: Introduction to Research in Nursing. Philadelphia, JB Lippincott, 1962
45. Myers J, Bean L, Pepper M: A Decade Later: A Follow-Up of Social Class and Mental Illness. New York, John Wiley & Sons, 1968
46. Myers J, Roberts B: Family and Class Dynamics in Mental Illness. New York, John Wiley & Sons, 1959
47. Ovesy L, Jameson J: Adaptational Techniques of Psychodynamic Therapy. In Rado S, Daniels G (eds): Changing Concepts of Psychoanalytic Medicine. New York, Grune & Stratton, 1956
48. Peplau H: Interpersonal Relations in Nursing. New York, GP Putnam, 1952
49. Pothier P: The Issue of Prevention in Psychiatric Nursing. Arch Psychiatr Nurs 1:143, 1987
50. Rapoport L: The state of crisis: Some theoretical considerations. Soc Serv Rev 36:211, 1972
51. Rappaport D: A Historical Survey of Psychoanalytic Ego Psychology. In Klein G (Ed): Psychological Issues. New York, International Universities Press, 1959
52. Riessman F, Scribner S: The underutilization of mental health services by workers and low-income groups: Causes and cures. Am J Psychiatry 121:798, 1965
53. Rusk T: Future changes in mental health care. Hosp Comm Psychiatry 22:7, 1972
54. Salzman L: Developments in Psychoanalysis. New York, Grune & Stratton, 1962
55. Sullivan-Taylor L: Policemen and nursing students: Crisis intervention teams. J Psychosoc Nurs Ment Health Serv 23:26, 1985
56. Tershakovek A: An observation concerning changing attitudes toward mental illness. Am J Psychiatry 121:353, 1964
57. Tyhurst J: Role of Transition Status—Including Disasters—in Mental Illness. Symposium on Preventive and Social Psychiatry, Walter Reed Institute of Research. Washington, DC, U.S. Government Printing Office, April 15–17, 1957
58. Wright B: Caring in Crisis. New York, Churchill Livingstone, 1986
59. Yamamoto J, Goin M: On the treatment of the poor. Am J Psychiatry 122:267, 1965

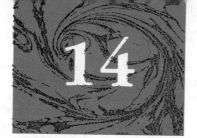

KATHLEEN L. PATUSKY

MILIEU THERAPY

Learning Objectives

Upon completion of this chapter the student should be able to do the following:

1. Define milieu therapy.
2. Differentiate between milieu therapy and the therapeutic community.
3. Identify five functional variables inherent in the milieu setting.
4. Describe three behavioral goals of the milieu and the related nursing roles.
5. Describe elements of milieu organization and related policies.
6. Discuss the role of discharge planning in the milieu setting.
7. Describe two specialized types of milieu therapy.
8. Identify four special problem areas in the milieu setting and discuss appropriate staff responses for each.
9. Discuss theoretical considerations that influence milieu therapy, with particular emphasis on communication theory.
10. Identify two major legal/political issues affecting the future of milieu therapy.
11. Identify three areas of future application for milieu therapy.

Introduction

The prospect of a first day on a psychiatric unit can be unsettling for a nurse. Getting used to this foreign environment engages all of one's energy—and it may be difficult to think of being therapeutic. But there is a method of dealing with this environment. The key lies in understanding *milieu therapy.*

This chapter explores milieu on two levels—the *concrete components* of the system, and the *conceptual framework* underlying the components. In the process, we will examine the historical roots of this therapeutic modality, related issues of the nursing role and system efficacy, and potential applications. Armed with this knowledge, the nurse will find the transition to inpatient psychiatry relatively painless and will understand what is observed.

First, it is helpful to know the nature of milieu therapy. Milieu is the French word for setting or environment. Hence, milieu therapy involves using and manipulating the environment in a therapeutic manner. A number of terms are used synonymously with milieu therapy, although controversy exists about whether these terms are actually interchangeable. Names such as therapeutic community, administrative therapy, social psychiatry, sociotherapy, socioenvironmental psychotherapy, and therapeutic milieu are frequently used.

Purists insist that two relatively distinct entities exist, namely milieu therapy and the therapeutic community. Using this distinction, *milieu therapy* refers to any program or setting that manipulates or exploits any part of the environment for therapeutic purposes. This generally alludes to behavioral aspects that influence psychological response, but is not limited specifically to psychiatric settings. For example, the physical make-up of most hospital medical units is not considered to be a therapeutic milieu, although the outcome for the client is certainly therapeutic. However, changes in a medical unit's make-up in order to influence the client's psychological response would be an application of milieu therapy.

The *therapeutic community,* in contrast, is a specific type of therapeutic technique. The basic concepts and philosophy of a therapeutic community are consistent with those of milieu therapy, but focus more on social interactions than on individual personality or response to the environment.[17] Further, the therapeutic community may rely primarily on a particular treatment modality (*e.g.,* psychoanalysis or transactional analysis), which influences its selection of treatment components and its interpretation of interactions.

Milieu therapy and therapeutic communities do share certain basic attributes. First, in both there is an emphasis on the conscious use of environment. This includes concern for the physical environment, the atmosphere of the psychiatric unit, attitudes and interactions among staff and clients, and social organization. Second, active participation is required of clients in the planning and implementation of their treatment. The focus is on clients' taking charge of changes that they will implement in their lives, rather than being passive recipients of the staff's absolute powers of healing. Third, there is a recognition that the psychiatric unit forms a community and culture of its own. As such, it acts as a microcosm of the outside world while developing its own rules and identity.[9]

Every psychiatric unit is comprised of a milieu in which the environment is used to promote health. The question is how deliberately and rigidly that milieu is structured. Consequently, the nurse can expect the attributes described above to be present in all cases, although the emphasis placed on the various attributes may differ between any two units. Once familiar with the basic elements, however, the nurse is prepared with reasonable expectations for the therapeutic environment. As with any new culture, once the nurse learns the basic rules and dynamics, and experiments with responding within this new culture, it will no longer seem foreign.

Historical Development of Milieu Therapy

Early Developments

The first milestone in the evolution of milieu therapy required a conceptual shift in attitude concerning the mentally ill and their right to the most basic standards of care. The work of Phillipe Pinel is generally noted as the introduction of humane reform. However, as far back as the 15th century, Spanish hospitals treating mental illness practiced an approach to care that influenced Pinel's thinking. Their environment included a good diet, adequate hygiene, activity programs, and the removal of shackles. For the first time, recipients of care were considered patients rather than inmates. Emphasis was placed on involvement in the hospital work force, from farming to caring for the sick. Capable patients were assigned to supervise more disturbed individuals. Patient occupation was considered an important factor in treatment outcome. Unfortunately, the decline of the Spanish empire following the Napoleonic Wars also saw the demise of this humane treatment for the mentally ill.[23]

Better known is the 18th century's era of "moral treatment," traditionally starting with Phillipe Pinel's recognition of the need for reform in France. This coincided with the spirit of the French Revolution. Pinel believed that the mentally ill were entitled to the same liberty, equality, and fraternity as were other citizens. His work at the Bicêtre prison-institution in 1793, and the Salpêtrière Hospital in 1795, improved care through the removal of shackles and the separation of violent patients from those who were calm. Pinel was rewarded by dramatic, positive changes in patient behavior.[7,23]

The United States, an amalgam of religious and egalitarian social concerns, entered its own era of "moral treatment" in the 1800s. In keeping with the social environment of rapid change, growth, and crude innovation, this era was inconsistent and fragmented. Individuals such as Benjamin Rush spearheaded limited efforts at humane care for the mentally ill, instituting change at only a few hospitals and only with the elite. Progress was complicated by growing social forces of urbanization, industrialization, and increased immigration. Mental hospitals grew in size and became custodial institutions, with increasing evidence of decaying facilities and neglectful care.[23]

By the mid-1800s, reform was again necessary. Dorothea Dix literally conducted a one-woman crusade to convince state legislatures of the need for improved conditions. While custodial care would remain the focus of treatment until after World War II, overall environmental conditions were improved. In a prophetic move made in the 1880s, the McLean Asylum for the Insane in Massachusetts opened a school for nurses and attendants. The curriculum emphasized the provision of individualized environmental adjustment as a part of patient treatment. However, the idea did not take hold until revived at the Menninger Sanitarium some 50 years later.[23]

Admittedly, reform in those days of "moral treatment" focused primarily on physical care and environment. It must be remembered that, prior to this movement, mental patients were seen as little better than criminals. Society did not accept these patients as human beings. That they deserved amenities like decent food and shelter, clothing, adequate heat, sanitation, or freedom from shackles was a new concept. However, the acceptance of these new standards was crucial to further advances in the development of milieu therapy.

The second milestone involved a conceptual shift in the etiology and treatment of mental illness. The late 19th century emphasis on organic disorders and the early 20th century advances in neurology set the stage for new attitudes toward treatment. Classifications of mental disease by Kraepelin and others helped sort out treatable dementias due to nutritional deficiencies or toxic effects. A clearer picture began to emerge of the sets of symptoms connected with specific diagnoses. At long last, mental illness was being presented in a manner similar to that of medical disorders. Its legitimacy gradually increased, and the possibility of treatment could finally be considered. In 1909, the work of Freud was introduced in the United States, providing an option for therapy as well as a model for intrapsychic mechanisms. The forces of scientific change rapidly gained momentum as treatment and individual psychology became active issues.[23]

The 20th Century

The beginning of the 20th century saw the first awareness that individuals exist in social environments, and should be dealt with accordingly. The work of Adolf Meyer and Ernest Southard in the early 1900s emphasized a holistic concept of human beings, a concern with past as well as present experiences, and a need to identify social forces interacting with individuals. The concurrent work of the National Committee for Mental Hygiene, under the leadership of Clifford Beers, fostered further improvements in hospital treatment of patients and in public education about mental illness.[23] While psychiatry continued its focus on psychobiology and organic theories of illness, psychosocial models, with emphasis on analytic theory, grew in importance.

Between 1900 and 1920, the little-known work of Hermann Simon in Germany incorporated the rudiments of milieu therapy in hospital settings. A system of treatment was established on the premise that patient behavior is responsive to expectations. Labeled by Simon as *activere behandlung* or *more active therapy,* the approach involved assigning patients to work and activities that were closely related to their status and background, and then encouraging success with increasingly demanding tasks. This mode of treatment spread to other German hospitals under the name *milieutherapie.* Alas, as with other prophetic innovations, this therapeutic movement succumbed to social forces, namely Hitler's rise to power.[3]

Ironically, military hospitals in the U.S. were among the first hospitals to use milieu concepts in psychiatry following World War I. However, this contribution actually had begun earlier with the historical focus of military medical settings. Emphasis on wellness and manipulation of the environment began as a means of maintaining discipline, but was inadvertently therapeutic. With the potential chaos of dormitory-style wards and low staff-to-patient ratios, a superstructure of authority and regulation was instituted as a functional necessity. The result was a program that worked.

Initially, this practice was not specific to psychiatry. Most military hospital wards observed the same basic rules, including units treating the families of active-duty personnel. (Officers and children, along with the gravely ill, were generally exempt from many ward rules.) Inpatients were expected to participate in their own treatment by attending to their own hygiene needs, making beds, keeping bedside areas clean, and even washing their own beds on discharge. Active-duty patients knew that "sick call" (the equivalent of staff rounds) meant that they were to stand at attention at the foot of their beds, address the doctors as if talking with their commanding officer, and give a clear accounting of their symptoms. By the same token, the patient's rank and seniority were observed appropriately and responded to by the staff. The senior enlisted person on each ward was designated Master at Arms. He was responsible for organizing "field day," using all ambulatory patients as his work crew. Once morning treatments were completed, these patients were put to work waxing floors, dusting, running errands, and carrying out an expanded definition of activities of daily living. Not only was the ward kept clean, but individual independence was maximized and problems with stasis were minimized.

Nursing emphasized helping patients to help themselves. Military hospitals have changed with the times, and this milieu-oriented system has been diluted on all but psychiatric or alcohol rehabilitation units. Many nurses who have experienced this system decry its erosion with the advent of semiprivate rooms and "civilianization" of medical care. Certainly, military nurses remember cases in which optimal functioning was achieved merely by expecting it.

The application of this lesson, combined with battlefield experiences of World Wars I and II, led to concepts of combat psychiatry that strongly influenced military psychiatric treatment. Concepts such as group cohesion, purposefulness of behavior, impact of labeling, expectancy of behavior, and brief interventions continue to influence modern military treatment.[10] As we will discuss later, many of these concepts are basic to milieu therapy.

In the civilian sector, the application of psychosocial theory, in the form of a rudimentary milieu therapy, began to emerge in isolated settings. Its primary competition lay in modalities such as insulin coma and electroshock therapies. Still, the emphasis was finally shifting from merely custodial care to treatment. In 1932, William Menninger described the need for hospitals to respond to patient needs, rather than forcing adaptation of patients to the institution. Employing psychoanalytic concepts at the Menninger Sanitarium, he advocated a total treatment environment, with scientifically-determined relationships between patients and staff, specially selected and trained staff, daily activity schedules, and individual contact for each patient.[23]

As psychosocial concerns became more prominent in institutions for the mentally ill, the first therapeutic social club was started in 1938 in England by Joshua Bierer. Providing rehabilitative social activities for mental patients, the program was initiated in a hospital setting and served acute and convalescing patients of various diagnoses. Following World War II, a similar club called Fountain House was started in the U.S. by a group of patients from Rockland State Hospital.[9] Socialization, patient involvement, and recreation were now recognized as important to treatment.

This, then, is the historical backdrop of milieu therapy. Changes in attitudes toward the mentally ill, knowledge of etiology and treatment options, and awareness of psychosocial factors were prerequisite to the first modern applications of a therapeutic environment. The rest is almost anticlimactic, yet it is at this point that milieu therapy is said to have begun.

Maxwell Jones is credited with the conceptual leap when, in 1953, he described an entire treatment modality centering on the psychiatric unit as a therapeutic environment.[14,15] The importance of this work lies in its identification of milieu as an adjunct to psychotherapy and medication, and in its emphasis on social interaction theory. *The Therapeutic Community* is a seminal work that fostered a new era of research and development in treatment. Studies based on Jones's work have explored topics such as patient behavior in response to staff conflicts[26] and the development of social systems in psychiatric hospitals.[11] Experiments with the application of milieu concepts have involved specific populations such as delinquents,[25] substance abusers,[6] and even entire families.[2,4] Today, research is more likely to address the efficacy of milieu treatment or its comparison with other modalities, but the proof of Maxwell Jones's work, and that of his predecessors, lies in the universal application of milieu concepts in psychiatric treatment settings.

Theoretical Framework

The Person as a System

In the course of individual therapy, the illusion may exist that the only partners in treatment are the client and the therapist. The fallacy of this illusion becomes abundantly clear once one has experienced the treatment process in a milieu setting. While individual client–therapist sessions are often conducted at set intervals, it is now recognized that the environment of the unit plays a crucial role in translating the clients' insights into concrete behavioral changes. The phrase, "The whole is more than the sum of its parts" is most poignant and meaningful when it is applied to human beings. Consequently, milieu therapy seeks to provide treatment by addressing all elements that make people who they are. To go one step further, however, milieu therapy does not merely manipulate or rearrange these elements. Milieu is itself a system of intricate processes that seeks to have a profound impact on that dynamic system we identify as the person.

System Components of the Person

While individuals cannot be understood solely by reducing them to a list of mechanical parts, the process they go through to define themselves as individuals can be viewed in terms of contributing components. Milieu therapy considers these components, and uses them realistically by setting up a microcosm of the forces that influence individuals outside of the therapeutic setting.

The physical and psychological make-up of individuals, as well as their cultural background, are elements they bring to the setting that are essential to an understanding of their world view. The societal and environmental components are equally important, although these components may have been altered temporarily by their removal (*e.g.*, absence of a negative peer influence or provision of a safe environment). Milieu therapy seeks to understand the individuals' perceptions of these components. The milieu process then introduces alternative views and options. Individuals are helped to formulate healthy and reasonable changes when necessary, while strengthening elements that already serve the individuals' welfare.

Nursing Process

The nursing process is closely intertwined with milieu therapy, and provides the expert dimension of the therapeutic use of self. All facets of the nursing process occur continuously. They are not applied in discrete increments (*e.g.*, assessment and planning on admission, evaluation on discharge). Rather, the process applies to each interaction, as well as to the overall progress of the client. Because milieu therapy generally occurs in settings that function around the clock, this means the nursing process also functions continually.

Levels of Prevention

Milieu therapy operates predominantly at a tertiary level of prevention, providing rehabilitative services. The aim is to return the client to a level of function that either is optimal or will permit continued outpatient treatment.

Milieu therapy also contributes to primary prevention by addressing potential problems identified through the nursing process. Patient teaching, focused on anticipated difficulties, can be readily incorporated into the milieu setting to use the clients' strengths in promoting problem-solving skills. Discharge groups, for example, may encourage clients to imagine how they might respond to questions about their illness during a job interview. This enables clients to build a repertoire of responses, thereby preventing a panic reaction during a real interview. Secondary prevention, or case-finding and early treatment, may be a part of milieu treatment, but is seldom applied when outpatient therapy will suffice.

The Therapeutic Process

Consider, for a moment, an individual who seeks treatment for a particular psychological or behavioral problem. When the person becomes a client in most outpatient or private-practice therapy settings, the client brings to each session a set of concerns and intrapsychic dynamics that have caused pain or discomfort in everyday life. The client and the therapist explore these concerns and dynamics, discuss alternatives for change, and arrive at a plan of action that the client is expected to implement between sessions. After the session, the therapist welcomes the next client as the first client leaves the therapy setting and reenters the outside world free to exercise the plan of action or not.

This is a very clean, neat, precise arrangement between two people—but a limited arrangement, based on a number of assumptions. It presumes honesty and openness on the part of the client, so that the therapist receives a true picture of the situation the client wishes to resolve. Denial, other defense mechanisms, or even blatant dishonesty muddle and lengthen the problem-solving process. The process presumes sufficient motivation on the part of clients to overcome the normal human impulse to resist change. It presumes a sufficient degree of ego strength on the part of clients to withstand pressure by significant others to continue unchanged. It further presumes that clients will avail themselves of opportunities to practice new skills and apply new insights. Most of all, it presumes that these clients possess sufficient impulse control to avoid creating a major disaster between sessions (*e.g.,* suicide or assaultive behavior).

Most practicing therapists are aware of these limitations, and use the therapeutic process to address them. But a therapist working on an intermittent basis may find it impossible to provide safe and effective treatment without hospitalization. Thus, the environment of the psychiatric unit becomes the means of dealing with an otherwise untenable situation.

Functional Variables of a Milieu

Ultimately, the purpose of a milieu program is to provide a treatment environment that enhances and contributes to therapy. Gunderson[12] described five functional variables that a milieu can offer. That is to say, he discussed the purpose of milieu in terms of five therapeutic activities that relate closely to the limitations of outpatient treatment described above. These variables include containment, support, structure, involvement, and validation.

Containment

Containment functions to preserve the physical integrity of the client. On a basic level, it entails the provision of food, shelter, and clothing. It also involves elements of the environment related to safety, such as screened windows, locked doors, and the use of nonbreakable materials. Unit policies and procedures address containment with the availability of medical care and special precautions against self-destructive or assaultive behavior. Danger exists, however, in interpreting this facet of the milieu approach as a license to exert strict control over behavior. The benefit of containment lies in providing the client with a sense of safety in a setting where self-control and personal power can be exercised with support and assistance. Containment is not meant to imply suppression. This aspect of milieu fails in its function when the emphasis turns to staff expediency rather than therapeutic necessity. At the same time, containment becomes of primary importance in crisis intervention or admission units, where clients are most likely to act on uncontrolled impulses.

Support

Support serves as a means of decreasing the client's level of anxiety, promoting trust, and increasing the ability to participate in therapy. It further acts to foster self-esteem. Support includes a wide variety of measures, from assistance with everyday behaviors, to actions designed for improving ego function, to verbal recognition of the client's reality and progress. Encouraging reluctant clients to participate in therapies and activities that are new, and therefore frightening to them, also comes under this heading. While an emphasis on nurturing is helpful to many individuals in crisis, this approach has its drawbacks. Carried too far, it can confirm the clients' beliefs that they are incapable of functioning autonomously and that dependency is the best option. It may also undermine the clients' acceptance of personal responsibility. Predominantly supportive environments are especially countertherapeutic for borderline and paranoid clients, who may feel smothered or threatened by the closeness. On the other hand, reasonable support is a part of most milieu programs and is particularly effective with special populations, such as autistic or developmentally-disabled individuals.

Structure

Structure provides a predictable framework within which a number of milieu concepts operate best. Consistency promotes a sense of trust and safety. Activities within the unit structure furnish opportunities for clients to practice adaptive behavior and test alternatives, while learning that their actions carry consequences and that they are capable of delaying gratification of impulses. Structure also sets up the rules for appropriate behavior. Unit organization is the primary focal point for this variable. Client governments, step or privilege systems, token economies, mandatory participation in meetings, and regulation of daily activities are a few means of achieving the desired structure. The problem with an overemphasis on structure is in its artificial and simplistic nature. Once the rules of this mini-society are learned, it is possible for clients to display appropriate behavior at the expense of their individuality. Pathology may lie dormant and untreated. As a result, the unit organization itself may compromise clients' ability to receive optimal treatment and readjust to the less structured environment outside the hospital. Still, the use of structure is quite helpful in the treatment of many psychotic or short-term disorders, and acts as a cornerstone for behavior modification units.

Involvement

Involvement fosters healthy initiative on the part of the client, supports adaptive function and social skills, and provides an arena for reality-testing and feedback. Involvement includes not only encouraging or requiring participation in activities, but also placing the client in a position of responsibility on the unit, as with an elected client representative who conducts community meetings. An important facet of this variable is the transmission of a clear message that individuals are important, and that they have an impact on everyone else around them. This is a two-sided coin, however. The community is there to share joys and triumphs, but the community also has a variety of responses to clients' negative experiences or self-destructive behaviors. This is quite a revelation to many clients. On the negative side, some clients may react with hostility to a perceived loss of privacy. Most units do not allow "secrets" between staff and clients, in order to maintain openness. This is dealt with by encouraging clients to reveal their "secrets" to the community, while insisting that suicidal (or similar) ideations will not be kept hidden from the people around them. Involvement is common in milieu programs, particularly with alcohol or drug abuse populations (Fig. 14-1).

Validation

Validation focuses on clients as individuals and affirms their individual identities. Gunderson uses the term validation in a manner that goes beyond merely agreeing with the clients' perceptions. A cause-and-effect relationship is implied, wherein acceptance and recognition of the clients' attributes and individuality by members of the community enable clients to perceive and experience these attributes as very real parts of themselves. It is in this area that the clients are encouraged to participate in their treatment planning, devise plans and alternatives that are specific to their style of being, and test the limits of their capabilities. One-to-one interactions and the observation of clients' rights are important here. The right to privacy is also an opportunity to exercise time alone in a positive manner. It can be difficult when individual rights of expression conflict with a need for containment; staff must be careful when choosing one variable over the other. The same is true when clients are involved in making obviously ineffective decisions. There is often a thin line between positive failure and negative success. Clients must be allowed to experience failure and loss if they are to grow. At the same time, caution must be exercised that an emphasis on individual choice does not overwhelm clients with indecision and frustration. Validation is another variable frequently evident in milieu, and is particularly useful in short-term treatments and step-down units, where clients are preparing for discharge to their former unstructured environments.

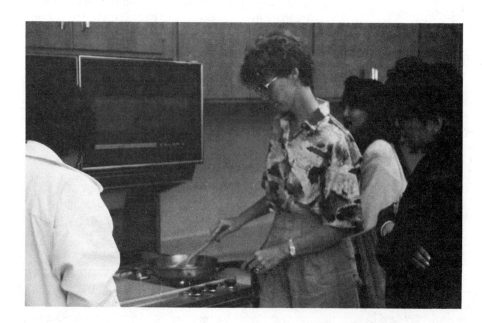

Figure 14-1. Client and staff in an inpatient milieu work together to prepare a meal.

Summary

Each milieu program is unique in its interpretation and application of Gunderson's functional variables. Certain variables may be primary areas of focus, while others are deemphasized. Ideally, an awareness of these variables and their relative merits and disadvantages will enable staff to construct an optimal treatment environment for the clients they expect to serve. No one milieu can do it all, however, and client needs may well change during the course of hospitalization. An attitude of flexibility and continual evaluation is imperative to a healthy milieu if it is to serve its purpose—that of providing a therapeutic environment through the use and adaptation of containment, support, structure, involvement, and validation.

The Therapeutic Use of Self

The key to the success of the functional variables described is the process of interaction, particularly the nurse's interaction with the client. In the milieu setting, the staff's therapeutic use of self occurs on two levels—individually and interpersonally. All staff members have individual impact through their personal contacts with each client. At the same time, the relationships and communication patterns modeled by staff among themselves serve as powerful interpersonal examples for good or ill. In both cases, individually and interpersonally, the staff members' experiences and personal styles cannot be divorced from each interaction. It is important for nurses to recognize that who they are has as much, if not more, of an impact on clients as the therapeutic techniques they choose to employ.

It must also be remembered that impact is mutual. Nurses have emotional responses to the clients, just as clients have responses to the nurses. The nurses' awareness and understanding of their own feelings and reactions supply important information about how others may react to the clients. If nurses are frustrated by their inability to engage the clients in discussions on other than an intellectual level, perhaps this same frustration is experienced by clients' friends and relatives. In this manner, nurses act as a barometer for the rest of the world.

Internal awareness is also imperative for nurses to be able to separate personal feelings from professional responses. Because an ability to reply nonjudgmentally to clients is fundamental to a successful milieu, nurses must cultivate this trait by clarifying their own values. Only then can they define the clients' behaviors as appropriate or not, without passing judgment on the clients themselves. Nurses must learn to discriminate between responses that relate to their own personal issues (see the discussion of countertransference in Chap. 20), and those that would be shared by many individuals who deal with the client.

Because psychiatric units vary in their focus and population, it is impossible and undesirable to provide a "cookbook" approach to interacting with clients. The therapeutic relationship must be fluid and dynamic if all clients are to receive optimal treatment. There are, however, certain characteristics of the therapeutic relationship that are especially important in the milieu context. Honesty, openness, and a sincere interest in the client foster an atmosphere of trust, and present a role model for the client. At the same time, nurses must be clear that they are operating in a professional capacity. It is detrimental and inaccurate to assume that the clients in a milieu setting can, or should, provide staff with friendship and recognition. This is not their function. Indeed, a blurring of role boundaries between clients and staff can have disastrous effects on the treatment process and the community trust level. This message may seem unnecessary, but remember it the first time a client asks for a favor—"because, after all, aren't you a friend?"

Keep in mind that clients usually don't know any of the staff personally. Consequently, although their complaints may be valid and should not be dismissed without proper consideration, it is just as likely that they are reacting to a stereotype or a transference (reacting to staff as the clients have done to significant people in their pasts). Nurses are encouraged not to take negative responses or insults personally. If they are inaccurate, the responses or insults become a part of the therapeutic process. If they are valid observations, they become a part of the nurse's self-evaluation and learning process.

The milieu offers a tremendous amount of data regarding how clients function with other people, and how other people respond. This first-hand information can be used to engage clients in very real negotiations of how to interact. Knowledge of the negotiation process is less important than willingness to engage in it. In the milieu setting, staff and clients participate in a continual process of interpersonal struggle in which the Self is the basic currency of exchange.

Goals

The five functional variables describing the purposes of milieu therapy can be viewed as a set of behavioral goals for the unit, to be achieved as staff work with clients. As discussed by a number of sources (Abroms,[1] Kraft,[17] Rosenbaum and Beebe[24]), the behaviors include reality testing, limit setting, and social skills training. The role of the nurse is to promote these goals through specific therapeutic actions. While this process will be described in some detail, it should be understood that staff members carry out their roles within the guidelines of the unit organization.

Reality Testing

Reality testing is the first goal to be considered. Some definitions might be helpful, since psychiatric settings are not necessarily scrupulous in their use of terminology. The *ego* performs a number of tasks in order to perceive and adapt to reality. These tasks are referred to as *ego functions.* Strictly speaking, reality testing is the ego function that assesses external reality and objectively evaluates what is happening in the environment. For example, when friends snap at us, we recognize that they are angry about something specific. Without accurate reality testing, we might perceive that they were plotting against us or that they disliked us. When the ability to test reality is missing, as with psychosis, or distorted, as with neurotic disorders, the clients' behavior appears inappropriate. After all, they are responding to a view of reality that is inaccurate.

Reality orientation is the process of calm, firm reminders to clients concerning what is happening around them. This may include repeated reminders of their name, the date, time, ward schedule, or other facts. It may also involve informing clients that their perception of hearing "voices" is not shared by anyone else in the immediate vicinity (but don't check with another hallucinating client for validation).

Reality orientation, which corrects the client's reality-testing as necessary, may intercede in any of three areas. The most obvious involves *external reality;* the realignment of the client's perceptions in keeping with social norms. Another area is *internal reality,* in which the client is assisted to identify accurately feelings and intrapsychic experiences. The third is *transactional reality,* in which the individual is helped to recognize the rules or interplay of power that guide interpersonal transactions.[24]

In the milieu setting, all staff participate in the reality-orientation process. Clients whose reality-testing ability is intact are encouraged and instructed to assist less capable clients with reality testing. Eventually, the clients with greater impairment are taught to stop in mid-thought, question the assessment of reality, and make any necessary corrections.

Limit Setting

Limit setting is the next goal used to help clients control or set appropriate limits on their behavior. Abroms[1] discusses five specific types of disordered behavior that are addressed in the milieu setting. The list is presented in priority order. That is, response to the more severe types or levels takes precedence over response to those that are lower on the scale.

Physically-destructive behavior is the most severe level of disturbance. This includes suicidal or homicidal actions as well as assault, vandalism, and self-mutilation. A number of preventive measures for such behavior exist on psychiatric units. Clients who display a potential for violence are placed in a special precautionary status. This alerts the staff to be cautious and to observe the individual closely. Admission may be made to a locked unit, if available. Staff are trained in safe restraint procedures to employ, if necessary. Medications are generally ordered to be used p.r.n. (as needed) in an acute crisis. Seclusion rooms may be available for clients to take a "time out" from the activity of the unit. Once clients have regained control of their impulses, their behavior may become the focus of community (unit) group therapy sessions. In this manner, clients are made aware of the impact of their ac-

tions, and the community is reassured that staff will respond appropriately if any other members lose control.

Disorganization, the second type of behavioral disturbance, involves a breakdown in the clients' ability to respond in an appropriate and goal-directed fashion. These disturbances include incoherence, regression, bizarre thought and actions, and intrusive hallucinations and delusions. Clients lose the ability to relate effectively within their environments or to attend to the activities of daily living. In this event, staff become involved in providing frequent, brief contacts with clients, and consistent direction to ensure meeting their basic needs. Disorganization is more common with organic diagnoses (*e.g.,* toxic psychosis secondary to drug ingestion), and may require the use of medications and seclusion. Subjecting these clients to community focus is generally not therapeutic, because the individuals usually become more disorganized under the stress of confrontation. However, the community may be mobilized as a resource to assist in structuring these clients' activities. The members may also appreciate an explanation of the clients' difficulties as reassurance that it isn't contagious.

Deviant or *rule-breaking behavior* is the third type of disorder, and can include anything from frequent violation of ward policies, to inappropriate sexual actions, to minor self-mutilation. These behaviors are also called "acting out." They represent expressions of anxiety in the present situation "as if" they were an earlier experience that caused the client conflict. For example, clients who have been hurt in previous attempts at close relationships may "act out" if they feel they are becoming too attached to other people on the unit. This type of behavior is particularly evident and problematic in clients with borderline personality disorders. Staff response is perhaps most difficult and sensitive in these cases. A united and well-coordinated team approach is crucial. Staff must maintain an accepting position toward clients while (1) holding them responsible for, and dealing with, the behaviors; (2) honoring their need for distance by not overwhelming or smothering them; and (3) honoring their need for closeness by not allowing anger to create too much distance. Does this sound like walking a tightrope? It is! As difficult as it is for the staff, it is even more confusing for the community members, who require guidance and support from staff in determining how to maintain their relationships with these clients.

Dysphoria, the fourth level of behavioral disturbance, refers to clients' withdrawal into themselves and isolation from their surroundings, including people. This is particularly seen with depression, hypochondriasis, and schizoid distancing. Obsessional and phobic anxiety states may also be considered in this category. Frequent, but brief, contacts for the client are provided within the milieu, while care is taken to avoid intrusive or overwhelming interactions. The staff enlists the aid of the community to increase gradually the client's involvement in unit activities. Community members may require guidance to ensure that they don't personalize the client's detachment and react with frustration, hostility, or dismissal. The staff also observes the client's capacity to perform activities of daily living and intervene, when necessary.

Dependency is the final type of behavioral disorder addressed by the milieu. This involves clients' attempts to avoid responsibility for their own actions and to manipulate others to provide unrealistic levels of nurturing and support. The milieu is used to promote a sense of personal competence and responsibility, as well as to confront and explore unrealistic demands on others. The clients' interactions with the staff and community members provide relevant examples for the therapeutic process. However, the staff must be cognizant of the potential for manipulation, without negating realistic requests by clients. The staff must also support efforts by the community to require responsible behavior from these clients. This last approach becomes particularly important when the community members themselves are dealing with dependency vs. care-taking issues.

Two comments remain to be made about this hierarchy of disordered behavior. First, it provides some guidelines for staff response. For example, in CPR, we know to establish a patent airway before assessing respiration, and this must be done before assessing cardiac function. Similarly, psychiatric treatment is most effective when the response to behavioral disorders takes place according to the priorities described. Discussing clients' dependency issues when they are slashing their wrists or tearing the unit apart is not effective.

Second, the descriptions (above) of response to behavioral disorders include involvement of the community. The milieu setting, a mini-society, acknowledges the impact people have on each other, even when the interaction is negative or seemingly nonexistent. The potential for positive and supportive connections among community members should not be underestimated. In fact, clients may be more receptive to feedback from their peers than from staff. At the same time, community members may identify with one client's difficulties and respond in one of two ways. They may see their own behavior more objectively and learn from the experience, or they may react with fear, anxiety, or even decompensation (a relapse of symptoms brought on by the breakdown of the defense system). Staff must be aware of these possibilities, and actively seek to anticipate them as a part of treatment.

Social Skills Training

Social skills training is the third goal of milieu therapy, after reality testing and limit setting. Psychiatric units may approach this area in a general manner or in a formal arrangement, or both. In the social microcosm of the unit, even if no formal program is used, interpersonal relationships are still part of unit activities and the community structure. As role models, staff act as guides for clients. The interventions of staff in the communication patterns among clients help to mold appropriate skills. The feedback process, in individual and group sessions, also provides learning experiences in the social skills. In addition to these informal and continuous activities, a unit may decide to include specific programs such as Personal Effectiveness Training (PET). PET sessions are designed to allow clients to practice in social situations they expect to encounter, while receiving detailed feedback about their verbal and nonverbal communication styles. Clients can also be videotaped to give them more vivid pictures of the impressions they create.

Teaching social skills in the areas of orientation, assertion, occupation, and recreation is particularly beneficial. *Orientation* means more than just being aware of person, place, and time. Acquainting clients with social roles and organizational functions can be accomplished in much the same manner. *Assertiveness training* introduces a new set of options for meeting individual needs without manipulating or submitting to other people in the environment. *Work-therapy programs* incorporate training and discussion around topics such as job hunting, interviewing, organizing time, and working cooperatively. *Recreation therapy,* often organized under an occupational therapy department, encourages the often-overlooked skill of using leisure time thoroughly and effectively.[1]

Other elements of social skills training are so much an integral part of a unit's fabric that they are not readily isolated. All interactions are potential learning situations for clients.

Techniques

Communication, facilitation of expression, and modification of behavior are techniques that make the potential a reality for all milieu goals.[24] Chapters 3 and 5 present basic skills in therapeutic relationships, with detailed descriptions of actual interactions. The section that follows will call the nurse's attention to specific applications in the milieu setting.

First and foremost is the importance these techniques have for staff interactions. The staff constitute their own subculture within the milieu, and as such must apply many of the same rules of relationships among themselves that they enforce for clients if they are to set an effective tone and example. For this reason, milieu settings tend to impress observers with their democratic atmosphere. Staff openness and interaction among themselves provide a necessary setting to work through differences in individual values, countertransference issues, and internal disagreements. In order to maximize the benefit of this process, all staff members must be committed to examining their own feelings and reactions on a continual basis, sharing them with other staff and accepting feedback, facilitating the same participation from others, and modifying their behavior when appropriate.

Staff interactions provide a role model for the client population, while group and individual techniques are used to enhance communication and facilitate the expression of feelings. Particular emphasis is placed on group process, because social context is of such importance in the milieu setting. For staff, the focus is on guiding the client through this process by supporting appropriate communication patterns. Modification of behavior can be effected in a variety of ways, depending on the treatment philosophy applied. The unit schedule and policies provide the framework. The client's style of adapting to this structure is the basis for intervention.

Organization

As previously indicated, the unit organization plays a crucial role in the success of the purpose, goals, and techniques of milieu therapy. We will discuss a number of the components generally found in milieu settings. However, the constituents and models described are meant only as a beginning guide to what the nurse can expect to find. Nurses must learn the particular elements operating on the unit to which they are assigned.

The role of nursing students in the milieu's policies and regulations is no less important than that of full-time staff members. On entering the unit, the nurses become a part of the mini-society. They also become authority figures, with responsibility for supporting the unit's structure. Sometimes psychiatric clients expect and seek lenience from nurses who are less familiar with the unit routines. An important rule to remember: when in doubt, defer a policy decision to the full-time staff. Until the student has become familiar with the regulations and how to respond to infractions, this will save a lot of confusion.

Policies and Procedures

Policies and procedures may be initiated by the hospital administration or by the unit itself, depending on the nature of the regulation. On most psychiatric units, particularly those within a general hospital, basic institution policies are given first priority. These include a range of requirements deemed necessary for hospital accreditation. Access to client records, documentation standards, staff and employment policies, fire and safety measures, and disposition of contraband on admission to the unit are just a few of the issues about which unit staff usually have little say.

These policies may be questioned by clients, especially regulations concerning the process for viewing their own charts or confiscation of their property when they are considered dangerous. In such cases, the issue becomes a part of therapy. Clients are helped to deal with their responses toward nonnegotiable rules.

The next level of priority involves policies that are negotiated with the hospital specifically for the psychiatric unit, and perhaps contrary to those enforced elsewhere. They may extend to visiting hours, smoking areas, unit furnishings, attire of clients and staff, and meal arrangements. Each is planned to support the unit milieu and enhance its operation. While there may be a bit more flexibility in changing these regulations as far as the hospital is concerned, they are presented by the unit staff as nonnegotiable, and may also become therapeutic issues as clients demonstrate their responses to structure.

Finally there are policies and organizational decisions that are generated specifically by the psychiatric unit to provide a safe environment or fulfill milieu objectives. The first consideration is to determine whether the unit will be open or locked. This is predominantly influenced by the type of clients that will be admitted. Hospitals with multiple units often designate one as a locked ward for crisis or admission clients, with a milieu constructed to provide maximum safety precautions against violence or acting-out behaviors. Such a unit is generally considered appropriate for short-term treatment, with clients transferred in or out (to less restrictive units) as their behavior warrants.

Despite the relative freedom of movement noted on most psychiatric units, several areas are designated as being off limits to clients, to ensure either safety or privacy and confidentiality. The nursing station is one area where traffic control is essential. In many institutions, clients are responsible for coming to the nursing station for medications. The presence of extra people at such times invites errors. Additionally, the presence of clients in the nursing station may allow them to see or hear communications regarding other individuals, thereby breaching confidentiality. Clients are also not allowed to enter staff offices unattended.

Making clients responsible for their own medications is a common policy, often included with the privilege system. While it is not advisable for clients to have direct access to their medications (at their bedside, for example), they are still required to know what they are receiving and at what time of day, and to present themselves at the nursing station accordingly. Clients are taught the actions of their medications, the major side-effects, and the circumstances under which p.r.n. medications will be given. They are then instructed to report side-effects or a need for medications to the staff. This differs from the procedure on medical units, not only in the requirement that clients present themselves physically for their medications, but also in the practice of including compliance as a therapeutic issue.

Client Government Systems

Client government systems, their structure and operation, influence a large portion of unit policies. A system of responsible client roles is implemented, with clients elected to office by all community members. At a minimum, a chairperson or president and an assistant are identified as the primary client representatives. They conduct meetings, assist in introducing new clients and making them comfortable, keep tabs on issues within the community, and report problems to the staff. Their role is not meant to supersede individual responsibility, but rather to facilitate it. Additional jobs may also be devised in keeping with milieu objectives.

Community meetings, a major component of the client government system, are conducted much like any formal meeting, following a prearranged structure with an agenda and times allotted for old as well as new business. The expectation is fostered that clients and staff alike may initiate action within the system. Democratic decision-making is encouraged whenever possible, although staff participants generally have veto power in special instances. One word of caution in this area. Staff must be careful to avoid using hidden rules and agendas, or limiting client actions through the staffs' own preconceived ideas of acceptable options. To avoid this difficulty, staff must clarify from the outset which decisions are within the clients' control and which are nonnegotiable, usually for therapeutic reasons or to maintain consistency with hospital policy. This approach prevents the unnecessary frustration of clients' putting time and energy into a project only to find that it would have been vetoed anyway. Many clients have learned not to trust or put forth their best effort because, although one message encouraged them to act independently, another conflicting message negated the first. If clients are to learn optimal autonomy and responsibility, rights and privileges must be clearly, fairly, and consistently applied.

At the same time, staff must be careful not to discount client options because of their own beliefs or prejudices. An example here should suffice to explain the point. On one military psychiatric unit, a group of clients had difficulty receiving paychecks. One of the clients with a diagnosis of passive-aggressive personality disorder was particularly angry. He had a reputation for acting out on the unit and had not endeared himself to the staff, nor had he benefited from attempts at learning to delay gratification. Much staff time had been devoted to discussing the advantages of utilizing the chain of command, however, and the young man came up with an idea. Military regulations stated that he had the right to "request Mast" (to bring any complaints to the attention of his commanding officer), and expect a resolution. Why couldn't he request Mast with the hospital CO, or even the CO of his original military unit, and secure his assistance in solving the problem? This idea challenged the comfort level of many staff members, who themselves would be reluctant to act in such an assertive manner. In fact, the Ward Medical Officer initially refused the request. The young man was within his legal rights, however, and not only was such an action preferable to his previous patterns, but the experience would be therapeutic! Authorization was eventually obtained, and the young man met with the CO to present respectfully the plight of the community. Within a week, the missing paychecks arrived. It should also be mentioned that the client's acting-out decreased and he became a unit leader. His success and newfound appreciation by fellow clients gave him the boost he needed to continue trying more appropriate methods of meeting his needs. A golden opportunity would have been lost if the staff's perception of limitations had been allowed to suppress the client's resourcefulness.

On a more detailed level, each unit has explicit rules concerning day-to-day operation. Because these may vary greatly among units, the general categories will be described, with few specifics. For example, meals are set up to allow independence as well as supervision. In some cases, clients may eat in a common hospital dining area along with staff. In other cases, home-style meals may be served in a dining room on the unit. Clients are rarely served in their rooms unless they are medically ill.

Appropriate clothing is usually determined by the level of a client's privileges. Pajamas may be required for clients that are restricted to the unit, or they may not be worn during the day at all, except during a period of medical illness. Otherwise, street clothes are worn to preserve individual rights, identity, and connection with the external environment.

Psychiatric units cannot restrict a client's right to telephone, mail, and visiting privileges because of inpatient status. Clients may, however, specify people they do not wish to have visit or call, including significant others. Occasionally, however, inappropriate client behavior dictates intervention in these areas. Client telephones are generally maintained separately from business phones. If use of them is abused, the community may be presented with the issue to determine fair and acceptable limits, with the clients then responsible for policing themselves. Mail may not be censored, but inappropriate letters (e.g., 50 a day written by a manic-depressive client) may become a treatment issue. The clients may then be helped to limit their own behavior. If clients become upset or violent after seeing certain visitors, the staff may ask those individuals to refrain from visiting until the client is better able to deal with any disturbed impulses. In any event, the need to limit client rights must be documented by the staff.

Each unit has its own time schedule for lights out, sleeping hours, and television hours. While these may seem to be minor issues, they are often the issues most contested by clients. The schedule exists to maximize appropriate use of recreational and therapeutic times and to minimize avoidance of treatment by clients. If allowed, some clients would stay up late watching T.V. and try to sleep late every morning, thereby evading unit activities. Clients are not allowed in their beds during the day unless they are ill, and this may require some attention to be sure the rule isn't being abused. The purpose of these rules is not to achieve a regimented atmosphere, but to help clients regulate their days in a more productive manner by maintaining a consistent schedule.

Community Meetings and Groups

Community meetings and groups are a significant part of milieu therapy.[1] The *Community* or *Morning Meeting* has already been mentioned. During this session, staff members share a report of ward events and client behaviors during the previous 24 hours. The community members are encouraged to discuss these events and add their own insights or problems for further examination. Clients are expected to present their requests for privilege changes or passes outside of the hospital, and receive feedback from the group regarding the merit of the request. Conflicts between clients or client and staff are legitimate topics for this meeting. Emergency Community Meetings may also be called to deal with unusual unit occurrences disturbing to clients, *e.g.,* a suicide attempt or the restraint of a violent client.

Small-group therapy is conducted several times a week, often during both the day and the evening shifts. These groups may be general problem-solving and discussion sessions, or may take on a specific theme. When Star Trek was popular, for example, one unit held voluntary groups after each show to discuss the philosophical messages presented in the episode and how they related to social awareness. Clients may be assigned to specific types of groups, based on the clients' level of function. Disorganized clients, for example, may participate in more structured groups, while clients functioning at a higher level are assigned to groups dealing with complex therapeutic issues. Other specialized meetings include *women's, couples',* or *family groups. Discharge groups* are useful for clients preparing to leave the hospital, and furnish a structured time to discuss their options, plans, and concerns. By virtue of the topics covered and the inclusion of family members, many of the small-group sessions have the added advantage of emphasizing that treatment and resulting behavior changes must extend beyond the hospital environment.

A variety of activities may be available to assist the client with appropriate time structuring or the development of leisure interests and social skills. Recreational, occupational, music, dance, or bibliotherapies come under this heading. Units may also incorporate weekly or periodic outings to provide social experiences outside the hospital. Shopping trips, picnics, and movies are a few such activities.

Staff meetings are also frequent in the milieu setting. *Staffings* involve the treatment team and client in planning individual goals and directions. *Team meetings* work out the daily treatment program, once the goals have been determined. *Staff sensitivity groups* provide a forum to discuss interpersonal differences and ensure teamwork on the unit. A *policy committee* may exist, with representation from each professional group, to negotiate changes in unit policies. All such groups are intended to increase staff effectiveness, but care must be taken that staff meetings don't overshadow the actual treatment program.

Step or Privilege Systems

Step or privilege systems are another important aspect in the overall scheme of unit organization. Frequently, clients are admitted to a unit with restrictions on their activities. Based on their behavior and their ability to convince the community of their reliability, they may receive increased privileges. These privileges may include hospital pass status (out of the psychiatric unit), a day pass away from the hospital, and overnight pass status. Each step may be modified to require a client or relative escort. Eligibility for step increase often entails compliance with unit regulations and responsible involvement in all activities. Violations of unit rules are generally tied closely to the step system. Infractions may result in a decrease in or removal of privileges, either for a specific time period or until reinstated by the community. In this manner, even

units that do not use a strict behavior modification regimen take advantage of behavior modification principles.

Often unit elements specific to expectations of client behavior are detailed in an orientation manual. The manual is useful for introducing clients to the unit and for providing staff with a ready reference to use to enforce unit regulations. A manual is also helpful for nurses to learn what they should expect from clients.

Discharge Planning

Discharge planning is a subject that pervades every area of the inpatient therapeutic process.[24] Clients are being prepared to leave the hospital from the first day they arrive. The initial assessment is geared toward having both nurse and client determine appropriate behavioral goals that will indicate readiness for discharge. Discussions with family and other members of the client's external support groups outside the hospital provide essential information concerning their ability to accept the client's return. Ongoing therapy constantly evaluates the client's progress toward meeting discharge goals, and the adequacy of the support system in light of that progress. About half-way through the process, decisions are made and implemented regarding community supports or alternative living arrangements necessary to maintain the client's anticipated level of recovery. In short, discharge planning does not begin with arbitrary behavioral improvements by the clients, followed by the staff's decision to include them in a discharge group. From the day of admission to the unit, the direction of treatment is determined and the milieu mobilizes to provide impetus in that direction.

Once clients' progress indicates readiness for trial returns to the external community, passes are arranged to test their responses outside the unit's safe milieu. If the clients' behavior has been seriously disturbed, the first passes may only be for a few hours' duration. Gradually, they are extended to encompass an entire day, and then a weekend. On their return to the unit, clients' behavior is carefully monitored and additional passes are contingent on the response to previous ones. It is generally most effective to have passes structured around an activity, like having dinner with the family. If the clients are capable of dealing with the stressors of their outside environments, they are ready to advance along the pass continuum to the point of discharge. Less seriously-disturbed clients may be guided through an abbreviated version of this system.

Ideally, once clients are ready for discharge, they will be returned to supportive family networks that will sustain the gains they have made in treatment. This is not always possible. An assessment of the individual's support group outside the hospital may indicate that it is ill-equipped to handle the degree of structure or assistance still needed by the client. It then becomes necessary to consider other options if the client is to avoid rehospitalization.

The introduction of new members into the outside support group is the least disruptive option. Outpatient follow-up and/or in-home psychiatric nursing visits will suffice in many instances. When they do not, it may become necessary for the client to enter a new support group. Daycare centers are frequently used for this purpose, and are preferable because they enable the client to remain within the family network. In extreme cases, when the individual lacks social resources or cannot sustain progress, the only alternative may be removal from the family and placement in a half-way house, residential care facility, or nursing home. The optimal approach is to implement the plan that is the least disruptive, yet the most effective at maintaining the client outside the hospital. The final role of the milieu is to prepare each client for adaptation to this plan.

Types of Milieu

While the environment of each psychiatric unit constitutes a milieu in the general sense, units may opt to incorporate a specific therapeutic model. This model then provides a theoretical framework for determining the most appropriate elements and organization of the milieu, as well as the particular emphasis of behavioral interpretation during the therapeutic process.

Behavior modification programs, for example, are especially effective with child and adolescent groups or severely disorganized individuals. These units are set up with a token economy system. A list of possible client behaviors is described in detail, from attending to each activity of daily living to social skills. Each desirable behavior is valued at an arbitrary number of tokens. When the clients perform the desirable behavior, they are rewarded with the appropriate number of tokens. These can be spent on privileges, or possibly on items in a hospital gift shop. Some programs focus only on rewarding desirable behavior, while others also subtract tokens for undesirable behavior.

In this type of program, the staff procedural rules described by Paul and Lentz[21] include: immediate reinforcement of desirable behaviors; no attention paid to undesirable behavior; compliments and explanations of the desired behavior that are given with the reinforcement; gradual shaping in the direction of the desirable behavior, using prompts and instructions; and conscientious recording of token exchange, behavior, and surrounding variables. Based on fairly strict behavioral theory, such a program requires much attention to detail. In fact, the client's behavior itself becomes less important than the specific environmental factors that precede or follow the behavior. Behavior is seen as occurring in response to particular stimuli, and is perpetuated by attention or reinforcement. If the stimuli or the reinforcement change, the behavior changes. The aim of the milieu is to create change in a positive direction.

Psychoanalytic programs are at the opposite end of the spectrum from behavior modification programs. The Menninger Sanitarium pioneered in this area in the 1930s.[24] Therapeutic discussions center around psychodynamics and defenses, rather than stimuli and reinforcement. This type of program is less detail-oriented and more concerned with understanding the intrapsychic position of the client as it is evidenced in the social environment.

While psychoanalytic deliberation is often difficult for students to understand, treatment approaches have been distilled to several specific types, formulated according to psychodynamic theory.[13] Also referred to as *attitude therapy,* these approaches are the closest one might come to a "cookbook model" of treatment. The attitudes are prescribed to meet individual clients' needs, and are useful in promoting consistency of treatment. Active friendliness, passive friendliness, matter-of-factness, kind firmness, and reality encouragement are some of the specific approaches involved. For example, passive friendliness is most useful with paranoid or withdrawn clients. Apart from common courtesy or ward routine, emphasis is placed on client initiative in approaching staff. The object is to avoid threatening the client while communicating that the staff is available to help when the client is ready. Kind firmness is used with depressed clients. The emphasis here is on clear, direct, confident statements with the expectation that requests are to be carried out; sympathetic, challenging, or overbearing messages are avoided. The object is to mobilize the clients' anger without becoming drawn into their complaints or feelings of hopelessness. If these approaches are used on a psychiatric unit, staff manuals thoroughly describe the attitudes and their application.

Other milieu programs lie on a broad continuum between the behavioral and the psychoanalytic approaches, and may lean in one direction or another or may be more eclectic. Specific modalities may be used, such as transactional analysis or rational emotive therapy. The approach used on any given psychiatric unit depends on the philosophy of the unit administrators, and the clients that are served.

Special Problems

Just as in society at large, psychiatric units are not without problems. However, because the therapeutic milieu is a controlled environment, problems are addressed more readily. For example, privilege and community systems are designed to deal with rule infractions. In order for these systems to work, staff must avoid overpermissiveness and must consider each piece of behavior seriously, without assuming that it is a one-time occurrence. In a similar manner, psychiatric units incorporate other methods to respond to dangerous situations or recurrent difficulties.

Self-destructive behavior is of primary concern. The role of the milieu in providing for basic needs, including safety, and in setting limits on disordered behavior, has already been discussed. It must be understood that, while the ultimate goal is to assist clients in controlling their own self-destructive impulses, the staff assumes the responsibility for providing control and protection during those periods when clients are unable to do so. The means to carry out this role is incorporated in unit policy.

Safety features include a number of regulations that must not be taken lightly, although they frequently become routine. Upon admission, all luggage is examined with both client and staff present. Sharp implements, breakable glass, weapons, and medications are taken away from the client. Depending on the resources at hand, these items may be sent home with a relative or inventoried and kept in a locker on the unit. The daily routine avoids potential risk by including supervised, limited, or no access to articles such as shaving equipment, scissors, and cleaning solutions or other poisons. Monitoring of eating utensils or use of plastic utensils may be indicated. Cigarettes, matches, and lighters may be restricted or used only under staff supervision. Client access to electrical fixtures is limited. Even water temperature on the unit is regulated, to prevent both accidental and intentional scalding. In short, every aspect of unit life is closely examined and modified to enhance safety.

Admission and ongoing assessments pay close attention to any self-mutilative or suicidal ideation, or history of them, on the part of a client. Minor client actions may respond to limit setting, while major occurrences require mobilization of the entire unit. If assessment or clients' behavior indicates the need, clients may be placed on a status called "suicide precautions," or may have portions of this status incorporated into their treatment plan. An example of one unit's suicide precaution policy is summarized in Table 14-1.

There is a saying in psychiatry that "the person who truly wanted to kill himself did so ten minutes ago." This statement is not made to emphasize the hopelessness of the situation, since most people who attempt suicide are actually ambivalent. However, it does point out the likelihood that suicide can occur on a psychiatric unit at any time, despite staff's best efforts to the contrary. Both clients and staff have an emotional response to such an occurrence. Particularly in the milieu environment, the method of handling the situation can have far-reaching effects. Staff must receive the support they need in order to provide adequate assistance for the rest of the community. Often this is best accomplished by using objective consultants during staff sessions. The remaining clients must be dealt with quickly and supportively. Suicide is a community issue, influencing the unit atmosphere and raising many doubts and fears for all concerned. Clients need to know that their safety is still of primary importance to the staff. A rash of minor, or even major, acting-out may follow a suicide in order to test staff's ability to respond. It is important for staff to be aware of this possibility and to deal with it appropriately, without acting out their own feelings toward the suicide. Once the situation stabilizes, it is also important that an evaluation of the occurrence be conducted, not to lay blame but to determine whether any modifications in the unit operation are necessary to improve safety in the future.

Violent behavior requires limit setting within the milieu. Specific policies for violent behavior are just as important as those for self-destructive behavior. However, contrary to popular belief, aggressive acting-out on a psychiatric unit that exercises proper awareness is the exception, rather than the rule. Conscious attention to changes in client behavior, environmental irritants, and provocative situations enables staff to intervene before an incident escalates to the point of physical force. Once again, the key is for staff to take any aggressive talk or behavior seriously.

TABLE 14-1.
SAMPLE SUICIDE PRECAUTIONS

1. Suicidal clients are to be restricted to the unit and wear pajamas. They are not allowed to leave the unit unless leaving is specifically ordered by a physician. If so ordered by a physician, clients may be required to participate in off-unit activities only with a one-to-one staff escort.

2. The community is to be informed of clients' suicidal precautionary status and instructed in appropriate ways of interacting with these clients.

3. If suicidal clients are voted an increase in privileges at community meeting and their doctors concur, suicide precautions are automatically discontinued.

   (*Note:* In this unit example, although suicide precautions are ordered by the psychiatrist, their removal is contingent upon community action as well as physician approval. Because clients must request consideration for a step increase, they are actually responsible for initiating a change in their precaution status. The same holds true for Elopement Precautions outlined in Table 14-5.)

4. Suicidal clients must be sighted by staff every 15 minutes. If necessary, one-to-one staff coverage may be instituted.

5. Suicidal clients are not allowed access to razor blades, scissors, or other sharp objects. Keep track of utensils on meal trays to make sure they are returned. Use paper trays and plastic utensils, as necessary. Observe for, and remove, potential sharp objects in the environment.

6. If suicidal clients are agitated or presenting a management problem, they may use the seclusion area to calm down.

7. As a last resort, restraint procedures and locked seclusion rooms may be used (see Tables 14-2, 14-3, and 14-4).

Unit rules address this area by clearly communicating that the expression of feelings is encouraged within appropriate limits. Screaming, even cursing, may be tolerated, although staff should quickly intercede to deescalate the situation and generate a positive resolution. However, the line is drawn at physical threat or contact. In fact, most units, except for those dealing with chemical dependence, discourage any touching among clients, in order to avoid misunderstandings of intent. Clients may also be encouraged to make use of seclusion areas by their own choice to give themselves a "time-out" from overstimulation on the unit. Both clients and staff are advised to avoid compromising situations in which they may be trapped alone with a potentially violent individual.

In the case of potential violence, as with possible self-destructive behavior, admission and ongoing assessments provide significant information for anticipating risk. The most effective responses to an identified danger include constant awareness, immediate recognition of risk factors, and implementation of an intervention hierarchy as described in Table 14-2. The goal is to control behavior using the least restrictive alternative. With an early response, the need for physical restraint can often be avoided. Once it becomes inevitable, however, unit staff must react as a team, calmly and quickly, with predetermined techniques of physical restraint.

One of the first issues addressed in the formation of a psychiatric unit is its response to violent behavior. Special call lights may be available, in addition to the usual room call bells, to notify the nursing station of emergencies. Phone lines directly connected with a security department may be used for back-up support. If a general hospital has had the foresight to recognize that it may require psychiatric support in other areas of the hospital, or that general units may need to send support to the psychiatric unit, an emergency paging system may exist to activate such a plan. In any event, each unit has its own means of summoning assistance to deal with violent behavior. Nurses should familiarize themselves with specific procedures during the orientation process as conscientiously as they do with cardiac arrest and fire procedures.

Although nursing students are not usually expected to participate in actual physical restraint of a client, the staff should be well trained in restraint techniques and maintain their ability to respond by practicing these techniques as a team. There are a number of alternate styles, most involving a multiple-member team approach and some including the use of blankets or mattresses. General principles for the use of restraint are given in Table 14-3. Nurses may find themselves in the position of providing crowd control, and will certainly participate in any community meetings after a restraint. Because violent behavior can be quite disturbing to the whole community, such a meeting may well be indicated. Paranoid clients, or those who doubt their own capacity for impulse control, are especially likely to question staff support and response.

Seclusion areas provide containment for restrained clients until their behavior can be brought under control. Typical policies observed during a period of restraint are described in Table 14-4. It is most important that the seclusion process be presented as a means of control, not as punishment. Clients frequently receive medications and

TABLE 14-2.
HIERARCHY OF RESPONSE TO VIOLENT BEHAVIOR

PHASE 1—TALK DOWN
Phase one is particularly important in order to avoid escalation of a potentially violent situation. Signs of disturbance or agitation are noted, and quickly responded to by staff. The client is guided away from extraneous stimulation in the environment and is continuously talked to, quietly but firmly. The client is encouraged to relax and calm down.

PHASE 2—CHEMICAL RESTRAINT
If the client is unable to regain or maintain self-control, p.r.n. medications are used in conjunction with a continuation of the talk-down phase. The medication is offered, then encouraged, before any ultimatum is issued.

PHASE 3—MANUAL RESTRAINT
If the other options have failed and the client poses a threat to self or others, a prearranged system of physical restraint is implemented. Staff may exercise approximate control (*e.g.*, holding the client's arms while walking the client to the seclusion area), or full control (*i.e.*, physical restraint of all limbs).

PHASE 4—MECHANICAL RESTRAINT
Depending on the degree of violence exhibited by the client, restraint devices may be required. These include leather or plastic bindings, a mattress, a blanket or sheet, or a litter. If the client is armed with any type of object that serves as a weapon, physical restraint may be initiated with a mattress or table as protection for the staff. Restraint procedures are used to provide external control for the client because of imminent self-harm, harm to others, destruction of property, or elopement (under circumstances in which staff are empowered to prevent the client, *e.g.*, a 72-hour hold). Restraints may also be necessary to provide treatment or enforce seclusion in order to control psychotic symptoms that are severe and causing serious psychological pain, *e.g.*, intense, hostile auditory hallucinations.

TABLE 14-3.
PRINCIPLES OF RESTRAINT

1. An ounce of prevention is worth a pound of cure. Don't delay in responding to a situation in the hope that it will resolve itself.

2. Never attempt to handle potentially violent situations alone or assume more responsibility than is necessary without assistance. Heroics lead to injuries. Always call for additional back-up support at the first sign of a possible problem.

3. Planning and teamwork are essential. The orientation of all staff and student nurses should include, at minimum: emergency response equipment, policies, and call systems; physical restraint techniques; roles to be assumed by restraint team members and assistance required from other available staff; and techniques for deescalating potentially violent situations. It is advisable for staff to practice mock restraint situations periodically to ensure a sense of teamwork and mutual trust among staff members.

4. When it appears that the necessity for a restraint procedure is imminent, make sure the environment is as safe as possible. Remove potentially dangerous objects from your person (*e.g.*, pens, jewelry) and from the surrounding area (*e.g.*, chairs, wastebaskets). Then concentrate on the restraint alone.

5. Response to a call for assistance, and to the directions of the procedure leader, must be prompt, in unison, and without question. Once a decision to react has been made, all questions or debate concerning the decision must be addressed afterward.

6. Once a restraint procedure has begun, it must never be interrupted or stopped until the client is under control with the restraint belt or the seclusion room door locked. Any hesitation allows the client time to take one extra swing that might injure someone, and gives the client the message that the staff is inconsistent in dealing with the client.

7. Throughout the procedure, one designated staff member should keep talking to the client calmly and reassuringly, explaining what is being done. This helps the client to relax and diverts the client's attention from planning a counterattack.

8. Use safe body mechanics in restraining and moving the client. During the restraint, maintain physical contact at all times to avoid allowing a free limb to cause injury. Use a cross-chest carry or stretcher to move the client to the seclusion area, if applicable.

9. During a restraint procedure, the client is never to be struck! Restraint techniques have been developed to prevent both staff and client injury, if applied properly. A violent response by staff is neither necessary nor appropriate.

10. Verbal interactions with the client should consist of calm, clear directions, explanations without judgment, and reassurance. Staff must remain in control of the situation and their own reactions. Once the point of restraint has been reached, do not bargain with the client, particularly if you have no intention of honoring the bargain. Do not threaten dire consequences. Do not respond to insults or provocation.

11. Be mindful of the need for crowd control. One staff member should clear other clients or visitors away from the restraint area to ensure that they are not injured or moved to interfere. A community meeting may be necessary after the client is controlled to assist the rest of the community in dealing with their reactions to what has happened.

require monitoring of their responses to the treatment. Seclusion in restraint is most effective when used only as a last resort, and for the least possible amount of time. The dehumanizing effect of any restraint procedure should not be underestimated. Hence, prevention is the best alternative, with minimization of seclusion time a poor second.

If the seclusion area is used for voluntary time-outs by clients, certain precautions are necessary. Client behavior and response should be observed frequently. Whenever possible, a staff member should remain with the client and use this opportunity to deal with therapeutic issues. Depending on the physical layout, it may be advisable not to allow voluntary time-outs while the seclusion area is occupied by an agitated client. Clients should never be allowed to enter the seclusion area without staff knowledge, or with personal articles that might be left behind to compromise the security of the room.

The preceding discussion of response to violent behavior is offered in support of prevention, not to frighten nurses. Much combativeness can be avoided if proper steps are taken quickly, and the quality of response can avert injury to clients and staff. The safety of all concerned is the paramount issue. Student nurses assist in this effort by maintaining an awareness of client behavior and reporting changes to the staff immediately.

Elopement or escape without authorization is another problem that arises occasionally. If the clients are restricted to the unit because of privilege status, concern about their level of confusion, or because they have been legally ordered into treatment, they may be placed on "elopement precautions" (see Table 14-5). The discussions of suicide and aggressive risks again apply here, in terms of prevention and awareness. In the case of mandatory treatment, known in the state of California as a *72-hour hold,* the police are notified if the client leaves. This

TABLE 14-4.
SAMPLE SECLUSION ROOM POLICIES

1. Seclusion rooms are used only for isolating clients for time-out, protection, or control of disruptive behavior. Otherwise, the rooms are to remain empty, locked, and frequently checked to ensure that no extraneous objects have been left there or brought in. The rooms must be available for use at a moment's notice.
2. When the rooms are used for time-out, the clients may remain in street clothes, but any items with which clients could injure themselves should be removed (*e.g.,* matches, hairpins).
3. After being placed in locked seclusion for restraint purposes, the client is reclothed in clean hospital pajamas. Nothing is left in the room with the client except a mattress and bedding, minus the pillow. Jewelry and other personal items are also removed.
4. During time-outs, clients should be observed frequently to ensure that they are safe and to offer an opportunity to discuss what they are experiencing. During locked seclusion, clients must be sighted, and observations charted, every 15 minutes. If necessary, an individual staff member may be assigned for continuous observation of the client.
5. If the client is intoxicated, under the influence of drugs, or being rapidly sedated, vital signs are taken at regular, frequent intervals, as ordered by the physician or the nurse.
6. It is the staff's responsibility to monitor clients' behavior, observe and evaluate responses to seclusion and medications, and anticipate needs in terms of activities of daily living (*e.g.,* meals, fluid intake, hygiene). Meals should be ordered on cardboard isolation trays, and any sharp utensils should be removed before trays are taken into the seclusion room. Liquids should be made available, a clean urinal should be provided, and bathroom trips should be offered periodically.
7. No less than two staff members are to be present whenever the locked doors are opened. With some clients, it may be advisable for a full restraint team to be present to prevent acting-out or escape.
8. Seclusion is not an optimal therapeutic mode unless control is mandatory; therefore, clients should be released as soon as they are willing to cooperate with the milieu, or are sedated and safe enough to be put to bed.
9. Cooperation of clients is more rapidly gained if they understand what is expected of them. Therefore, clients should receive frequent reality reminding and reassurance with explanation of why they are in a locked room and what behavior they must display in order to be released.
10. Clients in seclusion may not receive visitors unless visiting is specifically directed by their primary therapist.
11. Clients in restraints are checked for impaired circulation, friction burns, and abrasions every 15 minutes. Restraints are removed and passive range of motion is applied every four hours, unless otherwise ordered by the physician.

action is necessary because a 72-hour hold is used with clients who are deemed to be dangerous to themselves or others, or gravely disabled. In most other cases, it is sufficient to notify the family. If clients threaten to leave against medical advice, they cannot be prevented from doing so unless the conditions for a 72-hour hold exist. However, family members are usually called in for a conference to discuss the situation and determine a more

TABLE 14-5.
SAMPLE ELOPEMENT/ESCAPE PRECAUTIONS

1. Clients who are considered escape risks are restricted to the unit and to wearing pajamas. They are not allowed to leave the unit unless that is specifically ordered by a physician, and then only with a one-to-one staff escort.
2. The community is to be informed of these clients' precautionary status and instructed in appropriate ways of interacting with these clients.
3. If these clients are voted an increase in privileges at the community meeting, and their doctors concur, elopement precautions are automatically discontinued.
4. These clients are not allowed to go beyond the nursing station windows toward the unit doors. If so warranted by the degree of active intent, the clients may be required to check in with the staff at specific times, as deemed necessary. They must be sighted by the staff at least every 15 minutes.
5. If clients are agitated or present a management problem, they may use the seclusion room to calm down. At staff discretion, the unit doors may be locked to provide greater security. (This applies to open units with the ability to lock outer doors, as needed.)
6. As a last resort, restraint and seclusion may be used.

effective resolution for the client. It is advisable for units to have a policy concerning readmission for clients who leave against medical advice. Limit setting becomes necessary to prevent the avoidance or manipulation of therapy through threats to leave.

Certainly, potential problems on a psychiatric unit are not limited to self-destructive or violent behavior, or elopement; however, these are the major areas requiring immediate response by staff, and often mobilization of the entire community. Other issues arise that are best addressed in small-group or community meetings. The advantage of a therapeutic milieu is that the structure already exists within which these problems can be addressed and resolved for the benefit of the clients.

Clinical Considerations

The description of milieu elements provides a concrete working model for the operation of a psychiatric unit. On another level, this model can be explored in terms of underlying concepts contributing to milieu function. Many have already been alluded to in previous sections. This discussion will address a number of areas that go beyond organizational considerations, and relate to the basic philosophy of this text.

Theoretical Considerations

If one accepts the notion that each of us has an impact on the world and the people around us, then it becomes possible to believe that each of us is capable of using that impact to be therapeutic. In a milieu setting, this concept is not only enacted, but becomes a cornerstone for the therapy in which professionals engage. That cornerstone is highly individualized. To put it differently: what one believes about the world and how it operates will determine one's preference of therapeutic style. Herein lies the basic reason that there are psychoanalysts as well as behaviorists. All practitioners select a theoretical framework they believe to be therapeutic based on their personal philosophy.

Professionals who work with milieu therapy believe in ideas such as personal responsibility, group and individual impact, social dynamics and learning, democratic function, and positive expectation. All of these beliefs are apparent in the description of milieu elements. Milieu therapy also views the individual in a holistic sense. As discussed in this text's introduction, each client is more than the sum of a mind and a body. In the milieu setting, clients are whole human beings who are continually influenced by biological inclinations, psychological forces, and environmental factors. It should not be construed that because the milieu setting is structured and relatively static, the individual is viewed as two-dimensional. Rather, the authors' discussions of general systems theory become particularly relevant in understanding the client's position on the unit, as well as in the world.

Milieu therapy provides an opportunity to reframe or redefine the accepted medical model. Health and wellness are emphasized through their expectation. Additionally, when the nurse deals with relative realities, positions, and behaviors, it is difficult to label individuals and place them at one specific point along the health–illness continuum. When the nurse actually relates to a real live human being, categories and stereotypes become meaningless. Hence, a specific symptom is no longer a self-limiting piece of information, hypothetically referred to on page 391 of a medical text under the heading "Psychosis." It takes on new and much broader significance when understood, not only in a general systems context, but also in the context of the individual receiver. "I, the nurse therapist and human being, perceive you, the client and human being, in a complex manner that involves all of my feelings and beliefs, not just my preconceptions about psychosis. Further, in the process of our relationship with each other, we may both be changed." Not only is this a far cry from the attitude of "me therapist, you sick," but multiply this type of interaction by the number of staff members and other clients on the unit, and one can begin to comprehend the potential impact of milieu.

Communication

Communication is the vehicle through which milieu operates. On a basic level, this involves the sending and receiving of messages by individuals who filter the messages through their own previous experiences. On a more complex level, as discussed by Watzlawick, Beavin, and Jackson,[27] communication plays a specific role in maintaining or changing an individual's perceptions and behavior. While this aspect of communication theory is a topic unto itself, a look at some of its theoretical underpinnings might be useful in understanding cause and effect.

First is the concept that all behavior is communication and all communication affects behavior. Hence, any act, in or out of the milieu setting, carries a message. This extends to all types of verbal and nonverbal behavior. The trick is to understand behavior as if it were a language all its own, which it is. This goes beyond the popular notion of interpreting isolated bits of body language. Rather, behavior can be interpreted in terms of an individual's overall intention or priorities in the world.

An important corollary is the circular nature of communication. Not only does an action transmit a message, but that message is reacted to by the recipient, thereby having a direct effect on the receiver's response. This is known as *feedback*. In all human interaction, even the most impersonal, this process of message-sending and feedback occurs continuously, and is the basis for the idea of impact. In order to deny impact, one would have to construct a situation in which an individual operates in a vacuum. (Although some people live their lives as if this were the case, it is scientifically impossible.) Because we all insist on producing behaviors, we are always communicating. The question is not whether someone else receives the message, but how they react to it. Even ignoring a message is a response.

In the milieu setting, this background information is played out as the first axiom of communication theory: *there is no such thing as not communicating.* The role of the staff is to perceive behavior and read its message. Notice that perception is the first step. This includes the silent or withdrawn client whose seeming lack of communication may be saying, "I'm afraid to tell you about myself," or "I'm in so much pain that I've chosen to shut you out by not responding to your message." This also includes the psychotic client whose supposed gibberish may really be saying, "I'm not sure how to respond to you and I don't want you too close, so I won't make too much sense. That way I can always deny my message with more craziness." Communication can be used to get closer to people or to put distance between them; to make oneself clear or to obscure; to build a relationship or to destroy it. Understanding the message of the behavior enables one to gain a clearer picture of its underlying intent.

The second axiom of communication theory is that *there are two components of every message, content and command.* On one level, a message conveys information, referred to as "the content." This is the level we generally recognize, although it is the most simplistic and is often misleading. On another level, a message imposes behavior by addressing the relative relationship between individuals. In healthy relationships, the parties involved already have a reasonably clear and acceptable idea of the nature of their relationship. Friends relate spontaneously, as equals. Authority figures display a demeanor appropriate to their level of expertise, and subordinates demonstrate suitable awareness of their relative position. Sick relationships, on the other hand, involve constant struggle between the parties concerning the nature of their relationship. Often this is seen as a lack of congruence—for example, parents who tell their children to clean up their room, but do so in a whining tone, or the wife who orders her husband to be more spontaneous. In the first case, the parents are giving an authority-laden message in a nonauthoritative fashion. In the second instance, the wife is relating to her husband as if he were a subordinate rather than an equal. Further, it is a contradiction in terms to order someone to be spontaneous.

The milieu provides an opportunity for individuals to learn a way out of this nonproductive communication cycle. The answer lies in *metacommunication:* talking about how we communicate. To increase the efficacy of this process, staff address not only the presenting problems that the clients describe from the outside world, but also the interactions observed with other people on the unit. The problem-solving process is not limited to finding a specific answer or solution, but includes feedback and instruction in the methods of communication that make problem-solving easier.

The staff's position regarding communication makes or breaks the effectiveness of communication theory in the milieu setting. If the staff fail to perceive behavior, they are both missing the message and communicating that the message was also of dubious importance. While none of us is capable of registering every piece of information we receive in the course of a day, it is important for staff members to be as attentive as possible. At the same time, if staff members are struggling with the nature of their relationships with clients, they can expect difficulty with those relationships. It becomes the staff's responsibility to be clear in their understanding of their professional position while not abusing it, and to metacommunicate that position appropriately to clients.

Communication theory offers a number of other, more detailed, concepts regarding the manner in which people change each other through the process of behavior. Nurses are referred to Watzlawick[27] for a more detailed discussion of this area. For the purposes of this chapter, it is sufficient to introduce the definite cause-and-effect relationship between communication and behavioral change. The impact of this relationship within the milieu should not be underestimated.

Staff members will understandably expect that the newly-admitted client arrives fully motivated for behavioral change, but there are some additional issues to consider. Behavior, in the form of defenses, serves a purpose for clients. Therefore, nurses should not be surprised when clients don't respond immediately. It's bad enough that the staff expect the client to give up a well-established mode of operation; they generally expect clients to give up behavior that they consider protective, even effective! One note of optimism deserves attention, however. Although clients enter milieu settings in a state of chaos, professionals who have worked in these and other settings will attest to the remarkable resourcefulness of human beings. Given sufficient support and appropriate guidance, each client possesses the capacity to construct a new order out of that chaos. In fact, the milieu provides a safe, controlled environment within which staff deliberately capitalize on chaos to achieve therapeutic experiences and results.

Environmental Adjustment

Environmental adjustment or manipulation highlights the difference between a psychiatric unit and a glorified hotel. The goal is to be therapeutic, and the process of therapy is often painful. The psychiatric unit often foregoes the immediate comfort of the client in order to promote long-term gains. Hence, sleeping pills are often replaced by one-to-one interaction. Anxiety and psychic pain may be worked with rather than medicated. As a result, the behavior on the unit may appear less than orderly while the process of therapy takes place. The chaos of emotional pain may even be necessary before a higher level of behavioral change can take place.

Nursing Role

Whenever possible, this chapter has described the staff role in relation to the milieu elements discussed. It should also be mentioned that nowhere else in psychiatric nursing today will the interplay of nursing with other disciplines be as potentially close, collegial, and rewarding, as in milieu therapy. In part, this is due to the nature of milieu therapy. The emphasis on a social role-model of communication and cooperation accepts no less. The unique contributions of the nursing process and standards prove their efficacy daily on psychiatric units. Additionally, the milieu structure of around-the-clock treatment availability places the nurse in a central and powerful position as a therapeutic coordinator.

But these factors alone are not sufficient to secure the position of nursing in milieu therapy. It took years of effort and professional growth, contributed by psychiatric nurses who forged the role into what it is today. That role continues to grow, as nursing research and innovations become incorporated into the milieu setting.

Legal/Political Issues

The social microcosm of the milieu is not independent of society's forces. These forces have the potential of helping or hindering milieu therapy. With the understanding that knowledge is power, it behooves the professional to be aware of factors influencing society's impact on treatment modalities.

Client Rights

Client rights vs. options of treatment is one of the major issues continuously faced by psychiatric units. The psychiatric community has become sensitive about treatments that are considered inhumane or dangerous by society. For example, electroshock therapy and psychotropic medications have received much opposition for many years. Although these methods are still in use, it is with a great deal of caution and regulation. It might be argued that the result has been the limitation of options for appropriately treating clients' disturbed behaviors. This discussion is not meant to favor one side or another, for indeed there are two sides to the story. However, nurses should be aware that some unit policies currently exist and will continue to evolve in direct response to the issue of individuals rights vs. treatment options.

Many state legislatures have passed mental health acts that specify parameters of treatment. These acts dictate under what circumstances clients may be hospitalized against their will, and the process required to prevent abuse of the system. In response to concerns about overmedication and loss of client autonomy, most psychiatric units are prohibited from administering medications without the client's consent except under extreme circumstances. Restraint must be accomplished according to what is generally termed "least restrictive alternatives."[28] That is to say, documentation of the event must indicate that only the necessary amount of force was employed and that the client's freedom of movement was limited no more than required for safety or therapeutic purposes. Every effort has been made to protect the individual rights of the mentally ill. The future direction of

mental health care is, as yet, uncertain. However, the rights of clients are certain to be crucial issues.

Cost Concerns

Cost concerns are also crucial issues. It is rather ironic that society contradicts itself. At the same time that clients' rights are being enforced, political and financial considerations operate counter to this effort. In many cases it seems that cost considerations over-ride client rights to adequate treatment, at least in the political arena. It is only necessary to look at county mental health programs to see this reality in action. Milieu programs are especially affected, because inadequate funding for hospitalization and staffing severely compromises this modality's effectiveness, and fosters recidivism. The future of mental health care in this country depends, to a great extent, on the political machinery employed on its behalf. This will, in turn, rely on research and documentation that supports cost effectiveness. The needs of the mentally ill and the concept of quality of life must be addressed. However, these discussions are simply verbal exercise until ideals are translated into viable programs and funded action. Mental health professionals of all disciplines share the responsibility for political awareness and community education. The nursing profession in particular must become more politically astute and contribute its unique expertise in order to mold a solution.

Milieu Efficacy

While support from the political arena for mental illness treatment programs is largely influenced by the voting public, research findings from the professional community also play an influential role. Statistical proof of therapeutic efficacy supports the case for cost effectiveness. Unfortunately, much of the available research either yields ambiguous results or must be reworked to accept the scrutiny of cost–benefit analyses.

Separate studies[8,16,20] have explored milieu characteristics in an attempt to isolate indicators of a successful program. Client and staff perceptions along a number of dimensions, as well as treatment outcome, were measured. When the statistical results were adjusted and examined, it was found that the units fell into one of two categories: efficient, in which clients displayed shorter hospital stays and higher discharge rates; and effective, in which clients demonstrated higher community tenure (they remained in the community for at least 90 days after discharge). The studies suggested that the most efficient units (i.e., those having the highest discharge rates) fostered the least involvement and autonomy from staff and clients. The most effective units (i.e., those having the highest community tenure rates) emphasized both client and staff involvement.

In other words, the atmosphere and goals of the unit influenced treatment outcome. An emphasis on high discharge rates was most consistent with units that were more rigid, allowing less involvement and self-direction.

RELEVANT RESEARCH

Relationships between elements of the therapeutic milieu and treatment outcome were explored by examining the duration of non-hospital time after discharge. The atmospheres of 21 state hospital wards were assessed along 10 parameters, including support, autonomy, anger/aggression, and order/organization. Findings were compared with the amount of time clients remained out of the hospital after discharge.

It was found that the wards that kept the clients out of the hospital longer were those that were less tolerant of the expression of anger and aggression while at the same time placing greater emphasis on order and organization. The authors surmised that disorganized clients may internalize some of the unit structure, enabling them to remain in the community longer following hospitalization.

(Klass DB, Growe GA, Strizich M: Ward treatment milieu and posthospital functioning. Arch Gen Psychiatry 34:1047, 1977)

RELEVANT RESEARCH

This extensive project concerning chronically mentally ill clients contrasted the efficacy of milieu treatment with a social-learning approach on separate units of a mental health center. The two modalities actually have much in common, particularly for the purposes of this study. Both emphasize maximal use of actual treatment time, resocialization, and a reeducative rather than a disease model of client treatment. The difference lies in a greater emphasis on learning theory, reinforcement, and behavioral consequences in social-learning therapy. Milieu therapy concentrates more on group pressure and encouragement. In effect, using the most general definition of milieu, social-learning could be viewed as a specific type of milieu program. The hospital comparison group for the study was a large regional mental institution. Its normal program of operation was assessed but not modified. While it reportedly utilized some milieu elements (*e.g.*, activity therapies, ward meetings, group or individual therapy), the hospital group scheduled a minimal amount of formal treatment time and used a medical model of treatment, complete with white uniforms and more time spent with drug administration.

The project findings heavily supported the social-learning model over the milieu model, although both were more effective than was the hospital program. The same ranking applied in terms of cost savings, with social-learning therapy being the least expensive alternative and hospital treatment being the most expensive. Positive results were also determined to be a function of an effective aftercare program. Although this project dealt with chronic rather than acute populations, other findings with respect to staffing and program elements were similar to those in the studies cited earlier.

(Paul GL, Lentz R: Psychosocial Treatment of Chronic Mental Patients. Cambridge, Massachusetts, Harvard University Press, 1977)

On the other hand, an emphasis on keeping clients out of the hospital longer required the opposite approach. Additionally, clients responded well toward the units they perceived as having a practical orientation, with high emphasis on staff control and support. Control, in these instances, related to issues of organization and control of aggression. None of the units studied clearly indicated milieu characteristics that would promote both high discharge rates and high community tenure rates. A description of one of these studies is found in the first Relevant Research box above.

Some evidence has correlated decreased unit size and better staffing with positive milieu characteristics such as support, involvement, spontaneity, organization, and practical orientation. At the same time, staff control, in terms of rigidity and structure, was seen as deemphasized on well-staffed units.[19]

As with any research, findings differ as population variables change. An extensive project concerning chronically mentally ill clients contrasted the efficacy of milieu treatment with a social-learning approach on separate units of a mental health center, as is shown in the second Relevant Research box above.

It appears from the above studies that high discharge rates or high community tenure rates can be achieved through the manipulation of milieu, but not both at the same time. In other words, the cost of care is paid now or later. Given findings about size and staffing, the most therapeutically effective milieus require sufficient funding to ensure appropriate size and staff-to-client ratios. Another study that modestly supports the efficacy of step systems and restriction-coercion[5] makes the point that, in poorly staffed environments, abridgement of personal rights may be the only way to produce therapeutic results. This study is described in the following Relevant Research box. Milieu programs have displayed efficacy under specific circumstances. Further study is needed to provide cost–benefit analyses if these programs are to be

RELEVANT RESEARCH

This study examined the effects of ward policies utilizing restriction and coercion (*e.g.*, a step system of privileges). Comparisons were made between a unit with a formal step system, one without a formal step system but with significant use of restriction and coercion, and one in which most treatment modalities were voluntary. Seven dimensions of client behavior were assessed on admission, at discharge, and at one- and six-month intervals postdischarge.

Clients on the formal step system unit showed better adjustment

(on 23 of 35 ratings), but the degree was just short of clinical significance. The authors concluded that restriction-coercion may have therapeutic value, although the degree of value was not clearly indicated by the study, possibly due to imprecise measurement techniques. The issue was raised that abridgement of the freedom normally exercised in society may be necessary in a therapeutic environment in order to achieve certain therapeutic benefits.

(Bursten B, Fontana AF, Dowds BN et al: Ward polity and therapeutic outcome: II. Ratings of patient behavior. Hosp Community Psychiatry 31:33, 1980)

adequately funded. The alternative is a return to restrictive units that will be legally challenged by client rights activists. We are truly in the midst of a struggle between therapeutic and social forces. The solution will dictate whether mental health takes a step forward or backward.

There are initial indications that the solution will not be positive. In response to decreasing hospital stays and tighter third-party (*e.g.,* insurance company) reimbursement, many psychiatric units are moving back to a medical model of organization. This trend has been predicted to continue,[18,22] in direct contradiction of the research cited earlier that demonstrated the medical model as less effective than milieu and social-learning models. As a result, hospital alternative programs are emerging to implement milieu concepts and operate less expensively than hospital units.[18] The success of these alternative programs depends on their continued ability to demonstrate therapeutic effectiveness and convince third-party payers of the cost–benefit advantage of coverage.

Future Applications

At the very least, three areas of opportunity need attention with regard to milieu therapy: existing milieu programs, noninstitutional settings, and nonpsychiatric settings.

Milieu programs, as indicated in the previous discussion, still need research and justification of their existence. Additionally, milieu settings must be assessed to determine their present appropriateness and necessary modifications for specialized populations of mental health clients. These populations include children and adolescents, elderly and Alzheimer clients, as well as dually-diagnosed clients (*e.g.,* clients with the dual diagnoses of psychiatric disorder and chemical dependency or psychiatric disorder and medical illness). In some facilities, separate units have been established for these specialized populations, with the milieu being modified on an ongoing basis as additional theory or common sense dictates changes to accommodate clients' special needs. Other facilities lack the space or resources for specialized

units. In such cases, research on the relative effectiveness of specialized units could well indicate the need for client transfer to a more appropriate setting, changes in the existing milieu to accommodate a special group, or the cost–benefit advantages of seeking the space and resources for a new specialized unit. Concentration in these areas will have an important impact on hospital psychiatric treatment for both acute and chronic populations.

Noninstitutional settings are the next area requiring focus, particularly with the current emphasis on decreasing the length and frequency of hospital stays. Strides have already been made in daycare. Studies of the most appropriate application of milieu concepts in daycare, as well as outcome studies, are necessary to ensure maximum efficacy in maintaining clients outside the hospital environment. In addition, the new area of psychiatric home care is beginning to address the idea of bringing treatment to clients' own environments. This does not preclude the use of milieu concepts, with clients' cooperation, to restructure their environment along therapeutic lines. While present funding often requires that clients demonstrate some degree of homebound status before treatment is covered, research on home care outcomes may support this process as an adjunct to the hospital–daycare continuum. Research may show that quality care can best be accomplished by using hospitalization, followed by daycare and home care, either separately or in concert.

Nonpsychiatric settings are a final area that can derive benefit from milieu theory. Convalescent homes and board-and-care facilities would certainly benefit from a community approach to maintaining optimal client functioning. General hospital units as well would profit from certain milieu elements aimed at maximizing wellness and personal responsibility for medical care. The manipulation of any environment for the psychological benefit of the individual is a possibility. Milieu concepts that have already been applied and tested are certainly available for implementation.

When all of history is considered, it is difficult to imagine that a consistent focus on the scientific and humane treatment of mental illness has only occurred in the last 200 years. Indeed, most of the knowledge of human psychology currently considered valid has been amassed since the turn of the 20th century. In essence, psychiatric treatment is in its infancy and maturing at an ever-increasing pace.

When changes occur so rapidly in a field, it is often the unusual or the dramatic changes that stand out. Eventually, the unusual will drop away and the dramatic will become commonplace. It becomes difficult with time to imagine an era when a particular practice was considered radical, since the practice may have become so ingrained. Milieu therapy is just such a practice. At its beginning, it was regarded as an inconceivable and appalling alternative to the status quo. Today, it exists in a variety of forms on virtually every psychiatric treatment unit.

This chapter has attempted to describe milieu settings as most of them are or could be. The purpose, goals, and techniques form a foundation common to all milieu programs, and provide a basis for experimentation and innovation. The organizational elements described are less uniform from unit to unit, but offer some guidelines for what to expect. Additional differences are dictated by any specialized theoretical frameworks operating on an individual unit. All units have, incorporated into their policy structure, specific response directions for certain behavioral problems. The beauty of milieu therapy is that its effects and benefits are as holistic as its attitudes toward clients: both are far greater than the sum of any specific parts.

The point to be remembered by professional nurses is that, just as psychiatry continues to evolve, so will the concept and utilization of milieu. We can take it for granted and rest on our laurels, or we can test the limits. The discussion of issues related to milieu therapy merely provides a beginning. With a solid awareness of the principles and practices of milieu, we have a tremendous opportunity to study its effects and seek new applications in the service of client care. From this viewpoint, milieu becomes more than just "the way this unit is run." It is a dynamic and fluid treatment element with potential benefits for all areas of nursing.

Summary

1. Milieu therapy exists with any program that manipulates or capitalizes on the environment for therapeutic purposes, and need not be limited exclusively to psychiatric settings.
2. Milieu therapy emphasizes conscious use of the environment, active participation by the client in the planning and implementation of treatment, and a recognition that the milieu acts as a microcosm of the outside world.
3. Milieu settings capitalize on holistic concepts in their understanding of the individual, and consist of a dynamic interplay of processes between the milieu and the client.

4. Mutual personal impact is an essential part of the milieu, requiring a heightened level of awareness and an understanding of the principle that being authentic with the client is more important than technique.
5. The nursing process is an integral part of milieu therapy on a continual basis.
6. Milieu treatment operates primarily as a tertiary level of prevention, providing rehabilitative services.
7. Five therapeutic activities inherent in the milieu setting are containment, support, structure, involvement, and validation.
8. In working with clients, staff members aim to provide reality orientation, limit setting, and social skills training.
9. Disordered behaviors are responded to in order of priority, with more severe levels of disorder taking precedence.
10. The client or community government is a system that fosters responsible interactions and a sense of control over the environment, as long as hidden agendas are avoided by the staff.
11. The community participates on all levels of milieu functioning, and community members can be expected to have a variety of reactions to the setting and its occurrences.
12. Particular attention should be paid to community reactions when disturbing incidents occur, such as suicide or violence.
13. Communication, facilitation of expression, and modification of behavior are specific techniques that serve the milieu process.
14. Discharge planning begins when clients are admitted, and is a continual focus of the therapeutic process.

References

1. Abroms GM: Defining milieu therapy. Arch Gen Psychiatry 21: 553, 1969
2. Abroms GM, Fellner CH, Whitaker CA: The family enters the hospital. Am J Psychiatry 127:1363, 1971
3. Almond R: The Healing Community. New York, Jason Aronson, 1974
4. Barnes E: Psychosocial Nursing. London, Tavistock, 1968
5. Bursten B, Fontana AF, Dowds BN et al: Ward polity and therapeutic outcome: II. Ratings of patient behavior. Hosp Community Psychiatry 31:33, 1980
6. Daniels DN, Kuldau JM: Marginal man, the tether of tradition, and intentional social system therapy. Community Ment Health J 3:13, 1967
7. Dolan J: Goodnow's History of Nursing, 11th ed. Philadelphia, WB Saunders, 1967
8. Ellsworth R, Maroney R, Klett W et al: Milieu characteristics of successful psychiatric treatment programs. Am J Orthopsychiatry 41(3):427, 1971
9. Evans FMC: Psychosocial Nursing. New York, Macmillan, 1971

10. Glass AJ: Principles of combat psychiatry. Military Med July:27, 1955
11. Goffman E: Asylums. Garden City, New York, Doubleday, 1961
12. Gunderson JG: Defining the therapeutic processes in psychiatric milieus. Psychiatry 41:327, 1978
13. Hoblitzell DK: A psychiatric nursing care plan: Total care for the patient in military psychiatry. U.S. Navy Med 69:24, 1978
14. Jones M: The Therapeutic Community. New York, Basic Books, 1953
15. Jones M: Beyond the Therapeutic Community. New Haven, Yale University Press, 1968
16. Klass DB, Growe GA, Strizich M: Ward treatment milieu and posthospital functioning. Arch Gen Psychiatry 34:1047, 1977
17. Kraft AM: The Therapeutic Community. In Arieti S, Caplan G (eds): American Handbook of Psychiatry, 2nd ed, vol 2. New York, Basic Books, 1974
18. Mosher LR, Kresky-Wolff M, Mathews S et al: Milieu in the 1980s—a comparison of two residential alternatives to hospitalization. Bull Menninger Clin 50(3):257, 1986
19. Moos R: Size, staffing, and psychiatric ward treatment environments. Arch Gen Psychiatry 26:414, 1972
20. Moos R, Schwartz J: Treatment environment and treatment outcome. J Nerv Ment Dis 154:264, 1972
21. Paul GL, Lentz RJ: Psychosocial Treatment of Chronic Mental Patients. Cambridge, Massachusetts, Harvard University Press, 1977
22. Rabiner CJ: The impact of the emerging reimbursement systems upon professional roles. 38th Institute on Hospital and Community Psychiatry, 1986
23. Robbins LL: The Hospital as a Therapeutic Community. In Kaplan HI, Freedman AM, Sadock BJ (eds): Comprehensive Textbook of Psychiatry, 3rd ed, vol 3. Baltimore, Williams & Wilkins, 1980
24. Rosenbaum CP, Beebe JE III: Psychiatric Treatment. New York, McGraw-Hill, 1975
25. Slavson SR: Reeducating the Delinquent Through Group and Community Participation. New York, Harper & Row, 1955
26. Stanton AH, Schwartz MS: The Mental Hospital. New York, Basic Books, 1954
27. Watzlawick P, Beavin JH, Jackson DD: Pragmatics of Human Communication. New York, WW Norton, 1967
28. Wyatt vs. Stickney: 325 F. Supp. 781, M.D. Ala., 1971

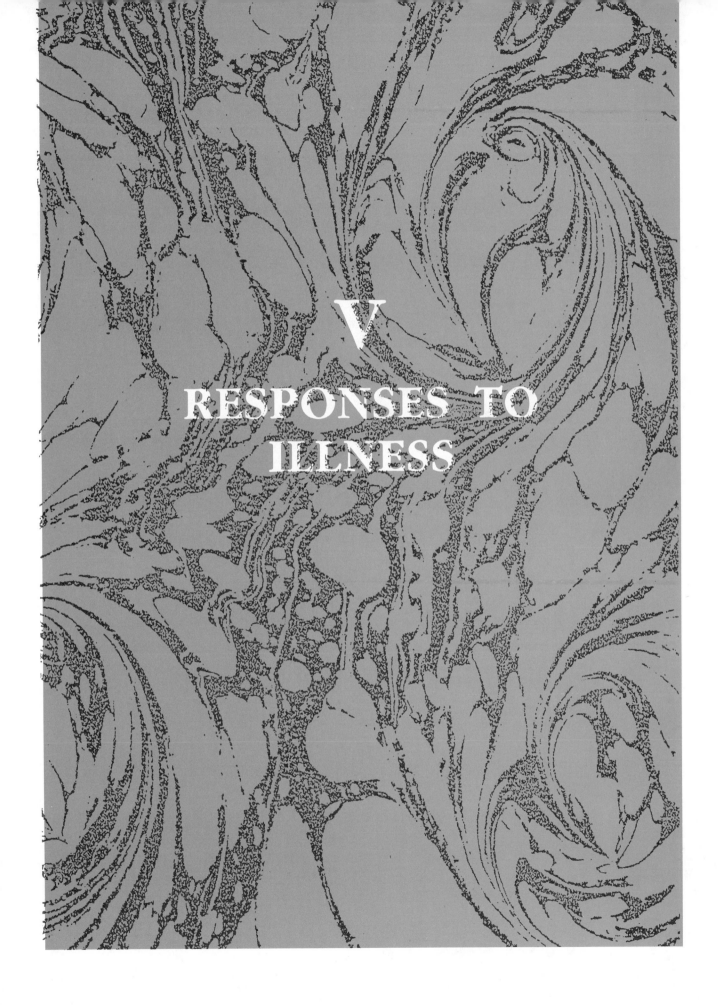

V
RESPONSES TO
ILLNESS

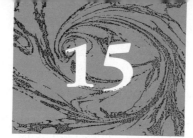

GWEN MARRAM VAN SERVELLEN AND ROBERTA NICHOLSON

DEPRESSIVE/MANIC DISORDERS

Learning Objectives

Upon completion of this chapter the student should be able to do the following:

1. Define depressive/manic disorders.
2. Differentiate between mild forms of impairment of mood and affect and more severe illness states.
3. Describe the work of several theorists who have been central in describing impairments of mood and affect as well as outlining the therapy for depressive/manic disorders.
4. Identify the stressors or precipitating events associated with these disorders.
5. Assess an individual with a depressive/manic disorder.
6. Plan specific interventions for a client who has a depressive/manic disorder.
7. Describe the impact of the nurse's use of therapeutic communication on the belief system and self-esteem of persons with a depressive/manic disorder.

8. Describe the importance of working with the family of the client with a mood disturbance.
9. Identify the primary somatic treatments used with depressive/manic disturbances and discuss the guidelines for their use.
10. Identify the possible side-effects of somatic therapies used with clients with depressive/manic impairment.

CLINICAL EXAMPLES

SHEILA

When the nurse walked into Sheila's room, Sheila was lying in bed with one arm slung over her eyes. When the nurse tapped her on the shoulder, Sheila turned to look long enough to allow an introduction, but then she rolled over and lay with her back toward the nurse. "Sheila," the nurse began, "we're getting a group of women together to do some stretching exercises in the activity room. I would like you to join us."

"I don't feel like being around other people."
"What do you mean?"

"Nobody wants to be around me," she said. "No stretching exercises are going to help; I'm way too fat. Fat and worthless."

The nurse walked around the bed, and sat in a chair at Sheila's bedside. Sheila had been crying.

"Have you been crying, Sheila?"
"I want to sleep. Leave me alone."

The nurse left the room feeling completely helpless about her inability to assist Sheila to feel like participating.

SERGIO

The nurse couldn't write half as quickly as Sergio talked. Later, after Sergio had been admitted as an inpatient, he became much more irritable. For two nights in a row he worked furiously into the morning writing lecture notes and letters, despite the sedative he had been given.

One morning the nurse walked into his room after he had had breakfast. There was paper all over the floor and the bed. "C'min!" he bellowed, as he quickly picked up the handwritten outlines. He shook a stack of paper at the nurse. "I hope it never stops," he said. He read a paragraph that sounded confusing and fragmented, and then shoved the paper into the nurse's hands.

"That, madam, is genius going nuts."
"You'd think I'd be dead after eating this hospital garbage for days, but it's gotta be doing something magic. Feed me more." He grabbed his papers from the nurse. "Ever occur to you that you're pretty damned lethargic?"
"Oh?," the nurse said.
"SLOTHFUL! You have taken days of my life, and consequently my money, to take a total of umpteen blood tests and run me through a couple of evaluation wringers, and you still can't decide what to do

with me. Why don't you lock me up? Never mind. You have already."
"We are here to help you, Sergio."
"Uh oh. I can see you're writing 'uncooperative' on my evaluation. Go ahead. I deserve a 'D.' You deserve a 'D+,' but only because you've got great legs. Don't talk. Just let me look at your legs."

Sergio was making the nurse nervous. As the nurse left the room, Sergio followed her into the hallway, "Okay. I just don't like it here," he said, panting.

Maintaining a professional bearing, the nurse said, "Let's go someplace where there's more space than there is in your room."

They arrived at the office. The nurse sat down, but Sergio remained on his feet.

"And in all this, I think what a crying shame it would be to be my little girl. God, I'm glad I don't have a father like me. I'm scared to death I'm gonna do something that could ruin her life. But you're going to set me straight, huh?"
"No, you are."

Introduction

Sheila and Sergio suffer from *affective disturbances,* or impairments of affect and mood. *Depression* is the more common manifestation of these disturbances, whereas *mania* (elation) comes to the attention of the health care professional less frequently, except in its severest state.

Both clients present a clinical picture typical of those that suffer depressive/manic disorders. As with thought disorders, depressive/manic disorders (also called affective disorders) are complex illnesses with a variety of proposed causes and a symptom picture that may indicate severe difficulties in living.

These clients present challenges to nurses because feelings of helplessness, low self-esteem, and frequently suicidal thoughts require skillful intervention. Nurses must provide relationships that are supportive and positive, and at the same time challenge the self-deprecatory thoughts of these patients.

This chapter will explore the various depressive/ manic impairments and their implication for nursing care.

The depressive/manic illnesses are characterized by disturbances in mood or affect. Although impairments of thinking, perception, and behavior may be evident with these individuals, the chief characteristic that receives ongoing attention is the disturbance in mood or affect. *Mood* refers to a feeling state—for example, a feeling of well-being or depression. *Affect* refers to an expressed feeling tone that is associated with an idea or mental representation. An individual may be unaware of affect, yet it may influence mood, result in physical manifestations, and not be clearly evident in a current mood or feeling state. This is why depressed individuals often do not recognize their depression. A change in affect or mood can be precipitated by a recurrent physical illness and medications taken for it. Mood and affect can also be influenced by multiple factors interacting in some combination to create a change in the individual's experience.

Oscillation between periods of feeling a sense of well-being and periods of depression is normal. The assertion that the normal population exhibits mood swings is supported by numerous studies.[1,2,5,30] All individuals experience mood swings, and it is customary for normal individuals to have "blue" hours or "blue" days. Mood swings, however, are more marked in individuals with depressive/manic disorders. The intensity and duration of mood states is a distinguishing feature in differentiating impaired states from periods of "normalcy," for both people with well-defined illnesses and those suspected of having their first recorded affective episode.

This chapter provides an overview of impairments of mood and affect, and details the nursing process used with people exhibiting these kinds of impairments. Because mood problems exist in a variety of clients, both those with defined emotional illnesses and those without, it is important that nurses understand what differentiates a condition needing further attention, what factors can contribute to the exacerbation or alleviation of symptoms, and how the nursing process is employed to address the specific symptoms associated with the impairments.

While depressive/manic disorders vary in type, one or more distinctive features are common in a given episode. Depression and/or exaggerated states of elation are most common, and the presence or absence of these phenomena distinguish the category of illness as described in the Diagnostic and Statistical Manual III-R (DSM-III-R).[3] According to the DSM-III-R, depressive/manic illnesses can be of two major types: *bipolar* or *unipolar* illness. This is to say that some clients with depressive/

manic illnesses exhibit exaggerated states of both depression and elation, while others present in single or recurrent episodes of depression only. Table 15-1 presents the major DSM-III-R diagnostic categories of depressive/manic disorders.

TABLE 15-1.
DSM-III-R DIAGNOSTIC CATEGORIES FOR DEPRESSIVE/MANIC DISORDERS

296.70   BIPOLAR DISORDER NOS

Bipolar Disorder, Depressed

296.56	In full remission
296.55	In partial remission
296.51	Mild
296.52	Moderate
296.53	Severe, without psychotic features
296.50	Unspecified
296.54	With psychotic features

Bipolar Disorder, Manic

296.46	In full remission
296.45	In partial remission
296.41	Mild
296.42	Moderate
296.43	Severe, without psychotic features
296.40	Unspecified
296.44	With psychotic features

Bipolar Disorder, Mixed

296.66	In full remission
296.65	In partial remission
296.61	Mild
296.62	Moderate
296.63	Severe, without psychotic features
296.60	Unspecified
296.64	With psychotic features

301.13   CYCLOTHYMIA

300.40   DYSTHYMIA

Major Depression, Recurrent

296.36	In full remission
296.35	In partial remission
296.31	Mild
296.32	Moderate
296.33	Severe, without psychotic features
296.30	Unspecified
296.34	With psychotic features

Major Depression, Single Episode

296.26	In full remission
296.25	In partial remission
296.21	Mild
296.22	Moderate
296.23	Severe, without psychotic features
296.20	Unspecified
296.24	With psychotic features

(American Psychiatric Association: Diagnostic and Statistical Manual of Mental Disorders III: Revised. Washington, DC, American Psychiatric Association, 1987.)

Theoretical Developments in Depressive/Manic Disorders

A review of scientific and nonscientific contributions to the diagnosis and treatment of depressive/manic disturbances requires an examination of how current theories have evolved, and how some notions may still pervade our thinking about these illness states. The following review will trace the evolution from very early notions to those that permeate current treatment practices.

History

As early as the fourth century, B.C., depression was identified as a problem requiring treatment. Hippocrates described a syndrome that he called "melancholia." He believed that it was caused by a predominance of black bile.[25] Subsequently, Aristotle observed the problem, and proposed wine and music as therapy for melancholia.[25]

From the first century B.C. through the early 1600s, scientists struggled with the differentiation of *depression* (still called melancholia) from what is now termed *mania.* Galen was the first to associate mania and melancholia with brain malfunction. In 1621, Burton wrote *The Anatomy of Melancholia,* describing melancholia as "a disease of the head or mind."[25]

Causes of melancholia were said to include God, witches, old age, poor diet, heredity, bad air, lack of exercise, and psychological states, including sorrow, fear, anger, and shame. These symptoms were thought to be alleviated by music, intellectual stimulation, good relationships, and drama. Treatment modalities for depression during this period included a wide array of activities, such as maintaining good hygiene, exercise, soothing music, the company of cheerful people, and the confession of shortcomings.

Kohlbaum made inroads on describing what was distinguished as not just depression but alternating states of moods.[25] He observed that individuals can have periods of sad mood that alternate with periods characterized by elated mood. In the late 1800s, Kraepelin defined various subdivisions of manic/depressive disorders. He believed, however, that these various manifestations were one disease process: manic/depressive "insanity."

Current Theories Explaining the Etiology and Manifestations of Depressive/Manic Disorders

Theorists continue to argue about whether depressive/manic impairments are chemically-transmitted, or are of psychological origin. Most agree that interpersonal relationships are very important in these disorders. Although the cause of depressive/manic disorders has been linked with biochemical research, there is still a great deal of credence given to psychosocial phenomena in the occurrence and resolution of depressive and manic episodes.

The two broad theories that address the origin of depressive/manic disorders are:

1. The *endogenous theory* suggests that the disorders are separate clinical entities. Thus, clinical depression is considered to be a well-defined disease quite different from the normal "depressed" mood. It is postulated that the observed depression or mania is caused by an internal biological defect. This hypothesis suggests that naturally-occurring depression results from a deficiency in one or more biogenic amines at receptor sites in the brain.

2. The *exogenous theory* postulates that depression or elation is caused by an individual's reaction to environmental or external factors, and may be experienced with varying degrees of intensity.

An episode of depression may also be termed *reactive.* Reactive disturbances consist of feelings and thoughts that range from elation to depression. Most people are susceptible to mood swings that are experienced as "highs" and "lows." Typical "Monday morning blues" and "holiday blues" are examples of mild and transient disturbances. Although depressive/manic disorders are primarily manifested as mood alterations, symptoms such as anorexia, insomnia, motor retardation, and motor excitation are also linked with milder forms of reactive disorders.

A common example of signs and symptoms exhibited in some depressive/manic disorders is found in the grief response. This naturally-occurring depression accompanying bereavement has been universally noted in almost all societies, and, unlike other forms of depression, is considered normal and even adaptive. Fatigue, dejected mood, reduction in gratification in activities previously enjoyed, and suicidal tendencies may all be exhibited. Most professionals view grief as different from clinical depression despite the similarity in symptoms. Delayed or absent bereavement has the potential to result in an impaired status. When these signs and symptoms persist for more than two weeks, they are considered beyond normal mood swings.

Another way of differentiating between clinical depression and a low normal mood is classifying this affective state by "neurotic" and "psychotic" manifestations. These terms were popularized in the 1960s and 1970s.

A *neurotic* episode is so labeled when the depression interferes with the individual's ability to meet the ordinary demands of life, but does not result in an impairment significant enough to alter the individual's ability to reality test.

Psychotic episodes, on the other hand, represent the extreme end of the continuum: impairment of the capacity to retain a sense of reality. Psychotic depressions are frequently accompanied by severe disturbances in perception, delusions, or paranoia. Likewise, psychotic manic episodes are frequently accompanied by delusions of grandeur. Such ideas permit individuals to believe that they are capable of great feats, beyond what they or anyone else could imagine.

Rather than view these disorders solely along lines of endogenous or exogenous disease processes, the more current approach, particularly to depression, is to view the disorder as a result of a multitude of interacting phenomena. Currently there are five dominant schools of thought that represent approximately ten models of depression.[1] These include the biological, psychoanalytic, behavioral, sociological, and existential points of view (see Table 15-2).

Biological Models

The psychiatric/mental health nurse with a biological point of view focuses on the genetic vulnerability of the central nervous system and the resulting behavioral pathology. According to biological theories, behavioral responses are dependent on electrical and neurochemical transmission in the brain. The electrical nerve impulse promotes release of chemical neurotransmitters from the synapse of a nerve-cell ending. These neurotransmission processes are further regulated by electrolyte concentration, brain metabolism, and hormones. Neurotransmitters, neuroendocrines, and electrolyte balance have been implicated in depression.[26]

Biogenic Amines. *Biogenic amines,* a class of chemical neurotransmitter, are thought to have a role in depressive/manic disorders. The biogenic amine hypothesis of depression states that too much norepinephrine is responsible for mania, while too little produces depression. Recent findings indicate that this hypothesis has been amplified, and that other neurotransmitters, such as serotonin, dopamine, acetylcholine, and several others, also may play a role in depression.[26]

Neurophysiological Factors. Associations between behavior and hormones, specifically neuroendocrine changes and depression, have been substantiated in many neuroendocrinology studies.[26] Several neuroendocrine disorders, including thyroid conditions and Cushing's disease, are associated with behavior similar to that in mental illness. Sex hormones are implicated in depression because decreased libido usually occurs in this disorder, and there are different prevalence rates for males and females. Cyclical mood changes occur in females. Significant findings in the neuroendocrinology of depression have been related only to unipolar depression at this time.

The electrolytes directly involved with nerve conduction and neurotransmission, such as sodium, potassium, calcium, and magnesium, are implicated in the neurochemistry of depressive/manic disorders.[26] Frequently, depressed clients complain of excess water retention. Some studies indicate that water retention is due to residual sodium. Both water retention and residual sodium usually subside after recovery from depression. Premenstrual tension has also been presented as a model to explain electrolyte imbalances in depression. Many women experience water retention and depressed mood prior to menstruation; with the onset of menstruation, these symptoms cease.

Each of the biological frameworks helps to clarify the relationship between behavioral pathology and biological abnormality. However, data from other schools of thought must also be integrated so that depressive illness can be conceptualized as an interaction among the chemical, experiential, and behavioral aspects of an individual experiencing depressive/manic disorder.

Psychoanalytic Models

The psychoanalytic school has considered the etiology and treatment of depression. This school proposed some of the first major theories of depression, which provided treatment guidelines for depression for decades. Many clinicians still use the psychoanalytic principles of depression. The psychoanalytic school encompasses four models: the ideas of Freud, object loss, loss of self-esteem, and negative cognitive set.

Aggression-Turned-Inward. Freud's aggression-turned-inward model viewed depression as dammed-up aggression that has not been directed at the appropriate object. The incident of depression, according to this hypothesis, is triggered by loss. Because individuals feel simultaneously love and anger toward an object, they are unable to express the feelings of anger or may think they are inappropriate or irrational. There may be lifelong patterns of containment of feelings that clients view as negative. These angry feelings are then *retroflexed*—turned inward and toward themselves. Suicide, according to Freud, is the ultimate act of retroflexed aggression. The self-destructive act is a strike against the ambivalent object as well as the self.[14]

This model does not lend itself to empirical verification, although this is the most widely quoted psychological conceptualization of depression. Some depressed clients actively express anger and hostility, and some who

TABLE 15-2.
MODELS OF DEPRESSION

SCHOOL	MODEL
Biological	Biogenic amine
	Neurophysiological
Psychoanalytic	Aggression-turned-inward
	Object loss
	Loss of self-esteem
	Negative cognitive set
Behavioral	Learned helplessness
	Loss of reinforcement
Sociological	Loss of role status
Existential	Loss of meaning of existence

(Akiskal H, McKinney W: Ten models of depression: Overview of recent research in depression. Arch Gen Psychiatry 32:286, 1975.)

RELEVANT RESEARCH

The authors pointed out that, while much research has been focused on biological factors related to the etiology of depression, there has been equally important concurrent research investigating the role of psychosocial factors in influencing the occurrence of milder depressive disorders. A number of demographic factors such as age, sex, marital status, social class, and education have been shown to affect the risk of depression. Four psychosocial factors were selected for study. These were: family history of psychiatric illness, early loss of a nurturing relationship, stressful life events, and low social support. The study used a cross-sectional design with a population of college students.

A depressed group (N = 160) of students attending a university psychiatric service was contrasted with a nondepressed group (N = 206). Depression was measured by the Beck Depression Inventory. It was found that family history of psychiatric illness, stressful life events, and a lack of confidants with whom to share problems all had significant, independent direct effects on the occurrence of depressive symptoms. However, early loss was not associated with a depressive disorder. The concept of interactional effects between social support and life events was not supported. The authors concluded that these findings can be generalized to other university student populations and, to a lesser extent, to other young adults.

(O'Neil MK, Lancee WJ, Freeman SJ: Psychosocial factors and depressive symptoms. J Nerv Ment Dis 174(1):15–23, 1985.)

learn to express their anger outwardly have not experienced clinical improvement. Thus, considerable doubt exists about the universality of the aggression-turned-inward model as the sole explanation of depression.

Object Loss. Object loss theory suggests that a history of traumatic separation events during early life may predispose an individual to adult depression. Separation is viewed as a traumatic event, capable of inducing dramatic behavioral changes. This hypothesis has been researched by Bowlby[9] and by Spitz.[24] Two important issues compose this theory: loss during childhood is a predisposing factor for the occurrence of adult depression, and separation in adult life can precipitate depression.

Spitz noted a deprivational reaction in infants separated from their mothers in the second half of the first year of life. This syndrome, known as *anaclitic depression,* is manifested by apprehension, crying, withdrawal, psychomotor slowing, dejection, stupor, insomnia, anorexia, weight loss, and gross retardation in growth and development. Bowlby noted a similar reaction, except in older children. The children reacted in three stages. During the first stage, the children searched for their mothers and appeared restless and tearful. Their next response was apathetic withdrawal. Last, some children became detached and felt rejected when reunited with their mothers.

Brown[11] studied 216 clients with depressive disorders, and two separate control groups. Forty-one percent of the depressed clients had lost a parent by death before the age of 15, compared to 16% and 12%, respectively, for the two control groups. Brown also noted that the loss of the mother was significant throughout earlier childhood. Other authorities have suggested that the loss of the father from ages 10 to 14 is the critical predisposing variable for adult depression. From a research standpoint, however, it is difficult to support the connection between early object loss and adult depression.

Loss of Self-Esteem. According to Bibring's model,[10] depression occurs when the ego suffers collapse, or loss of self-esteem, because it is aware of its goal yet simultaneously feels helpless to attain it. When clients cannot live up to their ego ideals, such as the wish to be loved, good, or human, for example, depression appears. Bibring believed that hostility is a secondary phenomenon that occurs with object loss or objects that prevent attainment of goals.

Negative Cognitive Set. According to cognitive theories, distorted views develop in early childhood that lead to susceptibility to depression in later life. These distorted views promote affective, motivational, and physical symptoms of depression. The disturbances in depression may be viewed in terms of the activation of a set of three major cognitive patterns that force individuals to view themselves, their world, and their future in a negative way. Beck referred to this as a *negative triad.*[5]

The first component of the triad is the pattern of construing experiences in a negative way. Clients consistently interpret their interactions with their environments as representing defeat, deprivation, or disparagement, and see their lives as obstacle-ridden and burdensome.

The second component is the pattern of clients' viewing themselves as inadequate and unworthy and tending to attribute these unpleasant experiences to some defect in themselves.

Last, clients view their futures in negative ways. They anticipate that their current difficulties or sufferings will continue indefinitely. Their futures will contain unremitting hardship, frustration, and deprivation. The cognitive approach emphasizes the role that thinking plays in determining emotional states. This theory has been supported by research data.

Depressed clients misinterpret events, and the range is from mild inaccuracies to total misinterpretations. The typical cognitions show a variety of deviations from logical thinking, including arbitrary inference (drawing conclusions in the absence of evidence); selective abstractions (conceptualizing a whole experience based on one detail); generalizations (drawing a conclusion on the basis of a single incident); magnification (assigning unusual weight to certain aspects of a situation); personalization (interpreting events in terms of self-reference); and dichotomous thinking (thinking in terms of extremes or opposites). Thus, clients automatically make a negative interpretation of situations even when more obvious and plausible explanations exist.[5]

Behavioral Models

The behavioral school focuses, not on internal mechanisms of the unconscious and defenses, but on behaviors of the individual who is depressed. The behavioral school also considers the traditional behavioral theory concepts of stimulus and response.

Two models from the behavioral school are presented: *learned helplessness*,[23] in which the mechanism is uncontrollable aversive stimulation, and *loss of reinforcement*,[1] in which the rewards of the "sick role" substitute for lost sources of reinforcement.

Learned Helplessness. Seligman[23] discovered a phenomenon termed *learned helplessness.* According to this theory, depression develops as a consequence of a history of failure to control the environment to one's advantage. According to Seligman, when individuals are confronted with aversive stimuli, they are not able to provide relief from such stimulation. Therefore, they see no relationship between their responses and relief from aversive events, and become "helpless." Seligman believed that depression-prone individuals have a life-long history characterized by relative failure in exercising control over the reinforcers in their environments. Depression then occurs when individuals perceive themselves as losing all control over such reinforcers and they are paralyzed by helplessness, passivity, and the inability to assert themselves.

Loss of Reinforcement. Lewinsohn and others[1] postulated that a low rate of response—*contingent positive reinforcement*—precedes depressive behaviors. The environment may repeatedly fail to provide reinforcement, which places the individual on an extinction scale, or the individual may fail to emit the appropriate responses to potentially reinforce the stimuli. The individual may receive rewards for the "sick role" and maintain depressive behaviors.

Sociological Theory

Becker[1] stated that the ego is a social phenomenon. He believed that the ego is rooted in social reality and is composed of socially-learned symbols and motives. Thus, a breakdown in self-esteem can lead to depression. Those with potential to become depressed not only experience object loss, but lose their sociological symbolic possessions such as power, status, roles, identity, and values, and perhaps their purpose for existence.

Existential Theory

The existential theories of depression explain depression as the loss of the meaning of one's existence. Ey[5] viewed depression as a "pathetic immobility, a suspension of existence, a syncope of time." Thus, depressed clients feel incomplete and impotent, and their lives have lost meaning.

Summary

In summary, these theoretical models stem from the biological, sociological, and psychological sciences. Some note that there is a common thread running throughout: namely, that an alteration in self-perception, caused by one or more factors, exists to yield a person who has given up hope in controlling environmental reinforcers. Circumstances like those of the individual's initial experiences with depression may exist and may bring these cognitions to the surface. The negative cognitions then translate into behaviors of a depressed individual—withdrawal and loss of interest in activities. Loss of motivation to obtain rewards is also impaired.

Stressors and Precipitating Events

The literature reveals that certain factors place persons at particular risk for depression. Factors include age, sex, family history, role strain, and recent life stresses.

Age

Although depression can strike at any age, there is evidence that it is more prominent in individuals over 30 years of age. One reason for this is that with age come more experiences of loss. Therefore, the incidence of depression increases with age. This is not to dismiss, however, early findings that depression is linked with behavioral disorders in young children and adolescents. Many of the injuries associated with children, *e.g.,* those run over by moving vehicles, are now being viewed as self-inflicted, purposeful events.

Sex

The preponderance of depression in women has been noted in the literature. The ratio of depression in women to that in men is believed to be 2:1. The high rate of depression among women has been associated with role strain, the premenstrual syndrome, and the general help-seeking behavior of women which differs from that of men. Studies have shown that, although work, marriage,

RELEVANT RESEARCH

A critical variable in research on depression, and one that has important clinical implications, is the presence of sex differences in the expression and frequency of occurrence of depressive symptoms.

The purpose of the study was to evaluate possible sex differences in the expression and intensity of depression. Large samples of college students indicated the extent to which they would use a number of behaviors or cognitions if depressed. The rated items were gathered, using procedures suggested by the behavioral-analytic model. The results augmented previous findings in this area. Men and women were shown to have distinct differences in the nature of their interpersonal behaviors as well as in cognitive styles for coping with depression. Women indicated that they would engage in expression of feelings to a greater extent than men. Also, women more often reported that they would be likely to avoid social situations involving large groups of people, yet would go to a close friend to discuss their problems.

(Funabike D, Bologna NC, Pepping M et al: Revisiting sex differences in the expression of depression. J Abnorm Psychol 89(2):194–202, 1980.)

and children can be sources of gratification, these factors may also predispose women to depression, especially when overload and conflict exist.

Family History

A history of depression or alcoholism in the family is generally known to increase the risk for depression. Still, this genetic link has not been confirmed, and there is much yet to be researched. There is stronger evidence that bipolar illness (manic/depressive illness) is genetically-transmitted.

In addition to genetically-transmitted disease, there is the question of the impact on depression of the quality of family relationships. For example, depressed, angry, hostile environments are more likely to produce depression in their members. Negative cognitions can also be taught to children. Regular exposure to negative attitudes, such as that the future holds no promise, or that one is unable to control the environment, or that one is not a worthwhile individual in one's own right, can be powerful forces.

Role Strain

Ilfeld[16] explored the relationship between role strain and depression. *Role* concerns how one functions in society. It is a set of expectations about how the person occupying one position behaves toward a person occupying another position. At times, the individual in a particular role is not able to accomplish all the tasks expected of the role and becomes overburdened. Role strain occurs. This may precede depression. Ilfeld found that chronic stressful experiences from the social role areas of neighborhood, job, financial affairs, homemaking, parenting, marriage, singlehood, unemployment, and retirement are significantly related to depressive symptoms.

Thus, certain factors, such as age, sex, family history, role strain, and chronic stressful experiences from the social role, place individuals at risk for depression.

Assessment of Depressed Clients

Depression has been called "the common cold" of psychopathology, and has touched the lives of all of us in varying degrees of severity (Fig. 15-1). Recognized for more than 2000 years, depression continues to rank as one of the major health problems today.[5] Up to 25% of the population will suffer from a significant depression during their lifetime.[29] A staggering eight to twenty million Americans need professional help for feelings of depression. It is also estimated that one out of 200 individuals affected will die from suicide.

The term depression has been used to designate a variety of illness states. As detailed by Akiskal and McKinney,[1] depression has been defined as an emotion of long- or short-term duration, as a significant mood state sustained over a long period of time, and as a syndrome characterized by a series of psychomotor retardative symptoms. Numerous studies depicting the incidence

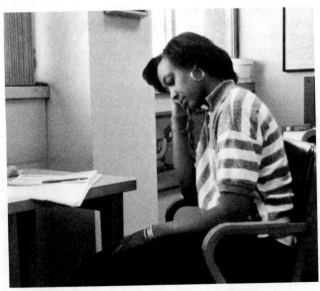

Figure 15-1. A depressed client at work finds it difficult to concentrate on her tasks.

and prevalence of depression in the population at large indicate that depression appears more frequently in women, in nonwhites more frequently than in whites, and in the very poor, the very rich, and the less educated.

Manifestations of Depressive Illness

The manifestations of depression depend on the severity of the episode. The continuum notion of affective illness holds that depression can be manifest in a variety of states, from a normal to a severe or a psychotic episode.

Depression, when classified as an illness of either neurotic or psychotic nature, is accompanied by a cluster of somatic and psychological symptoms (see Table 15-3). Some of these symptoms relate to the impairment itself, and others to the nature of the disability generated by the impairment. The major impairments in mood and affect are evidenced by the following:

1. A dejected mood
2. Feelings of helplessness
3. Hopelessness
4. Negative feelings about self

Disturbances in functioning exhibited by individuals include:

1. Decreased energy
2. Fatigue
3. Loss of appetite
4. Difficulty in sleeping

Beck's Signs and Symptoms

Beck[4] offers one of the most comprehensive lists of signs and symptoms of depression. These include three categories of symptoms, encompassing emotional and cognitive impairment and volitional functioning.

1. *Emotional:* dejected mood, negative feelings toward self, reduction in gratification, loss of emotional attachments, crying spells, and loss of mirth responses
2. *Cognitive/motivational:* low self-evaluation, negative expectations, indecisiveness, distorted self-image, paralysis of will, avoidance, escapism, withdrawal, suicidal thoughts, increased dependency, thought retardation, and unusual content
3. *Vegetative and physical manifestations:* loss of appetite, sleep disturbances, loss of libido, fatigability

Diagnostic Classification: Depression

The American Psychiatric Association's Classification of Depression (DSM-III-R) isolates core signs and symptoms of depression to be used in the diagnosis of depression. Four types of depressive disorders are recognized:[3] Major Depression (Single Episode—296.2x; Recurrent—296.3x; see the following box); Dysthymic Disorder (300.40); Adjustment Disorder With Depressed Mood (309.00); and Depressive Disorder Not Otherwise Specified (311.00).

1. *Major depression:* Major depression is clinically illustrated by dysphoric mood and loss of interest and/or pleasure in activities. The following box lists diagnostic criteria for a major depression.
2. *Dysthymic disorders* (depressive neurosis) are defined as a set of signs and symptoms that have affected the individual most or all of the time but are not of sufficient severity and duration to meet the criteria for a major depressive episode.
3. *Adjustment disorder with depressed mood* is the category used when signs and symptoms are those of the depressed mood, coupled with an adjustment disorder.

TABLE 15-3.
SYMPTOMS ASSOCIATED WITH THE DEPRESSIVE CONTINUUM

NORMAL	NEUROTIC DEPRESSION OR DYSTHYMIC DISORDER (Presence of two of the following:)	PSYCHOTIC DEPRESSION (May have five or more symptoms associated with neurotic depression, plus:)
Transient feelings of fatigue	Notable appetite and/or weight change	Depressive stupor/moodiness or unresponsiveness
Temporary reduction in gratification	Sleep disturbance	Delusions or hallucinations that are mood-congruent or -incongruent
Minor alterations in sleeping/eating patterns may or may not be present.	Fatigability, energy loss	
	Psychomotor agitation or retardation	
	Reduction in gratification	
	Feelings of self-reproach or excessive or inappropriate guilt	
	Crying	
	Slowed thinking and ability to concentrate	
	Pessimistic attitude	
	Brooding regarding past or current unpleasant events	
	Preoccupation with feelings of inadequacy	
	Recurrent thoughts of death or suicide	

DIAGNOSTIC CRITERIA FOR MAJOR DEPRESSION

MAJOR DEPRESSION, SINGLE EPISODE

For fifth digit, use the Major Depressive Episode codes to describe current state.
A. A single Major Depressive Episode
B. Has never had a Manic Episode or an unequivocal Hypomanic Episode
Specify if seasonal pattern

MAJOR DEPRESSION, RECURRENT

For fifth digit, use the Major Depressive Episode codes to describe current state.
A. Two or more Major Depressive Episodes, each separated by at least two months of return to more or less usual functioning. (If there has been a previous Major Depressive Episode, the current episode of depression need not meet the full criteria for a Major Depressive Episode.)
B. Has never had a Manic Episode or an unequivocal Hypomanic Episode
Specify if seasonal pattern.

4. *Atypical depression* is a category for individuals with depressive symptoms who cannot be diagnosed as having major depressive or adjustment disorders.

Primary vs. Secondary Depression

Categorization into primary and secondary depression is another method of diagnosing and classifying depression when a second illness entity is present. This classification is based on the idea that depression has a different basis and outcome when it occurs in conjunction with another psychiatric or medical condition. The feelings of sadness, self-deprecation, and despair that occur in conjunction with other illness states—psychiatric illness or medical problem—are said to be secondary to the original diagnosis. Primary depression is that group of symptoms that presents for the first time as a disorder of mood or affect. The *primary disorder* is frequently the first entity to present itself, with the *secondary disorder* usually being caused by the primary disorder.

It is often difficult to differentiate primary from secondary depression. Primary depression can be seen in clients with somatic signs and symptoms, thus confusing the psychological disease with a physiological one.

Psychiatric problems, such as depression, may have somatic signs and symptoms such as headaches, back pain, abdominal pain, loss of appetite, weight loss, chest pain, and fatigue. In these cases, depression can go undiagnosed.

Differentiation between primary and secondary depression is important for the recovery of the patient. Many primary medical problems create or present with symptoms of hopelessness and helplessness and the somatic symptoms occurring with grief. Brain tumors, cancer, viral pneumonia, arthritis, alcoholism, and many other diseases typically include these signs and symptoms of depression. Thus, the differentiation between primary and secondary depression is crucial to the diagnosis, treatment, and recovery of the patient.

The manner in which signs and symptoms present themselves can be a key component in the recognition, diagnosis, and successful treatment of depression. When depression surfaces as somatic complaints, the clinical picture becomes much more complicated. Somatic manifestations of depression are so common in everyday life that they are often not recognized as characteristics of illness. Therefore, these somatic symptoms often mask the depressed mood, resulting, as indicated previously, in nonrecognition of a depressed state. Health care practitioners should be attentive to clues that may enable them to readily recognize and distinguish the presence of clinical depression. The following signs and symptoms may reveal impairment of affect and mood in individuals:

- Physical signs and symptoms that elude a physiological explanation
- Physical signs and symptoms that resist treatment by usual methods
- Physical symptoms involving many body systems
- Complaints of chronic fatigue and loss of energy
- Changes in the appetite or body weight
- Alcoholism and patterns of drug abuse
- Change in sexual interest or performance
- Change in interpersonal relationships

In the assessment of impaired clients, high-risk factors should be considered. An increase in age, pregnancy, increased use of alcohol, and times of grief or loss are risk factors for depression. Disturbances in family group relationships that can alter self-perception may also precipitate moderate to major depressive episodes. The idea that certain individuals may be more sensitive to depressive episodes will be addressed later in this chapter when the theories of impairment in affect are reviewed in more detail.

The diagnosis of depression is aided by the existence of several instruments or scales that are sensitive to this problem. Among these are the Hamilton Depressive Scale,[15] the Beck Depressive Inventory,[7] and the Zung Self-Rating Depressive Scale.[31]

Assessment of the Manic Client

Depression is more common than mania, and has probably caused more anguish and suffering than any other medical or psychiatric illness. Because of the pleasurable effect of elation in manic states, this illness is less often addressed as a problem; when it is recognized, it is usually in its most severe manifestation. Nonetheless, it is regarded as an impairment of mood and affect with a very important potential to disable and handicap.

Manifestation of Mania

Like depression, the manifestations of mania depend on the severity of the condition. Mild states of elation are normal and are commonly termed "highs." The sense of euphoria felt periodically (experienced as feelings of well-being) is termed *euthymia*, and is not associated with a disorder *per se*. However, two additional states, *hypomania* and *mania*, are considered indicative of illness or impairment and therefore considered problematic manifestations of elated states. The normal, hypomanic, and manic states occur on a continuum, as depicted in Table 15-4.

Table 15-4 presents the symptoms most frequently associated with normal, hypomanic, and manic manifestations of elation. As illustrated in this table, mania, when classified as an illness of either hypomanic or full-fledged manic proportions, is also accompanied by a cluster of psychological and somatic signs and symptoms. The major psychological components are feelings of well-being, grandiosity, and inflated self-esteem. Somatic symptoms include increased energy, increased activity, little need for sleep, and impulsivity. Specifically, hypomania and mania are usually differentiated by the number of symptoms present and the duration of these symptoms.

Hypomania is a state of euphoria accompanied by two or more of the following manifestations: increased talkativeness, pressured speech, flight of ideas, grandios-ity, increased spending, hyper-sexuality, impulsivity, and reckless driving. *Mania* is more persistent and is regarded as a more severe state of the same condition. At least three of the following symptoms are present: increased activity, accelerated speech, flight of ideas, inflated self-esteem, decreased need for sleep, distractibility, and excessive activity. With the manic client one may notice that meaningful conversation is impossible, thus seriously impairing the individual socially. Manic features usually last at least one week. As suggested here, mania, like depression, can be conceptualized on a continuum from mild to severe states.

Diagnostic Classifications: Mania

The DSM-III-R specifies three major diagnostic categories in which mania or hypomania (single episodes or recurring states) can be found:[3]

1. Manic Episode
2. Bipolar Disorder: Mixed (296.6x), Manic (296.4), or Depressed (296.5x)
3. Cyclothymic Disorder (301.13)
4. Bipolar Disorder Not Otherwise Specified (296.70)

The following boxes describe the diagnostic criteria for a manic episode and for a bipolar disorder.

1. *Bipolar disorders*[3] always involve manic and depressive mood swings, indicative of both manic and depressive episodes. The mood shifts may be intermixed or may alternate rapidly every few days. With a diagnosis of mixed mood states, depressive symp-

TABLE 15-4.
THE MANIC CONTINUUM

MILD	MODERATE	SEVERE
"High" "Up" "In seventh heaven"	Hypomania	Mania of psychotic proportions

THE CONTINUUM OF SYMPTOMS ASSOCIATED WITH MANIA

MILD ("HIGH")	MODERATE (HYPOMANIA)	SEVERE (MANIA)
Transient feelings of elation; a "high" feeling Feelings of well-being; confidence Minor alterations in habits; different eating and sleeping patterns may or may not be present.	Clear sense of euphoria (yet not as severe as in mania) Two or more of the following: Talkativeness Pressured speech Flight of ideas Grandiosity Excessive spending Hypersexuality Impulsivity Reckless driving	Euphoria Three or more of the following: Activity Talkativeness Flight of ideas Inflated self-esteem Need for sleep Distractibility Excessiveness (buying, driving, sexual indiscretions)

DIAGNOSTIC CRITERIA FOR MANIC EPISODE

Note: A "Manic Syndrome" is defined as including criteria A, B, and C below. A "Hypomanic Syndrome" is defined as including criteria A and B, but not C, *i.e.,* no marked impairment.

A. A distinct period of abnormally and persistently elevated, expansive, or irritable mood

B. During the period of mood disturbance, at least three of the following symptoms have persisted (four if the mood is only irritable) and have been present to a significant degree:
  1. Inflated self-esteem or grandiosity
  2. Decreased need for sleep, *e.g.,* feels rested after only three hours of sleep
  3. More talkativeness than usual or pressure to keep talking
  4. Flight of ideas or subjective experience that thoughts are racing
  5. Distractibility, *i.e.,* attention too easily drawn to unimportant or irrelevant external stimuli
  6. Increase in goal-directed activity (either socially, at work or school, or sexually) or psychomotor agitation
  7. Excessive involvement in pleasurable activities that have a high potential for painful consequences, *e.g.,* the person engages in unrestrained buying sprees, sexual indiscretions, or foolish business investments

C. Mood disturbance sufficiently severe to cause marked impairment in occupational functioning or in usual social activities or relationships with others, or to necessitate hospitalization to prevent harm to self or others

D. At no time during the disturbance have there been delusions or hallucinations for as long as two weeks in the absence of prominent mood symptoms (*i.e.,* before the mood symptoms developed or after they have remitted).

E. Not superimposed on Schizophrenia, Schizophreniform Disorder, Delusional Disorder, or Psychotic Disorder NOS

F. It cannot be established that an organic factor initiated and maintained the disturbance.

MANIC EPISODE CODES: Fifth-digit code numbers and criteria for severity of current state of Bipolar Disorder, Manic or Mixed

1. *Mild:* Meets minimum symptom criteria for a Manic Episode (or almost meets symptom criteria if there has been a previous Manic Episode)
2. *Moderate:* Extreme increase in activity or impairment in judgment
3. *Severe, Without Psychotic Features:* Almost continual supervision required in order to prevent physical harm to self or others.
4. *With Psychotic Features:* Delusions, hallucinations, or catatonic symptoms. If possible, specify whether the psychotic features are *mood-congruent* or *mood-incongruent.*

    Mood-congruent psychotic features: Delusions or hallucinations of which the content is entirely consistent with the typical manic themes of inflated worth, power, knowledge, identity, or special relationship to a deity or famous person.

    Mood-incongruent psychotic features: Either (*a*) or (*b*):
    a. Delusions or hallucinations of which the content does *not* involve the typical manic themes of inflated worth, power, knowledge, identity, or special relationship to a deity or famous person. Included are such symptoms as persecutory delusions (not directly related to grandiose ideas or themes), thought insertion, and delusions of being controlled.
    b. Catatonic symptoms, *e.g.,* stupor, mutism, negativism, posturing
5. *In Partial Remission:* Full criteria were previously, but are not currently, met; some signs or symptoms of the disturbance have persisted.
6. *In Full Remission:* Full criteria were previously met, but there have been no significant signs or symptoms of the disturbance for at least six months.
0. *Unspecified*

---

toms are prominent and last at least a full day. With a diagnosis of Bipolar Disorder, Manic Episode, the manic phase of the illness is most recent. With Bipolar Disorder, Depressed, the depressed phase is most recent.

Manic episodes are evidenced by one or more distinct periods in which an elevated, sometimes irritable mood is present. This elevation in mood must be persistent and sufficiently evident even if depressed moods are also observed. In addition, at least three of the following symptoms must be present for at least one week:

a. Increased activity (socially, at work, and/or sexually) or physical restlessness
b. Increased talkativeness or incessant talking
c. Flight of ideas or the feeling that one's thoughts are racing
d. Inflated self-esteem that may be so grandiose as to be delusional in the psychotic phase of the illness
e. Decreased need for sleep
f. Distractibility, *i.e.,* attention too readily drawn to unimportant or irrelevant external stimuli
g. Excessive involvement in activities that frequently have negative consequences, *e.g.,* buying sprees, sexual indiscretions, foolish business ventures, reckless driving

Neither mood-incongruent delusions nor hallucinations dominate the clinical picture. Symptoms are not due to a schizophrenic disorder or an organic

DIAGNOSTIC CRITERIA FOR BIPOLAR DISORDERS

BIPOLAR DISORDER, MIXED

For fifth digit, use the Manic Episode codes to describe current state.

A. Current (or most recent) episode involves the full symptomatic picture of both Manic and Major Depressive Episodes (except for the duration requirement of two weeks for depressive symptoms), intermixed or rapidly alternating every few days.

B. Prominent depressive symptoms lasting at least a full day

Specify if seasonal pattern.

BIPOLAR DISORDER, MANIC

For fifth digit, use the Manic Episode codes to describe current state.

Currently (or most recently) in a Manic Episode. (If there has been a previous Manic Episode, the current episode need not meet the full criteria for a Manic Episode.)

Specify if seasonal pattern.

BIPOLAR DISORDER, DEPRESSED

For fifth digit, use the Major Depressive Episode codes to describe current state.

A. Has had one or more Manic Episodes

B. Currently (or most recently) in a Major Depressive Episode. (If there has been a previous Major Depressive Episode, the current episode need not meet the full criteria for a Major Depressive Episode.)

Specify if seasonal pattern.

---

disorder. Manic episodes can be accompanied by psychotic features in which hallucinations or delusions are present. For this reason manic disorders are frequently confused with thought disorders.

2. *Cyclothymic disorders* are disorders in which periods of depression and hypomania are evident but these episodes are not sufficient in severity or duration to warrant a diagnosis of Bipolar Disorder, Major Depression or Manic Episode. The periods of depression and hypomania may be intermixed with periods of normal mood. Psychotic features are never a characteristic of this disorder.

3. *Atypical bipolar disorder* is a category of diagnosis that represents a residual disorder. Individuals may have previously had a major depression. Now their illnesses exhibit hypomanic features, but not of sufficient severity or duration to meet the criteria for a manic episode.

To summarize, depression and elation may occur together, and when this happens there are two possibilities:

1. A client experiences depression with mania, thus meeting the criteria for symptoms of a manic, as well as a depressive, disorder.

2. Depression and hypomania may occur together. Clients' histories may indicate that they meet the criteria for a hypomanic disorder and major or minor depression, yet they may never have had a clear manic attack requiring hospitalization.

Mania and depression are well-recognized entities that have, in the past, been confused with schizophrenia.

This is particularly true when referring to the psychotic manifestations of a manic/depressive disorder. It has recently been learned that many state hospital patients diagnosed as incurable schizophrenics are actually manic/depressives who can improve significantly with therapy.

Mania, in its singular sense, is not lethal. Coupled with depression in the *manic/depressive bipolar illness,* the depressive states can yield suicidal gestures and attempts. Hypomanic clients frequently have car accidents, give away valuable possessions, drive others to and away from them, and have difficulty concentrating. They may devise wild, creative schemes, yet be unable to take the steps necessary to bring the plans to fruition.

There are positive aspects of hypomania. Clients, while experiencing "high" episodes, report increased productivity and creativity bordering on genius. Some very gifted artists, musicians, composers, comedians, and poets have suffered from manic/depressive illnesses in which the manic stage assisted them in their achievements. These same gifted people often lapsed into severe depression between hypomanic episodes, alerting them that a health problem existed and causing them to seek professional treatment.

There are genetic factors in the transmission of manic/depressive disorder. It is reported that relatives of clients with manic/depressive disorders or mania show a higher prevalence of mood disorders than does the general population. The age at onset for manic/depressive disorders is fairly evenly distributed throughout life, although manic and bipolar disorders tend to begin in early adulthood. Manic/depressive disorders do not appear to be sex-linked; there are not more females than males exhibiting this disorder.

A stressful lifestyle is not clearly linked with the occurrence of manic/depressive episodes. Characteristic life events have not been known to precipitate manic/depressive symptoms. Although individuals with manic/depressive illness may exhibit a number of stressors, these stresses seem to be more a consequence of the illness than precipitants of the disorder.

Assessment of the Depressed Client for Suicide

One of the antecedents of suicide is depression. Most individuals who engage in suicidal behaviors suffer from mental disorders. Suicidal individuals are most commonly classified by outcome—the *completers* and the *attempters*. The suicide completers are affectively ill or alcoholic, whereas the attempters are personality-disordered.[17] Suicides due to primary depression account for 30% to 70% of all suicides, depending on the study (see Table 15-5).

One out of every 10,000 people kills him or herself. Suicide is the tenth leading cause of death in the United States for the general population, and is ranked third for the age 15 to 24 group.[17] Table 15-6 compares the demographic characteristics of completed and attempted suicide. White, elderly men most commonly complete suicide, and young, nonwhite women attempt it more frequently.

Khuri and Akiskal indicated that interpersonal and/or economic loss often precedes suicidal behavior. They stated that the majority of suicide completers communicate their intent through direct or indirect statements or acts. An indirect client statement, such as "It's more than I can bear," might be coupled with indirect behavioral clues such as buying a casket, giving away cherished belongings, or "putting my affairs in order."

Khuri and Akiskal suggested that 70% to 90% of suicide attempts are drug overdoses, with alcohol and drug

TABLE 15-5.
PERCENTAGES OF CLIENTS WITH DEPRESSIVE/MANIC DISORDERS WHO COMPLETED SUICIDE

	CLIENTS WITH DEPRESSIVE/MANIC DISORDERS*	TOTAL PERCENT OF CLIENTS WITH PSYCHIATRIC ILLNESS
Robins et al, 1959	55%	94%
Dorpat and Ripley, 1960	30%	100%
Barraclough et al, 1974	70%	93%
Kraft and Babigian, 1976	37%	96%

* Combines manic/depressive illness and psychotic and neurotic depressions.
(Modified from Khuri R, Akiskal H: Types and percentages of mental disorders in completed suicide. Psychiatr Clin North Am 6:197, 1983.)

TABLE 15-6.
CHARACTERISTICS OF INDIVIDUALS WHO ATTEMPTED AND COMPLETED SUICIDE

	ATTEMPTED	COMPLETED
Annual incidence	160–730/100,000	11/100,000
Peak age risk	20–30	45–65
Sex predominance	Female	Male
Marital status	Separated, divorced	Single, widowed, divorced
Race predominance	Nonwhite	White

(Khuri R, Akiskal H: Differences between attempted and completed suicide. Psychiatr Clin North Am 6:194, 1983.)

combinations increasing. Wrist-cutting constitutes 10% to 20% of suicide attempts. Violent methods, such as shooting, hanging, or drowning, are chosen by men more often than by women. Five high-risk suicide groups have been identified:

1. Suicide is the leading cause of death among previous attempters. This group has an 80 to 100 times increased risk relative to the general population.

2. People with the demographic characteristics of suicide completers are at high risk (see Table 11-6). White, elderly males with disrupted interpersonal bonds are statistically a high-risk group.

3. Clients diagnosed as suffering from primary depression or chronic alcohol abuse are in the highest-risk groups.

4. People who communicate their suicidal intent are at high risk, because the majority of completed suicides were preceded by communicated intent.

5. Clients with chronic interpersonal conflicts and psychosocial problems are at risk, because hopelessness and negative expectations correlate highly with suicidal behavior.

Most suicidal behaviors stem from a sense of isolation and from feelings of some intolerable emotion, with suicide seen as a way to interrupt an intolerable existence. A common intolerable emotion is rejection, which may lead to suicide if not overcome by a feeling of acceptance.

Suicide may be an act of revenge to elicit guilt and remorse from others. It may also be self-punishment to handle guilt or to control one's fate. There is an element of extreme hostility in a suicidal act. Suicidal attempts are not only intended to be self-destructive, but are also hostile impulses against significant others or even the therapist. Frequently the nonlethal suicide attempt is meant to communicate more severe suicidal intentions.

A significant principle for the psychiatric nurse to keep in mind is that the recovery period from depression may be more dangerous than the depression itself. While clients are recovering they may have the energy to act on their suicidal thoughts and feelings.

RELEVANT RESEARCH

The authors reported a clear association between depression and suicide. They stated that 45% to 70% of those who commit suicide can be found retrospectively to have had a syndrome of depression. They conducted a follow-up study of suicide and suicidal behaviors in those patients receiving ECT or antidepressants.

Suicide, attempted suicide, and relapse rates were examined in 519 cases of depression. After six months, suicide attempts were seen significantly less frequently in the ECT group (0.8%) than in the antidepressant group (4.2%) or the "adequate" antidepressant subgroup (7.0%).

It was found that fewer suicide attempts occurred in the ECT group compared to those in the antidepressant group, among both those who had attempted suicide prior to admission (0% vs. 10%) and those who had not (1.1% vs. 3.6%). Those who had made a previous suicide attempt were more at risk for suicide in the following year and for a subsequent suicide attempt. The authors concluded that a depressive disorder may be as good a predictor of suicidal behavior as a history of suicide attempts.

(Avery D, Winokur, G: Suicide, attempted suicide, and relapse rates in depression. Arch Gen Psychiatry 35(6):749–753, 1978.)

The challenge for the psychiatric nurse is determining which depressed clients are at risk for committing suicide. Once this group has been identified, nurses face the burden of assessing which clients act out with more overt suicidal intent and are more characteristically suicidal rather than acutely so. The treatment and management of these clients is difficult, especially in the hospital setting.

Nurses behave in nurturing ways in the interest of preventing suicide. The more suicidally the clients behave, the more parental the nursing staff becomes. Once the suicide risk subsides, nurses can relax their precautionary style. However, for the characteristically suicidal person, the risk does not abate. In fact, the parental or "mothering" behavior may enhance the risk of suicide. This nurturing behavior creates a secondary gain for suicidal behaviors and may foster the suicidal characterology of the individual.[22]

For the person in acute and painful despair, desperately in need of nurturing, suicide becomes the admission ticket to fulfillment of that need. The psychiatric nurse is faced with a dilemma. If the nurse's response to this regressive behavior is nurturing, and the intervention relieves the immediate distress and offers strength to the client, it does so at the cost of having "rewarded" the regressive behavior. The nurse has intervened by offering a prominent secondary gain. Thus, the psychiatric nurse must assess the value of nurturing responses and compare the advantages of short-term support with the disadvantages of the secondary gain.

A *no-suicide contract* could be developed between the client and the nurse. A contract such as

"No matter what happens, I will not kill myself accidentally or on purpose, at any time"

could be written by the client, signed by the nurse or the treatment team,[27] and placed in the client's chart. The client who confidently makes this statement and shows congruent behavior is at less risk than the individual who refuses to make a contract, or alters the contract.

Alterations of the contract frequently occur in three areas. The most common alteration of the contract is made in relation to time. To the contract, the client may add the statement "for one day" or "for a week." This gives the nurse a time frame for working with the client. The individual must be reevaluated for suicide potential before the contract expires. The date and time of the contract must be recorded initially and each time it is renewed. If the contract has not been renewed before it expires, it may provide the patient with a sense of "free reign" to commit suicide.

The second condition a client may make is in the "no matter what" part of the statement. The client may add a conditional statement, such as "unless my husband leaves me." There are innumerable possibilities. Suggest to the client that this is another issue requiring further intervention.

The third qualification a client may make is, "I will try not to kill myself" rather than "I will not kill myself." Avoid accepting nebulous decisions. Counter the client's variation with, "But will you?" This forces the individual to reconsider and make a definite decision by either saying no or stating a time limit.

The word "accidentally" is essential in the contract. The client may take unnecessary risks under the guise of normal routine or recreation. Accidents can be unconscious decisions and have the advantage of being socially acceptable.

The "no-suicide contract" is a tool that provides the psychiatric nurse with a margin for safety in dealing more effectively with suicidal clients. Table 15-7 lists appropriate nursing interventions for working with suicidal clients.

Issues for Client Teaching

Clients must be informed that suicidal thoughts are self-limiting, and that there are other options available to deal with the crisis. Often clients are unable to determine other options by themselves. The important point in

TABLE 15-7.
NURSING INTERVENTIONS FOR DEPRESSED,
SUICIDAL CLIENTS

GENERAL NURSING APPROACHES TO SUICIDE

1. Observe the client closely at all times, for direct and indirect verbal and behavioral clues indicating suicide potential.
2. Emphasize the need to protect the client against self-destruction rather than punish the client.
3. Support the part of the client that wants to live.
4. Remove environmental objects that could be used to injure self.
5. Elicit what is meaningful to the client at the moment.
6. Avoid imposing your own feelings of reality on the client.
7. Listen with empathy, but let the client know there are other alternatives to suicide.
8. Structure a plan that the client can use to cope with future suicidal ideation or acts (*e.g.*, call therapist, go to nearest emergency room).
9. Demonstrate concern for the client as a person.

teaching is to explain to clients that they are teetering between a wish to live and a wish to die, and that an option can be chosen that emphasizes the drive toward life and living. Ultimately it is a choice, or a decision, that rests with the client. It is crucial that clients know that they are expected to accept a major share of the responsibility for their own lives. The temptation to relinquish this responsibility to nurses and/or other therapists is strong. Nurses can help clients to fulfill their responsibilities but can't be responsible for them—only clients can do that.

Nursing Interventions With Depressive/Manic Impairments

The DSM-III-R framework used to depict categories or classifications of impairments of mood and affect is a paradigm for viewing mental illness. Nurses should be aware that classifications are particularly useful in establishing diagnostic parameters, but tend to underemphasize some important principles, including: (1) the idea that mental illness or health is a dynamic process that can be charted on a continuum, and (2) the fact that the diagnostic label is highly contingent on the judgment of those evaluating the client's condition. Because the client's condition is the outcome of many factors interacting together (as suggested by systems theory), it is somewhat misleading to look at pathology only as it rests in the individual. Rather, the nurse examines how societal, cultural, and environmental factors may foster dysfunction in the individual.

The general aim of the next section of this chapter is to identify major symptoms in categories or classification of impairments of mood and affect, and to depict nursing interventions pertinent to these symptoms or clusters of symptoms. Major factors that contribute to client recovery

will be cited, along with implications for primary, secondary, and tertiary prevention.

Nursing Process and Depression

The precise symptoms and symptom clusters in depression are reintroduced now with an emphasis on care planning, intervention, and evaluation. Only the major symptoms are addressed in the model that follows.

As was discussed earlier, impairments in mood and affect can be seen in a variety of diagnoses, including major depression, dysthymic personality, and bipolar affective disorder with depressed mood. Depression can also be manifest in symptoms of sleep disturbance, weight loss, loss of interest in pleasurable activities, and in a number of related problems that do not meet criteria for inclusion in the DSM-III-R diagnosis of depressive illness.

The following two clinical examples demonstrate the nursing process. Both individuals were hospitalized with a diagnosis of impairment of affect: one had a diagnosis of major, recurrent depression, and the other was diagnosed as having a mixed bipolar disorder. Phases of the nursing process will be addressed, and sample care plans will be utilized to display this information.

The Use of Therapeutic Communication With Depressive/Manic Impairments

Nurses begin the therapeutic process with depressed individuals by using themselves as tools to deal with clients' major symptoms, namely lowered self-esteem, worthlessness, guilt, negativity, and irrational beliefs. Nurses prepare clients for the many steps and risks that will be taken to effect the desirable changes. Carefully and patiently nurses proceed, making sure not to add any new injuries to clients' self-esteem. The nurse's goal is to preserve and enhance depressed clients' self-esteem while challenging the irrational beliefs that perpetuate the depression.

Rogers believed that growth potential of any individual will tend to be released in a relationship in which the helping person is experiencing and communicating realness, caring, and nonjudgmental understanding.[10] He stated that, if certain conditions are present in the attitudes of the person designated as the "therapist," then growthful change will take place. These conditions are congruence, positive regard, and empathic understanding.

The most basic of the three conditions, *congruence* or genuineness, is the ability of therapists to be themselves. The words spoken by nurses must be congruent with their present experiences. They must attempt to be fully present to the clients.

To demonstrate *unconditional positive regard,* therapists must avoid any behavior that is overtly or covertly judgmental. This attitude comes partly from therapists' trust in the inner wisdom of their clients and the belief that clients will discover the resources and directions the growth will take.

Accurate, *empathic understanding* implies that therapists, in the fullness of their own personalities, try to immerse themselves in the feeling world of the clients, and then experience that world within themselves. Therapists experience both clients' feelings and their own inner responses to those feelings. Being understood effects growth change in clients.

The congruent, empathic nurse next faces the challenges of dispelling the irrational beliefs of clients that are perpetuating the depression. Ellis[13] believed that virtually all serious emotional problems stem directly from magical, empirically unvalidatable beliefs, and that they can almost invariably be eliminated or minimized with the therapist's use of logical and empirical thinking to refute them.

Ellis indicated that, no matter how defective a client's heredity is or how traumatic the client's experience has been, the main reason for over- or under-reaction to obnoxious stimuli is a dogmatic, irrational belief system. Thus, depressed people do not merely believe it is undesirable to reject their children, but believe it is awful, and that they are entirely worthless people if they do so. The following therapeutic communication clarifies this issue.

A single, working mother with four children was hospitalized with a unipolar depression. She felt guilty and blamed herself because she was rejecting her children.

Client: "I feel guilty about not wanting the children. I don't apply the rules to myself. It's wrong for everybody else to reject their children, but here I am wanting to leave my kids."

Nurse: "So you suspect that you are feeling guilty because of your feelings of not wanting the kids?"

Client: "Yes."

Nurse: "What do you mean when you say you don't want them?"

Client: "I don't know. I don't like the responsibility of the children. If they could just all play together. But you have to discipline them . . . you have to teach them . . . you have to do this . . . and that."

Nurse: "It gets to be a heavy burden. Is that what you mean?"

Client: "Yes. I am mature enough to have them, so I should be mature enough to take care of them."

Nurse: "When you notice that sometimes you are not fully the mother that you want to be, then you blame yourself. Is that it?"

Client: "Yes, I do . . . it can't be anybody else's fault."

Nurse: "I didn't say fault. I said blame. Do you know what I mean by blame? By blame I mean that you are not only dissatisfied with yourself as a mother, but you are dissatisfied with you as a person and as a woman. You're telling yourself, 'I'm not a good mother, and that makes me an awful, worthless, good-for-nothing human being.' You get depressed when you admit that you are not a good mother. You convince yourself that you are not a good person because you happen not to be a good mother. Do you follow me?"

Client: "Yes."

Nurse: "Explain it to me, then."

In this interaction, the nurse identifies the essence of the client's problem of depression—it is not the activating event (the disinterest in the children), but her irrational belief system. She clearly is telling herself that she should be a good mother, and that if she is not she is an awful, worthless person.

In this situation, the nurse's use of therapeutic communication challenges the irrational belief system of this depressed client. The nurse's ultimate goal during this interaction is to assist the client with logical and empirical thinking in order to refute the client's irrational belief. The client will then accept a belief that she is a good person who does both good and bad deeds. She can choose to focus on enjoying herself even if she has undesirable traits, because she does not have to "rate" herself by the number of good vs. bad deeds.

Satir[19] explained that it is possible to enhance feelings of self-esteem when there is "the willingness to be open to new possibilities, to try them on for size, and then, if they fit us, to practice using them until they are ours." She described five freedoms to develop emotional honesty and enhance self-esteem:

1. The freedom to see and hear what is here instead of what should be, was, or will be
2. The freedom to say what one feels and thinks, instead of what one *should* say
3. The freedom to feel what one feels, instead of what one *ought* to feel
4. The freedom to ask for what one wants, instead of always waiting for permission
5. The freedom to take risks on one's own behalf, instead of choosing to be only "secure" and not "rocking the boat"

During therapeutic interactions nurses can, one piece at a time, teach clients methods to increase emotional honesty that will enhance self-esteem and communication skills, and decrease depressive symptoms. Each change affects the other parts.

Kraines[18] suggested that a direct approach works best with depressed clients. They are comforted with a straightforward explanation of their illness and positive reassurance of their eventual recovery. A possible approach might be, "You will need to be patient and you will need to cooperate. It won't be easy; it will take time; but you will recover."

Another technique that counteracts clients' low self-esteem and hopelessness is a discussion of positive achievements. If allowed to follow their inclinations, clients will dwell on past failures and traumatic experi-

CLINICAL EXAMPLES (CONTINUED)

SHEILA

Later that afternoon, the nurse approached Sheila again. The nurse wanted to talk to Sheila, hoping to clarify in her own mind what was bothering Sheila so much.

Sheila was sitting in a corner of the day room watching a T.V. game show, but the volume was turned off. The nurse sat near her.

"How come no sound, Sheila?"
"I don't like to hear people talk when they're happy."
"Then why do you have the TV turned on at all?"
"If I watch it, I won't think so much about why I feel so bad."
"What is the reason you think you feel bad?"
"Why do you want to know?"
"Sometimes it helps just to talk about things."

Her eyes fell from the television set, and she turned toward the window. "I . . . ," she began. Her voice was barely audible. The nurse heard her sigh, but then she continued:

"I have no family, no friends, and no life. My husband left me five years ago, and my son is married and has a life of his own."
"Which loss seems the most difficult for you?"
"Sometimes I wish I were anybody else but me. If I were somebody else, I couldn't stand to be around me. Either I just lie in bed all morning, or if I get up I eat ice cream or bake blueberry muffins from a can because I don't feel like getting dressed to go to the store. And I'm so fat! I can't stand the thought of people seeing me—especially if they're people I know. I've gained ten pounds in a month. And it's been a whole month, a MONTH since my only son came to see me."
"Does he live very far away?"
"Three blocks. He could easily walk three blocks." Sheila held up three fingers.
"Do you walk over to see him?"
"That neighborhood is unsafe for an old woman like me. Besides, if I wanted to be hurt, I'd just hurt myself. I think about that all the time. Hurting myself. I'm scared I might do it. It's so easy, that kind of thing, you know? I'm scared I'll go out of control one day."
"Whom do you see during the day?"
"I can't be around my friends anymore without feeling worse. Every single one of them is happy with life, while I just can't stand living."

Sheila is diagnosed as having a Major Depressive Episode and meets the following criteria: a dysphoric mood and at least five associated symptoms present for at least two weeks—fluctuation in appetite

with weight gain, hypersomnia, loss of interest in usual activities, feelings of worthlessness, and, most recently, thoughts of death and suicide. Sheila does not exhibit any other phenomena suggesting a primary psychiatric or medical disorder other than depression. The Nursing Care Plan suggested uses the cardinal symptoms of major depression as a format for nursing diagnosis and intervention. Sheila's problems, as identified by the DSM-III-R and standard diagnoses, are addressed in the following Nursing Care Plan.

Choosing one example from the Nursing Care Plan, we can discuss the range of nursing activities. Sheila exhibits a decreased interest in pleasurable activities that represents a problem in coping. Sheila has withdrawn from her family and friends, and no longer shops, takes walks, or sews for her grandchildren. She has a great deal of time on her hands but, rather than interesting herself with her hobbies, she dwells on her dysphoria, sleeps too much, and becomes more depressed. She assumes that withdrawal from others, whom she believes expect things from her, is the answer to managing her depression. But, as she has begun to realize, this withdrawal has merely made her condition worse.

Appropriate nursing interventions for a decreased interest in pleasurable activities or the problem of coping include the nurse's discussing with Sheila her feelings of rejection (and behavior of withdrawal) in relationships with her son and friends. The nurse would encourage Sheila to join the group activities on the unit. If these nursing interventions are instituted and the program is consistent, Sheila will develop increased awareness of her depression, feelings, and reactions to her son and friends, and will modify these relationships to include more contact and communication. The modification of Sheila's current symptoms is important, but attention must also focus on the environment to which she will return after hospitalization.

In planning for early discharge, the nurse should note various points from the personal history taken at admission. Sheila's pre-illness condition included preexisting impairments of mood and affect. However, her symptoms, up to this time, did not warrant hospitalization. Two additional points can be made about her prognosis. It is likely, given Sheila's improvement, that her status will return to some level of "health." It is also possible, if she continues to have acute illness episodes, that her impairment of mood and affect and corresponding interpersonal disabilities will produce a chronic illness state. To the extent that Sheila's condition becomes a nonreversible health deviation, and

(Continued)

ences. Nurses can foster a more realistic appraisal of the past and improve clients' self-evaluation by skillfully guiding them into describing successes in detail.

Nurses should draw clients into discussions of life situations and relationships that bother them. Nurses then should model the techniques to enhance self-esteem and honest communication, and challenge the irrational beliefs. Most importantly, nurses should stress that depression is a self-limited disorder—"The thing for you to remember is that this exhaustion can, and will, be overcome."

The Therapeutic Use of Self With Clients With a Depressive/Manic Disturbance

Nursing care of the client with depressive/manic disturbance is challenging. Nurses must view clients as unique individuals and follow clients' leads in interchanges that strive for positive, healing relationships.

CLINICAL EXAMPLES (CONTINUED)

SHEILA (CONTINUED)

exacerbations and remissions depict her clinical picture, she will be judged as having a chronic illness, impairment in mood and affect.

Sheila's awareness of her illness is as important in planning her discharge as is her actual clinical history. The client's perception of disturbance in functional performance or activity is as important as the actual disturbance. Illness behavior, or reactions to the expectations others have of her, will influence her recovery from this acute illness episode. The disadvantages experienced by Sheila as a result of her impairment and disabilities can be seen in the withdrawal of her family when they suspect she is ill. Sheila can not readily adapt to an environment that includes nonsupportive relationships. Therefore, as is impor-

tant with most discharge planning, it is essential that Sheila's family, and the potential for support, be assessed and targeted for change. It is commonplace for the hospital to reinforce the role of a single identified patient, and respond as such from the client's admission to discharge. Current approaches to inpatient treatment suggest, however, that the family be seen on admission, or shortly thereafter, with the understanding that the crisis and/or hospitalization presents a special opportunity for change that, if not acted upon, will pass quickly. Chapter 12 includes a detailed description of the use of family intervention in the treatment of both psychiatric and nonpsychiatric clients.

SERGIO

The second clinical example of impairment of affect and mood is that of Sergio. Sergio was diagnosed with Bipolar Disorder, Mixed (DSM-III-R, 296.6x). The nursing process with Sergio, which will be discussed in detail, will focus on the aspects of mania that are another component of illness of this type.

Sergio is a 32-year-old Hispanic husband and father of an infant, aged 6 months. He is a college professor at a nearby university where he received his doctorate in history. Sergio has been married for three years; currently his wife is pursuing a degree in psychology. The couple live in a modest apartment in a college community. They rely heavily on Sergio's parents to babysit with their infant daughter while they work and/or go to school. Sergio currently appears agitated and reports feeling "high"; at times he feels that he can negotiate "big deals" with the college to have him teach more courses. He admits to having had sexual intercourse with some of his female students, but explains that they were really "one-night stands." He also expresses concern that he has not slept for several nights, and that, without his wife's knowledge, he has spent most of this month's paycheck on sports equipment he had wanted since he was in high school. He indicates that he had had one episode of depression in his lifetime for which he had had to seek medical attention. He had stayed in counseling for two to three months, and had then terminated because he was "feeling better." Sergio describes his relationship with his wife as "rocky"; "rocky" refers to the fact that they have fought a lot lately and are talking about separation.

Sergio is hospitalized to assess his symptoms further and gain control of his spending and sexual behaviors, which appear out of control. The symptoms shown by Sergio that are diagnostic of Bipolar

Disorder are increased activity, decreased need for sleep, sexual indiscretions, and some indications of inflated self-esteem.

Sergio has no delusions or hallucinations, and his symptoms are not due to a schizophrenic disorder. Because Sergio has had at least one episode of depression lasting longer than two weeks and requiring treatment, his illness is believed to combine facets of depression and mania or hypomania (Bipolar Disorder, Mixed).

Each of Sergio's problems is identified by standard nursing diagnosis terminology (see Nursing Care Plan). Each problem or diagnosis is addressed in the formulation of goals and specific interventions. These goals later form the basis for the nurse's evaluation criteria.

Depression and mania produce significant disabilities that eventually become obvious to others. To the extent that Sergio's condition represents a nonreversible health deviation, he too will be judged to have a chronic illness. Sergio's perception of his disability as well as the perceptions of others will influence the course of his chronic illness. The present disadvantages to Sergio are the beginnings of marital discord and the disability status activated by his absence from his teaching job at the university. Sergio's discharge planning and follow-up care should include attention to the marital discord that currently exists. Marital or couple's therapy should be considered.

Clients who exhibit primary impairments of mood and affect may have a wide array of symptoms, ranging from categories of mood disturbance to behavioral syndromes. The obvious symptoms present the basis on which nursing diagnoses are made and interventions are implemented. Goals linked to these symptoms or symptom clusters later form the criteria for expected outcomes.

However, when confronted with depressive/manic clients, nurses frequently have a reserve of life experiences that inhibit their therapeutic potential. They may be crippled by their own occasional depression, be overwhelmed with the responsibility of caring for someone who may have plans to commit suicide, or get caught up in the typical euphoria of hypomanic clients. Nurses must recognize that their own unique backgrounds will contribute to their abilities or inabilities to focus on clients' unique selves, and follow the lead of clients in interactions with them. They must concede that their own depressions and those of clients can be frightening, and

may contribute to avoidance of thoughts and feelings in the therapeutic exchange. Sometimes these fears will cause nurses to want to "cheer up" the clients, to ridicule the clients for not having the courage to face life, or to believe in the grandiose plans of manic clients.

At certain times nurses may view clients as individuals to be pitied, and who should control their self-destructive potential. However, nurses should first attempt to understand clients for who they are. Understanding the theories of depression and mania will assist nurses to bring about change in clients. Nurses will come to the interchange with a way of seeing these clients from a ho-

NURSING CARE PLAN—MAJOR DEPRESSIVE EPISODE: Sheila

ASSESSMENT	NURSING INTERVENTIONS	EVALUATION CRITERIA
NURSING DIAGNOSIS: Hypersomnia (25.01.03)		
SUBJECTIVE Client states, "I stay in bed a lot." OBJECTIVE Prolonged resting periods	Awaken client at scheduled time each morning.	Client will obtain adequate sleep, not to exceed 7–9 hours in 24 hours.
NURSING DIAGNOSIS: Alteration in nutrition: More than body requirements (NANDA)		
SUBJECTIVE Client states, "I have gained 10 pounds recently." OBJECTIVE Rapid weight gain	Assess client's recent eating habits and current food preferences. Establish a regular, well-balanced diet incorporating food preferences. Oversee eating patterns, weight gain/loss.	Client's subcutaneous fat is sufficient to pad bones and muscles, but no more than a one-inch fold.
NURSING DIAGNOSIS: Withdrawal/social isolation (23.02.01)		
SUBJECTIVE Client states she talks to no one. OBJECTIVE Decreased ability to relate to others	Discuss the following with client: pressure in interpersonal relationships, fear of rejection by significant others, and fear of anger toward others. Encourage group activities to decrease isolation.	Client will achieve productive interpersonal relationships.
NURSING DIAGNOSIS: Impaired self-esteem (50.07.04)		
SUBJECTIVE Client states she feels low. OBJECTIVE Client feels worthless.	Assist client to focus on the positive aspects of self and experiences. Clarify with client negative over-generalizations and alter negative abstractions.	Client will achieve positive expressions, feelings, and reactions.
NURSING DIAGNOSIS: Suicidal (21.03.04)		
SUBJECTIVE Client states she has thoughts of suicide OBJECTIVE Client feels hopeless.	Place client on suicide precautions.	Client will achieve positive expressions, feelings, and reactions. Client will enter into a no-suicide contract.

listic perspective. The nurse uses a bio-psycho-social perspective, viewing the environment and culture as integral components in shaping the current experience of the client.

The use of a limited perspective would be exemplified in the nurse's point of view that clients' depression is too overwhelming to change. This perspective assumes that clients cannot use their own growth potential and respond to the therapeutic communications of nurses.

Nurses do not automatically label a problem as an "affective disturbance." Nurses first notice that clients' moods are "blue," that their movements are slowed, and that clients use self-accusatory remarks when describing themselves. Nurses then apply labels to these percep-

NURSING CARE PLAN—BIPOLAR DISORDER, MIXED: Sergio

ASSESSMENT	NURSING INTERVENTIONS	EVALUATION CRITERIA
NURSING DIAGNOSIS: Insomnia (25.01.04)		
SUBJECTIVE Client states he has not slept in several nights. OBJECTIVE Sleep deficit	Sleeping medications PRN. Monitor sleep disturbance and impact of medication(s).	Client will obtain adequate sleep: not less than 6 uninterrupted hours in 24 hours.
NURSING DIAGNOSIS: Hyperirritability (15.04.03)		
SUBJECTIVE Client states he fights with his wife. OBJECTIVE Agitated, hyperactive	Maintain medications and monitor activity/agitation. When client presents agitated communications, reflect underlying feelings and set limits.	Client will have activity/exercise periods alternated with relaxed states and rest until client returns to normal activity pattern.
NURSING DIAGNOSIS: Alterations in Conduct/Impulse Control (21)		
SUBJECTIVE Client has overspent and engaged in random sexual activity. OBJECTIVE Poor judgment in finances and sexual behavior	Confiscate credit cards, personal cash. Establish rules of hospital client/client relationships.	Client will achieve positive expressions, feelings, and reactions and productive interpersonal relationships.
NURSING DIAGNOSIS: Elation (30.01.11)		
SUBJECTIVE Client states he is working on the university's most important project. OBJECTIVE Grandiosity	Establish with client that his plans are unrealistic and assist in setting realistic goals after hospitalization.	Client will view activities and projects realistically.

tions. A particular client is depressed, is showing vegetative signs of depression, and suffers from low self-esteem. In this way a beginning understanding of the client evolves.

Nurses then stay with these observations, focusing on these and the medical diagnosis of affective disorders. The nurse aims to change presently experienced phenomena of the client. If the nurse continues to focus on the medical diagnosis, medications would seem to suffice. There are very effective psychopharmacological agents to alter mood and affect, but, for the purposes of nursing the client at a specific point in time, these agents are self-limiting. The nurse is an expert in human nature—in responses to illness, and in responses to treatment. To respect the client as a unique individual, and not just a clinical syndrome, has a healing quality.

By this focus on the uniqueness of clients, they are truly appreciated for themselves. A basic need of human nature is to be appreciated for one's individuality and, at the same time, to be viewed as similar to others who have commonalities with oneself.

The Importance of Working With the Family

The anxiety and awkwardness of not knowing what is happening to a loved one is tremendously debilitating. When a family member with a mental illness is hospitalized, a severe disruption of the family system can occur.

It is easy to understand this anxiety-filled situation. Not only is the family confused about the behaviors associated with the affective disorders, but they may also feel perplexed about the foreign setting of the hospital.

At this point nurses enter into the family system, serving as vital communication links between the open systems of the family and the hospital. Nurses explain their roles and functions as well as developing a therapeutic alliance with the family. They build rapport by working with families' immediate concerns, and take those concerns very seriously. An attitude of interest prevails.

Why work with the family? Traditionally, the family has been viewed as the place in which love, understanding, and support can be found when all else fails, the place in which members can be refreshed and recharged in order to cope more effectively with the outside world. For millions of troubled families, this is a myth. Families accept a troubled path only because no other way is known.

Nurses work with families to offer another way—the path to a nurturing family life. If the family works *with* the nurse, they can be taught the skills required to maintain homeostasis for the client and the family during a mental health crisis.

Upon admission, the client may be angry, hostile, and/or dependent. Anger is a response to anxiety—specifically, anxiety related to powerlessness, helplessness, and devalued self-esteem. It is an unconscious psychological process employed to obtain relief from anxiety produced by a sense of danger. The hospital culture removes the identity and status from clients and their families, making anger an inevitable part of the hospital experience. The family is dependent on the staff for information, and at times this engenders helplessness.

If families take pride in being able to care for "their own," but must relinquish this care to "experts," they usually have painful feelings of helplessness, uncertainty, and powerlessness. Anger is a natural outcome of these feelings. Families experience their own powerlessness and helplessness as well as those of their loved ones.

The saying "You only hurt the ones you love" depicts another type of anger experienced by family members. The trust and familiarity in family relationships make them easy targets for displaced anger in the hospital setting. A husband may find a hostile and complaining wife when he comes to visit. She complains about the way he dresses and is managing the children. Her husband is the target for her unexpressed anger about hospitalization. The husband feels hurt and bewildered. She feels guilty and unsatisfied by the interaction.

From another perspective, a wife may find herself angry and resentful toward her depressed and helpless husband because he is not the way he used to be or the way she needs him to be. Resentment and anger are difficult to acknowledge toward a depressed, helpless person. Because these feelings exist, they will be expressed, perhaps indirectly.

Family members may feel responsible for the illness. "If only I had been more perceptive, or responsive, this wouldn't have happened." The guilt that results from the "shoulds" of family life, in combination with anxiety due to the crisis, creates increased risk for unreasonable behavior.

Anger is similar to hostility. Horney defined hostility as "a response to subjectively-experienced humiliation." When individuals feel or think that others do not have the expected respect for them, they feel and/or express hostility.[18] Clients project or displace the blame onto someone in the environment. Clients often feel that other individuals have become the "harmful agents" that produce feelings of lowered self-esteem or respect. The "harmful agents" become the object of hostility. When a person is admitted to the hospital, the "agent of harm" can be a family member, a nurse, or another significant person.

There are several factors that lead to feelings of hostility: frustration, loss of self-esteem, or unfulfilled needs for status and prestige. When depressed clients experience forced hospitalization and restriction, frustration ensues. Self-esteem becomes threatened as clients are thrust into a forced dependency role, especially if they are socially prestigious individuals. Clients now experience dependent relationships with their families and care-givers.

Clients' families can also feel hostility, since they too are placed in a dependent relationship with the care-givers. Hostility and anger will manifest themselves in some manner. Nurses can teach family members what to expect during hospitalization, prepare them for the myriad of feelings involved, and intervene as necessary. When family members talk together, energy can be channeled constructively rather than converted into anger. Nurses can facilitate families' verbal expression of feelings and assist them to examine realistically the threatening aspects of their current situations. The recognition of the threatening aspects affords a measure of cognitive control and the beginning of problem solution by constructively channeling the families' energies. Once the threats have been recognized, the nurse can ask, "What are your plans for managing?" This will help the family focus positively on reorganization and mastery.

Responses such as "Why bother?" or "Nothing" indicate the presence of repressed anger. In this case, the nurse can employ exploration and clarification, with a focus on the realistic threats of the situation. "This illness is certainly a challenge for the family," followed by, "What will help most?"

The following are guidelines for the nurse working with the angry client and/or family:

1. Determine what factors in the situation may have precipitated the anxiety that led to anger.
2. Emphasize and acknowledge the precipitant, not the anger—remember that anger is evidence of anxiety. "You were surprised when the doctor extended your involuntary stay."
3. Do not press for direct expression at this time. "Are you angry?" can be threatening to a family who has

difficulty expressing feelings directly. To make the family more emotionally comfortable, use a less threatening term such as "annoying" and focus on the situation's stresses.

4. For overt, hostile outbursts, it is necessary to set limits without prohibiting the expression of anger. Destructive actions are not permitted. The present outburst may be the result of an accumulation of anxiety and anger, and thus the present precipitants may not represent all of the factors responsible for the present demonstration of hostility. It is not possible to reason with the client or the family at this time. The nurse might say, "I know you're upset but you can't scream at me."

5. Focus on the situation that caused the anger and allow ventilation and expression of feeling. Nurses should beware of the risks of their becoming angry, when being threatened by an angry, hostile person.

6. Suggest physical expression such as sports, exercise, or creative endeavors as a way for the client and family to dissipate anger. The nurse can suggest, "While visiting, walk and talk for 15 minutes in the courtyard."

Somatic Therapies for Depressive/Manic Disorders

Monoamine Re-uptake Inhibitor Antidepressants (Tricyclics and Related Compounds)

Tricyclic antidepressants are rapidly absorbed and extensively metabolized. Absorption is usually complete within ten hours of oral ingestion, and maximal plasma concentrations are attained after one to two hours. However, absorption after intramuscular injection is slower. Tricyclic antidepressants are extensively metabolized in the liver, and only small amounts of the drugs are excreted unchanged.

It appears that the clinical effects of tricyclic antidepressants are related to their activity in blocking the reuptake into the presynaptic vesicles of serotonin, noradrenaline, and dopamine. These uptake pumps are located in the cell membranes.

Antidepressants are indicated for the following:

A. A diagnosis of depression as evidenced by the following vegetative signs:
1. Appetite disturbance (increase or decrease from normal)
2. Sleep disturbance (increase or decrease from normal)
3. Low energy
4. Anhedonia

5. Feelings of guilt or worthlessness
6. Decreased concentration
7. Psychomotor agitation or retardation
8. Suicidal ideation or behavior
B. Panic attacks with or without phobias and/or free-floating anxiety attacks
C. Certain pain–depression syndromes (somatic depressions)

Prior to administration of antidepressant medications, baseline vital signs are taken, a physical examination is performed, and laboratory tests (CBC, M-300, UA) and ECG are usually ordered. Initially antidepressants are given in low, divided doses which may be increased daily. After a period of time, the entire dose can be given at bedtime to decrease side-effects and take advantage of its sedative effects. Therapeutic levels are not reached before 10 to 14 days. A full trial requires four weeks. The drug card for imipramine outlines its uses and effects.

Tricyclic antidepressants and related compounds are potentiated by other anticholinergic medications, alcohol, central nervous system depressants, and antiparkinsonian drugs. Other drug interactions include those with hypnotics, which affect monoamine re-uptake inhibitor levels, and those with sympathomimetic amines, antianxiety agents, and MAO inhibitors, which increase the effects of antidepressants.

Other contraindications and cautions include:

1. Guanethidine and methyldopa are contraindicated.
2. Propranolol is the antihypertensive of choice while a client is on antidepressants.
3. Clients with prostatic hypertrophy are at high risk for urinary retention and paralytic ileus.
4. Tricyclic antidepressants are contraindicated in clients with narrow-angle glaucoma, increased ocular pressure, and cardiovascular disease.
5. Use of other drugs with anticholinergic properties will increase the anticholinergic side-effects.

Table 15-8 lists common antidepressants used as well as common and uncommon side-effects of antidepressant medications. Nursing interventions for these side-effects are addressed in Table 15-9.

Issues for Client Teaching

It is important to stress that tricyclic antidepressant medication is not effective for 10 to 14 days and may take three to four weeks to effect a good response. Clients become discouraged, so positive reassurance and support throughout this time are usually needed. The client can be told that the medication can and will be effective. Also, the nurse may choose to enlist the support of significant others in helping the client maintain a positive attitude toward therapy. The psychiatric nurse must assess closely for ideation of suicide throughout the pretherapeutic period.

The psychiatric nurse must emphasize the importance of medication follow-up. The medication must be

imipramine

(tricyclic antidepressant)

Janimine, Presamine, Ropramine, Tipramine, Tofranil

Action: Blocks reuptake of neurotransmitters (norepinephrine, serotonin) into nerve endings, increasing action of norepinephrine, serotonin at postsynaptic receptors.

Uses: Depression, adjunctive therapy for treatment of enuresis in children

Side-effects: Dizziness, drowsiness, confusion; diarrhea, dry mouth; urinary retention; postural hypotension; ECG changes, tachycardia

Toxic effects: Agranulocytosis, thrombocytopenia, eosinophilia, leukopenia; paralytic ileus; hepatitis (extremely rare); acute renal failure

Contraindications:
- Recovery period of myocardial infarction

Precautions:
- Prostatic hypertrophy
- History of seizures
- Cardiac/hepatic/renal disease
- Urinary retention
- Glaucoma

Interactions:
- Sympathomimetics (decreased effects)
- CNS depressants (increased effects)
- MAO inhibitors (may cause hyperpyretic crisis, convulsions)
- Clonidine (decreased effects)

Nursing implications:
- Monitor for daily bowel activity.
- Assess for urinary retention by palpation.
- Evaluate mental status—suicidal tendencies, mood.
- Monitor for withdrawal symptoms: headache, nausea, vomiting, muscle pain, weakness.

Client teaching:
- Therapeutic effects may take 2 to 3 weeks.
- Maintain ample fluid intake.
- Avoid alcohol.
- Exercise caution in driving or operating machinery.

titrated and monitored for maximum effectiveness. The client must be aware that tapering should take place under close supervision to avoid serious withdrawal responses. At times, once clients begin to "feel well," they want to stop taking the medication on their own. Clients need to be cautioned against doing this, because another episode of depression can be precipitated. Clients need to be given some general guidelines about antidepressant medications. The recommended treatment with antidepressant medication lasts for approximately one year, with tapering off of the medication during the last three to six months. Encourage clients to continue with ongoing psychotherapy, because medication is most effective when combined with this second treatment modality.

The client is "captain of the ship." If the client is at the helm, the client must know the signs and symptoms of the disorder that indicate an exacerbation of the illness. Clients will receive indications at least several weeks before a depressive episode begins, and they must be taught to intervene and deal appropriately with these signs and symptoms at that point. Nurses must teach not only clients, but also significant others, the signs and symptoms of depression and early intervention techniques.

MAO Inhibitors

MAO inhibitors are used less frequently than tricyclic antidepressants. For clients who are on MAO inhibitors, particular attention is given to the vital signs of the client because there is a danger of hypertensive crisis when this medication is combined with other drugs and tyramine-containing foods.

TABLE 15-8.
ANTIDEPRESSANT MEDICATIONS

GENERIC NAME	TRADE NAME	DOSAGE RANGE (mg/24 hr, dependent on dose form)	DOSE FORM	SIDE-EFFECTS	OTHER CONSIDERATIONS
TRICYCLICS					
Amitriptyline	Elavil	75 to 300	Tablet, parenteral	Dry mouth, blurred vision, constipation, drowsiness (except protriptyline), jitteriness, nausea, heartburn	Caution needed with suicidal patients; avoid hazardous activities; potentiated by alcohol; not to be combined with MAO inhibitors
Desipramine	Norpramin, Pertofrane	75 to 300	Tablet		
Doxepin	Adapin, Sinequan	75 to 300	Capsule, concentrate		
Imipramine	Presamine, Tofranil	75 to 300	Tablet, capsule, parenteral		
Nortriptyline	Aventyl, Pamelor	50 to 100	Capsule, liquid		
Protriptyline	Vivactil	15 to 60	Tablet		
Trimipramine	Surmontil	75 to 300	Capsule		New antidepressant, second generation
MAO INHIBITORS					
Isocarboxazid	Marplan	10 to 30	Tablet	Hypertensive crisis if combined with tyramine-containing foods; severe headaches, dry mouth, constipation, insomnia, over-stimulation, dizziness	Not to be combined with tricyclics; inhibited by alcohol; potentiates amphetamines, barbiturates, chloral hydrate, antiparkinsonian agents, antianxiety drugs, phenothiazines, sympathomimetics
Phenelzine	Nardil	15 to 75	Tablet		
Tranylcypromine	Parnate	10 to 30	Tablet		
OTHERS					
Amoxapine	Asendin	100 to 300	Tablets	Anticholinergic, extrapyramidal signs, tardive dyskinesia, galactorrhea	New antidepressant
Trazodone	Desyrel	150 to 600	Tablets	Sedation, hypertension, priapism	New antidepressant
Fluoxetine	Prozac	10 to 20	Capsule	Nausea, anxiety/nervousness, insomnia, drowsiness	New antidepressant unrelated to all others

(Based on data from Cain RM, Cain NN: A Compendium of Psychiatric Drugs, Part 1, January, 1975; and Veterans Administration: Drug Treatment in Psychiatry, Washington, DC, 1970. Chart of new antidepressants contributed by Jambur Ananth, M.D., Psychopharmacologist at U.C.L.A., 1986.)

Dietary interactions constitute the best-known untoward effect. This syndrome takes the form of a severe occipital headache with a hypertensive crisis. The headache is sudden and severe and can be accompanied by vomiting, chest pain, hyperpyrexia, and restlessness. Death may occur. Many foods have been implicated in dietary reaction. All foods containing the amino acid tyramine must be avoided. Serious reactions are unlikely if clients avoid meat and yeast extracts, red wine, matured cheese, and food that is not fresh.

Drug interactions are very important. Any sympathomimetic agent can cause a hypertensive reaction, as does tyramine. Such agents are ephedrine, amphetamine, phenylephrine, and phenylpropanolamine, some of which are found in cough medicines and nasal decongestants. Alcohol, ether, the barbiturates, pethidine, morphine, cocaine, procaine, and insulin can cause dangerous, or even fatal, interactions. In the United States, tricyclic antidepressants and MAO inhibitors are never administered at the same time. The FDA prohibits the use of both drugs simultaneously, and considers this a dangerous method of treatment.

Nursing interventions include medication teaching, providing clients with a list of foods containing tyramine,

TABLE 15-9.
NURSING INTERVENTIONS FOR ANTIDEPRESSANT SIDE-EFFECTS

I. Common anticholinergic responses
  A. Dry mouth

    1. Frequent sips of water
    2. Mouth swabs
    3. Thorough and frequent mouth rinsing
    4. Hard, sugarless lemon candies

  B. Constipation

    • Mild to moderate

    1. Encourage adequate roughage in diet.
    2. Ensure adequate fluid intake.
    3. Stool softeners
    4. Encourage daily exercise.

    • Severe

    1. Hold medication.
    2. Notify physician.
    3. Bethanechol may be necessary for prevention of paralytic ileus.

  C. Blurred vision

    1. Reassure client this is a temporary condition with no pathological effects on the eyes.
    2. Inform client that this side-effect should resolve within three weeks as the body becomes adjusted to the medication.
    3. If condition persists beyond three weeks, notify physician regarding necessity of an eye consult.
    4. Check with physician regarding the possible use of physostigmine eye solution if noncompliance related to this side-effect seems likely.
    5. Blurring is related to near vision changes, and clients who wear glasses to correct such a problem may experience less blurring if they do not wear their glasses during the initial weeks.

  D. Nasal congestion

    1. Reassure client that this side-effect will also resolve as the body becomes adjusted to the medication.
    2. Moisturizer as needed
    3. Decongestants and/or nose drops as ordered
    4. Close observation to be sure congestion is not due to a developing physical illness

II. Uncommon anticholinergic responses
  A. Urinary retention and/or delayed micturition

    1. Monitor intake and output.
    2. Check for abdominal distention.
    3. If client is unable to void, hold medication and notify physician.
    4. Catheterization and/or bethanechol as necessary

  B. Diaphoresis

    1. Assess electrolyte imbalance.
    2. Encourage high noncaloric fluid intake.
    3. Encourage good personal hygiene.

  C. Atropine psychosis—a serious side-effect with central and peripheral symptoms.

    • *Central* (resembles organic brain syndrome): Confusion, disorientation, short-term memory loss, hallucinations, insomnia, agitation and restlessness, picking behaviors, inappropriate affect
    • *Peripheral:* Fever, flushed skin, dry mucous membranes, dilated pupils, poorly reactive pupils, thirst, blurred vision, photophobia

    1. Hold medication—symptoms will worsen if medication is continued.
    2. Notify physician.
    3. Monitor urinary output closely.
    4. Monitor vital signs closely.
    5. Provide safe, protective environment.
    6. Provide frequent reassurance to patient.
    7. Administration of physostigmine as ordered for diagnosis and/or treatment.
    8. ECG monitoring and medical observation for one week following anticholinergic psychosis that is a result of antidepressant therapy
    9. Awareness that risk of psychosis increases as number of anticholinergic medications increases
    10. Alert patient not to use drug again.

III. Common cardiovascular responses
  A. Orthostatic hypotension

    1. Take blood pressures while client is lying down and after one full minute of standing.
    2. Hold medication and notify physician if there is a systolic drop of more than 30 mm or blood pressure is lower than 90/60.
    3. Reassure client that this side-effect will subside over one to two weeks as the body adjusts to the medication.
    4. Caution client against getting up quickly after sitting or lying.
    5. Instruct client to sit for one full minute when getting up from a supine position and to stand stationary for one full minute before attempting to walk.
    6. Elastic stockings may be used initially, as ordered, to control side-effects.

(Continued)

TABLE 15-9 (CONTINUED).
NURSING INTERVENTIONS FOR ANTIDEPRESSANT SIDE-EFFECTS

B. Arrythmias and T-wave abnormalities
1. Monitor pulse for irregularities.
2. Check ECG prior to initiation of antidepressant therapy.
3. Check serial ECGs if client has a history of conduction defects.
4. Review cardiology consult in chart, if completed.
5. If client expresses concern, reassure that minor changes are expected and indicate that there is no serious medical problem.

C. Tachycardia
1. Monitor pulse.
2. Hold medication and notify physician if resting pulse is greater than 120.

IV. Common negative psychiatric responses
A. Hypomania (*Note:* Symptoms will evidence a progressive shift from depressive symptomatology to increased activity, social aggression, talkativeness with increased emotional tone, irritability and/or impatience, distractibility, loosening of associations, and increased seductive behaviors.)
1. Hold medication and notify physician because the client may be bipolar; continued administration of antidepressants may precipitate a manic episode.
2. Give neuroleptics, as ordered, to control hypomanic behavior.
3. Give lithium, as ordered, for treatment of bipolar disorder.
4. Provide protective environment until behavior is controlled.

B. Anxiety, restlessness, and/or irritability
1. Assess closely to determine if this is part of the client's psychiatric condition or a response to the medication.
2. Notify physician—an increase or decrease in medication may be necessary.
3. Request that physician change medication schedule in order to control symptoms.
4. Request that physician change to a more sedating antidepressant, if possible.
5. Provide a protective environment.
6. Give neuroleptics, as ordered, to control behavior.

V. Common neurologic responses
A. Lowering of seizure threshold
1. Observe seizure precautions on any client with history of seizures.
2. Clients may need an increase in their seizure medication when psychotropic drugs are added to their regimen.
3. If seizure activity occurs, notify physician immediately as medication adjustments will be necessary.

B. Drowsiness
1. Reassure client that this side-effect will generally disappear after five to seven days as the body adjusts to the medication.
2. Advise client to participate in physical activity to offset sedative effects.
3. Caution client not to engage in hazardous activities (*e.g.,* driving or operating machinery).
4. Notify physician regarding a change in schedule, with all medication given at bedtime.
5. If symptom persists beyond two weeks, request that physician adjust dosage or change to less sedating antidepressant.

C. Fine tremor and/or mild ataxia
1. Reassure client that this is expected and should decrease over time.
2. If it is severe, hold medication and request that physician adjust dosage.
3. If problem interferes with client's work, notify physician—client may not comply with medication regimen.

VI. Common reproductive or genitourinary responses
A. Decreased libido (in rare cases, increased)
1. Assess closely to determine if problem is related to medication or is manifestation of ongoing psychiatric condition and/or marital conflicts.
2. Reassure client that this side-effect is transitory and should decrease in one to two weeks.
3. If symptom persists or inferferes with compliance, notify physician regarding change in dose or medication.

VII. Common metabolic problems
A. Weight gain
1. Monitor weight.
2. Counsel client to maintain a well-balanced, nutritionally adequate diet.
3. Recommend diet tray, if necessary, to maintain normal weight.
4. Encourage exercise.

VIII. Uncommon reproductive responses
A. Ejaculatory and/or erection disturbances
1. Refer to libido disturbances (VI above).

(Modified from Leslie Groenwald, R.N., Medication Module. Unpublished manuscript, 1984.)

and instructions not to take any other medication without consulting the physician. Clients are informed that any incidence of headache should be reported immediately.

Antimania Medication: Lithium Carbonate

Lithium carbonate quiets manic behaviors and is most commonly used for treatment of manic and hypomanic episodes in bipolar affective disorders. Other indications include long-term prophylaxis against manic episodes and, to a lesser extent, depressive episodes.

Lithium is absorbed well from the intestine and is excreted by the kidney. Lithium excretion is linked to sodium balance in the body. If sodium intake is lowered and blood pressure drops, lithium excretion is reduced and toxicity can supervene.

The exact mode of action of lithium in preventing affective episodes is not known. Lithium affects various neurotransmitters and receptor processes and also influences the electrolyte and neuroendocrine systems.

Lithium has a low therapeutic index, and therapeutic levels can be reached easily and with unexpected rapidity. Serum lithium levels must be monitored at appropriate intervals. Monitoring is important when treatment is first begun or when dosage regimens are changed, particularly during exacerbations of the illness. While clients are hospitalized, blood samples may be checked two or three times weekly and then, perhaps, on the seventh, fourteenth, twenty-first, and twenty-eighth days of treatment. Subsequently, lithium levels may be checked monthly, depending on the reliability of the clients and the variability in their lithium concentrations. Blood samples must be drawn at the same time each day. Usually the blood is drawn before the first morning dose. The usual therapeutic range is a blood level of 0.5 to 1.5 mEq/L. Toxicity generally occurs at concentrations greater than 2.0 mEq/L. Effects, precautions, interactions, and nursing implications for lithium are listed in the drug card.

About 85% of manic clients respond well to lithium therapy. However, highly overactive manic clients respond best to neuroleptics initially, because the therapeutic effects of lithium are often not apparent for at least a week. Combinations of neuroleptics and lithium are commonly used. Thus, an antipsychotic medication is initiated to effect initial control, and lithium is added with the expectation that the initial medication can then be carefully withdrawn. Because lithium is prescribed prophylactically to prevent future episodes of manic/depressive behavior, the client will probably take it indefinitely.

During the pretreatment phase, laboratory work is ordered, especially a CBC, M-300, T³, T⁴, T⁵, and urinalysis. Baseline vital signs are obtained, and a physical exam is completed. Usually an ECG is performed.

Lithium is administered orally only. Initially it is given in small divided dosages, TID or QID, to offset common gastrointestinal side-effects until a therapeutic level is obtained. Maintenance dosages of lithium range from 600 to 1200 mg per 24 hours.

Lithium is contraindicated with electroconvulsive therapy (ECT), the presence of renal failure or tubular disease, hyperthyroidism, goiter, and pregnancy.

Several unfavorable drug interactions can occur. Diuretics cause an increase in lithium excretion. Lithium potentiates the effects of digoxin. The combination of lithium, digoxin, and diuretics can be dangerous. Some clients have developed toxicity to a regimen of tetracyclines and/or spectinomycin. Lastly, Indocin and Butazolidin can cause lithium retention and toxicity.

Side-effects of some kind, even at therapeutic levels, are experienced by most clients, and can begin anytime after the first dose. However, most side-effects subside after one to two weeks of treatment.

Development of side-effects tends to parallel blood levels. Table 15-10 lists toxicity levels of lithium, with their side-effects. Table 15-11 lists the nursing interventions for the side-effects of lithium.

Issues for Client Teaching

Because most clients experience some side-effects during lithium therapy, psychiatric nurses must stress that the effects will generally subside within one to two weeks, and that all side-effects are reversible. Clients might be tempted to change their medication, but they should be cautioned to notify their physician if symptoms worsen or become severe. Clients should be aware of all recurrent symptoms of mania (e.g., euphoria, decreased sleep, increased verbosity, increased motor activity, grandiosity, increased sexual behavior, increased distractibility, spending sprees, racing thoughts). Clients should be instructed to intervene by notifying the clinical nurse specialist/practitioner or physician.

Clients need to be aware of the signs and dangers of lithium toxicity and what should be done if these symptoms become apparent. Advise clients of common precipitants of toxic reactions (e.g., fever, weight loss, diaphoresis, loss of appetite).

At an appropriate time the nurse will discuss the chronic nature of this disorder, and the necessity of taking medication even if the client feels "well."

Lastly, positive, achievable results must be emphasized with maintenance medication and therapeutic intervention. Whenever possible, family members and significant others are included in the teaching.

Electroconvulsive Therapy

Electroconvulsive therapy (ECT), or the use of electrically-induced seizures for psychiatric purposes, is a controversial treatment modality. For this reason, psychiatric nurses must understand each of the pertinent issues involving ECT and be fully aware of the following topics: the historical perspective, indications, mechanisms of action, risks and side-effects, contraindications, informed consent, techniques, and nursing interventions.

Historical Perspective. During the late 1930s, Bini[8] studied the effects of electrically-induced seizures in animals in an effort to understand the mechanism of epilepsy. During this period, it was believed that epilep-

lithium

(antimanic)

Lithane, Eskalith, Lithonate, Lithobid

Action: Alters sodium, potassium, calcium, and magnesium transport across cell membranes in nerve and muscle cells.

Uses: Prevention and treatment of manic episodes of bipolar disorder

Side-effects: Polyuria, polydipsia, hypotension, headache, drowsiness, mild nausea, dizziness

Toxic effects: Acute toxicity characterized by seizures, oliguria, circulatory failure, coma

Precautions:
- Hepatic disease
- Renal disease
- Brain trauma
- Pregnancy and lactation
- Cardiovascular disease
- Severe dehydration

Interactions:
- Haloperidol (may result in brain damage)
- Neuromuscular blocking agents (increased effects)
- Theophyllines (decreased effect of drug)
- Indomethacin, thiazide diuretics (increased toxicity)

Nursing implications:
- Weigh daily and check for edema.
- Monitor sodium intake.
- Assess skin turgor.
- Monitor serum lithium levels.
- Assess neurological status.
- Administer with meals to avoid GI upset.
- Monitor for increased urine output.

Client teaching:
- Watch for signs of toxicity: diarrhea, vomiting, drowsiness, poor coordination, muscular weakness.
- Avoid intense physical activities.
- Report excessive sweating or diarrhea—may indicate need for supplemental fluids or salt.

tics were rarely schizophrenics, and that convulsions improved schizophrenia. Bini learned to transfer this seizure induction technique to humans. Thus, ECT became the dominant somatic method used to treat schizophrenia during the 1940s. Later, it was discovered that ECT was more effective for severe endogenous (vegetative) depressive disorders rather than for schizophrenia.

During the 1950s and 1960s, pharmacologic agents for the treatment of affective disorders and thought disturbances were developed, which reduced the use of ECT. However, a survey undertaken in 1975–1976 by the American Psychiatric Task Force on ECT, questioning 4,000 members, indicated that 72% of the respondents felt that there are clients for whom ECT is the safest, least expensive, and most effective form of treatment.

Indications. In actuality, ECT is generally used when medications are not therapeutic or are contraindicated. Thus, the typical client receiving ECT is severely depressed and has failed to respond to antidepressant medications. ECT may also be used as an emergency treatment for an extremely suicidal patient to avoid the weeks it may take for the antidepressant medications to take effect. Evidence strongly suggests that, for acutely ill, nonchronic schizophrenic clients, particularly those who are paranoid, catatonic, or display a major affective component, ECT is comparable to major tranquilizers.[26] ECT can be used for mania, but should never be used concurrently with lithium. This diminishes its therapeutic effects and increases side-effects. Neurotic conditions, psychophysiological problems, and personality disorders do not respond to ECT.

Mechanism of Action. The monoamine hypothesis, for some, explains the action of antidepressants and ECT. This theory suggests that the hypothalamus controls the vegetative features of depression and is affected by norepinephrine levels. As levels of norepinephrine increase, vegetative signs diminish. According to this theory, ECT increases norepinephrine turnover, which has a palliative effect on vegetative symptoms.[28] Ottosson suggested that the induction of a series of seizures spaced

TABLE 15-10.
TOXICITY LEVEL OF LITHIUM AND SIDE-EFFECTS

TOXICITY LEVEL	SIDE-EFFECTS
Mild: less than 1.5 mEq/L	Metallic taste in mouth
	Fine hand tremor
	Nausea
	Polyuria
	Polydipsia
	Diarrhea or loose stools
	Muscular weakness or fatigue
Moderate: 1.5–2.5 mEq/L	Severe diarrhea
	Nausea and vomiting
	Mild to moderate ataxia
	Incoordination
	Dizziness, sluggishness, giddiness, vertigo
	Slurred speech
	Tinnitus
	Blurred vision
	Increasing tremor
	Muscle irritability or twitching
	Asymmetrical deep-tendon reflexes
	Increased muscle tone
Severe: 2.5–7.0 mEq/L	Nystagmus
	Coarse tremor
	Dysarthria
	Fasciculations
	Visual or tactile hallucinations
	Oliguria, anuria
	Confusion
	Impaired consciousness
	Dyskinesias—chorea, athetoid movements
	Grand mal convulsions
	Coma
	Death

(Leslie Groenwald, R.N., Medication Module. Unpublished manuscript, 1984.)

out over time may cause the subcortical structures in the reticular core of the brain stem, along with the specific and nonspecific nuclei of the thalamus, to be involved in the mediation of ECT's therapeutic effect.[28]

Risks/Side-Effects. The risks and side-effects of ECT include four categories: (1) those related to seizures, (2) the electrical stimulus itself, (3) anesthetic and relaxant drugs, and (4) the effects of the above on cardiovascular, cerebrovascular, and metabolic functioning.

Mortality figures for ECT are one per 10,000 clients, and death is usually a result of cardiac complications. The most common cardiac complication—premature ventricular contractions—happens as a result of vagal hyperactivity. Atropine is administered to alleviate this problem. Clients commonly complain of memory disturbances, headaches, and muscle aches.

During a seizure, the brain has increased metabolic needs. Without oxygenation and muscular relaxation, anoxia can occur. Usually 100% oxygen is administered prior to the seizure. This hyperoxygenation prepares the client for the period of apnea that will result from the muscle relaxant and the convulsion.

Memory deficits associated with ECT have been well established in the literature. Because depression itself is also associated with memory loss, it is difficult to measure objectively memory loss associated with a standard course of ECT compared to memory loss resulting from depression. Attempts have been made to diminish memory loss. Acute memory losses associated with unilateral ECT to the nondominant hemisphere are much less apparent that those observed with bilateral treatments.[28]

The pretreatment phase for ECT includes a history, physical exam, laboratory tests, urinalysis, chest x-ray, ECG, EEG, and x-rays of the spine.

Contraindications. ECT is usually contraindicated for clients with severely compromised cardiac status, those suffering from severe hypertension, those with a cerebral mass lesion such as a tumor, and those with musculoskeletal injuries, especially within the spinal column. The presence of organic brain syndrome is not a contraindication for ECT.[28]

Informed Consent. A major component of preparing the client for ECT is informed consent. The formal aspects, such as the specific information that must be imparted to the client by law and obtaining the client's signature on the consent form, are the responsibility of the physician. Nurses prepare clients psychologically for the treatment. Certain topics may need clarification. Nurses can use themselves as a therapeutic tool for the benefit of the client and the family.

Involuntary clients may receive ECT. The nurse acts as the client's advocate, explaining the legal documents and protocols as they occur, in addition to physical and psychological preparation of the client and family.

Techniques. The usual technique includes premedication with an anticholinergic agent to prevent cardiac arrhythmias and aspiration. A fast-acting general anesthetic is administered to induce a light coma. This reduced dose of anesthetic lowers the seizure threshold and reduces the apneic period. A muscle relaxant is given immediately after the onset of anesthesia to modify the convulsive activity of the induced seizure.

Electrodes are placed on the scalp. This permits the electrical stimulus to pass through the scalp to the brain to evoke a seizure. Electrodes may be placed unilaterally or bilaterally. With unilateral electrode placement, both stimulus electrodes are placed over the same cerebral nondominant hemisphere. With bilateral ECT, each electrode is placed over a separate cerebral hemisphere.

Concurrent with the passage of the electrical stimulus is a period of muscular contraction, which is followed by the tonic phase of a seizure. Last, the clonic phase occurs. After the seizure, the client spontaneously begins breathing within 60 to 120 seconds. Consciousness is regained shortly thereafter.[28]

For depression, a client may receive six to ten treatments. Schizophrenic clients usually receive more.

TABLE 15-11.
NURSING INTERVENTIONS FOR LITHIUM SIDE-EFFECTS

I. Edema of feet and/or hands	1. Monitor intake and output, check for possible decreased urinary output.
	2. Test for specific gravity of urine, if ordered. If not, request that the test be ordered.
	3. Monitor sodium intake.
	4. Client should elevate legs when sitting or lying.
	5. Monitor weight.
II. Fine hand tremor	1. Provide support and reassurance, if it does not interfere with daily activities.
	2. Notify physician if it interferes with client's work and compliance will be an issue. Discuss alternatives with physician, *e.g.,* possible change to Inderol.
III. Mild diarrhea	1. Provide support and reassurance.
	2. Provide for fluid replacement.
IV. Muscle weakness and fatigue and/or metallic taste in mouth	1. Provide support and reassurance.
	2. Suggest sugarless candies.
	3. Encourage frequent oral hygiene.
V. Nausea and/or abdominal discomfort	1. Consider dividing the medication into smaller doses, or give it at more frequent intervals.
	2. Give medication with meals.
VI. Polydipsia	1. Reassure client that this is a normal mechanism to cope with polyuria.
VII. Polyuria	1. Monitor intake and output.
	2. Provide reassurance and explain nature of side-effect. Also explain that this causes no physical damage to kidneys.
VIII. Toxicity Symptoms of the impending development of lithium toxicity are listed under the "Moderate" section of Table 16-10. In assessing a client for the development of toxicity, the most important indication is the observation that initial side-effects are gradually becoming more severe, or that the symptoms are beginning to occur in clusters. Either of these observations requires immediate medical attention.	1. Hold medication.
	2. Notify physician.
	3. Use symptomatic treatments.

(Modified from Leslie Groenwald, R.N., Medication Module. Unpublished manuscript, 1984.)

Nursing Interventions.   Nursing interventions begin once the client and family have been informed of the possibility that ECT may be used as a treatment modality. Nursing interventions can be divided into three stages. Table 15-12 explains the nursing actions during the preoperative, administration of ECT, and postoperative phases.

Electroconvulsive therapy is a means of treating severe endogenous depressions and, in some instances, thought disturbance disorders. Its continued use reflects its helpfulness to many psychiatric patients.

A variety of somatic therapies play a vital role in psychiatric treatment. Psychiatric nurses must have a complete knowledge and understanding of the nursing skills required for each of these modalities.

Primary, Secondary, and Tertiary Prevention

The role of the nurse in working with depressed/manic clients can be very specific or can be very broad. As nurses work with family and client simultaneously, they deal with illness prevention as well as with treatment and rehabilitation.

Primary prevention is the promotion of mental health and the prevention of illness. By teaching clients and families, nurses can prevent episodes of illness. Striking relationships exist among families' abilities to cope with members and the occurrence of symptomatology in these same individuals. We noted in the clinical example that the course of Sergio's illness will be affected by the perceptions and reactions of others. Sergio and Sheila's development and primary family relationships may have had a significant impact on their current state of health and illness. If ways in which parents treat children can be traced to eventual illness states, then early family teaching about effective parenting skills is important. The provision of screening for affective disorders is still another approach to primary prevention. With thought disturbances, the social support network of the client prone to affective disorders is important. Provision of counseling and support groups at various junctures in a client's psychosocial development can prove to be an effective measure of primary prevention.

Secondary prevention refers to early case-finding

TABLE 15-12.
ELECTROCONVULSIVE THERAPY PHASES AND NURSING INTERVENTIONS

I. Preprocedure phase

    A. Day preceding ECT

       1. When discussing ECT treatment, do not use emotion-laden words (*e.g.,* "shock treatments").

       2. Conduct preoperative teaching throughout the day(s). The definition of informed consent varies, depending on the state's mental health act. The physician will provide information at the time informed consent is obtained; however, the nurse will review and reinforce this information and ask clients to repeat what has been explained to help identify areas of confusion.

       3. Encourage clients to verbalize concerns and feelings; listen for misconceptions and clarify information about which clients are confused.

       4. Inform clients that they will be NPO after midnight, and explain the three phases of ECT therapy.

       5. Check to make sure that all emergency equipment, including oxygen, suction, and cardiac resuscitation equipment for use during ECT, is functioning.

       6. Make sure the ECT machine and IV equipment are readily available.

    B. The morning of ECT

       1. Vital signs are taken.

       2. Ask client to void.

       3. Remove client's nail polish, hair pins, dentures, and contact lenses.

       4. Be certain consent has been signed and client understands procedure.

       5. Allow time for client to express concerns and/or feelings.

       6. Atropine sulfate is frequently given subcutaneously or intramuscularly 30 minutes prior to treatment. May be given intravenously with the other premedications.

       7. A quick-acting barbiturate, such as sodium methohexital, is administered intravenously to induce anesthesia.

       8. A muscle relaxant is administered after the anesthetic.

       9. Medications may be injected directly into the vein or through tubing of a previously started intravenous infusion.

II. During ECT

       1. ECT may be given in the operating room or in a specially equipped room in the inpatient or outpatient psychiatric section.

       2. Client lies supine on bed and is hyperoxygenated, usually while IV infusion is being started, and medications are given. When paralysis occurs, the treatment is given.

III. Postprocedure phase

       1. Vital signs are taken and monitored closely until client is conscious, usually within 15 to 30 minutes.

       2. Close nursing observation is required immediately after ECT, and emergency equipment should be readily available.

       3. Nurse will maintain a patent airway for unconscious client. This may require suctioning, appropriate positioning, and like steps.

       4. Nurse will orient client to date, time, place, and situation, because most clients are confused immediately following a treatment and become frightened if they are not oriented.

       5. Observe the client every 20 minutes for the first two hours after returning to the unit from ECT.

       6. Agitation occasionally occurs. Client may require restraints.

       7. Once clients are ambulatory, they should continue their usual daily routine.

       8. Assess for physical discomforts (*e.g.,* headaches, muscle soreness, nausea) and intervene accordingly.

and treatment of illness states. The training of human service professionals to detect the symptoms of disorders early is an example of secondary prevention. The provision of highly effective outpatient and inpatient services for people with these disorders is still another step. Finally, the early detection of secondary problems in people suspected of having primary problems with other origins is important.

Finally, *tertiary prevention* is the return of clients to their highest level of functioning prior to the onset of illness. Many of the discharge interventions suggested for Sergio and Sheila lie in this domain. Providing psychiatric care that is geared toward early discharge planning is important. A focus on treating the predictable remissions of individuals suffering from bipolar illness or chronic depression is needed. Finally, the provision of adequate follow-up of persons in the community on antidepressant and lithium medications is important.

Summary

1. The major affective illnesses are characterized by primary disturbances of mood or affect.

2. Affective disorders were recognized as early as the fourth century B.C. with the description of melancholia believed to be caused by the presence of black bile.

3. To this day, theorists continue to argue about whether affective impairments are transmitted chemically or are of psychological origin. A combined view suggests that many factors, including bio-psycho-social phenomena, are important in understanding the precipitation and course of affective illnesses.

4. Current theories of causation include the following causes:
   - The biogenic amine

- Neurophysiological
- Psychoanalytic
- Object loss
- Loss of self-esteem
- Negative cognition
- Learned helplessness
- Loss of reinforcement
- Sociological
- Existential

5. The literature indicates that age, sex, family history, role strain, and recent life events place individuals at risk for depression.

6. The continuum notion of depression holds that depression can be manifest in a variety of states, from normal to severe cases of mood impairment.

7. Depression includes emotional, cognitive, vegetative, and physical manifestations.

8. A method of classifying depression when a second illness is present is categorization into primary and secondary forms. It is often difficult, although important, to differentiate between the two.

9. Because of the pleasurable effect of elation in manic states, this illness is less often addressed. Major components include feelings of well-being, grandiosity, inflated self-esteem, increased energy and activity, impulsivity, and little need for sleep.

10. A clear antecedent for suicidal gestures or behavior is the depressed mood. Interpersonal and/or economic loss often precedes suicidal behavior.

11. The challenge for the nurse is predicting which clients are at risk for suicide, and then developing effective methods of management. This includes development of the "no-suicide contract."

12. Nursing care with these problems involves working with observable behavioral manifestations. An individual's self-esteem is a frequent target of the nurse's communications with clients. The nurse's use of self prevents unnecessary labeling and allows the nurse to enter into an authentic here-and-now exchange with the client.

13. Medications are useful in altering mood and affect states. ECT is used in cases in which medications have been unsuccessful at relieving the individual's depression.

14. The role of the nurse can be viewed as very narrow and specific, as in dealing with suicidal gestures in the inpatient setting, or as very broad, involving the full range of primary, secondary, and tertiary prevention approaches.

References

1. Akiskal HS, McKinney WT: Overview of recent research in depression. Arch Gen Psychiatry 32:285–305, 1975
2. Akiskal HS, Rosenthal RJ, Kashgarian M et al: Differentiation of primary affective illness from situational symptomatic and secondary depressions. Arch Gen Psychiatry 36:635–643, 1979
3. American Psychiatric Association: Diagnostic and Statistical Manual of Mental Disorders, 3rd ed revised (DSM-III-R). Washington, DC, American Psychiatric Association, 1987
4. Asnis G, Fink M, Soferstein S: ECT in metropolitan New York hospitals: A survey of practice. Am J Psychiatr 135:479, 1978
5. Beck AT: Depression: Causes and Treatment. Philadelphia, University of Pennsylvania Press, 1980
6. Beck AT: Depression: Clinical, Experimental, and Theoretical Aspects. New York, Harper & Row, 1967
7. Beck A, Ward C, Mendelson M: An Inventory for Measuring Depression. Arch Gen Psychiatry 4:561–571, 1961
8. Bini L: Experimental researches on epileptic attacks induced by the electric current. Am J Psychiatr Suppl (May):172, 1938
9. Bowlby J: Grief and mourning in infancy and early childhood. Psychoanal Study Child 15:9–52, 1960
10. Bibring E: Mechanism of Depression. In Greenacre P: Affective Disorders. New York, International University Press, 1965
11. Brown F: Depression and Childhood Bereavement. J Ment Sci 107:754–777, 1961
12. Corsini RJ: Current Psychotherapies, 2nd ed. Itasca, Illinois, FE Peacock, 1979
13. Ellis A: Reason and Emotion in Psychotherapy. Secaucus, New Jersey, The Citadel Press, 1977
14. Freud S: Mourning and Melancholia, standard ed. In The Complete Psychological Works of Sigmund Freud, vol 14. London, Hogarth Press, 1957
15. Hamilton M: Development of a rating scale for primary depressive illness. Br J Soc Clin Psychol 6:278–296, 1967
16. Ilfeld F: Current social stressors and symptoms of depression. Am J Psychiatry 134:161, 1977
17. Khuri R, Akiskal HS: Suicide Prevention: The necessity of treating contributory psychiatric disorders. Psychiatr Clin North Am 6:193–207, 1983
18. Kraines SH: Mental Depressions and Their Treatment. New York, Macmillan, 1957
19. Leavett M: Families at Risk: Primary Prevention in Nursing Practice. Boston, Little, Brown & Co, 1982
20. Roberts S: Behavioral Concepts and Nursing Throughout the Life Span. Englewood Cliffs, New Jersey, Prentice-Hall, 1978
21. Satir V: Making Contact. Millbrae, California, Celestial Arts, 1976
22. Schwartz D, Flinn D, Slawson PF: Treatment of the Suicidal Character. Am J Psychother 28:194–207, 1974
23. Seligman M: Helplessness: On Depression, Development, and Death. San Francisco, WH Freeman, 1975
24. Spitz R: Anaclitic depression: An inquiry into the genesis of psychiatric conditions in early childhood. Psychoanal Study Child 2:313–342, 1942
25. Taska R, Sullivan J: Depression. In Cavenar J, Brodie HK: Signs and Symptoms in Psychiatry. Philadelphia, JB Lippincott, 1983
26. Teuting P, Koslow S, Hirschfeld R: Special Report on Depression Research. Washington, DC, Alcohol, Drug Abuse, and Mental Health Administration, 1981
27. Twiname B: No-suicide contract for nurses. J Psychosoc Nurs Ment Health Serv 9:11–12, 1981
28. Weiner RD: The psychiatric use of electrically-induced seizure. Am J Psychiatry 136:1507–1517, 1979
29. Weissman MM, Klerman G: Epidemiology of mental disorders. Arch Gen Psychiatry 35:705–712, 1978
30. Weissman MM, Myers JK: Affective disorders in a U.S. urban community: The use of research diagnostic criteria in an epidemiological survey. Arch Gen Psychiatry 35:1304–1311, 1980
31. Zung W, Durham W: A self-rating depression scale. Arch Gen Psychiatry 12:63–70, 1965

16

LORETTA M. BIRCKHEAD

THOUGHT DISORDER AND NURSING INTERVENTIONS

Learning Objectives

Upon completion of this chapter the student should be able to do the following:

1. Define *thought disorder*.
2. Describe the work of several theorists who have been central to the development of ideas in the study of the psychotherapy of thought disorder.
3. Describe the major theories about the etiology of a thought disorder.
4. Identify the alterations commonly found during a nursing assessment of an individual with a thought disorder.
5. Plan interventions for a client who has a thought disorder.
6. Describe the relationship between the nurse's use of language and the client's thoughts.
7. Describe the importance of working with the family of the client with a thought disorder.
8. Identify the medications used with a thought disorder and give guidelines for their use.
9. Identify the possible side-effects of medications used with clients with a thought disorder.

Phil

The notes on Phil's history and admission interview contained little more than a skeletal picture of his problem. The note stated, "20-year-old Caucasian male, college student, brought to psychiatric unit by police who found him on a street corner talking and shouting incoherently to himself."

The nurse checked his bag of belongings, and found several religious pamphlets, a pair of running shoes, a small wallet containing nothing but an expired library card, and a tiny gold crucifix.

After Phil's admission, the nurse walked into his room to introduce herself and to invite him to a music program offered in the unit. Lying on the bed, Phil let his gaze roam around the room; he made little eye contact. The nurse couldn't tell whether Phil was listening to her, watching her, or looking straight through her.

The nurse said, "Phil?"

She realized that Phil was looking at her in the same way he would stare at a wall or out the window. She asked him again if he would like to join the group, but he didn't acknowledge her presence in the room. He blinked, examined his hands, and then rolled over.

Introduction

Although clients with a medical diagnosis of schizophrenia show varying symptom patterns, the above description of Phil shows how many individuals cope with this disease. This complex disorder has various proposed causes and a variety of symptoms that may include severe difficulty in carrying on activities of daily living that provide personal safety. People with the disorder may also have difficulty establishing satisfactory interpersonal relationships with others.

These clients represent a challenge to the nurse. The demands on nurses in establishing professional relationships with these clients are difficult. The nurse must be able to reach out without being threatening, and to be natural and honest while maintaining a professional role. This chapter explores the illness of schizophrenia and the implications of this disorder for nursing care.

There is no single definition of schizophrenia or thought disorder that precisely fits what is observed in any one client. Even the symptoms of a thought disorder are not well defined. *Schizophrenia* is the medical term for this disorder, whereas *thought disorder* is the nursing term. The terms are interchangeable.

It is best to consider a thought disorder as an *open* (although scientific) label or concept. A thought disorder cannot be observed directly like germs under a microscope, but *symptoms* of the illness can be observed, and these symptoms can be related, in many cases, to specific occurrences in the environment. For example, Phil was talking incoherently on the street corner just prior to admission, yet on the psychiatric unit he became withdrawn. Phil was unable to relate to others (talking with others incoherently on the street corner and not at all with the hospital staff).

These maladaptations are the observable events that are related to a thought disorder. The concept of a thought disorder is *inferred from what can be observed.* We must make this inference because it helps us know what may best assist Phil in his recovery.

A thought disorder can best be defined as an illness in which an individual experiences disturbances in thoughts, such as delusions, hallucinations, and illogical thoughts. Inappropriate affect may occur as a consequence of the disorder of thought. The person with a thought disorder has excessive anxiety and usually fails to manage anxiety.[14,26]

This definition highlights the *internal processes* of a thought disorder (such as thought difficulties and anxiety), yet it would be impossible to identify consistently someone who has a thought disorder by using this definition alone. The Diagnostic and Statistical Manual of Mental Disorders-III-R (DSM-III-R)[3] provides a definition more tied to observable behaviors or symptoms of the disease, which will be discussed later in the chapter.

Theoretical Developments in Thought Disorders

The history of scientific contributions to the study of thought disorders can help students understand current treatment and key symptoms of clients who have a thought disorder.

The Early Work[28]

The contributions that led to today's understanding of thought disorders began with the publications of Kraepelin, a physician in Europe. Kraepelin worked in a number of mental institutions and observed what he called *dementia* (a progressive intellectual deterioration) *praecox* (early onset). Among the major symptoms that Kraepelin observed were hallucinations, delusions, negativism, attentional problems, stereotyped (repeated) behaviors, and emotional difficulties.

Bleuler, also a European physician, attempted to define the essence of the disorder. He proposed the term *schizophrenia* for the breaking of associative *thoughts* that occurs in the illness (meaning the occurrence of thoughts, expressed in language, that show no logical connection among the thoughts). Normally, thinking is described as logical and purposeful. In clients with a thought disorder the normal thought patterns are broken, and can be observed in clients as a loss of purposeful direction of thought, or what appears to be a stoppage, or passivity, in thought.

Because the illness process includes *thought* disturbances (and language that reflects thoughts), schizophrenia is often referred to as a "thought disorder." The label *thought disorder* is useful because it identifies the focus of the nurse's work with the client: the client's *language* and the *thoughts* expressed by this language.

Bleuler proposed the following four fundamental symptoms of schizophrenia:

- An *associative disturbance* (the occurrence of thoughts expressed in language that shows no logical connection among the thoughts)
- *Autism* (a tendency toward fantasy and withdrawal from reality)
- *Affective disturbance* (flat affect or affect that is not congruent with the circumstance)
- *Ambivalence* (the experience of incompatible thoughts or feelings at the same time)[28]

Sullivan, an American psychiatrist, was the first major theorist to develop an extensive approach to the psychological treatment of schizophrenia. Sullivan emphasized the emotional and intellectual factors that precipitated the client's withdrawal from interpersonal relationships.

Peplau, the founder of modern psychiatric nursing, built on Sullivan's concepts in formulating her *interpersonal approach* in working with clients. Many of Peplau's ideas concerning working with clients with thought disorders are included in this chapter.

In the 1960s and 1970s the terms *process schizophrenia* and *reactive schizophrenia* were key concepts. In process schizophrenia there is slow onset and a poor premorbid condition of the client. These clients typically do not fully recover. In the reactive group the clients have a sudden onset of illness due to a precipitating cause and the course of illness is relatively short. The concepts of "reactive" and "process" remain in use today.[28]

Etiology

For years there has been a "nature or nurture" question of the etiology of thought disorders. Is a thought disorder caused by genetic inheritance (nature) or by the early environment (nurture) of the individual who, later in life, develops a thought disorder? There is no indication that there is a single cause of the disorder, but rather that there are multiple causes, each of which will be reviewed.

Genetic and Constitutional Factors

Genes differ in their *penetrance,* the degree to which the presence of the gene alone leads to the expression of a characteristic in an individual. The gene itself may be influenced by the prenatal and postnatal environments, including psychological and physical stress and drugs.

One genetic theory is the *diathesis–stress model.*[36] This model emphasizes the idea that a liability, or a "diathesis," for a thought disorder is inherited, rather than the disease itself. An individual receives an inherited component, such as a central nervous system deficit or a high anxiety of responsiveness (the diathesis). Thought disorder behaviors are then learned, or become expressed, under the influence of stress.

Geneticists have studied and compared morbidity or risk rates in first-degree relatives (parents, siblings, and children) of individuals with thought disorders who have a 50% genetic overlap; second-degree relatives (grandparents, half-siblings, uncles, nephews, and grandchildren) who have a 25% genetic overlap; third-degree relatives (cousins) who have a 12.5% overlap; and monozygotic twins, with identical genes, who have 100% overlap. The risk rates for developing a thought disorder increase proportionately with the increase in genetic overlap, or with the degree of blood relationship to the person with a thought disorder.

Also, *concordance rates* (the occurrence or absence of a trait) are higher among monozygotic twins than among dizygotic twins. These studies support the presence of a genetic factor in the occurrence of a thought disorder. This correlation holds, regardless of whether or not the monozygotic twins were raised together or apart.

A thought disorder, however, is not a "simple" or Mendelian genetic disorder. In Mendelian disorders there are consistent ratios of dominant-to-recessive features. In albinism, for instance, a gene is expressed *unequivocally.* If individuals have the albinism gene, they will invariably exhibit the trait of albinism. The unequivocal expression of a thought disorder does not occur as in albinism.

Although research supports the idea that there is a genetic component to the display of a thought disorder, scientists do not know the exact nature of the genetic transmission. Research in the area is complicated by factors such as the definition of a thought disorder used in the study, and the nature of the individual cases. For instance, some studies have used very ill clients with thought disorders and studied the presence of the disorder in their siblings. The researchers found low concordance rates. Such low concordance rates, however, may be expected, because it would be unlikely to find two such extremely ill siblings in the same family.

Constitution and *temperament* are factors that are present in individuals at birth. These factors are products of infants' genetic makeup and intrauterine experiences. Some studies indicate that people with thought disorders have unusual sensitivities at birth, such as a hypersensitivity to sound. These hypersensitivities place an unusual demand on caregivers to understand the hypersensitivity and to moderate their own behavior according to the infants' needs. The inability of caregivers to moderate their responses places a stress on the infants to adapt—a requirement that may be beyond the adaptive resources of the infants.[36] While these studies have definite implications for the caregiver–child relationship, more emphasis is placed on research into the genetic and biochemical theories of thought disorders than on constitutional factors.

Several studies have examined genetics and other factors thought to be involved in the etiology of constitutional factors. The researchers[22,37,39] studied 100 Israeli boys and girls, half of whom were at risk for developing a thought disorder (they had a parent with a thought disorder), and the other half of whom had parents with no pathology. Also, half of the subjects were raised in an Israeli kibbutz, out of the home, and half were raised in an

Israeli town, at home. The subjects were tested over a period of 13 years to determine which factors were most likely to promote the development of a thought disorder. The causative factors of concern were (1) genetic and biochemical, (2) diathesis–stress, and (3) the life experience factor.

In one study few differences were found in the subjects regardless of whether the children were reared on a kibbutz or in a town setting. However, subjects who had a parent with a thought disorder generally (1) were more distractible, (2) had poorer visual–motor coordination, (3) had poorer cognitive integration, and (4) had lower self-esteem ratings and a higher level of personality maladjustment. The researchers supported the idea of a developmental (diathesis–stress) model, in which subjects are at risk for developing a thought disorder early in life, and then do not have sufficient competencies to cope with stressful conditions later in life.

Environmental factors were also found to influence the development of a thought disorder. Same-sex offspring (*e.g.,* a male child who develops a thought disorder with a male parent who also has the disorder) exhibited greater psychopathology *only* in town settings.

Biochemical Factors

Some evidence supports the idea that a thought disorder reflects a deficiency of endorphins. Berger[5] reviewed a number of studies that examined thought disorder symptoms and endorphin activity. When administered to individuals with a thought disorder, various endorphins have each decreased thought disorder symptoms.

Several studies have indicated that an increase in endorphin activity occurs in a thought disorder. In one study subjects became worse after the administration of an endorphin. In other studies hallucinations decreased in subjects with a thought disorder after administration of an endorphin antagonist, naloxone.

Shapiro[36] highlighted the role of dopamine in the occurrence of a thought disorder. Dopamine is one of two principal catecholamines in the brain, with norepinephrine being the other; both are major neurotransmitters. Usually dopamine is converted into norepinephrine. It is thought that an excess of dopamine promotes thought disorders. Phenothiazines (drugs used in the treatment of thought disorders) block the effects of dopamine, which supports the idea that an excess of dopamine promotes a thought disorder.

Not all clients with a thought disorder respond to phenothiazine treatment with a reduction of symptoms. Some individuals may have been incorrectly diagnosed, or perhaps there are other unclassified subtypes of a thought disorder, each with a different underlying biochemical disturbance and response to medication.

Cornblatt and others[9] studied clients who were depressed or had a thought disorder, and compared them with "normal" or control subjects, in order to assess negative and positive symptoms of a thought disorder within the same individuals. Positive and negative dimensions have figured prominently in recent discussions of the cause of a thought disorder.

Positive symptoms include hallucinations and delusions and are thought to be caused by disturbances in dopamine transmission. *Negative symptoms,* such as apathy and a "flat" or bland affect, are thought to be caused by a structural abnormality of the brain. Negative, rather than positive, symptoms are thought to indicate a chronic course of the illness rather than a favorable prognosis.

The authors found that the contrasting patterns of cognitive processing found in the subjects supported the idea of a distinction between positive and negative symptoms. The hypothesis of the presence of two distinct disease processes involved in a thought disorder, one biochemical and the other structural, was also supported.

Goldberg[13] also studied structural brain changes (with subsequent biochemical changes) that may cause a thought disorder. He reported that some manifestations of a thought disorder, such as slowed information processing, resemble the symptoms found in clients with frontal lobe damage. Hence, it can be concluded that frontal lobe damage plays a role in the formation of a thought disorder. The author also reported, however, that there may be more than one cause, or a chain of events, leading to such symptoms: other brain areas, in addition to the frontal lobes, may promote the occurrence of a thought disorder. The discovery of a more specific link between symptoms and brain areas affecting these symptoms will assist in the classification of the type of thought disorder present in a specific client.

Psychophysiological Factors

In psychophysiological tests, the electrical activity of various biological systems is studied, while the person either is performing a task or is at rest. The activity of the autonomic nervous system is studied by measuring electrodermal activity and heart rate. Clients with a thought disorder have a higher frequency of spontaneous fluctuations in skin conductance, a measure of electrodermal activity. These findings may indicate a left-hemisphere dysfunction in the temporal lobe.

Analyses of electroencephalograms (EEGs) show that clients with a thought disorder have fewer alpha rhythms than clients without such a disturbance. During sleep some clients show less rapid-eye-movement (REM) time and less stage-4 (deep) sleep. EEGs also show that clients with a thought disorder have excessively slow delta waves and increased fast beta activity. These findings may indicate an impairment in the subcortical gating and filtering processes. However, no electrophysiological findings are sufficiently consistent and specific to serve as a diagnostic indicator of a thought disorder.[26]

Orienting responses to simple stimuli and smooth-pursuit eye movements (when the eye tracks a moving object) are also areas of research interest. It has been found that clients show no (or slow) habituation to an orienting response. (*Habituation* means that the subject no longer responds to a specific stimulus.) Also, some clients with a thought disorder change their classification from no habituation to fast habituation, perhaps as a result of influence by the environment. Clients with a thought disorder, and their first-degree relatives, appear to have problems in following a moving target. This difficulty may be linked to a reticular formation deficit.[26]

Language and Information-Processing Factors

Individuals with a thought disorder demonstrate a disruption in communicating—hence the diagnostic label thought disorder. By hearing the disruptions in a client's *speech or language* (as in the example of the client rapidly changing from one topic to another), *the inference is made that there is a disturbance in the client's thinking processes.* This inference also works in reverse: by assisting clients to alter their language, the nurse can influence clients' thoughts.[31] Thus, it is important for nurses to be consistent in their verbal interchanges with these clients. Examples of the use of the nurse's language to affect the client's language (and subsequent thought) are provided later in this chapter in the section on interventions. Figure 16-1 depicts this circular process.

Research indicates that many clients with a thought disorder have difficulty controlling their information-processing abilities. On tasks that necessitate short-term recall, clients are not efficient in organizing perceptions into manageable pieces of information. Also, clients with a thought disorder often hesitate before stating sentences. They may experience this difficulty because of an excess of environmental stimuli and their inability to block out the stimuli.[30] Automatic operations of thought are not as markedly affected (such as when a person sings a well-known song).[29] Clients with a thought disorder are generally unable to plan their verbal discourses. This inability may be explained by the neural mechanisms of the frontal, subcortical, or localized left-hemisphere language system.[26]

Problems with information processing are not unique, however, to clients with a thought disorder.

Manic clients sometimes display similar communication problems, and people who are depressed sometimes have difficulty performing information-processing tasks, as indicated by long pauses in speech. These deficiencies may be more closely tied to particular symptoms, such as the inability to attend, or to concentrate, than to specific diagnostic categories.[29]

Intrapsychic and Interpersonal Factors

In the past individuals with a thought disorder have endured poor treatment and ridicule. At times they were considered to be possessed by the devil. Historically, psychiatry was the first discipline to view them as people to be understood, rather than shunned or merely controlled.

Psychoanalysts have many ideas about the nature of a thought disorder. One description views the illness on a continuum with other states of psychiatric illness, all of which represent a response to conflict. The person with a thought disorder differs from other individuals who have a mental illness in terms of degree, being more severely ill than, for example, someone with a fear of open spaces.

Psychoanalysis also views a thought disorder as indicative of a problem in the early maturation of the individual. This is viewed as a constitutional weakness that may not be amenable to corrective experiences (such as conversation with a clinician) in adulthood. Freud held this belief. He thought that, because individuals with a thought disorder had weaknesses that began in early periods of their lives, they could not relate to reality sufficiently to form an alliance with a clinician, and thus their conflicts could not be resolved. This belief prevailed among Freudians until recently, and these early opinions are partially responsible for the lack of psychotherapeutic work done with clients with a thought disorder.

Psychoanalytic theorists view an individual's problems as stemming mainly from their internal drives, which they do not know how to manage (the *intrapsychic* perspective). *Interpersonal* theorists view mental illness as a result of the interactions among people, not what occurs only within one individual. Sullivan, an interpersonal theorist, worked extensively with clients with a thought disorder.

Sullivan viewed a thought disorder as a failure of the self of the client to maintain appropriately a reality perspective that can be shared in communication with others. He also described the development of a thought disorder as a process in which the anxiety of those caring for the individual, such as a child, was communicated to the individual, who later developed a thought disorder. In periods of high anxiety, the individual could not focus on reality and actually learned a distorted picture of reality.

Sullivan described the individual with a thought disorder as having low self-worth, and also as being especially afraid of cultural rules that can no longer be followed because of the illness. Such an individual would probably be ridiculed by others in public when talking incoherently, or by other clients in a hospital, once admitted. Although many people relate to others in the best

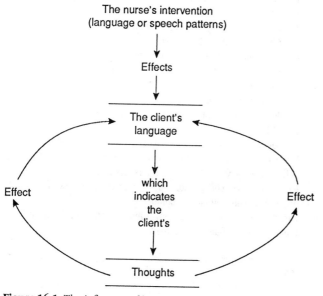

The nurse's intervention
(language or speech patterns)

↓

Effects

↓

The client's language

which indicates the client's

↓

Thoughts

Effect

Effect

Figure 16-1. The influence of language on thought.

way they are able, appropriate cultural rules are validated. Clients may fear, and be confused about, cultural rules because they have been hurt by them so often.

Work has been done to further the ideas of the interpersonal theorists, particularly in the field of family therapy. Family theories provide a means of understanding the cause or early development of a thought disorder, and give some direction for its cure. These theories propose that behavior in people with a thought disorder is caused by specific patterns found in the family system. At times these theories are weak because they are based on observations after the thought disorder has occurred. Thus, there is some question as to whether the observable behaviors are a consequence of the illness or a cause of the illness.

Treating the intrapsychic and interpersonal dynamics of a thought disorder with psychotherapy is currently considered essential. However, psychotherapy is generally not used to treat the illness itself. Therapy is done to (1) foster adaptive ways for clients to communicate with others, (2) help clients work on their feelings about having a thought disorder, and (3) support clients in adapting to everyday living expectations (such as living with others in a home setting and taking medications).[26] It is unfortunate that few can afford psychotherapy on a consistent basis.

Family Factors

Until the 1950s there were few studies of the families of individuals with a thought disorder. Interest in studying the families grew as a result of the work of Sullivan and Fromm-Reichmann,[12] a psychoanalyst. Both Sullivan and Fromm-Reichmann spent an extensive amount of time treating clients with a thought disorder using psychotherapy. They showed that clients with a thought disorder *were treatable.* It is unfortunate that today it is too expensive to treat clients with a thought disorder in a way that assists them to understand their lives and the nature of their illness, and to improve the quality of their lives. Instead, medication and a safe haven (the hospital) are used when clients are too ill to take care of themselves. Although medication can assist in decreasing some symptoms of a thought disorder, it does not help individuals to understand their lives or to form relationships with others. This assistance is obtained through work with a trained professional, such as a psychiatric nurse, social worker, psychologist, or psychiatrist.

Fromm-Reichmann[12] was the first theorist to apply the term *schizophrenogenic* to the mothers of schizophrenic people. In that construct, a schizophrenogenic mother is domineering but insecure. From Fromm-Reichmann's work, attention was placed on understanding families with a schizophrenic member.

T. Lidz. In one study Lidz[36] extensively interviewed 17 families, each with one member between the ages of 15 and 30 who was unmarried and had a thought disorder. The families also had both a mother and a sibling of the member with a thought disorder.

Lidz differentiated between two basic types of families that have a member with a thought disorder. In the *skewed* family, one parent is seriously disturbed psychiatrically, but the other parent does not acknowledge the emotional problems of the disturbed spouse. For example, if the mother has psychiatric problems, she may not nurture her child but may expect her child to fulfill her own dreams. She may be overprotective or seductive. In this case the father tends to be passive, is also not nurturing, and offers no counterbalance towards "normalcy" in opposition to the mother. Lidz's findings about families with a schizophrenic member are summarized in Table 16-1.

In the example of Phil mentioned at the beginning of this chapter, the student nurse observed a pattern of marital skew on the second day of Phil's hospitalization. A woman, approximately 45 years old, came onto the unit and looked around, as if seeking directions. The student introduced herself and the visitor said that her name was Phyllis, and that she had come to visit Phil, her son. She also remarked that she had cookies for Phil, as well as Phil's favorite shirt. The student told Phyllis Phil's room number. Phyllis entered the room.

The student left Phyllis alone with her son for about five minutes. She wanted to talk with Phyllis and Phil about Phil's hospitalization and what had happened at home just prior to Phil's hospitalization, and she also wanted to observe the mother–son interaction. The student knocked on the door, and when she entered Phil's room she observed Phyllis and Phil sitting across from each other looking into each other's eyes but saying nothing.

TABLE 16-1.
LIDZ'S CONCLUSIONS ABOUT THE NATURE OF FAMILIES WITH A SCHIZOPHRENIC MEMBER

1. All schizophrenics come from families with serious emotional strife.
2. Schizophrenics' mothers tend to
   a. Be unaware of their child's needs
   b. Be extremely intrusive
   c. Confuse their children's needs with their own
   d. Give conflicting verbal and empathic signals
   e. Live their lives through their children
   f. Be either too restrictive or insufficiently firm
3. Fathers are often
   a. Insecure in their masculinity
   b. In need of constant admiration to bolster their self-esteem
   c. Mildly paranoid
4. Schizophrenics' families tend to have unclear sexual and generational boundaries. Parents are often seductive with their children, act like children themselves and, at times, reverse sex roles.
5. Parents are often more tied to, and identified with, their own families of origin than with their current families.
6. Parents do not provide a secure environment for their children. Some promote a sense of distrust of those outside the family.

(Adapted from Lidz T, Fleck S, Cornelison A: Schizophrenia and the Family. New York, International Universities Press, 1965)

The student asked why they were staring at each other. Phyllis responded, "I am telling him all he needs to know." Phyllis and Phil remained silent and motionless. The student said, "I need for you, Phil and Phyllis, and myself to sit in a conference room for a while and discuss Phil's hospitalization." At this point Phyllis patted Phil on the knee and said "O.K., Phil, you don't want your father to come with us, though, do you? He is concerned about you, but he is so tired. He's in the lobby. You don't want him to come." She shook her head indicating "no." Phil answered "No" obediently.

In this situation the student observed the pattern of interaction, hypothesizing that marital skew was occurring. She noted in the treatment plan the need to observe for marital skew, with the father being left out of the family unit. She also noted the relationship between mother and son. Since this type of interaction was repeatedly noted, it was seen by the treatment staff as a family pattern.

This pattern had difficult implications for Phil. He was drawn into a nonverbal, mystical, and obscure pattern of relating to his mother. She identified herself as *the one* who defines reality for Phil. She also encouraged Phil not to interact with his father, thus leaving the mother–son dyad intact and not threatened, although overinvolved. The student tried, in her brief interaction, to engage the mother and son in an open, verbal dialogue.

In families with *marital schism,* the parents are in continuous conflict and compete for the child's loyalty. The child is caught in a difficult situation: showing love to one parent may promote jealousy in the other parent. The jealous parent may vent frustrations either toward the child or toward the spouse, thus initiating conflict. In marital schism, there is general, overall, continuous disruption and chaos.

One difficulty with families showing either skew or marital schism is that the child becomes the focus in the family, rather than carrying on its own life. A child cannot easily escape from the family; the child is forced continually to be a part of the problems in the family. The child and family are overinvolved, to the detriment of the growth of the child and the strengthening of the family unit.

The child is so trapped that ways to escape the family are developed—to escape not bodily, but by altering the child's perceptions of needs and motivations. The child abandons logical thinking or adopts a pattern of behavior that is below expected behavior for the age of the child or adolescent. Although this escape offers some relief from the pain felt in the family, this form of adaptation also limits the growth of the individual.

Gregory Bateson.   Bateson[36] studied conditions in a family with a schizophrenic member that foster the abandonment of a perspective on reality within the ill member. He identified a frequent pattern in such families called the *double bind.*

In a double bind, a positive message is sent at the same time as a negative message. The messages may be verbal or nonverbal, but can include one of each, and al-

ways contradict one another. The receiver of the messages is usually a child who is incapable of deciding which message warrants a response—the child seeks the positive message and, at the same time, fears the repercussions of the negative message, which usually carries an implied threat. When double binds occur frequently, over a long period of time, disturbed communication patterns are reinforced.

An important element of the double bind is that the child cannot run away from the situation or from the parents. Most children *want* to understand what is being communicated by those who provide for the necessities of daily life, even if it is confusing. However, even if the child or adolescent wants to understand what is being communicated, this cannot happen because the child does not yet have the intellectual skill to untangle the grossly disordered communication of the adults.

In the above interaction between Phil and Phyllis, her last statement to Phil was a double bind. Phil is exposed to two different messages, one of which contradicts the other. Phyllis stated that Phil's father was concerned, and at the same time she said that his father was waiting in the hospital lobby. A truly concerned father would not remain apart from his son during the son's first hospitalization on a psychiatric unit.

Another example of a double bind occurred when Phyllis brought up the question of whether the father should visit the son, while telling Phil that he does not want his father on the unit and at the same time shaking her head as if to say "no" in unison with Phil's anticipated negative response. The son would wonder on some level whether or not the mother really is bringing up the question of the father's coming onto the unit as an open question that can be answered *either* "yes" *or* "no."

Phil is involved in an intense relationship with his mother. Phyllis *is* his mother, so Phil has all the inclinations children usually have to understand what the parent is saying, especially in such a serious circumstance as being on a psychiatric unit. Also, *Phyllis has helped Phil learn their intenseness* by presenting to him on many occasions in his life the requirement (demand) that he exist in an intense relationship with her.

L. Wynne and M. Singer.   Wynne and Singer[36] investigated the relationship between thought disturbances of young adults and the family environment in which they were reared. Specifically, Wynne and Singer examined possible links between disturbed family communication patterns and styles of focusing attention, and the effects that this type of family disorganization may have on young adults adopting the same type of disruptive communication.

Although an interchange among family members of only a few sentences may appear normal, if the therapist looked at a much longer family exchange the *family-wide* communication would appear very much like that of the disordered communication of the single family member with a thought disorder. Much more disturbed communication in the family-wide group would be observed in situations involving anxiety (especially when related to

RELEVANT RESEARCH

This study compared populations of black, white, and Puerto Rican Hispanic depressed clients for a previous misdiagnosis of a thought disorder. The project was conducted in the outpatient department of an inner-city hospital.

The clients' hospital records were reviewed for previous occasions of a diagnosis of a thought disorder (schizophrenia). There were no significant differences among the ethnic groups in mean age, sex, marital status, or income level.

It was found that 68.4% of the clients had previously been *misdiagnosed* as having a thought disorder. Blacks were significantly more often misdiagnosed as paranoid schizophrenic than were either whites

or Hispanics. The authors had difficulty explaining this because there were no significant differences among the ethnic groups in persecutory delusions, ideas of reference, anger, or violent behavior. Every black and Hispanic client shown to have bizarre delusions was misdiagnosed, while only four of seven whites with similar symptoms were misdiagnosed.

Mukherjee and others concluded that there was an ethnicity-related factor in the misdiagnosis of depressed clients as having a thought disorder, with blacks and Hispanics at a higher risk than whites for misdiagnosis. The authors could not explain the nature of the ethnic effect, and encouraged further research.

(Mukherjee S, Shukla S, Woodle J et al: Misdiagnosis of schizophrenia in bipolar patients: A multiethnic comparison. Am J Psychiatry 140:1571, 1983)

intimacy), separation, and loss. This disturbed communication may not be seen in a fact-oriented, history-taking individual interview.

Further examples of disturbed family communication patterns observed by Wynne and Singer include: (1) reactions in very literal or concrete terms to threatening situations, (2) severely blurred or unclear meanings, (3) confused sex roles, (4) confused generational roles (the child may act as a parent to the adult), and (5) pervasive enmeshment of family members with each other (denying the individual identity development of members) and looking to each other to fulfill all needs.

The authors also gave some attention to the so-called "well" siblings of the person with a thought disorder, and found that these siblings characteristically have fewer emotional problems, are less likely to be overinvolved in family struggles, and achieve considerable psychological health from experiences outside the family, although at the cost of an emotional shallowness and intellectual constriction. The well siblings may become identifiably ill when they are in an unstructured environment and experience stress.

Research and study in the use of family therapy in families with a member with a thought disorder has declined in recent years due to the reliance on drug therapy to decrease symptoms and the failure of earlier family therapy methods to affect the illness process significantly. Traditionally, the family therapy that was performed with families in which there was a member with a thought disorder included assisting family members to understand their own underlying personalities and to gain insight into the disturbed ways in which they related. There was also some inclination to rescue an ill member from the disturbed family, thereby blaming the family. This approach did not produce useful results.

Family therapists have sought new approaches to working with the family. The family is now seen as a crucial part of treatment of the member with a thought disorder because (1) families can be effective in preventing frequent client relapses and in promoting more productive lives for their members, (2) the family may be able to assist in safely reducing drug dosage, and (3) families have become *the* support group for clients after the closing of many state hospitals and community homes where clients with a thought disorder lived at one time.

Also, the family therapy done today involves a treatment *team* rather than a single therapist. The team can consist of the family therapist(s), psychiatrist, occupational therapist, and social skills trainer. Nurses, because of their preparation, can take a number of directions in their roles with family work. They can specialize in this area of family treatment and provide counseling in the home or the hospital, so that the family can experience alternate ways to cope with the illness.

The function of current therapies is to enlist the family as adjunct helpers to the treatment team. The job of the family is to help rehabilitate the client and to relieve symptoms within the family, not *cure* an ill family. The family is helped to compensate for their difficulties in definite ways.

It is important to assist the family in areas that they have identified as problems. The treatment team assists by relieving the family of the suffering and confusion, as well as by decreasing the family's sense that they are alone with their problem. In a later section of this chapter, specific family interventions will be discussed.

Cultural Factors

As with other types of mental health problems, thought disorders have been studied from a cultural perspective. Durham[10] discussed the process whereby cultural factors affect the personality and emerge as mental disorders. In a study by Mukherjee and others,[27] the records of clients from various ethnic groups were studied to determine if there was a history of misdiagnosis of a thought disorder. The Relevant Research at the top of this page describes their findings.

In a study by Skilbeck and others,[38] low-income psychotherapy clients from various cultures were assessed

RELEVANT RESEARCH

This study examined the relationship between client self-reported severity of symptoms and therapist-reported severity evidenced by psychiatric diagnoses. Client applicants for outpatient psychotherapy in a large urban medical center were asked to complete questionnaires that assessed psychiatric symptoms. The applicants were also interviewed by a psychotherapist in an initial therapy session. The therapists were asked to diagnose each applicant.

Black clients reported fewer symptoms than Hispanics or whites.

White and Hispanic clients self-reported symptoms that were similar to the severity of the therapist-reported diagnoses. This parallel, however, did not occur for black clients: black clients received diagnoses that indicated a greater level of severity than their self-reported symptoms would have predicted. The best correlation between client-reported and therapist-diagnosed severity was obtained for the white clients. The authors cautioned that prejudice may influence diagnostic labeling and encouraged further research.

(Skilbeck W, Acosta F, Yamamoto J, Evans L: Self-reported psychiatric symptoms among black, Hispanic, and white outpatients. J Clin Psychol 40:1184, 1984)

for differences in the diagnostic labels applied to them. The Relevant Research on this page describes their findings.

Environmental Factors

Klein and others[20] described their findings in a study that attempted to identify social, psychological, and environmental variables related to a client's adjustment in the community after hospitalization. They also assessed factors associated with readmission to the psychiatric hospital.

The researchers compared the environmental qualities of the psychiatric hospital with those of the client's home. They compared qualities such as the amount of space per person, heating of the client's home in the winter and cooling in the summer, toilet and bath facilities, quality of furnishings, safety of the neighborhood, and cleanliness and esthetic qualities of the neighborhood.

The data collector made a professional judgment of whether the home or the hospital had a greater adequacy of such qualities. These physical attributes were not significant for all of the cultural groups they studied. Rehospitalization was not related to these environmental factors.

The authors noted that the relationship between the client's home environment and community adjustment or rehospitalization is not as strong as is often believed in clinical practice. It is possible that the client's deep lack of self-esteem is a stronger factor in determining rehospitalization than is the home environment.

Acosta and others[1] noted that a significant part of our population falls into the poor or working-class categories. They live in economically disadvantaged environments, and more frequently come to mental health centers than do people from the middle and upper classes.

Many clients with a thought disturbance are poor or working-class and live in substandard housing. This environment is typically impoverished and in high-crime areas. At times the nurse can assist clients in coping with the problems that occur in substandard living environments. More research is needed to document the effects of inadequate living environments that decrease the sense of well-being in clients with a thought disorder.

There may be an association between environmental conditions, perinatal factors, and the occurrence of a thought disorder. Substandard environmental living conditions promote poor nutrition in pregnant women. Higher rates of thought disorder are found in children of women with a poor nutritional state at the time of birth.[26]

The Therapeutic Use of Self With Clients With a Thought Disorder

The first responsibility of the nurse is to obtain a comprehensive view of the client who needs therapeutic work. The nurse assesses the nature of the client in a "pure" form rather than viewing the client with a preset (and limited) framework with which to categorize the client.

For example, one may come to the client with a thought disorder with the framework that proposes that an improvement in the quality of life for the client is impossible and hopeless. According to this framework, the client needs or has the capacity to make use of only a secure, limited environment, such as a psychiatric unit or halfway house. This secure environment is all that will or should be provided and consists mainly of a setting that will *control* the client and prevent others from being harmed by the client. This view is similar to the antiquated theories that psychiatric hospitals should be built in a secluded area or in an area that could be easily observed in case the clients should come too close to affecting the outside society. Lock clients up and *control* them.

Psychiatric/mental health nurses, however, should not have such a restricted view. They should first perceive the client in the client's "pure" form, meaning that whatever characteristics the client has about himself the nurse will perceive them, and then determine the particular needs of the client in an initial review of those perceptions. The nurse does not, for instance, view the client as only someone who must be controlled. The nurse first attempts to understand who the client "is," and then works within the selected theoretical framework to assist the client in bringing about change.

The use of a limited perspective is exemplified by the clinician's question, "This person is so sick, what can I possibly do?" This perspective assumes that the client cannot capitalize on the growth potential remaining in the client and respond over time to the consistent input of the nurse.

In the case of a client with a thought disorder, the nurse does not first think "thought disorder." The nurse first notices that the client is withdrawn and frequently moves the lips as if talking to someone when no one is around. The nurse then applies labels to these perceptions (such as "withdrawn behavior" and "hallucinations") to begin to derive a summary of what the client is experiencing and what problems need attention.

In intervening with the client, the nurse focuses on these relevant perceptions, not on the medical diagnosis of schizophrenia. The nurse may learn quite a bit by reviewing the writings on schizophrenia, but the nurse works with the presently experienced phenomena of the client to bring about change. The nurse intervenes through the therapeutic use of self.

If the nurse focuses on the medical diagnosis of schizophrenia, the priority becomes the administration of medications for hallucinations, rather than determining the relevance of the content of the hallucination to the client's life. In the mental health treatment system, the nurse must take a primary role in assisting the client to examine these aspects of the client's life or the examination will not occur, especially because of the difficult nature of clients with a thought disorder.

Obtaining a view of the "pure" client from observable behaviors, rather than from a preconceived idea of expected behaviors, is challenging for the nurse. The variety of client characteristics and behaviors is as large as the uniqueness of the person. The nurse, as an expert in the study of human nature, takes the numerous qualities and nuances presented by clients to determine *their* needs. Clients generally welcome this approach because

TABLE 16-2.
DIAGNOSTIC CRITERIA FOR SCHIZOPHRENIA

A. The presence of characteristic psychotic symptoms in the active phase has been noted: either (1), (2), or (3) below for at least one week (unless the symptoms are successfully treated).
   1. Two of the following
      a. Delusions
      b. Prominent hallucinations.
      c. Incoherence or marked loosening of associations
      d. Catatonic behavior
      e. Flat or inappropriate affect
   2. Bizarre delusions
   3. Prominent hallucinations
B. During the course of the disturbance, functioning in such areas as work, social relations, and self-care is markedly below the highest level achieved before onset of the disturbance (or, when the onset is in childhood or adolescence, failure to achieve expected level of social development).
C. Schizoaffective Disorder and Mood Disorder with Psychotic Features have been ruled out.
D. Continuous signs of the disturbance have been seen for at least six months.
   Prodromal phase: A clear deterioration in functioning before the active phase of the disturbance that is not due to a disturbance in mood or to a Psychoactive Substance Use Disorder and that involves at least two of the symptoms listed below.
   Residual phase: Following the active phase of the disturbance, persistence of at least two of the symptoms noted below, these not being due to a disturbance in mood or to a Psychoactive Substance Use Disorder.
   Prodromal or residual symptoms:
   1. Marked social isolation or withdrawal
   2. Marked impairment in role functioning as wage-earner, student, or homemaker
   3. Markedly peculiar behavior (*e.g.,* collecting garbage, talking to self in public, hoarding food)
   4. Marked impairment in personal hygiene and grooming
   5. Blunted or inappropriate affect
   6. Digressive, vague, overelaborate, or circumstantial speech, or poverty of speech, or poverty of content of speech
   7. Odd beliefs or magical thinking, influencing behavior and inconsistent with cultural norms, *e.g.,* superstitiousness, belief in clairvoyance, telepathy, "sixth sense," "others can feel my feelings," overvalued ideas, ideas of reference
   8. Unusual perceptual experiences, *e.g.,* recurrent illusions, sensing the presence of a force or person not actually present
   9. Marked lack of initiative, interests, or energy
E. It cannot be established that an organic factor initiated and maintained the disturbance.
F. If there is a history of Autistic Disorder, the additional diagnosis of Schizophrenia is made only if prominent delusions or hallucinations are also present.

(American Psychiatric Association: Diagnostic and Statistical Manual of Mental Disorders-III-R. Washington, DC, American Psychiatric Association, 1987) they usually feel relief in being understood in terms of their exact nature, rather than as mere examples of categories of mental illness.

To employ the therapeutic use of self, the nurse must be aware of the illness process of a thought disorder as well as have a sensitivity toward, and a respect for, the client as a person. Other challenges for nurses working with these clients include:

1. Messages from other professionals who work with the therapeutic benefit of medications (or some other aspect of treatment), rather than professional interpersonal relationships with clients. At times other professionals may seek to establish policies that mitigate the interpersonal relationship philosophy of nurses in working with clients. Nurses must ensure that their professional role is protected so that the client's problems can be investigated. Nurses do not need permission to perform interpersonal relationship interventions—that is a professional obligation.

2. The ability to maintain the energy for consistent relationships with clients despite (a) negative client behaviors and (b) what may seem to be "small" client changes.

3. The ability to maintain hope for client changes despite the willingness of many treatment facilities to discharge clients who are still ill.

Classifications of Thought Disorders

The Diagnostic and Statistical Manual of Mental Disorders (DSM-III-R)[3] identifies the observable behaviors found in clients with schizophrenia. It also identifies five types of thought disorders: *catatonic, disorganized, paranoid, undifferentiated,* and *residual.* The diagnostic criteria for schizophrenia, as well as the five types, are presented in Tables 16-2 through 16-7. Nursing diagnoses for a thought disorder are included in the nursing process section of the chapter.

TABLE 16-3.
DIAGNOSTIC CRITERIA FOR CATATONIC TYPE SCHIZOPHRENIA 295.2x

A type of Schizophrenia in which the clinical picture is dominated by any of the following:
1. Catatonic stupor or mutism
2. Catatonic negativism
3. Catatonic rigidity
4. Catatonic excitement
5. Catatonic posturing

(American Psychiatric Association: Diagnostic and Statistical Manual of Mental Disorders-III-R. Washington, DC, American Psychiatric Association, 1987)

TABLE 16-4.
DIAGNOSTIC CRITERIA FOR DISORGANIZED TYPE SCHIZOPHRENIA 295.1x

A type of Schizophrenia in which the following criteria are met:
1. Incoherence, marked loosening of associations, or grossly disorganized behavior
2. Flat or grossly inappropriate affect
3. Does not meet the criteria for Catatonic Type

(American Psychiatric Association: Diagnostic and Statistical Manual of Mental Disorders-III-R. Washington, DC, American Psychiatric Association, 1987)

TABLE 16-5.
DIAGNOSTIC CRITERIA FOR PARANOID TYPE SCHIZOPHRENIA 295.3x

A type of Schizophrenia in which the following criteria are met:
1. Preoccupation with one or more systematized delusions or with frequent auditory hallucinations related to a single theme
2. *None* of the following: incoherence, marked loosening of associations, flat or grossly inappropriate affect, catatonic behavior, grossly disorganized behavior

(American Psychiatric Association: Diagnostic and Statistical Manual of Mental Disorders-III-R. Washington, DC, American Psychiatric Association, 1987)

TABLE 16-6.
DIAGNOSTIC CRITERIA FOR UNDIFFERENTIATED TYPE SCHIZOPHRENIA 295.9x

A type of Schizophrenia in which the following criteria are met:
1. Prominent delusions, hallucinations, incoherence, or grossly disorganized behavior
2. Does not meet the criteria for Paranoid, Catatonic, or Disorganized Type

(American Psychiatric Association: Diagnostic and Statistical Manual of Mental Disorders-III-R. Washington, DC, American Psychiatric Association, 1987)

TABLE 16-7.
DIAGNOSTIC CRITERIA FOR RESIDUAL TYPE SCHIZOPHRENIA 295.6x

A type of Schizophrenia in which the following criteria are met:
1. Absence of prominent delusions, hallucinations, incoherence, or grossly disorganized behavior
2. Continuing evidence of the disturbance, as indicated by two or more of the residual symptoms listed in criterion D of Schizophrenia.

(American Psychiatric Association: Diagnostic and Statistical Manual of Mental Disorders-III-R. Washington, DC, American Psychiatric Association, 1987)

The Nursing Process

Assessment

Nursing diagnoses associated with a thought disorder are found in Table 16-8. These diagnoses are useful because they identify the behaviors the nurse observes in the client. Not all listed diagnoses will be discussed here. A few of the diagnoses need particular description to help the nurse determine accurately their presence or absence in the assessment phase of the nursing process.

Alterations in Communication (20)

Impaired Verbal Communication (20.02). Because of the central effect of language on thought, the client's language is important in directing the statements made by the nurse. The language of the client cannot be overlooked, but rather can be identified as an area for interventions. It is also important in assessment because it has significant interpersonal ramifications. If a client does not speak, the distortions of the client cannot be clarified in the relationship with the nurse. The client's interpersonal relationships are also hampered when there are distortions in the client's language because others do not have a clear sense of what the client is trying to communicate. Clients learn nothing about themselves and their relationships with others, and thus no changes occur.

Alterations in Conduct/Impulse Control (21)

Regressed Behavior (21.07.02). Clients with a thought disorder may behave in ways similar to earlier growth and development stages. This could be demonstrated by an adult client who comes up to a nurse with a pen in one hand and the pen cap in the other, asking the nurse, "What do I do with these?" Adults demonstrating appropriate developmental behaviors of adulthood would know what to do with a pen and cap.

Alterations in Motor Behavior (22)

Clients may demonstrate unusual motor behaviors as a side-effect of medications or as a result of disordered thoughts. For example, clients who believe that their food is poisoned may gesture with their hands over the food before eating it. Motor behavior alterations can severely limit social acceptance by others. They can also be frightening and embarrassing to the client. The client can be aware of the behaviors, but unable to stop them.

Alterations in Role Performance (23)

Impaired Social/Leisure Role (23.02). Clients may be unable to maintain interpersonal relationships, and may have painful feelings of loneliness. Because of the loneliness they may be driven to establish interpersonal contact, yet the contact may fail in part because of the client's loss of social competence. A client, for example, may believe that one can establish meaningful friendships at a bus stop.

Excess or Deficit in Dominant Emotions (30)

The client with a thought disorder has many emotional problems, and perhaps the most difficult is anxiety. The ordinary techniques of containing and managing anxiety do not work for the person with a thought disorder. Attempts to contain anxiety are so exhausting that the client has little energy for other things. Because there is frequently a high degree of anxiety, the person's thoughts become more disorganized. The anxiety is not only psychologically painful and exhausting, but isolating. Others around the client find themselves uncomfortable with such anxiety and avoid the client.[25]

Alterations in Perception/Cognition (50)

Clients with a thought disorder may show an impairment in attention, evidenced by decreased concentration, a narrowed attention span, an inability to shift the focus of attention from one topic to another, and blank spells (when the client seems to be experiencing an absence of thought). The client with blank spells may be experiencing hallucinations or general anxiety. These impairments severely limit the ability of the individual with a thought disorder to communicate with others.

Alterations in Perception (50.06). False perceptions (including hallucinations and pseudohallucinations) are untrue or abnormal perceptions that are not based on objective sense data. Pseudohallucinations are experiences that the person does not perceive with the same vividness as hallucinations. Pseudohallucinations are not actually seen by the client as true perceptual experiences; they appear more as ideas, having no more intensity than ordinary thoughts. The client is aware that they are part of the imagination and not reality, although the client may not be able to ignore these ideas because of their intrusive, obsessive quality.

Hallucinations (50.06.02). Hallucinations are false sensory perceptions that occur in the absence of any actual stimulus. For example, a client may hear a voice telling him that he is a bad person when, in fact, there is no such person talking. The hallucinations most frequently experienced are auditory. Other possible forms of hallucinations include visual, olfactory, gustatory, tactile (clients may report that insects are crawling under their skin, although this type of hallucination is more frequently seen in toxic states and in certain drug addictions), kinesthetic (false perceptions of movement), hypnagogic (occurring in the drowsy state preceding deep sleep), and hypnopompic (occurring after deep sleep). Hypnagogic and hypnopompic hallucinations may occur in "healthy" individuals.

Some researchers feel that hallucinations are a response to disturbed biochemical functions of the body.[7] Further research on the neurological mechanisms of thought disruption may lead to refinements of the psychotropic medications developed to assist in controlling the symptoms of a thought disorder.

Other writers have considered the interpersonal dynamics of hallucinations. Peplau[30] stated that hallucinations result from an accumulation of difficulties in living that have been experienced but handled ineptly. Hallucinations begin in experiences of anxiety and panic—emotions that set the stage for the client's inability to understand what is occurring.

Peplau described hallucinations as a process whereby a client derives comfort during a stressful period by recalling memories of a person who had offered comfort when the client had experienced stress previously. As the client continues to experience anxiety, memories of the individual become more frequent, to the exclusion of real people in the client's environment. Because the imaginary friend does not respond as a real person would, the client does not feel threatened and seeks to spend more time with the imaginary friend. Ultimately the client begins to relate to the imaginary person while real people are present, causing embarrassment for the client. The client eventually experiences terror at the inability to control the experiences, and attempts to compromise with the imaginary figure: in return for the client's not telling anyone about the figure, the client expects not to be harmed by the figure. If the client's safety is threatened by the imaginary figure in spite of the compromise, the client experiences extreme panic and anxiety. Panic can occur, for example, when the hallucinatory voice says to the client, "Kill yourself."

In addition to Peplau's psychodynamic theory, Walker and Cavenar[40] theorized that there are three possible causes for hallucinations. The *perceptual release theory* maintains that hallucinations occur either when sensory stimulation is significantly decreased from previous levels or in situations of panic or marked arousal. *Impaired information processing* is found when the central nervous system's ability to maintain an appropriate associative chain among thoughts is lost, such as in cases of anxiety. *Biochemical factors,* including dopamine, transmethylation, monoamine oxidase, and endorphins, can also be involved in the occurrence of hallucinations.

Psychotropic medications have been very effective in decreasing the occurrence of hallucinations in clients with thought disorders. Additional nursing interventions for working with clients with hallucinations will be discussed later in the chapter.

Illusions (50.06.03). *Illusions* are misinterpreted perceptions of actual external stimuli. Clients with a thought disorder may experience illusions, especially during periods of high anxiety. A relevant theme may be present for the client in the illusion. For example, the client may mistake a moving curtain for a menacing figure coming to harm the client. This theme of self-destruction may be present in the psychic life of the client.

Alterations in Thought Content (50.08)

Delusions (50.08.02). Peplau[31] defined a *delusion* as an idea that is an inadequate conclusion or explanation of an experience in which the client experienced panic. The false conclusion serves to lessen the anxiety because at least some explanation has been derived, even if it is false.

The individual experiencing panic may go from focusing on one detail of a subject to arriving at a conclusion about the meaning of the detail. Since the individual feels some relief in deriving this conclusion, the individual does not seek other information in order to compare the conclusion with reality in the presence of others.

The delusional idea is *fixed*—the same idea reoccurs. In a true delusion, this must involve a fairly extensive or elaborate story. It is not a fleeting, fragmented idea stated by the client that is not true, but rather it is a strong conviction, held by the client even if evidence is presented to the contrary. The delusion may be based on fact, yet the intensity with which the idea is held and the manner in which the individual uses other ideas to support the delusion indicate that a delusion is present. There is a potential for mislabeling clients as delusional when, in reality, they may have had a fleeting mistaken notion.

Religious delusions include beliefs that are morbid and serve to justify difficulties in life. The ideas may also serve as a rationalization or way to verbalize what the client experiences as a disintegration of personality. A client, for example, stated that God punishes her and would do so again if the client left the hospital room. The client used her religious delusion to maintain her isolation and remoteness from feelings and experiences.[11]

It should be noted that if a nonbizarre delusion (*i.e.,* involving situations that happen in real life, such as being followed) occurs, and the person has never met the medical criteria for schizophrenia,[3] the person should be given the medical diagnosis of Delusional (Paranoid) Disorder, not schizophrenia. Nursing diagnoses and interventions for delusions, however, are similar to those for schizophrenia.

Because of the variety of possible symptoms presented, it is recommended that different nurses on a unit, or in a particular organization, develop expertise in one or two areas of their work according to their interests. For example, one nurse could study the side-effects of medications, another could study measures to assess the unit environment or mood, and still another could specialize in the phenomena of delusions. In this manner nurses can have easy access to fellow professionals with whom to discuss the meaning of their observations. This use of the nursing staff can also assist in maintaining current use of research on thought disorders.

Nursing Diagnosis

In addition to the diagnoses defined in the Assessment section above, the American Nurses' Association has identified a broad range of nursing diagnoses related to a thought disorder. These can be found in the working draft of the *Taxonomy for the Classification of Human Responses of Concern for Psychiatric/Mental Health Nursing Practice,*[2] and are included in Table 16-8.

TABLE 16-8.
NURSING DIAGNOSES RELATED TO A THOUGHT DISORDER

SOCIO/BEHAVIORAL HUMAN RESPONSE PATTERNS	EMOTIONAL HUMAN RESPONSE PATTERNS
20. Alterations in communication	30. Excess of or deficit in dominant emotions*
20.01 Impaired nonverbal	30.02 Impaired appropriateness of emotional expression
20.01.01 Incongruent	30.03 Impaired congruence of emotions, thoughts, behavior
20.01.02 Inappropriate	30.04 Impaired range of expression
20.02 Impaired verbal*	PERCEPTUAL/COGNITIVE HUMAN RESPONSE PATTERNS
20.02.02 Bizarre content	50. Alterations in perception/cognition*
20.02.03 Circumstantial	50.01 Alterations in attention
20.02.07 Echolalia	50.01.01 Distractibility
20.02.09 Incoherent	50.01.02 Hyperalertness
20.02.10 Mutism	50.01.03 Inattention
20.02.11 Neologisms	50.01.04 Selective inattention
20.02.12 Nonsense/word salad	50.03 Alterations in judgment
20.02.14 Perseveration	50.03.01 Blocking of ideas
20.02.18 Severe delay	50.03.02 Circumstantial thinking
20.02.20 Volume too loud	50.03.03 Constructional difficulty
20.02.21 Volume too soft*	50.03.04 Flight of ideas
21. Alterations in conduct/impulse control	50.03.05 Impaired abstract thinking
21.04 Bizarre behavior	50.03.06 Impaired concentration
21.06 Disorganized behavior	50.03.07 Impaired judgment
21.07 Age-inappropriate behavior	50.03.09 Impaired logical thinking
21.07.02 Regressed behavior*	50.03.11 Impaired thought processes
21.08 Unpredictable behavior*	50.03.13 Loose associations
22. Alterations in motor behavior	50.05 Alterations in orientation
22.01.01 Bizarre gesturing	50.05.01 Autism
22.01.02 Catatonia	50.06 Alterations in perception*
22.01.04 Dystonias	50.06.02 Hallucinations*
22.01.05 Echopraxia	50.06.03 Illusions*
22.01.06 Extrapyramidal symptoms	50.07 Alterations in self-concept
22.01.10 Muscular rigidity	50.07.01 Impaired body image
22.01.11 Psychomotor retardation	50.07.03 Impaired personal identity
22.01.12 Restlessness	50.08 Alterations in thought content
23. Alterations in role performance	50.08.01 Ideas of reference
23.02 Impaired social/leisure role*	50.08.02 Delusions*
23.02.01 Withdrawal/social isolation	50.08.04 Magical thinking

* See discussion of these diagnoses in Assessment section.
(Adapted from American Nurses' Association: Taxonomy for the Classification of Human Responses of Concern for Psychiatric/Mental Health Nursing Practice. Kansas City, American Nurses' Association, 1986)

Intervention

Therapeutic Communication With a Client With a Thought Disorder

The psychiatric/mental health nurse needs to know the names of the various patterns of disorganized language and thought demonstrated by clients with a thought disorder. Only a few of the possible patterns are mentioned in the sections above. The nursing staff may want to designate a nurse who is especially expert at identifying language and thought disturbances to assist other staff members.

Peplau[31] stated that thinking is a process by which experience is incorporated, organized, and recalled by way of thought events that are linked with one another. The thoughts are then expressed in language. Hence, underlying disorders of the thought processes are observed in the language of the client.

Labeling the pattern of a thought disorder is only one part of the interaction between nurse and client, and it is not the most difficult. Correcting the thought disorder starts with the clinician. The corrective aim of the clinician is summarized in the steps in the case study below. These steps occur over a period of several weeks of work with the client:

1.   The same client and nurse are assigned to work together in individual relationship counseling throughout the client's stay on the treatment unit.

Example:

The student nurse introduces herself to Phil, the client, and states that she will meet with Phil twice a week when she is on the unit in order to allow Phil time to talk about his concerns.

2. The client says something to the nurse.

Example:

At the designated time and place, the student nurse and Phil sit together. The student waits for Phil to begin. Phil does not begin, but stares at the wall.

Student: "Talk about what concerns you."
Phil: "Nothing much."
Student: "What was it like for you to come to the hospital?" Phil remains silent.
Student: "What was happening just prior to coming to the hospital?"
Phil: "I was out of the hospital. This hospital is sure a strange place."

3. The nurse hears the statement and infers the nature of the client's difficulty.

Example:

The student infers that:

a. The client needs to talk about his thoughts and feelings about being in the hospital or about the hospital itself, though he finds this difficult, or
b. The client feels "strange" himself, or
c. The word "strange" is vague and the client may have his own private (autistic) meaning for this word, that another person would not easily understand.

If the student has not worked extensively with the client, she may not be certain which inference to pursue, yet she has confidence that Phil's statement falls within one of her inferences.

4. The nurse makes a statement that serves as a task for the client to consider. This leads the client closer to clarifying the concern.

Example:

The student replies, "In what way is the unit strange?"

The student is asking the client to do the "work" of the interview. While the nurse sets the form and structure of the work with the client, the client must verbalize the meanings and descriptions of what is occurring.[31]

For the student to respond "yes" to Phil's statement that the hospital unit is strange would have been to validate and approve of the client's vagueness and possibly to validate an inappropriate meaning attached to the hospital unit by the client. The student would have been agreeing with the pathology and not serving as a pull counter to the pathology.

5. A corrective effect is achieved.

Example:

Phil: "Some people here are evil."
Student: "Talk about one person with whom you have had difficulty."

The client continues to talk about the word evil.

Phil: "There's badness here."
Student: "Name someone with whom you have had a difficult time."

Through persistent and consistent work with the client, the nurse, by use of her language, exerts a corrective effect on the ability of the client to engage in a discussion that can be understood by the other person. This takes more than one interview, but can be achieved with a consistent approach.

Example:

In the third interview, Phil states, "No one here likes me."

Student: "Who is one person whom you believe does not like you?"
Phil: "Well, Margaret."
Student: "Tell me what happened with Margaret."
Phil: "Margaret doesn't like me." (Margaret is a nurse.)
Student: "Did she tell you that?"
Phil: "She told me she doesn't like the way I eat."
Student: "What did she say about the way you eat?"
Phil: "She said I eat like a bird."
Student: "Tell me what happened from the beginning."
Phil: "It's not what she said. Not just that. I could hear her thoughts, too, the way I hear my mother's thoughts."
Student: "Phil, no one I know can hear anyone's thoughts but his or her own. Ask Margaret the reason that she said you eat like a bird. Listen to Margaret tell you what she's thinking."

The student met Margaret in the nurses' station a few minutes later, and asked her to stop by Phil's room. Margaret was concerned to hear that Phil had misinterpreted her comment about his eating habits. The student met her again at the end of the shift.

"I told him he'd feel better if he ate better, but whether he ate like a bird or a bull, he'd be a fine young man either way," asserted Margaret.

The student met with Phil the next day and asked, "Did you and Margaret have that talk?"

He nodded. Phil and the student later discussed his conversation with Margaret and what happens when each person states openly what they are thinking.

Through the purposeful effort of the student, the client talked about real events that presented a difficulty for the client. The client and the student continue to talk about what happened between Phil and Margaret.

6. The language of the client changes.

   Example:

   The student meets with Phil and waits for him to begin.

   Phil: "Well, this morning we met in group therapy and Margaret was there."

   Here, because of the effort of the student, the client demonstrates, through his language, that he can talk in a manner that can be understood by another person, that is not vague, and that relates to something occurring in reality.

7. The language change affects the thoughts of the client.

   Example:

   The student observes that Phil's language is much more direct and clear. He talks in a way that can be understood by others. Because of the language of the student in requesting understandable language from the client, the thoughts of the client have become understandable, direct, and clear.

8. Changes in the client's thoughts affect the client's feelings and actions that are guided by the thoughts.

   Example:

   In working with the student, Phil states that he has talked with Margaret and clarified his difficulties with her. He describes the difficulties to the student, and states that he is more comfortable when Margaret is around him.

9. Changes in the client's language, thoughts, feelings, and actions facilitate participation in society.

   Example:

   The student observes Phil being less withdrawn on the unit. The group leader who also works with Phil states that he is more willing to talk in the group and stays on the same train of thought as the group for most of the length of the group. Phil begins to discuss with the student his feeling responses to a number of events that he had previously distorted or dismissed.

   In conclusion, the communication and personhood of the nurse involved in a professional relationship with the client can have an immense benefit to the client.

   In the example, Phil experienced, at some point during his hospitalization, a number of the problems associated with a thought disorder. The problems mentioned below are listed, with examples of Phil's behavior that led to the particular nursing diagnosis.

1. *Impaired logical thinking.* Phil had difficulty progressing from one thought to another. Phil did not attempt to clarify his mother's statement that he was obtaining all he needed to know from her thoughts.

2. *Inattention.* Initially, Phil did not answer statements made to him by the student nurse. He seemed preoccupied.

3. *Autism.* Phil referred to "badness" on the psychiatric unit. The use of this word was unclear to the nurse.

4. *Blocking of ideas.* Phil made statements and then suddenly stopped talking.

5. *Inappropriate nonverbal communication.* Initially, Phil's body language did not indicate that he was engaged in conversation with the nurse.

6. *Mutism.* Initially, Phil refused to talk with the student nurse.

7. *Impaired social/leisure role.* Phil did not ask Margaret to clarify her statement about his eating habits; he simply avoided the topic. Phil would not engage in an interview with the student nurse in the beginning stages of his hospitalization.

Other problems associated with a thought disorder that were not evident in Phil's care might include the following:

1. *Severe delay in verbal communication.* This is usually evidenced by silence and a lack of effort to take a more comprehensive view of experiences.

2. *Impaired personal identity.* This is apparent when clients state that they have no sense of who they are.

3. *Impaired social/leisure role.* In addition to the example above, this can be seen when clients are silent and removed from what is happening around them (Fig. 16-2).

In working with clients with a thought disorder, the nurse would not include all of the above problems on the nursing care plan. The nurse would work with the most severe problems, or those that seem to be of most concern to the client.

Nursing Interventions for Alteration in Attention (50.01).

Impairments of attention can be distracting to the nurse who is working with the client. For instance, while working with Phil the student noted that there were often long pauses in his speaking. At times he forgot the topic being discussed prior to the pause. The nurse can exert a significant pull on the client toward reality. Part of the art of interviewing a client with blank spells is to know the difference between normal silences (used to consider what is being said) and blank spells. Blank spells are nonproductive time with the client. The nurse could say, "Say some more about. . . ." and mention the topic the client was talking about prior to the blank spell. The client may be anxious and need to talk, but the silence allows the client to spend more time in a disturbed state while not relating with others. Most beginning clinicians will be (1) shocked by the degree of loss of language and thought competencies of the client, and then, (2) surprised (and pleased) with the changes the client makes with the nurse's *consistent* pull toward relating with others.

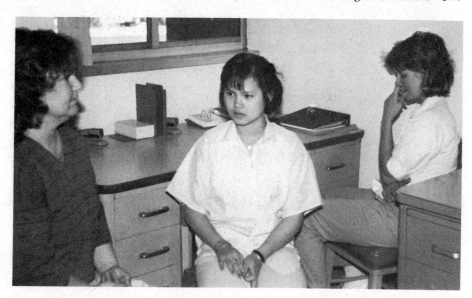

Figure 16-2. A client with a language and thought disorder (at the right) may seclude herself from interaction with others. The psychiatric nurse can facilitate the client's inclusion with others.

Nursing Interventions for Delusions (50.08.02).
In working with a client who is delusional, the nurse needs to obtain the content of the delusion from the client while never agreeing that the delusion is factual. The nurse can use this information to determine the theme the client is considering.

One client, for instance, stated that the mayor had called her many times to serve on various commissions. The client mentioned this a number of times during the day, especially when others attempted to get to know her. The nurse asked if the client had anything else to say about her comment that the mayor had called her. The client described that she was supposed to serve on a housing commission and elaborated on the housing situation. The nurse wondered if the client was delusional and grandiose, since no other client behaviors had indicated the possibility that the client was on such a commission.

The nurse then did not challenge the delusional idea—a nurse can not so easily "take away" such pathology. Also, the client must find new ways to handle anxiety so that the delusional ideas are no longer needed to provide comfort. The nurse could ask, however, "When did you first think that the mayor called you, as you said?"

Eventually this client related the real life experience that she had been forced to leave her family home because she was unable to pay the property taxes. She now lived alone in another city. The nurse focused on the topic of this real content in order to help the client understand her experiences and to help her achieve a sense of well-being while being able to relate to others.

There are a number of types of delusions. In *paranoid delusions,* individuals believe that events in their surroundings are happening especially in connection with the client. The delusions may originate logically, but then the ideas become more bizarre. For example, a client became anxious and immobilized and stated that her husband was having an affair. The client stated that she knew this because there were often new cars around the house that belonged to all his friends. She stated that a woman in one of the cars wanted to kill her, so that she could have her husband "all to herself." In actuality the husband was having an affair, but the wife, in the presence of isolation and panic, developed an understanding that reflected a delusional system.

Somatic delusions include false beliefs concerning a body part or function. For example, a client may believe that his brain is corroded and may visualize a brown film covering the brain.

Delusions of *control* or *influence* are unrealistic beliefs about magical ("telepathic") communication and control of a person's thoughts or behavior by another. An alternate form of this delusion occurs when clients believe that they control or influence others.[14,33] The Relevant Research box on page 328 identifies various other types of delusions.

Nursing Interventions for Hallucinations (50.06.02).   Clients who hallucinate may seem preoccupied, or may pause for a long time before responding during a conversation. They may also move their lips as if talking with an illusory figure, or look toward an area of the room as if relating to someone, when no one is there.

The nurse can ask the client what is happening by saying, "I noticed your lips moving as if you are talking to someone, and I wonder what is going on with you." This response leaves the client an open field in which to respond, while indicating to the client what the nurse observed that led the nurse to make the statement. However, the client may not respond.

Then the nurse can ask, "I saw your lips moving and I thought you might be talking to someone you believe is present." This narrows the nurse's response somewhat ("talking to someone"), while noting that the illusory figure is what the client believes, not what the nurse believes. The nurse should never validate the reality of an illusion. Nonvalidation keeps the hallucinatory experience with the client, not with the nurse, and not shared

RELEVANT RESEARCH

In this study the authors described how delusional clients viewed their world and how best to treat clients with delusions. The data for the study were collected, in journal form, from the observations and impressions of researchers who were staff nurses or instructors with students. The field notes were then analyzed with the help of other professionals.

Five categories of delusions emerged from data analysis:

1. *Persecutory delusions.* Example: A depressed female client believed that the Catholic church was conspiring against her every Sunday in mass.

2. *Negative delusions.* Example: A depressed client stated that she was worthless and that the devil was in her.

3. *Grandiose delusions.* Example: A former electrical engineer stated that he was the long-lost pregnant daughter of a Czar of Russia and that Stalin had impregnated him.

4. *Sexual delusions.* Example: A 19-year-old client stated that the book *The Joy of Sex* was written about her life. She was frightened of males and believed men were missiles waiting to be ejected.

5. *Difficult to understand delusions*, which occur without an *immediately* recognizable basis. Example: A client stated that he felt that he was being bombarded with signals from outer space. Such a delusion may mean that the person feels burdened with external pressures. The authors of this research noted that the client with this delusion had recently been confronted with a large promotion.

The authors noted that a central theme emerged from the five categories of delusions: delusions reflected either low self-esteem or a need for increased self-esteem. For example, clients may feel inadequate, so they shift internal feelings away from the actual problem to decrease anxiety.

On the basis of their research, the authors recommended several interventions for dealing with clients' delusions:

1. Avoid agreeing with or arguing about the delusion.

2. Avoid debating the logic of the delusion. Arguing may increase the client's agitation.

3. Humor may seem demeaning to the client.

4. Avoid focusing on the delusion beyond ascertaining its content. Instead, focus on the feelings of the client that are reflected in the delusion.

(Rosenthal T, McGuinnese T: Dealing with delusional patients: Discovering the distorted truth. Issues Ment Health Nurs 8:143, 1986)

---

by the nurse and client. In no instance should the nurse join in the client's pathology, such as by saying, "Well, I'll be the voice and say something pleasant to you," nor should the nurse claim to be able to take the voices away.

When the nurse uses the above response, the client's anxiety may increase. The client may fear that the nurse will deprive the client of what seems to be comforting and familiar (the voice). Typically, this anxiety is tolerable.

If the client then describes the hallucinatory experience, the nurse should carefully note what the client believes the experience involves. In the case of a hallucinatory voice, for instance, the client would describe what the voice said, when it seems to occur most frequently (possibly during stressful experiences), and how the client feels when the so-called voice is heard.

The nurse uses this information to gain some insight into the client's emotional life. For instance, if the voice tells the client what a terrible person the client is, one theme the client is probably working with is a low sense of self-esteem or self-worth.

Having obtained such a description, however, the nurse then leaves the topic of the hallucinatory experience. Challenging the reality of the hallucinatory experience may force the client to grasp for it even more tightly, or to elaborate on the experience so that it pervades the life of the client to an even greater extent.

The nurse, however, can begin to work with the client in developing the professional relationship between the client and the nurse. In this relationship the nurse exerts a definite pull toward reality and toward the client's expression of what is troublesome in reality. As the client works on these real concerns, the hallucinatory experience occurs less frequently as the client finds other, less pathological, ways to deal with anxiety and loneliness.

In the next section, nursing care plans address several of the problems frequently associated with a thought disorder.

Levels of Prevention

Schizophrenia is a dreaded illness. Although no one knows for certain whether or not a person with a particular mental illness can improve, the words "There is no cure" are frequently heard in reference to schizophrenia. The nursing profession believes that each individual, regardless of degree of illness, deserves professional treatment. Examples of nursing actions related to a thought disorder and to the client's degree of illness are as follows:

Primary prevention in a thought disorder can be accomplished by:

1. Providing parent training in which expectant parents learn ways of forming a healthy family. In this manner patterns of family functioning that contribute to precipitating a thought disorder in a child may be alleviated.

2. Providing genetic screening whereby those who have a thought disorder can obtain counseling regarding their likelihood of having a child with a thought disorder. The purpose of this counseling is not to pressure these adults into not having children, but rather to (1) assist them in becoming aware of their likelihood of producing a child with a thought disorder, and (2) make appropriate referrals to parent training classes if they decide to become parents.

3. Providing support groups for adolescents and parents of adolescents. Adolescence is the age when many individuals develop the obvious symptoms of a thought disorder. However, support services are not always available for the adolescent population.

Secondary prevention in a thought disorder may be accomplished by:

1. Appropriate application of the nursing process whereby psychological aspects of the total person are assessed, regardless of the setting in which clients are seen. This process facilitates early case-finding. The development of the active phase of a thought disorder is usually preceded by a prodromal phase[3] in which there is clear deterioration in functioning. Prodromal signs are listed in Table 16-2.

2. Increased research into the treatment methods whereby clients experiencing their first episode of a thought disorder are treated in order to prevent further illness and to regain their former level of health

3. Training school teachers and counselors to recognize early signs of a thought disorder in pupils with whom they work

4. Training health personnel in use of referral sources for those showing symptoms of a thought disorder

5. Providing special "crisis units" on inpatient psychiatric units where clients and their families can be treated quickly and intensely

Tertiary prevention in a thought disorder can be accomplished by:

1. Providing adequate numbers of professional psychiatric nurses to work on long-term psychiatric inpatient units

2. Providing nationwide support for home care of clients with a thought disorder after hospital discharge

3. Increased funding for psychiatric nurses doing psychotherapeutic interventions with clients in board-and-care homes

4. Increased research on how best to treat the severely ill client with many remissions

5. Increased research on the effectiveness of the psychiatric nurse in working with the severely ill client

The Family Environment

The family environment has a powerful influence on the course of a thought disorder. Clients must cope with the illness process and their reactions to having the illness, as well as with the usual tensions involved in being a part of a family. Family members may find it difficult to support the client because of the client's behavior or because of the family members' own feelings about the client's diagnosis. Family members may feel guilt, for example, for what they perceive as provoking the client's breakdown.[21]

It is not unusual for a client with a thought disorder to be vulnerable to family intrusions into the client's life. The client may react to family criticism with increased anxiety or too much emotional stimulation. On the other hand, too little emotional stimulation promotes apathy and withdrawal from others.[8,35]

The Family During Hospitalization

It is important for professionals to include the family in the care of a client who has a thought disorder.[32] Indeed, the family itself can often be viewed as needing treatment, and not simply the person with the diagnosis of a thought disorder. However, the member with a thought disorder is referred to as the identified patient (IP) because of the convention of hospitalization or treatment of one family member rather than the total family.

It is important to intervene and work with the family from the first moment of admission of the client to the hospital. At the time of admission the client will probably be very anxious. The nurse should obtain all possible information from the client, as is usually done in an initial assessment. However, some of this information can be obtained a number of hours after admission when the client's anxiety has decreased. The family can be contacted at the time of admission, preferably in a face-to-face interview, to gain additional information.

It is important for the nurse to tell the client that on the unit families of clients are included in treatment. If the client is too upset on admission to join in meeting with the nurse and the family, the client is told what occurred in the family meeting at a later time.

Initially the nurse informs the family that the unit considers the family to be an important part of treatment, and then talks with the family to gather information about the precipitating event before hospitalization, subsequent behavior of all family members, and how the decision to hospitalize the client was made and carried out. After determining the family members' reactions to the client's illness, and offering emotional support to them, the nurse tells the family about the part they will play in the client's treatment. They are also informed of the unit's policy on confidentiality of conversations between one (or more) family members (including the client and treatment staff) when other family members are not present. The nature of this confidentiality agreement is established as a treatment principle or policy among the hospital staff for use with all families.

Thus, on admission nurses attend to the needs of the client as well as of the family members. As an understanding of and alliance with the family increases, the nurse

(Text continues on p. 336.)

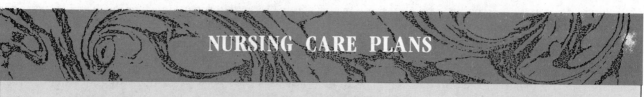

NURSING CARE PLANS

ASSESSMENT	NURSING INTERVENTIONS	EVALUATION CRITERIA

I.   Alterations in Communications (20), Impaired Verbal Communication (20.02)

NURSING DIAGNOSIS: Volume (speech) too soft (20.02.21)

SUBJECTIVE DATA Client: "Umm. Well. . . ." (Client whispers inaudibly.) **OBJECTIVE DATA** Indistinct speech	1. Label the voice or speech problem and also indicate an appropriate response for the client. Say, "Mr. Jones, I could not hear you. Please talk louder. What did you say about the meeting this morning?"	Client will demonstrate a significant increase in voice volume after prompting.
	2. Maintain a focus on receiving client's message.	Client will remain with nurse while nurse continues to assist client to increase voice production.
	3. Avoid blaming client. Instead say, "Mr. Jones, what you are saying is important. I can't hear you. Please repeat what you said."	Client will appear more willing to talk so that others can hear.
	4. Ask the reason the client is talking so softly. Discuss client's experience further (*e.g.,* low self-esteem, fear, apathy)	Client will become aware of the use client makes of soft voice.

II.   Alterations in Role Performance (23), Inspired Social/Leisure Role (23.02)

NURSING DIAGNOSIS: Withdrawal/social isolation (23.02.01)

SUBJECTIVE DATA
Client: "I don't need to talk with anyone in this hospital. I only need myself."
 	
OBJECTIVE DATA
Client stays by self. Is irritable, alienated from others, and questions other's intentions towards self. Is overly sensitive to interpersonal trauma, *e.g.,* perceived rejection
	(It is assumed that the primary nurse will meet daily with the client to establish a relationship with the client).
	1. Encourage client to join in events on unit where other people are present.
	2. Explore with client the nature of difficult relationships client has had in past which led to self-isolation. Assist client in seeing a repeated pattern of how client was during past difficult relationships, and how client presently relates with the nurse and other clients on the unit.
	3. Assist client in identifying what client and nurse can do differently to keep from repeating previous patterns of behavior that severed social relationships.
	4. Provide graded expectations for relating to others, one at a time, including:
	   a. Be with others.
	   b. Listen to others.
	   c. Make one verbal response to another person.
	   d. Make more than one verbal response in succession to another (conversation).
	   e. Label thoughts about conversation.
	   f. Label feelings about conversation.
		Client will attend, of own volition, at least one event on the unit where others are present.
		Client will label at least one difficult pattern of interpersonal behavior that the client repeats today.
		
		Client and nurse will test and evaluate one different pattern of interpersonal behavior that promotes client's and other's sense of well-being.
		Client will report significant increase in ease of relating to others.

(Continued)

NURSING CARE PLANS (CONTINUED)

ASSESSMENT	NURSING INTERVENTIONS	EVALUATION CRITERIA
	g. Repeat steps *a–f* several times with the same person. h. Label the nature of the relationship with person in *g* (such as pleasant, distant, supportive). i. Practice several times changing the pattern of relating to others, as needed.	

III. Excess of or Deficit in Dominant Emotions (30)

NURSING DIAGNOSIS: Impaired congruence of emotions, thoughts, behavior (30.03)

SUBJECTIVE DATA Client states, "I have no sense of myself." Facial expression indicates no concern. **OBJECTIVE DATA** Incongruity of facial expression and meaning of what is said	1. Point out a behavior that is incongruent with what client has said or what has happened to client. Ask client if the reality of the event is in accord with this (incongruent) behavioral response of the client.	Client will describe one present experience when displayed behavior is incongruent with a particular event.
	2. Ask client to define what has interfered with clear awareness of what is occurring. (Is client preoccupied? Anxious?)	Client will describe what interferes with awareness that keeps thoughts/feelings/actions from being congruent.
	3. Assist client to define what an appropriate behavioral response would be. 4. Assist client to define what happened in the past when client displayed event-appropriate behavior. (Was client told that he or she was "crazy," wrong, or inappropriate for congruent behavior so that the others protected their own interests rather than those of the client?)	Client will describe an appropriate behavioral response to the situation being discussed. Client will describe the inappropriate response client received from others when client made an *appropriate* response to an interpersonal situation.
	5. Discuss true feelings masked by incongruent thoughts, feelings, and actions.	Client will demonstrate congruency in thoughts, feelings, and behavior.

IV. Alterations in Perception/Cognition (50), Alterations in Judgment (50.03)

NURSING DIAGNOSIS: Blocking of ideas (50.03.01)

SUBJECTIVE DATA Client suddenly becomes silent during a conversation. **OBJECTIVE DATA** Client seems preoccupied.	1. Say, "You were talking and then became silent. What happened that you became silent?"	Client will label blocking pattern.
	2. Ask, "What were you thinking just before you became silent?"	Client will demonstrate ability to label blocked topic.
	3. Ask, "What were you feeling just before you became silent?"	Client will label feeling that promoted a blocking response.
	4. If client cannot identify thoughts or feelings, ask, "Were you anxious just before you became silent?"	Client will label underlying anxiety if other feelings are not present.

(Continued)

NURSING CARE PLANS (CONTINUED)

ASSESSMENT	NURSING INTERVENTIONS	EVALUATION CRITERIA
	5. Facilitate client's discussion of anxiety, thoughts, or feelings that promoted blocking.	Client will demonstrate decreased need for blocking after emotional release and clarification.

V.   Alterations in Perception/Cognition (50), Alterations in Judgment (50.03)

NURSING DIAGNOSIS: Circumstantial thinking (50.03.02)

SUBJECTIVE DATA Client (after being asked the reason for not relating to other clients): "Well, it doesn't matter. I want a cigarette. Probably no one smokes here, huh?"	1. Ask direct questions about the topic. For example: "What is it that does not matter?"	Client will elaborate on the topic of concern. Client will provide at least one statement that provides useful details about the topic of concern.
OBJECTIVE DATA Client does not deal directly with the experience.	2. Bring client back to topic without damaging client's self-esteem. Say "Phil, before you and I talk about your cigarette, what is the reason you aren't with the other clients?"	Client will converse about the topic of concern.
	3. Inquire as to what may be keeping client from providing more details about the experience.	Client will provide an explanation of reasons for not talking directly about the concern.
	4. Suggest what may come next in client's description but only after (a) asking client for further description, and (b) making sure that such an intervention will promote your alliance with the client rather than irritation. Avoid guessing about the client's experiences: ask the client to provide information.	Client will provide a description after prompting about the concern.
	5. Build on words client uses to talk about the concern. Say "What about relating to others on the unit doesn't matter?" or "When did you first think relating doesn't matter?"	Client will continue on topic of concern with prompting.

VI.   Alterations in Perception/Cognition (50), Alterations in Judgment (50.03)

NURSING DIAGNOSIS: A. Constructional difficulty (50.03.03)

SUBJECTIVE DATA When asked to begin to talk about something of concern in the interview with the nurse, the client says, "Nothing. I don't know."	1. Ask client to identify event (or experience). Provide clues if needed, such as, "Well, Phil, what was it like for you to come to the hospital?"	Client will identify an experience.
OBJECTIVE DATA Client cannot interpret and state the meaning of what has been perceived.	2. Identify an event for client if client cannot do so with clues. Say, "I imagine it's not easy for you to be in the hospital."	Client will identify an experience after prompting.
	3. Ask if client is anxious. If so, intervene accordingly.	Client will identify specific feelings interfering with identification of an experience.
	4. Provide and encourage daily opportunities for meaningful dialogue and socialization.	Client will engage in dialogue with others in which understandable meaning is attributed to events.

(Continued)

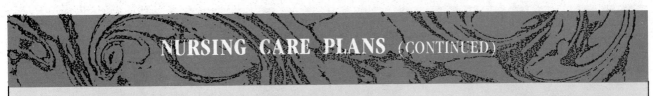

NURSING CARE PLANS (CONTINUED)

ASSESSMENT	NURSING INTERVENTIONS	EVALUATION CRITERIA
	5. Provide opportunity to discuss what it is like for client to review experiences. Say, "What is it like to talk with someone about your life?"	Client will describe the internal unique experiences that occur when talking about self.

VII.   Alterations in Perception/Cognition (50), Alterations in Judgment (50.03)

NURSING DIAGNOSIS: B. Impaired abstract thinking (50.03.05)

SUBJECTIVE DATA Nurse: "What was happening just prior to your coming into the hospital?" Client: "I was out of the hospital." OBJECTIVE DATA Client cannot understand the more general meaning of communication other than what is concrete.	1. Do not deviate from topic, but ask for a description in a more concrete fashion, such as, "Where were you just before coming to the hospital?" 2. If client still does not respond, do not deviate from topic but ask for a response to another concrete question, such as, "Whom were you with just before coming to the hospital?" 3. Provide information for client if client shows no response to the more concrete requests for a description, such as, "Sometimes a person has been having family difficulties just before coming to the hospital." 4. When client is in group therapy and another client makes a reply indicating an ability to abstract, ask client if the other client's experience is similar.	Client will respond appropriately to concrete statements. Client will respond appropriately to concrete statements when prompted about one topic. Client will talk about abstract topic when led into the discussion. Client will be able to relate abstract statements others make about their lives to client's own life when prompted.

VIII.   Alterations in Perception/Cognition (50), Alterations in Judgment (50.03)

NURSING DIAGNOSIS: C. Impaired logical thinking (50.03.09)

SUBJECTIVE DATA Client (Phil) labels others on unit as "evil." OBJECTIVE DATA Client maintains irrational ideas.	1. Determine whether the content of the expressed thoughts denotes another true concern. 2. Ascertain if client is anxious and if anxiety is promoting such relief behavior. 3. Label what may be client's concern if client cannot state it.	Client will talk about a true concern in a way that can be understood by others. Client will name a feeling that requires the relief behavior. Client will discuss the true concern with the nurse.

IX.   Alterations in Perception/Cognition (50), Alterations in Orientation (50.05)

NURSING DIAGNOSIS: Autism (50.05.01)

SUBJECTIVE DATA Client (Phil) states "There's badness here." OBJECTIVE DATA Client uses words with a private meaning.	1. Indicate to the client that you do not understand the client's use of a word. Say, "Phil, you stated that there is *badness* here." Ask client to express that thought in a way that you can	Client will alter speech and talk about true concerns in order to be understood by others.

(Continued)

NURSING CARE PLANS (CONTINUED)

ASSESSMENT	NURSING INTERVENTIONS	EVALUATION CRITERIA
	understand. ("Tell me in another way that I can understand.")	
	2. If client does not respond, say, "My idea is that this is a psychiatric unit. In what way is there badness here, as you said?"	Client will talk in ways understood by others with prompting.
	3. If client does not respond, decode client's statement. Say, "I still don't understand you. Do you mean that something has happened on the unit and you are uncomfortable?"	Label what may be client's experience if the client cannot.
	4. Intervene accordingly if anxiety is present.	Client's anxiety will decrease such that client can talk in ways understood by others.

X. Alterations in Perception/Cognition (50), Alterations in Perception (50.06)

NURSING DIAGNOSIS: Hallucinations (50.06.02)

SUBJECTIVE DATA Client: "A voice is telling me to leave." **OBJECTIVE DATA** Client glances about and moves lips as if talking to someone.	1. Obtain description of the so-called voice. (Say, "Exactly what is the so-called voice saying?")	Client will describe to the nurse what the hallucinatory voice is saying.
	2. Intervene if the client is anxious.	Client's anxiety will decrease to the point that the hallucinatory experience does not interfere with everyday functioning.
	3. Determine the "context" of the hallucinatory experience: When did the client first hear a so-called voice? What was occurring in the client's life at the time? What circumstances promote the occurrence of hallucinations? Is the so-called voice similar to the voice of someone the client knows?	Client will have some element of an objective view of the hallucinatory experience (will identify the association between increased anxiety and loneliness, and hallucinations).
	4. Remain with client or encourage client to join others (to socialize).	Hallucinations will decrease in frequency as client is around others.

XI. Alterations in Perception/Cognition (50), Alterations in Perception (50.06)

NURSING DIAGNOSIS: Illusions (50.06.03)

SUBJECTIVE DATA Client: "That is my mother walking." (Curtain is moving.) **OBJECTIVE DATA** Client mistakes an environmental event for a personalized event.	1. Intervene if client is anxious.	Client's anxiety will decrease to the point that client does not experience illusions. Client will recognize the actual event that was distorted.
	2. State to client what you think really occurred: "Do you think you mistook the moving curtain for your mother?"	
	3. Ask the client to talk about the true concern: "My idea is that you mistook the	Client will more readily describe the anxiety-provoking experiences.

(Continued)

NURSING CARE PLANS (CONTINUED)

ASSESSMENT	NURSING INTERVENTIONS	EVALUATION CRITERIA
	moving curtain for your mother. Say some more about your mother."	
	4. Remain with client or encourage client to join others (to socialize).	Illusions will decrease in frequency as client is around others.

XII.   Alterations in Perception/Cognition (50), Alterations in Self-Concept (50.07)

NURSING DIAGNOSIS: Impaired body image (50.07.01)

SUBJECTIVE DATA Client (Phil): "My body feels alien to me" or "My arms and legs are not attached to me." **OBJECTIVE DATA** Relationship of client to own body (or environment) is altered or considered foreign.	1. Obtain description of disturbance. 2. Intervene if client is anxious. 3. Decode meaning of the disturbance.	Client will provide a description of how client perceives own body. Client's anxiety will decrease such that body focus is appropriate. Client will talk about the true concern promoting the impaired body image.

XIII.   Alterations in Perception/Cognition, Alterations in Self-Concept (50.07)

NURSING DIAGNOSIS: Impaired personal identity (50.07.03)

SUBJECTIVE DATA Client states, "I have no sense of Self." **OBJECTIVE DATA** Client has no sense of purpose or direction, cannot make decisions alone.	1. Ask client to describe when an absence of a sense of Self was first felt. What in the client's life promoted such an experience (an interpersonal problem)? 2. Ask client to describe a time when sense of Self *was* felt. Based on this description, define, in concrete terms, what *client* means when using the word "Self." 3. Ask client to set one goal to establish this sense of Self. For example: if client describes having a sense of Self when working, ask client to think of a way to occupy time in a work-like fashion after hospitalization (through volunteer work or part-time employment).	Client will describe when sense of Self decreased. Client will describe what sense of "Self" means. Client will set one goal to establish a sense of Self, and complete actions to meet goal. Client will describe effect of working on goal on sense of Self.

XIV.   Alterations in Perception/Cognition (50), Alterations in Thought Content (50.08)

NURSING DIAGNOSIS: Delusions (50.08.02)

SUBJECTIVE DATA Client: "I am the Queen of Scotland." **OBJECTIVE DATA** Client has grandiose false ideas.	1. Get a description of the delusion. 2. Intervene if client is anxious. 3. Ascertain the real life experience related to delusion. 4. Facilitate understanding of the real life experience for client.	Client will give details of delusion. Delusions will decrease as anxiety decreases. Client will describe true concerns that may promote a delusion. Use of delusion will decrease as true concerns of client are considered.

RELEVANT RESEARCH

This study compared the quality of life of care providers (spouse and/or blood relatives) of a schizophrenic client before and after the discharge of the schizophrenic family member to the home of the providers. This research arose from the question of whether the discharge of clients with schizophrenia from hospital care had inhumane effects on the family with whom the client lived after discharge.

The researchers measured the quality of life of the family members using two scales that measured the level of gratification of basic needs, as defined by Maslow. It was thought that fulfillment of these basic needs is linked to the quality of human life. Each scale contained 25 Likert-scale items, such as "I decide when to share my feelings, thoughts, and beliefs." This item measured a growth need to exercise control over the self. The scales were formulated by the researchers, administered to a panel of 18 nursing experts for content validation, and then administered to ten heads of households to determine clarity of the scales.

A total of 212 family members responded to the scales, at least three weeks after the placement of the client with schizophrenia into the family home. Family members responded to the *Present Quality of Life* scale at the same time that they responded to the *Past Quality of Life* scale. While responding to the *Past Quality of Life* scale, the family members were asked to take a retrospective view and to describe how they had felt during the client's last hospitalization.

Findings indicated that there was a difference in the total quality of life of care providers when the schizophrenic family members were at home, compared to when they were hospitalized (t test, $p < 0.0005$). Quality of life scores decreased when the clients returned home. The widest variation occurred in the category of safety needs of family members, including freedom from actual or threatened physical, social, or emotional abuse.

The study highlighted the need for psychiatric and community nurses to understand the effects that discharged schizophrenic clients may have on their family and care providers. The nurse can foster both the client's and the family's adjustment to the schizophrenic illness process. The nurse can guide the adjustment process both in the hospital setting (when the family attends family conferences) and in the community (when the home care nurse provides care to the client and family).

(Seymour R, Dawson N: The schizophrenic at home. J Psychosoc Nurs Ment Health Serv 26:28, 1986)

can serve as a clarifier to the family of events on the unit. This alliance also maintains the perspective for the client, the family, and the nurse that the client has come to the hospital from a context of ongoing ties with others (the family), and the client will maintain and return to these ties once discharged.

It is not therapeutic to blame the family for what has happened to the hospitalized client. The client, the family, the nurse, the physician, the social skills trainer, and the occupational therapist all work as a team to improve the quality of life of the family and the client. The family and the client probably have had serious problems managing the illness and coping with the changes it has necessitated in their lives. The idea is not to rescue the client from the family, but to promote a quality of kinship among all the family members by easing the burden of the illness wherever possible.

Family members are involved in various treatment programs while the client is hospitalized; examples are given below.[4,23] The hospitalized member should attend with the family when not occupied with individual psychotherapy or group psychotherapy. Several families can attend the programs at the same time to promote sharing and learning from each other.

Programs for the Family During the Member's Hospitalization

Program 1: a discussion of topics to be included that family members feel are important. Staff members add their ideas. These ideas are compiled into a schedule of programs (several suggestions are included below).

Program 2: educative meeting about the nature of a thought disorder. Topics include onset, course, outcome, theories of etiology, prognosis (including the risk of relapse on and off medication), forms of treatment, and the use and impact of psychotropic drugs (and their side-effects).

Program 3: the management of the illness by the family. In this program families are told that, given the nature of a thought disorder, the response of many families may not be the most helpful. To promote alliance with the families, the staff may want to describe what the families probably have done to cope with the illness. They have probably tried to understand the client's strange behavior, to ignore the behavior, to avoid hurting the client by not setting limits on the client's behavior, to curtail their own lives, and to punish the client.

The negative role that stress plays in the illness is discussed to help family members understand the role they play in the course of the disease. Relapse is related to increased interpersonal and intrapsychic stress. *Interpersonal stress* is exemplified by conflict, simultaneous multiple conversations, confusing power structures, unclear boundaries between adults and children, criticism, and the family's extreme involvement (positive and negative) with the client. *Intrapsychic stress* includes not sharing thoughts and feelings, not establishing a support system, and oversensitivity.

The staff can help the family maintain greater family stability by maintaining appropriate expectations, setting reasonable limits in a confident and matter-of-fact way, guiding family members to stay involved in activities outside the family, and establishing a friendship/support network outside the family.

Program 4: establishing the family's aftercare program (see section below)

Each program listed above can best be done in a group setting of three to four families. During this time members feel less isolated as they hear others share similar experiences. The group itself can be a source of strength beyond that of individual members.

Despite attempts not to threaten families by insisting that they examine their own psychic functioning, the family cannot withhold its pathology. The nurse will see such pathology demonstrated. Table 16-9 lists examples of such pathology and recommended interventions.

Aftercare

Continued care after hospitalization is an important component of the health care services provided for clients with a thought disorder. Hospitalization is used to manage the acute phase of the illness. Clients are usually hospitalized for one to three weeks, and are discharged in a fragile state.

Aftercare provides clients with psychological and pharmacological support to (1) prevent regression, (2) further restore clients to their prehospitalization competency levels, (3) facilitate the process of growth, and (4) facilitate integration into the community.

Pharmacological treatment is helpful to clients with a thought disorder as part of their aftercare program. However, noncompliance with recommended dosages can occur. Injections of fluphenazine enanthate (Prolixin) can be used in cases of noncompliance by clients: these injections can be given biweekly, thereby eliminating the need for daily oral medications.

The need for aftercare services is indicated from several statistics. Approximately one out of every two clients with a thought disorder regresses to the point of requiring rehospitalization within six months of discharge from an inpatient unit. The highest risk of relapse occurs during the six weeks immediately after discharge.[21] It is useful if aftercare services assist the client in coping successfully with the elements of the client's day-to-day experience that promote anxiety. These elements include the families and environment of clients with a thought disorder and the clients themselves.

Table 16-10 summarizes frequent problems of clients and families after discharge, as well as interventions the nurse can use to facilitate coping with these problems.

Relapse may be preceded by an increase in the symptoms listed in Table 16-7. The client, the client's family, and health care providers must be familiar with these symptoms to prevent further decompensation and hospitalization.

TABLE 16-9.
FAMILY PROBLEMS DURING A MEMBER'S HOSPITALIZATION

PROBLEM	INTERVENTION
1. Family members are over-involved and intrusive. They attempt to monitor and protect clients.	Show appreciation to family members for their attempts to care. Remind family members of the Self/Other/Relationship model (see the discussion in Chapter 5). Emphasize the idea that, although clients must have their own individual lives, this does not eliminate the need for family units.
2. Family members become frustrated, angry, and withdrawn from the client and staff.	Maintain an educational approach when speaking with the family. Make educational programs enjoyable to the greatest degree possible by including films, refreshments, a friendly and welcoming atmosphere, and remembering family members' names. Call and/or write to family members and encourage their participation. Do not agree with any family member's attempt to place blame on the client. Maintain the focus on *all* family members.
3. Family members engage in vague communication patterns.	Do not make (what could be interpreted as) negative comments about family communication patterns. Maintain a simple, concrete focus on content to obtain clarity. Reward the family for their efforts in verbalizing. Return to the topic later, if needed.

TABLE 16-10.
AFTERCARE PROBLEMS OF THE CLIENT AND FAMILY

CLIENT PROBLEMS	INTERVENTIONS FOR THE FAMILY TO USE WITH THE CLIENT
1. Establishing a sense of equilibrium when first at home	Encourage client to obtain or avoid stimulation, as needed; avoid conflict; and take medications, as prescribed.
2. The occurrence of stressful events	Promote anticipatory planning by identifying potentially stressful upcoming events and devise coping strategies.
3. Lack of competence in behaving in ways that are acceptable to others and safe for the client (such as the client using matches and cigarettes inappropriately)	Assist family and client to arrive at appropriate limits for behavior.
4. Lack of a range of responses to use in coping with anticipated stresses (when client returns to work, or begins to date)	Work with family and client to define stressors and typical stress responses. Plan with client so client can understand stress management strategies and maintain willingness to perform the strategies, once learned.

FAMILY (OR SIGNIFICANT OTHER) PROBLEMS	INTERVENTIONS FOR THE NURSE TO USE WITH THE FAMILY
1. Inappropriate expectations (e.g., the client should be fully functional immediately after hospitalization)	Assist family to understand the stress placed on the client with such demands; discuss that full recovery takes 6 months to one year.
2. Inappropriate expectations: the client will never improve	Bolster hope for growth over time; assist family to set reasonable short-term expectations; acknowledge positive changes, however slight.
3. Lack of clarity about reactions to the client's illness and hospitalization	Ask family about subjective reactions to client's illness (e.g., shame, fear, anxiety, guilt); assist family to understand the nature and meaning of the illness; assist family to understand warning signs of client decompensation.
4. Family interactions promote stress	Assist all members in defining what events (not individuals) are stressors (to avoid blame, guilt, and defensiveness); explain rationale of stress management techniques to avoid increased tension in the family; review the use of stress management techniques in the family; assist the family to become comfortable with (what may appear to be) artificially simplistic ways to communicate; help family learn ways to maintain artificially low levels of emotionality.

(Adapted from Anderson C: A Psychoeducational Program for Families of Patients With Schizophrenia. In McFarlane W (ed): Family Therapy in Schizophrenia. New York, Guilford Press, 1983)

Somatic Therapies

Harris[15] stated that antipsychotic medications such as those used with a thought disorder assist in reducing symptoms of agitation, rage, overreactivity to sensory stimuli, hallucinations, delusions, paranoia, combativeness, insomnia (as a symptom of the psychosis), hostility, negativism, and thought disturbances. These drugs, however, *do not change a person's personality or help the client improve poor judgment.* These elements can only be corrected with work in an interpersonal relationship with a professional person, such as a nurse.

Table 16-11 lists the antipsychotic medications and the potency of each medication relative to chlorpromazine, a low-potency antipsychotic. Medications with a high potency have a greater likelihood of producing side-effects.

All antipsychotic medications are thought to provide some relief from thought disorder symptoms by blocking the dopamine receptors in the brain. The antipsychotic medications also have anticholinergic effects that are re-

sponsible for some of their side-effects. (Drugs used with clients with a thought disorder may be called either *antipsychotic, psychotropic,* or *neuroleptic* medications.) Effects, interactions, and nursing implications for chlorpromazine are outlined in the drug card.

Antipsychotic medications are not addictive. They do not produce euphoria, and no tolerance is acquired for their antipsychotic effects.

Acute treatment refers to therapy provided for a client experiencing high anxiety who poses a safety risk for self or others. For instance, a client experiencing a suicidal hallucinatory voice for the first time would probably feel extreme anxiety and panic. The client is extremely uncomfortable, and can find no relief. The client cannot be calmed through a verbal discussion.

Reid,[32] and McGinnis and Foote[24] recommend rapid neuroleptization for such a client. In this treatment regimen, the client is first assessed for findings that would eliminate the possibility of using medication for a thought disorder, such as hepatic damage. Information is also obtained about the sequence of events prior to the

TABLE 16-11.
ANTIPSYCHOTIC MEDICATIONS

GENERIC NAME	TRADE NAME	APPROXIMATE POTENCY RELATIVE TO CHLORPROMAZINE	IM FORM
PHENOTHIAZINES			
Aliphatics			
Chlorpromazine	Thorazine	100 mg	Yes
Triflupromazine	Vesprin	25–50 mg	Yes
Piperidines			
Thioridazine	Mellaril	100 mg	No
Mesoridazine	Serentil	25–50 mg	Yes
Piperacelazine	Quide	10–15 mg	No
Piperazines			
Trifluoperazine	Stelazine	5 mg	Yes
Acetophenazine	Tindal	20 mg	No
Fluphenazine	Prolixin	1–4 mg	Yes
Fluphenazine enanthate	Prolixin Enanthate	No reliable correlation	Yes
Fluphenazine decanoate	Prolixin Decanoate	No reliable correlation	Yes
Perphenazine	Trilafon	8–12 mg	Yes
Prochlorperazine	Compazine	15–50 mg	Yes
Butaperazine	Repoise	10–15 mg	No
Carphenazine	Prokelazine	25–50 mg	No
THIOXANTHENES			
Chlorprothixene	Taractan	50–100 mg	Yes
Thiothixene	Navane	2–10 mg	Yes
BUTYROPHENONES			
Haloperidol	Haldol	1.6–2 mg	Yes
DIHYDROINDOLONES			
Molindone	Lidone Moban	10–15 mg	No
DIBENZOXAZEPINES			
Loxapine	Loxitane Daxolin	10–20 mg	No
DIPHENYLBUTYL PIPERIDINES			
Penfluridol	Both are experimental.		
Pimozide			

(Harris E: Antipsychotic medications. Am J Nurs 81:1316–1323, 1981)

distress, recent ingestion of any drugs, and recent trauma. The severity of agitation should be documented to establish a baseline. Baseline information includes the degree and nature of agitation, anxiety level, delusions, hallucinations, tenseness, and cooperativeness. The client would probably be hospitalized because the client is unable to care for self and perhaps even a danger to self or to others. Once the client is admitted to the hospital unit, the rapid neuroleptization schedule begins, as does milieu treatment to provide a safe and therapeutic environment for the client.

The most commonly used medication in rapid neuroleptization is haloperidol, which should be given intramuscularly initially, 0.5–10 mg every 60 minutes. This schedule is continued unless the symptoms improve, se-

dation begins, medical complications arise (such as hypotension), or the total dose of medication received over a 12-hour period approaches 100 mg. Most clients will not require this level of medication, however.

Thiothixene or loxapine may be used in place of haloperidol, although these less potent neuroleptic medications may result in increased client discomfort, sedation, or tissue damage.

Rapid neuroleptization has also been performed with oral medications. Examples of these agents include liquid haloperidol and fluphenazine. However, the absorption and peak concentrations of the medication in the body are significantly delayed and a higher dose may be required than when the medications are given intramuscularly. The treatment team may, however, decide to

chlorpromazine HCl

(antipsychotic)

Clorazine, Ormazine, Promapar, Thorazine

Action: Antagonizes dopamine neurotransmission at postsynaptic receptors.

Uses: Acute and chronic psychoses; mania; schizophrenia. Relief of intractable hiccups. Acute intermittent porphyria.

Side effects: Extrapyramidal symptoms; dizziness; rash; dry mouth; nausea; orthostatic hypotension

Toxic effects: Laryngospasm; agranulocytosis

Contraindications:
- Severe cardiovascular disease
- Bone marrow depression
- Hypersensitivity
- Liver damage
- Comatose states
- Alcohol and barbiturate withdrawal

Interactions:
- Other CNS depressants, including alcohol (may cause oversedation)
- Epinephrine (may cause toxicity)
- Lithium, levodopa (may cause decreased effects)
- Anticholinergics (effects increased)

Nursing implications:
- Assess for urinary retention by palpation.
- Monitor blood pressure for hypotension.
- Monitor for early signs of tardive dyskinesia.
- Provide increased fluid to prevent constipation.
- Monitor for extrapyramidal symptoms.
- Supervise ambulation until stabilized.

Client teaching:
- Rise slowly from sitting or lying position.
- Avoid abrupt withdrawal from long-term therapy.
- Report sore throat, malaise, fever, bleeding, mouth sores.
- Avoid use with alcohol or CNS depressants.

use oral medications with a client when the client's anxiety is significantly raised by the issues of invasiveness or powerlessness (which may occur when receiving an injection). The client should be offered reassurance and orientation. The client should be told that the medications are not a punishment and are only given until control is restored.

When the rapid neuroleptization regimen is used, nursing care must include, among other elements, close observation for side-effects of the medications. Vital signs should be taken prior to the administration of medications, and then every 15 to 30 minutes.

If the treatment team decides that rapid neuroleptization is not the treatment of choice (if the staff needs more time for observation, if the client has a high potential for feeling side-effects of the medication, or if the hospital follows a treatment plan that does not include rapid neuroleptization), the client may be started on

lower doses of antipsychotic medication. The medication will then be increased every several days until improvement occurs.

Nonacute Treatment in Early and Brief Hospitalization

The use of antipsychotic medication alleviates or decreases many symptoms of a thought disorder. Medications can also significantly decrease the time needed for hospitalization. Sufficient medication increases the chances of successful progress once the client is discharged. Because of the decrease of symptoms, the client is more likely to integrate interpersonal relationships successfully. The accompanying drug card lists the side-

thiothixene

(antipsychotic, neuroleptic)

Navane

Action: Inhibits postsynaptic dopamine receptors at subcortical levels of reticular formation, hypothalmus, and limbic system, interrupting impulse movement.

Uses: Psychotic disorders, schizophrenia, acute agitation

Side-effects: Dry mouth, constipation, blurred vision, rash, extrapyramidal symptoms, orthostatic hypotension, tachycardia, akathisia, dystonia

Toxic effects: Laryngospasm, agranulocytosis, cardiac arrest

Contraindications:
- Comatose states
- Hypersensitivity
- Blood dyscrasias

Precautions:
- Severe cardiovascular disorders
- Pregnancy
- Lactation
- Seizure disorders
- Hypertension
- Hepatic disease

Interactions:
- CNS depressants (oversedation)
- Epinephrine (toxicity)
- Anticholinergic, hypotensive agents (increased effects)
- Alcohol (oversedation)

Nursing implications:
- Monitor intake and output.
- Provide increased fluids to prevent constipation.
- Assess for urinary retention.
- Evaluate skin turgor daily.

Client teaching:
- Change position slowly to avoid orthostatic hypotension.
- Report visual disturbances.
- Report sore throat, malaise, fever, bleeding, mouth sores.
- Avoid abrupt withdrawal of drug.
- Avoid exposure to sun and heat.

effects, precautions, interactions, and nursing implications for thiothixene.

The client may recommend a useful medication that has been taken in the past. The drugs of choice may come from the drug groups phenothiazines, butyrophenones, or thioxanthenes. Medications used when a high-potency drug is desired include fluphenazine, haloperidol, and thiothixene.

If rapid neuroleptization was used with a client in the acute phase, this drug may be continued after the acute phase. The initial dosage level can be reduced by 50% once the client has been stabilized. In the nonacute phase of treatment, oral medication is usually prescribed.

The response to most antipsychotic medications peaks in several weeks, except in cases in which rapid neuroleptization is used. Serum levels of the medication are *not* well correlated with client response to the medication.

Maintenance Treatment

A client whose illness is tied to specific stressors and who has a temporary illness can be taken off psychotropic medication once the client has regained the pre-illness competency level. For clients whose tendency toward a thought disorder is high, the client should be removed from medication only with caution.

The treatment team may examine variables such as the stability of the social environment of the client in order to determine when to remove clients from medication. Some clients remain on medications for years with supervision. Most clients can remain on half the dosage of the medications received during the acute phase of treatment.

Side-Effects

Harris[16] reported that about one third of all clients receiving antipsychotic medications experience extrapyramidal side-effects (EPS). These side-effects are difficult to prevent, but they are also relatively easily controlled when diagnosed and treated.

Extrapyramidal side-effects are uncomfortable and frightening to clients. Many times the client does not comply with recommendations for antipsychotic medications because of these symptoms. The side-effects may resemble depression, hysteria, malingering, epilepsy, and other conditions. EPS are more pronounced in stressful situations, and their presence is not an indication that the antipsychotic medications are helping the client.

Harris[16] lists four classes of extrapyramidal symptoms:

Parkinsonism

This type of parkinsonism is drug-induced. It is thought to be caused by the dopamine blockade created by the antipsychotic medication. This syndrome consists of akinesia, muscular rigidity, alterations of posture, tremor, masklike faces, shuffling gait, loss of associated movements, and drooling.

This side-effect usually begins after the first week but within two months of the start of the medication. Clients can accommodate to parkinsonism symptoms so that the symptoms fade over two or three months, with or without treatment.

1. *Akinesia* is often experienced as fatigue, lack of interest, slowness, heaviness, a lack of drive or ambition, or vague bodily discomforts. These symptoms may be confused with depression, demoralization, or negativism. It is important for the nurse to understand that symptoms of akinesia may occur as a side-effect of medication, not as a personality trait (such as negativism) of the client. The client with akinesia will report feelings of being slowed down, weak, and less spontaneous. Clients may also report feeling like a "zombie" or like being "under water." Clients are painfully aware of the side-effects as they occur.

2. *Rigidity* is a plastic hypertonicity that affects axial and limb muscles. The rigidity can be assessed by holding a client's elbow in the palm of your hand with your thumb positioned over the flexor tendons. Flex and extend the arm with your other hand, asking the client to relax the arm and allow you to do the moving. You may find a smooth resistance to the move-

ment, known as "lead-pipe" rigidity, or a ratchetlike phenomenon, known as "cog-wheel" rigidity. Either of these findings is evidence of drug-induced rigidity.

3. The *tremor* seen in parkinsonian symptoms usually begins in one or both upper extremities and, when severe, involves the tongue, jaw, and lower extremities. This symptom is most discouraging for clients who wish to maintain fine motor movements.

4. The *masklike faces* associated with this type of side-effect can be mistaken for the flat affect of a client with a thought disorder. A client with masklike faces, however, employs means other than facial gestures to indicate a wider range of emotion.

5. The *loss of associated movements* is seen most easily in a decreased or absent arm swing. The client walks with the forearms perpendicular to the trunk. It is important to recognize that these symptoms are side-effects of the antipsychotic medications, not necessarily an element of some "bizarreness" of a thought disorder.

Parkinsonian symptoms induced by antipsychotic medication can usually be controlled by decreasing the dose or by administering an antiparkinsonian agent. These drugs are listed in Table 16-12.

Dyskinesias and Dystonias

Dyskinesias are coordinated, involuntary, stereotyped, rhythmic movements of the limbs and trunk that are commonly seen in males. The *dystonias* are uncoordinated, bizarre, jerking or spastic movements of the neck, face, eyes, tongue, torso, arm, or leg muscles. Also included are backward rolling of the eyes in the sockets (oculogyric crisis), sideways twisting of the neck (torticollis), protrusion of the tongue, or spasms of the back muscles (opisthotonus). These symptoms occur suddenly, and are frightening and painful to the client. The client may experience difficulty in breathing or swallowing.

Dystonic reactions can be treated with benadryl. An intramuscular injection usually decreases symptoms within 15 minutes. The antiparkinsonian agent used may be continued for two or three months to prevent the reoccurrence of the symptoms. Clients experiencing these side-effects should be reassured that they are, indeed, side-effects, and can be reduced with specific antiparkinsonian medication.

Akathisia

Akathisia is a feeling of restlessness and agitation. This side-effect most frequently leads to client noncompliance with recommended drug regimens. The client may not be able to stand still, and may sit or stand repeatedly with an obvious inability to stop. The client may rock or constantly shift weight from one side to the other, or the client may experience this side-effect as sexual excitement. Typically the emotions experienced with this side-effect are anger, fear, and desperation.

TABLE 16-12.
DRUGS USED AS ANTIPARKINSONIAN AGENTS

GENERIC NAME	TRADE NAME	USUAL DAILY DOSE (mg)
ANTICHOLINERGICS		
Benztropine mesylate	Cogentin	1–6
Trihexyphenidyl hydrochloride	Artane (and others)	2–15
Procyclidine hydrochloride	Kemadrin	5–20
Cycrimine hydrochloride	Pagliane	3.75–15.0
Biperiden hydrochloride	Akineton	2–6
Ethopropazine hydrochloride	Parsidol	50–600
ANTIHISTAMINES		
Diphenhydramine hydrochloride	Benadryl (and others)	25–200
Chlorphenoxamine hydrochloride	Phenoxene	150–400
Orphenadrine hydrochloride	Disipal	50–250
OTHERS		
Amantadine hydrochloride	Symmetrel	100–300

(Harris E: Extrapyramidal side-effects of antipsychotic medications. Am J Nurs 81:1324, 1981)

Akathisia may be mistaken for psychomotor agitation or for a symptom of a thought disorder. If the antipsychotic medication is increased, the akathisia will worsen. However, treatment with an antiparkinsonian medication will curtail the akathisia side-effect.

To differentiate akathisia from anxiety or agitation, the nurse can ask the client if the client had ever felt like this before taking the medication. A "no" answer suggests akathisia. The nurse can also ask if the client feels more comfortable moving around or lying down. If the client responds that moving around is more comfortable, the client is probably experiencing the side-effect of akathisia.

Tardive Dyskinesia

Tardive dyskinesia (*TD*) is the onset of involuntary movements of the buccolingual masticatory area (mouth, tongue, and jaw) and/or choreoathetoid movements of the extremities after treatment with neuroleptic medications.

The movements: (1) are *decreased* by voluntary activity of muscles in the affected areas and temporarily by volition, and *increased* by stress; (2) disappear during sleep; (3) are resistant to treatment with antiparkinsonian drugs; (4) are accompanied by no neurological problems similar to (but not) tardive dyskinesia; and (5) accompany a history of treatment with neuroleptics.[18]

The assessment of TD is complex. Several screening tools exist to determine the presence or absence of involuntary abnormal movements in clients. These tools include the Abnormal Involuntary Movement Scale (AIMS) and the Rockland Simpson TD Rating Scale.

The AIMS tool examines the three major areas where abnormal movements appear: the facial and oral area, the extremities, and the trunk. Each of these three areas is then divided into specific muscle groups (such as those

involved in jaw biting, or lateral jaw movements). Each muscle group is rated from 0 to 4, with 4 representing "severe."[34]

Scrak and Greenstein[34] reported that TD is the most difficult side-effect to identify accurately because involuntary muscular activity occurs in normal populations.

Harris[16] reported that 10% to 20% of patients receiving antipsychotic drugs for a year or more develop TD. To date, no cure has been found for it. Guidelines for prevention include using the lowest possible dosage of antipsychotic medication and, when possible, discontinuing the drug no more than three months after the initiation of therapy. All clients on antipsychotic medication should be screened for TD at least every three months.

Early case-finding, *secondary prevention,* cannot be stressed enough. TD can be observed by the nurse before it becomes obvious to family and friends. With the advent of TD symptoms, the neuroleptic medication can be changed, reduced in dosage, or stopped.

In one study,[34] 81 clients with chronic schizophrenia were treated with the neuroleptic Prolixin decanoate (IM) and were observed over a three-year period. Clients attended a structured educational program stressing medication side-effects and discussion with health care providers about the side-effects.

During the first year of the study, 18% of the clients had a mild AIMS rating and 10% had moderate ratings. In the second year of the study, 10% of the sample had mild AIMS ratings and 6% had moderate ratings. In the third year, a drop to 3% in both mild and moderate ratings was seen as a result of close monitoring of medication dosage and effects.

Harris[16] also mentioned that general principles of treating EPS include giving all clients a drug-free trial after remaining on antipsychotic medication for six to twelve months. Half of all clients should be able to function without beginning medication again.

All antipsychotic medications can produce changes in the client's symptoms, yet some work with clients while others fail. Also, all psychotropic medications have the potential to produce side-effects, yet some may produce more of one side-effect than others. For instance, while chlorpromazine does not produce the greatest incidence of EPS among the antipsychotic medications, it commonly causes sedation.

Because EPS are so uncomfortable and frightening to clients, some clinicians treat all clients on antipsychotic medications with prophylactic doses of antiparkinsonian drugs (AP). Precautions for the use of AP drugs are listed in Table 16-13, and other contraindications and interactions are outlined in the drug card.

In addition to extrapyramidal side-effects, other possible side-effects of antipsychotic medications include: sedation, orthostatic hypotension, alterations in sexual function (decreased sex drive or ejaculatory difficulty), depression of hypothalamic functions, seizures, decreased tolerance to alcohol, anticholinergic side-effects (dry mouth, nasal congestion), photosensitivity, cholestatic jaundice, agranulocytosis, pigmentation of the skin and eyes, pigmentary retinopathy, hyperglycemia, cardiac changes, and gastrointestinal distress.

Various precautions exist for administering psychotropic medications. For example, the administration of oral liquid psychotropic medications along with other liquids (such as juice) is a frequent practice. However, many of the medications used with psychiatric clients are prone to incompatibility reactions when mixed with other liquids, due to the drugs' acid–base characteristics. This unintended reaction may cause serious underdosing of the client. Thioridazine (Mellaril), for example, is incompatible with orange "drink." Chlorpromazine (Thorazine) is incompatible with cranberry juice.[19]

Psychotropic medications are given because the symptoms of a thought disorder are troublesome to clients, and promote a sense of discomfort that can reach acute proportions. Medications are administered as part of a treatment program, and clients take part in planning this program.

Medications are not given solely to control clients. In some instances clients may be experiencing a thought disorder and threatening to harm others. In these cases, the clients may receive psychotropic medication against their wishes. These are seen as temporary situations, and

are overcome as clients experience relief from the anxiety and panic of the experience.

The client should understand the nature of the medication, the benefits of taking the medication, and possible side-effects. Client compliance with the prescribed medication regimen is a major factor in the client's being able to remain out of the hospital once discharged. Staff can promote client compliance with the medication regimen by adopting the perspective that clients can and will actively participate in their treatment and will be treated as partners in the treatment-planning process.

Coordination of Treatment Modalities

Heinrichs and Carpenter[17] developed a model for use in selecting from the various options for a therapeutic approach to use with a client with a thought disorder. Some clients manifest "excessive activation" in the form of hallucinations, delusions, and emotional chaos. Other clients, however, manifest "deficit" symptoms of apathy, social withdrawal, reduced energy level, narrowed fields of interest and thought, decreased motivation, and dampened emotions. Deficit symptoms result from inadequate activation.

As shown in Figure 16-3, clients function best (75% on the vertical axis) when there are intermediate levels of arousal (50% on the horizontal axis). For example, students may experience this relationship when taking an exam: the student must have some arousal to take the exam in order to perform well, but too much arousal can lead the student to panic during the exam and perform poorly.

All individuals with a thought disorder have varying patterns of arousal and functioning. Phil, for instance, typically spent days alone in his room. His parents altered their life (by not leaving Phil alone) in an attempt to prevent the more bizarre behaviors of Phil's thought disorder from happening. At times, however, when Phil's parents argued and fought, he became anxious and wandered around the neighborhood talking to himself. His typical state demonstrated the deficit symptoms of a thought disorder.

TABLE 16-13.
PRECAUTIONS FOR THE USE OF ANTIPARKINSONIAN (AP) AGENTS

Prophylactic AP medications have not been shown to prevent all EPS.
Not all patients develop EPS.
Excess doses of AP drugs can cause atropine psychosis.
Use of AP medications may decrease the blood level of antipsychotics by interfering with absorption.
AP medications may worsen the symptoms of TD or may add to the risk of developing TD.
AP medications have their own side-effects.
AP medications add to the patient's expense.

(Harris E: Extrapyramidal side-effects of antipsychotic medications. Am J Nurs 81:1324, 1981)

benztropine mesylate

(anticholinergic, antiparkinsonian)

Cogentin

Action: Blocks cholinergic receptors in CNS and may lower reuptake and storage of dopamine in nerve endings. Reduces tremor.

Uses: Treatment of parkinsonism; also, dystonia associated with drugs used to treat neuroleptic diseases

Side-effects: Dry mouth, blurred vision, mild nausea, constipation, drowsiness, nervousness, urinary retention

Toxic effects: CNS depression preceded or followed by CNS stimulation

Contraindications:
- Hypersensitivity
- Glaucoma
- GI obstruction
- Prostatic hypertrophy
- Myasthenia gravis

Precautions:
- Pregnancy
- Elderly
- Lactation
- Tachycardia

Interactions:
- Haloperidol, phenothiazines (effectiveness decreased)
- Tricyclic antidepressants (adverse effects increased)

Nursing implications:
- Monitor daily bowel activity.
- Monitor intake and output for urinary retention.
- Assess blood pressure and temperature.
- Administer with food to decrease GI symptoms.
- Evaluate mental status.

Client teaching:
- Maintain ample fluid intake.
- Avoid OTC medications unless directed by physician.
- Avoid abrupt withdrawal from drug therapy.

A focus of treatment for Phil would include social stimulation, such as in a day treatment program, occupational counseling, social skills training, and therapy (counseling) that would assist Phil to better understand his life, his coping strengths, and his weaknesses. Phil's arousal or even his anxiety level may initially increase when he first labels and discusses problems. Individual, group, and family therapy would be recommended for Phil.

Other clients, however, may be over-aroused. These clients actively hallucinate, engage in extreme physical movements, and seem very active in many areas of their lives, although in ways that do not contribute positively to their quality of life and their relationships with others. These clients may need a more controlled environment and decreased environmental stress.

Clinicians can provide over-aroused clients with specific times for large muscle movement, rest, and medications. With these clients, counseling may include family and client education about the nature of the illness and similar topics (see the section of this chapter on The Family Environment for a description of these programs). Individual and group work with the client can also help the client establish rapport and trust with the staff and begin to regain the intellectual and interpersonal competencies the client has lost or has never had the opportunity to develop.

Nurses have a unique opportunity in working with clients with a thought disorder because they can intervene with clients immediately when problems arise or when clients communicate in a disturbed manner. This is a significant and responsible role for nurses, since it is often the first time clients have experienced a relationship with another person who will assist in their development.

Nurses are also in an excellent position to develop and coordinate treatment plans tailored to individual clients. They talk with the family when they come to visit,

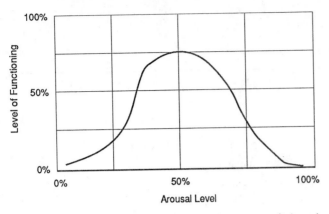

Figure 16-3. The effect of arousal on client functioning. (Adapted from Heinrichs D, Carpenter W: The Coordination of Family Therapy With Other Treatment Modalities for Schizophrenia. In McFarlane W (ed): Family Therapy in Schizophrenia. New York, Guilford Press, 1983.)

they can make home visits, and they can talk with and observe clients in the hospital unit or day treatment unit. Nurses have the opportunity to evaluate their own reactions to clients as clients behave in the presence of the nurse. Nurses have the best opportunity to observe and assess clients for possible distortions in daily living and thought.

Birckhead[6] outlined techniques for the nurse to use in working with clients with a thought disorder in group therapy, a much-needed form of treatment. Clients can make use of this modality, and often state their appreciation for the opportunity to talk with others.

The nurse can also provide opportunities for clients to obtain or regain social skills competencies. "Personal Effectiveness Training"[23] is one way to accomplish this goal. These skills include goal-setting, behavioral research, prompting, positive feedback, and reporting back to the nurse.

Summary

1. The initial work in identifying thought disorders as an illness began in the late nineteenth and early twentieth centuries.
2. Emil Kraepelin and Eugen Bleuler, European physicians, developed many early ideas about what they termed *schizophrenia* (thought disorder). They viewed a thought disorder as including symptoms such as hallucinations, delusions, an illogical connection among thoughts expressed in language, problems with maintaining attention, and an affect that is not congruent with the circumstance.
3. Harry Stack Sullivan, a psychiatrist, and Hildegard Peplau, the founder of modern psychiatric nursing, emphasized the client's withdrawal from, and difficulty with, interpersonal relationships.
4. A thought disorder is complex, and defies succinct definition.

5. Current theories of the etiology of a thought disorder include:
   a. Genetic and constitutional factors
   b. Biochemical factors
   c. Psychophysical factors
   d. Language and information-processing factors
   e. Intrapsychic/interpersonal factors (including family factors)
6. Family-related factors include alliances of some family members against others. In these families there are unclear communication patterns and an over-involvement of parents in the lives of the children who later develop a thought disorder. Typically, family members have a great deal of unresolved conflict with each other.
7. Nurses can assist clients in coping with the impoverished environment in which clients with a thought disorder may live.
8. Nurses work with clients on observable problems, many of which can be inferred from clients' use of language. Clients may also demonstrate poor interpersonal relationships. Nurses' therapeutic use of self facilitates clients' learning more about their present circumstances and methods for dealing with their problems.
9. Medications can decrease clients' symptoms, thereby helping clients maintain some level of functioning. However, medications do not help clients regain intellectual and interpersonal competencies, such as the ability to label feelings and the ability to establish satisfactory interpersonal relationships. These competencies may be regained with psychotherapeutic intervention with a psychiatric/mental health nurse.
10. Many psychotropic medications have permanent side-effects, so the use of medications requires careful monitoring.
11. Many clients can benefit from continued intervention after hospitalization. These programs include assisting the family to work with the member who has a thought disorder, as well as day treatment or home care.

References

1. Acosta F, Yamamoto J, Evans L: Effective Psychotherapy for Low-Income and Minority Patients. New York, Plenum, 1982
2. American Nurses' Association: Taxonomy for the Classification of Human Responses of Concern for Psychiatric/Mental Health Nursing Practice (Working Draft). Kansas City, American Nurses' Association, 1986
3. American Psychiatric Association: Diagnostic and Statistical Manual of Mental Disorders-III-R. Washington, DC, American Psychiatric Association, 1987
4. Anderson C: A Psychoeducational Program for Families of Patients With Schizophrenia. In McFarlane W (ed): Family Therapy in Schizophrenia. New York, Guilford Press, 1983

5. Berger PA: Endorphins in Emotions, Behavior, and Mental Illness. In Temoshok C, Dyke C, Zegans L (eds): Emotions in Health and Illness: Theoretical and Research Foundations. San Diego, Grune & Stratton, 1983

6. Birckhead L: Techniques for group psychotherapy on inpatient units. Issues Ment Health Nurs 6:127, 1984

7. Brain/Mind Bulletin: Universal forms of hallucinations aid brain research. Brain/Mind Bull 5:1, 1980

8. Brown G: Expressed emotion and life events in schizophrenia and depression. J Psychosoc Nurs Ment Health Serv 24:31, 1986

9. Cornblatt B, Lenzenweger M, Dworkin R et al: Positive and negative schizophrenic symptoms, attention, and information processing. Schizophr Bull 11:397, 1985

10. Durham W: Society, culture, and mental disorder. Arch Gen Psychiatry 33:147, 1976

11. Field W: Religiosity as a psychiatric symptom. Perspect Psychiatr Care 11:100, 1978

12. Fromm-Reichmann F: Notes on the Development of Treatment of Schizophrenics by Psychoanalytic Psychotherapy. In Bullard D (ed): Psychoanalysis and Psychotherapy: Selected Papers. Chicago, University of Chicago Press, 1959

13. Goldberg E: Akinesia, tardive dysmentia, and frontal lobe disorder in schizophrenia. Schizophr Bull 11:255, 1985

14. Gregory I, Smeltzer D: Psychiatry. Boston, Little, Brown & Co, 1977

15. Harris E: Antipsychotic medications. Am J Nurs 81:1316–1323, 1981

16. Harris E: Extrapyramidal side-effects of antipsychotic medications. Am J Nurs 81:1324, 1981

17. Heinrichs D, Carpenter W: The Coordination of Family Therapy with Other Treatment Modalities for Schizophrenia. In McFarlane W (ed): Family Therapy in Schizophrenia. New York, Guilford Press, 1983

18. Jeste D, Potkin S, Sinha S et al: Tardive dyskinesia—reversible and persistent. Arch Gen Psychiatry 36:585, 1979

19. Kerr L: Oral liquid neuroleptics. J Psychosoc Nurs Ment Health Serv 24:33, 1986

20. Klein H, Mosberger M, Person T et al: Transcultural nursing research with schizophrenics. Int J Nurs Stud 15:135, 1978

21. Kopeikin S, Marshall V, Goldstein H: Stages and Impact of Crisis-Oriented Family Therapy in the Aftercare of Acute Schizophrenia. In McFarlane W (ed): Family Therapy in Schizophrenia. New York, Guilford Press, 1983

22. Lifshitz M, Kugelmass S, Karov M: Perceptual, motor, and memory performance of high-risk children. Schizophr Bull 11:74, 1985

23. McFarlane W: Introduction. In McFarlane W (ed): Family Therapy in Schizophrenia. New York, Guilford Press, 1983

24. McGinnis J, Foote K: Rapid neuroleptization. J Psychosoc Nurs Ment Health Serv 24:17, 1986

25. Mendel W: Schizophrenia: The Experience and Its Treatment. San Francisco, Jossey-Bass, 1979

26. Menuck M, Seeman M: New Perspectives in Schizophrenia. New York, Macmillan, 1985

27. Mukherjee S, Shukla S, Woodle J et al: Misdiagnosis of schizophrenia in bipolar patients: A multiethnic comparison. Am J Psychiatry 140:1571, 1983

28. Neale JM, Oltmanns TF: Schizophrenia. New York, John Wiley & Sons, 1980

29. Oades R: Attention and Schizophrenia. Boston, Pitman Advanced Publishing Program, 1982

30. Peplau H: Hallucinations and Delusions (Audio Tape). New Braunfels, TX, PFS Productions, 1973

31. Peplau H: Language and Its Relation to Thought Disorder (Audio Tape). New Braunfels, TX, PSF Productions, 1973

32. Reid W: Treatment of the DMS-III Psychiatric Disorders. New York, Brunner/Minzel, 1983

33. Rosenthal T, McGuinnese T: Dealing with delusional patients: Discovering the distorted truth. Issues Ment Health Nurs 8:143, 1986

34. Scrak B, Greenstein R: Tardive dyskinesia: Evaluation of a nurse-managed prolixin program. J Psychosoc Nurs Ment Health Serv 24:10, 1986

35. Seymour R, Dawson N: The schizophrenic at home. J Psychosoc Nurs Ment Health Serv 24:28, 1986

36. Shapiro S: Contemporary Theories of Schizophrenia. New York, McGraw-Hill, 1981

37. Silberman E, Nagler S, Ayalon M et al: Clinical–subjective evaluation of high-risk children: Integration and discussion. Schizophr Bull 11:121, 1985

38. Skilbeck W, Yamamoto J, Acosta F et al: Self-reported psychiatric symptoms among black, hispanic, and white outpatients. J Clin Psychol 40:1184, 1984

39. Sohlberg S: Personality and neuropsychological performance of high-risk children. Schizophr Bull 11:48, 1985

40. Walker J, Cavenar J: Hallucinations. In Walker J, Cavenar J, Brodie H (eds): Signs and Symptoms in Psychiatry. Philadelphia, JB Lippincott, 1983

17

JANET A. CIPKALA-GAFFIN AND GERALD L. CIPKALA-GAFFIN

DEVELOPMENTAL DISABILITIES AND NURSING INTERVENTIONS

Learning Objectives

Upon completion of this chapter the student should be able to do the following:

1. Define the term developmental disability.
2. Define the five major conditions classified as developmental disabilities.
3. Describe two major developmental disabilities.
4. Define the term "dual diagnosis." Give one example of a client with a dual diagnosis.

5. Describe the nurse's role during primary, secondary, and tertiary prevention of developmental disabilities.
6. Name and describe the usefulness of one screening tool and one assessment tool used with the developmentally disabled.
7. List the components of a comprehensive assessment.
8. Describe the impact on the family of having a developmentally disabled child.
9. Define the terms normalization and deinstitutionalization and discuss how these concepts relate to the social integration of the developmentally disabled.
10. Describe the interdisciplinary approach and the nurse's role as a member of the treatment team.

CLINICAL EXAMPLES

BERNIE

John and Susan bring four-year-old Bernie to an emergency room; Bernie is crying. The nurse notes a reddish area on Bernie's hand. The parents report that he had placed his hand in a cup of hot coffee.

The parents also report many concerns about Bernie. He is not social. He does not smile and has a fixed stare. He has a monotonous tone to his voice, and is accident-prone. The nurse takes a complete history and notes other problems. Bernie is referred to a psychiatric hospital with a diagnosis of autism.

FRANK

The school nurse has a conference with Frank's elementary school teacher during which the teacher states that Frank is disruptive in the classroom. He also has a very short attention span. The nurse visits the classroom to observe Frank and suspects that Frank has an attention deficit disorder. The nurse asks the parents to come to the school to discuss Frank, and to suggest a referral to a psychiatric outpatient clinic.

JOHN

John and his mother come to the admitting area of a psychiatric hospital. John is 19 years old and is mentally retarded. His mother is concerned about his depressed mood and his declining interest in taking care of himself. Later, John is admitted with a dual diagnosis of mental retardation and depression.

Introduction

Each of these individuals has a developmental disability. Developmentally disabled persons experience a chronic disability that substantially limits their functioning in broad areas of major life activity central to independent living.[46] These individuals are found in a variety of settings such as homes, hospitals, outpatient clinics, psychiatric institutions, schools, and residential centers. The discipline of nursing plays an integral part in the delivery of care to developmentally disabled individuals as nurses provide numerous services in these varied settings. Also, nurses bring a holistic approach to health care in this special area. Clients and their families are viewed from biological, sociological, psychological, environmental, and cultural perspectives.

The purpose of this chapter is to enable an understanding of the field of developmental disabilities and to contribute to the promotion of healthy adaptation of disabled individuals and their families. Because most developmental disabilities occur early in life, this chapter focuses primarily on the child. Some references will be made to the adult population.

Theoretical Development

What does the term developmental disability mean? The term was coined in 1970 after several legislative debates focused on services being provided to the mentally ill and mentally retarded. During that year, the Developmental Disabilities Service and Facilities Construction Amendments of 1970 law was passed. One of the key amendments of that law was to replace the term "mental retardation" with "developmental disabilities." Numerous definitions have been recommended since then. The current definition for the developmentally disabled, established in 1978, follows.

The Definition of Developmental Disability

A *developmental disability* is a severe, chronic disability that is attributable to a mental or physical impairment or combination of mental and physical impairments; it is manifest before age 22; it is likely to continue indefinitely; and it results in substantial functional limitations in three or more areas of major life activity. These areas are: self-care, receptive and expressive language, learning, mobility, self-direction, capacity for independent living, and economic self-sufficiency.

A developmental disability also reflects the need for a combination and sequence of special, interdisciplinary, or generic care, treatment, or other services that are of lifelong or extended duration and are individually planned and coordinated.[46]

The current concept of developmental disabilities originated with President Kennedy's appointment in 1961 of a President's Panel on Mental Retardation. The purpose of this panel was to propose and plan a national action to combat mental retardation. In 1963, based on the panel's recommendations, President Kennedy appealed to Congress, asking for legislative support. Congressional efforts and the legislative process were instrumental in defining the population designated as developmentally disabled. As a result, several laws were enacted (see Table 17-1).

The major physiological conditions that impede human development and limit functioning are mental retar-

dation, autism, epilepsy, learning disabilities, and cerebral palsy. At times these are linked with emotional disorders, resulting in a dual diagnosis of developmental disability and emotional disorder. In the following sections, these conditions will be defined, the Diagnostic and Statistical Manual of Mental Disorders (DSM-III-R) diagnostic criteria will be presented, and etiology and epidemiology will be discussed.

While epilepsy and cerebral palsy are not psychiatric disorders, they are developmental disorders, which are the focus of this chapter. Children with these disorders often obtain needed psychosocial services when diagnosed as having cerebral palsy or epilepsy. For these reasons, these two disorders are included in this chapter, although they are not psychiatric or nursing diagnoses *per se.*

Mental Retardation

The current definition of mental retardation is that adopted by the American Association on Mental Deficiency. *Mental retardation* is defined as "significantly subaverage general intellectual functioning with deficits in adaptive behavior manifested during developmental periods."[17]

The general consensus among clinicians is that the I.Q. range for mental retardation is 70 or below. The DSM-III-R lists four subtypes of mental retardation (see Table 17-2). However, I.Q. should never be the sole determinant of a diagnosis of mental retardation. Impairment in adaptive behavior must also be present.

The two basic types of mental retardation are clinical and sociocultural.[45] *Clinical retardation* has the following characteristics: impairment is generally moderate to

TABLE 17-1.
LEGISLATION AFFECTING DEVELOPMENTALLY DISABLED PERSONS

P.L. 88-156:	This law amended the maternal and child health provisions of the Social Security Act by adding comprehensive maternity and infant care projects targeted toward high-risk mothers. Additionally, this bill authorized grants for state support for mentally retarded persons.
P.L. 88-164:	The Mental Retardation Facilities and Community Mental Health Centers Construction Act of 1963 provided federal funds for the construction of facilities for mentally ill and mentally retarded persons.
Title 1 (a component of P.L. 88-164):	This act provided money for constructing research centers for the study of mental retardation, as well as facilities for mentally retarded persons.
Part A, Title 1:	Matching grants were allocated for up to 75% of the cost of construction of research centers on mental retardation and related aspects of human development.
Part B, Title 1:	Matching grants were provided for construction of university-affiliated facilities for the mentally retarded. Up to 75% of the costs of construction of facilities for research and training of persons to work with the mentally retarded were allocated.
Part C, Title 1:	Matching grants were provided for the construction of facilities focusing on mental retardation.
P.L. 91-517:	The Developmental Disabilities Service and Facilities Construction Amendments were passed in 1970. In this bill, the term *mental retardation* was replaced by the term *developmental disabilities.*
P.L. 94-103:	The Developmentally Disabled Assistance and Bill of Rights Act added autism to the list of developmental disabilities.
P.L. 95-602:	The Rehabilitation, Comprehensive Services, and Developmental Disabilities Amendments of 1978 provided the current definition of developmental disabilities.

TABLE 17-2.
SUBTYPES OF MENTAL RETARDATION BASED ON I.Q.

SUBTYPES OF MR	I.Q.
Mild	50–55 to approximately 70
Moderate	35–40 to 50–55
Severe	20–25 to 35–40
Profound	Below 20 or 25

(American Psychiatric Association: Diagnostic and Statistical Manual of Mental Disorders III, Revised (DSM-III-R). Washington, DC, American Psychiatric Association, 1987.)

profound, it is usually established at birth or at a young age, the condition is stable, and the clinical diagnosis remains essentially unaltered through life.

Sociocultural retardation, however, is highly class-dependent. It is usually not diagnosed until the child enters school, and the diagnosis is usually removed when the person reaches adulthood. The retardation is mild, with the I.Q. ranging between 50 and 70. Economically, educationally, and socially disadvantaged groups are most commonly represented.

Epidemiology

The number of mentally retarded individuals in the United States is estimated at 3% of the population, or approximately 6 million affected individuals.[25] Tarjan[45] argues, however, that in reality the overall prevalence of retardation is closer to two million, or 1%. He states that the "standardization" of I.Q. tests contributes to inaccurate results for individuals scoring 70 or below. In addition, many individuals are diagnosed as retarded on the basis of I.Q. only. Many more males than females are mentally retarded, by a ratio of 65 to 35.[45]

Etiology

According to the American Psychiatric Association, 30% to 40% of cases of mental retardation have no clear etiology. In the remaining cases, approximately 5% involve hereditary factors (such as genetic abnormalities); 30% result from early alterations in embryonic development; and 10% are associated with pregnancy and perinatal problems. In approximately 5% of cases, the mental retardation is caused by a physical disorder acquired in childhood (such as an infection). Fifteen percent to twenty percent of cases are associated with environmental influences and mental disorders (such as poor parenting or an early-onset language and thought disorder in individuals with borderline-level I.Q.s).

As described above, etiologic factors may include biological, psychological, or environmental factors, or a combination. The prevalence of mental retardation is the same in upper and lower socioeconomic groups. Specific causal factors are linked, however, to the lower socioeconomic groups, in which lead poisoning and premature births are more common. The age of diagnosis of mental retardation depends on the degree of severity; those with the more severe illness are usually diagnosed earlier.

Autism

For many years there have been varied definitions and descriptions of autism. As early as 1911, Bleuler[6] defined *autism* as a thought process disorder in the schizophrenic syndrome. Kanner[19] believed that autism occurs before the second or third year of life, and thus called the syndrome infantile autism. He defined *infantile autism* as "an inborn autistic disturbance of affective *contact*." Kanner's premise was that autistic children are unable to relate to others, and thus possess an abnormality in social development (the disturbance of affective contact). Kanner's definition was highly controversial, however, because he saw autism as a disease that affects normal children. Today, the term *pervasive developmental disorders* is used to identify a general class of disorders in which many areas of psychological development are severely affected at the same time.[2] A pervasive lack of responsiveness may be observed in the autistic child's lack of eye contact, lack of separation anxiety, lack of development of peer relationships, and apparent abhorrence of physical contact.[40] Autism is the only recognized subtype of pervasive developmental disorders. Future research may confirm that autism is merely the most severe form of the pervasive developmental disorders.

Clinical Features

The primary manifestations of autism are a lack of responsiveness to others, gross impairment in language skills, and bizarre responses to the environment. These mani-

---

DIAGNOSTIC CRITERIA FOR AUTISTIC DISORDER

1. Qualitative impairment in reciprocal social interaction
2. Qualitative impairment in verbal and nonverbal communication and in imaginative activity
3. Markedly restricted repertoire of activities and interests
4. Onset during infancy or childhood

Note: The DSM-III-R includes specific criteria within each category above.

(American Psychiatric Association: Diagnostic and Statistical Manual of Mental Disorders III, Revised (DSM-III-R). Washington, DC, American Psychiatric Association, 1987.)

festations occur first during infancy or childhood.[2] A *lack of responsiveness* may be noted in a child who fails to make eye contact with its mother. Likewise, a child may fail to develop cooperative play and friendships. *Language impairment* may be demonstrated, both verbally and nonverbally. The child may use pronominal reversal, *i.e.,* use the pronoun "you" instead of "I," or may exhibit delayed or immediate echolalia (the repetition of words or sounds). *Bizarre responses to the environment* may be seen in ritualistic routines, hand flapping, rocking motions, a fascination with spinning objects or flicking fingers, or an unusual interest in inanimate objects, such as a paper wrapper. The diagnostic criteria (DSM-III-R classification) for autistic disorder are listed in the box on page 352.

Epidemiology

Autism is more frequently seen in boys than in girls. However, the disorder is very rare, occurring in only four to five children out of 10,000.[2] The incidence of autism in siblings is more common than in the general population.[2] According to the National Society for Children and Adults With Autism, there are approximately 80,000 children and adults in the United States who may be autistic.[25]

Etiology

As with the definition of autism, there is also controversy over the etiology of the syndrome. Several general theories have been suggested, including psychogenic, biological, and deficit theories that include biochemical, viral, and genetic factors. A single etiologic factor has not yet been identified.

Epilepsy

Although epilepsy is not a psychiatric disorder, it is a developmental disability. The word "epilepsy" originated from the Greek word that means "to seize" or "to halt." Epilepsy is frequently labeled a "hidden" disease because the symptoms, *i.e.,* seizures, are often intermittent and the condition is not as debilitating as mental retardation or autism. There are several types of epileptic seizures, including grand mal seizures, petit mal seizures, and jacksonian seizures. The terms *seizure disorders* or *convulsive disorders* are used interchangeably for the condition of epilepsy.

Epileptic seizures are divided into two major subdivisions: (1) generalized seizures, and (2) partial seizures. *Generalized seizures* are characterized by loss of consciousness. During a generalized seizure, both hemispheres of the brain are affected at once, thereby involving all of the body and its functioning.[5] *Partial seizures* begin in a specific part of the brain and are usually limited to a single function.[5] Partial seizures are further classified based on whether or not consciousness is lost.

Epidemiology

It is difficult to determine accurately the number of individuals who are affected with epilepsy. The Epilepsy Foundation of America notes that a major reason for this is inconsistency in defining epilepsy. Other reasons for not obtaining accurate reports are that (1) people do not always seek medical care because of the stigma associated with the condition, and (2) individuals may be controlled on medication, and therefore less likely to admit that they have epilepsy. In the U.S. there are approximately four million people with this condition.[44] The incidence of epilepsy is particularly high in newborns. In 1984, Sugarman[44] reported a rate of 560 cases per 100,000 newborns. As children grow older, however, the incidence decreases. Epilepsy is found in males at a slightly higher rate than in females.

Etiology

Most epileptic seizures are classified as idiopathic or of unknown cause. However, according to Sugarman,[44] some general causes for seizure activity include the following:

1. Degenerative diseases, structural abnormalities, syndromes, and hereditary disorders
2. Birth injuries (*e.g.,* birth trauma and anoxia)
3. Infections
4. Vascular abnormalities
5. Head trauma
6. Tumors of the brain and central nervous system
7. Metabolic imbalances
8. Exposure to toxins

Cerebral Palsy

Like epilepsy, cerebral palsy is not a psychiatric problem *per se.* However, because some of its manifestations include psychiatric problems, it is included here. *Cerebral palsy* is a nonprogressive disorder characterized by "aberrations of motor function (paralysis, weakness, incoordination) and often other manifestations of organic brain damage, such as sensory disorders, seizures, mental retardation, learning difficulties, and behavioral disorders."[16]

Epidemiology

Estimates of the incidence of cerebral palsy vary. In 1980, it was reported that the incidence ranged from 1:500[3] to 1:650.[24] The United Cerebral Palsy Association reports a rate of 0.3%, or approximately 700,000 to 750,000 Americans who have cerebral palsy.[25]

Etiology

Prenatal, perinatal, and postnatal factors have been identified in the etiology of cerebral palsy.[3,14,24] Examples of these factors are listed in the box below.

Learning Disabilities

The field of learning disabilities is a relatively new one from the standpoint of being a discrete area of investigation and remediation. Although children with learning disabilities have always existed, it was not until the early 1960s, when Kirk[21] called attention to this problem and Cruickshank[9] first used this term, that the field of learning disabilities was born. Initially concerned with school-based academic difficulties, it is now a discipline involved with the educational, psychological, and social aspects and causes of learning disabilities, and their behavioral concomitants.

Many terms have been used to designate a learning disability. Among these are learning disorder, specific learning disorder, attention-deficit hyperactivity disorder, dyslexia, alexia, perceptual handicap, brain damage, neurologic impairment, dyscalculia, and minimal brain dysfunction. Learning disabilities are not a single homogeneous entity. In fact, there is considerable disagreement about the classification and etiology of learning disabilities. Most simply, a learning disability exists when there is a significant discrepancy among several areas of an individual's cognitive functioning. Many more comprehensive definitions have been proposed, but they have suffered from being definitions of what learning-disabled persons are not, rather than what they are. At present, the definition most frequently cited is from P.L. 94-142 (Education For All Handicapped Children Act):

> Specific Learning Disability means a disorder in one or more of the basic psychological processes involved in understanding or in using language, written or spoken, which may manifest itself in an imperfect ability to listen, think, read, write, spell, or do mathematical calculations. The term includes such conditions as perceptual handicaps, brain injury, minimal brain dysfunction, dyslexia, and developmental aphasia. The term does not include children who have learning problems that are primarily the result of visual, hearing, or motor handicaps, of mental retardation, or of environmental, cultural, or economic disadvantage.[12]

The DSM-III-R specifies a list of conditions commonly placed in the category of learning disabilities. The box on page 355 lists diagnostic criteria for several such diagnoses.

Epidemiology

While it is difficult to determine the exact prevalence of learning disabilities, federal agencies estimate that about 12% of the public school population alone may be in need of some type of special education.[12] Approximately 75% of these students exhibit some type of learning disorder. It is obvious that learning disabilities require major attention from health care providers and educators.

Etiology

The greatest difficulty in identifying and defining specific learning disabilities has been the inconsistency in etiologies and behavioral manifestations present in this population. The most notable question is whether learning disabilities are a result of minimal brain damage. Because many learning disabled students show no demonstrable neurologic dysfunction, this question remains unanswered. Another major complication is the large number of learning-disabled children who also exhibit emotional and/or behavioral problems in school settings, thus making it more difficult for investigators to sort out exactly what is involved in this disorder. Behavioral correlates of learning-disabled students, as seen by educators and research investigators, include academic retardation, language-use problems, attention deficits and impulsivity, memory and problem-solving difficulties, social adjustment problems, and an external locus of control.

The field of learning disabilities also suffers from a lack of well-demonstrated means for helping these children. Widely accepted teaching practices such as perceptual training, modality preference, and diagnostic-prescriptive teaching have been shown to be of limited effectiveness. Although considerable hope is held out for techniques such as cognitive behavior modification or a task-training model, more research is needed. Remediation is further hampered by the large number of individuals who are "dually-diagnosed" (learning-disabled children whose functioning is limited by a secondary

ETIOLOGIC FACTORS IN CEREBRAL PALSY

PRENATAL FACTORS	PERINATAL FACTORS	POSTNATAL FACTORS
• RH incompatibility	• Prolonged labor	• Head trauma and other neurologic problems
• Intrauterine infection	• Birth injury	• Kernicterus
• Nutritional disturbances		• Meningitis
• Hypoxia		
• Prenatal and congenital infections		

DIAGNOSTIC CRITERIA FOR SELECTED DEVELOPMENTAL DISORDERS

DIAGNOSTIC CRITERIA FOR 315.80 DEVELOPMENTAL EXPRESSIVE WRITING DISORDER

A. Writing skills, as measured by a standardized, individually administered test, are markedly below the expected level, given the person's schooling and intellectual capacity (as determined by an individually administered I.Q. test).
B. The disturbance in A significantly interferes with academic achievement or activities of daily living requiring the composition of written texts.
C. The disturbance in A is not due to a defect in visual or hearing acuity or a neurologic disorder.

DIAGNOSTIC CRITERIA FOR 315.31 DEVELOPMENTAL EXPRESSIVE LANGUAGE DISORDER

A. The score obtained from a standardized measure of expressive language is substantially below that obtained from a standardized measure of nonverbal intellectual capacity (as determined by an individually administered I.Q. test).
B. The disturbance in A significantly interferes with academic achievement or activities of daily living requiring the expression of verbal (or sign) language.
C. The disturbance in A is not due to a Pervasive Developmental Disorder, a defect in hearing acuity, or a neurologic disorder (aphasia).

DIAGNOSTIC CRITERIA FOR 315.31 DEVELOPMENTAL RECEPTIVE LANGUAGE DISORDER

A. The score obtained from a standardized measure of receptive language is substantially below that obtained from a standardized measure of nonverbal intellectual capacity (as determined by an individually administered I.Q. test).
B. The disturbance in A significantly interferes with academic achievement or activities of daily living requiring the comprehension of verbal (or sign) language.
C. The disturbance in A is not due to a Pervasive Developmental Disorder, a defect in hearing acuity, or a neurologic disorder (aphasia).

DIAGNOSTIC CRITERIA FOR 315.40 DEVELOPMENTAL COORDINATION DISORDER

A. The person's performance in daily activities requiring motor coordination is markedly below the expected level, given the person's chronological age and intellectual capacity.
B. The disturbance in A significantly interferes with academic achievement or activities of daily living.
C. The disturbance in A is not due to a known physical disorder, such as cerebral palsy, hemiplegia, or muscular dystrophy.

(American Psychiatric Association: Diagnostic and Statistical Manual III, Revised. Washington, DC, American Psychiatric Association, 1987.)

psychiatric disorder). Clearly, major remedial and therapeutic interventions are still needed in order to ameliorate this difficult situation.

Other Developmental Disabilities

In addition to the five disabilities just presented, two other conditions, *blindness* and *deafness,* can also be included because they meet the criteria for being a developmental disability. Both conditions are continuous, frequently occur during the developmental period, and may limit a person's physical, intellectual, and social development.

Further, it should be mentioned that many clinical manifestations of developmental disabilities overlap. For example, a child with cerebral palsy may also have seizures, or a mentally-retarded child may become psychotic. Figure 17-1 illustrates the overlapping of clinical manifestations.

Dual Diagnosis

In recent years, it has become evident that many children and adults have developmental disabilities in addition to emotional and behavioral problems. These individuals have a *dual diagnosis*—for example, mental retardation coupled with an affective disorder, such as major depression. Russell[36] stated that it is clear that we do not know enough about individuals with a dual diagnosis. Cushwa, Szymanski, and Tanguay[10] also recognized this problem in the mentally retarded populations they studied. They noted that many health professionals are not well trained in mental retardation, and that care-givers of the mentally retarded lack sufficient knowledge and resources to provide psychiatric care to these clients. As with other mental health professions, these problems create serious implications for the psychiatric nurse working with the dually-diagnosed client. The mental health nurse must become knowledgeable about and sophisticated in recognizing these clients and providing appropriate interventions.

CLINICAL EXAMPLE: JENNIFER

Jennifer, a 14-year-old, somewhat overweight, Mexican-American female, is brought to a psychiatric facility for "help" by her mother. She was diagnosed as mentally retarded at the age of 7, and has been in a special school since she was diagnosed. On her most recent Wechsler Intelligence Scale for Children (WISC-R) evaluation, she obtained a Full Scale Score of 66. Jennifer is unable to get to and from school without close supervision, and has difficulty in getting along with the other children in her class.

Within the past month, Jennifer's parents have noticed a change in her behavior and, being very concerned, brought her to the outpa-

tient clinic. Jennifer has refused to go to school, and has not been the cheerful and happy child they have been accustomed to. She has slept more and eaten only one small meal a day. Her mother reports that "she doesn't want to do much around the house." Also, the toys she used to love to play with have gone untouched. At the clinic Jennifer appears to be a quiet, withdrawn, and sad adolescent. Her hair hangs down in her face, and she avoids any eye contact. No thought disorder is present. After a thorough assessment, the therapist recommends further evaluation to rule out a major depression.

Mental Retardation

Most of the literature on dual diagnosis has been associated with the mentally retarded population. It is estimated that the incidence of psychiatric disturbances in mentally retarded children ranges from 25% to 100%.[48] Webster[48] reported that, in very young preschool children, he was unable to find a child who was simply retarded without any emotional disturbance. O'Connor[29] added that, in severe forms of psychopathology, retardation and behavioral disorders develop concomitantly from a point very early in life.

Numerous research studies have examined the relationship between mental retardation and psychiatric dis-

orders.[22,38] It is beyond the scope of this chapter to examine these studies. However, at some point, the nurse may find further exploration of these studies to be useful in clinical practice.

Others at Risk

Mentally retarded people are not the only developmentally disabled individuals at risk for psychopathology. Individuals with cerebral palsy, epilepsy, and language disorders are also vulnerable. In one study,[7] 53 out of 100 children between the ages of 2 and 13 who were referred to a community speech and hearing clinic were also found to suffer from an emotional disorder. A variety of

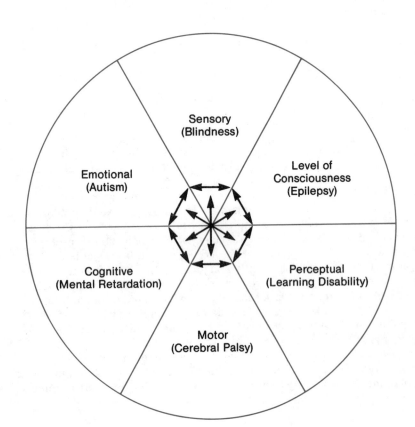

Figure 17-1. Overlapping of clinical manifestations of disabilities. (Seidel M: Career Development in the Health Professions: Nursing Care of Children With Mental Retardation and Other Developmental Disabilities. University of Washington School of Nursing and Child Development and Mental Retardation Center, 1976.)

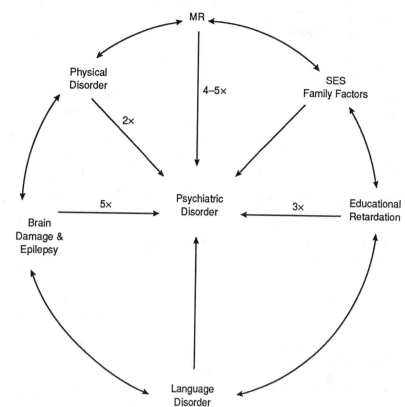

Figure 17-2. Association of psychiatric disorder in children with other handicaps. Rates of psychiatric disorder shown as multiples of prevalence figures for normal or comparison population. Approximately 50% of language-disordered children have associated psychiatric and behavioral disorders. (By permission: Russell A: The Mentally Retarded, Emotionally Disturbed Child and Adolescent. In Sigman M: Children With Emotional Disorders and Developmental Disabilities: Assessment and Treatment. Orlando, Grune & Stratton, 1985.)

factors may influence this high rate of emotional disturbances among developmentally disabled children. Some of these factors and their influences on the genesis of psychiatric disorders are depicted in Figure 17-2.

Assessment

Child Assessment

A complete, comprehensive assessment is essential when determining the diagnosis of a child with a developmental disability. The components of a comprehensive assessment are listed in the following box. The nurse is not expected to be able to complete all areas of assessment alone. In fact, even Master's-prepared nurses work in collaboration with other team members to provide a comprehensive assessment of clients. Nevertheless, the nurse can provide valuable information in many of the assessment areas.

The assessment should always begin with a *parent interview.* The parents are most knowledgeable about the child, and can provide a wealth of information. Initially, the child's presenting problems are explored. The interviewer attempts to elicit specific information about the behaviors exhibited by the child. For example, the parents are asked, "What exactly does the child do? Tell me when it happens? What time of day? What are the circumstances around the change in behavior?" Ample time should be allowed to complete the initial interview in

order to get a good data base. Other areas that should be assessed at this time are the developmental history of the child, including the mother's pregnancy, labor, and delivery. Information about the child's developmental milestones is also essential. Sometimes questionnaires are used to gain additional information about the child's development—for example, the Adaptive Behavior Scale (AAMD) or the Alpern-Bohl Development Profile (see Table 17-3).

COMPONENTS OF A COMPREHENSIVE ASSESSMENT

A. Parent interview
B. Medical examination
C. Child interview
   1. Behavior
   2. Cognition
   3. Mood and affect
   4. Language
   5. Play
   6. Social interactions
   7. Gross/fine motor movements (skills)
D. Assessment of family functioning
E. Assessment of the environment
F. Other testing

TABLE 17-3.
ASSESSMENT TOOLS

TOOL	PRIMARY OBJECTIVE	AGE RANGE	ADMINISTRATION TIME
Brazelton Neonatal Behavioral Assessment Scale	Measures reflexes, motor responses, and interactive behavioral responses of newborns. The main emphasis is on observation and rating of infant interactive behavior. Also provides stimulation assessment of neurologic adequacy and estimates of attentional excitement	3 days–1 month	30 minutes
Alpern-Bohl Developmental Profile	Assesses gross motor, fine motor, language, conceptual, social, and self-help skills	0–12 years	30–40 minutes
Home Observation for the Measurement of the Environment	Identifies children at risk for developmental problems due to inadequate home environments	0–3 years	Varies
Adaptive Behavior Scale (AAMD): for infants and early childhood and for school-aged children	Measures independent functioning, physical development, communication skills, conceptual skills, play, self-direction, personal responsibility, and social skills	0–6 years ≥7 years	Approximately 30 minutes
Peabody Individual Achievement Test (PIAT)	Measures school readiness and academic achievement	2½–18 years	30–40 minutes
Stanford-Binet Intelligence Scale*	Measures intelligence. Primarily verbal items, with some performance items for preschool years. Strongly predictive of academic achievement	2 years–adult	30–90 minutes
Wechsler Preschool and Primary Scale of Intelligence (WPPSI)	Measures intelligence from the standpoint of verbal and performance scores	4–6½ years	Varies
Cattell Infant Intelligence Scale*	Measures intelligence. Better for exceptional children	3–30 months	20–40 minutes
Bayley Scales of Infant Development: Motor Scale, Mental Scale, and Infant Behavior Record	Evaluates gross and fine motor skills, language, and other areas of cognitive development. Evaluates interpersonal, affective, motivational, and interest levels of sensory experience	2–30 months	45–60 minutes

* Primarily diagnostic.
(Abstracted from Roberts PH: Nursing Assessments—Screening for Developmental Problems. In Krajicek M, Tearney-Tomlinson A: Detection of Developmental Problems in Children: Birth to Adolescence, pp 9–30. Baltimore, University Park Press, 1981.)

The *medical examination* usually follows the initial interview. As always, it should include an exam of all of the systems. This is usually performed by the physician with the assistance of the nurse. Particular attention is given to hearing and vision testing to determine if the problem is related to a sensory deficit. The nurse can perform visual screening, such as the Denver Eye Screening Test (DEST), and assist the physician or nurse practitioner in obtaining a health history.

Time should always be allotted in the assessment process for the *child interview*. The child is observed for *behavior, cognition, mood* and *affect, language, play,* and the *ability to interact* with the interviewer. The child's play is an extremely useful medium for evaluation of the child's ability to interact with others, including the parents. During the child interview, an assessment of *gross and fine motor movement* should also be made.

The next essential component of the comprehensive assessment is the *assessment of family functioning.* When assessing family functioning, it is crucial to assess the parent–child relationship. The way the child and parents relate to one another is a major area of concern in relation to developmental disability. For example, children with developmental disabilities are at great risk for secondary emotional problems. If there appear to be problems in the parent–child relationship, the clinician must address the problems and institute interventions accordingly. Observations of the parents' perceptions of the child should also be included. For example, the clinician should assess how the parents speak of their child. Do they speak of him/her in a positive manner? Additional areas, such as discipline and the parents' allowance for the child's autonomy, are important to assess. Who disciplines the child? Is the discipline consistent? How does the child respond? Do the parents feel guilty when disciplining? Do the parents allow the child freedom to play or to go to others? Must the child be with a parent at all times? All of these questions and observations should be included when assessing parent–child relationships. (A more detailed discussion of family functioning in response to having a developmentally delayed child will be presented later in this chapter.)

The assessment is not complete without exploring the child's *environment.* Here the nurse can contribute important information from home and school visits. Children may act very differently in school and at home than when they are examined in an office. Therefore, it is necessary to observe the child further in his or her natural environment. Areas assessed in the child interview should also be included here, *e.g.,* social functioning in-

CLINICAL EXAMPLE: JOSHUA

Joshua is a three-year-old black male who is first seen in a pre-school setting by a student nurse working with the Head Start Program. She had been asked to come and observe Joshua for the following reasons: (1) he is inattentive, (2) he has difficulty "keeping up" with the other children, especially on the playground, and (3) his speech is limited and difficult to understand. The student nurse administers a Denver Developmental Screening Test under the supervision of her instructor. The findings point out delays in two areas, language and gross motor development. The instructor recommends that Joshua be retested in three weeks to be certain that the initial findings were accurate.

The results of the second screening are the same. The nurse explains the results to Joshua's parents and provides information about where further examination can be performed. When they arrive at the outpatient child psychiatric clinic, Joshua and his parents are seen by a nurse who begins to obtain further information on the presenting problems.

The father reports that the family is intact and includes his wife and two additional children, ages seven years and six months. The father had worked as a car salesman until two months ago, when he was laid off. The mother, a part-time teacher, was forced to go back to teaching. These changes have made it very difficult and stressful at home, as reported by the mother. The father now assumes many roles that he previously did not fulfill, and he states adamantly that he doesn't like women's work. There appears to be good communication between the parents, however, and they state in the interview that they have always been able to talk to each other.

Observations of Joshua relating to his parents are positive. Both mother and father are very affectionate toward their son and speak of him in a positive manner. Joshua has some difficulty, however, in separating from his mother. When this occurs, she reassures him that she will be back, and leaves with the father until asked to return.

The clinician, in reporting on the interview, states that Joshua appears to have difficulty focusing on one toy during play, *i.e.*, he played with five different toys in one minute. During the interview he was very active, climbing on chairs and counters (*behavior*). He was able to say his full name, and responded accurately to most questions. There was no indication of any disturbance in thought processes (*cognition*). He was happy and smiling during the interview, and cried appropriately when he fell once (*mood and affect*). There did appear, however, to be an expressive language difficulty that necessitated further exploration. Sentence structure was limited to three words (*language*). Joshua's play was also very scattered; his attention span appeared limited. Occasionally he threw a toy across the room. He was engaging with the clinician, and asked her to play with him, yet he initiated interactions only a few times (*social*). He appeared to like the blocks the most, but became very frustrated when he could not stack them (*play*). Joshua further seemed to have difficulty in both gross and fine motor movements. He had difficulty unbuttoning his coat, and was very awkward at holding and throwing a large ball (*gross and fine motor movements*).

Depending on the findings of the initial components of the assessment, especially the child interview, *additional testing* may be needed. In Joshua's case, a more thorough examination in the areas of speech and language is indicated. Further testing in the area of adaptive behavior is also ordered, *i.e.*, the Adaptive Behavior Scale (AAMD) and the Alpern-Boll Developmental Profile. The psychologist, after being apprised of the case, also recommends I.Q. testing utilizing the Stanford-Binet Intelligence Scale (1972) and the Wechsler Preschool and Primary Test of Intelligence (WPPSI). These tests are listed in Table 17-3.

---

teractions, behavior, play, gross and fine motor movements, and language. One assessment tool used by nurses in the home is the Home Observation tool.

The above Clinical Example illustrates the components of a comprehensive assessment. An assessment report by the clinician is included.

Infant Assessment

Because special attention is being paid to infant assessment of developmental disabilities, it is important that the nurse be knowledgeable about neonatal assessment. A few of the infant assessment and screening tools used most widely are the Brazelton, the Cattell, the Gesell, and the Bayley scales. To explore these tools in detail is beyond the scope of this chapter. Only the Brazelton and Bayley Scales will be discussed.

The Brazelton Neonatal Behavioral Assessment Scale measures 27 behavioral responses, including the neonate's inherent neurologic capacities, as well as the neonate's responses to certain sets of stimuli.[32] The items of

the scale are repeated several times, and the neonates receive a score based on their best performance. This tool is valuable for teaching parents about their child's behavioral patterns and temperament.

The Bayley Scales of Infant Development is regarded as "the best researched and standardized infant test available."[29] The test is divided into two areas, one evaluating the infant's mental age and the other evaluating psychomotor development. This tool also includes behavioral observations of the child.

Both of these tests can be administered by nurses, after they have received specific training and instructions.

Many screening and assessment tools have been discussed in this section. Assessments at regular intervals to observe patterns of development and adaptation are extremely helpful when working with developmentally disabled children. Longitudinal assessments help nurses to organize individual programs and to assist children in reaching their maximum potential. Individuals with developmental disabilities should be reassessed during infancy, childhood, adolescence, and adulthood.

ASSESSMENT	NURSING INTERVENTIONS	EVALUATION CRITERIA

Inpatient hospitalization of an autistic child

NURSING DIAGNOSIS: Potential for elopement and increased level of anxiety due to a new environment

SUBJECTIVE DATA

"I'm not sure if he'll stay with you—he may try to run away." (mother's statement)

OBJECTIVE DATA

Bernie does not have a sense of environment. Changes in his routines create anxiety.

(Rationale for nursing interventions is provided if it is not self-evident.)

1. The primary nurse will give the parents and Bernie a tour of the Unit.

2. Bernie will be introduced to staff members and other patients slowly. No more than 3 individuals will be introduced per day. (*Rationale:* A limit was placed on interactions with others to decrease anxiety and change for Bernie.)

3. Prepare a routine that includes a schedule of daily activities as similar to those at home as possible, *e.g.,* meals, naps, and playtime, to ensure consistency in his daily life. (*Rationale:* Autistic children resist change and need very structured programs.)

4. Inform Bernie of activities in his daily routine, such as when it is time to get dressed. Encourage independence, but remain available for assistance. (*Rationale:* Communicating with Bernie is essential to allay anxiety while modeling the use of language. Hospitalization may cause regression. Independence is encouraged to maintain the child's present level of functioning.)

5. Obtain baseline data for one week. Observe and record behavior every shift until treatment planning on December 11. Pay particular attention to:
   a. Attempts to run away
   b. Self-abusive behavior
   c. Abilities to complete activities of daily living (*e.g.,* toileting, eating).
   d. Tantrums
   e. Stereotypic behavior (hand flapping, spinning objects, rocking)
   (*Rationale:* Data is needed to formulate appropriate nursing interventions and to evaluate the client's progress.)

Bernie will become familiar with his surroundings on the ward, including his room, by December 11. By December 28, Bernie will adjust to the Unit and his primary nurse.

By December 11, data collection will be completed.

NURSING DIAGNOSIS: Alterations in Conduct/Impulse Control (21.)

SUBJECTIVE DATA

"No, no, no!" (client, while biting his hands)

1. Ignore tantrums when the client is not engaging in life-threatening or

By December 11, Bernie's temper tantrums will decrease in number to 5 per day. By

(Continued)

ASSESSMENT	NURSING INTERVENTIONS	EVALUATION CRITERIA
OBJECTIVE DATA The client demonstrates self-mutilating behavior and tantrums.	mutilating behaviors. (*Rationale:* Ignoring tantrums decreases their frequency. Self-injurious behavior is similarly ignored unless it is life-threatening, in which case a totally different approach should be used, *e.g.,* stopping the abusive behavior and ignoring the tantrum. Paying attention to the behavior, even if it is negative, is still reinforcing.)	December 18, temper tantrums will decrease to 2 per day.
	2. If the tantrum is accompanied by hand biting, continue to ignore the tantrum.	By December 11, handbiting will decrease to 4 times per day. By December 14, handbiting will decrease to 2 times per day.
	3. Record what happens before the tantrum, what exact behavior Bernie demonstrates, and what the nurse did afterward. (*Rationale:* Precise record-keeping is essential in data collection.)	
	4. Label Bernie's feelings, *e.g.,* "You were angry or mad because. . . ." (*Rationale:* Labeling of feelings is done to assist Bernie in learning about feelings and to increase language.)	
	5. Supervise on 1:1 (nurse-patient ratio) basis for 48 hours to determine if there is any aggression toward staff or other clients.	By December 6, the need for close supervision will be determined.
	6. If Bernie strikes out at others, hold his hands down and say "No hitting." Then put him in time-out for 2 minutes. (Time-out should be in a quiet area where there is no stimulation or distraction.)	

NURSING DIAGNOSIS: Withdrawal/Social Isolation (23.02.01)

SUBJECTIVE DATA "He usually plays alone." (mother) **OBJECTIVE DATA** Bernie is observed playing alone in a corner in a room full of children.	1. Schedule 1:1 time with a primary or associate care-taker, *e.g.,* 2 hours each shift daily. Interactional time should be the same each day, such as 9–10 a.m. and 1–2 p.m. (*Rationale:* Consistent staff and meeting times assist in developing trusting relationships.)	By December 11, the client will demonstrate trust with the primary caretaker.
	2. When speaking to Bernie, gently hold his head so that he looks at staff and makes eye contact. (*Rationale:* It is important to help the client become aware of those interacting with him.)	By December 11, Bernie will turn his head when his name is called. By December 18, he will tolerate having the staff make contact and not try to run away.
	3. Schedule Bernie during the second week to partake in one play group activity with	By December 14, Bernie will tolerate playing with other children for 10 minutes. By

(Continued)

NURSING CARE PLAN: BERNIE (CONTINUED)

ASSESSMENT	NURSING INTERVENTIONS	EVALUATION CRITERIA
	other children in the age range of 2–5 years. Increase as tolerated. (*Rationale:* Play helps client become aware of peers and learn to interact with them.)	December 21, Bernie will stay in group play for 20 minutes.

NURSING DIAGNOSIS: Impaired Verbal Communication (20.02)

ASSESSMENT	NURSING INTERVENTIONS	EVALUATION CRITERIA
SUBJECTIVE DATA "He seems to be losing ground; he doesn't talk that often." (mother) **OBJECTIVE DATA** Bernie says about 20 words.	1. A speech therapist is scheduled to see Bernie every day from 2–4 p.m. 2. Give praise when Bernie puts names to activities, people, and the like. Also reinforce this achievement with stickers. Record language gains, *i.e.,* which words he has learned. 3. Be sure that Bernie's attention is gained before speaking to him. Speak in short, concise sentences.	By December 11, Bernie will repeat words said to him by staff related to his daily activities. By December 21, Bernie will begin to say words (on his own) related to his care. By December 11, Bernie will listen to staff's directions after the 2nd prompt. By December 21, Bernie will begin to listen to staff when first prompted and demonstrate receptivity.

NURSING DIAGNOSIS: Alterations in Sensory-Acuity (15.02)

ASSESSMENT	NURSING INTERVENTIONS	EVALUATION CRITERIA
SUBJECTIVE DATA "This worries me—it's new." (mother) **OBJECTIVE DATA** Bernie does not pay attention to where he's walking. This has been observed especially at night.	1. Maintain 1:1 supervision for up to 48 hours. Provide extreme caution when Bernie is involved in activities that are potentially dangerous, *e.g.,* bathing (check temperature of water), eating meals (check food for temperature consistency first), or playing with toys (examine for safety).	By December 11, Bernie will play safely and perform activities of daily living with supervision. By December 22, Bernie will not require close 1:1 supervision.

(Continued)

Nursing Assessment: Bernie

Bernie, an attractive four-year-old Asian-American male, is brought to the inpatient psychiatric hospital on December 4. He is accompanied by his biological parents, John and Susan. The presenting complaints include severe language delay and behavior problems, *e.g.,* running away, tantrums, hand biting, face slapping, hand flapping, and being "generally unmanageable at home." The parents also describe Bernie as a child who plays in "his own world." They state that he often sits on a favorite chair rocking from side to side for hours, and loves to play with the wheels on his cars. His mother reports that he gets very upset if certain rituals aren't followed, *e.g.,* holding his favorite car when he eats. He makes little or no eye contact. Lately, he has been accident-prone, *e.g.,* getting burned and bumping into walls.

The family consists of mother, father, and two sisters, ages two and one. The family lives in a three-bedroom house in a middle-class neighborhood. Both parents work full time, managing their own paper company. The parents report moderate marital conflict that primarily centers around Bernie's care. They state that they have no family in the area, and little social support.

The mother states that the pregnancy with Bernie was unplanned. The pregnancy was uneventful, and Bernie's Apgar score was 9. As an infant, Bernie had several

NURSING CARE PLAN: BERNIE (CONTINUED)

ASSESSMENT	NURSING INTERVENTIONS	EVALUATION CRITERIA
	2. Have visual screening and testing done. 3. When hand flapping occurs, use diversional tactics, *e.g.*, call his name and engage him in another activity. Record when hand flapping occurs and if redirection was successful.	By December 11, results will be back. By December 28, Bernie will be able to be redirected when hand flapping occurs. By January 4, Bernie will have less hand flapping activity.

NURSING DIAGNOSIS: Ineffective family coping

SUBJECTIVE DATA "It's not that bad." (father) **OBJECTIVE DATA** Both parents demonstrated a considerable amount of anxiety and stress during the initial interview.	1. Discuss the need for family therapy with the case coordinator. 2. The primary nurse will meet weekly with the parents to inform them of Bernie's progress. (*Rationale:* Providing information and allowing time for discussion will help to alleviate stress.) 3. Give positive feedback to the parents when they spend time with Bernie.	By December 11, Bernie's parents will have 1 family therapy session. By December 28, the primary nurse will begin to discuss alternatives in Bernie's care in order to decrease family and marital stress.

NURSING DIAGNOSIS: Alteration in Self-Care (24.)

SUBJECTIVE DATA "I can't believe how much work he requires." (mother) **OBJECTIVE DATA** Bernie needs help to cut up food and is unable to dress himself. He can toilet himself with close supervision, however.	1. Assist Bernie with all activities of daily living for 1 week to assess his strengths and deficits. 2. Praise Bernie for demonstrating independence, *e.g.*, if he picks up his shirt to put it on, praise him verbally. Increase expectations accordingly. 3. For reinforcement, put a sticker on Bernie's shirt when he is actively involved in activities of daily living. (*Rationale:* Autistic children need immediate reinforcement.)	By December 11, data will be collected. By December 15, Bernie will assist in dressing himself. By December 30, he will put on his pants. By December 28, Bernie will receive 1 sticker per day.

bouts of colic and had noticeably delayed speech: by age 15 months, he spoke only four words. His present vocabulary is very limited. While he says a few words on his own, he mostly repeats what he hears. His mother also reports that Bernie seemed to withdraw at age two, and did not want to be held or cuddled. This coincided with the birth of the second child. Bernie needs assistance with the activities of daily living.

This is the first psychiatric admission or hospitalization for Bernie. Its purpose is to conduct an intensive diagnostic evaluation of the presenting problems and his autistic behaviors. Previous outpatient evaluations were completed at ages 2½, 3, and 3½ years. The care plan for Bernie, an autistic child, begins on page 360.

Nursing Assessment: Frank

Frank is a seven-year-old Caucasian child who is being seen in the psychiatric outpatient clinic for school problems. Reports from his teacher indicate that Frank has been having difficulty in the classroom. He is always on the go, frequently laughs out loud during the lessons, and has difficulty taking turns with his peers.

The teacher's primary concern is that he is not paying attention and that he is apt to fall behind in his classes. The parents say that Frank was always a very active child, and that they didn't realize that his behavior was abnormal until he started school.

NURSING CARE PLAN: FRANK

ASSESSMENT	NURSING INTERVENTIONS	EVALUATION CRITERIA

Outpatient treatment of a child with attention deficit hyperactivity disorder

NURSING DIAGNOSIS: Alterations in Conduct/Impulse Control (21.)

SUBJECTIVE DATA

"The teacher says that he acts quickly without thinking." (mother)

OBJECTIVE DATA

During the initial interview, Frank spoke out of turn and laughed inappropriately.

(Rationale for nursing interventions is provided if it is not self-evident.)

1. Discuss with the parents the format in which information will be collected on Frank's behavior to determine a baseline.
2. Contact Frank's school teacher to determine the extent of his impulsivity. Also, inform the teacher of the need to collect data for a baseline, which includes type of behavior, frequency of behavior, duration of behavior, and circumstances surrounding the behavior.
3. In addition to collecting baseline information, it is also important to have both the parents and the teacher complete daily behavior rating scales, *e.g.,* the Connors' Behavior Rating Scale. If standardized scales such as the Connors' are not available, the nurse may devise a rating scale; it should include questions relating to impulse control, attention span, and activity level. Using a Likert scale with responses such as "not at all, some of the time, most of the time, or always" gives a good account of observable behavior. This type of data-gathering can be especially useful during the administration of medication because it is aimed at providing valuable information on the effectiveness of drug therapy.
4. When behaviors are determined, assist the parents to construct a behavioral program. Encourage communication between the school and the parents in order to provide consistency. (*Rationale:*

By January 15, baseline data will be collected.

By January 30, a behavioral program will be established.
By February 10, Frank will begin to display less impulsivity.

(*Continued*)

There are no other children in the family. Both parents work full time. The father is a physician and the mother is a nurse practitioner. The family resides in an upper-class neighborhood. There are many family and friends available for support. The parents deny any marital stress. Before the interview ends, the father asks if perhaps Frank may need to be on Ritalin.

The care plan that begins on this page is based on contact with the nurse therapist.

Nursing Assessment: John

John is a 19-year-old, mildly mentally retarded, Filipino male who is admitted to an inpatient psychiatric facility to be evaluated for a major depression. His mother, a psychiatric nurse, reports that for approximately the past month he has been significantly dysphoric (depressed mood) and has lacked interest in the activities that used

NURSING CARE PLAN: FRANK (CONTINUED)

ASSESSMENT	NURSING INTERVENTIONS	EVALUATION CRITERIA
	Behavioral programs are useful in providing structure and in setting limits for children who present with impulsive behavior. However, this approach is most effective when combined with other therapies, *e.g.*, Ritalin.)	

NURSING DIAGNOSIS: Hyperactivity (22.01.07)

SUBJECTIVE DATA "I get bored if I'm not doing something." (Frank) OBJECTIVE DATA Frank stood up and sat down 10 times during the session.	1. Follow previous nursing interventions. 2. Encourage the parents and Frank's teacher to provide stimulation for Frank, as well as set limits on times for rest, *e.g.*, at bedtime and at school lunchtime.	By January 30, a behavioral program will be established. By February 10, Frank will show less hyperactivity. By February 3, the parents and Frank's teacher will indicate that Frank is resting at designated times of the day.

NURSING DIAGNOSIS: Inattention (50.01.03)

SUBJECTIVE DATA "I'm concerned that he won't keep up with the class." (teacher) OBJECTIVE DATA Frank watched TV for 10-minute intervals but appeared restless (childcare worker's observation).	1. Inform the parents and Frank's teacher to collect information on Frank's attention span in order to establish baseline data. 2. Instruct the parents and Frank's teacher to provide praise when Frank pays attention for designated periods of time. Caution the parents and his teacher to be realistic in their expectations. Set limits for a minimum time that Frank must pay attention. Let Frank know the consequences for not complying. 3. Administer Ritalin as ordered (Ritalin trial to begin on February 10). 4. Review with the parents and Frank's teacher the side-effects, times of administration, and record-keeping involved in Frank's receiving medication. (Refer to the section on pharmacology for additional information on Ritalin and other drugs used in treating hyperactivity.)	By January 15, baseline data will be obtained. By January 30, the parents and Frank's teacher will report their expectations for Frank's behavior. By February 10, Frank will pay attention for 15-minute intervals. By February 10, Ritalin trial will have begun. By February 10, the parents and Frank's teacher will discuss the implications of the Ritalin administration. By February 15, Frank will be able to pay attention in the classroom, demonstrating less hyperactivity and less impulsivity.

to excite him, such as playing ball. Other symptoms she has recognized are increased weight gain, disinterest in his physical appearance, increased sleeping, and fatigue. When the mental status exam is performed, John appears sad and lethargic. He has poor eye contact, and only responds when asked questions. His long-term memory is intact, but he has some difficulty with short-term recall. Once during the initial interview, when he cannot remember information, he picks up his chair and threatens the nurse with it. His mother notes that John has also been aggressive at other times in the last month. Outbursts consist mainly of throwing objects. Additionally, in the past week John has begun to use sexually provocative language.

John's mother recalls that her pregnancy, labor, and delivery with John were all normal, but that he did not begin walking until he was 15 months old. At age five there was a noticeable language delay, even after being

(Text continues on p. 370.)
(*Text continues on p. 370.*)

NURSING CARE PLAN: JOHN

ASSESSMENT	NURSING INTERVENTIONS	EVALUATION CRITERIA

Inpatient hospitalization of the dually-diagnosed adolescent (mental retardation, depression)

NURSING DIAGNOSIS: Abuse—Physical (21.02.01)

SUBJECTIVE DATA

"He's been aggressive, throwing things at me and at the walls." (mother)

OBJECTIVE DATA

John picked up a chair and threatened the nurse during the initial interview after becoming frustrated when he could not remember certain facts.

(Rationale is provided for nursing interventions if it is not self-evident.)

1. The primary nurse will check John and his belongings for harmful or sharp objects. This is to be repeated every shift for the first 24 hours. (*Rationale:* Safety is a major issue because John has demonstrated violent behavior. Depressed clients should be examined for any possessions that might be used to injure themselves.)

2. During the first week, the staff will assess John's environment and the circumstances in which his aggressive behaviors occur. (*Rationale:* In designing a behavior modification program, it is necessary to collect information in order to establish baseline data.)

3. The staff will record specifically what happened before each aggressive behavior (antecedent), what the exact behavior was, and the staff response to the behavior (consequence). (*Rationale:* In developing a program, information relating to the antecedent, the behavior, and the consequence provides valuable information in order to develop a plan of care.)

In collecting specific information about John's behaviors for baseline information, it is also important to look for any organic causes for his behaviors and be aware of symptoms such as seizures. (*Rationale:* Sometimes, organic disorders are manifested by symptoms that may mimic those of behavior problems.)

4. During the first 24 hours, the staff will assess John's developmental and cognitive abilities. (*Rationale:* In using a behavioral approach, it is essential to determine the client's developmental and cognitive functioning levels. In John's case, this is even more important because he is mentally retarded.)

5. At treatment planning, the primary nurse will identify a target behavior, and later will discuss the behavior with John. (A target behavior is a behavior that hopefully John will achieve.)

John will be in a safe environment and will adjust to his surroundings by March 16.

By March 22, John will exhibit a pattern of behavior related to his aggressive outbursts.

By March 16, John will demonstrate his cognitive and developmental levels.

By March 22, John will verbalize the target behaviors.

(Continued)

ASSESSMENT	NURSING INTERVENTIONS	EVALUATION CRITERIA

	6. After treatment planning, a program will be constructed and developed for John.
	7. Program for aggressive behavior:
	  a. John will be informed of the targeted behavior, namely, that he is to express his anger and frustration appropriately in words.
	  b. When John communicates his feelings of anger or frustration, the staff will praise him verbally, and he will gain two points that can be applied toward special activities, *e.g.,* staying up one half hour later in the evening (10 points), or playing basketball during quiet-time (20 points).
	  c. For any throwing of or attempts to throw objects, John will be isolated from others or sent to his room.
	  d. After 10 minutes of quiet-time, the staff will discuss his behavior with John at a level that he can understand. (*Rationale:* Because John is mentally retarded, staff should take into consideration his cognitive ability and assess his level of understanding.)
		By March 22, John will verbalize an understanding of the program.
		By March 29, John will express his anger and frustration verbally once every other day.

NURSING DIAGNOSIS: Impaired Range of Expression of Emotions (30.04)

SUBJECTIVE DATA "He's been very dysphoric—he doesn't like to do much any more. He's always sleeping." (mother) **OBJECTIVE DATA** John has exhibited a major depressive episode lasting one month in duration. Further, his mental status exam is consistent with a history of depression.	1. The staff will assess John's level of depression and initiate suicide precautions for the first 24 to 48 hours. (*Rationale:* With any depressed client, suicide precautions should be taken until it is determined that the client is not suicidal.) Remove all harmful objects from John's possession and explain to him the purpose for this. Examine John's room and remove any dangerous objects. 2. The primary nurse or designee will reschedule half-hour sessions with John in order to develop trust between them and begin to establish a nurse–client relationship. 3. John will be included in a minimum of one unit activity per shift, *e.g.,* boys' group, for the first week. The number of activities will be increased over time. (*Rationale:* Clients who are depressed	By March 17, John will exhibit a beginning baseline of mood and affect that will be used to assess his depression. By March 17, John will initiate conversation with the primary nurse. By March 28, John will demonstrate a trusting relationship with his primary nurse. By March 18, John will participate in one unit activity per shift. By March 22, John will participate in two unit activities per shift. By March 28, John will indicate a desire to

(*Continued*)

ASSESSMENT	NURSING INTERVENTIONS	EVALUATION CRITERIA
	lack the desire and energy to be physically active and need support and structure.)	participate in ward activities without prompting.
	4. The primary nurse will give feedback to the physician in the event that antidepressant medication may be indicated.	By March 30, John's affect and mood will improve, indicating that antidepressants are not necessary at this time.

NURSING DIAGNOSIS: Impaired Verbal Communication (20.02)

ASSESSMENT	NURSING INTERVENTIONS	EVALUATION CRITERIA
SUBJECTIVE DATA "John's language is embarrassing." (mother) OBJECTIVE DATA During the past week, John has increasingly used provocative language.	1. When John uses provocative language, give him a verbal warning, stating that "that language is not permitted." (*Rationale:* Limit-setting is necessary for inappropriate milieu behavior.)	By March 18, John will stop using sexually provocative language after one warning. By March 27, John will decrease sexually provocative language from one time per day to 0 times per day.
	2. If John continues to use sexually provocative language, give him a second warning and state, "If you do not stop talking like that, you will have to go to your room for 15 minutes." (*Rationale:* Consequences are added if provocative language persists.)	
	3. After John's purpose for using sexually provocative language is determined, John may be included in a sex education class for the developmentally disabled clients on the Unit. (*Rationale:* As with any teenager, there is a need to be informed of sexual development. Developmentally disabled individuals require special education in this area because their cognitive level is lower than that of normal individuals.)	By March 2, John will be able to tolerate participation in a sexual education class for developmentally disabled clients.

NURSING DIAGNOSIS: Alterations in Self-Concept (50.07)

ASSESSMENT	NURSING INTERVENTIONS	EVALUATION CRITERIA
SUBJECTIVE DATA "He doesn't want to take care of himself like he used to." (mother) OBJECTIVE DATA John's appearance is disheveled and unkempt.	1. John will be given instructions for Unit rules regarding activities of daily living. (*Rationale:* Because of John's mental retardation, particular attention should be given to assist John in understanding Unit rules).	By March 19, John will understand the Unit's expectations for activities of daily living.
	2. John will be given verbal praise for maintaining cleanliness.	By March 19, John will dress neatly.

(Continued)

ASSESSMENT	NURSING INTERVENTIONS	EVALUATION CRITERIA
	3. To build self-esteem, initially praise John for attempts to complete self-care. Continue to praise John for increasingly taking responsibility for his care. 4. Provide opportunities to explain things to John in greater detail, especially related to developmental changes. (*Rationale:* Mentally retarded individuals have more difficulty dealing with adolescent issues and bodily changes. This occurs because they have neither the cognitive ability nor the coping skills of normal adolescents. Consequently, mentally retarded people have more pronounced problems with their self-concept.)	By March 22, John will dress neatly and bathe daily. By April 2, John will dress neatly and bathe without prompting. By April 4, John will talk with his primary nurse about adolescent issues.

NURSING DIAGNOSIS: Impaired Sensory Integration (15.04)

ASSESSMENT	NURSING INTERVENTIONS	EVALUATION CRITERIA
SUBJECTIVE DATA "He's been diagnosed as mentally retarded since the age of five." (mother) **OBJECTIVE DATA** John exhibits cognitive deficits for a 19-year-old.	1. Approach John on his level and be certain that he is comprehending information, *e.g.*, have him repeat what was said if he does not seem to understand. 2. John will attend special education classes during the school period. 3. Arrange for John to have successes that are realistic for his intellectual level. Praise him when successful. (*Rationale:* Modified activities should be planned that are appropriate for a mildly mentally retarded adolescent in order to enhance self-esteem.)	By March 22, John will demonstrate an ability to understand information from staff. By March 17, John will attend special education classes. By April 2, John will actively participate in his classes. By March 2, John will demonstrate an increased ease with participating in activities. By April 2, John will accept praise for his accomplishments.

NURSING DIAGNOSIS: Alterations in parenting

ASSESSMENT	NURSING INTERVENTIONS	EVALUATION CRITERIA
SUBJECTIVE DATA "I haven't thought of looking into group homes." (mother) **OBJECTIVE DATA** John will soon be approaching a developmental stage at which he can live independently with supervision.	1. The primary nurse will explore future plans for John with the mother. 2. The primary nurse will present the option of group living for John, and will assess the mother's readiness for this. Cultural beliefs and values will be explored. 3. The social worker will give the mother information about appropriate facilities for John. 4. The primary nurse will help in communication between the mother and John regarding future plans.	By April 15, the mother will begin to talk about future plans for John. By April 18, the mother will discuss with John his feelings about living away from home.

in preschool. At that time he was seen in an outpatient psychiatric facility for a complete evaluation, and was diagnosed as being mildly mentally retarded.

There are two other siblings in the family, Jane, age 23, and Paul, age 21. Both are married and have their own homes near the house in which John and his mother live. John's father died when he was six years old. He and his mother live in a condominium in a middle-class Filipino neighborhood. There are several extended family members who live nearby and who are actively involved with John. John attends a special education school program.

During the parent interview, John's mother voices concern about his aggressive behavior and suggests that a behavioral approach be utilized, because he has been very responsive to behavior modification in the past. She also discusses her concern about the possibility of John's hurting himself, although there has not been any apparent incidence of this yet. The care plan for John begins on page 366.

The Family and Systems Theory

As previously stated, one component of a comprehensive individual assessment is the overall assessment of family functioning. Nursing has long recognized the importance of the family unit and has practiced under the standard of providing family-centered care.[1] In working with developmentally disabled persons, the philosophy of family-centered care is especially important. The family is the "core" unit for the developmentally disabled child. It is where the child functions, finds love and attention, and is physically cared for. The family provides a bridge between the child and society.

The family, a complex group of individuals, has a profound effect on the adjustment of the developmentally disabled child. Similarly, having a developmentally disabled child has serious implications for the family. In order to sift out the reactions that occur, it is helpful to examine how the family works as a system.

General systems theory[47] provides a framework for understanding families as a system. The family is viewed as a dynamic system that cannot operate in isolation. For example, in the case of the family with a disabled child, all family members are called on to assist in the child's care. All of the individuals in the family, working together, provide strength to endure hardships associated with delivering care to the disabled child. Further, the family system interacts with larger systems outside of itself. Some of these are hospitals, clinics, school systems, the community, and society in general (see Fig. 17-3). Families often find their interactions with these systems to be difficult and painful. It is not uncommon for families to be rejected by society because they do not have a "normal" child. The nurse is encouraged to examine how the family functions on its own in society during family assessments.

Family Stress/Family Crisis

The family system experiences frequent periods of stress when there is a developmentally disabled member. The

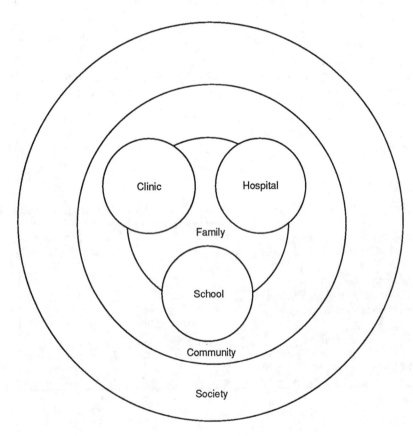

Figure 17-3. Family interactions with other systems.

stress varies from social isolation to increased demands on the care-takers. Some situations may overwhelm the family completely, such as when a family is first informed that their child is mentally retarded. When family coping is greatly impaired, the family is said to reach a crisis state.

Farber[11] described the crisis experienced by the family with a developmentally disabled member as an induction into a new distortive process in family life. This process is divided into the following crisis phases:

Phase 1. The family attempts to handle the disability. There is usually no crisis here because the family is usually successful at maintaining normalcy.

Phase 2. The initial crisis surfaces. For example, family relationships are so distorted that the family concedes that the child is disabled.

Phase 3. Distorted relationships within the family mandate that changes be made. Activities outside the family are restricted. The family realizes that it needs help from other sources.

Phase 4. There are rearrangements in the family. Ages and sex roles are rearranged to balance the deficiencies of the developmentally disabled child. For example, older children assume additional responsibilities.

Phase 5. In this phase, the family is unable to cope with the crisis, and places the child outside of the home.

Many others have also investigated the crises experienced by the disabled family. Hill,[18] in his ABCX (crisis) Model, eloquently described the process families experience when in crisis. He posited this process as a function of A (the stressor event), B (the family's crisis-meeting resources), and C (the definition the family makes of the event). McCubbin and Patterson[26] added to Hill's model and also investigated what happens after the crisis. Their model provided insight into how families cope with such developmental disabilities as cerebral palsy.

There are 10 developmental crisis points for families with disabled children:[30,49]

1. Diagnosis
2. Time for walking
3. Time for talking
4. Occasions when siblings surpass the disabled child
5. When alternative placement is considered
6. Entry into school
7. Management of crises, *e.g.,* behavior problems
8. Puberty
9. The child's 21st birthday
10. When guardianship is needed

In the following sections, the impact of having a developmentally disabled child on the parents, the siblings, and the grandparents will be discussed.

Effects on Parents

With the birth of a developmentally disabled child, parents immediately experience the loss of their expected "normal" child. Parental reactions to the birth have been linked to the influence on and meaning the child has for the parents. Rykman and Henderson[39] enumerated a number of these common meanings:

1. The child is viewed as a physical and psychological extension of the parents.
2. The child enables the parents to experience vicarious satisfaction.
3. The parents experience some measure of immortality with the birth of a child.
4. The child represents a personalized love object.
5. The child provides the parents with the opportunity to experience a sense of worth by meeting the child's dependency needs.
6. Children evoke in parents negative feelings about the limitations and demands of child rearing.

All but the last of these influences are very closely associated with the parents' self-concepts. Therefore, it is understandable that the loss of the expected "normal" child has a profound effect on the parents.

How parents react to the birth of a disabled child is difficult to describe precisely. There are many variations due to the individual characteristics of each parent, *e.g.,* the emotional adjustment of the parents, or their own life experiences. Some authorities say, however, that one of the most common initial reactions is denial. It can be hypothesized that parents use this defense mechanism to lessen the blow to their own self-image of having a disabled child. As with any crisis, many different periods of "ups and downs" are experienced. A mixture of emotional responses such as anger, grief, despair, and acceptance may be experienced by parents at various times during the course of their adjustment. The nurse can find descriptions of the stages associated with this grief process in the works of Kennedy,[20] Goodman,[13] Cohen,[8] and Solnit and Stark.[42] When the parents reach a point of self-awareness, this usually signals that they are beginning to deal with the fact that their child is disabled. This is considered a time of progress. However, if parents fail to reach this stage, serious parental adaptation problems can be anticipated.

A classic, but controversial, description of the ways in which parents respond to having a developmentally delayed child is what Olshansky[30] called "chronic sorrow." In 1962, he proposed that parents having a mentally retarded child suffer from a pervasive psychological reaction, and that this reaction, chronic sorrow, is a natural and understandable response to a tragic event. Olshansky's *chronic sorrow* can be defined as an intermittent, recurrent feeling of sadness that parents experience. The intensity of the sorrow and how it is expressed by parents are based on individual characteristics of the parents. For example, it has been noted that Anglo-Saxon parents tend to try to "cover up" their sorrow. Olshansky stated that chronic sorrow is only alleviated through the death of the child.

Professionals have long debated whether parents really experience this chronic sorrow, or whether they experience progressive stages of adjustment moving toward complete adjustment. Bearing on this issue, a comparative study[49] was conducted to evaluate which pattern

RELEVANT RESEARCH

The goal of this study was to determine which pattern, *i.e.,* chronic sorrow or time-bound grief, best reflected the experiences of parents with retarded children. The subjects in the study were from two groups, social work practitioners and parents of retarded children. One hundred social workers were randomly selected from a county social service department. In addition, 100 parents were selected from among those who had received evaluation services between 1975 and 1977 from a Diagnostic and Treatment Unit for Mental Retardation.

Questionnaires were mailed to the participants. A total of 32 responses to the questionnaires were obtained from each group. The questionnaire consisted of three parts: a free-form graph for depicting the adjustment process, a structured graph, and a direct question, *i.e.,* "Do you experience chronic sorrow?"

From the free-form graph, only one fourth of the parents indicated that they had time bound grief. Interestingly, parents' and social workers' free-form graphs did not differ significantly.

From the structured graphs, data were obtained relating to the parents' and social workers' evaluation of the degree of upset involved at specific developmental points in the child's life, such as birthdays. The results indicate that social workers were very accurate in their perceptions of the parents' feelings about having a retarded child, but that they tended to overestimate how the parents would react to their child's early developmental experiences, while underestimating the impact of later experiences. It is interesting to note that social workers considerably underestimated how upsetting the child's 21st birthday was for the parents.

In response to the question "Do you experience chronic sorrow?" 63% of the parents and 65% of the social workers said yes. Thus, this study tends to support the view that parents do experience chronic sorrow. However, the results are not totally conclusive because continuous sorrow does not appear to exist, but rather, periodic crises occur that are associated with the developmental stages of the child.

Many limitations plague this study. The non-random sample of parents may contribute to a possible bias. Likewise, the sampling of parents from one treatment center may have skewed the results. Also of concern was the very small respondent rate from both groups. Finally, the accuracy of the interpretations of the graphs must be questioned. Despite these limitations, however, there are clinical implications from this study that suggest that chronic sorrow does not seem to be an abnormal response, but is rather a normal reaction of parents who have mentally retarded children. Further, because parents seem to experience crisis at different developmental stages, a continuum of services over the life span must be provided.

(Wikler L, Wasow M, Hattfield E: Chronic sorrow revisited: Parent vs. professional depiction of the adjustment of parents of mentally retarded children. Am J Orthopsychiatry 51:1, 1981.)

of adjustment best reflected the parents' experience of having a retarded child.

See the Relevant Research Box above.

Effects on Mothers

The mother's reaction to a disabled child has received considerable attention in the studies of parental response. Solnit and Stark[42] explored mothers' responses by first looking at maternal responses to child-bearing and then analyzing mothers' experiences following the birth of a child with a defect. Their research provided insight into the anticipatory process of pregnancy. They found that mothers view their expected baby as a composite of representations of "the self" and love objects, *e.g.,* mother, husband, and siblings. Further, the composite representation includes an image of the expected child that was conveyed to the mother-to-be by her mother. During this anticipatory process, basic conflicts and identifications that the expectant mother had had with her own mother are resolved. When a child with a disability is born, this preparatory and, more important, adaptive aspect of the process is interrupted.

Two extreme reactions to the birth of a disabled child were also identified by Solnit and Stark. One extreme reaction was guilt feelings leading to the mother's unend-ing dedication to the child. The other extreme reaction was an intolerance for the child, and an inclination to deny a relationship with the son or daughter.

Some mothers with a disabled child also, at times, fail to relate adequately to other family members when they respond with a guilty, depressed attachment to the disabled child. Other mothers respond by identifying with their disabled child. When this occurs, the mother is narcissistically wounded. This identification is often intolerable for the mother. Moreover, it may be compounded by the mother's need to mourn the loss of the "wished-for child" and to meet the demands of the new baby.

Effects on Fathers

Much less reference is made in the literature to the impact of a disabled child on the father. One study[53] interviewed fathers and found that they often have a more difficult time adjusting to the reality of having a disabled child than do their wives. Fathers may be particularly stressed by the financial burden of caring for a child with a disability, and by having to assume "foreign" roles at home. For example, fathers may assume many new domestic tasks, like cooking and shopping. Thus, fathers do not go unscathed. They too experience the loss of the "normal" child.

Impact on Siblings

A new focus in the field of developmental disabilities is the sibling. Clinicians are aware that siblings are also at risk when there is a disabled child in the family. In fact, it has been reported that psychiatrists treat more siblings of disabled children than disabled children themselves.[33] The siblings most affected in these families are (1) those who are in a developmental transition (*e.g.,* starting school), (2) those who have few or ineffective coping skills, and (3) those who have poor parental relationships.[41] Additionally, older sisters and those closest in age to the disabled child have been identified as being most vulnerable.

Siblings often respond to having a disabled child in the family by expressing anxiety, *e.g.,* nightmares, jealousy, school problems, and behavioral problems. Often the siblings are expected to assume surrogate parent roles. Moreover, siblings struggle with the ambivalence of feeling ashamed of their disabled brother or sister while at the same time feeling a love for them.

Many interesting findings have surfaced from the research on siblings. Grossman[15] found that younger siblings and siblings from lower socioeconomic backgrounds are most affected. Other results from his work indicate that sibling reactions are related to parental reactions and the parents' ability to cope. As well, a major concern of normal siblings is how *not* to identify with their affected siblings.

The research substantiates the grave impact of a child's disability on siblings, and the need for nursing interventions. The nurse is encouraged to refer to Siemon's work[41] for further information when working with this sibling population.

Each family member is touched by the birth of the child with a disability, both individually and as a part of the "whole" family. The family's vulnerability to stress is dependent on variables such as degree of handicap, sex, and birth order of the disabled child, and the family's socioeconomic status, religion, marital stability, and available supports. Obtaining information about these variables provides valuable data in assessing family function, and therefore should be included in the family assessment process.

As can be seen, a complete family history and report of family functioning are central. Chapter 12 provides guidelines for and insight into obtaining a comprehensive family assessment. The nurse is strongly encouraged to evaluate the family as a "whole" or system, while simultaneously assessing each member individually. Through this approach, all family members are likely to receive the attention they need.

Levels of Prevention

Nursing plays a salient role in the prevention of developmental disabilities. One major task of nursing is the prevention of handicapping conditions, not only through counteracting conditions that cause these handicaps, but also through circumventing the secondary problems that result from improper management.[4]

In the first of the three areas of prevention, *primary prevention,* there is a concerted effort to prevent the initial impairment, defect, or illness that may lead to a developmental disability. In *secondary prevention,* the early discovery and treatment of the condition, with the goal of halting the disability, is paramount. *Tertiary prevention* is aimed at providing the best possible care and treatment of the established disability.[28]

Primary Prevention

Primary prevention of developmental disabilities focuses on the areas of immunization, nutrition, education, and genetic counseling. Nurses working in pediatric clinics have a unique opportunity to teach mothers about the necessity for immunization while simultaneously administering these medications to their children. Nurses have also become a vital source of nutritional information delivered to families. The nurse's involvement with the nutritional aspect of pregnant women's care has had a major impact on fetal growth and development. Similarly, nurses have contributed significantly to prevention of child abuse through educational programs on parenting and child-rearing.

Prevention in Various Phases of Pregnancy and Childhood

The most logical time for primary prevention of developmental disabilities is during pregnancy. North[28] suggested that primary preventative efforts may take place during various cycles of pregnancy. Maternal child nurses can intervene with preventative efforts in the following stages:

1. Prevention prior to pregnancy
2. Prevention during pregnancy
3. Prevention at the time surrounding birth
4. Prevention in infancy and early childhood
5. Prevention in the preschool and school years

Prevention prior to pregnancy involves the identification of individuals at risk, *e.g.,* older parents who are at risk for having a child with Down's syndrome, and setting up plans for following these individuals closely. As can be seen in Table 17-4, the risk of having a child with Down's syndrome increases noticeably when a woman reaches the age of 35. With the help of sophisticated tests, such as amniocentesis, and nursing support, combined with education and information, parents can make choices that result in prevention.

Prevention during pregnancy can also be achieved. In this area, nurses can provide general information about proper prenatal care. Protection from chemicals, drugs, and stress is extremely important.

At the time of birth, primary prevention may take the form of nurses assisting mothers to enhance affectional bonding with their infants. Further, this is an opportune

TABLE 17-4.
RISK OF HAVING A BABY WITH DOWN'S SYNDROME ACCORDING TO MATERNAL AGE

AGE OF MOTHER (years)	APPROXIMATE RISK (per pregnancy)
29	1 in 3,000
30–34	1 in 600
35–39	1 in 280
40–44	1 in 70
45–49	1 in 40
All mothers in the population	*1 in 665*

(Reproduced by permission from Motalsky A, Hecht F: Genetic prognosis and counseling. Am J Obstet Gynecol 90:1227, 1964.)

time for nurses to teach mothers who may lack parenting skills and guide individuals who have fewer financial and emotional resources.

Prevention in infancy and early childhood is also crucial. Ensuring that children have immunizations is paramount in this phase. The development of infant stimulation programs has proven to be extremely beneficial in this area of primary prevention. Similarly, it is essential that parents and teachers receive instruction during this phase.

Last, *prevention in the preschool and school years* should not be discounted. School nurses are challenged to guide teachers and parents regarding discipline and educational approaches to children with special needs. Nurses assume the role of advocate for children, and model appropriate approaches to enhance the self-esteem of school-aged children.

Genetic Counseling

A further focus of primary prevention is found in the area of genetic counseling. The genetic counseling field is growing rapidly, primarily in response to advances in technology. Tremendous strides have been made over the years with the advent of gene therapy. The reality exists, however, that the pain of having a child with a congenital anomaly is still being experienced by numerous couples. It has been reported that healthy couples have a 2% to 4% chance of having a child with a birth defect, of which many have a genetic basis.[51] Genetic counseling is indicated when there is a family history of a genetic disorder, a family history of developmental disabilities (with or without a known genetic etiology), a previous child born with a developmental disability, a history of excessive fetal wastage (*i.e.,* miscarriages), or a mother who is 35 years old or older.[40]

Nursing recognizes genetic counseling as a major component of primary prevention. Although nurses working in the area of genetics are usually Master's-prepared, there are still opportunities for other nurses to provide services in this area. Nurses trained in genetics can assist physicians in screening procedures and can con-

tribute by obtaining information for family and individual assessments. Additionally, nurses can collect data for pedigrees, perform physical exams on children, and provide support and counseling to family members. Finally, nurses can be the vital liaison between physicians and families when reinforcement of genetic information and encouragement are needed.

Secondary Prevention

The main area that warrants exploration in this section is the screening for developmental disabilities.

Screening

Often the term "case-finding" is used when discussing screening. *Screening* simply means the process by which children are identified who exhibit suspicious or positive findings, and who, therefore, need further diagnosis and assessment.

Screening Tools. Screening tools can be administered by nurses who are well trained in the procedures for administration. It is suggested that nurses maintain proficiency by practicing administration of the tools with different children at various levels of development. Initial administration under the supervision of someone who is already proficient is strongly recommended. Examples of screening tools are The Washington Guide to Promoting Development in the Young Child, The Denver Developmental Screening Test (DDST), The Gesell Developmental Schedules, and the Developmental Screening Inventory.

Caution must be exercised when using screening tools so that the results are not interpreted nor utilized as diagnostic measures. Rather, they are used to assess a child's developmental level before intervention, and at periodic intervals during intervention or treatment. When there are abnormal findings, a second evaluation is recommended two to three weeks later. If the subsequent findings are abnormal, then a referral is made for further diagnostic evaluation. For example, if the results of a DDST are abnormal, a child may be referred to an outpatient clinic for further evaluation and diagnosis.

Roberts[35] identified a particular type of screening, mass screening, that is particularly important in the prevention of developmental disabilities. *Mass screening* is the examination of large numbers of individuals for a particular syndrome or characteristic, *e.g.,* an enzyme deficiency. Mass screening is often done with newborns. The purpose of newborn screening is to detect genetic disorders and, ultimately, to decrease disorders such as mental retardation. The three tests most frequently performed in neonatal screening are those for phenylketonuria, hypothyroidism, and galactosemia. Other screening programs, such as testing for biofinidase deficiency and Maple Syrup Urine disease, are becoming more common.

Tertiary Prevention

Tertiary prevention is the stage in which rehabilitation occurs and in which nurses assist families to adapt to the presence of a chronically disabled child. As in secondary prevention, nursing care plans are very useful in establishing strategies for action in the delivery of comprehensive care. To assist the nurse in formulating plans of care for the developmentally disabled, examples of care plans for an autistic child, a child with attention deficit disorder, and a dually-diagnosed adolescent have been presented. During tertiary prevention, the nurse combines nursing theories and the nursing process to construct standards of care with the ultimate goal of helping the child and family function to their fullest capacity. The nursing care administered during tertiary prevention is most effective when the nurse uses information from former interactions with families during the primary and secondary prevention stages.

Social Integration of Developmentally Disabled Persons

Included in the interventions provided during tertiary prevention is the social integration of developmentally disabled individuals. Beyond the general acceptance of disabled persons, social integration provides residential placement, rehabilitation, special education, and support services, such as respite care. Obtaining these services and gaining the acceptance of the larger social system outside of the family, namely, the community, can be an arduous process. As one mother of a child with cerebral palsy noted,

> We have become executive managers of our child's care, which includes being astute consumers of the many services provided. The struggle continues day in and day out. And probably the greatest challenge of all is trying to live a normal family life like everyone else in our neighborhood.[31]

The two major philosophical principles that have contributed to the socialization of disabled individuals into the community are deinstitutionalization and normalization.

Deinstitutionalization began in 1970 when a plan was made to reduce the number of individuals living in institutions. Included in this mandate were two additional concepts, habilitative services and the least restrictive alternative. *Habilitative services* are community services such as educational programs, case management, and respite care. *Least restrictive alternative* refers to an "environment that provides the minimum supervision necessary in the smallest living unit possible with the maximum integration into the mainstream of the community."[50] Although the social policy of deinstitutionalization has been widely accepted by many, it has been under debate for many years for the following reasons. First, it has been difficult to establish a uniform definition of deinstitutionalization. Second, there is confusion over the exact meaning of institutionalization for the develop-

mentally disabled. As a result of these confusions, a more salient issue has surfaced in the form of a debate over deinstitutionalization vs. noninstitutionalization.

Advocates of *noninstitutionalization* have proposed that there should be a reduction in the number of individuals living in institutions (deinstitutionalization), and that there should be a systematic plan for discouraging institutionalization in the first place. Further, they suggest that the most appropriate care for developmentally disabled individuals can be provided in community-based residential programs that allow for normal activities of daily living, including the use of facilities and services available to all members of the community. As one might expect, there is still much debate and work to be done in this area.

Normalization was first defined by the Scandinavians as allowing the mentally retarded to attain an existence as close to normal as possible. Others, such as Nirje,[27] have added to the definition of this term. He defined normalization as "patterns of life and conditions of everyday living that are as close as possible to the regular circumstances or ways of life of society . . . a normal rhythm of the day, with privacy activities and mutual responsibility; a normal rhythm of the week, with a home to live in, a school or work to go to, and leisure time with a modicum of social interaction. . . . If retarded persons cannot or should not live in their family or own home, the homes provided should be of normal size and situated in normal residential areas."[27]

"Normalization does not focus on the services or programs provided, but rather describes the goals, standards of treatment, and process of integration for devalued groups of people."[16] The concept of normalization counteracts previously held beliefs in segregated treatment programs for the developmentally disabled.

Normalization can also be referred to as a cultural issue. The end goal of normalization is to establish and/or maintain personal behaviors and characteristics that are as culturally normative as possible.[52] The concept of normalization has also been supported through legislative and court proceedings.

In conjunction with enactment of normalization and deinstitutionalization is the assumption that many families will keep disabled members in their homes. This means that families will need community support to maintain the disabled relative. *Respite care,* in which the individual is taken care of temporarily to relieve the caretakers, is a service that has proved successful. Examples of respite care are sitters coming into the home and temporary placement of disabled members in a foster home. Currently, legislative support exists that provides financial reimbursement in many cases for these services.

Families need guidance and assistance in discerning the options for community services and in integrating their disabled relatives into society. Nurses can provide such information. Often referrals to regional centers enable families to obtain guidance in selecting services. Nurses can also help families gain entry into specific programs, such as Head Start, a provider of preschool education for handicapped children. Moreover, nursing interventions that make families aware of advocacy organizations have proved to be extremely useful.

It is evident that the social integration of disabled persons is an ongoing crusade. Great strides have been made, yet much work remains. In this struggle, the nurse may become involved in the efforts to provide a place for the disabled in society. If and when nurses participate in placing the developmentally disabled, however, it is strongly recommended that they examine their beliefs regarding the ethical and moral issues involved, and look at how these beliefs may affect their work.

The Interdisciplinary Approach

Developmentally disabled clients have a multitude of problems that necessitate the collaborative work of several disciplines. Therefore, nurses must function as members of "a team" of skilled individuals when providing care. The unified efforts of the interdisciplinary team make comprehensive treatment possible.

The unique characteristic of the interdisciplinary team is that case management rests neither with one person nor with one discipline, but rather rotates among team members or is given to the team member who is best qualified for a particular case.[46] For example, the clinical nurse specialist with a background in early child development and chronic diseases may be selected as the case coordinator for a young child with cerebral palsy. Often an audiologist will direct the care of a child whose primary problem is language-related, while an educational psychologist will direct the care of a child with learning disabilities. The responsibility of diagnosis, treatment planning, formulating interventions, and conducting treatment evaluations, however, rests on all of the individuals involved.

The disciplines involved in an interdisciplinary approach include nursing, medicine, linguistics, nutrition, dentistry, education, occupational therapy, physical therapy, social work, psychology, and psychiatry. For the team to function smoothly, each member must have a clear understanding of, and respect for, his or her own and other team members' expertise and role function.[40] If and when there is an overlap of functions among disciplines, the team profits most by combining resources rather than delineating boundaries. For example, the nurse with advanced training in child psychotherapy may possess the same skill in doing therapy as does a psychologist. Hence, both disciplines, nursing and psychology, may work in close collaboration with each other.

The output of the group is dependent on the quality of their interactions. Critics of the interdisciplinary approach have voiced concern over the poor dynamics among team members resulting from conflicts or territoriality. This must be avoided as much as possible. It is essential that team members be confident in their own abilities and, likewise, accept the beliefs and recommendations of others. No matter what one's philosophical beliefs are, it is vital that members be open to the approach that is most beneficial to the client.

Nursing Research

As in any aspect of nursing practice, with the developmentally disabled client there is a need for continued nursing research. Nurses can contribute a wealth of knowledge to the field by studying the effects of interventions on these individuals. Longitudinal outcome studies are recommended, with a particular emphasis on prevention and assessment of family strengths.

Recently, studies have been conducted exploring the concerns of parents with disabled children[43] (see Relevant Research below), as well as focusing on parents' expectations of professionals providing services to their handicapped children.[34] These and other studies geared toward assessing family strengths have produced valuable information for improving the delivery of care to the developmentally disabled.

Collaborative research within the discipline of nursing and in conjunction with other disciplines is also suggested. Just as the team works together in diagnosis, treatment planning, and evaluation, the team approach should extend into the area of research. The combined skills and knowledge of individuals from other disciplines assist in producing high-quality research studies.

Somatic Therapies

Pharmacology

Depending on the condition being treated, medication may be a component of the treatment plan. In most cases, medications are only prescribed after a comprehensive evaluation of the developmentally disabled individual. Because there are many disorders that qualify as developmental disabilities, there may be a wide variety of pharmacologic agents selected. For example, with an epileptic child, a wide array of anticonvulsants may be given, ranging from phenobarbital to sodium valproate. Also, many of these drugs may be given in combination with one another, depending on the type of seizure activity. Also, it is common for epileptic children to have their medication adjusted numerous times throughout their lives.

With a small number of children diagnosed as hyperactive, drugs such as dextroamphetamine, methylphenidate hydrochloride (Ritalin), and pemoline may be used. These drugs have a mechanism of action that promotes attention to tasks. This results in better school performance as well as improved ability to complete tasks. Specifically, methylphenidate hydrochloride acts on the cerebral cortex with mild CNS and respiratory stimulation. This drug has been used most frequently as an adjunctive therapy for hyperactive children.

Prior to administration of medication for hyperactivity, and with parental consent, a child is tested to determine the appropriate use of the medication through a series of drug trials. For a period of several days or weeks, the child may be alternated on and off a given medication

RELEVANT RESEARCH

This study investigated the concerns of 16 parents regarding their developmentally delayed infants and toddlers. The sample was composed predominantly of developmentally delayed children, ranging in age from 4 weeks to 26 months, with a variety of etiologies, such as prematurity and Down's syndrome. The project was conducted with 10 parents in their homes, while the other 6 were involved with infant stimulation program centers. All of the parents were involved in infant stimulation programs.

This descriptive study consisted of a brief interview with several open-ended questions about parents' present and future concerns, as well as an assessment of their support systems. The majority of the interviews were conducted with the mothers, and lasted from 30 minutes to an hour.

Responses to questions regarding parents' sources of support, current involvement in infant programs, and future worries were clustered into three major areas: (1) grieving and depression, (2) difficulties in obtaining adequate services for the parents and their children, and (3) fears about the future.

In more closely examining the area of grieving and depression, all of the parents indicated that some grieving and depression occurred after learning that their children had a disability. However, the expressions of grief and its intensity varied, especially between mothers and fathers. It was also found that current and past life experiences influenced the parents' grief experiences.

The parents reported that parents of other delayed children, developmental program staff, ministers, and the parents' own religious faith were most helpful sources of support. Conversely, delayed referrals for services and negative experiences with health care providers were the most problematic experiences.

Although the findings of this study raise some important points for work with families of developmentally delayed children, one must keep in perspective the small sample size and the sample selection criteria utilized before generalizing these results to other families with disabled children.

(Strauss S, Munton M: Common concerns of parents with disabled children. Pediatr Nurs 11:371, 1985.)

without the knowledge of the parents, staff, and teachers, who are asked to report on the child's behavior. This is known as a double-blind study. If it is determined that the medication is useful and should be continued, several nursing implications arise. Methylphenidate should be administered 30 to 45 minutes before meals to avoid nausea. Blood pressure and pulse should be monitored at appropriate intervals, and side-effects must be noted, *e.g.,* insomnia, nervousness, and weight loss. Finally, this medication regimen necessitates close monitoring and

continued supervision by the physician, parents, and teachers. Table 17-5 lists primary medications used for hyperactivity.

The Therapeutic Use of Self

The psychiatric nurse is challenged to be critically more perceptive and creative when caring for developmentally

TABLE 17-5.
MEDICATIONS FOR HYPERACTIVITY

DRUG	DOSAGE (mg/day)	ACTION	SIDE-EFFECTS
Dextroamphetamine (Dexedrine)	2.5–20	Stabilizing effect on behavior	Used with caution in children Not recommended for children under 5 years. Long-term effects of amphetamines in children have not been established. Growth delay is possible. Other effects include palpitation, tachycardia, elevation of blood pressure, overstimulation, restlessness, insomnia, dryness of mouth, diarrhea, weight loss.
Methylphenidate (Ritalin)	15–45	Stabilizing effect on behavior	Should not be used in children under 5 years Effects include nervousness, insomnia; less common—skin rash, urticaria, fever, arthralgia, anorexia, nausea, dizziness, dyskinesia, elevation in plasma corticosteroids; growth delay is possible.
Pemoline (Cylert)	37.5–150	Stabilizing effect on behavior	Not recommended for use in children under 6 years. Insomnia is the most frequently reported side-effect. Effects include anorexia, weight loss, stomach ache, skin rashes, increased irritability, mild depression, nausea, headache, dizziness, and elevation of SGOT, SGPT, and LDH.

(Reproduced by permission from Waechter E, Phillips J, Holaday B: Nursing Care of Children. Philadelphia, JB Lippincott, 1985.)

disabled clients. The nurse's ability to work with and through the client's disability is critical. Problem-solving becomes a fine art as the nurse implements interventions that are unique for this population.

An empathic approach in working with disabled persons is paramount. However, the nurse is cautioned to maintain an empathic approach rather than a sympathetic one. In doing so, the nurses assist clients to strive toward utilizing their strengths and capabilities.

The nurse contributes to the sense of self-worth of persons with developmental disabilities when independence is encouraged. The psychiatric nurse is often presented with the opportunity to affect the client's growth and development. Assisting clients to reach their fullest potential is probably the most important goal in working with these clients. Nurses are instrumental in setting parameters for clients and monitoring their individual levels of achievement. Another crucial component in working with disabled persons is recognizing clients' limitations. Nurses must be careful not to lose sight of individual clients' competencies, thus preventing "setting the client up" for failure.

The nurse must maintain a positive therapeutic approach in addition to coping with special problems presented by clients who are developmentally disabled. For example, these clients may demonstrate slow progress. Client teaching is difficult because many clients have impaired language skills. Many of these clients will never be "normal." Often in their care there is not the instant gratification of seeing immediate progress.

On the other hand, clients can be helped to lead more productive lives. The nurse can observe the family coping with stress with renewed resources. The nurse receives the rewards of the disabled client's affection and the family's appreciation.

In all, the nurse brings to the clinical setting a sense of respect, sensitivity, and creativity when working with people who are developmentally disabled. The psychiatric nurse helps to build both the sense of hope and the endurance that clients will need in order to become functional individuals in society. Last, the clinician views clients with disabilities as unique individuals who have special qualities and characteristics that supersede their disability, and works with them in that framework.

Summary

1. A developmental disability is a severe, chronic disability that is attributable to a mental or a physical impairment, or both; is manifest before age 22; continues indefinitely; results in a limitation of function in self-care, language, learning, mobility, self-direction, independent living, or economic self-sufficiency; and requires special care.

2. Autism, epilepsy, cerebral palsy, mental retardation, and learning disabilities are five major conditions that meet the criteria of developmental disabilities.

3. A developmentally disabled child who also has a psychiatric condition is said to have a dual diagnosis.

4. Public Law 94-142, the Education for All Handi-

capped Children Act, was directly responsible for increasing public awareness of the rights of mentally retarded individuals and others with disabling conditions.

5. Nursing has been instrumental in advocating for the rights and needs of developmentally disabled people.

6. In primary prevention, nurses focus on preventing initial impairments or defects through genetic counseling and educational programs.

7. In secondary prevention, the early discovery and treatment of the disability, nurses are instrumental in case-finding, screening, and assessment of the handicapping conditions.

8. In tertiary prevention, consisting of care and treatment of the disability, nurses deliver high-quality medical and psychosocial care, as well as developing programs and providing community services for developmentally disabled people.

9. A distinctive characteristic of nursing practice with developmentally disabled clients is that nurses employ a holistic approach, viewing the client and family from biological, psychological, social, and cultural perspectives.

10. Diagnosis of developmentally disabled individuals is made after a comprehensive assessment that includes a child and a parent interview, a medical exam, an assessment of family functioning, and an assessment of the child's environment.

11. The entire family is greatly affected when there is a member who is developmentally disabled.

12. Social integration is defined as providing residential placement, rehabilitation, special education, and support services for developmentally disabled persons.

13. Deinstitutionalization of developmentally disabled people began in the early 1970s, with the intention of reducing the number of individuals living in institutions.

14. Normalization occurs when an effort is made to assist developmentally disabled persons to live a life as close to normal as possible.

References

1. American Nurses' Association, Division of Maternal and Child Health Nursing Practice: Standards of Maternal and Child Health Nursing Practice. Kansas City, American Nurses' Association, 1983
2. American Psychiatric Association: Diagnostic and Statistical Manual of Mental Disorders III, Revised (DSM-III-R). Washington, DC, American Psychiatric Association, 1987
3. Anderson FM, Klarke I: Disability in Adolescence. London, Methvin, 1982
4. Barnard K, Erickson M: Teaching Children With Developmental Problems: A Family Care Approach. St Louis, CV Mosby, 1976
5. Black R, Herman B, Shope J: Nursing Management of Epilepsy. Maryland, Aspen Publications, 1982
6. Bleuler E: Dementia praecox oder Gruppe der Schizophren-

ien. Leipzig, Franz Deuticke, 1911. Zimpkin J (trans). New York, International Press, 1952

7. Cantwell D, Baker L: Psychiatric and behavioral characteristics of children with communication disorders. J Pediatr Psychol 5: 161–178, 1980
8. Cohen P: The impact of a handicapped child on the family. Soc Casework 43:137, 1962
9. Cruickshank WM, Bentzen FA, Ratzeburg FH et al: A Teaching Method for Brain-Injured and Hyperactive Children. Syracuse, Syracuse University Press, 1961
10. Cushwa B, Szymanski IL, Tanguay PE: Professionals' Roles and Unmet Manpower Needs. In Szymanski LS, Tanguay PE (eds): Emotional Disorders of Mentally Retarded Persons. Baltimore, University Press, 1980
11. Farber B: Family Organization and Interaction. San Francisco, Chandler, 1964
12. Federal Register, August 23, 1977
13. Goodman L: Continuing Treatment of Parents with Congenitally Defective Infants. Soc Work 9:92, 1964
14. Gordon N: Pediatric Neurology for the Clinician. London, Heineman, 1976
15. Grossman HJ: Classification in Mental Retardation, p 163. Washington, DC, American Association on Mental Deficiency, 1983
16. Grossman FK: Brothers and Sisters of Retarded Children: An Exploratory Study. Syracuse, Syracuse University Press, 1972
17. Grossman JH: Manual on Terminology and Classification in Mental Retardation. Washington, DC, American Association on Mental Deficiency, 1977
18. Hill R: Families Under Stress. Connecticut, Greenwood Press, 1949
19. Kanner L: Autistic Disturbances of Affective Contact. Nerv Child 2:217–250, 1943
20. Kennedy JF: Maternal reactions to the birth of a defective baby. Soc Casework 51:411, 1970
21. Kirk SA: Educating Exceptional Children. Boston, Houghton-Mifflin, 1962
22. Koller H, Richardson SA, Katz M et al: Behavior disturbance in childhood and the early adult years in populations who were and were not mentally retarded. J Prevent Psychiatry 1:453–468, 1982
23. Lakin C, Bruininks R: Social Integration of Developmentally Disabled Persons. In Lakin C, Bruininks R (eds): Strategies for Achieving Community Integration of Developmentally Disabled Citizens. Baltimore, Paul H. Brooks, 1985
24. Lansdown R: More than Sympathy: The Everyday Needs of Sick and Handicapped Children and Their Families. London, Tavistock Publishers, 1980
25. Lippman L, Loberg D: An Overview of Developmental Disabilities. In Janicki M, Wisniewski H: Aging and Developmental Disabilities: Issues and Approaches, pp 41–58. Baltimore, Paul H. Brooks, 1985
26. McCubbin H, Patterson J: Family Transitions: Adaptations to Stress. In McCubbin H, Figley C (eds): Stress and the Family: Coping With Normative Transitions, Vol 1. New York, Brunner-Mazel, 1983
27. Nirje F: The Normalization Principle. In Kugel RB, Shearer A (eds): Changing Patterns in Residential Services for the Mentally Retarded (rev), pp 231–232. Washington, DC, US Government Printing Office, 1976
28. North AF: The Developmentally Disabled Child: Preventative Efforts and Governmental Programs. In Gabel S, Erickson M (eds): Child Development and Developmental Disabilities. Boston, Little, Brown & Co, 1980
29. O'Connor M: Assessment and Treatment of the Child With Dual Disabilities. In Sigman M (ed): Children With Emotional Disorders and Developmental Disabilities: Assessment and Treatment, pp 193–228. New York, Grune & Stratton, 1985

30. Olshansky S: Chronic sorrow: A response to having a mentally defective child. Soc Casework 43:190–193, 1962
31. Personal communication with an anonymous parent, December 1985
32. Powell M: Assessment and Management of Developmental Changes in Children. St Louis, CV Mosby, 1981
33. Poznanski E: Psychiatric difficulties in siblings of handicapped children. Pediatrics 8:232–234, 1969
34. Redman-Bentley D: Parent expectations for professionals providing services to their handicapped children. Phys Occup Ther Pediatrics 2(1): 1982
35. Roberts P: Nursing Assessments Screening for Developmental Problems. In Krajicek M, Tearney-Tomlison A: Detection of Developmental Problems in Children. Baltimore, University Park Press, 1981
36. Russell A: The Mentally Retarded, Emotionally Disturbed Child and Adolescent. In Sigman M (ed): Children With Emotional Disorders and Developmental Disabilities: Assessment and Treatment, pp 111–135. New York, Grune & Stratton, 1985
37. Rutter M, Graham P, Yule W: A Neuropsychiatric Study in Childhood. London, Spastics International Medical Publications, 1970
38. Rutter M: Psychotic Disorders in Early Childhood. In Cooper AJ, Walk D: Recent Developments in Schizophrenia. Ashford, Kent, Headley Bros, 1967
39. Rykman D, Henderson R: The meaning of a retarded child for his parents: A focus for counselors. Ment Retard 3:4–7, 1965
40. Savino A: Developmental Disabilities 1980. Unpublished manuscript, 1980
41. Seimon M: Siblings of the chronically ill or disabled child: Meeting their needs. In Nurs Clin North Am 19(2):295–307, 1984
42. Solnit AJ, Stark M: Mourning the Birth of a Defective Child. In The Psychoanalytic Study of the Child, vol 16. New York, International University Press, 1961
43. Strauss S, Munton M: Common concerns of parents with disabled children. Pediatr Nurs 11:371–375, 1985
44. Sugarman G: Epilepsy Handbook: A Guide to Understanding Seizure Disorders. St Louis, CV Mosby, 1984
45. Tarjan G, Keeran C: Overview of Mental Retardation. Psychiatr Ann: 1–7, 1974
46. Thompson R, O'Quinn A: Developmental Disabilities: Etiologies, Manifestations, Diagnosis, and Treatments, p 14. New York, Oxford University Press, 1979
47. Von Bertalanffy L: The Meaning of General Systems Theory. In Von Bertalanffy L (ed): General Systems Theory, pp 30–53. New York, Braziller, 1968
48. Webster TG: Unique Aspects of Emotional Development in Mentally Retarded Individuals. In Menolascino FJ (ed): Psychiatric Approaches to Mental Retardation. New York, Basic Books, 1970
49. Wikler L, Wasow M, Hatfield E: Chronic sorrow revisited: Parents vs. professional depiction of the adjustment of families of mentally retarded children. Am J Orthopsychol 51:63–70, 1981
50. Willer B, Schecrenberger RC, Intagliata J: Deinstitutionalization and mentally retarded persons. Comm Ment Health Rev 3: 3–12, 1976
51. Wilson M: Medical Genetics: Health for Future Generations. Report from the Genetics Division, Los Angeles County–USC Medical Center, 1978
52. Wolfensberger W: Normalization: The Principle of Normalization in Human Services, p 28. Toronto, National Institute on Mental Retardation, 1972
53. Zelle R: The Developmentally Disabled Child and the Family. In Hymovich D, Barnard M (eds): Family Health Care. Vol II: Developmental and Situational Crisis. New York, McGraw-Hill, 1979

18

NANCY K. ENGLISH, REBECCA A. VAN SLYKE-MARTIN, SHIRL A. SCHEIDER, AND DAYA RAO

PSYCHOPHYSIOLOGICAL DISTURBANCES AND NURSING INTERVENTIONS

Learning Objectives

Upon completion of this chapter the student should be able to do the following:

1. Describe the relationship between systems theory and psychophysiological disturbances.
2. Describe the effects of various forms of stress on the breakdown of human systems.
3. Identify disease lifetypes, their components, and eclectic (holistic) interventions.
4. Explain the systems model of disease manifestation.
5. List patterns of behavior that describe psychosomatic disease.
6. Describe the role of the nurse in planning interventions for individuals with psychophysiological disturbance.
7. State three nursing diagnoses that reflect alterations in mind–body harmony.
8. State two nursing interventions that facilitate mind–body harmony.
9. Cite the rationale on which relaxation training is based.
10. Cite the rationale on which breath awareness is based.
11. Give two examples of client situations in which deep breathing, relaxation, or other holistic interventions can be utilized.

12. Apply the nursing process to a client exhibiting behaviors that reflect psychophysiological disorders.
13. Explain levels of prevention in relation to psychophysiological disease.
14. State areas for further research in psychophysiological disease management.

CLINICAL EXAMPLES

MARY

A tense and thin figure sits in the dayroom, flipping through the pages of a textbook. Mary, 32 years old, appears much older, and her body language supports her emotional tension. As the student nurse approaches her, Mary leans forward and puts her book aside, not making any eye contact.

The student nurse introduces herself and begins her therapeutic interventions. She smiles and says, "What are you studying? It looks difficult."

Mary snaps back without looking up, "No. Just for me." She then shyly explains that she is finally doing something to meet her goal of becoming a writer. She comments that she has been a devoted housewife and mother for the past 15 years, and wanted to succeed at something else. After the first quarter at the community college, she began to experience severe abdominal cramps that hindered her progress.

"I've had x-rays and all kinds of tests, and there's no sign of an ulcer. But the pain is there. My doctor tells me to relax, as if I could turn my pain off and on at will." Mary's eyes become moist as she turns inward: "Why does this happen to me, anyway?"

MRS. REED

Mrs. Reed, a slim, attractive woman of 50, is admitted to the medical unit for current evaluation of a diagnosis of rheumatoid arthritis. For the past five years, the condition has been relatively under control, until a few weeks ago. Shortly after beginning a new position as an office manager, her joints began to swell more than usual, especially in her fingers; movement became progressively painful and limited.

"I am so *nervous!*" Mrs. Reed says during the first interview with the student nurse. "I finally win the job I've worked toward all my life, and now I can't . . . I can't. . . ." She slowly closes her hand into a weak fist, which obviously takes too much effort. "I can't even move my fingers."

Introduction

This chapter examines the nature of psychophysical disturbances, and nursing interventions used with clients who have psychophysiological illnesses. Psychophysiological disturbances are thought to begin as emotional stimulation that influences the biological structures to such an extent that pathology results. The emotional stimulation is intense or sustained.[19] Because of the connection between the emotional stimulation and biological changes, the disturbance can be affected (reversed or decreased) by providing physiological intervention along with psychological intervention.

In the past 10 to 15 years there has been an increasing interest in wellness, as evidenced by the focus on preventive medicine, holistic medicine, and lifestyle medicine. We have become aware of specific behavior mechanisms that develop obstructions to the lives we seek to live. We eat healthier diets; we recognize and address the physiologically negative effects of nicotine, drug, and alcohol overindulgence; and we exercise our bodies, minds, and wills more consciously. We have become enlightened about the various concepts of stress and the immense impact it has on our sense of homeostasis, while learning numerous methods and techniques to modify our reactions to stress. Key factors in health and longevity have been enumerated, such as job satisfaction, overall happiness, involvement with life, minimizing negative stressors, and careful moderation in lifestyle choices. We have come to accept the fact that people maintain a responsibility for their own state of health or disease, and have considerable conscious command over it.[11,18]

In this chapter, the nature of psychophysiological disturbances is explored. When do they begin? What triggers them? How can beliefs predict physiological manifestations? Is there a recognizable formula for a psychosomatic breakdown? Are there specific psychosomatic disorders and personality types? What are the distinctions among organic illnesses, conversion reactions, and psychosomatic disorders? What are specific key factors in health and longevity? What role do nurses have in working with clients with psychophysiological disturbances? What nursing interventions are useful and appropriate in working with clients with psychophysiological problems?

Theoretical Perspectives on Psychophysiological Disturbances

Historical Developments

The term *psychosomatic* (which will be used interchangeably with *psychophysiological*) is derived from two Greek words, "psyche" (soul) and "soma" (body). These words reflect the influence of the mind on the body and on general physical health. The theory of psychosomatic medicine dates back to the beginning of Chinese medicine. Today the "Nei Ching",[36] the classic work of internal medicine by the Yellow Emperor, Huang Ti, continues as one of the Asian physician's most important references. Freud[12] demonstrated that certain specific, unconscious mental events are symbolically expressed in the "body language" of somatic symptoms. Rorschach[3] tests indicate that clients have an unconscious knowledge of their diseases.

Lifetypes

Recent medical and behavioral research has shown that particular personality types, evidenced during times of stress, demonstrate specific and predictable manifestations of life-threatening or chronic physiological conditions. These conditions will be referred to as *lifetypes.*[2]

Each individual displays unique characteristics based on his or her internal and external variables. Figure 18-1 illustrates this concept. Specific patterns of psychophysi-

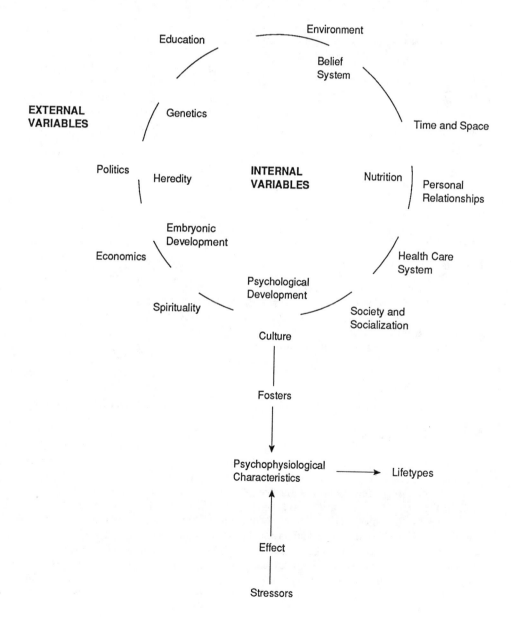

Figure 18-1. Etiology of lifetypes.

RELEVANT RESEARCH

Thirty male volunteers were designated as Type A or Type B on the basis of a standard structured interview. Fifteen were classified as Type A (mean age 37.2 years) and 15 as Type B (mean age 32.4 years). The purpose of the research was to determine if Type-A men had exaggerated changes in ventricular repolarization, compared to changes in a sample of Type B men. These changes would be measured by changes in ECG T waves.

The experimental task was to state out-loud answers to subtraction problems. Twenty task trials were presented, with intertrial intervals varying between 40, 50, and 60 seconds. Subjects were told that their performance was expected to improve over successive trials, and that they should strive to improve their proficiency. Before the task trials, subjects completed the Today Form of the Multiple Affect Adjective Checklist. This form was again administered following the last trial task.

The results of this experiment were that Type-A men showed greater reductions in TWA (ventricular performance). This TWA hyper-responsivity may be attributable to CNS influences, which suggests why these individuals may be predisposed to acute myocardial infarctions. These responses could be elicited by simple mental work.

(Scher H, Hartman L, Furedy J et al: Electrocardiographic T-wave changes are more pronounced in Type-A than in Type-B men during mental work. Psychosom Med 48:3–4, 1986.)

ological functioning can be identified. Some examples of patterns are Type-A and Type-B personalities.

Type A

Some individuals externalize their stress. Examples include driving, excitable, volatile, success-oriented career people who are "engaged in a chronic struggle against time and other people."[29] They are continually bombarded with short-term stress and, because they allow no time for relaxation, their short-term stress becomes long-term. They become likely candidates for myocardial infarctions and other cardiovascular diseases, as well as at high risk for the development of obesity and ulcers.

Type B

Other individuals are able to adjust to the extremes of short- and long-term stress. Type-B personalities learn to rest after each stressful period. These individuals seem to have an adequate amount of serenity and optimism, and a sense of moderation. When a stressor is presented, these types know how to control their response in a calm way.

Systems Theory

Some guiding principles of systems theory help nurses to understand the wholeness of the individual with psychophysiological problems. Systems theory explains that each individual interacts with a complexity of components: self, family, and environments. The principle of a change in any part of the system affecting the whole can be important in psychopsysiological disease. Disturbances in one organ system do exert stress on other organ systems, resulting in a variety of organic complaints that must be considered. Change in the status of a family member at one point in time also effects change in other members, which indicates the need for complete data in the areas of psychosocial history, as well as in the physical assessment.

The principle that each system has boundaries with varying degrees of openness to external influences is also relevant to these clients. The nurse may encounter selective communication patterns and themes in the verbal and nonverbal behaviors of clients with specific psychosomatic disorders.

Systems are continuously changing and growing. The application of systems theory to nursing interventions with psychophysiologically-compromised clients is great. We must be aware of the need for frequent reassessment, because individuals can change their coping patterns to be more harmonious with healthy outcomes. This principle promotes the belief that individuals strive toward their optimum level of harmony, and are capable of physiological and psychological balance.

The Differentiation of Psychophysical Disorders

Demonstrated conditions may be considered organic illnesses, conversion reactions, or psychosomatic illnesses. Psychosomatic disorders and organic illnesses both involve physical changes in the body. Psychosomatic illnesses are evoked by psychological stimuli, whereas organic illnesses are evoked by a "physical" cause, such as a laceration. Conversion reactions are motor or sensory displays of internal conflict. Both psychosomatic disorders and conversion reactions are evoked by psychogenic factors. However, psychosomatic illnesses involve tissue pathology.

Table 18-1 presents the differentiating characteristics of organic illnesses, conversion reactions, and psychosomatic disorders.[19]

TABLE 18-1.

DIFFERENTIATING CHARACTERISTICS OF ORGANIC ILLNESSES, CONVERSION REACTIONS, AND PSYCHOSOMATIC DISORDERS

Organic illnesses, as indicated by:

1. *Biogenic changes* caused by microorganisms, lacerations, abrasions, contusions, or concussions, or
2. *Structural changes* that are nonspecific, and may involve any part of the individual, including:
   Obvious tissue pathology
   Major/minor physical incapacity
   Observable changes that are effects of physical or medical treatment
   Clients' attitudes of concern rather than indifference
   Consistent and anatomically-logical symptoms in accordance with the severity of injury or assault

Conversion reactions, as indicated by:

1. The occurrence of a psychogenic factor(s), such as a traumatic psychological experience, and conscious knowledge of the conversion symptoms
2. An absence of tissue pathology
3. A specific and highly selective functional incapacity
4. Little or no appreciable effect elicited by physical treatment
5. Indifferent or detached client attitudes towards self
6. Symptoms that do not correspond to logical stimulus–response anatomic patterns

Psychosomatic disorders, as indicated by:

1. Physical changes evoked by internal or external psychological stimuli (a psychogenic cause)
2. The involvement of the autonomic nervous system or analogous structures
3. The frequent presence of tissue pathology
4. Limited physical capacity or potential
5. A consistent set of symptoms and logical anatomical involvement

Specific Disease Lifetypes

Psychophysiological disturbances can be classified into two general categories, related both to specific organ system functions or involvement and to exhibited lifetypes.[2,3]

The following case histories will facilitate an understanding of this complex categorization. Some clients exhibit patterns of reflecting more than one lifetype; however, a predominant pattern is distinguishable with a thorough investigation of sensitizing and triggering agents.

The histories that are presented feature lifetype categories, assessment data with physiological components, psychosocial history, and interventions based on considering the person holistically. The results sections cite how the psychological and physiological variables work together to manifest disease states, as well as to help resolve disease states.

I. *Cancer Lifetype*[20]

  A. *Physiological:*

    Carcinoma, a malignant growth, a morbid swelling or enlargement, a mass of new tissue biologically detrimental to the organism. The mass persists and grows, independent of surrounding structures.

  B. *Psychogenic:*

    Childhood trauma (most frequently loss of a significant other), followed by continuous feelings (with eventual repression) of despair, grief, or loneliness. Those feelings trigger limbic and hypothalamic functioning, resulting in suppression of the immune system by elevating adrenal steroid hormone secretion. Similar later trauma produces acute immune suppression, resulting in increased susceptibility to carcinogens (viral, radical, or chemical).

  C. *Case History:* Oat-cell carcinoma of the diaphragm

    Alice is a 63-year-old Caucasian woman, widowed, without children. The onset of her illness was six months prior to being evaluated by her physician.

  D. *Presenting Symptoms:*

    1. *Physical:* Labored breathing, insomnia, nocturnal dyspnea, orthopnea, debilitating pain, poor appetite, diaphragm partially paralyzed

    2. *Psychosocial:* Extreme anxiety, fearfulness, hopelessness, resignation. Alice was told that the tumor was inoperable, and that she would die soon.

  E. *Intervention:*

    1. *Physical:* Radiation and chemotherapy

    2. *Psychosocial:* Relaxation training, visualization training, autogenic training, therapeutic touch

  F. *Results:*

    Alice's initial response to radiation and chemotherapy was minimal and disappointing. At the time of her diagnosis, the recovery rate from oat-cell carcinoma was less than 1%. Alice soon began to show improvement and an abatement of symptoms. A systems approach was used in planning and carrying out her care. It was noted that, as her psychological, emotional, and spiritual needs were identified and met, she improved dramatically. To date, Alice is currently classified as free of cancer.

II. *Cardiovascular Lifetype*

  A. *Physiological:*

    Coronary disease; heart attack; coronary occlusion due to embolus or thrombus; irritable myocardium syndrome; functional dysrhythmias, *e.g.,* tachycardia, bradycardia, paroxysmal atrial tachycardia; palpitations; essential hypertension; vascular spasms; angina syndrome

  B. *Psychogenic:*

    Childhood demands to achieve successfully and compete with deadlines result in a lifelong attitude of competitiveness and the habitual setting of unattainable personal goals. The body is in a chronic state of preparation for "fight or flight." These unabated stressors result in pathologically elevated adrenaline and norepinephrine levels that may stimulate and elevate circulating fatty acid titers, while raising blood pressure and increasing the probability of embolus formation. Increased serum lipid levels clog coronary arteries and limit the myocardial oxygen absorption. Later life trauma can result in a sudden and acute stress response which, if left untreated, will eventually result in cardiovascular disease.

Emotional responses often affect cardiac rate, tonicity, stroke volume, peripheral vascular resistance, pulse regularity, blood pressure fluctuation, and blood chemistry.

C. *Case History:*
George is a 59-year-old Caucasian man, divorced, father of two living children. He is a prominent corporate attorney and a classic Type A personality. The length of his illness prior to treatment was five years.

D. *Presenting Symptoms:*
1. *Physical:* Tachycardia, palpitations, severe angina, exertional dyspnea
2. *Psychosocial:* Anxiety, dissatisfaction with self-image and physical limitations, high motivation to succeed and maintain "self-control"

E. *Intervention:*
1. *Physical:* Cardiac stress test with follow-up cardiac catheterization
Aortic valve replacement followed in three years by triple coronary artery bypass
2. *Psychosocial:* Time management technique training, relaxation training, autogenic training, biofeedback, therapeutic touch

F. *Results:*
Counseling revealed that at an early age George began to compete with his image of his father's success. He chose the same occupation as his father and needed to surpass his father's accomplishments. His need to appear masculine and virile stemmed from an early bout with asthma that severely restricted his childhood physical activity and expression.

When an understanding of the triggering agents and motivators of the past became clear, George changed many of his ideas about himself and his life's work. Physically, he gained control of the tachycardia and began feeling and acting more energetic. His level of psychological stress was greatly reduced, allowing George a more relaxed and accepting attitude about himself and life in general.

III. *Endocrine Lifetype*[4,13]
A. *Physiological:*
Hypo/hypersecretion of hormones with under/overstimulation of the target organ and resultant imbalance and pathological tissue deterioration (*e.g.,* diabetes, goiter, hyper/hypothyroidism)

B. *Psychogenic:*
A traumatic childhood frequently includes the loss of an authority figure, stringent parental requirements, or neglect, thus producing unmet dependency feelings and self-pity. These may result in chronic emotional stimulation of the autonomic nervous system, including extreme changes in blood chemistry due to adrenal secretion of epinephrine and norepinephrine; gonadal secretion of testosterone or estrogen; pituitary secretion of pituitin or other trophic hormones; and pancreatic secretion of insulin.

Endocrine disorders exhibited in adult life generally are preceded by a traumatic childhood event that stimulated the initial metabolic shift in an already psychophysiologically-predisposed individual.

C. *Case History:* Diabetes Mellitus
Maria is a 34-year-old Filipino-American, married, and mother of three healthy children. The length of her illness prior to treatment was one year.

D. *Presenting Symptoms:*
1. *Physical:* Elevated blood glucose, weight gain, general weakness, frequent headaches
2. *Psychosocial:* Extreme anxiety, feelings of helplessness, feelings of isolation

E. *Intervention:*
1. *Physical:* Insulin administration for elevated glucose, plus dietary management instructions, supervised exercise, and diabetic teaching
2. *Psychosocial:* Relaxation and visualization therapy, autogenic therapy to facilitate pancreatic functioning, therapeutic touch

F. *Results:*
Counseling revealed that, when Maria was seven years old, her mother died, leaving several younger brothers and sisters for whom Maria provided care. She assumed the maternal role for her siblings and provided a normal home life for her father. This created conflicting dependency needs in Maria, because she was a child in need of parenting yet had siblings dependent on her as a parent figure. As a result, Maria's autonomic nervous system may have begun to react to the chronic emotional stimulation by producing changes in her blood chemistry. The secretion of adrenaline and norepinephrine, gonadal and pituitary secretions, and pancreatic secretion of insulin

may have begun the gradual process of endocrine imbalance.

When she was at age 33, Maria's husband was transferred to the United States, and her struggle to reestablish a home and community support system for herself and her family restimulated her childhood feelings of displacement and insecurity. These feelings may have been the triggering agents for the diabetes.

Maria's understanding of the emotional triggers in her life became clearer through counseling. Relaxation techniques and visualization of a harmonious endocrine system facilitated control of her imbalances. Maria has been free of diabetic crises as a result of her regulated and positive approach to her life-long condition.

IV. *Gastrointestinal Lifetype*
  A. *Physiological:*
   Emotional responses can affect the rate of digestion, intestinal diameter, peristalsis, and quantity of secretions. Emotions can stimulate reverse motility and involuntary defecation. Gastrointestinal disorders include ulcers, ulcerative colitis, anorexia nervosa, obesity, and others.
  B. *Psychogenic:*
   An emotionally disturbed childhood, with the threat of loss of a significant other, can create conflicting and often unsatisfied dependency needs resulting in limbic and hypothalamic activity. Intense, ambivalent emotional reactions (and/or possible inherited propensities) may affect the vagal nerve. Pituitary and adrenal hormones react to the same stimuli, eventually causing chronic increases in secretion of stomach acids. These increases raise the possibility of breaks in the mucoid lining that allow for irritation and corrosion of the intestinal tract. Traumatic events in later life create acute acid production and, if left untreated, stimulate gastrointestinal diseases.
  C. *Case History:* Crohn's disease, regional ileitis, regional enteritis
   Jason is a 24-year-old Caucasian man, unmarried. The length of his illness prior to treatment was five years.
  D. *Presenting Symptoms:*
   1. *Physical:* Inflammatory bowel syndrome; excessive weight loss; lower abdominal pain; continuous, severe diarrhea
   2. *Psychosocial:* A feeling of tension, anxiety, depression, self-consciousness, introversion
  E. *Intervention:*
   1. *Physical:* Surgical ileostomy and dietary management
   2. *Psychosocial:* Relaxation, autogenic therapy, visualization of soothing and healing action and functioning of the intestinal tract and alimentary canal, therapeutic touch
  F. *Results:*
   Jason came from a family of tense, nervous individuals. His early behavior patterns were very likely influenced by consistently internalizing the feelings of both parents. Inconclusive studies have shown the possibility of both genetic and infectious transmission of Crohn's Disease.[17] Jason's father was a career military officer and was often absent for extended periods of time. The demands Jason felt to be the "man of the house" while his father was away, the necessary adjustments when he returned, and Jason's normal desire to be dependent may have chronically stimulated the secretion of stomach acid and eventually corroded the intestinal tract lining.

Jason's disease was diagnosed shortly after he entered college. The stress of separation from his family, and his need for personal reliance, may have been aggravating factors.

Through holistic interventions, Jason was able to change his behavioral patterns and lower his stress levels. He now is able to cope normally with his independent life at college, and is enjoying his emotional freedom. He is anticipating a career in political science, and has found much fulfillment in a nurturing relationship with a woman undergraduate.

V. *Genitourinary Lifetype*
  A. *Physiological:*
   Impotence, hypomenorrhea, frigidity, vaginismus, disturbances of reproductive functioning, amenorrhea, spontaneous abortion, pseudocyesis, disturbances of urinary function, involuntary micturition
  B. *Psychogenic:*
   Trauma in childhood and a dominant parental figure with rigid requirements can evoke emotional reactions that produce patterns of endocrine and/or autonomic activity. These patterns can interfere with micturition and/or glandular secretion.

Events of similar stress in later life may retrigger childhood feelings of insecurity and personal ambivalence, particularly genitourinary-related events, resulting in sexual, reproductive, and/or urinary dysfunction. Emotional responses may cause enuresis, incontinence, priapism, or ejaculation praecox.
  C. *Case History:* Primary severe dysmenorrhea
   Ellen is a 23-year-old Caucasian woman, married for one year, with no children. Length of illness prior to treatment was nine years.
  D. *Presenting Symptoms:*
   1. *Physical:* Chronic painful menses
   2. *Psychosocial:* Chronic depression, defensiveness, difficulty in maintaining a nurturing relationship

E. *Intervention:*
1. *Physical:* Generalized abdominal pain treated with nonnarcotic analgesics
2. *Psychosocial:* Relaxation, autogenic therapy, therapeutic touch
F. *Results:*
Counseling revealed that Ellen's childhood with alcoholic parents generated extremely strong feelings of insecurity. Her father was a quiet and reserved man, while her mother was excessively domineering and demanding. Ellen needed to please and manipulate others. Her difficulty in relationships mirrored her parents' alcoholic dependence and ambivalent, insecure, unstable behavior.

Therapy supported Ellen's acceptance and nurturance of self as she developed self-reliance skills. Her struggle with the need to be taken care of vs. independence resulted in life-changing insight. Control of her painful menses became an actual means of self-empowerment.

Since she learned self-management skills, Ellen has stopped addictive behaviors such as drinking and smoking without intervention or therapy. Her marital relationship has become an avenue for her self-expression and interdependence.

VI. *Musculoskeletal Lifetype*[4,5]
A. *Physiological:*
Changes in muscle tonicity, elasticity, and reflex arc result in aberrant twitching, tremor, clonus, tonus, convulsions, cramping, and spasmaticity; joint limitations; and pain.
B. *Psychogenic:*
Because of genetic predisposition, all rheumatoid patients and an estimated 25% of their closest relatives demonstrate the autoimmune phenomenon of elevated RA factors in their serum. Coupled with a traumatic childhood, this genetic predisposition results in immune system impairment that may eventually permit the RA factor molecules to penetrate the joint linings and connective tissues.

Helpless emotional responses to later life trauma do not stimulate the production of the adrenal corticosteroid hormones that prevent rheumatoid arthritis, but further depress the immune response through parasympathetic activity. It is likely that the acute, final effort of the immune system to destroy the RA factor actually produces rheumatoid arthritis.
C. *Case History:* Rheumatoid arthritis
Sandy is a 38-year-old Caucasian woman, unmarried. Length of illness prior to treatment was 3½ years.
D. *Presenting Symptoms:*
1. *Physical:* Fatigue, anorexia with accompanying weight loss, low-grade fever, morning stiffness, pain, and tenderness in joints of hands and feet
2. *Psychosocial:* Inability to express normal anger or anxiety, difficulty with control, sensitivity to criticism
E. *Intervention:*
1. *Physical:* Cortisone therapy
Daily mega-dose of vitamin C (minimum 5 grams/day)
Range of motion therapy
2. Psychosocial: Relaxation training with emphasis on self-appreciation and normal emotional reactions to stress, autogenic therapy, visualization training in reconstructing collagen, counseling involving issues of anger, separation, and autonomy
F. *Results:*
Sandy's early childhood environment made excessive demands on her to meet unattainable expectations of others. Although she was always conscientious and responsible in her school work, her parents criticized her from an early age. After repeated negative feedback, she withdrew, still remaining angry at her parents. Six months prior to the onset of her stiffness and joint tenderness, Sandy's father died unexpectedly. Conscious recognition of childhood psychophysiological conditioning allowed Sandy to take an active role in changing her attitudes about herself. Her self-image improved as she became able to validate herself and her accomplishments. Control of her disease progression was achieved within three months of psychosocial counseling and holistic therapies.

VII. *Respiratory Lifetype*
A. *Physiological:*
Changes include disruption of inspiratory/expiratory pattern, apnea, frequent sighing, aerophagia, gasping, crying with resulting changes in membrane potentials, production of secretion, and/or airway diameter fluctuation. Respiratory disorders include bronchial asthma, hay fever, and chronic rhinitis.
B. *Psychogenic:*
Frequently one dominant parent and one weak parent, or rejecting parents, cause the development of unmet dependency needs, repressed emotions, hypersensitivity to environments, and immune system dysfunction. In asthma, for example, the hypothalamus stimulates the parasympathetic nervous system (particularly the vagus nerve), creating bronchial constricture through the release of acetylcholine. Excessive contractions and spasms stimulate mast cells to produce histamine, which engorges mucous membrane linings, producing respiratory disturbances.

Traumas in later life may trigger learned/adaptive patterns of emotional response, resulting in stimulation or activation of respiratory ailments.

C. *Case History:* Bronchial asthma
Amy is a three-year-old Caucasian girl. The length of illness prior to treatment was one year.

D. *Presenting Symptoms:*
1. *Physical:* Acute asthmatic attacks with wheezing, dyspnea, poor appetite, and disrupted sleep patterns
2. *Psychosocial:* Shyness, withdrawal, and whiny behavior

E. *Intervention:*
1. *Physical:* Immunization, desensitization, epinephrine
2. *Psychosocial:* Relaxation and visualization therapy (through story-telling); imagery for condition control

F. *Results:*
Counseling revealed that, when Amy was at age 1½, her parents divorced. Her father moved out of the state, and her mother began working away from home. Being cared for by several different sitters may have resulted in unmet dependency needs and repression of emotional expression.[9] Therapy involved training Amy's mother to help her daughter develop imaginary helpers inside her chest. Amy chose tiny rainbow-colored ponies. Whenever Amy felt an impending asthma attack, she was encouraged to call upon her helper ponies who "know just what to do" to help her feel better. Within three weeks, Amy was better able to control her physical symptoms and appeared more self-assured and communicative in her relationships with others. As Amy sensed her own abilities to control her inner world, she seemed to gain the strength to deal with her outer world.

In an examination of psychophysiological disturbances, we understand the basic physiological involvement of the person stimulated by various psychological antigens or triggering agents. Various organic symptoms are produced by emotional factors that evoke responses through mediation of the autonomic nervous system. Prolonged maladapted physiological states of visceral function, stimulated by emotional factors, lead to organic, molecular, and cellular structural changes, if left untreated.

Psychophysiological maladaptations may result from challenges of living. A holistic assessment of the individual's growth and development, working conditions, interpersonal relationships, motivations, security structures, significant others, economic structure and dependency, frustration tolerance, and overall coping mechanisms is mandatory in order to evaluate psychophysical maladaptations.

Many clients rarely complain of anxiety, depression, sexual dysfunction, embarrassment, or resentment. Their complaints are physical, such as anorexia, vomiting, diar-

rhea, backaches, headaches, insomnia, hyperventilation, or cardiac palpitations.

It takes a skilled healthcare-giver to anticipate that organic symptoms may have psychophysiological components, and to pay attention to all areas of assessment.

Emotional Arousal and Physiological Function

Individuals are capable of responding to experiences with a multitude of emotional behaviors: fear, surprise, sadness, disgust, anger, anticipation, joy, acceptance, receptivity, and love. An individual's body image develops from one's emotional experiences. Negative, as well as positive, ideas of body image have an impact on the physiological functioning of the body. People need to be aware of their emotional patterns. Emotion results from a complex series of events, including motivations, cognitive appraisal, and overt behavior that meets the demands of an initial sensitizing agent or situation.

The research of Cannon[15] demonstrated that emotional arousal resulting in the induction or inhibition of organ functioning could be a learned conditioned response. For example, feelings of dejection and frustration are associated with hypofunctioning of the large intestine; aggressive emotions, including resentment and hostility, stimulate increased mucosal secretion and vascularity; sadness, self-reproach, and discouragement lead to continued mucosal pallor and hyposecretion. Emotions and self-image have a great potential for establishing disruptive patterns of physiological functioning. Similar to the client with neurosis, the client with a psychophysiological disturbance remains resistant to relinquishing defense mechanisms. The objective of therapy is to assist the client to understand the relationship of the anxiety reaction and personality restraints or maladjustments. When emotional disorders are identified incorrectly or treated as isolated entities, the client does not improve, or begins to change symptoms into chronic physiological disorders.[22]

A client frequently experiences several emotions simultaneously. As Darwin found while developing his theory of evolution, emotions are appropriate adaptive reactions to emergencies and concurrently increase the individual's chances of survival when faced with a threat to the integrity of body, mind, spirit, or emotions.[22]

Emotions and Pathophysiology

Psychophysiological breakdown results from a variety of events. Early life trauma, lack of positive emotions, lack of an emotionally supportive atmosphere, and repressed negative, destructive, or self-negating emotions are prime examples. The perception of these events and accompanying negative emotions override the strength of the individual's basic and acquired biological assets. A breakdown of physiological and psychological systems then occurs.

Initially, emotional reactions are constructive, defensive, and adaptive in nature. Emotional overreactions are destructive; when they occur chronically, physiological damage, disease, or death can follow. The effects of emotional overactivity and psychobiological breakdown can impinge on any body system. However, the body systems that are directly innervated and regulated by the autonomic nervous system are the primary targets.

An emotion is evoked by a sequence of events. Thoughts and feelings are elicited. The resulting physiological reaction is the end product of this chain of phenomena.

Cognitive and emotional processes enable the client to construct a mental map of the immediate environment. This map guides future responses required for basic survival.[27]

Despite the significance and importance of defense mechanisms provided by emotions, few attempts have been made to provide a theoretical framework for understanding and measuring these defenses. This is evidenced by the inability of the mental health sciences to define or describe the structure of emotions—the basic elements of human personality.

Historically, psychological factors have been recognized as "triggers" for the development of psychosomatic disturbances. Clients need to be taught how various negative emotions can release endotoxins (components of bacterial catabolism) that affect the brain and immune system. The brain is capable of sorting and storing infinite particles of information that, when transmitted via the psychophysiological links or emotional language, can be evoked in subconscious or conscious states to insulate or protect the individual from insult or injury. When considering possible triggering mechanisms for psychophysiological disturbances, it is essential to remember that the individual's totality is not merely physical, mental, emotional, spiritual, magnetic, or electrical, but an integration of all of these aspects.

The basic circuit by which we communicate our sense of being is our belief system—our particular organization of self-image. A *belief system* is a set of assumptions and values that restricts our perceptions of the surrounding environment. A key to health, therefore, is belief. Belief engages the electro-magnetic-chemical circuitry of our mind, automatically establishing a pattern within the basic physiology of health, homeostasis, or disturbances. It is important to understand the circuitry of consciousness and the mechanisms by which we create our experience of life and reality.

Soviet scientist Victor Inyushin[3] demonstrated in 1970 his belief that the human body is a three-dimensional "virtual image," formed in our mind by our self-image. Inyushin hypothesized that we continually "self-organize," depending on the image we hold of ourselves within our mind. This unconscious self-image can be transmitted from the brain to the nucleus of each cell to reform our basic cellular structure. A state of homeostasis or disequilibrium results, depending on the individual's self-image. This research demonstrates the stimulus for psychophysiological disturbance or disease manifestation.

It has become accepted that the unique manifestations of a physical illness are overshadowed by the client's personality structures. Numerous clients, who have well-established chronic diseases experience recurrent exacerbations of symptoms in relation to severe life stress. The outcome of any physiological process will be greatly influenced by the mental attitude of the client.

A recent health survey report illustrates an orientation to traditional medicine fostered by the holistic health movement. Franz Ingelfinger, former editor of The New England Journal of Medicine, estimated that 80% of all patients are unaffected by medical treatment. Only 10% actually experience "dramatically successful" medical intervention, while 9% are made sicker by the cure than by the disease. This report demonstrates that the traditional medical model of care may not be meeting the holistic needs of a large proportion of clients in the general population.

It is easily demonstrated that a client experiencing a serious and/or progressive physical malady is prone to developing various psychological responses to it (*e.g.,* denial, repression, conversion reactions). Note also that the particular insult experienced emotionally by the client may be more serious and permanent than the physical manifestations of psychophysiological imbalance.

In the individual experiencing a psychosomatic state of disequilibrium, there may be expressed a conscious desire for a release from a particular physical disability, while the person unconsciously maintains a desire for the symptoms to continue unabated. The client's unconscious needs for self-depreciation, self-punishment, self-importance, protest, jealousy, or even revenge can precipitate a resistance to change. Subsequently, if this is left untreated, the client may exhibit a prolonged convalescence or chronic invalidism as a subconscious attempt to seek further treatment of the root cause for the disease process (*i.e.,* chronic invalids may suffer more from diseased family relationships than from the disease processes themselves).

Physicist Fred Alan Wolf stated in his book, *Taking the Quantum Leap:*

> "The experiences we often call 'reality' depend upon how we make life choices. Each act we perform is a choice, even if we are unaware that we have made a choice. Our unawareness of choice at the level of electrons and atoms gives the illusion of mechanical reality. In this way, we continue to appear as mere victims subject to the whims of a 'higher being.' We appear to be victims ruled by a destiny we did not create."[38]

The Psychosocial Perspective

At a very early age, individuals formulate personal attitudes and self-concepts that affect their health. In the succeeding years of personal development, coping strate-

RELEVANT RESEARCH

Cassileth and others tested the ability of selected factors to predict survival and relapse in recently diagnosed clients with advanced malignant disease. Two groups of clients were studied. Group I had advanced malignant disease associated with poor prognoses. They were followed for length of survival.

Group II clients had cutaneous malignant melanomas or Stage II breast cancer. Group II clients were followed for recurrence of disease. The treatment process for each client was recorded, as was the level of activity.

All clients completed a questionnaire concerning seven variables found in previous studies to predict longevity, including: social ties and marital history, job satisfaction, use of psychotropic drugs, general satisfaction, general health, hopelessness/helplessness, and adjustment required to cope with the illness.

Findings indicated that psychosocial variables (mentioned above) do not predict longer survival in clients with advanced metastatic disease (Group I). Also, these factors did not predict the recurrence interval of disease in clients with high-risk primary melanoma or Stage II breast cancer (Group II).

The authors concluded that the inherent biological process of malignant disease alone determined the prognosis. The authors noted that their study did not address the possibility that psychosocial factors or events may influence the cause of the disease or the recurrence of disease in patients with more favorable cancer diagnoses.

(Cassileth C, Lusk E, Miller D et al: Psychosocial correlates of survival in advanced malignant disease. N Engl J Med 312:1551, 1985.)

---

gies are created consciously and unconsciously. Coping strategies are unique to each individual's internal and external experiences. In some persons, coping mechanisms serve as a mask for true inner feelings.[22]

Thomas conducted a study of 17 successive classes of medical students over a 40-year period at Johns Hopkins Medical Institute. She found that students who were cold or dispassionate were not close to their parents, or that frequently the father figure had been absent. Thomas also found that generally the middle child in birth order demonstrated a strong predisposition to major illnesses, including heart disease, cancer, obesity, and ulcers.[35]

Using a "life change" theory of disease, Rahe found that a pattern of significant life changes generally preceded mental and physical illness.[30] (See discussion in Chap. 9.)

Stewart has shown that polio and other viruses can be carried by individuals for months or years with no appreciable effects. He states that "the resulting disease is, in fact, determined by the host, rather than by the bacillus."[34]

Research by Gray and LaViolette[14] into the specifics of personality structure and mechanics presents an integrative psychological and neurophysical model. This model suggests that, when an emotional stimulus is transmitted to the memory sector of the brain/mind, this stimulus serves as a coded label for a specific mental experience. Thus, when the memory tracts later react, they elicit an emotional transmission in its originally-recorded form. The ideas of Gray and LaViolette provide a viable explanation for the occurrence and recurrence of psychophysiological disorders.

The literature is full of numerous studies by leading authorities in nutrition, psychiatry, medicine, and physiology reinforcing the theories of how mental beliefs and the interactions of physiological and psychological factors create states of health or disease.[21] Williams[37] found that emotional states leading to psychophysiological diseases may be predisposed by poor nutrition, resulting in impaired brain functioning. Pauling[26] cites the body's specific needs for adequate daily intake of ascorbic acid, thiamine, niacinamide, pyridoxine, vitamin B_{12}, folic acid, magnesium, glutamic acid, and 1-tryptophane for the maintenance of psychophysiological health. A counter to the theories postulating a propensity of psychological factors to promote physiological illness has been presented by Cassileth[8] in the following Relevant Research.

The Biological Perspective

To understand better the nature of human psychophysiology, we must concern ourselves with the functioning of three distinct biological structures: receptors, integrators, and effectors.

Receptors are energy-sensitive organ structures. Receptors include light-sensitive components of the eyes, sound-sensitive structures in the ears, chemical-sensitive structures on the surface of the tongue, temperature-sensitive structures in the skin, and pressure-sensitive structures in the muscles and joints.

Effectors are response mechanism structures. The two kinds of effector structures are muscles, specialized for contracting, and glands, specialized for secreting.

Integrators are mediators between receptors (sense organs) and effectors (muscle and glands). The nervous system in its entirety is a specialized integrator.

The stimulation of any sense organ results in electrochemical impulses, conveyed via afferent neurons to the central nervous system. The stimuli are effectively or ineffectively interpreted and autonomic activity is initiated, which causes changes in the cardiovascular, endocrine, and gastrointestinal systems. According to Selye's stress theory, an individual can react in different ways to stressors. When the severity of a stressor is within an individual's tolerance, the person can adjust to the stress over a long period of time. When a stressor exceeds the individual's tolerance, the period before the body's resources are exhausted is shorter, and physical deterioration begins. If a period of adjustment or tolerance is followed by a period of disorganization, physical disorders develop. Exhaustion then ensues which, if untreated or uninterrupted, can result in death.[33]

The Therapeutic Use of Self

It seems ambiguous that, even with the openness of mental health education today, so many people are still afraid of mental illness. Nursing students also exhibit some of the apprehension found in the general lay population. Nursing instructors and peers can gently help nursing students to focus on the concept that the quantity of illness symptoms, and the degree to which they interfere with one's life, are more significant than having some unhealthy thoughts, symptoms, or beliefs. This understanding aids in separating the nursing student from the role of client. Nursing students can be reassured in ways that validate that they have successfully learned to navigate their responses to crises and unpleasant situations in a predominantly healthy manner. Once fear and anxiety on the part of the student subside, the nursing student emerges as a role model for healthy resolution of problems; the student emerges as a self-responsible person and as a self-healer. All of these qualities are necessary for therapeutic intervention with the special clients who are the focus in this chapter. The role of the student nurse must also encompass an attitude of reality tempered with optimism. The encouragement and nurturing posture of the student are vital, and inseparable from a regimen of psychotropic medicines, counseling, history-taking, and other therapeutic interventions.

One needs to act on the definition of nursing as both an art and a science in order to interact therapeutically with clients displaying psychophysiological disorders. The nursing student has the challenge of synthesizing theory from a variety of disciplines, such as anatomy, physiology, motivation theory, sociology, psychology, communication, and spirituality, in order to use the nursing process effectively with these unique clients.

Another aspect of the therapeutic use of self involves listening freely without judgment, and going beyond personal limits of "right or wrong." Nurses must examine their own belief systems in such a vigilant manner in order not to role-model personal prejudices or circumscribed beliefs to vulnerable clients.

It is important to emphasize that clients are faced with a frightening dilemma: they need to *change* their behaviors, thought patterns, or even involuntary responses in order to become more healthy. However, they do not really know what their new "harmonized" self will be, and so there exist two poles: the comfort of remaining the same (even when this alternative is unhealthy and self-destructive), and the risk of change. Health care providers need to address this dilemma in an empathic style.

Nurses can only hope to shift the fulcrum of decision-making on the part of clients toward taking the risk of moving into what is, for them, the healthy unknown.

Classifications of Psychophysiological Disturbances

The Diagnostic and Statistical Manual of Mental Disorders (DSM-III-R)[1] describes a category of psychological factors affecting physical conditions. Diagnostic criteria, as stated in the DSM-III-R, include:

A. The presence of psychologically meaningful environmental stimuli that are related to the initiation or potentiation of a physical condition.
B. The presence of a physical condition that occurs either with demonstrated organic pathology (*e.g.,* rheumatoid arthritis) or with a known pathophysiological process (*e.g.,* migraine headache, vomiting).
C. The condition is not due to a Somatoform Disorder (as hypochondriasis).

The Nursing Process

New frontiers of psychophysiological research offer nurses ways to integrate the nursing process and many innovative interventions to promote the client's awareness of how to harmonize the mind, body, spirit, and emotions. The essential role of the nurse as a teacher and facilitator for change is addressed through the use of the systems model discussed throughout this text.

Assessment

The first step in the nursing process is assessment of psychophysiological behaviors. In the psychophysiological realm, it is particularly important to assess the psychological state by:

1. Determining the client's definition of the present problem
2. Identifying the client's understanding of the presenting problem and any contributing factors, stresses, or conflicts that may have caused the problem
3. Evaluating the client's self-concept and sense of self-worth and how these fit in with the client's relationship with his or her environment
4. Identifying the client's belief system that has influenced behaviors
5. Evaluating environmental, social, and psychological variables that have influenced the client's behavior
6. Evaluating the client's readiness to change behaviors that have a negative effect on psychophysiological functioning

7. Helping the client to identify support systems that can reinforce appropriate and healthy new behaviors

Nursing Diagnosis

Nursing diagnoses are summary statements based on the nurse's initial and ongoing assessment. The following are examples of nursing diagnoses[24] that may be useful for clients with psychophysiological problems:

1. *Knowledge deficit:* There is a lack of information regarding stress-producing environmental factors.
2. *Self-concept disturbance:* Self-esteem is threatened by feelings of powerlessness and helplessness when client is confronted with conflict.
3. *Anxiety:* Increased cardiovascular responses when client is informed of hospital procedures are secondary to feelings of loss of control because of past experience with hospitalization.
4. *Ineffective coping:* The individual is unable to function in former roles.

Nursing Interventions and Case Examples

Once clearly stated nursing diagnoses are made, along with outcome criteria (evaluation) statements, the interventions are outlined. Interventions are the tools used to meet the goals of client care. The nurse's role extends beyond the behaviors presented by the client. The interpersonal relationship is used as a therapeutic tool in the interchange with clients. This is done through further therapeutic communication and through teaching clients new ways of coping. The following format is the basis on which nursing interventions are planned.

Rationale for Intervention:

1. Clients come fully equipped to heal themselves. The nurse's role is as an educator and facilitator of the clients' learning to initiate the self-healing properties within the body.
2. The emotional conflict that the client has not chosen to deal with previously now takes the form of a physical distress, *i.e.,* pain or discomfort. The nurse's role is to employ the therapeutic use of the self through communication and interpersonal skills. The client's awareness is enhanced.
3. The client's emotional conflicts are based on false beliefs that are maintained as part of the self-concept. The nurse's role is to build a consistent, trusting relationship whereby the client may redefine some personal beliefs regarding the self.

Interventions will be addressed here that research has shown can help an individual learn new ways to reduce stress and to develop greater self-awareness in order to create changes in feelings and behavior.

Intervention

Interventions may include:

1. *Visualization* is forming a mental picture or vision of what is not actually present to the sight. One achieves a "focused awareness, while minimizing thoughts, emotions, and physical pain."[10] *Example:* client closes eyes and visualizes a cool color in order to relax.
2. *Guided imagery* includes listening to a recorded or actual voice describing a relaxing scene or experience.
3. *Autogenic training* uses the bodily sensations of heaviness and warmth to relax the body and then expand this relaxed state to the mind. *Autogenic* means self-generating or doing a procedure oneself to self-heal.[15] *Example:* client repeats calming phrases, such as "I am quiet," while reclining.
4. *Therapeutic touch* is the use of techniques such as massage or the laying on of hands to promote healing and relaxation.[7,16]
5. *Time management* increases decision-making and priority-setting skills in order to decrease frustrations, fatigue, and feeling overwhelmed.[10]
6. *Biofeedback* is a technique for measuring physiological stress by means of instruments, and using this information as feedback to the client who is learning to control body processes.[15]
7. *Meditation* is a mental exercise used to facilitate control of attention rather than being bombarded by environmental stimuli. Attention is focused, or opened up.[15] *Example:* A client assumes a comfortable position and silently repeats a calming word.
8. *Relaxation* and *breath awareness* are additional techniques that will be discussed in greater depth later in this chapter.

Application of the Nursing Process in Psychophysiological Disorders

Case I: Mary. Mary and the student nurse sit in the day room talking about Mary's abdominal pain. Mary begins to cry.

"It's okay to cry, you know," the nurse says. Mary avoids eye contact.

"I *hate* to cry. It serves no purpose. God, I wish my body would just let me do all I have to do. There's so much, and I have to do every bit of it myself."

The student responds: "So neither your husband nor your children help you with the housework or meals, and on top of managing a household you have your own obligations to yourself and your career, right?"

"Not exactly," Mary responds after a few seconds of thought. "The kids help when they can. I just . . . well . . . it's done faster and better if I do it myself. It's done right." She grasps her waist more tightly and begins to rock in her chair, with a barely audible moan.

"What is the reason you are grabbing your waist?"

NURSING CARE PLAN

ASSESSMENT	NURSING INTERVENTIONS	EVALUATION CRITERIA

NURSING DIAGNOSIS: Ineffective Individual Coping

SUBJECTIVE DATA

Client states, "I hate to cry. It serves no purpose."
"I have to do everything myself."
"I am my job at home."

OBJECTIVE DATA

Client has stomach pain; it hurts when she attempts to hold in feelings.
Client does not ask for help. Has Type-A personality.
Client has unclear definition of her own identity.

1. In a structured one-to-one session with the client, *facilitate* awareness of the relationship between gastric pain and the inability to ask for help.
2. In a 20-minute session, teach breathing exercises. Request feedback and return demonstration 8 hours after initial instruction. Have client perform the exercise 3 times daily: mid-morning, mid-afternoon, and bedtime.
3. Ask client to describe daily routine at home. Assist in time management. Observe for willingness to ask for help and to include relaxation and breathing exercises in daily routine.

Client will state relationship between feelings and pain. By May 14, will have a 60% decrease in requests for pain medication.

Client will independently offer feedback to nursing staff on breathing exercises. Will state increasing insight into self and personal feelings in group sessions and in one-to-one sessions.

Client will present time management plan for post discharge in group meeting.

The nurse watches Mary's jaws tense before she responds. "Because my stomach hurts and because I'm angry. There's so much expected of me."

"Who expects you to do all you tell me you have to do?" Mary doesn't answer. "Then you can quietly answer that question in your own mind. Now consider this: if you don't do it all yourself, are you scared things at home might be able to run well without you?"

"No . . . well . . . yes." The student nurse watches Mary's hands knot into fists.

"Looks like you're getting mad because you *Want* to be the perfect mother and at the same time you want to start a career. You get mad when your family doesn't take care of itself, and again when it does. That's an awful lot of stress to handle, and your body has to cope with it as well as your emotions."

"I never saw things that way," Mary whispers. She bites her upper lip.

"Does your stomach hurt right where your diaphragm is, right under your ribs?" Mary nods. "I want you to relax," the student says. "Take a deep breath. You're holding a lot inside, and that's hard on both your mind and your body. Now, take a *really* deep breath."

Mary inhales, sighs, and begins to cry.

"Go, Mary. C'mon. Be Mary, now. You don't have to be the perfect mother. You don't have to be the perfect student. Just be who you are this second."

"I'm really scared. For so long, what made me who I was—am—was my job at home. If I give up that part of

my identity, and if I fail at school, I'll be nobody." She chokes, takes another deep breath, and then begins to cry freely. "But yes, this is who I am right now. I am worried and frightened, and have to cry."

"You're doing fine. Now, just release that tension instead of locking it in and carrying it around."

"I can't believe how . . . well, it feels . . . I feel better. I'm still scared, but it feels good just to be here. . . ." Mary's arms unravel from around her waist, and she leans back in her chair.

Summary: Mary's goals were met. During her treatment she incorporated breathing exercises into her daily routine, and stated that this helps her become more "together." She was able to express feelings of guilt and resentment. Her gastric pain was almost nonexistent on discharge. She planned to continue working part-time and to take one class, one evening per week.

Case II: Ms. Reed.   Ms. Reed talks with the student nurse during their interview.

"Look at these hands." She forces a smile. "They used to fly across a keyboard. Before word processors were even heard of, I could type 90 words a minute."

The student asks, "Is typing a primary part of your job now that you've been promoted?"

"Well, no. But I have to set an example. There are reports and letters to be written, and plenty of charts to do. And I don't know . . . I just don't know if I can do it *all* now. I could if it weren't for this arthritis."

NURSING CARE PLAN

ASSESSMENT	NURSING INTERVENTIONS	EVALUATION CRITERIA

NURSING DIAGNOSIS: Potential Alteration in Self-Concept, Role Performance

SUBJECTIVE DATA

Client: "Look at these hands." (smiles)
Client talked about job and pain, and blood pressure increased
Client showed facial distress when moving hands.

OBJECTIVE DATA

Inappropriate affect may indicate anger.
Anxiety related to role performance
Pain

1. In a structured one-to-one session, teach 20 minutes in "layman's terms" the benefits (*i.e.,* autonomic nervous system response) of relaxation training, and correct procedure.
   a. Guide the client through a 20-minute relaxation session.
   b. Assess heart rate, respiratory rate, and blood pressure before and after exercise.

Client will fill out menus for next three meals without increase in pain.
Client will have increased R.O.M. in both hands without increasing pain.
Client will discuss role performance with the nurse. B/P will not increase more than 10 mm between pre- and post-intervention.
Client will state that the relaxation exercise has benefited her medical regimen.

"Think of the worst that could happen," the student suggests. (The student notes that Ms. Reed begins to massage the backs of her hands and grimace.)

"If I lost this job, I'd be at home all day. Financially, we're okay. . . . But I'd just go crazy at home doing nothing, thinking about where I could be instead—in the office."

The student asks if she'd be angry at herself.

"Not really angry, just disappointed. All my life, I've wanted to be in charge. I knew how to make people work for me. I just never expected that something like arthritis would keep me from being the person I wanted to be."

The student comments, "It sounds like you have a tough job, even for someone who doesn't have arthritis."

"I do!" Ms. Reed's face flushes. "It *is* tough, and I'm scared to death every morning when I sit behind that desk. The only way to learn to do things right is to *do* them. I wish I had never seen a typewriter in my life. I wish I could have been happy just being a mother and a wife." She raises her voice, and her words seem to spill out of her mouth. "My whole life has just been an accident. I let things happen, or waited for them to happen, and I've never had any control or worked toward any real goal, until a couple of years ago when I saw that I might be able to make a dream come true."

The student interrupts her, "Slow down, Ms. Reed. You are very hard on yourself." The student nurse checks Ms. Reed's blood pressure. It has increased from resting 102/62 to 160/80 during their conversation.

Summary: Ms. Reed is very receptive to the relaxation training. She uses the suggestions without any difficulty and without having to be reminded. She states that she really enjoys feeling relaxed. Her condition improves. Blood pressure recording shows a consistent,

near-normal value, before and after conversation. Her arthritis pain diminishes in her hands, and her function increases, after the use of relaxation techniques. On discharge, Ms. Reed plans to take extended medical leave for two more weeks and then, hopefully, to return to work.

Evaluation

The client and the nurse formulate mutually-accepted goals after making the initial assessment. Long-term outcome criteria are those that are attainable before discharge from the acute care setting or in terminating care. The following are examples of outcome criteria written as evaluative statements:

1. The client will demonstrate relaxation techniques after two instructional periods.
2. The client will demonstrate a significant decrease in cardiovascular measures after utilizing the above method of relaxation for three days.
3. The client will independently demonstrate a breathing method after three instructional periods.
4. The client will show a definite reduction in physiological parameters that have indicated the psychophysiological disorder (*i.e.,* decreased pain, decrease in heart rate, lowered blood pressure).
5. The client will express three "I" statements that reflect how stress is contributing to the present physical condition.
6. The client will express three ways to cope with future stresses. These three ways will be based upon new learning experiences.

Specific Interventions

Relaxation Training

The mind–body relationship was explored by Miller, a well-known learning theorist who showed that visceral and glandular responses could be learned. He demonstrated experimentally that individuals can learn to decrease, as well as increase, the heart rate. Individuals learn to increase or relax intestinal contractions, decrease or increase stomach contractions, change blood pressure (independent of the heart rate), and change brain wave patterns.[25]

This opened new vistas for a multitude of innovative modalities, and created new ways in which individuals can learn to bring the autonomic nervous system under self-control.[23,28]

Herbert Benson was a pioneer in relaxation response research, *i.e.,* relaxation training. The relaxation response is now defined as an integrated hypothalamic reaction, resulting in a generalized decrease in sympathetic nervous system activity.[6]

Intrigued by studies on transcendental meditation, Benson noted that physiological changes elicited during meditation differed from the changes that occurred while subjects were sitting quietly or sleeping. The meditators showed a decrease in their body metabolism and in their heart and respiratory rates. Further, Benson found four commonalities in different modes of relaxation with meditation:

1. A comfortable position
2. A quiet environment
3. Repetition of a word, a prayer, a sound, or a phrase
4. Adoption of a passive mode when other thoughts came into consciousness

The implication of Benson's research concerning relaxation is vital for individuals with cardiac problems or essential hypertension. His work supports the theories of mind–body interaction outlined in this chapter.

From this initial research, various relaxation exercises have been developed. In 1982, the California Nurses' Association adopted a position that there is clearly a role for registered nurses as providers of relaxation therapies to health care consumers.[32]

Benson's relaxation method is summarized as follows:

Breath Awareness

Controlling the breath, and thus calming the nerves, is a prerequisite to controlling the mind and the body.[31] One simple intervention is *breath awareness.* Through the breath, one can learn to relax and be cognizant of body–mind interaction. It is essential to help clients become intensely aware of their bodily signals of stress and anxiety.

The focus of breath awareness as a nursing intervention is the quality of the breath as it relates to stressful events. Normally, a full exhalation and inhalation begin when the diaphragm muscle contracts. This results in a slight expansion of the lower ribs and protrusion of the upper abdomen. The middle portions of the lungs expand with outward chest movements in the thoracic phase as inhalation proceeds further. At the end of inhalation, still more air is admitted when the clavicles rise and the uppermost region of the lungs is expanded. Each

---

RELAXATION EXERCISES

EXERCISE 1

The following seven basic elements in a simple mental procedure can evoke the relaxation response:

1. Choose a quiet environment.
2. Sit in a comfortable position.
3. Close your eyes.
4. Deeply relax all of your muscles, beginning at your feet and progressing up to your face (feet, calves, thighs, lower torso, chest, shoulders, neck, and head). Allow them to remain deeply relaxed. Breathe through your nose. Become aware of your breathing.
5. As you breathe out, say the word "one" silently to yourself. Then breathe in. Then breathe out with "one," in, and out with "one."
6. Continue this practice for 20 minutes.
7. You may open your eyes to check the time, but do not use an alarm. When you finish, sit quietly for several minutes, at first with your eyes closed and later with your eyes open.

Remember not to worry about whether you were successful in achieving a deep level of relaxation. Maintain a passive attitude and permit relaxation to occur at its own pace. When distracting thoughts occur, ignore them and continue to repeat "one" as you breathe. This technique should be practiced at least once a day; do not do it within two hours of any meal because the digestive processes seem to interfere with the elicitation of the expected changes.[6]

EXERCISE 2

The second exercise, which is a little easier to practice and takes about three to five minutes, is appropriate when time is limited. The client repeats slowly after the nurse:

I close my eyes gently and take a calming breath.
I empty my mind of all thoughts and feelings and distractions.
As these leave my mind I notice and let them go.
I let all thoughts flow like a river through my mind.
My mind empties and the cool rivers calm me.
I allow my mind to rest.
I notice what it is like to empty my mind.
I appreciate the deep rest and peace.
I take a slow and energizing breath and go about my day with calm efficiency.

RELEVANT RESEARCH

Benson studied the effects of relaxation training on 126 manufacturing employees. Three small groups, labeled A, B, and C, were observed. Group A was taught a technique for initiating a relaxation response. Group B was instructed to sit quietly. Group C received no instructions, in order to act as a control group. Groups A and B took two 15-minute relaxation breaks daily. After eight weeks they showed great improvement in every index: illness, performance, sociability, job satisfaction, and happiness. Little improvement was shown by Group C, and blood pressure was significantly lower in Group A. It was interesting to note that those with the highest blood pressure readings prior to the study experienced the greatest decrease in blood pressure.

(Benson H: The Relaxation Response. New York, William Morrow, 1973.)

phase of inhalation acts on one particular area of the lung. When exhaling, the opposite process occurs. The chest relaxes, the abdomen flattens, and the breath is fully expelled.

The most natural way of breathing can best be seen in a child under age six. The abdomen is fully expanded on inhalation, the chest is held up and out and the shoulders are relaxed as the child exhales. A common request of a parent to "stand tall and hold the tummy in" alters the breathing pattern. The child begins to breathe with the costal muscle only. This alteration in the breathing pattern can result in a decreased vital lung capacity. This creates a shallowness in the breathing pattern that results in a restricted, controlled breath. It also results in a disproportion between the inhalation phase and the exhalation phase.

As feelings are repressed, the breathing restriction becomes more severe. One clinician observed that, when individuals are afraid, breathing becomes more shallow and rapid, i.e., anxiety promotes hyperventilation. When individuals are depressed, breathing becomes slow, heavy, and labored. When the client is aware of the restrictions in breathing, the first step in becoming more in tune with the body and the breath has been accomplished.

Learning to take in a full breath is comparable on a physiological level to receiving love and nourishment on a psychological level. Restriction of inhalation may imply that the individual fears receiving attention or caring from others, and may enjoy giving to others rather than receiving. This individual must learn to receive as well as to give, in order to create the body–mind harmony.

Restriction on exhalation is comparable on a physiological level to fears of fully expressing the self and letting go on a psychological level. Individuals may be afraid to express fully who they are because of intense fears of rejection. Thus, they are observed to hold on to the breath. The child learns to stifle sobs and inhibit crying. Later the child may develop the habit of holding on to the breath, which may develop into asthma or a chronic lung condition.[31]

The client's attention must be directed to conscious breathing. The nurse's role is as a facilitator and teacher in assisting clients to become more aware of their breath, and more aware of where their feelings were repressed. This can be the beginning of a therapeutic exchange.

Breath Awareness Exercise

The ideal times for the breath awareness exercise are early in the morning prior to breakfast, at mid-morning, or just before retiring in the evening. The exercise should not be done immediately following a meal because the exercise slows the digestive processes of the body. A simple explanation to the client of the benefits of diaphragmatic breathing is essential prior to beginning the exercise. The following box provides some guidelines and instructions that can easily be given in approximately 10 to 15 minutes:

Notice the difference in the heart and respiratory rates before and after the exercise. If clients have difficulty with the repetitions, have them perform the repetitions until they are comfortable. Be sure to tell clients that they are relearning the breathing process, and that it will soon become easier.

A variation of this exercise is to place the hands below the sternum and above the umbilicus. Focusing the

BREATH AWARENESS EXERCISE

Give the client the following instructions:
1. Lie in a comfortable supine position.
2. Place your hands over the lower part of the abdomen, below the umbilicus and above the pubic crest. The right hand should be over the left.
3. Breathe through the nose.
4. Inhale on the count of 5, slowly and silently. (First your abdomen expands, and then your chest.)
5. Exhale through the nose on the count of 5. First your abdomen retracts, and then your chest relaxes.)
6. Repeat the complete exercise 5 times.
7. When finished, take a full, deep breath.

hands and the breath on a particular part of the body helps to relax that area. Placing the hands in this area when doing this breathing exercise is especially helpful to clients with acute gastric distress, nausea, vomiting, anorexia, or ulcers. A simplified version of the breathing exercise can be especially helpful in helping clients to relax during intrusive procedures, such as venipuncture and lumbar puncture. Because these procedures increase feelings of anxiety, this intervention may be appropriately introduced in a shortened form. Instruct clients to:

1. Take a deep breath—inhale. (Abdomen expands.)
2. Exhale slowly. (Abdomen deflates.)
3. Focus the mind elsewhere (*e.g.,* past pleasant experience or activity).
4. Repeat three times.

Levels of Prevention

Primary prevention concerns the promotion of mental health and the prevention of illness. Nurses practicing primary prevention help people to understand the pervasive effects of undue stress on their psychological and physiological status. The nurse also works with clients to help them understand the importance of planning and developing lifestyles that promote psychological and physiological health. Do clients have a balance in their lives? Do they engage in health practices conducive to wellness in each of the components of the person as a system (societal, environmental, cultural, psychological, and biological)? Do the environmental systems of the clients promote wellness in each of the components?

Primary prevention is an important focus for health care providers and consumers in the fast-paced 1980s. We have identified types of people who may demonstrate psychosomatic illness due to high stress levels, poor coping strategies, dysfunctional reactions to childhood traumas, and the like. Type-A and Type-B personalities are familiar concepts for the consumer, who is cognizant of the impact these behaviors play on psychological and physiological functioning. Mental health is being promoted by the media through commercials teaching us how to recognize mental illness in adolescence and young adulthood. Business and industry have taken a giant step in mitigating the effects of stress through building wellness programs at the workplace. Many nurses work in such programs.

Secondary prevention concerns early case-finding and treatment. Education is an important aspect of this intervention. *Many* individuals do not believe that there is a psychological component to their psychophysiological illness. What is the best approach in working with clients to discuss the psychological and physiological connections in their illness? Some clients deny any psychological aspect of their illness when the topic is presented to them in a way that indicates that the client has a "mental" issue or concern. Clients can respond to an approach that introduces concepts about a healthy lifestyle. Problematic lifestyle patterns are seen as deviations from health rather than illnesses per se.

The media are in the forefront as communicators about agencies, places, and people who can be used for those in mental crisis. The range of treatments are unlimited today, and include modalities as contrasting as psychotropic medicines and laying on of hands, and all combinations in between.

The case studies and nursing process examples used in this chapter illustrate that many clients exhibiting psychophysiological disorders enter the health care delivery system at the tertiary prevention stage. *Tertiary prevention* in reference to these clients encompasses a broad spectrum of rehabilitation techniques. Counseling, visualization, imagery, biofeedback, exercise, and nutrition may be used singly or concurrently to aid the client to return to, or discover, an optimum level of functioning.

In many cases, clients at the tertiary level of care require deliberate and consistent feedback as they work on lifestyle changes. Clients need encouragement and support: one relaxation exercise session will not produce a lifestyle change or tension release. Clients need to practice recommended interventions consistently to feel the effects. During the period in which there is little felt effect, clients may believe that they are expending wasted effort and may not engage in the tertiary-level work. Many clients at the tertiary level of care also need help to understand that their illness needs constant and long-term effort. A client with asthma, for example, who believes that the illness has gone away after a period of intense treatment, may become depressed upon return of the illness.

Summary

1. Increasing public interest in wellness contributes to the emergence of a new awareness of personal health maintenance.

2. Current concepts of diagnosis and intervention involve a view of the total person, including the individual's physical and psychological concerns and the manner in which the two can interact to produce illness.

3. Many chronic and acute physical disturbances are the result of early environmental factors that influence psychoemotional perceptions and reactions that prompt physiological stress. Such physiological stress promotes a predisposition to disease.

4. Health care professionals whose work addresses the whole person may recognize the "lifetype" of clients, and search for causative psychosocial/emotional factors in the development of disease processes.

5. Clinical use of relaxation, breath awareness, visualization, and touch therapies have proved to be powerful and effective tools for healing of psychophysiological disturbances.

6. Beginning mental health nurses can use relaxation training and breath awareness in caring for clients with psychophysiological disorders.

7. Relevant research in the area of psychophysiological functions has aided nurses in understanding the dynamics of mind–body interactions.

References

1. American Psychiatric Association: Diagnostic and Statistical Manual of Mental Disorders, Revised (DSM-III-R). Washington, DC, American Psychiatric Association, 1987

2. Arehart-Treichel J: Biotypes. San Diego, Harcourt-Brace-Jovanovich, 1972

3. Arehart-Treichel J: The mind–body link. Sci News 20:393, 1975

4. Bahnson C, Bahnson M: Personality Variables and Life Experiences Predicting Specific Disease Syndromes. Paper presented at the 82nd American Psychological Association meeting, 1974

5. Bennett C: Family Stress May Trigger Childhood Arthritis. The Arthritis Foundation, 1978

6. Benson H: The Relaxation Response. New York, William Morrow, 1973

7. Brallier L: Successfully Managing Stress. Los Altos, California, National Nursing Review, 1982

8. Cassileth B: Patient outlook plays no role in cancer recurrence or survival. Brain Mind Bull 10:1, 1985

9. Coddington R: The significance of life events as etiologic factors in the disease of children. J Psychosom Res 16:7, 1972

10. Davis M, Eshelman E, McKay M: The Relaxation and Stress Reduction Workbook. Oakland, California, New Harbinger, 1982

11. Flynn P: Holistic Health: The Art and Science of Care. New York, Robert Brady, 1980

12. Freud S: Project for a Scientific Psychology. In The Origins of Psychoanalysis. New York, Basic Books, 1954

13. Garrity T, Marx M, Somes G: The relationship of recent life changes to seriousness of later illness. J Psychosom Res 22:7, 1978

14. Gray G, LaViolette T: The Great Ravelled Knot. Sci Am 179:27, 1948

15. Greenberg J: Comprehensive Stress Management. Dubuque, Iowa, William C. Brown, 1983

16. Krieger D: The Therapeutic Touch: How To Use Your Hands to Help or to Heal. Englewood Cliffs, New Jersey, Prentice-Hall, 1979

17. Krupp M, Chatton M: Current Medical Diagnosis and Treatment. Los Altos, California, Lange Medical Publications, 1982

18. Kurtz R, Prestera H: The Body Reveals. New York, Harper & Row, 1976

19. Lachman S: Psychosomatic Disorders: A Behavioristic Interpretation. New York, John Wiley & Sons, 1972

20. LeShan L: You Can Fight for Your Life—Emotional Factors in the Causation of Cancer. New York, Evans, 1977

21. Leukel F: Introduction to Physiological Psychology. St Louis, CV Mosby, 1972

22. Lewis H, Lewis M: Psychosomatics: How Your Emotions Can Damage Your Health. New York, Viking Press, 1972

23. Lowan A: Bioenergetics. New York, Penguin, 1976

24. McFarland G, Wasli E: Nursing Diagnosis and Process in Psychiatric/Mental Health Nursing. Philadelphia, JB Lippincott, 1986

25. Miller N, DiCara L, Solomon H: Learned modification of autonomic functions: A review and some data. Circ Res 26:1, 1970

26. Pauling L: The new medicine. Nutr Today 7:18, 1972

27. Paulley J: Cultural influences on the incidence and pattern of disease. Psychother Psychosom 26:2, 1975

28. Pelletier K: Mind as Healer: Mind as Slayer. New York, Dell Publishing, 1977

29. Powell L, Friedman M: Alteration of Type-A Behavior in Coronary Patients. The Psychosomatic Approach: Contemporary Practice of Whole-Person Care. New York, John Wiley & Sons, 1985

30. Rahe R: Life Change and Illness Studies: Past and Future Directions. J Human Stress 4:3, 1978

31. Rama S, Ballentine R, Hymes A: Science of Breath. Honesdale, Pennsylvania, Himalayan International Institute, 1980

32. Schwartz G: Position Statement. California Nurs 56:5, 1982

33. Selye H: The Stress of Life. New York, McGraw-Hill, 1956

34. Stewart G: Infection and immunization. Scott Med J 24:47, 1979

35. Thomas C: Prospective study of the Rorschachs of suicides: The predictive potential of pathological content. Johns Hopk Med J 132:334, 1973

36. Vieth I: Huang Ti Nei Su Wen: The Yellow Emperor's Classic of Internal Medicine. Berkeley, University of California Press, 1972

37. Williams R: Immunopathology of rheumatoid arthritis. Hosp Pract 13:53, 1978

38. Wolf F: Taking the Quantum Leap: The New Physics for Nonscientists. San Francisco, Harper & Row, 1981

SUSAN CRAMER

PERSONALITY DISORDERS

Learning Objectives

Upon completion of this chapter the student should be able to do the following:

1. Enumerate significant causal factors in the development of personality disorders.
2. Discuss the principle of object constancy in the child who eventually develops a Borderline Personality Disorder.
3. Describe the most common characteristics of the Borderline Personality Disorders.
4. Discuss how the defense mechanism of *splitting* causes difficulties in the treatment program of the client with a Borderline Personality Disorder.
5. Plan nursing interventions for a client with a Borderline Personality Disorder.
6. Enumerate the necessary therapeutic techniques and interventions for suicidal clients.

7. Discuss the merits of family therapy in the treatment of clients with a Borderline Personality Disorder.
8. Describe the most common characteristics of the Narcissistic Personality Disorder.
9. Describe the nurse's therapeutic use of self in the treatment of the client with a Narcissistic Personality Disorder.
10. Make an assessment of a client with an Antisocial Personality Disorder.
11. Discuss the use of behavioral techniques in the treatment of clients with an Antisocial Personality Disorder.
12. Describe the significant factors in the prevention of personality disorders.

CLINICAL EXAMPLES

MICHAEL (BORDERLINE PERSONALITY)

Michael, a 26-year-old delivery person, was referred to the clinic by his family because of his thoughts of suicide. At times he thinks of jumping off a bridge, and he frequently wants to hit others with his delivery van. In the interview with the nurse, he does not seem concerned about what he is saying.

Michael says that he hates his job, but that he wants to keep it because of the good retirement benefits. He does not see any value in changing jobs, because he always ends up hating whatever he is doing. Michael has a few male acquaintances, but feels lonely much of the time. He has had a few affairs but, because he feels that he can not assert his wishes with women, he soon resents their way of doing things and leaves them. At present he gets drunk on occasion.

MR. WILSON (NARCISSISTIC PERSONALITY)

Mr. Wilson, a 48-year-old married professional man with three daughters, came for treatment at the substance abuse treatment center because he was not chosen to be president of his company. He is depressed and angry. His family agrees with Mr. Wilson's employer that he is selfish and self-involved and that he is unaware of the needs of others.

Mr. Wilson maintains that they all are wrong, and that it is his family and employees who are cold, incompetent, and unloving. He reports that both with people at work and with his family he feels he knows better how to manage situations, and he is critical and intolerant of their opinions. Mr. Wilson drinks heavily and has had many affairs throughout his 20-year marriage. He is admitted to the substance abuse unit.

Introduction

Personality disorders originate from immature and/or disturbed personality development. In the client with a personality disorder, traits have been developed that are rigid and do not assist the client to function optimally in the world.

While a personality disorder generally is not as debilitating as is a major depression or a language and thought disorder, a personality disorder can result in moderate to severe limitations for the client in the areas of (1) forming close and lasting relationships that serve to enhance the growth of the individuals involved, and (2) scholastic, work, and career development.

Personality disorders are generally recognizable in early adolescence; however, according to the Diagnostic and Statistical Manual of Mental Disorders (3rd edition, revised: DSM-III-R), the diagnosis of personality disor-

der may not be made until the age of 18 years. In addition, a diagnosis of personality disorder is made only when the characteristic features of the disorder are part of the individual's long-term functioning, and are not merely related to episodes of illness.[3]

The box on page 403 provides a list of personality disorders.[3] The spectrum of behavior problems is broad, and levels of functioning vary in severity. Mildly- to moderately-impaired individuals may appear gifted, gregarious, and professionally accomplished, but complain of feelings of emptiness and ennui with the inability to give or receive love in interpersonal relationships. Others around the individual may label the person "difficult." Severely-impaired individuals may demonstrate "acting out" behaviors that are self-destructive or are perceived as unethical by society. Severely-impaired individuals are often incarcerated in prisons or maximum security hospitals.

Because the behavior of clients suffering from personality disorders is generally not problematic to the individuals themselves, they often do not seek treatment for psychological problems, but come for help only when significant others insist, or when their behaviors are in conflict with the legal system. It is estimated that a high percentage of incarcerated individuals could be classified as having personality disorders.[9]

A differential diagnosis is often difficult for the clinician because many of the characteristics of personality disorders are similar to those of the psychoses to which they are related. An examination of personality disorders reveals a unique clinical picture with many common characteristics. While all personality disorders are important, in this chapter a more extensive description is offered of the Borderline Personality Disorder and Narcissistic Personality Disorder—two disorders currently receiving much discussion.

Precipitating Factors of Personality Disorders

Genetic and Constitutional Factors

Generally, the research on genetic and constitutional factors in personality disorders is not as extensive as the research that has been done on the depressive and language and thought disorders. One study in the area of personality disorders sought to answer the question of whether Schizotypal Personality Disorder and Borderline Personality Disorder cluster in families with members who have the same diagnosis.[4]

The researchers screened 310 college students and hospital employees to select normal subjects as well as subjects with various types of psychopathology, including Borderline Personality Disorder and Schizotypal Personality Disorder. Screening tools included the Schedule for Affective Disorders and Schizophrenia, and the Schedule for Interviewing Borderlines.

Student subjects were white. Those considered to have a personality disorder were 21 to 34 years of age. Seventeen subjects had Borderline Personality Disorder, and 29 had Schizotypal Personality Disorder. The researchers studied 576 first-degree relatives of the students with a personality disorder.

The risk for definite and probable Borderline Personality was significantly greater in the relatives of the students with Borderline Personality Disorder when compared with the relatives of normal subjects. A similar finding occurred for relatives of the Schizotypal Disorder students: these relatives had a significantly greater risk for Schizotypal Personality Disorder than did the normal students.

The data supported the ideas that Schizotypal Personality Disorder and Borderline Personality Disorder are familial disorders. However, several limitations of the

---

PERSONALITY DISORDERS: DSM-III-R CATEGORIES (CODED ON AXIS II)

CLUSTER A

301.00	Paranoid Personality Disorder
301.21	Schizoid Personality Disorder
301.22	Schizotypal Personality Disorder

CLUSTER B

301.70	Antisocial Personality Disorder
301.83	Borderline Personality Disorder
301.50	Histrionic Personality Disorder
301.81	Narcissistic Personality Disorder

CLUSTER C

301.82	Avoidant Personality Disorder
301.60	Dependent Personality Disorder
301.40	Obsessive/Compulsive Personality Disorder
301.84	Passive/Aggressive Personality Disorder
301.90	Personality Disorder Not Otherwise Specified

(American Psychiatric Association: Diagnostic and Statistical Manual of Mental Disorders, 3rd ed, revised. Washington, DC, American Psychiatric Association, 1987.)

---

research should be noted. The sample of affected students did not consist of identified patients. One could argue that the student sample is not comparable to a patient population. Also, family members of the students were not interviewed directly, and the interviewers collecting family data from the students were not blind with respect to the diagnostic status of the affected students.

There is some evidence that genetic factors may predispose individuals to the development of an Antisocial Personality Disorder. It is also believed that attention deficit disorders, or learning disabilities, in childhood may increase the possibility of the development of an Antisocial Personality Disorder in adult life.

Some researchers report a high incidence of abnormal EEGs among antisocial personality clients.[9] In fact, most Antisocial Personality individuals do not have abnormal EEGs, and the increase in abnormalities is probably the result of interactive factors rather than a primary determinant of the formation of the Antisocial Personality. Other researchers postulated that there is a marked deficit in emotional arousal in individuals with an Antisocial Personality. While this may be based on deficiencies in the physical constitution, it is more likely the result of learned behavior.

Reich[32] has studied the sex distribution of personality disorders in psychiatric outpatients. The author mentioned that, except for the Borderline and Antisocial Per-

RELEVANT RESEARCH

In this pilot study, the ethnic and sex distribution of clients with Borderline Personality Disorder in a psychiatric inpatient population was examined. A total of 1,583 charts of clients hospitalized for a psychiatric illness in New York City were reviewed. The clients were classified as white, black, Hispanic, and other. Of the 101 clients classified as having Borderline Personality Disorder, 32 were male and 69 were female. Their mean age was 21.5 years, and the mean length of stay in the hospital was 14 days.

It was determined that, in the sample studied, three times as many women as men among whites and blacks were diagnosed as having Borderline Personality Disorder; no difference in prevalence between men and women was found among Hispanics. More Hispanic men were diagnosed as having Borderline Personality Disorder than white and black men. There were no significant differences among the women of the different ethnic groups, or among the ethnic groups overall.

The authors stated that the greater prevalence of Borderline Personality Disorder among women may be due to the perception by those diagnosing such cases that identity problems (found in Borderline Personality Disorder) are more acceptable in men than in women; hence, the clinicians may underdiagnose Borderline Personality Disorder in men.

Women were more frequently diagnosed as having Borderline Personality Disorder than were men among whites and blacks. However, Hispanic men and women were diagnosed with the disorder in equal numbers, suggesting a different sex distribution of the disorder in this ethnic group. This finding concerning Hispanic men and women may be explained by the fact that most clinicians diagnosing the cases were white and did not speak Spanish. The clinicians may misdiagnose the Hispanic clients.

Also, behavior considered as normal within the Hispanic culture may be regarded as deviant in white culture. For example, the display of enthusiasm and dramatic behavior on the part of a Hispanic man may lead a white clinician to classify him as having a Borderline Personality Disorder. On the other hand, the stresses accompanying the immigration of the Puerto Rican and other Hispanic population may have had a detrimental impact on the stability of male identity, leading to a higher prevalence of the Borderline Personality Disorder among Hispanic men.

The authors concluded by stating that additional research is needed on the differences in prevalence rates among ethnic and gender groups. Such research can enhance the understanding of factors that promote the expression of the disorder.

(Castaneda R, Franco H: Sex and ethnic distribution of borderline personality disorder in an inpatient sample. Am J Psychiatry 142:1202, 1985.)

sonality Disorders, no data exist to document the sex distribution among persons with personality disorders.

The researcher interviewed 170 psychiatric outpatients to determine their DSM-III-R psychiatric diagnosis. The author found more women diagnosed with Histrionic Personality Disorder and more men diagnosed as having one of the following personality disorders: Paranoid, Obsessive/Compulsive, and Antisocial. Women did not have the Borderline Personality Disorder or the Dependent Personality Disorder more frequently. In the sample, there were too few Narcissistic Personality Disorder and Passive/Aggressive Disorder clients to include in the data analysis.

The author found that the lack of difference between men and women in prevalence of Borderline Personality Disorder was due to the fact that predictions of the preponderance of women having the disorder, as noted in the DSM-III-R, are based on an inpatient sample rather than on an outpatient sample, as was used in this study. The author also found that some studies reporting a greater prevalence in women of Borderline Personality Disorder may not have adjusted for a baseline preponderance of women in their patient samples.

Some experts theorize that, because the characteristics of clients with Schizoid Personality Disorders are so similar to those of clients with a psychotic diagnosis, there may be genetic or constitutional factors involved. Except for these examples, however, experts feel that additional evidence is needed to link heredity or constitu-

tional factors to the development of personality disorders.

Environmental and Cultural Factors

Some clinicians believe that the incidence of personality disorders has increased in recent years. This may be true, or it is possible that individuals with personality disorders are more evident because they find it increasingly difficult to cope with growing numbers of cultural and environmental stressors.

In the present space age and computerized environment, many youth feel overwhelmed by the amount of knowledge and scientific data they are expected to absorb. Concerns about pollution and the dangers of atomic energy use require a stressful adjustment of people of all ages. Society is far more mobile than ever before, which adds to the lack of stability in traditional family roles. There is greater mixing of cultures, which adds another adjustment stress for many families. Rapid advances in medical science have lengthened the expected life span and increased the population. As the number of people in the environment increases, so does the need to interact, both personally and professionally, with more people. Most clients with personality disorders suffer from an inability to interact appropriately with others, and to derive satisfaction from their interpersonal relationships. Hence, they have an increase in their level of stress.

Clearly a case can be made for the influence of cultural and environmental factors on stress levels and behaviors. However, more research is needed to indicate that these factors lead to the development of personality disorders. The following Relevant Research box demonstrates additional cultural and sex-related factors that may have an impact on diagnoses of Borderline Personality Disorders.

Psychological Factors

Much of the discussion of psychological causal factors seems relevant to an understanding of the personality disorders. Psychological factors are influenced by learned behaviors and social expectations. Individuals need security, self-esteem, identity, love, and approval. A lack of satisfaction in meeting these needs is the significant factor in the development of many personality disorders.

The outcome of the individual's relationships with others influences personality formation. Factors such as parental deprivation, maladaptive family systems, and dysfunctional parent–child relationships directly influence the formation of personality disorders. Although there is no consensus among experts, it is the opinion of most that psychosocial factors are the most influential antecedent of the development of personality disorders.

The Therapeutic Use of Self

The treatment of clients with a personality disorder takes a long time, and is marked by frequent remissions. This slow process is discouraging at times because it is difficult for nurses to realize how they may be contributing to the client's improvement. It is important to examine nurses' personal feelings regarding their need to be helpful and productive. Values regarding gratification for work accomplished may need to be modified to adjust to the long course of therapy.

The treatment course is often marked with intense responses of anger and devaluative and manipulative behavior directed toward nurses by the clients. This creates an intense milieu in which nurses must function.

The Nurse as a Real Person

As previously mentioned, the nurse must be a "real person," conveying an expression of genuine human interest in the client, as well as maintaining consistency in supporting the client. The nurse must be positive regarding the client's efforts to individuate, to become autonomous, and to establish an identity. The nurse must project expectations that the client will act in a realistic and healthy fashion.

At times, clients with a Borderline Personality Disorder will respond with "pseudo-helpless" attitudes. The nurse might say, "I see you as a responsible person—why do you act that way? You don't look helpless to me." The nurse's confrontation focuses on the client's strengths, and offers tangible emotional support. The nurse's attitude of sincerity and positive regard helps the client to gradually develop a sense of trust and emotional investment in the treatment.

Supporting the Growth of Self-Identity

It is expected that clients with a Borderline Personality Disorder will vacillate in their feelings regarding the nurse. Because of their difficulties with closeness and trust, clients may respond to the nurse with splitting, manipulation, devaluation, and anger in order to push the nurse away. The intolerance of ambivalent feelings (good or bad) is so great that clients vacillate between idealizing and devaluing the nurse. The nurse should respond with an attitude of curiosity, genuine concern, and investigation of the client's behavior. It is appropriate to commend the client for realistic achievements and to empathize, with genuine disappointment, with failures.

Confrontation

When faced with self-destructive behavior, the nurse has a two-fold responsibility. First, accurate observation and assessment of the behavior are essential, and then steps must be taken to provide as safe an environment as possible. It is important to note that clients may quickly lapse into unpredictable behavior; acting-out behaviors often occur in rapid sequence.[11]

Second, the rules and regulations of the milieu, and appropriate sanctions for breaking rules, should be clearly defined and enforced: kindly, firmly, and consistently. Although this limit-setting may elicit an angry response from clients, it will provide a definite structure that is vital to the treatment plan. Because clients often deny the destructiveness of their behavior, it is necessary to point out emphatically the obvious destructiveness of their actions.

Clients may participate in their treatment by engaging in a verbal contract not to be self-destructive. How often this contract is renewed will depend on the individual client. The general consensus among authors is that contractual interventions are effective.[28]

Nurses must help clients to become aware of inconsistencies and nonproductive aspects of their thinking and behavior. "It must be awful to have these feelings and to want to hurt yourself, but you do have a choice," the nurse might say. This statement both conveys support to the client and is a gentle form of limit-setting. Never encourage or reward regressive behavior.

Helping Clients to Understand Their Own Feelings

Nurses must try to model limit-setting. Because clients have difficulty expressing feelings, try not to intellectualize; rather, focus on the affect, the mood, that clients are projecting. It is important to assist clients with a Borderline Personality Disorder to read their own feelings. "You say you don't feel anything right now, but you look very sad to me," might be an appropriate response by the nurse to help a client get in touch with sad feelings.

Role-Modeling

Clients with a Borderline Personality Disorder have an uncanny ability to sense the feelings of others. When the client's angry, frustrating, and helpless feelings are projected onto the nurse and the nurse responds with anger, this confirms the client's distrust of the nurse's therapeutic role and increases the client's feelings of rejection. The nurse must be able to tolerate the client's aggression and to establish the limits of the immediate reality within which the client is expected to conform. The nurse's focus should be on the "here and now."

How, then, do nurses deal with their own human fallibilities? They must be able to reassure themselves that every human being makes mistakes, and remind themselves to examine their own feelings of anger, separation, and the need to rescue. After a therapeutic nurse–client relationship has developed, nurses may use humor occasionally in dealing with their frustrations, except when the client is in a psychotic state. A sense of humor is a sign of an observing ego, and the sharing of humor with clients provides good role-modeling. "I see I've put my foot in my mouth again," would be an appropriate response to an error in observation or assessment of behavior by the nurse.

Somatic Therapies

To date, research on the use of medications for personality disorders is limited. However, there is a growing tendency "to medicate psychotic-like symptoms in personality disorders."[17] Clinical understanding promoting the use of medications in personality disorders includes the ideas that psychotic symptoms are difficult to treat with psychotherapeutic intervention alone, and that psychotic symptoms are the result of a biological deficit and, hence, treatable with medication, a biological agent.

Klar and Siever[17] reported that medications prescribed for personality disorders are not prescribed according to the particular type of personality disorder present, but according to the individual symptoms present. Hence, a specific personality disorder may be treated with one drug in one instance and treated with a different drug at another time or with another client, according to

the specific symptoms present. Table 19-1 lists several symptom patterns and medications used to treat these patterns. Specific personality disorders in which the symptoms occur are also listed, if the information is available. For some symptoms, specific drugs are listed. For other symptoms, only categories of drugs are included. This difference is due to the manner in which the relatively scarce literature occurs.

Borderline Personality Disorder

Precipitating Factors

Differences of opinion exist among clinicians regarding causal factors in the development of the Borderline Personality Disorder. Most agree that growth and development are the single most influential factors.

According to Mahler,[23] during the rapprochement phase (16–25 months) the child attains a sense of individuation, autonomy, and object constancy. McDevitt defined object constancy as "the ability of the child to maintain a relatively nonchanging emotional image of the mother as being basically good but having both good and bad qualities, an emotional image that changes little under frustration or during absence."[27]

Children who eventually develop a Borderline Personality Disorder do not achieve object constancy, and thus develop a mutually exclusive view of reality as either all good or all bad. They continue to use splitting behavior to cope with frustration and anxiety for the rest of their lives.

Because children who eventually develop a Borderline Personality Disorder have not been allowed to explore the world and seek self-expression, they do not learn to be careful, to delay gratification, or to establish priorities. According to this theory, their mothers have always performed these tasks for their children, and because they do not allow their children to individuate they must continue to perform the tasks for the children. This accounts for the poor impulse control and poor choosing skills, as well as fears of rejection and of closeness, seen in clients with a Borderline Personality Disorder. Usually, concomitant with the emotional withdrawal of the mother from the child is the absence or unavailability of the father.

According to Kernberg, the presence of an excessive amount of aggressive drive in the earliest years of life (the pregenital phase) interferes with the separation/individuation process.[12] This results in splitting being reinforced and object constancy never being obtained. Complementing Kernberg, and in accord with Mahler, are Masterson[25,26] and Rinsley.[33] In their view, the mother, often a Borderline Personality Disorder herself and deriving much gratification from the symbiotic involvement with the child, withdraws her emotional availability when the child begins to make an effort to separate and individuate.

TABLE 19-1.
MEDICATION USE WITH SYMPTOMS OF PERSONALITY DISORDERS

SYMPTOM OR SYMPTOM CLUSTER	TYPE OF PERSONALITY DISORDER	MEDICATION
1. Has massive anxiety; reports few pleasures in life	Schizotypal Avoidant Borderline	Antidepressants
2. Reports few pleasures in life	Schizotypal Avoidant Borderline	Imipramine
3. Reports few pleasures in life; compulsions, obsessions, phobias	(Not available)	Tricyclic antidepressants, monamine oxidase (MAO) inhibitors
4. Mild, persistent thought disorder; debilitating anxiety	(Not available)	Neuroleptics
5. Reports few pleasures in life and is anxious due to an underlying chronic depression	(Not available)	Antidepressants
6. Dangerously impulsive	Borderline Antisocial Histrionic Narcissistic	High-potency, low-dose neuroleptics
7. Impulsive during periods of intense affect; emotionally labile, with unexplained episodic violence	Borderline Antisocial Histrionic Narcissistic	Lithium (serum levels of 0.9 to 1.2 mEq per L provide therapeutic dosage with minimal sedation.)
8. Impulsive behavior in clients with abnormal electroencephalograms (EEGs)	(Not available)	Diphenylhydantoin
9. Episodic violence in clients with abnormal EEGs	(Not available)	Carbamazepine
10. Episodic violence in clients with normal EEGs	(Not available)	Carbamazepine (6 to 8 μg per ml)
11. Impulsive; overly aroused	(Not available)	Methylphenidate
12. Aggressive outbursts	(Not available)	Propranolol (100–300 mg per day)

(Adapted from Klar H, Siever L: The psychopharmacologic treatment of personality disorders. Psychiatr Clin North Am 7: 791, 1984.)

Common Characteristics

Clients with a Borderline Personality Disorder exhibit a great deal of anger and depression. The anger is diffuse, and the depression is not a true depression but a feeling of loneliness and isolation. Because there is little tolerance for these unpleasant feelings, the client with this personality disorder may be demanding, sarcastic, and hostile. The relevant diagnostic criteria in the DSM-III-R are found in the box on page 408. Although the client with a Borderline Personality Disorder displays a wide range of behaviors, the following are typical.[21,29,30]

Self-Concept

Clients with a Borderline Personality Disorder are constantly searching for an identity, and readily yield to the influence of others. Their suggestibility conceals a great deal of hostility, anger, and general aggressiveness. The clients never quite know who they are or what they want. They repeatedly, knowingly, and unavoidably feel hurt and victimized, yet seem unable to recognize their part in the process.

Typically, clients with a Borderline Personality Disorder have a poor frustration tolerance and lack the ability to control impulses. Although their general intent is not to be self-destructive, impulsiveness often causes behavior that is self-destructive. Such impulsive behavior might take the form of episodic acts of self-mutilation, drug overdose, or more chronic behavior patterns of drug dependency or promiscuity. At times the self-destructive behavior may be a manipulative effort to exact a "saving" response from a significant other.

Interpersonal Relationships

Although clients with a Borderline Personality Disorder may appear to be amiable, attractive, and personable, underneath there is a lack of genuineness and a poverty of ideas and feelings. Clients experience free-floating anxiety and emptiness or despair. They are self-centered, with a hypersensitivity to failure and rejection. There is a pattern of unsatisfying relationships. Characteristically, relationships vacillate between being transient and superficial and being intense and dependent. Clients with a Borderline Personality Disorder may fall madly in love, and just as quickly terminate their relationships in spells of anger and disappointment. This dissatisfaction in relationships extends to family, friends, and co-workers.

There is an inability to integrate positive and nega-

DIAGNOSTIC CRITERIA FOR 301.83 BORDERLINE PERSONALITY DISORDER

A pervasive pattern of instability of mood, interpersonal relationships, and self-image, beginning by early adulthood and present in a variety of contexts, as indicated by at least *five* of the following:

1. A pattern of unstable and intense interpersonal relationships characterized by alternating between extremes of overidealization and devaluation
2. Impulsiveness in at least two areas that are potentially self-damaging, *e.g.,* spending, sex, substance use, shoplifting, reckless driving, binge eating
3. Affective instability: marked shifts from baseline mood to depression, irritability, or anxiety, lasting usually a few hours and only rarely more than a few days
4. Inappropriate, intense anger or lack of control of anger, *e.g.,* frequent displays of temper
5. Recurrent suicidal threats, gestures, or behavior, or self-mutilating behavior
6. Marked and persistent identity disturbance manifested by uncertainty about at least two of the following: self-image, sexual orientation, long-term goals or career choice, type of friends desired, preferred values
7. Chronic feelings of emptiness or boredom
8. Frantic efforts to avoid real or imagined abandonment

(American Psychiatric Association: Diagnostic and Statistical Manual of Mental Disorders, 3rd ed, revised. Washington, DC, American Psychiatric Association, 1987.)

tive feelings. Thus, when conflicts arise they are interpreted by clients as negating all positive aspects of the relationship. To avoid closeness, the individuals choose to isolate themselves, or to select partners who do not demand intimacy or commitment.

Social Adaptation

Clients with a Borderline Personality Disorder acutely experience the stress of accomplishing developmental tasks with each stage of life. The adolescent years and the search for identity are characterized by rebelliousness and acting-out behavior. During young adulthood, there is difficulty with intimacy and the resulting loneliness. Middle age is characterized by depression because real life opportunities for satisfaction typically decrease. Much of the individuals' lives have been spent fantasizing that their needs will be met rather than actually working constructively toward fulfillment of the needs. Old age brings the reality of change and loss, and the inflexibility of the clients makes it extremely difficult to deal with either of these.

Work and Productivity

Clients with a Borderline Personality Disorder may defend themselves well by splitting, projecting, acting out, denial, clinging, and distancing. The price for the use of these defenses is high, and they generally derive little satisfaction from their work.

Frequently, clients with a Borderline Personality Disorder are talented or artistic and gravitate to professions such as acting, writing, law, medicine, journalism, and photography. Masterson[24] considered this best explained by the fact that these professions contain only the illusion of closeness, or closeness with limits. These occupations allow clients to experience emotions that are inhibited in their personal lives, but within safe limits. Often the experience is vicarious.

Cognitive Style and Thinking

Under extreme stress, clients with a Borderline Personality Disorder may experience brief psychotic experiences. Unlike the experiences of psychotic clients, these episodes are distinguished by their brevity, their reversibility, and their obvious relationships to precipitating events.[12]

The psychological testing performance of these clients may reveal bizarre, unrealistic, illogical, or primitive responses on unstructured tests, such as the Rorschach, but not on the more structured Wechsler Adult Intelligence Scale (WAIS).[13] This lends support to the theory that clients with a Borderline Personality Disorder perform much better in a structured environment.

The idea that the information processing of clients with a diagnosis of Borderline Personality Disorder is similar to that of psychotic clients was not supported by the research of Schubert, Saccuzzo, and Braff.[35] These investigators found, in a task measuring the speed of information-processing, that Borderline clients were similar to normal subjects in doing the task, and that both Borderline clients and normal subjects were superior in doing the task to clients with diagnoses of major depressive, manic, or schizoaffective illness. The findings supported the idea that clients with Borderline Personality Disorder have normal-range information-processing abilities and perform better at these tasks than do clients with a major psychiatric illness.

The Nursing Process

Assessment

Kaplan[15] identified a number of characteristics that signal the presence of a Borderline condition. These characteristics include "negativistic, demanding, self-destructive"[15] behaviors, as well as a number of acting-out behaviors (such as leaving a hospital unit without permission). The client may have little capacity for "anxiety, frustration, delay, and impulse control."[15] Clients with a Borderline Personality Disorder may frequently request special attention, and have a sense that everyone else should respect their wishes. Such clients are sensitive to criticism, have a difficult time trusting others, and demonstrate sexual promiscuity and a low frustration tolerance.

Clients with a Borderline Personality Disorder may briefly show psychotic symptoms. Chopra and Beatson[8] studied 13 clients with Borderline Personality Disorder. The researchers administered the Diagnostic Interview for Borderline Patients to determine symptoms of the clients. They found that the most common psychotic symptoms experienced by the clients were derealization and depersonalization. The former was present in 12 cases studied, and the latter in 11 cases. Other symptoms experienced included: brief paranoid experiences (in 10 cases), brief psychotic depressive experiences (10 cases), and hallucinations or delusions (7 cases). The hallucinations appeared to be "manifestations of the intense anxiety resulting from the patients' inability to cope with their stresses."[8] The hallucinations would last for a few hours and disappear after the anxiety decreased. Nurses can observe such symptoms and understand them, not as evidence of a worsening condition, but as a possible accompaniment to the Borderline Personality Disorder.

Clients with a Borderline Personality Disorder frequently engage in what is known as *splitting behavior.* Gallop[11] stated that, in splitting, the client related to persons in the environment as if they were "part" of a person. For example, one nurse would be considered by the clients to be "all good" while another nurse would be considered "all bad." These traits indicate that the client must "split" a whole perception of a person (a combination of both good and bad, which most people typically see) into part of a perception. The client will see only good attributes in one nurse and bad attributes in another. Other combinations can exist: one nurse can be beautiful, and the other ugly; the doctor can be "all-knowing," and a nurse knows nothing; the family can be uncaring, and the staff caring, and so on. The particular way in which the client characterizes individuals may change impulsively. Splitting behavior can cause deep conflicts among the staff if they are not aware of the splitting phenomenon.

Braverman and Shook[7] discussed the case of a Borderline client in the emergency room, and emphasized the importance of quickly identifying the client with a diagnosis of Borderline Personality Disorder. According to the authors, a client, Ms. L., came into the emergency room after she had slashed her wrists. Her boyfriend accompanied her. She was crying and demanded immediate attention. In the admission interview Ms. L. stated that she had slashed her wrists after her boyfriend had threatened to leave her if she did not stop her alcohol abuse. The authors stated that Ms. L. represents one of the 33% of clients who come to emergency rooms with psychological, as well as physical, problems.

As Ms. L. continued her stay in the ER, she continued to demonstrate characteristics of a client with a Borderline diagnosis. She clung to her boyfriend, yet continued to argue with him. She did not demonstrate psychotic behaviors (such as hallucinations), and was uncooperative at first. She later calmed down when the triage nurse explained her admission in matter-of-fact terms.

As the client waited for the treatment team, she complained about several of the nurses and asked for one particular nurse whom she had seen on the unit. Later, when the physician was suturing one of her wrists, Ms. L. refused further treatment and swung at the nurse, missing her. The staff had to restrain the client so that treatment could be completed.

Although beginning clinicians may picture clients with a psychological problem as being only in a psychiatric hospital, the above client's behavior, demonstrating the Borderline Personality Disorder, may occur in any health care setting. Ms. L. could have easily disrupted the ER if the nursing staff had not been aware of Borderline client dynamics, and useful interventions.

Clients with a Borderline Personality Disorder are found, not only in psychiatric hospitals and in the ER setting, but also among populations not generally regarded as having Borderline pathology. Little is known about the Borderline condition among elderly persons. Siegel and Small[36] report that little attention has been given in the literature to this condition in the elderly. To date there is no "clear theoretical framework to predict the natural history of the disorder."

The authors reported on one case involving a 69-year-old woman who was admitted to the hospital after ingesting 20 Haldol tablets. The client had previously experienced mood swings of anger and sadness, and had chronically abused alcohol. She periodically gambled, and had lost a considerable amount of money. She was widowed five years prior to the hospital admission; her marriage had been unstable, with frequent fights. Her symptoms had gradually increased following a six-month mourning period after the death of her husband. Siegel and Small[36] concluded their work by stating that "Borderline Personality Disorder may continue throughout the life span, and may in fact worsen with age."

Nursing Diagnosis

Psychiatric/mental health nursing diagnoses[2] that may be of concern in working with clients with a Borderline Personality Disorder are listed in the box on page 410.

Planning

Because of the difficult behavior of the client with a diagnosis of Borderline Personality Disorder (such as splitting), treatment planning must be thorough and all team members treating the client must be aware of, and follow, the treatment plan. Kaplan[15] advocated a plan composed of all treatment modalities: "milieu, individual, family, occupational, and group therapies."[15]

For the client with a Borderline diagnosis, the *milieu* in an inpatient unit offers containment to protect the client's physical safety. Support is offered to decrease anxiety and maintain self-esteem. The milieu offers structure in which the client is expected to function in activities

NURSING DIAGNOSES RELATED TO BORDERLINE PERSONALITY DISORDER

21. Alterations in Conduct/Impulse Control
    21.02   Aggression/violence toward others
        21.02.03   Abuse—verbal
    21.03   Aggression/violence toward self
        21.03.02   Self-mutilation
        21.03.04   Suicidal
23. Alterations in Role Performance
    23.01   Impaired family role
    23.02   Impaired social/leisure role
30. Excess of or Deficit in Dominant Emotions
    30.01   Impaired emotional experience
        30.01.01   Anger/rage
        30.01.12   Loneliness
    30.02   Impaired appropriateness of emotional expression
    30.04   Impaired range of expression
    30.99   Excess of or deficit in dominant emotions
50. Alterations in Perception/Cognition
    50.07   Alterations in self-concept
        50.07.03   Impaired personal identity

during the day. The milieu also offers the opportunity for relating to others in a healthy manner, or to discover ways in which one does not relate to others in an adaptive fashion. Milieu therapy can offer a balance in emphasizing social integration of clients, while individual therapy can help solidify with clients what their experiences are, and how they can make better use of the environment.

Occupational therapists can work with clients to assess work histories. Many Borderline clients have experienced "inconsistent work patterns, intense involvement followed by precipitous termination of employment, troubled relationships with bosses and co-workers, procrastination, and lack of satisfaction with work."[12] Occupational therapy can assist the client to learn new behaviors to facilitate a positive work experience.

It is generally accepted that *family therapy* is beneficial for clients with a Borderline Personality Disorder. Some therapists recommend family therapy because there is a belief that contributions from the entire family system affect the development of the Borderline Personality Disorder. The role of the nurse in family therapy is to support the family, provide stability, and set limits on chaotic interactions among members.

However, a more widely accepted view is that, because the family is seriously disturbed, the early initiation of family therapy increases the difficulty the nurse therapist will have in developing a trusting relationship with the client.[16] Early family therapy can increase the client's anxiety, which may ultimately provoke the client into leaving therapy. If family therapy is undertaken, it should be started later in the client's treatment process.

Group therapy provides an opportunity for clients to identify with peers and to learn social skills. Group therapy may also help to increase clients' sense of identity in social situations, as well as help to soften and control abrasive behavior.[22]

The role of the nurse is to make the group "safe." When group members project their anger onto other members, an appropriate response might be, "I wonder if anyone has ever spoken to you like that before?" This validates the reality of the anger, but also helps to diffuse the projection and focus the anger back onto the member who is experiencing this feeling. If the group is not a safe place, the possibility of some clients decompensating (*e.g.,* later making a suicide gesture, eloping, or becoming verbally or physically abusive in the milieu) is great.

Intervention

The treatment of clients with a Borderline Personality Disorder is directly related to the basic deficits of the disorder:

1. Lack of a definitive self-identity
2. A limited range of affects, dominated by anxiety and anger
3. Deficient impulse controls
4. Depressive loneliness
5. Deficient interpersonal relationships

The treatment of clients with a Borderline Personality Disorder places extreme demands on the resourcefulness, adaptation, and energy of the nurse. The nurse must adopt a wide range of therapeutic techniques, specific to each individual client and to the different phases of each client's therapy. Most clients will require ongoing or intermittent therapy over a period of months or years. In general, nurses take a more active, "real person" role while working with clients with a Borderline Personality Disorder than in work with many neurotic clients or individuals with other personality disorders.

General interventions for use in working with the client with a Borderline diagnosis are listed in the boxes on page 411. In the first box, interventions to use with the client are suggested. In the second box, elements of team functioning in working with the client with a Borderline diagnosis are described.

Evaluation

As previously indicated, the course of treatment for clients with a Borderline Personality Disorder is usually long. How, then, does the nurse know when clients are improving? The following are suggested guidelines:

1. Clients are better able to tolerate confrontation.
2. Clients are better able to tolerate disappointments.
3. There is a decrease in anger and depression.

INTERVENTIONS FOR WORKING WITH CLIENTS WITH A DIAGNOSIS OF BORDERLINE PERSONALITY DISORDER

1. Promptly evaluate and treat physical and psychological problems, to prevent the client from splitting the staff.
2. Closely monitor the behavior of the client when the client is stressed, because the client may rapidly lose touch with reality.
3. Assess for substance abuse.
4. Provide care for the client in a quiet area, because auditory and visual stimulation may increase the potential for labile affect and acting-out.
5. Give specific information and expectations in a clear, firm manner.
6. If the nurse notes rising anxiety or a loss of touch with reality, use repeated, simple explanations to subdue the client's fears or suspicions.
7. Provide clear and quick responses to the client's questions to promote a sense of trust. However, do not let the client overwhelm the staff with demands; set appropriate limits.
8. Because clients with a Borderline diagnosis are sensitive, avoid facial expressions that express annoyance or a body stance that conveys impatience.
9. If limit-setting does not control the client's behavior, use physical restraints, with proper explanation to the client; physical restraints are preferable to medications if the client is suspected of recent substance abuse.
10. Develop a contract for care with the client, stipulating client expectations to assist in: engaging the client in structured participation in the nursing care process, minimizing regression, and providing the desired elements of control.
11. Provide a predictable and scheduled treatment environment.
12. Include the client in the interpersonal environment of the treatment program so that the client can learn interpersonal skills.

(Kaplan C: The challenge of working with patients diagnosed as having a borderline personality disorder. Nurs Clin North Am 21:429, 1986; and McEnany G, Tescher B: Contracting for care. J Psychosoc Nurs Ment Health Serv 23:1, 1985; and Gross B, Shook J: Spotting the borderline personality. Am J Nurs 87:200, 1987.)

GUIDELINES FOR TEAM FUNCTIONING WHEN WORKING WITH CLIENTS WITH A DIAGNOSIS OF BORDERLINE PERSONALITY DISORDER

1. While providing for containment of the client's behavior to ensure the safety of the client and others, also offer support to reduce anxiety and bolster the client's self-esteem.
2. Maintain an awareness within the treatment staff of the nature of the splitting done by the client. For example, some staff may believe that the client is manipulative and mean, or needs more structure, or simply needs punishment. Other staff may believe the client is in pain and needs support. Some staff may react to the client with fear, hostility, and rigid, controlling limits, while others may react with overprotectiveness, masochistic tolerance, and excessive solicitousness. Team members may become suspicious of each other and begin to undermine their colleagues' work. Staff experiencing such splits should make it clear to clients that they are considered responsible for their behavior and that they must respect treatment rules.
3. Maintain an awareness of the need of the client for control. Recognize that the staff may become locked into attempts to control the client inappropriately.
4. Work toward a team structure that emphasizes firm but shared leadership, clear individual boundaries among team members, high reliance on negotiation, team closeness, and adaptive responses to stress. A well-functioning team can more easily deal with the pathology demonstrated toward the staff by the client with Borderline pathology.
5. Develop a clearly-defined philosophy of care that is shared by all team members.
6. Hold frequent team meetings to discuss client care.
7. Provide a treatment atmosphere in which individual team members can become aware of their own responses to clients without receiving judgmental feedback from other staff members.

(Kaplan C: The challenge of working with patients diagnosed as having a borderline personality disorder. Nurs Clin North Am 21:429, 1986.)

CLINICAL EXAMPLE: NURSING CARE PLAN

The nurse (Nurse A.) who has been assigned to work with Michael (introduced at the beginning of this chapter) has daily individual sessions with him. In these meetings, the nurse and Michael discuss his concerns as well as his participation in unit activities. Nurse A. states that Michael has not attended the last two unit meetings held each morning for all clients and staff. Michael states that he was there and that the nurse must be mistaken.

Later that day, after Nurse A. has left for the day, Michael approaches the head nurse and states that he wants to be assigned to work with a different primary nurse during his hospital stay. He states that "it's no big deal, but some nurses have only a few clients assigned to them. Nurse A. is coordinator of all the therapy groups on the unit and has too much to do." The head nurse remarks that she will review client-nurse assignments as soon as she can.

The next day, Michael attends the unit meeting of all clients and staff. He remarks that the clients on the unit would prefer to have more occupational and recreational therapy (O.T., R.T.), and less group therapy, since O.T. and R.T. are more active. He encourages other clients to agree. The O.T., R.T., and nursing staff look confused and say nothing. Michael asks the clients to vote on his proposal.

Nurse A. states that group therapy is needed as part of the program because it gives clients therapy that is needed as part of the program and because it gives clients the opportunity to examine their relationships with others. Michael becomes angry and states that the clients can learn about relating in O.T. and R.T., because there they are "doing rather than talking." He encourages other clients to support him. The R.T. and O.T. staff remain quiet. Nurse A. states that the matter cannot be decided before a discussion by the staff in their afternoon team meeting. Michael storms out of the meeting room.

The nursing care plan for Michael is shown on page 413.

4. There is a decrease in self-destructive, and other impulsive, behaviors.
5. Clients are hospitalized for shorter periods of time during crises.

Narcissistic Personality Disorder

Precipitating Factors

Causal factors in the development of personality disorders were discussed earlier in this chapter. However, major research in the field of growth and development has confirmed that these factors have the most influence on the formation of the Narcissistic Personality Disorder.

According to Mahler,[23] during the *practicing subphase* (8–16 months) of the separation and individuation stage, children begin to explore their environment in search of autonomy. Children return to their mothers periodically for "emotional refueling." The chief characteristic of this subphase is children's great narcissistic investment in their own bodies and functions, as well as in the objects and loved ones in their expanding reality. The child seems relatively impervious to life's frustrations.

Toward the end of the practicing subphase, the toddlers begin to lose their sense of grandiosity and an increased separation anxiety is observed. They begin to realize that they must cope with life on their own. In the development of the Narcissistic Personality Disorder, there is a failure of the primary parental figure to support and participate in the child's achievements. Rather, the parental figure exploits the child's weaknesses. The parent is generally threatened by the child's accomplishments and sees them as demonstrations of weakness in the parent. Thus, children's grandiose self-appraisal is reinforced and they are expected to be more than they are capable of being.

According to Kohut,[20] the essential feature of clients with a Narcissistic Personality Disorder is their need for "self objects" to help them regulate their self-esteem and feel complete. The self object is someone who performs necessary functions for the child while being experienced as part of the child. Contrastingly, Kernberg[12] postulates that the children's sole defense is to take refuge in some aspect of themselves that the parents have valued. Thus, the grandiose self develops. Clinically, this can best be understood by picturing these clients as persons who have combined only what they want from an ideal other person (such as a parent) and all they grandiosely want for themselves with only a few aspects of their real selves.

The reason that the fixation occurs at this level is complex and poorly understood. The children have not yet developed a separate sense of self, and thus their fantasy, that the world revolves around them, persists. In order to protect this fantasy, the children must seal off, by avoidance, denial, and devaluation, those aspects of reality that do not fit with their images of their grandiose selves.

Common Characteristics

Clients with a Narcissistic Personality Disorder typically have an exaggerated sense of self-importance or self-uniqueness, with an excessive focus on themselves. Behaviors may include grandiose fantasies and highly unrealistic goals. There is a general lack of interest in or empathy for others. At the same time, there is an obvious pursuit of others in order to obtain admiration and approval. Occasionally, clients with a Narcissistic Personal-

NURSING CARE PLAN: Michael

ASSESSMENT	NURSING INTERVENTIONS	EVALUATION CRITERIA
NURSING DIAGNOSIS: Splitting		
SUBJECTIVE DATA Michael talks with head nurse rather than Nurse A. about his assigned nurse. He attempts to align clients with him during times of staff indecision. He states that O.T. and R.T. are "good" and group therapy is "bad."	1. Observe every 15 minutes to determine that client is controlling anger. 2. Discuss countertransference in staff meeting. Identify the pattern in the countertransference. 3. Develop and use a consistent approach to deal with Michael's splitting the staff.	Client will not harm self or others. Staff will spontaneously identify their counter-transference when client tries to split staff. Staff will feel more confident in knowing when client is splitting and will channel client toward healthier ways of dealing with sensitivities or disappointments when the client's splitting behavior is occurring.
OBJECTIVE DATA Client reacts to some in his environment as "good" and some as "bad."	4. Maintain Nurse A.'s regular sessions with Michael. Other staff should direct Michael to Nurse A. for discussion of Michael's concerns. 5. Emphasize with Michael the choices he can make concerning his activities that are within the program structure. 6. In regular individual sessions, discuss oversensitivity, such as when Nurse A. questioned Michael about his unit meeting attendance and he began to treat Nurse A. as if she were "all bad."	Staff support Michael's work with Nurse A. Client will sense a greater degree of control and make fewer attempts to manipulate others to attain control. Client will seek clarification in interactions when he senses that he is not being helped by another person.
NURSING DIAGNOSIS: 30.01.01 IMPAIRED EMOTIONAL EXPERIENCE, ANGER		
SUBJECTIVE DATA Michael leaves unit meeting abruptly with an angry expression and voice tone. **OBJECTIVE DATA** Client becomes angry when he does not get his way.	1. Assist client to identify his feeling when he left the unit meeting. 2. Assist client to describe the sequence of events leading up to his expression of anger. 3. Work with client to identify the target of his anger and why that particular target was selected. 4. Ask client to identify other ways he can express himself, other than by anger/rage. Develop written contract with client to try new ways of dealing with anger. 5. Encourage client to attend relaxation training class on unit.	Client will identify his rage or anger experienced before leaving the unit meeting. Client will describe his sequence of oversensitivity to Nurse A.'s questioning him about his unit meeting attendance. Client will state that Nurse A. was the target for his anger because he perceived Nurse A. as insensitive to him. Within one day, client will state two other ways in which he can deal with his anger and will place these ideas in the form of a written contract. Client will learn relaxation techniques.

ity Disorder present themselves as shy, timid, inhibited, and ineffective—only to reveal their omnipotent selves later. Typically, clients are driven by an unremitting need for perfection, brilliance, power, and beauty, and attempts to find others who will admire them. There is an intense envy of the others admired by the client, and as a result the client attempts to devalue the admired ones. The relevant diagnostic criteria occurring in the DSM-III-R are found in the following box. Although not all clients display all of these characteristics, the following patterns are typical of clients with a Narcissistic Personality Disorder.

DIAGNOSTIC CRITERIA FOR 301.81 NARCISSISTIC PERSONALITY DISORDER

A pervasive pattern of grandiosity (in fantasy or behavior), lack of empathy, and hypersensitivity to the evaluation of others, beginning by early adulthood and present in a variety of contexts, as indicated by at least *five* of the following:

1. Reacts to criticism with feelings of rage, shame, or humiliation (even if not expressed)
2. Is interpersonally exploitative: takes advantage of others to achieve his or her own ends
3. Has a grandiose sense of self-importance, *e.g.,* exaggerates achievements and talents
4. Believes that his or her problems are unique and can be understood only by other special people
5. Is preoccupied with fantasies of unlimited success, power, brilliance, beauty, or ideal love
6. Has a sense of entitlement: unreasonable expectation of especially favorable treatment
7. Requires constant attention and admiration
8. Lacks empathy: shows inability to recognize and experience how others feel
9. Is preoccupied with feelings of envy

(American Psychiatric Association: Diagnostic and Statistical Manual of Mental Disorders, 3rd ed, revised. Washington, DC, American Psychiatric Association, 1987.)

Self-Concept

Often, clients with a Narcissistic Personality Disorder are profoundly angry in response to what they perceive as an injury to their self-esteem. They may respond with coldness, self-consciousness, stilted speech, or hypomanic episodes in response to a threat to their self-esteem.[20] Unlike clients with affective disorders, clients with a Narcissistic Personality Disorder maintain insight and general integrity of personality during hypomanic episodes. They generally feel that anything that humiliates them is not appropriate to their personality, and so they reject it. They keep away anything that would diminish their ego by using denial.

Interpersonal Relationships

Clients with a Narcissistic Personality Disorder show a lack of empathy for others while maintaining an adequate external adaptation to reality. There is an attitude of condescending superiority, and exploitation of others. This is often apparent in sexual matters, with partners viewed or treated as less than people and simply a means of obtaining physical pleasure. Relationships are often "stormy" because there is a tendency toward sexual promiscuity, perversions, and substance abuse. These behaviors are manifested because the clients are uncertain of their own identity and are always ready and willing to shift values quickly in order to gain favor from admired others.

Social Adaptation

These clients may appear to be superficially adaptive and even quite successful professionally. However, they experience chronic feelings of boredom, emptiness, and uncertainty about their identity.

Work and Productivity

Work and productivity are most often in the service of exhibitionism, and are really "pseudo success." These individuals seem to lack genuine, serious professional interests. Clients with a Narcissistic Personality Disorder do little because they want to. Rather, their actions are constantly influenced by their perceptions of what will make others like them. Their pursuit of admiring attention is a means to undo feelings of inferiority.

Cognitive Style and Thinking

Although frequently intelligent, clients with a Narcissistic Personality Disorder use language for well-being and self-esteem, rather than for communicating or understanding. There is a peculiar gap between words and perceptions, and clients give the impression that they are talking to themselves or that their words circle endlessly. Because their perspectives are inflexible, they tend to be either abstract or overly concrete, or they fluctuate between these extremes. They think for the sake of thinking and often use impersonal subjects, such as, "they say that," or "the thought occurred."

The Nursing Process

Assessment

The client with a diagnosis of narcissism is typically free of any obvious symptoms such as hallucinations or delusions. In most instances, the diagnosis of a Narcissistic Disorder is derived after assessing the history and daily life habits of the client.

Stanton[38] reports that these clients' anxiety tolerance is low. Anxiety is handled by either (1) acting as if they were completely undisturbed by what is occurring, or (2) showing surprise that any event could affect them, because they consider themselves invulnerable and above, or immune to, life stresses.

Impulse control is another area in which the client with a Narcissistic Disorder demonstrates an inadequacy. The individual is intolerant and does not have sufficient "organization and flexibility available in the pursuit of goals."[38] If the individual's wishes are blocked, the response is self-blame, or blaming others, for the lack of fulfillment.

The client with a diagnosis of narcissism may show a low sense of self-esteem and feel insignificant. The client may be overly influenced by what others are doing. Importantly, the person "tends to govern his relations according to a perception of others as like himself (a mirror image), as a source of satisfaction of his own special needs, or as someone he wants to be like."[38] If an idealized person in the client's life disappoints the client in some way, the client may respond with anger, fear, or a "rapid replacement by someone else."

The relationships of the person with narcissism are superficial. Instead of intimacy, the client feels a "sense of inadequacy, envy, futility, emptiness, or aggressive triumph"[38] over the other. Because clients feel uncertain about their own selves, they may respond to others as (1) a "potential threat,"[38] or (2) someone to mistrust, since the clients cannot trust closeness. Such clients are "constantly alert"[38] to what the other is doing, and frequently test the other person in the relationship to determine if the other cares. The other finds this a suffocating and controlling pattern. Because the client has such problems in relating to others, the client does not attain the usual boost to self-esteem that can come from social interaction.

Nursing Diagnosis

Clients with a diagnosis of Narcissistic Personality Disorder present with varying diagnoses, depending on what their particular array of traits is. Some clients may idealize one person and impulsively act indignant toward another. Therefore, the nursing diagnoses listed in the box below may seem contradictory. Some explanation is given below specific diagnoses, if needed.

Many specific diagnoses listed under this classification do not relate specifically to the clinical picture of the narcissistic client (because typically these clients are not "assaultive"). However, the client may frequently demonstrate impulsive behavior toward others whom the client perceives as slighting the client in some way. Clients may impulsively isolate themselves from others whom they perceive as not fulfilling their narcissistic wishes. This impulsivity can be troublesome in supposedly intimate relationships.

Planning

As stated earlier, clients with a diagnosis of Narcissistic Personality Disorder may also have had problems of substance abuse, criminality, and promiscuity. Clinicians working with these clients must coordinate the treatment program, especially if a number of professionals are working with the client. For example, one clinician may do individual psychotherapy to assist with the problem of narcissism, while another clinician(s) works on substance abuse issues.

The treatment plan may also include group and/or family therapy. These therapies can assist clients to understand better their relationship difficulties.

Interventions

The grandiose self-image, the potential for acting-out behavior, and the defense mechanisms of projection, de-

NURSING DIAGNOSES RELATED TO NARCISSISTIC PERSONALITY DISORDER

21. Alterations in Conduct/Impulse Control
   21.07 Age-inappropriate behavior
      21.07.01 Pseudomature behavior
      21.07.02 Regressed behavior
   21.08 Unpredictable behavior
23. Alterations in Role Performance
   23.01 Impaired family role
      23.01.03 Enmeshment
      23.01.04 Role loss/disengagement
   23.02 Impaired social/leisure role
      23.02.01 Withdrawal/social isolation
24. Alterations in Self-Care
   24.05 Impairment in solitude/social interaction
26. Alterations in Sexuality
      26.01.02 Excess seductiveness
      26.01.03 Excess sex play/talk/activity
      26.01.07 Inappropriate sexual objects
30. Excess of or Deficit in Dominant Emotions
   30.01 Impaired emotional experience
      30.01.01 Anger/rage
      30.01.02 Anxiety
      30.01.03 Disgust/contempt
      30.01.05 Envy/jealousy
      30.01.12 Loneliness
      30.01.15 Shame/humiliation
   30.02 Impaired appropriateness of emotional expression
   30.04 Impaired range of expression
   30.05 Impaired range of focus
40. Excess of or Deficit in Defenses
   40.01 Impaired functioning of defenses
      40.01.01 Denial
      40.01.04 Introjection (identification/incorporation)
      40.01.05 Isolation
      40.01.06 Projection
      40.01.10 Repression
50. Alterations in Perception/Cognition
   50.06 Alterations in perception
      50.06.05 Impaired self-awareness
   50.07 Alterations in self-concept
      50.07.04 Impaired personal identity
      50.07.05 Impaired self-esteem
      50.05.05 Impaired social identity

(American Nurses' Association: Taxonomy for the Classification of Human Responses of Concern for Psychiatric/Mental Health Nursing Practice. Kansas City, American Nurses' Association, 1986.)

nial, and splitting are the core problem areas to be addressed in the treatment of the Narcissistic Personality Disorder. The therapeutic technique of interpretation, rather than confrontation, is the most effective approach

CLINICAL EXAMPLE: NURSING CARE PLAN

The following data were obtained from the nursing assessment and talking with Mr. Wilson and his family (continued from beginning of chapter):

Ms. Wilson reports that Mr. Wilson has resisted previous attempts to attend marital therapy. She says he is selfish and unloving, drinks too much, and makes unusual sexual demands on her. Ms. Wilson feels that he views her and the children as possessions, and is insensitive.

Mr. Wilson admits that he is absorbed in other people. He plays tennis, sails, and exercises daily. He feels that he needs structured daily activities, as well as a constant supply of friends; otherwise he becomes bored, angry, and depressed. Although active in outside interests, he always experiences anxiety when he has to perform.

He admits that he needs constant connection with, and continuous admiration from, other people. Without them he feels anxious, insecure, and alone. Mr. Wilson is aware that he gives little to his relationships, but feels that he always tries to please others. This makes him feel frustrated and isolated.

Mr. Wilson feels that his professional life is considered successful by others, but that he does not yet have enough knowledge in his field to achieve his goal, to be company president. At work he is extraordinarily sensitive to, and intolerant of, criticism, and feels a poor work performance by his employees directly reflects upon him. He constantly criticizes his employees for not meeting his every need, although much of the time he does not directly identify his needs.

Recently, Mr. Wilson has increased his drinking to the point of daily intoxication after returning home from work. Mr. Wilson speaks angrily and rapidly, while jumping from one topic to another. Mr. Wilson projects a general attitude of not being taken care of. He is tremulous at times, with bouts of perspiration.

Nursing diagnoses most pertinent at the time of admission are those related to substance abuse. The reader is referred to the chapter on substance abuse for a discussion of the nursing process related to substance abuse.

Later in Mr. Wilson's hospitalization, he continues to demonstrate a critical and angry attitude. The nurse identifies anger as a problem area for work.

---

in the nurse's interaction with these clients. Confrontation is most often viewed by these clients as an attack on their grandiose self-image.

Initially, clients are allowed to display their grandiosity and to idealize the nurse. The nurse then empathically points out the clients' and nurse's realistic limitations. The purpose is to begin role-modeling good parenting, with the nurse acting in the parent role, in order to diminish some of the grandiosity and to illustrate the reality of parental limitations. The nurse points out aspects of reality that the clients are avoiding or devaluing because they do not see this avoidance as harmful to their interests.

It is important for nurses to examine their own feelings regarding dealing with the projected anger of the clients as well as the clients' idealization of the nurse. While flattering, this experience can be frustrating, but nurses must remember that clients with a Narcissistic Personality Disorder are merely using them as a mirror for their own feelings.

Although it is tempting to confront clients' self-destructive behavior, the nurse should interpret to these clients that their acting-out behavior leaves them vulnerable to disappointment. An appropriate interpretation would be, "Even though these interactions with other clients, who are critical, are disappointing to you, you seem compelled to seek them out to feel good about yourself." Only then can the nurse begin to show how this behavior interferes with the clients' true self-interest, and begin to assist them in choosing other, healthier behaviors to deal with disappointments.

Evaluation

In treatment, the clinician and client work with the more specific problems of Narcissistic Personality Disorder.

For example, the problem of an inability to achieve intimacy could be evaluated by examining whether or not the client gives personal information to another person and receives personal information from another, on a continuing basis. Other evaluation criteria indicating resolution of specific concerns related to the Narcissistic Personality Disorder include an ability to:

1. Identify personal strengths and weaknesses.
2. Establish realistic relationship and career goals.
3. Express self empathically.
4. Value self and others in a genuine fashion.
5. Maintain a sense of self-esteem despite some failures.

Antisocial Personality Disorder

Common Characteristics

The Antisocial Personality Disorder is marked by an apparent inability to adhere to socially acceptable modes of behavior. There is a history of chronic antisocial behavior prior to age 15, including delinquency, lying, substance abuse, truancy, and a violation of family and societal rules. If these behaviors continue after age 18, the client with an Antisocial Personality Disorder will be unable to work productively, to function as a responsible parent, to comply with societal laws, and to form satisfactory, loyal interpersonal relationships. Interactions are characterized by impulsiveness, recklessness, and lying.

Clients with an Antisocial Personality Disorder are grossly selfish, irresponsible, callous, and unable to feel guilt or to learn from experience and punishment. This

NURSING CARE PLAN: Mr. Wilson

ASSESSMENT	NURSING INTERVENTIONS	EVALUATION CRITERIA

NURSING DIAGNOSIS: 30. Excess of or Deficit in Dominant Emotions
30.01 Impaired Emotional Experience
30.01.01 Anger/rage

ASSESSMENT	NURSING INTERVENTIONS	EVALUATION CRITERIA

SUBJECTIVE DATA
Client states that no one knows what they are doing on the unit and that no one knows how to help him.
 	
OBJECTIVE DATA
Client is angry.
Client does not take advantage of treatment program.
	1. Ask client to describe what he wants. Ask more than once if client cannot label needs.
	2. When client is angry, ask him to:
	  a. Label his behavior or feeling.
	  b. Describe what he wanted that was not fulfilled.
	  c. Describe what he did to relieve his feelings of anger and disappointment.
	  d. Describe what he could do differently to relieve the anger.
	3. Facilitate a discussion in group therapy about anger when client is present. Discuss how anger interferes with relationships.
	4. Examine countertransference feelings of impatience and anger toward client.
		Within one week, client will describe at least two appropriate needs/wants a day.
		
		Within two weeks, client will describe his angry behavior pattern and test a new way of dealing with anger.
		
		In two weeks, client will understand how others in group experience and cope with anger.
		
		Staff in team meetings will identify feelings in response to client.

NURSING DIAGNOSIS: 21.02.03 Aggression Toward Others—Verbal Abuse

ASSESSMENT	NURSING INTERVENTIONS	EVALUATION CRITERIA
SUBJECTIVE DATA Client verbalizes anger when disappointed in others or when alone. Client has an attitude of "not being taken care of." OBJECTIVE DATA Client speaks in angry, demanding tone of voice.	1. Help client identify his needs. 2. Do not avoid client or respond with anger. 3. Encourage attendance at unit activities.	Within one week, client will make one self-disclosure per day. Within two weeks, client will ask only for necessities. By the end of the first week, client will attend 60% of all unit activities.

group includes individuals such as unprincipled business people, drug dealers, and criminals.[9] Although many of these individuals are confined to penal institutions, the majority are not, because of their highly-developed skills of manipulation.

Clients with an Antisocial Personality Disorder tolerate frustration poorly. When frustrated they may be dangerous to others, since internal controls do not exist. They are often highly intelligent but use their intelligence to deceive or defraud. Immediate gratification is a stronger motive for behavior; there is little consideration of realistic expectations. Clients with an Antisocial Personality Disorder are predominantly men.

Leading theories of etiology support the effect of parents' emotional deprivations and failures to set standards and instill values. The antisocial child has little guidance in dealing effectively with frustration. In many cases, the father is absent and the mother either does not want the child or is not vested in her parenting. Clients with an Antisocial Personality Disorder are often from low economic groups, and from broken homes. There is often a direct correlation between antisocial behavior on a parent's part, e.g., prostitution or alcoholism, and the development of an Antisocial Personality Disorder in the adult client. There is also some evidence that genetic factors may predispose individuals to the development of an Antisocial Personality Disorder. Children who have a learning disability or an attention deficit disorder may have increased risk of developing an Antisocial Personality Disorder in adult life.[9]

RELEVANT RESEARCH

One hundred clients were referred to Johns Hopkins Hospital for follow-up psychiatric evaluation for unexplained somatic complaints. The group consisted of 77 women and 23 men, with a mean age of 41.4 years. Fifty-seven clients were referred from medical services, 32 from neurology, and 11 from surgical services.

Each referring physician was given a 16-item checklist about the client. Although some characteristics of clients with Histrionic Personality Disorders were omitted, the checklist was designed to be completed easily and was intended to be relevant to the referring physician's clinical concerns.

The results indicated that many clients referred for psychiatric evaluation of medically-unexplained somatic complaints are judged by their physicians to have histrionic personality traits. Furthermore, the attribution of these traits to clients by their physicians does not necessarily entail the opinion that clients are malingering, have fictitious illnesses, or are misappropriating the benefits of the sick roll.

As psychiatrists more clearly define the relationship between histrionic traits and medically-unexplained somatic complaints, they can better advise their medical and surgical colleagues about the care of clients who provoke uncertainty, frustration, and concern.

(Slaveny P, Teitlebaum M, Chase G: Referral for medically unexplained somatic complaints: The role of histrionic traits. Psychosomatics 26:103, 1985.)

Nursing Diagnosis and Interventions

It is difficult to treat clients with an Antisocial Personality Disorder because of the issues surrounding authority, ethics, and moral values. Nurses must be firm, consistent, and constantly aware of their own countertransference in clients' acting-out behavior. If nurses find themselves responding with provocative behavior, inconsistent limit-setting, or feelings of anger or pleasure, they should see these as warning signs that they are not responding objectively to a client's behavior.

Because clients with an Antisocial Personality Disorder have often successfully avoided punishment, they experience little anxiety or guilt about their behaviors, and thus have little motivation to change. This may be difficult for nurses who feel the need to rescue clients, or assist in significant changes in behavior. Nurses can effectively deal with issues of countertransference by exploration of their behaviors and feelings (along with those of the client) with other treatment team members.

Fortunately, many clients with Antisocial Personality Disorders improve after the age of 40, even without treatment. Possible explanations include weaker biological drives, better insight into their own self-defeating behavior, and the cumulative effects of social conditions.[9] Because of their significant impact on society, both prior to and after the age of 40 it is reasonable to suggest that effective treatment programs are important for clients with Antisocial Personality Disorders.

Effective treatment for clients with Antisocial Personality Disorders must include a strict and consistent behavioral program, with clear limits. Appropriate behavior is rewarded, while inappropriate behavior results in withdrawal of privileges and opportunities for desired activities. The emphasis of treatment should gradually shift from the application of external controls to allowing clients to assume responsibility for their behavior when internal controls are manifested. Nurses should always role-model acceptable behavior.

Histrionic Personality Disorder

Common Characteristics

Typically, clients with a Histrionic Personality Disorder are immature, excitable, and emotionally unstable. They crave excitement and are dramatic in a seductive, attention-seeking manner. Relationships tend to be chaotic because the individuals are intimately superficial, have strong reactions to disapproval, and use physical closeness as a substitute for emotional closeness.

Sexual adjustment is usually poor, and there is a constant striving for emotional rapport. These clients use their bodies as instruments to obtain approval, admiration, and protection. They are often hostile and competitive with members of their own sex, and are frequently promiscuous. Clients with a Histrionic Personality Disorder require a great deal of attention from others, are unable to entertain themselves, and are frequently loud and disorderly. The Histrionic Personality Disorder is much more common in women. Work productivity suffers because clients with a Histrionic Personality Disorder find mundane tasks a burden, need immediate gratification, are poor financial planners, and are prone to extravagance.

Frequent somatic complaints are common, including headaches, backaches, and other problems. In severe cases conversion reactions, disassociation, and suicide attempts, may occur. Suicide attempts are the result of extreme frustration and depression, with an intent to influence others rather than to die. The following research was undertaken to assess unexplained somatic complaints and the role of histrionic traits.[31]

Clients with a Histrionic Personality Disorder have an intense fear of loss of love that subsequently makes them dependent on those who withhold love. These clients, unlike those with a Narcissistic Personality Disorder, retain the capacity for empathy, concern, and love for

CLINICAL EXAMPLE

Harry, a 27-year-old, has been married to Mary for two years. Mary has been a faithful wife and a good housekeeper, yet Harry is suspicious that Mary has been seeing other men during their brief marriage. Harry demands that Mary stay at home unless he goes out with her.

Mary returns from the supermarket one day with packages. Although she pleads that she has only been shopping, Harry becomes angry and accuses her of meeting a lover. He saw the manager of the supermarket helping her with packages last week, and is convinced that they are having an affair. Although Mary pleads her innocence, Harry contends that Mary is looking for someone who is richer and more important than he is.

others.[1] The level of functioning may be extreme, with individuals at higher levels being competitive, ambitious, and energetic while lower-functioning individuals are more passive and helpless, with low self-esteem.

Nursing Diagnosis and Interventions

Nurses should use a firm and empathic approach, while setting limits on manipulative behavior. Therapy should be directed at a decreased focus on somatic complaints and an increased focus on alternate coping mechanisms. Group and family therapy should be encouraged.

It is important for nurses to be comfortable with their own sexuality in order to interact effectively with the seductiveness, competitiveness, and manipulation of clients with a Histrionic Personality Disorder. Acceptance of some of the client's dependence is appropriate, and communication of caring, with firm limits, is important. Nurses' responses should originate from an understanding of the clients' need to search for love, and not from the nurses' need to react to clients' behaviors.

Paranoid Personality Disorder

Common Characteristics

Clients with a Paranoid Personality Disorder have a pervasive and unwarranted suspiciousness, are hypersensitive, and have restricted affect. They have a sense of excessive self-importance and are argumentative, with a tendency to blame others for their mistakes. Family and friends find them difficult to get along with, and feel ineffective in attempting to communicate with them. These clients feel that others are "out to get them"; even when evidence proves them wrong, they cannot accept it. Feelings of envy of those in power are noted, as well as a general hatred for those who show weakness. They instill feelings of inadequacy in others through hostility, intimidation, and rigid controls.

The absence of delusions and hallucinations found in schizophrenia and not in paranoid disorders is a significant difference, and is essential for the diagnosis of Paranoid Personality Disorder. The example above gives a picture of a client with a Paranoid Personality Disorder.

Nursing Diagnosis and Interventions

It is difficult to form a therapeutic relationship because clients with a Paranoid Personality Disorder lack trust and fear closeness. Nurses must not overwhelm clients, but they should be direct and straightforward. Nurses must monitor their body language at all times, because clients may suspect that smiles mean that the nurses are laughing at them.

Nurses should encourage active involvement in the milieu activities to decrease clients' isolative behavior and reestablish communication. Direct and straightforward verbal and nonverbal communication should be practiced by nurses to avoid misinterpretations. Nurses must also be consistent with all commitments made to clients. Meetings with clients throughout the day should be brief if prolonged contact increases their anxiety.

Schizotypal Personality Disorder

Common Characteristics

The primary feature of Schizotypal Personality Disorder is the presence of thoughts that are not sufficiently distorted to meet the criteria of schizophrenia. Clients with a Schizotypal Personality Disorder may be seclusive, overly sensitive, and avoidant. They are self-centered, because they frequently see chance events as related to themselves. Superstitious or magical thinking is common, although reality contact is usually maintained. Speech patterns may be vague, digressive, or overly elaborative, but there is no evidence of loose associations or incoherence.

As the disorder progresses, there is a gradual reduction of external attachments and interests. These clients are apathetic and indifferent, and have few interpersonal relationships. Unlike clients with an Avoidant Personality Disorder, who fear rejection from others, clients with a

Schizotypal Personality Disorder show no apparent desire for interpersonal relationships. Generally, their functioning is at a lower level than that of persons with avoidant behavior.

Nursing Diagnosis and Interventions

Because these clients have never felt accepted since childhood, and they suffer from a basic lack of trust with anxieties and fears, the gentle formation of a therapeutic alliance is essential for effective treatment. Treatment is usually sought when a crisis disrupts these clients' minimal functioning.

Nurses must assess the clients' level of functioning and assist them with basic needs, such as nutrition, hygiene, and the like. Nurses need to encourage clients with a Schizotypal Personality Disorder to become involved in the structured activities of the milieu. This is essential in order to increase the clients' social interactions. Nurses must also support these clients when anxieties increase.

Schizoid Personality Disorder

Clients with a Schizoid Personality Disorder are characterized by an inability to form social relationships, and a lack of interest in doing so. There is an absence of warm feelings for others and an indifference to praise or criticism. These clients are viewed as cold and distant, and often lack social skills. Although some clients with a Schizoid Personality Disorder are capable of high occupational achievement, they are usually classified as "loners," with solitary interests and occupations.

By their own standards these clients feel content, and function reasonably well, when given tasks that isolate them from others, *e.g.,* housekeeper or night watchman. They rarely seek treatment unless it is insisted upon by others. In some cases, under extreme stress, these individuals may become worse and display more serious withdrawals or even psychotic symptoms.[14]

The treatment for clients with a Schizoid Personality Disorder is the same as that for clients with a Schizotypal Personality Disorder.

Avoidant Personality Disorder

Clients with an Avoidant Personality Disorder are extremely sensitive to potential rejection, and fearfully watchful for any sign of social unacceptance. They expect a guarantee of acceptance before they are willing to enter a relationship, and will isolate themselves despite their desire for affection and approval. Unlike clients with a Schizoid Personality Disorder, they do not enjoy being alone. The inability to relate socially results in low self-esteem. Clients with an Avoidant Personality Disorder desire affection and acceptance and feel depression, anger, and anxiety for their inability to develop social relationships. There is a tendency to devalue their own achievements. The Relevant Research box on page 421 shows some of the traits that are commonly seen in individuals with Avoidant Personality Disorder.

Dependent Personality Disorder

Characteristically, clients with a Dependent Personality Disorder passively allow others to be responsible for their lives because they lack self-confidence and the ability to function independently. They experience discomfort—even panic—when alone. They sacrifice their own needs in an effort to keep others involved with them. Although they may have good professional skills and talents, they are unable to utilize these talents if required to do so independently or alone.

Some researchers[31] have investigated the association between Dependent Personality Disorder and Panic Disorder. This association could be anticipated: a clinician may suspect that clients with agoraphobia (a fear of open spaces), for example, have Dependent Personality traits. Because a person with agoraphobia has a restricted ability to go outside the house, others must do at least some things for the agoraphobic client, such as buy groceries. This could be seen as being dependent on others for meeting one's needs. It should be noted that Panic Disorder is classified as an Anxiety Disorder, not a Personality Disorder as is Dependent Personality Disorder.

Reich, Noyes and Troughton[31] studied 88 clients admitted to a drug treatment study of Panic Disorder. All had a Panic Disorder. Subjects were excluded if they had schizophrenia, mental retardation, depression, or drug or alcohol abuse. Subjects were tested with measurement tools used in assessing personality disorders.

Results indicated that 50 out of the 88 subjects with a Panic Disorder had no personality disorders. Of the remaining 38 subjects, the most prevalent personality disorder was the Dependent Personality Disorder. Results from one measure of personality disorders indicated that 22 clients who had a Panic Disorder also had a Dependent Personality Disorder.

The researchers could not conclude which disorder comes first: the Panic Disorder or the Dependent Personality Disorder. A Dependent Personality Disorder may be a predisposing factor to Panic Disorder. On the other hand, a dependent personality may be secondary to a Panic Disorder. The researchers stated that some clients report living "independent and self-confident" lives before the onset of a Panic Disorder. After developing the Panic Disorder, the client would cling fearfully to a close friend or family member. Panic Disorder behavior (as in agoraphobia) "may well have contributed to an unwelcomed dependence."[31]

This study is an example of how personality disorders may occur along with other psychiatric diagnoses. Indeed, it is not unusual for a client to have multiple problems.

RELEVANT RESEARCH

Researchers Greenberg and Stravynski studied 46 outpatient clients in a psychiatric clinic. The purpose of the study was to describe clients who were seen in the clinic for more than three years, and whose "main clinical problem was lifelong difficulties and associated anxiety in establishing social contacts." Through the years, the clients had adopted a pattern of living that included social withdrawal and poor occupational performance in order to prevent "rejection and humiliation." One reason that the researchers performed the study was to give proper focus to the Avoidant Personality—a disorder typically overlooked when the client is also anxious or depressed.

The 46 clients in the study were selected from more than 300 clients who had various diagnoses. The criteria for inclusion in the study included lifelong difficulty in initiating and maintaining social interaction, and a life-style that precluded social and occupational integration or achievement.

All clients in the research project responded to the Social Situations Questionnaire, used to obtain a description of social problems of the subjects. The clients also participated in a face-to-face interview used to assess Avoidant Personality Disorder pathology.

The clients ranged in age from 18 to 63 years. Thirty-five of the clients were male, and the remaining 11 clients were female. Seventy-six percent of the clients were unmarried, while 39% of the clients at the same clinic without an Avoidant Personality Diagnosis were single.

Early social problems had occurred for many of the clients. Sixty-one percent of the clients reported having no friends as children. Eighteen of the clients had never had an intimate social relationship. More than half of the sample had never had any sexual experience. Fifty-four percent had had sexual intercourse, with 12 cases reporting sexual problems.

More than 60% of the sample had had previous psychiatric care. Complaints had included depression and difficulties in establishing social contact with others. None of the clients had a history of schizophrenia. "The treatments they received included psychotherapy (41.3%), medication (37%), behavior therapy (17.4%), ECT (4.3%) and psychosurgery (2.2%)."

At the time of the study, 63% complained of "social dysfunction and related anxiety as their only problem." Twenty-six percent reported sexual dysfunction, one client had alcoholism, and another had a specific phobia.

Most clients in the study had begun to have problems in their twenties. The problematic behavior had lasted from 2 to 38 years. More than 53% had had the problem for 2 to 8 years.

The clients stated that the places they found most difficult were parties, dances, and rooms full of people. They found meeting people of their own age more difficult than meeting others older or younger. They found it difficult to initiate a social interaction, and could not keep the interaction going once it had begun. They could not get to know others in depth.

The authors stated that, although the above reactions can be experienced by many individuals (not only those with an Avoidant Personality Disorder), the reactions are different in several ways. The clients in the study experienced the above reactions with a higher rating of anxiety than that of a separate group of outpatients who were not severely ill and who did not have Avoidant Personality Disorder. Also, the experience of anxiety limited the clients: in general, they withdrew from social interaction.

When asked what they feared would occur in a social situation, the answer they gave most frequently was a reaction from others of ridicule or hostility (10 out of 46). They also feared that they might look silly (5), have a panic episode (5), or not know what to say (4).

In discussing their findings, the researchers stated that social skills training should not be reserved for the younger population (such as teenagers). According to the findings in this study, social problems can occur at any age. Other needed interventions include insights and practice in dealing with criticism, rejection, and embarrassment.

When clients attended social skills-training sessions, 21% did not complete the classes for fear of ridicule. The researchers suggested "cognitive" techniques for use by clinicians to help clients dispel the idea that they will be made to feel shame in working on their skills. The authors concluded their work by stating that more emphasis should be placed on the distinct diagnosis of Avoidant Personality Disorder in clients, because this disorder can be differentiated from other disorders.

(Greenberg D, Stravynski A: Patients who complain of social dysfunction as their main problem: Clinical and demographic features. Can J Psychiatry 30:206, 1985.)

Obsessive/Compulsive Personality Disorder

The characteristic features of clients with an Obsessive/Compulsive Personality Disorder are the inability to express warm and tender emotions and a preoccupation and concern with rules, order, and work. These clients insist that others do things their way, and are excessively devoted to work, to the exclusion of pleasure. When they are unable to control others, a situation, or their environment, they often become angry, although the anger is not expressed directly. These clients are overly inhibited and conscientious, with an obsession for trivial details and an inability to prioritize.

Van den Hout and Hessels[39] studied eight mildly to severely obsessive/compulsive clients. The researchers examined the contention that compulsive rituals should elevate anxiety and are associated with a deterioration of mood. Ritualistic behavior included actions such as compulsive hand washing, in which clients repeatedly wash their hands although they are clean.

Each subject was interviewed to determine the compulsive behavior, the level of anxiety before and after doing the compulsive ritual, and the mood before and after the ritual. Results indicated that anxiety decreased after performing the ritual and increased if subjects expected to be prevented from engaging in the ritual.

Also, ritualizing is accompanied by depressing thoughts about self. These depressive thoughts are more pronounced after ritualizing than before, and are less likely to occur if the individual does not engage in ritualistic behavior.

The authors concluded that, when a client feels the urge to ritualize, the compulsive client faces a dilemma. The client can "either perform the ritual or refrain from doing so."[39] In the latter case, the "client will experience anxiety, but will be less troubled by depressing"[39] thoughts about self. If the client does engage in the compulsive behavior, the client will reduce or prevent anxiety, but "accomplish this at the expense of raising depressive ideas about self."[39] The authors suggested that more on-the-spot research be done on this client dilemma.

Passive/Aggressive Personality Disorder

Clients with a Passive/Aggressive Personality Disorder are characterized by a hostile attitude that is expressed indirectly and nonviolently in resistance to demands for adequate performance in both social and occupational functioning. Typical hostile behaviors include procrastination, stubbornness, or intentionally "forgetting." They are generally ineffective both socially and occupationally. These clients are pessimistic regarding the future, but generally do not see that their behavior is responsible for their difficulties.

Nursing Diagnosis and Interventions for the Avoidant, Dependent, Obsessive/Compulsive, and Passive/Aggressive Personality Disorders

Clients with these disorders suffer from anxiety and fearfulness and are more likely than others to seek help. Because these clients acknowledge the need for help, nurses can take an active role in the treatment program.

Nurses should actively involve clients in milieu activities in order to overcome isolative behaviors, when this is a problem. Empathic support and encouragement should be given to address issues of low self-esteem. At the same time, active role-modeling by the nurse is essential to improve social skills. Nurses should assign tasks that provide opportunities for the clients to succeed. The degree of difficulty of these tasks should increase as the client moves from dependence to independence. Family therapy, and possibly recommendations for clients to be involved in structured living situations and day treatment programs, might be considered when family conflicts consistently exacerbate clients' symptoms.

Multiple Personality Disorder

Multiple Personality Disorder is not, in the strictest sense, an official personality disorder as listed in the DSM-III-R. Multiple Personality Disorder is listed in DSM-III-R[3] as a dissociative disorder. Multiple Personality Disorder is described here with personality disorders because it is similar to them in causing distress but not including symptoms of a major psychosis.

All dissociative disorders involve some disturbance in an individual's sense of "identity, memory, or consciousness."[3] In the case of Multiple Personality Disorder, the "person's customary identity is temporarily forgotten and a new identity may be assumed or imposed."[3]

In some cases, each personality state has "unique memories, behavior, or social relationships. In other cases, there may be varying degrees of sharing of memories and commonalities in behavior or social relationships. . . . Approximately half of recently reported cases have ten personalities or fewer, and half have over ten."[3]

The transition among personalities may occur because of stress or conflict. The "personalities may be aware of the existence of the other personalities." "At any given moment, only one personality interacts with the external environment . . . , though more than one personality may understand what is occurring."[3]

"Most of the personalities are aware of lost periods of time."[3] One or more of the personalities may function well in society. Also, the different personalities in the same individual may have varying physiological responses, as well as varying responses to psychological tests. One personality may be male, while the individual in whom the personality resides is female.[3]

The typical onset of Multiple Personality Disorder is in childhood, although in many cases a diagnosis of Multiple Personality is not made until adulthood. "Several studies indicate that, in nearly all cases, the disorder has been preceded by abuse (often sexual) or another form of severe emotional trauma in childhood." The disorder is "three to nine times more frequent in females than in males."[3]

Kluft reported that the prognosis for Multiple Personality Disorder is excellent when "intensive and prolonged psychotherapy with an experienced clinician is available."[18] Research in progress by Birckhead,[5] consisting of interviews with more than 35 female survivors of incest, includes five individuals who have self-reported multiple personalities. All five also reported difficulties in obtaining effective clinical help. All were misdiagnosed, and one reported being hospitalized when "one of my more angry personalities came out and the therapist couldn't deal with the emotions. I did not have to be hospitalized. It was the clinician's problem."

Kluft stated that "the impact of feminism and the increasing numbers of women in the mental health professions have encouraged serious attention to Multiple Personality Disorder. . . . Females with Multiple Personality Disorder report a 75% to 88% prevalence of sexual abuse during childhood."[18] The author believes that

RELEVANT RESEARCH

Bliss and Jeppsen performed a survey of 50 psychiatric inpatients and 100 psychiatric outpatients to determine the presence of Multiple Personality Disorder. The authors conducted the study based on their belief that the disorder is "relatively common, though most cases go undetected and are usually labeled as schizophrenic" or some other mental illness.

All inpatients admitted to two acute units of a university hospital were asked to complete a self-report questionnaire to determine those who had symptoms suggestive of Multiple Personality Disorder. Those who did have such symptoms were interviewed. Outpatients in the sample came from clients drawn randomly from the files of one of the principal investigators in private practice. Their records of these individuals were reviewed to determine patient diagnosis.

Of the 50 inpatients interviewed, 13% were found to have Multiple Personality Disorder. Of the 100 outpatients interviewed, 10% had the disorder.

The researchers stated that approximately 10% of the patients in the study had Multiple Personality Disorder despite the fact that many clinicians believe the disorder is rare. They concluded that, although the study included a small sample size, there is an indication that the "presence of multiple personality . . . is overlooked frequently among inpatients and outpatients. Such patients then receive inappropriate or inadequate therapy."

(Bliss E, Jeppsen A: Prevalence of multiple personality among inpatients and outpatients. Am J Psychiatry 142:250, 1985.)

---

nurses can make a valuable contribution to the field of Multiple Personality Disorder by assessing inpatients and outpatients for the illness, and by working in the area of sexual abuse at primary, secondary, and tertiary levels of prevention. The above Relevant Research box shows the prevalence of Multiple Personality Disorder in two sample populations.

The Nursing Process

Assessment and Diagnosis

Schafer reported on the difficulty in diagnosing Multiple Personality Disorder. Clients typically do not state that they suffer from the disorder. Many fear being made fun of, or fear being thought of as "crazy." Others believe that "everyone has similar experiences."[34] One or more of an individual's personalities may not want anyone else to know about the existence of the number of personalities, thus perhaps repeating the aura of secrecy and terror associated with an earlier period of sexual abuse.

The main relevant diagnostic criteria from the DSM-III-R[3] include "the existence within the person of two or more distinct personalities or personality states" (each with its own personality pattern), and the occurrence that "at least two of these personalities . . . take full control of the person's behavior."[3] Additional assessment criteria mentioned by Schafer[34] include the following:

1. Amnesic periods
2. Child abuse
3. A psychiatric history with different diagnoses at different periods of time and difficult treatment histories; previous treatment with electroconvulsive shock therapy
4. The use of dissociation as a defense of any group of mental processes from the rest of the psychic capabilities. For example, an individual's memory may be lost concerning particular events. The use of dissociation allows the client "to survive and to escape psychosis." The defense allows for a "complete repression of unacceptable memories from an earlier period."
5. "Head voices" should be differentiated from the "voices" heard by schizophrenic clients. In multiple personality clients, the voices are those of "the various personalities talking to each other or to the dominant personality. . . . Much of what is heard is conversational." The voices of schizophrenics, however, usually concern "a vague 'they'." Unlike the voices of a client with a Multiple Personality Disorder, the voices of a schizophrenic client may become derogatory or persecutory to the client.
6. The finding of a high I.Q.

Related to the finding of a high I.Q. (point 6) is the report of Kluft[19] describing a number of high-functioning individuals who had diagnoses of Multiple Personality Disorder. These clients performed major social and professional activities with consistent competence. In reference to the organic diagnoses found in Multiple Personality Disorder, Schafer reported that approximately 50% of clients with Multiple Personality Disorder also carried a diagnosis of "Petit Mal Epilepsy, Fugue States" (a condition in which the client suddenly stops previous activity and begins to wander, and later is amnesic about the wandering behavior), "alcoholic blackouts, or some cerebral organic diagnosis."[34] It is unclear which organic diagnoses were appropriate and which were substituted for an undiagnosed Multiple Personality Disorder.

In assessing for Multiple Personality Disorder, the clinician should be alert for varying moods of clients. The client may also wear extremely different styles of clothing and report spells of "not remembering." A client may suddenly develop a headache, heralding the emergence of another personality. The clinician can ask, "Is there another part of you that wants to say something?"[34]

Planning

In planning care for the client with Multiple Personality Disorder, it is important for the clinician to determine immediately that the client is not suicidal, and is not currently in an abusive situation. In many instances, the spouse may need individual therapy or counseling with the client. Group therapy with other clients who have the disorder, or with other clients who are incest survivors, may be helpful, as described by Coons and Bradley.[10] Clients may also need referrals to assertiveness training groups or vocational counseling.

Intervention

Because dissociation is often used as a defense by clients, much work in therapy concerns this "fragmentation or compartmentalization process" of the client as clients begin to reintegrate those aspects of their selves that had been separated from others. Special concern should also be taken to show caring and genuine concern for these clients. Clients resort to developing many personalities as a way to deal with the terror of their past (such as in cases of abuse). Clients can easily distort clinicians as individuals who will also hurt them.

Braun[6] presents other interventions that may help in working with clients with multiple personalities. These include (1) developing trust with the client; (2) making and sharing the diagnosis of Multiple Personality Disorder with the client; (3) communicating with each of the client's personality states, as required; (4) contracting with the client (such as a "no harm" contract); (5) gathering the client's history, including the history of abuse and the use of the dissociation process; (6) achieving integration of the personalities; (7) developing new behaviors; and (8) using support systems (including group therapy).

All of the above interventions will not be discussed in this chapter, but a nursing care plan will be presented for the third intervention listed above, "communicating with each of the client's personality states, as required." Related to this behavior, the nurse can serve a pivotal role by assisting the client to describe what is currently happening with a particular personality state. This is important because the client usually has not had the opportunity to communicate with others who know of the existence of alternative personalities. Describing what is happening with the alternative personalities can be a rewarding experience for the client. According to Birckhead's research,[5] one client with multiple personalities stated: "I'm a multiple. When I told a friend about my sexual abuse it was kind of like, I'm the weird one. Now, I'm trying to work through this. I'm a multiple personality because of my abuse, and if others can't take it, that's their problem. Before, I haven't been a complete person. Now that the personalities are being verbalized, I'm a complete person."

The clinician needs a thorough description of each personality. The description can provide an enormous amount of data. The client typically has difficulty describing the personality states since emotional and physical responses accompanying the states can emerge while describing the personalities. The client may fear humiliation or rejection while talking about the personalities. However, some sense of congruence and understanding can occur about the states as they are depicted. Mapping or charting the personalities can help with these clients.[34]

Evaluation

The resolution of a Multiple Personality Disorder is best achieved through the counseling process. A successful overall treatment plan would result in development of one personal identity and an absence of intrusive personalities occurring within the person's consciousness.

The evaluation of the overall treatment of clients with Multiple Personalities would also indicate the clients' ability to identify their thoughts and feelings, understanding of the life experiences that necessitated the formation of multiple personalities, and ability to deal effectively with their thoughts and feelings. Birckhead's research[5] concerning incest survivors (many of whom have a Multiple Personality Disorder) has included accounts of several subjects who have successfully resolved their Multiple Personality Disorder.

Other Personality Disorders

When clients meet the DSM-III-R requirements for a specific personality disorder, even if features of other disorders are noted, the specific diagnosis should be made. However, some clients demonstrate symptoms of two or more personality disorders; in these cases, multiple diagnoses should be made.

Past experiences of resolving conflict within the nurses' own families and other relationships should be recounted in order for nurses to deal effectively with the issues of anger, criticism, and manipulation that arise with these clients. In the professional setting, the nurse's objective is to respond to these feelings of the client, but not to react with personal feelings. An awareness of the impact of clients on nurses is most helpful in separating personal from professional feelings.

Frequent acting-out behavior on the part of the clients, which may include suicide attempts, creates a sense of urgency for nurses to provide a safe environment for clients. The impact of this self-destructive behavior on the milieu necessitates a response to these clients, and often to other clients in the milieu who may identify with the clients' distress and react in a similar fashion.

The intense emotions of nurses in dealing with self-destructive behavior present a tremendous challenge in psychiatric nursing. Lifelong feelings and ideas regarding pain, respect for the decisions of others, and death must be dealt with on a daily basis when treating clients with personality disorders. Exploring feelings and values with other treatment team members is essential for nurses in order to provide professional and objective nursing care.

NURSING CARE PLAN: MULTIPLE PERSONALITY DISORDER

DSM-III-R Diagnosis: Multiple Personality Disorder

ASSESSMENT	NURSING INTERVENTIONS	EVALUATION CRITERIA
NURSING DIAGNOSIS: Impaired Verbal Communication (20.02)		
SUBJECTIVE DATA Client states, "I don't want to talk about my selves—no one will understand."	1. Establish rapport with client.	Client will show willingness to meet regularly with nurse. Client will agree to common objective.
OBJECTIVE DATA Client fears rejection upon sharing information about personalities.	2. Have a meeting of not more than two staff members (*e.g.*, the nurse and the psychiatrist) with client to discuss the common objective of describing personality states.	
	3. Do not encourage emotional discharge related to personality states prior to completion of their description.	Client will not become severely anxious while describing personalities.
	4. Provide a controlled environment if client's description of child personality precipitates childlike behavior.	Client will not harm self or others.
	5. Develop a "map" of the personality states showing age of state, trauma event precipitating state development, state description, purpose served by state.	Client and staff will complete "map."

Levels of Care

Primary Prevention

As previously discussed, the origins of the personality disorders begin early in life. If preventive measures are to be implemented, interventions must be considered early, possibly even before birth. Prospective parents might consider prenatal parenting classes and parent effectiveness training courses shortly after birth.

For those who are experiencing adjustment difficulties in their relationships, relationship skills education or training is advocated to increase awareness of their own individual and family interpersonal behaviors. Desire to change is an important factor in breaking the multigenerational effect of disordered personality development.

Secondary Prevention

Because individuals with a personality disorder are often reluctant to seek early treatment on their own, it is difficult to implement early case-finding and treatment. Increased education of teachers and school nurses will help to identify maladaptive child behaviors early, and can influence the degree of severity of the personality disorder if early treatment for the child and family is imple-

mented. Nurses and educators should be well-informed regarding the mental health services available in their communities.

Although the level of functioning in the personality disorders may be mildly to severely impaired, there is potential for rehabilitation at most levels. Hospitalization is recommended for periods of crisis and anxiety. This provides safety from self-destructive behaviors, as well as a supportive environment in which to deal with issues of stress. Students' effective use of empathy and positive regard for clients, as well as their skills of observation and accurate assessment, will contribute to relieving the stressful crisis and to the return of the client to the community.

Tertiary Prevention

For clients whose level of functioning requires constant monitoring, it may be necessary for nurses to assist the individual in adapting to a hospital.

Summary

1. The therapeutic use of self is best described as the use of "the real self" of the nurse in working with clients with personality disorders.

2. Masterson, Mahler, Kohut, and Kernberg emphasized the influence of developmental object relations and psychosocial influences on the development of the Borderline and Narcissistic Disorders.

3. Individuals with a Borderline Personality Disorder have extreme mood shifts and behavior problems. They are impulsive and angry, and may be prone to brief and reversible psychotic episodes.

4. Clients with a Narcissistic Personality Disorder possess a grandiose sense of self and are exploitive of others, without empathy.

5. Antisocial and Histrionic personalities tend to be dramatic, forceful, and erratic.

6. Paranoid, schizoid, and schizotypal personalities appear "different," unusual, and eccentric to others.

7. Avoidant, dependent, obsessive/compulsive, and passive/aggressive personalities are afraid and anxious, and most likely to seek help.

8. A central component of prevention of personality disorders is early identification and adjustment of personality difficulties. Intervention at the primary level can take the form of education concerning interpersonal relationships and can prevent the need for more difficult intervention at the secondary level.

References

1. Akhtar S: Overview of narcissistic personality disorder. Am J Psychiatry 139:1, 1982

2. American Nurses' Association: Taxonomy for the Classification of Human Responses of Concern for Psychiatric/Mental Health Nursing Practice. Kansas City, American Nurses' Association, 1986

3. American Psychiatric Association: Diagnostic and Statistical Manual of Mental Disorders 3rd ed, revised (DSM-III-R). Washington, DC, American Psychiatric Association, 1987

4. Baron M, Gruen R, Asnis L et al: Familial transmission of schizotypal and borderline personality disorders. Am J Psychiatry 142:927, 1985

5. Birckhead L: The Psychotherapy Process with Incest Survivors (research in progress), 1988

6. Braun B: Issues in the Psychotherapy of Multiple Personality Disorder. In Braun B (ed): Treatment of Multiple Personality Disorder. Washington, DC, American Psychiatric Association, 1986

7. Braverman B, Shook J: Spotting the borderline. Am J Nurs 87: 200, 1987

8. Chopra H, Beatson J: Psychotic symptoms in borderline personality disorder. Am J Psychiatry 143:1605, 1986

9. Coleman J, Butcher J, Carson R: Abnormal Psychology and Modern Life. Glenview, Illinois, Scott-Foresman, 1984

10. Coons P, Bradley K: Group psychotherapy with multiple personality patients. J Nerv Ment Dis 173:515, 1985

11. Gallop R: The patient is splitting. J Psychosoc Nurs Ment Health Serv 23:6, 1985

12. Goldstein W: Understanding Kernberg on the borderline patient. NAPPH 13:52, 1984

13. Gunderson J: Defining borderline patients: An overview. Am J Psychiatry 132:1, 1975

14. Johnson S: Characterological Transformation: The Hard Work Miracle. New York, WW Norton, 1985

15. Kaplan C: The challenge of working with patients diagnosed as having a borderline personality disorder. Nurs Clin North Am 21:429, 1986

16. Katz S: Office management of borderline personalities. Psychiatr Ann 12:6, 1982

17. Klar H, Siever L: The psychopharmacologic treatment of personality disorders. Psychiatr Clin North Am 7:791, 1984

18. Kluft R: An update on multiple personality disorder. Hosp Comm Psychiatry 38:363, 1987

19. Kluft R: High-functioning multiple personality patients. J Nerv Ment Dis 174:722, 1986

20. Kohut H: The Analysis of the Self. New York, International Universities Press, 1971

21. Kolb J: Diagnosing borderline patients with a semi-structured interview. Arch Gen Psychiatry 37:31, 1980

22. Kretsch R, Goren Y, Wasserman A: Change patterns of borderline patients in individual and group therapy. Int J Group Psychother 37:95, 1987

23. Mahler M: On Human Symbiosis and the Viscissitudes of Individuation. New York, International Universities Press, 1970

24. Masterson J: Psychotherapy of the Borderline Adult: A Developmental Approach. New York, Brunner-Mazel, 1976

25. Masterson J: The Narcissistic and Borderline Disorders. New York, Brunner-Mazel, 1981

26. Masterson J: Treatment of the Borderline Adolescent: A Developmental Approach. New York, Brunner-Mazel, 1985

27. McDevitt J: Separation-individuation and object constancy. J Am Psychoanal Assoc 23:713, 1975

28. McEnany G: Contracting for care. J Psychosoc Nurs Ment Health Serv 23:11, 1985

29. Pechlaner I: The Borderline Syndrome. Vancouver, British Columbia, Continuing Education Electives Program, 1981

30. Pfeiffer E: Disordered Behavior: Basic Concepts in Clinical Psychiatry. Oxford, Oxford University Press, 1975

31. Reich J, Noyes R, Troughton E: Dependent personality disorder associated with phobic avoidance in patients with panic disorder. Am J Psychiatry 144:323, 1987

32. Reich J: Sex distribution of DSM-III personality disorders in psychiatric outpatients. Am J Psychiatry 14:485, 1987

33. Rinsley D: An Object Relations View of Borderline Personality. In Hartocollis P: Borderline Personality Disorders: The Concept, the Syndrome, the Patient. New York, International Universities Press, 1977

34. Schafer D: Recognizing multiple personality patients. Am J Psychother 15:500, 1986

35. Schubert D, Saccuzzo D, Braff D: Information processing in borderline patients. J Nerv Ment Dis 173:26, 1985

36. Siegel D, Small G: Borderline personality disorder in the elderly: A case study. Can J Psychiatry 31:859, 1986

37. Slaveny P, Teitlebaum M, Chase G: Referral for medically unexplained somatic complaints: The role of histrionic traits. Psychosomatics 26:103, 1985

38. Stanton A: Personality Disorders. In Nicholi A: The Harvard Guide to Modern Psychiatry. Cambridge, Massachusetts, Harvard University Press, 1978

39. van den Hout M, Hessels K: Deterioration of mood and elevation of anxiety in compulsive ritualizing. Can J Psychiatry 29: 390, 1984

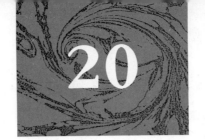

MADELINE A. NAEGLE

SUBSTANCE ABUSE

Learning Objectives

Upon completion of this chapter the student should be able to do the following:

1. Assess personal attitudes and behaviors in relation to substance abuse and dependence.
2. Define substance abuse and substance dependence on alcohol and other psychoactive substances.

3. Describe major etiologic perspectives in the development of drug-related problems.
4. List components of the nursing assessment specific to alcoholism and other substance dependence.
5. Identify nursing diagnoses and nursing interventions with the substance-abusing client.
6. Identify appropriate nursing interventions at primary, secondary, and tertiary levels of prevention in substance abuse and dependence.
7. Plan nursing interventions appropriate to the role of the nurse generalist.
8. List the components of a comprehensive approach to the case of the client who is abusing or is dependent upon alcohol and/or other psychoactive drugs.
9. Describe the role of the nurse generalist in relation to the substance-dependent client and family.
10. Describe nursing actions appropriate for the nurse generalist in relation to colleagues or other health professionals who are practicing while impaired.

CLINICAL EXAMPLES

AMY

Amy is a 28-year-old critical care nurse. Her history of drug and alcohol abuse began in high school, where she used a variety of "recreational drugs" including marijuana, and drank with friends on weekends. While studying for an associate degree in nursing, she occasionally used cocaine, continued drinking, and used marijuana in social settings. After graduating from the local community college, Amy married her high-school sweetheart and moved to a large Midwestern city, where her husband taught elementary school. Amy began a part-time program to study for a baccalaureate degree while working in the ICU of a busy city hospital. She worked long hours, frequently working double shifts, while attending school.

Over a five-year period, Amy's use of alcohol increased steadily. After work she generally had two or three drinks to "unwind," and several cognacs before bed because she had trouble sleeping after studying. Amy strained her back while lifting an obese client, and her doctor prescribed Valium. Within a short period of time, she was medicating herself during the day with Valium and drinking in the evening until she fell asleep. On the weekends, without access to the unit supply, she drank wine during the day and continued her usual drinking habits in the evening.

Amy's drinking was the source of many disagreements with her husband, who expressed concern over the drinking, and resentment over her lack of emotional availability and her overinvolvement with work and school. She failed one course and took an incomplete in the other. One evening, the head nurse on the ICU called to ask her to work a double shift the next day. She agreed, but did not recall the conversation when she reported to work the next day. Her failure to remember the conversation and her groggy response on the telephone concerned the head nurse, so she reviewed Amy's recent job performance evaluation. The number of absences, her charting errors, and numerous late arrivals for work alerted the head nurse to Amy's deteriorating job performance. She scheduled a conference with Amy for the following day.

TONY

Everything seemed too quiet when the nursing students were receiving report. All the clients were doing better than last week, and there had been no assaultive or angry disturbances in weeks.

However, around 10 a.m., while the clients were gathering for recreational therapy, there was a scuffle and pounding outside the main entrance to the unit. Three security guards and an emergency room nurse were battling to bring what appeared to be a slightly overweight, young man of medium height onto the unit. He was yelling obscenities and giving the large, strong security guards quite a struggle. This young man began yelling, "Bring on the troops! I'll fight you all if I have to! I'm Rambo and Cobra put together! You're history, man! History!!!"

Frightened clients on the unit began to back away from their regular lineup area near the door. A staff member asked that the clients all stay together in the dining room with two staff members and the students. The dining room door was then closed and locked. The rest of the nursing staff moved to assist the security guards in bringing this young man onto the unit. Because he was very aggressive and resistant to settling down, the staff made the decision to place him in 5-point restraints in the special restraint room until he calmed down. The nurse was then able to receive the admission information. Tony was a 16-year-old Hispanic male who had recently become very aggressive. He had attacked his sister with a baseball bat when she wouldn't give him any money. That morning his mother had found a bag full of marijuana in his jeans pocket. The emergency room report stated that the marijuana had been heavily laced with PCP.

Introduction

These clients have something in common. Amy chose to experiment with mind-altering substances that can become addictive, while Tony experienced a frightening yet powerful surge of chaotic energy as a result of taking drugs. Yet Amy and Tony are not alone in choosing drugs as a means of coping with pressures and responsibilities. Substance abuse disorders are a major public health problem in the United States today. While patterns and trends of drug use vary, the chronic problems of alcoholism and long-term effects of substance abuse will continue to be important issues at least until the end of this century.[23]

Many factors influence patterns of drinking and drug use: the individual's social milieu with its expectations and rituals; the subculture of which the individual is a member; and constitutional traits, both physical and psychological. These interact to determine whether the individual will use certain drugs, and to what extent. This complex interaction of factors determining drug use is key to nursing assessment and interventions at all phases along the continuum of substance abuse.[14]

The nurse's participation with client and family systems is altered by the attitudes and beliefs of the practitioner about substance abuse. Old beliefs about the immorality of drunkenness and the ability of the individual to exercise control over compulsive drinking or drug-taking persist, and are expressed even by health professionals such as students and practitioners.[29] Despite new research evidence about the onset and progression of addiction as a disease, substance dependence continues to be considered a stigma, that is, an attribute that is deeply discrediting to the individual and those associated with that person.[13] Drinking behaviors that deviate from socially-acceptable patterns contradict our assumptions about what an individual ought to be.[26] The subsequent stigma influences the alcoholic by reinforcing the experienced alienation and isolation that support continued ingestion of substances.

Alcoholism is so widespread that it is the third cause of mortality after cancer and heart disease. Consequently, there is a high probability that the health practitioner knows alcoholic family members and friends.[42] Because 25% to 35% of all clients in non-psychiatric health care settings have an alcohol-related illness, the graduating nurse will certainly encounter the alcoholic in practice. If the nurse believes that substance dependence is a disease that can be treated and arrested, attitudes will be characterized by hope, and hope is essential to recovery.

Research on substance abuse has advanced in all areas during the 1970s and 1980s. In basic science research, expanded efforts have sought to identify the etiology of alcoholism, and to isolate biological markers that might indicate susceptibility of certain individuals to the illness. The effects of alcohol on all organs and body systems are being studied in detail, and the impact of alcohol on the developing human fetus has been delineated. Endorphin receptor sites that may influence the individual's response to psychoactive drugs have been more clearly delineated, and their influence on drug effects has been explored. Research goals have also been identified in the area of treatment modalities and effectiveness.

The Diagnostic and Statistical Manual of Mental Disorders, 3rd edition, Revised (DSM-III-R)[5] identifies 11 classes of drugs associated with substance abuse and dependency, as seen in Table 20-1. Substance abuse and dependence describe mental disorders involving the use of drugs in ways that are markedly different from use of drugs in a recreational manner or for medical purposes. The behavioral changes associated with such use are maladaptive, and recognized as dysfunctional by the health care professional. With this differentiation in mind, this chapter provides an overview of substance abuse and dependence, and details the nursing process for individuals exhibiting these signs and symptoms.

Theories of Drug and Alcohol Use and Abuse

Theories on the etiology of substance abuse include models that attempt to explain the development and continuation of drug use patterns that result in psychological and physiological dependence on alcohol and other drugs. Early notions of an "alcoholic" or "addictive" personality type explored by some researchers have been set aside because research and clinical data have failed to support the notion of one personality style that explains the development of substance abuse illness. Four major groups of theories have been suggested to explain drug dependence: psychoanalytic theory, the disease model, sociopsychologic theory, and the interactional model.

The Psychoanalytic Theory

The *psychoanalytic theory*, as described previously in Chapters 6 and 7 is one major etiologic model in the psychological framework. It focuses on early developmental experience and unconscious dynamics as the sources of such disturbances. Disruptions in the normal stages of psychosexual development are believed to explain the individual's personality traits and the abuse of and dependence on drugs. Dependency needs and unresolved feelings about them are identified as motives for withdrawal into passive drug-induced states that restrict movement toward independence and limit social learning and emotional maturation.

In psychoanalytic theory, self-destructive motives and negative feelings about the self that arise from an overly punitive "superego" or conscience are also implicated in alcoholism and drug dependence. The development of a harsh superego results from overly punitive parenting during childhood. When the superego surfaces in the adult, feelings of guilt, shame, and negativity prevail. These feelings are so intolerable and painful that the individual seeks relief through drug experimentation and use.

TABLE 20-1.
DSM-III-R CATEGORIES: PSYCHOACTIVE SUBSTANCE-INDUCED ORGANIC MENTAL DISORDERS

I. ALCOHOL	VI. HALLUCINOGEN
Intoxication	Hallucinosis
Idiosyncratic intoxication	Delusional disorder
Uncomplicated withdrawal	Mood disorder
Withdrawal delirium	Posthallucinogen perception disorder
Hallucinosis	VII. INHALANT
Amnestic disorder	Intoxication
Dementia associated with alcohol	
II. AMPHETAMINE OR SIMILARLY-ACTING SYMPATHOMIMETIC	
	Withdrawal
Intoxication	
Withdrawal	
Delirium	Intoxication
Delusional disorder	Withdrawal
III. CAFFEINE	X. PHENCYCLIDINE (PCP) OR SIMILARLY-ACTING ARYLCYCLOHEXYLAMINE
Intoxication	Intoxication
IV. CANNABIS	Delirium
Intoxication	Delusional disorder
Delusional disorder	Mood disorder
V. COCAINE	Organic mental disorder NOS
	XI. SEDATIVE, HYPNOTIC, OR ANXIOLYTIC
Intoxication	Intoxication
Withdrawal	Uncomplicated withdrawal
Delirium	Withdrawal delirium
Delusional disorder	Amnestic disorder

Another component of the psychoanalytic view is the concept of regression to an earlier stage of development, along with the behaviors associated with these stages. These behaviors include narcissistic preoccupation, self-indulgence, and unrealistic beliefs about need fulfillment. Early loss of a loved object (person) results in a constant sense of deprivation and the intense need to find love in other relationships, including that with the drug. The mood-altering effects of alcohol and its effects on thought patterns provide an escape from reality that allows one to achieve gratification but also evokes the expression of hostile antisocial behaviors and self-destructive activities. Similarly, opioids are chosen as drugs of addiction because they facilitate the individual's preferred mode of coping with stress by promoting indifference and withdrawal, and reinforcing passive/dependent traits.

The Disease Model of Alcoholism

The *disease model* of alcoholism is the most clearly developed model of substance abuse illness. It is most widely used as a source of criteria for diagnosis and treatment of alcoholism, and has greatly increased the acceptance of the syndrome as a medical illness that is responsive to treatment.

E. M. Jellinek[31] articulated and described the disease concept of alcoholism in 1960. By emphasizing that alcohol abuse leads to addiction, including *tolerance* of alcohol and *physical dependence,* Jellinek made it possible to regard alcoholism as a medical disease. Jellinek further attempted to explain variations in drinking patterns and in disease as a genus with many species. In addition to describing five species or types of alcoholism, Jellinek delineated four phases in the disease process through which the alcoholic progresses. He further described drinking phenomena central to recognition of the disease, loss of control, inability to abstain, and tolerance.

Loss of control denotes a stage in drinking in which one alcoholic drink sets up a chain reaction of repeated drinking, contrary to the will of the drinker. The *inability to abstain* varies, according to Jellinek, with the types of alcoholism, and has different meaning to each type. For example, some individuals may be unable to abstain from daily intoxication and others from a state of controlled, but constant, consumption. *Tolerance,* as defined earlier, refers to the increasing amount of alcohol required for effect. Tolerance may be a characteristic of physical constitution or may be acquired by habitual drinking of consistent amounts.

In delineating five "species," Jellinek attempted to explain the wide variation in drinking patterns and their influences on the lives of alcoholics. *Alpha alcoholism* was thought to involve psychological dependence but not physiological dependence. The *Delta* alcoholic cannot abstain from drinking and drinks at a steady pace to maintain intoxication. This type varies from the *Gamma* alcoholic, who can abstain for given periods but who cannot control drinking once it has begun. Jellinek used the term *Epsilon* for periodic drinking, to describe the individual who goes on drinking sprees or binges even after a period of abstinence. The term *Beta* alcoholism was used to refer to physical problems associated with alcoholic drinking. While each type of alcoholism includes specific drinking behaviors, Jellinek's rigid delineation of types does not conform to the observed realities of alcoholic behaviors, wherein behaviors overlap and vary. Drinking problems are manifested in different degrees by all alcoholics. The problems are not mutually exclusive, and are not consistently present in the same individual or in groups of alcoholics in such a way as to allow standardization.

Jellinek's four-phase model of alcoholic progression corresponds most closely to the tradition of medical disease, and describes the alcoholism phenomenon itself, apart from variations in individuals. Jellinek's four phases are described as:

Phase I, prealcoholic phase: Alcohol is used frequently to relax and deal with the anxieties of everyday life.

Phase II, early alcoholic stage: This phase is initiated by a blackout (a brief period of amnesia occurring during or directly after a drinking episode). Other signs include (1) further blackouts, (2) sneaking drinks, (3) growing preoccupation with drinking, (4) defensiveness about drinking, and (5) feelings of guilt leading to excessive denial.

Phase III, frank addiction: Physiological dependence is evidenced by loss of control over drinking. Job loss, marital conflict, and interpersonal and legal difficulties usually occur.

Phase IV, chronic illness: Physical illnesses secondary to alcoholism develop, including cirrhosis of the liver. On abrupt withdrawal of alcohol, the individual may experience the hallucinations, tremors, paranoia, and agitation of delirium tremens.

Jellinek's pioneering work was an early attempt to standardize and interpret the signs and symptoms of alcoholism. While aspects of his model are relevant today, the rigid delineation of phase-related symptoms can sometimes interfere with diagnosis. Not all signs appear consistently in alcoholics, and signs vary in occurrence from time to time, in severity, and in number. Not considering that alcoholism may be present because all criteria are not met may mean that the illness goes undetected and untreated. Jellinek's model, however, greatly decreased the stigma associated with alcoholism by stressing the physiological dependence and the limited control that the addicted individual can exert over the process.

The increasing acceptance of alcoholism as a disease process has advanced research on causative factors in the biological framework. This framework emphasizes the nature and relevance of individual constitutional factors in the development of the disease. Research on *constitutional factors* suggests hereditary predisposition to alcoholism, as well as *familial patterns* of alcoholism. In studies of families of 6,251 alcoholics and 4,083 nonalcoholics, Cotton noted that alcoholics were more likely than nonalcoholics to have an alcoholic father, mother, sibling, or distant relative.[18]

In two separate studies, Goodwin looked at the incidence of alcoholism in twins and adopted males. These studies suggest the strongest evidence of genetic predisposition. A 1972 study of 164 half-siblings of 69 hospitalized alcoholics found that 20% of the half-siblings were also alcoholic.[27] Goodwin's work on adoptees (N = 5,483) found that adopted sons of alcoholics were three times more likely to become alcoholics than were the adopted sons of nonalcoholics. Bohman's work included men (N = 1,125) and women (N = 1,199), and again the incidence of alcoholism supports a genetic factor.[9] Results of studies of environmental vs. genetic predisposition in women are more conflicting. Goodwin found that adopted-away control subjects, nonadopted daughters of alcoholics, and adopted-away daughters all had 2% to 4% higher rates of alcoholism than the population norm.[27] Bohman[9] et al examined 1775 Swedish adoptees, of whom 913 were women, with mixed results. The frequency of alcohol abuse was more than three times higher in adopted daughters of alcoholic biological mothers than in the daughters of nonalcoholic parents: 10.8% of the daughters of alcoholic biological mothers were alcohol abusers, compared to 2.8% of daughters who did not have an alcoholic biological parent.[7]

Sociopsychological Models

The *sociopsychological models* include the idea that behaviors associated with alcohol and drug abuse are learned in a variety of ways involving social experiences, cognitive processes, and reinforcement of drug-taking behaviors.

An early and commonly investigated learning model was that of *tension-reduction*. It was based on the premise that alcohol influences conflict resolution and avoidance behavior in animals. The first theory proposed that alcohol reduces tension within the biophysiological system, and that alcohol is consumed for tension-reducing effects. Repeated achievement of this effect might establish a cycle of psychological and behavioral reinforcement. It was later hypothesized that alcohol should suppress the avoidance component of conflict and allow an animal to approach a goal that otherwise presents a conflict. Other research shows that the tension-reduction hypotheses (TRH) do not sufficiently explain drinking or alcoholism in humans.

Modeling, as a factor in the development of drinking habits, has been noted in various situations involving social forces. According to social learning theory, models serve to teach new behaviors, strengthen or weaken previously learned behaviors, or increase the value of particular behaviors.

Cultural norms about drinking patterns and styles of drug use are transmitted to individuals by socializing agents, including family members, peers, and the media.[25] Patterns of drug use, particularly drinking by parents, have been reported as predictive of drinking by adolescents. The use of drugs as coping mechanisms within the family system connotes an acceptability of drug use, as well as demonstrating a maladaptive method of coping. One sociopsychological perspective on alcohol use includes the views that: (1) drinking behavior is functional, and is an instrumental action that has meaning for the drinker; (2) drinking practices and their meanings are learned; (3) social experience relevant to alcohol use is patterned by the individual's social environment, including norms and regulations about drinking; and (4) social experience leads to beliefs, attitudes, values, and personal controls regarding alcohol use.

These perspectives appear to apply also to drug use, because the experimental use of nonalcoholic drugs becomes an addiction for particular individuals and not for others, precisely because of the effects achieved. At the same time, the social culture that surrounds the use of drugs is learned and reinforced by activities involved with procuring the drug, evading criminal prosecution, and maintaining peer networks associated with the drug-taking culture. Peer use of drugs appears to be a strong factor for the experimenter who later becomes addicted to drugs other than alcohol.

The Interactional Model

The individual's development of alcoholism or substance dependence results from the interaction of many factors, and cannot be clearly predicted by the presence of one or more constitutional, social, or other traits. The presence of certain traits, such as genetic predisposition, may place the individual at risk, but are not necessarily causative in nature. Similarly, while the presence of both psychological traits and disorders such as depression contribute to the development of substance dependence and complicate the course of the illness, they do not contribute in a cause-and-effect manner to the disease onset.

Research on an interactional model in which constitutional, environmental, and psychological factors are assessed for their contributions to substance abuse has only recently been implemented in relation to alcoholism. Dependence on addicting drugs other than alcohol has long been recognized, however, as a multidetermined phenomenon. Dependence is greatly influenced by social environment, peer relationships within the drug culture, and exposure to and use of particular substances. Life-style is a particularly important aspect of drug use patterns, and must be addressed with therapeutic interventions designed to alter the progress of the disease.

When substance abuse illness is seen as multidetermined, greater understanding of the interactional nature of causative factors, as well as of circumstances supporting the progress of the illness, can develop. Clearly, the individual with certain constitutional traits develops an addiction because these traits interact with the socioenvironmental system and result in behavioral patterns that include the development of disease.

Precipitating Factors in Drug Use

Environmental Factors

The prevalence of alcohol and other drug use is highly determined by the interaction of social, biological, genetic, cultural, psychological, and environmental systems. The social milieu, characterized by peer pressures, accessibility of certain drugs, and the social function that drug-taking serves, influences the choice of drugs and the frequency of use. Many cultures have used drugs over the centuries to alter psychological patterns and feeling states. In social contexts, drug use has been part of community life, religious rituals, and ceremonies. Since 1900, hundreds of new and important drugs have been manufactured and made available in the U.S. Their therapeutic effects have revolutionized medical practice, and the use of drugs for convenience and pleasure has become commonplace. The use of illicit drugs for recreational purposes is more common in the U.S. than in any Western society.

Many factors influence decisions to use drugs and choices about which drugs will be used. These factors include the characteristics of individuals' physical and psychological systems, including health, past history, and expectations of what a drug will do. Patterns of use are influenced by the social context in which use occurs. The cultural milieu determines the types of drugs available and their acceptability and accessibility. Over a lifetime, an individual may use one or more drugs in four major classes:

1. Prescription drugs
2. Over-the-counter (OTC) medication
3. Mood- and consciousness-altering chemicals that are legally available, including alcohol, nicotine, and caffeine
4. Psychoactive compounds

Anthropological studies and survey research identify patterns and trends in alcohol and drug use that vary over time and are observed to be different in groups by gender, race, age, and cultural subgroup.

Patterns also occur in the continuum from use to abuse. Drinking alcohol, for example, is practiced by 68% of the U.S. population. This population can be described by drinking categories as *infrequent* (less than once a month) 15%, *light* (once a month in small quantities) 3%, *moderate* (several times a month but no more than three to four drinks per occasion) 13%, and *heavy* (almost every day, consuming five or more drinks on occasion) 12%. Approximately 1 in 10 drinkers will become alcoholics.[8]

Family History

The recurrence of a number of characteristics in the lives of individuals who become alcoholic suggest that certain factors predispose the drinker to the development of difficulties. Ewing[24] discussed the interaction of social, psychological, and constitutional factors with availability of alcohol in the development of the disease. He contended that the presence of particular interacting factors predisposes individuals to alcoholism and enhances the probability of illness. Ewing and other investigators[1,24,28] identified factors in each of these categories, including:

1. Being a child of an alcoholic or of alcoholic parents
2. Leaving home environments where teetotalism is extolled, to enter permissive social settings
3. Being born last in a large family
4. Early death or loss of a parent
5. Frequent parental marital discord, divorce, or separation
6. History of alcoholism in members of the immediate or extended family
7. Belonging to a cultural group in which the incidence of alcoholism is higher than that in other cultural groups
8. Transgenerational history of depression in female relatives

Sex

The prevalence of alcoholism in men has consistently exceeded that in women, as indicated in measures of daily, heavy, and hazardous use of alcohol.[13] Problem drinkers, whose drinking is accompanied by interference with aspects of their life and the evidence of symptoms of early alcoholism, are rated as between 10% and 15% for men and between 3% and 5% for women.[13]

As with alcohol, gender differences in drug use and addiction are apparent.[40,41] Men's use of drugs differs in frequency, choice, and amount from that of women. Heroin or morphine, PCP or PCP combinations, and alcohol in combination with other drugs are used more frequently by men. Women more frequently use and become addicted to minor tranquilizers such as Valium and Librium. When these drugs are taken with alcohol or in alternating dosage, these women rapidly develop a use pattern of "dual addiction" to both drugs. Differences between men and women in symptom development and the illnesses of substance abuse are evident. Treatment approaches and available drug treatment services reflect these differences.

Age

Age is an important determinant of drug use and drug effects. Metabolic capacity changes with age, and the capacity to break down and excrete drug metabolites decreases over time. Aging individuals metabolize alcohol and other drugs less rapidly and efficiently, and generally respond to these changes by modifying intake and use. Metabolic changes are particularly important in relation to alcohol and other drugs used concurrently with alcohol. Heavy drinking, for example, is most common in men in the youngest (18–20) and oldest (65+) age groups studied. While fewer women drink heavily, those who do fall into two major age groups, 21 to 24 and 41 to 49.[6] Failure to modify drinking behaviors in relation to changes in metabolism indicates problem use of alcohol. Heavy drinkers tend to continue the pattern into old age, and constitute the majority of elderly alcoholics (10%–20%).[42]

These are not the only elders, however, who develop problems with alcohol. The increasing number of men and women living beyond age 65 have health problems and health care needs that include issues of substance use. Because older people are usually less involved in social networks, not employed, and often not married, assessment of problem drinking becomes difficult. Greater numbers of middle-aged and older women, for example, are drinking in light to moderate amounts. While these changed patterns expose some to the risk of alcohol dependence, criteria for identifying problems are different from those used for younger populations, such as occupational impairment or marital disharmony. For the most part, individuals drink less or give up drinking as they get older. Aging individuals who develop problems fall into two categories: (a) reactive alcoholics, or (b) long-time heavy drinkers or alcoholics who continue drinking into old age.

Reactive alcoholism is a significant alcohol syndrome associated with events like retirement, loss, and aging. It is frequent in midlife as well as in old age, and may occur in individuals without a history of problem drinking.

Just as age and developmental phases interact in relation to alcohol use by the elderly, drug use in adolescence is related to developmental tasks, life circumstances, and constitutional factors. Drug use is a common social phenomenon at this stage in the life cycle, but nowhere in the world is this as true as it is for U.S. youth. Survey research on high school seniors in the last nine years indicates that nearly 62% of American youth try an illicit drug before they finish high school, and 93% have used alcohol, with 39% reporting occasional heavy drinking.[32] Despite recent declines in the use of marijuana, tranquilizers, and barbiturates, the levels of substance abuse remain disturbingly high in this group. While experimentation with cocaine by all age-group users doubled between 1979 and 1982, accessibility of this drug to adolescents and preadolescents has increased markedly. Of considerable concern is the increase in mortality rate for the 18- to 24-year-old age group. While drug use is not the only contributing factor, suicide, homicide, and motor vehicle and other accidents occur frequently in relation to alcohol and drug use.

Drug use, especially marijuana use, is being initiated at increasingly younger ages, and its use increases the likelihood of involvement with more serious drugs.[32]

RELEVANT RESEARCH

Research to assess the social consequences of drinking was conducted from the perspective of the drinker's victims. A sample of 1022 respondents were selected from the general population of Berkeley, California. Subjects were asked 15 questions, from six scales, about something that had happened to them in the last 12 months because of someone else's drinking. The scales identified obnoxious behavior, property damage, problems with family and friends, violence, accidents, and threats to employment. Quantitative and qualitative data were sought for the items, along with related information. The degree to which respondents experienced alcohol-related social victimization and the context in which it occurred were reported.

The majority (87%) of the subjects had encountered obnoxious behavior among other drinkers in the previous year; 42% had had property littered or damaged by someone who had been drinking; and 31% had a "significant other" whose drinking problem caused them difficulty or affected the friendship. Subjects' experience of violence (13%), accidents (4%), and employment problems as a result of someone else's drinking (1%) was relatively rare.

These victims tend to resemble problem drinkers in this population, especially in terms of their own drinking and drinking-related problems. Women are at higher risk for being victimized, especially those who are heavy, frequent, or problem drinkers. Findings suggest that heavier and more frequent drinking by victims puts them at increased risk for suffering the consequences of other people's drinking behavior. Further, sex differences demonstrated in this study should be taken into consideration in societies in which a woman's roles and drinking behavior have changed in the last 40 years.

(Fillmore K: Social victims of drinking. Br J Addict 80(3):307-314, 1985.)

Many high school seniors polled (34%) reported beginning marijuana use in junior high.[32] The changes and demands associated with accomplishing the psychological tasks of adolescence create emotional turmoil and discomfort. Attempts to solve life problems may be restricted to withdrawal or denial of the need to develop active coping skills appropriate to maturation.

Sociocultural Factors

Life-style is a sociocultural factor that influences drug use through exposure to drugs and peer pressure.[37] Drinking patterns have long been of concern to the gay community, for example, because of the degree of socializing that occurs in bars and restaurants. Members of the gay community are also at risk because of the same characteristics that predispose others to drug and alcohol problems. The AIDS epidemic has focused new attention on exploring the impact that alcohol has on the immune system. Evidence suggests that alcohol and amyl nitrate, inhaled to alter consciousness at the time of sexual orgasm, act directly on the hematologic and immune systems to cause anemias and increase susceptibility to infection, including the HTLV-III virus that causes AIDS. At the same time, intravenous drug users in homosexual and heterosexual populations are at risk for this disease.

Racial and cultural subgroups manifest changing but discernible patterns in the types of drugs used. Alcohol, accessible and legal, is widely used among Native Americans and Eskimos, who have high incidences of alcoholism. The use of inhalants by youths 12 to 17 years old and young adults 18 to 25 years old is more common among Hispanics and Native Americans. The recent use of cocaine and crack by 10 million Americans crosses all gender, socioeconomic, and racial lines and is second in popularity only to use of marijuana.

Alcohol use is a multidetermined phenomena. Genetic, psychological, and constitutional factors as well as the familial, cultural, and social systems of which the individual is a member must be considered in understanding the origins of alcohol use and abuse. These factors and circumstances contribute to its perpetuation, and the response of the individual to treatment.

Alcohol and drug abuse can have extremely negative impact on society. The following Relevant Research box shows the impact on victims of alcohol abusers.

Substance Use and Dependence

The most widely abused drugs in the world are caffeine, nicotine, and alcohol. All are legal, and all are used in greater or lesser degrees by vast numbers of people. Although many people are psychologically, if not physically, dependent on these drugs, they are not readily regarded by the lay public as "dangerous." In fact, cigarette smoking is the largest single preventable cause of illness and premature death in the United States, and alcoholism afflicts between 10 and 15 million men and women.

Alcohol use and abuse occur at points along a continuum. Assessment of dependence on alcohol is related to the amount and frequency of drinking and to its behavioral and social consequences. The National Commission on Marijuana and Drug Abuse has identified five patterns that provide a framework for understanding use. They apply primarily to nonprescription, psychoactive drugs, and can be found in Table 20-2. It is important to note that none of these categories includes the concepts of loss of control over drug-taking or physiological dependence. Continued use despite the loss of control and associated problems is central to addiction or dependence as defined by the DSM-III-R.

TABLE 20-2.
THE USE–ABUSE CONTINUUM

VARIABLES	EXPERIMENTAL USE	SOCIAL/ RECREATIONAL USE	CIRCUMSTANTIAL/ SITUATIONAL USE	INTENSIFIED USE	COMPULSIVE USE
LENGTH OF CONDITION	Short-term	Short-term	Long-term	Long-term	Long-term
PRESENCE OF A PATTERN	No	No	Variable; task-specific	Once a day	High-frequency, high-duration
MOTIVATION	Peer-inspired; curiosity and desire for an effect	Peer-inspired; social acceptability/fitting in	To cope with a specific condition or situation	Relief from a problem or stressful situation	Psychological dependence; physiological discomfort if tries to stop

(Adapted from Wilford B: Drug abuse: A Guide for the Primary Care Physician. Chicago, American Medical Association, 1981.)

Addiction

Definitions of substance abuse are general as well as specific for particular drugs. The World Health Organization (WHO) defines addiction as a point on a continuum where the degree of drug use affects the total life quality of the drug user. *Addiction* is the degree to which circumstances associated with procuring and administering the drug control the behavior of the substance abuser. This definition refers to the *extent* of involvement with the drug and the scope of the impact of its use. The actual WHO definition of addiction further describes associated behaviors: addiction is a behavioral pattern of drug use characterized by *overwhelming involvement* with the use of a drug, *compulsive* drug-seeking behavior, and a high tendency to *relapse* after withdrawal.[17]

Pathological use of drugs is described in patterns of substance abuse or dependence.[15] A pattern of pathological use varies by substance, but may be manifested by: intoxication throughout the day; inability to cut down or stop use; repeated efforts to control use through periods of temporary abstinence or restriction of use to certain times of the day; continuation of substance use despite a serious physical disorder that the individual knows is exacerbated by use of the substance; need for daily use of the substance for adequate functioning; and episodes of a complication of the substance intoxication (*e.g.*, alcoholic blackouts, opioid overdose).[19]

Pathological use is also characterized by impairment in social or occupational functioning. Social relations can be disturbed by: the individual's failure to meet important obligations to friends and family; erratic and impulsive behavior; and inappropriate expression of aggressive feelings. The individual may have legal difficulties because of complications of intoxication (*e.g.*, car accidents), or because of criminal behavior related to arrests while intoxicated. However, legal difficulties due to possession or use of alcohol or other drugs are highly dependent on local customs and laws. For this reason, singular legal difficulties (for example, one conviction for driving

while intoxicated) should not be considered in the evaluation of impairment in social functioning.[16]

Occupational functioning deteriorates when the individual misses work or school, or is unable to function effectively because of intoxication. When impairment is severe, the individual's life is totally dominated by obtaining and using the substance, with marked deterioration in physical and psychological functioning. Incapacitation is most frequently associated with alcohol and other psychoactive dependence rather than abuse.

Frequently, individuals who develop substance abuse disorders have preexisting personality disorders and affective disorders with concomitant impairment in social and occupational functioning.[19] It is therefore necessary to determine that the impairment associated with the diagnosis of substance abuse or dependence is actually due to the use of the substance. A change in functioning that accompanies the onset of a pathological pattern of substance use or the development of physiological dependence, is a good indicator.

Duration of the abuse is also a factor. Abuse, in this definition, requires that the disturbance last at least one month. Signs of the disturbance need not be present continuously throughout this period, but should appear sufficiently frequently to constitute a pattern of pathological use. For example, several episodes of binge drinking causing family arguments during a one-month period would be sufficient, even if the individual's functioning between binges was apparently not impaired.

Dependence

Substance dependence is generally a more severe form of substance use disorder than substance abuse, and includes physiological dependence, evidenced by either tolerance or withdrawal. Almost invariably there is also a pattern of pathological use that causes impairment in functioning, although in rare cases the manifestations of the disorder are limited to physiological dependence. An example would be an individual's inadvertent physiological dependence on an analgesic opioid prescribed for the relief of physical pain.

To establish that substance dependence exists requires only evidence of tolerance or withdrawal symptoms, except for alcohol and cannabis dependence. These require, in addition, evidence of social or occupational impairment from use of the substance or a pattern of pathological substance use.

Tolerance

Tolerance means that markedly increased amounts of the substance are required to achieve the desired effect, or that there is a markedly diminished effect with regular use of the same dose. Tolerance occurs as a result of adaptation to a drug at the cellular level. When the substance used is illegal and mixed with various diluents or with other substances, tolerance may be difficult to determine. In the case of alcohol, it should be noted that there are wide individual variations in the capacity to drink large quantities of alcohol without intoxication. Because some people have the capacity to drink large amounts despite limited drinking experience, the distinguishing feature of alcohol tolerance is that the individual reports that the amount of alcohol he or she can drink before showing signs of intoxication has increased markedly over time.

Withdrawal

In withdrawal, a substance-specific set of symptoms follows cessation of, or reduction in, intake of a substance that was previously used regularly by the individual to induce a physiological state of intoxication. When drugs produce physiological as well as psychological dependence with chronic use, a *withdrawal syndrome* develops when the individual ceases taking the drug. The signs and symptoms of withdrawal vary according to the class of drug on which the individual is dependent. For example, a cold- or flu-like syndrome develops in response to withdrawal from opioids; alcoholic hallucinosis may result when the chronic drinker suddenly ceases consumption.

Many heavy coffee drinkers are physiologically dependent on caffeine and exhibit both tolerance and withdrawal. However, because such use generally does not cause distress or impairment, and because few if any of these individuals have difficulty switching to decaffeinated coffee or coffee substitutes, the condition does not appear to be of clinical significance. Therefore, caffeine dependence is not included in this classification of abuse disorders.

The individual who abuses or is dependent on drugs rarely limits use to one class or kind of drug. Table 20-3 lists the two types of behavioral addiction and one type of physiological tolerance that occur with drug dependence. The symptoms of intoxication vary with the drug that is used. For example, central nervous system depressants, such as alcohol and sedative hypnotics, produce ataxia and slurred speech. The toxic effects of LSD and mescaline are similar, and range from extreme agitation to panic.

Behavioral Responses to Drugs: Manifestations of Human–Environment Interaction

Nurses seek to modify the interaction between the substance-abusing individual and the sociocultural environment, the system in which drug use and abuse occur. Nurses must understand the manifestations and patterns that are the results of a person's interaction with a drug-using environment, and the behaviors of drug use and abuse, in order to intervene appropriately. Behavioral manifestations are a function of the pharmacologic effect on the psychological, cognitive, and physiological systems of the drug user. Constitutional traits, as well as changing biological states, influence the function that drug-taking serves and the individual's response to drugs.

TABLE 20-3.
BEHAVIORAL AND PHYSIOLOGICAL PATTERNS OF SUBSTANCE DEPENDENCE

PATTERNS	VARIABLES		
	DEPENDENCY	DESCRIPTION	EXAMPLE
BEHAVIORAL			
Mixed Addiction	Dependence on more than one substance	Alternating use of one class of drugs with another that counteracts the effects of the first drug	Use of cocaine (a stimulant) with a sedative-hypnotic
Dual Addiction	Dependence on more than one substance	Use of drugs with similar effects	Use of alcohol and barbiturates or alcohol and heroin
PHYSIOLOGICAL			
Cross-Tolerance	Dependence on one substance	Tolerance to other drugs in the same class with similar pharmacological action.	Tolerance to alcohol and to sedatives

Table 20-4 contains basic facts on classes of drugs, their effects, and their potential for dependence. This information assists nurses to identify signs, symptoms, and syndromes specific to particular drug classes.[21,50]

Hallucinogenic Drugs

Hallucinogenic drugs alter perception and cognition, thereby inducing syndromes characterized by changes in thought and feeling. These syndromes may include the secondary symptoms of psychosis, such as delusions and hallucinations. LSD, psilocybin, and mescaline are three of these drugs. LSD is synthetically made in illicit laboratories, and was commonly used in the 1960s to induce pleasant brain states. Psilocybin and mescaline are far less potent drugs found in mushrooms and cacti, respectively. 2,5-dimethoxy-4-methylamphetamine (DOM) and methylenedioxyamphetamine (MDA), also in this class, are synthetically-produced compounds marketed illicitly and available as street drugs. These compounds are less potent than LSD but are more potent than mescaline or psilocybin.

The above hallucinogenics are ingested orally and produce somatic sensations, but few induce physiological effects. Negative outcomes of LSD use include accidents due to altered perception, and dramatic and uncomfortable psychic effects in the psychologically unstable or uninitiated user. "Bad trips," which include frank hallucinations, are treated with major tranquilizers, a quiet environment, and interpersonal support. "Flashbacks," or spontaneous recurrences of these drug effects, may occur if the user has experienced hallucinogenic intoxication. These are transient but severe psychological states, and should be treated. In high doses, MDA has been associated with severe intoxication, confusion, and convulsions. Its recent availability on the illicit drug market and its unsupervised therapeutic use are causing current problems.

Phencyclidine

Phencyclidine (PCP) is a chemical synthetic that is estimated to have been used by six and one half million people in the United States, particularly low-income and minority adolescents and young adults.[48] It is easily synthesized in home laboratories and is sold as a liquid, a slightly discolored powder, or in a cube or tablet. It may be sprinkled on tobacco or marijuana, taken intravenously, or inhaled. PCP has potentially severe toxicity, producing multiple and dramatic physiological and behavioral effects. Ingestion of the drug at relatively low doses produces euphoria as well as bursts of anxiety, emotional lability, and hostile and aggressive expressions. Clarity of thought and perception are impaired, and panic attacks or psychosis may occur. Reports of antisocial acts, assaults, and homicide in association with its use have recently increased.

The PCP-intoxicated individual requires treatment in a controlled environment, and may vacillate rapidly between an agitated, combative state and one of withdrawal and possible coma. The "talking down" procedures, often effective with people experiencing toxicity to psychedelics, does not work with PCP because of the degree of confusion and impaired sensory processing. The chronic PCP user requires ongoing treatment and may experience hypertension, seizure, coma, and psychosis at various times.

Marijuana and Hashish

Marijuana, or cannibis sativa, grows naturally as hemp. The dried flowering tops and leaves of the plant are smoked to produce euphoric effects probably due to THC (Δ-9-tetrahydrocannabinol). *Hashish* is a derivative of the resin from the marijuana plant's leaves, and may contain even higher concentrations of THC.

Marijuana is smoked or ingested to produce rapid psychoactive effects on the central nervous and cardiovascular systems. Changes in mood, time, sensorium, and memory occur, as well as feelings of well-being. Physical dependence on marijuana is not supported by research evidence; however, psychological dependence has been observed clinically. An "amotivational syndrome" characterized by apathy and poor concentration may occur in chronic smokers.

Stimulants

Stimulants that are used and abused in this country include caffeine and nicotine, amphetamines, cocaine, methylphenidate, and phenmetrazine. While caffeine and nicotine are the most common stimulants, they do not produce the same behavioral changes as other stimulants, and will not be discussed here. Most stimulants have legitimate medical uses, especially for treatment of narcolepsy, diet control, and hyperkinesis. All have a high potential for inducing psychological dependence and may also cause physical dependence. Amphetamines stimulate the central nervous system to produce the signs and symptoms listed on Table 20-4. With intoxication, these symptoms may progress to the development of a delusional disorder in which the client becomes argumentative, and may experience ideas of reference, aggressiveness, hostility, marked anxiety, and psychomotor agitation. Psychotic symptoms may occur as a function of acute toxicity or may be drug-precipitated. Some reactions continue following the clearing of amphetamines from the body. Long-term psychoses generally occur in individuals with latent symptoms then activated by the drug. Psychopharmacologic interventions with antipsychotic drugs produce the best response, and may need to be continued. Individuals using amphetamines recreationally develop tolerance of the drug, although there is no proof of physical dependence and no clear withdrawal syndrome. The cessation of drug-taking results in depression, anxiety, and sleep difficulties.

TABLE 20-4.
CLASSIFICATION OF COMMON DRUGS

CLASS OF DRUG	NAMES	FORM AND ROUTE OF ADMINISTRATION	DRUG EFFECTS	HOURS OF DURATION OF EFFECT	POTENTIAL FOR DEPENDENCE
HALLUCINOGENS	Lysergic acid diethylamine (LSD) Acid Blotter Sunshine	Oral: Cubes Tablets Liquid	Illusions, hallucinations, altered perceptions, euphoria, poor judgment, dizziness, tremors, weakness, nausea, psychotic-like symptoms, suspiciousness, bizarre behavior, increased blood pressure, mood swings	12	Degree unknown
	Psilocybin Magic Mexican Mushrooms	Tabs Oral	Same as other hallucinogens	6	Degree unknown
	Mescaline Mescal Cactus	Tabs Oral		4	Degree unknown
	Methylene dioxyamphetamine (MDA) 2,5-dimethoxy-4-methyl-amphetamine (DOM) Ecstacy Peace pill Serenity	Oral Tabs		May last days	Degree unknown
PHENCYCLIDINE	PCP Angel dust Killer weed Crystal Sernyl	Powder Smoked Liquid Inhaled	Nystagmus, increased blood pressure, tachycardia, numbness and diminished sensation, ataxia, dysarthria, euphoria, body-image changes, psychomotor agitation, anxiety, emotional lability, grandiosity, sensation of slowed time, maladaptive behavioral effects	Dose-related flashbacks	Degree unknown
CANNABINOIDS	Marijuana Hashish MJ Mary Jane Hash	Pressed weed Smoked Ingested	Poor judgment, poor memory, mild intoxication, euphoria, relaxation, reddened eyes, tachycardia	3-7	Psychological dependence
STIMULANTS	Amphetamines Benzedrine Dexedrine Daro Obotan	Capsules Oral Injected	Psychomotor agitation, euphoria, stimulation, relief from fatigue, suppression of appetite, increased sense of power and energy, sweating, dilated pupils, increased blood pressure, tremors, hypervigilance	4	High

(Continued)

Cocaine

Cocaine is a purified extract of the coca plant. It is illicitly marketed as a crystalline powder diluted with sugars and local anesthetics. It is inhaled through the nose and absorbed through the nasal mucosa; it is also applied to mucosal tissues of the nipples and vagina. Cocaine may also be mixed with heroin to produce a "speedball," which is injected intravenously. *Crack* is a category of cocaine known as *freebase*. It is produced by processing cocaine using ether, baking soda, and heat. The final product contains some impurities and, when heated, makes a crackling sound. Crack looks like small lumps or shavings of soap, and has the texture of porcelain.

The stimulating effects on the central nervous system of cocaine and crack are described in Table 20-4. The effect is a rapid and intense, but brief, high. Crack produces the more dramatic high, as smoking allows high doses of cocaine to reach the brain almost instantly. The pleasurable effects of the drug, including euphoria and expanded thinking, are so intense that the user is driven to reexperience them. The compulsive need to repeat the

TABLE 20-4 (CONTINUED)
CLASSIFICATION OF COMMON DRUGS

CLASS OF DRUG	NAMES	FORM AND ROUTE OF ADMINISTRATION	DRUG EFFECTS	HOURS OF DURATION OF EFFECT	POTENTIAL FOR DEPENDENCE
	Cocaine	Powder	Same as other stimulants	2	High and rapid
	C, coke, toot,	Oral	As with other stimulants, but response is more		
	snow, blow,	Inhaled	rapid.		
	nose candy				
	Crack, rock,		May cause heart seizures, grand mal seizures		
	ready rock,				
	ridges, teeth				
	Methylphenidate	Oral	Same as other stimulants	4-6	High
	Ritalin		Same as other stimulants	4-6	High
	Phenmetrazine		Same as other stimulants	4-6	High
INHALANTS	Benzene	Vapor	Euphoria, headache, fatigue, elevated blood	Rapid	Degree unknown
	Nitrites	Inhaled	pressure, tachycardia, organ damage		
	Freons				
	Nitrous oxide				
DEPRESSANTS	Barbiturates	Tabs	Euphoria, reduction of sexual and aggressive drives,	4	High to moderate
	Nembutal	Capsules	drowsiness, sedation, respiratory depression,		
	Seconal	Oral	constricted pupils, nausea		
	Barbiturate-like	Oral	Emotional instability	4	High
	Doriden	Tabs			
	Quaalud				
	Benzodiazepines	Oral		4-6	Low
	Librium	Capsules			
	Valium				
OPIOIDS	Codeine	Oral	Euphoria, escape, reduction of sexual and	3-6	Moderate
		Tabs	aggressive drives, drowsiness, respiratory		
		Liquid	depression, constricted pupils, nausea		
		Injection			
	Heroin	Oral	Same as for other opioids	3-6	Very high
		Injection			
	Methadone	Oral: liquid	Same as for other opioids	12-24	High
		Injection			
	Morphine	Injection	Same as for other opioids	4	High
		Oral			
	Opium	Oral	Same as for other opioids	4	High
ALCOHOL	Beverage alcohol	Oral: liquid	Relaxation, sedation, release of inhibition,	20 min.–1 hr.	High
			incoordination, nausea, vomiting, slurred speech		

experience suggests that addiction occurs rapidly and progresses to lack of control in a short time. Susceptible users soon develop an expensive cocaine habit and an overwhelming involvement with the drug. Repeated use leads to the need for more frequent "snorting" to achieve the feelings that were originally experienced. With the need for escalating doses to achieve a high, there are intense and morbid depressions following such elation. Suicide is a serious concern in the periods of withdrawal or discontinued use. In recent years, cocaine and crack experimentation and use have become increasingly popular in adolescent and young adult age-groups. Cocaine has replaced heroin as the second most frequent cause of drug toxicity and drug overdose cases treated in emergency rooms throughout the country.

Inhalants

Inhalants describe a variety of psychoactive substances inhaled as gases. They are quickly absorbed through the pulmonary system into the central nervous system, and produce euphoria or giddiness. *Benzenes* and related compounds are found in gasoline, aerosol sprays, paint thinners, and rubber cement. *Nitrites* are found in room deodorants and are diverted to street sale from legitimate sources of prescription drugs for angina. *Freons* are active chemicals found in aerosol sprays, degreasers, and paint thinners. *Nitrous oxide* or "laughing gas" is available through legitimate pharmaceutical sources and is most widely abused by dentists, whose practice allows access to the drug. It is inhaled to produce a high similar to those produced by inhalants mentioned previously. The use of inhalants in behaviors such as "glue sniffing" appears highly determined by social forces and peer activities.[43] Because products that are inhaled to produce psychoactive effects are inexpensive and commercially available, preadolescents and adolescents without economic resources are the greatest users. All inhalants have varying degrees of toxicity and potential to damage the central nervous system. The initial response to an inhalant is euphoria, which progresses to headache, and sometimes to physical collapse as a result of central nervous system depression. The effects of the chemical in combination with other product ingredients have been linked to sudden death. More frequently, changes occur in the central nervous system, primarily the brain and peripheral nerves, as a function of chronic use.

Depressants

Depressant medications are a class of drugs primarily obtained by prescription, but frequently abused and thus available through illicit channels. These drugs depress the central nervous system as does alcohol, and consequently *cross-tolerance* and *cross-dependence* develop among the various types of drugs and alcohol. All depressants are synthetic drugs manufactured for medical use to induce sleep or to produce a calming effect (minor tranquilizers). The ultimate effect of these drugs is sedative; they initially induce responses of euphoria, especially in high doses. Users ingest the drugs to produce euphoria or relieve chronic or acute dysphoria. *Barbiturates* are rapidly-acting compounds absorbed through the gastrointestinal tract, and are rapidly taken up in the central nervous system. They, and the barbiturate-like *hypnotics,* produce an alcohol-like depressant effect and have a high potential for abuse in combination with alcohol. *Benzodiazepines* are widely used to reduce anxiety, produce muscle relaxation, and induce sleep.

When used over a period of time, all these drugs have diminished effects. That is, the user becomes *tolerant* of the medication and psychoactive effects become a function of escalating dosage. In the dependent individual, sudden abstinence from the drug produces withdrawal syndromes that can be life-threatening and require knowledgeable medical management and nursing care. Such syndromes include psychotic delirium and agitation, seizures, hyperpyrexia, dehydration, cardiovascular collapse, and death. The barbiturates and barbiturate-like medications have the ability to depress the central nervous system in degrees from tranquilization to stupor to respiratory depression and death. In combination with alcohol, they are frequently the cause of suicides. There are no antidotes or antagonists that counteract the drug

effects, so emergency life support services must be quickly implemented and maintained.

Opioids

Opioids are drugs, similar in action to morphine, that are widely used as analgesics. Heroin, morphine, codeine, and opium are purified or extracted from the poppy, while other drugs such as Demerol, Dilaudid, and Dolophine (methadone) are synthetically manufactured. All drugs in this class are popular drugs of abuse. Because heroin is not legally available in this country and the others are only available by prescription, the social and legal ramifications of their use are complex aspects of the client's health problem.

Opioids are taken orally or injected intravenously. Absorption after oral ingestion is slower, and users may prefer the sudden effect from injection of heroin intravenously ("the rush"). Other active and recovering addicts prefer methadone. Methadone, when taken in low doses as part of a drug rehabilitation program, provides pharmacologic maintenance considered to be a helpful adjunct to treatment of addiction. The central nervous system effects of opioids result from the interference with pain perception and a direct effect on the medullary structures of the brain. Respiratory suppression may result in death from overdose. Coma can be reversed and depressed respiration can be stimulated by the administration of naloxone, a narcotic antagonist.

Other medical problems of heroin use result from the mode of ingesting or injecting the drug. When it is injected subcutaneously, infections and subcutaneous abscesses are frequent complications. Veins become scarred, sclerosed, and otherwise damaged as a result of intravenous injections. The user is at risk for the development of emboli as well as infections from unclean equipment. These infections include hepatitis, bacterial endocarditis, and other blood-borne infections. The transmission of the AIDS virus by unclean equipment has been the primary mode of transmission of the virus to heterosexual adults, pregnant women, and subsequently their offspring. Health professionals frequently become addicted to opioid analgesics obtained by prescription. Percodan, Demerol, and Dilaudid are diverted from hospital supplies by chemically-dependent nurses, pharmacists, or physicians to self-medicate.

Tolerance and dependence, with the associated withdrawal syndrome, occur with all opioids. Dependence occurs fairly rapidly, after even a brief course of analgesics. The need for increasing amounts of the drug to forestall the withdrawal syndrome, however, is less of a health risk than that associated with dependence on a combination of barbiturates and alcohol. When drugs are not accessible, individuals addicted to opioids frequently withdraw themselves and substitute alcohol as the drug of choice. Opioid withdrawal syndrome consists of a symptom similar to a generalized viral infection or flu. While uncomfortable, it is not life-threatening. On withdrawal, four to eight hours after the last use, the individual will undergo rhinorrhea, tearing, abdominal cramps, diarrhea, muscle cramps, chills, sweating, and general anxiety and irritability. Symptoms grow worse and peak in 24 to 48 hours, with the acute phase generally ending within 72 hours.

During acute withdrawal, medical and nursing personnel must be aware of the interpersonal and pharmacologic needs of the client. Dependence on heroin, methadone, and prescription drugs is closely related to social issues and the individual's life-style. Obtaining the drug, on the street or from hospital supplies, constitutes an illegal act. Networks, connections, and the secrecy associated with drug-seeking activities have meaning and importance for the user. Consequently, these individuals are frequently labeled deviant, antisocial, or undesirable as a function of the type of drug to which they are addicted.

Alcohol

Alcohol is the most frequently used and abused drug in the Western world.[44,47] In the U.S. alone, alcoholism ranks among the four major health problems. It is consumed as a beverage in a variety of forms. Alcohol (ethanol) is the product of fermentation of various carbohydrate sources with yeast. It is marketed as wine, beer, distilled spirits, and liqueurs, and is manufactured both legally and illegally. The psychoactive effects of alcohol result from the type and amount of beverage consumed, as seen in Table 20-5.

The term "proof" refers to the doubling of the percentage of alcohol by volume. A 50% solution of alcohol in water is referred to as "100 proof."

Increased concentration of alcohol speeds up the gastrointestinal absorption of the substance and increases the blood alcohol concentration achieved by the drinker. The degree of impact of alcohol is assessed by measuring *blood alcohol concentration (BAC)*. The amount of alcohol present in the blood is reported as the number of grams of alcohol present in 100 ml of blood. For example, 200 mg of alcohol per 100 ml of blood equals .2 gm per 100 ml, or .2%. In most states, a concentration greater than .1% while operating a motor vehicle is indicative of driving while intoxicated. Central nervous system responses are slowed at .10% to .15% BAC, and a

BAC of greater than .2% is thought to be strong supportive evidence of alcoholism. At levels of .3 and .4, coma and death ensue.[51]

Alcohol is metabolized to acetaldehyde and further oxidized to CO_2, primarily in the liver. Alcohol can also be metabolized to acetaldehyde by another enzymatic system, the microsomal mixed-function oxidase system (MEOS). This system goes into full function primarily when large amounts of alcohol are consumed. Even then it can only metabolize about 25% of the alcohol consumed.

Alcohol alters cellular function and increases salivary flow, vasodilation, heart rate, urine flow, and temperature. The behavioral effects of alcohol result primarily from its depressant effect on the central nervous system. Behavior, cognition, judgment, respiration, and sexuality are all affected by alcohol consumption. The psychoactive effect is described primarily as one of creating euphoric feelings or relieving uncomfortable feelings such as dysphoria or anxiety. As consumption increases, however, the buoyant, upbeat response decreases and psychomotor activities, as well as mood, are slowed down or depressed.

Tolerance

Tolerance of the psychoactive effect develops in individuals who drink large amounts of alcohol, and is caused by adaptational changes of CNS cells. These individuals are also *cross-tolerant* to other CNS depressants such as opioids, barbiturates, and the benzodiazepines. This does not mean, however, that intoxication is not a problem. Toxic states are achieved with high doses of alcohol even for tolerant individuals. In other instances, combinations with other drugs result in *addictive* pharmacologic effects, such as increased CNS depression. In combination with barbiturates, alcohol reduces the amount of barbiturate sufficient to produce death by aspiration of stomach contents, respiratory depression, cardiovascular failure, and severe hypothermia. Other drugs that produce addictive effects when combined with alcohol include the phenothiazines, non-opioid sedative hypnotics other than barbiturates, and cannabis sativa. Other drugs act *synergistically* with alcohol, and these include the opioids (heroin, morphine, Demerol) and the benzodiazepines (Valium, Librium, Ativan).

Withdrawal

In the individual who has become physiologically dependent on alcohol, sudden abstinence produces a withdrawal syndrome or *delirium tremens,* which can be life-threatening if not treated. The onset of an alcohol withdrawal syndrome frequently goes unrecognized by nurses and other health practitioners because the widespread incidence of alcoholism is generally not acknowledged. Also, many practitioners accept the client's report of the amount of alcohol he or she consumes. Because denial is a key element in the illness, the drinker minimizes or underestimates consumption. Physiological de-

TABLE 20-5.
ALCOHOL CONTENT IN VARIOUS BEVERAGES

BEVERAGE	1 oz. alcohol is contained in:	PERCENT ALCOHOL
Beer	8 oz.	4%–6%
Wine	4 oz.	12%–14%
Dessert wines	3 oz.	18%
Liqueurs	1½ oz.	20%–30%
Distilled spirits	1½ oz.	40%–50%

pendence rarely develops in individuals without at least three years of chronic alcoholism. Withdrawal syndrome from alcohol usually occurs within 24 to 48 hours after the last drink, but can occur as much as seven days later. The symptoms are due to a rebound response of the central nervous system following prolonged depression by alcohol. The increased sensitivity of the CNS results in:

1. Loss of appetite (anorexia)
2. Nausea
3. Irritability, restlessness, hyperactivity
4. Tremor and weakness, increasing in severity
5. Diaphoresis, increased pulse rate (100–120/min), hyperpyrexia 37.2–27.8° C
6. Anxiety and depression
7. Insomnia, confusion, disorientation progressing to delirium, illusions, and hallucinations
8. Grand mal seizures may occur.

While hallucinations, along with general disorientation, may occur as part of delirium tremens, *alcoholic hallucinosis* is a disturbing syndrome that occurs in the individual who is not disoriented (except for time), and in whom other signs of alcohol withdrawal have disappeared. The client may experience visual or auditory hallucinations intermittently, and may also demonstrate paranoid ideation. This transient disturbance tends to occur within 24 hours after the client has stopped drinking, and the client is, unlike clients with other psychosis, aware that he or she is hallucinating. The client requires supportive interpersonal nursing care, including the administration of benzodiazepines or sedative-hypnotic drugs.

Long-Term Effects of Alcohol

The ingestion of alcohol over a long period of time affects the psychological/social system of the individual, and has clear impact on all organ systems of the body.[23] Alcohol affects the brain and the entire nervous system and results in loss of brain tissue (atrophy) and nerve cells (neurons). The mechanisms by which alcohol affects the brain, however, are not clearly understood, nor are the other factors that increase the individual's susceptibility to damage to the brain and other organs. In the past, neurologic and other system effects of alcohol were felt to be the result of poor nutrition, as a result of alcohol's impact on nutrient absorption and metabolism or undernutrition. Research suggests that apart from these factors alcohol has a toxic effect through direct exposure to the cells, as a chemical irritant, and through interaction with a combination of other factors. The combined effects of alcohol on the functions of all body systems is to reduce life expectancy by 10 years from that of the nondrinking individual.

Table 20-6 describes the mechanisms of damage to the body systems as well as the short- and long-term effects on them as a result of chronic ingestion of excessive amounts of alcohol. Cause-and-effect relationships between the duration of drinking and amount consumed and the actual effects on the body cannot be postulated

because a multitude of variables increase or decrease the vulnerability of the individual. Susceptibility is influenced by constitutional factors such as heredity, sex, and physical attributes. Women, for example, appear to develop cirrhosis of the liver with a higher incidence and in a shorter period of time than do men.[20,31] The National Council on Alcoholism describes these signs on two tracks: (1) physiological and clinical, and (2) behavioral, psychological, and attitudinal. The Council also identifies diagnostic criteria. Table 20-6 also describes signs of alcoholism in a modified form.

The effects of heavy alcohol consumption on the total human system and psychological as well as physiological dependence are best described in phases that permit combining physiological and behavioral changes. These changes are classified according to early, middle, and late stages of the illness. From its onset, alcoholism is a chronic, progressive disease in which physiological, psychological, and social changes occur in relation to one another over a period of time. Whether physiological or psychological signs indicate that the individual is alcoholic can be decided only in the context of the total behavioral profile, supported by objective signs identified by health and laboratory assessments shown in Table 20-7.

The Impaired Professional

Assessment

Practicing as a health professional while impaired by alcohol or drugs is usually, but not always, associated with the middle or late stages of drug dependence, although heavy drinking and drug use while off duty also affect cognitive and psychomotor function. Assessment of impaired practice problems is based on objective signs manifested by the health professional in the work setting,[11] and includes the following:

A. Variations in record-keeping and documentation
 1. Deterioration of handwriting throughout the course of the day
 2. Discrepancies in drug count that occur consistently when one nurse is on duty
 3. Falsification of records, including borrowing drugs from other floors and/or the use of fictitious client names
B. Changes in interpersonal behavior
 1. Excessive irritability with clients and staff
 2. Angry outbursts that seem unprovoked
 3. Sudden changes in behavior from congenial to argumentative
 4. Increasing social isolation; lack of attendance at staff meetings and/or social gatherings
C. Changes in professional and community activities
 1. Withdrawal from professional activities
 2. Failure to complete assumed responsibilities
 3. Withdrawal from social participation outside the home

TABLE 20-6.
DIAGNOSTIC CRITERIA FOR ALCOHOLISM

MAJOR DIAGNOSTIC CRITERIA

PHYSIOLOGICAL AND CLINICAL	BEHAVIORAL, PSYCHOLOGICAL, ATTITUDINAL
PHYSIOLOGICAL DEPENDENCE	
1. Evidenced by withdrawal syndrome when intake is stopped or decreased	1. Continued drinking despite strong medical contraindication known to the client
2. Evidenced by tolerance, manifested by blood alcohol concentration (BAC) over 150 mg/100 ml without signs of intoxication or BAC over 300 mg/100 ml at any time	2. Drinking despite strong social contraindications such as job loss for intoxication, marital disruption related to drinking, DWI arrest
3. Presence of a major alcohol-associated illness in a person who drinks regularly	3. Client may or may not complain of loss of control over alcohol consumption.
4. Blackouts may or may not occur.	

MINOR PHYSIOLOGICAL CRITERIA IN EARLY, MIDDLE, AND LATE PHASES

	EARLY	MIDDLE	LATE
DIRECT EFFECTS OF ALCOHOL	Alcohol is frequently on breath at time of medical evaluation.	Client often has alcoholic facies, vascular engorgement of face, peripheral neuropathy. Client may manifest toxic amblyopia; increased incidence of infection; cardiac arrhythmia.	*Definitive signs:* alcoholic hepatitis, alcoholic cerebellar degeneration *Frequent manifestations:* fatty liver, Laennec's cirrhosis, pancreatitis, Wernicke-Korsakoff's syndrome, cerebral degeneration in the absence of Alzheimer's disease, peripheral neuropathy, alcoholic myopathy, alcoholic cardiomyopathy
INDIRECT EFFECTS	Client may manifest tachycardia, flushed face, nocturnal diaphoresis	Client may manifest bruises, scars, injuries to extremities; cigarette or other burns; hyporeflexia while drinking.	Client may manifest chronic gastritis, anemias and clotting disorders, toxic amblyopia, beriberi, pellagra, decreased tolerance to alcohol.

(Adapted from Estes N, Heinemann E: Alcoholism: Development, Consequences, and Interventions. St Louis, CV Mosby, 1982.)

D. Impaired professional judgment
   1. Inappropriate decision-making regarding client care
   2. Problems in relationships with colleagues and other health professionals
   3. Failure to complete assignments at the minimum level of performance
E. Impaired psychomotor skills
   1. Problems preparing and administering medications
   2. Inability to complete technical nursing procedures safely and competently
F. Changes in personal conduct
   1. Deterioration in grooming
   2. Excessive drowsiness
   3. Frequent absences from the unit

Assessment of impaired practice proceeds in the context of the job setting and the nursing role. A co-worker, alert to the signs of impaired practice, may be the first to notice that a peer is experiencing difficulty. The decision about whether or not to intervene is based on the co-worker's awareness of the individual's level of comfort with expressions of concern, and the ethical con-

TABLE 20-7.
LABORATORY SIGNS INDICATIVE OF CHRONIC ALCOHOL CONSUMPTION

SERUM OSMOLALITY	Every 22.4 increase over 200 mOsm/L reflects 50 mg/100 ml alcohol.
LIVER ABNORMALITY	Frequent presence of elevated SGPT, BSD, bilirubin, urobilinogen elevation, serum A/G ratio reversal. Client may manifest SGOT elevation.
RESULTS OF ALCOHOL INGESTION	Frequently manifests low magnesium level; hypoglycemia, hyperchloremia, alkalosis, lactic acid, transient uric acid elevations, potassium depletion
HEMATOLOGIC PROBLEMS	May manifest anemias, especially macrocytic hemolytic; clotting disorders, such as thrombocytopenia, prothrombin elevation
ECG ABNORMALITIES	May manifest tachycardias, T-wave irregularities, atrial fibrillation, premature ventricular contractions, abnormal P waves
EEG ABNORMALITIES	May manifest decreased or increased REM sleep, depending on phase, loss of delta sleep
OTHER ABNORMALITIES	May manifest decreased immune response, chromosomal damage

RELEVANT RESEARCH

Qualitative research methods were used to explore and describe the process through which nurses become chemically dependent. Using the grounded theory method, the researcher sought to identify a specific shared social-psychological problem underlying the self-destructive behavior manifested in addiction. Reviews of case histories, interviews, and participant observation were used to collect data, which were then analyzed using the constant comparative method. The sample was composed of 20 registered nurses. Their behavior was compared by categories of race, gender, age, educational degree, and clinical assignments.

Findings included the observation that physical and psychological pain, in varying degrees, is the basic problem for nurses who become chemically dependent. A trajectory of self-annihilation was delineated and described as occurring in three sequential stages: experience, commitment, and compulsion. Unless the process is aborted, its negative consequences include social losses, illness, and ultimately death.

(Hutchinson S: Chemically-dependent nurses: The trajectory toward self-annihilation. Nurs Res 35:196, 1986.)

straints the co-worker feels in relation to the risks presented to clients' well-being and standards of professional practice. Peers are often reluctant to confront friends or co-workers, knowing that the response will be defensive, unpleasant, or possibly threatening. It is common for colleagues or co-workers simply to deny the problem and fail to take action. This generally results in changes in work patterns, such as assuming extra work loads to compensate for the frequently absent colleague, or "covering up" for the nurse who is intoxicated or nonfunctional. These responses "enable" the ill individual to continue a pattern of drug use that becomes progressively serious and can end in job loss, reporting of the individual to the State Board of Nursing, and possibly the death of the nurse by suicide or drug overdose. The following Relevant Research box outlines some of the causes and outcomes of chemical dependence of nurses.

ANA Code on Addictions and Psychological Dysfunctions

The ANA Code details the ethics that guide nursing practice, and states that the nurse "acts to safeguard the client and the public when health care and safety are affected by incompetent, unethical, or illegal practice of any person."[4] Acting according to the code, however, necessarily has implications for professional and employment relations that are complex and perhaps bewildering. For example, how can one *act* when the impaired nurse is the immediate supervisor? What are the risks involved in confronting a co-worker who is also a friend? What are the legal implications of falsely accusing a colleague? What are the legal implications of not reporting a practitioner who is functioning incompetently? These and similar questions are rarely addressed in common exchanges in the work setting, and yet these questions arise with increasing frequency. As knowledge of the ethical, legal, and professional implications of impaired practice increases, decisions and choices will become easier. At the present time, many questions remain unanswered.

The nursing supervisor bears responsibility for the well-being of clients and personnel. The decision to intervene when impaired practice occurs cannot be dependent on the supervisor's level of comfort or ambivalence about decision-making. The supervisor's action has legal and ethical determinants.

When deteriorating job performance occurs for any reason, the supervisor must address the issue with the employee.[6] Certain guidelines can help the first-line manager, whether head nurse or supervisor, to intervene with the goal of removing impaired nurses from clinical settings in which they pose a threat to client well-being, co-worker safety, and standards of practice. The well-being of the nurse and minimization of the impact of illness on his or her career are also important reasons for action. Once the nurse enters a treatment program appropriate to the illness, the process of rehabilitation is begun. Successful progress in a program of recovery then allows the nurse the option of returning to practice.

Guidelines for Intervention in the Employment Setting

Departments of nursing and peer assistance programs have developed progressive steps that provide a general action guide for nursing administrators when deteriorating job performance is observed.[36] The goal is to gather and present documentation of a problem that is affecting work. It is important not to diagnose the problem or suggest that a particular illness is occurring.

1. Document changes in job performance with objective observations.
2. Review medication records and charts for errors and other indications that record-keeping is inaccurate.
3. Meet with the nurse to discuss the observations of deteriorating job performance.
4. Require the nurse to seek consultation with the institution's employee assistance program or health service, or a health professional of the individual's choice.

5. Establish a time frame within which the consulting professional will provide relevant data concerning the facts that consultation was sought and that the individual is undertaking treatment or is well enough to continue practice.
6. Establish a time limit for job performance improvement.
7. Communicate clearly to the nurse that he or she cannot continue to practice if job performance does not improve.
8. Comply with the stated outcome: that, if the nurse with a drug or alcohol problem does not seek treatment, employment cannot be sustained.
9. If the nurse who is practicing incompetently does not seek treatment and states the intention to leave the employment setting, inform the nurse of what will happen and then implement proceedings to report the nurse to the state's agency that licenses nurses.

Rationale for Action

Nurses who practice incompetently because of drug or alcohol dependence practice in the professional microcosm of nursing: they practice in a professional community as peer and co-worker. The level of practice demonstrated by an impaired nurse has an impact on the image of nursing and on the professional group as a whole. Nurses who practice while using alcohol or other drugs experience an altered state of consciousness that compromises cognitive function and impairs professional judgment. Because of the consequences, practicing while impaired becomes more than a personal problem: it becomes a professional issue.

Intervention in the problem of impaired nursing practice is determined by nursing roles and settings, but also in accord with the resources at the disposal of the individual who is planning to take action. It is only in recent years that the health professions have acknowledged that their members develop problems with alcohol and drugs. Old beliefs associated with the care-taking role and the notion that knowledge of drugs somehow protects against addiction perpetuate the illusion that alcoholism or drug dependence do not occur in doctors, nurses, dentists, and other health care providers. With the recognition that denial and old beliefs have interfered with action, medicine, dentistry, and nursing have taken steps to provide assistance to their members with such problems, and to teach professionals how to respond when these problems occur.

Professional Group Action

Action by professional groups takes a variety of forms. The most common first step has been the passage of a resolution or the formulation of a policy statement. These statements identify the existence of drug, alcohol, and psychiatric problems within the professional population and state the intent to assist these individuals through actions listed in the resolution. The American Nurses' Association passed such a resolution in its House of Delegates in 1982, and by doing so established a model for state nurses' associations that sought to address the problem. Even before that, state nurses' associations had passed resolutions and/or established peer assistance programs to aid practitioners of nursing with drug and alcohol problems. *Peer assistance* is one nurse reaching out to another with the intention of providing help. Peer assistance can take the forms of consultation, education, or efforts to motivate the nurse to seek treatment. If the nurse acknowledges having a problem, a peer may be useful in facilitating a referral to a treatment facility or in assisting the individual in initiating therapy.

Organizational efforts by state nurses' associations and other nursing groups include the following:

1. *Peer assistance programs* that reach out to nurses observed to be experiencing problems related to practice. These programs attempt to motivate individuals to seek treatment. The nurse has the option to enter into a contract with the program that designates methods for monitoring progress after acute treatment and during rehabilitation.
2. *Networking activities* that put recovering nurses in touch with one another, facilitate collaboration among health professionals who are working in this area, and promote the sharing of political and educational efforts
3. *Educational activities,* ranging from formal curriculum development to informal seminars and workshops, sponsored by nursing groups or derived from collaborative interdisciplinary efforts
4. *Referral and information services* that maintain hotlines or telephone resources to provide information and/or guidance to nurses experiencing difficulty or to others involved in the situation
5. *Peer support groups,* composed of recovering nurses who meet regularly to discuss issues related to recovery and the maintenance or reinstitution of nursing practice. Attending these groups is not considered treatment, but provides for support on shared concerns.

Much of this activity is based on the commitment of recovering nurses to action by the profession on these issues, and their belief in the importance of such action. In addition to providing assistance to individuals and groups, the American Nurses' Association and 48 of its constituent state associations have established committees or task forces that oversee the conduct of activities related to impaired nursing practice and address its professional implications. The American Nurses' Association Committee on Impaired Nursing Practice, convened in 1986, has the responsibility of delineating professional action and policies that relate to this issue and that support the provision of assistance to nurses with drug, alcohol, or psychiatric problems.

Association efforts at state and national levels are directed toward changing employment conditions and legal statutes about incompetent practice resulting from substance abuse illness. Conditions of employment can negatively influence the treatment of addictive illness in a number of ways. These include the absence of employee assistance programs or substance abuse counseling services in employee health services, lax monitoring of narcotics and other controlled substances, limited health care benefits for treatment of substance abuse illness, and a tradition of firing nurses for alcoholism or drug dependence without recommending resources or providing benefits for treatment. Nurses within institutions are acting to change policy and practice so that addictions are regarded in the same way as other illnesses, and employment provisions and treatment benefits are uniform.

Diversion legislation has been passed in a number of states, and represents an alternative to legal disciplinary action against nursing licensure. This legislation provides options by which a nurse can voluntarily agree not to practice nursing. Such an agreement, when substance abuse illness occurs, means that the nurse will not be disciplined for incompetent practice. The bill provides for a nurse who is addicted to voluntarily surrender licensure and be diverted from the usual disciplinary process, which often takes a year or more and may result in probation or the revocation of the nurse's license for many years. Voluntary surrender allows the nurse to begin treatment immediately while the license is inactive. This legislation does not, however, remove the individual's need to respond to criminal charges as a result of drug theft.

The problem of impaired practice has only recently emerged as one of many current professional issues. While the problem within the profession occurs in relatively few nurses, it poses a threat to professional standards, consumer well-being, and the professional image. The profession of nursing has chosen to address and regulate this problem internally, that is, through various activities that derive from professional policy and organized activity.

The Nursing Process and Substance Abuse

Caring for the client who is dependent on or abusing substances proceeds according to the systematic steps of the nursing process, beginning with *assessment* and progressing to the formulation of a nursing diagnosis. Several *nursing diagnoses* are applicable to the substance-dependent client, and the formulation of these from collected data reflects an understanding of the many facets of the client's health that are affected by such illness. *Planning* processes that reflect the comprehensive nature of the nursing approach include the client and family in the formulation of realistic long- and short-term goals.

Working within the family system and participating with the client are essential to implementing *interventions*. *Evaluation* of interventions is a process involving the client and the care-giver, and extends over time. These steps of the nursing process form the scientific framework for nursing care of the substance-abusing client at primary, secondary, and tertiary levels of prevention.

Nursing care plans for Amy and Tony, the cases described in the clinical examples at the beginning of this chapter, follow below.

The Therapeutic Use of Self With Substance-Abusing Clients

Negative attitudes about drug and alcohol problems dominate the thinking of the lay public and health professionals.[34] Before the nurse or the nursing student initiates a relationship with the alcoholic or drug-dependent client, consideration must be given to personal attitudes and societal beliefs. The old belief suggests that continued drug use is willful, and that the addict lacks the discipline or strength to stop using the drug. Another commonly-held view is that drug use reflects a moral flaw, or an impoverished upbringing. These views are impediments to the development of the therapeutic social milieu necessary to the recovery of the addicted person, and interfere with the formation of a therapeutic alliance between the nurse and the client.

It is important for students and practitioners of nursing to acknowledge the ways in which their family history, life experiences, skills, and attitudes influence their appraisal of the client. Beyond assessment skills, personal qualities such as insight and empathy can constructively contribute to the quality and therapeutic potential of the nurse–client relationship. When the helping professional is aware of the influence of attitudes, personal characteristics, experiences, and family and sociocultural factors, this self-knowledge can contribute to the capacity to focus on the unique qualities of the client and to work more objectively toward treatment goals.

Self-assessment and an honest appraisal of personal beliefs are complex, but should be considered as an important first step in learning. Drugs and alcohol are widely used in society, and most students will have some history of alcohol and/or drug use. Some may even be recovering from addiction. For the most part, students' drug use is recreational and by choice, rather than of a longstanding and compulsive nature. Given these circumstances, students need to consider personal views in the following areas:

1. What is my personal drug-taking history? What function does drug-taking serve for me?
2. What are my views on why people take drugs? Do I believe in a particular theory of drug use?
3. How do my personal experiences with alcohol and drugs, and the experiences of my family and friends, influence my developing relationships with clients?

4. How do I perceive my ability to help a client who leaves a drug treatment program, resumes drinking, or refuses to admit to having a problem?
5. How do my own behaviors and the behaviors of family members support the client's continued denial of a problem or continued drug use?[35]

When students are able to address these questions and consider the answers as important shaping factors in relationships, they will be better able to develop therapeutic relationships. Understanding how personal attitudes and behaviors influence nurse–client interactions related to drug use and a drug-using life-style may require participation in self-help groups and/or student support groups and in guidance sessions with nursing instructors. Attendance at open Alcoholics Anonymous, Narcotics Anonymous, or Al-Anon meetings can increase students' understanding of the difficult tasks faced by individuals working to achieve a drug-free recovery.

The interpersonal difficulties encountered by health professionals working with drug- or alcohol-dependent clients also result from the nature of these illnesses and the patterns of relapse characteristic of these diseases. When clients "slip" and begin using drugs or alcohol again, the care-taker's response is often one of *anger and frustration.* The nurse may assume personal responsibility for the client's failure and interpret a setback as an indication that the nursing assessment or care plan was somehow faulty. The client, struggling to disengage from the drug and its compulsive use, may behave in ways that provoke the anger of nursing, medical, and other professional staff members by violating the treatment contract or hospital rules about the use or sale of drugs in the treatment setting. Because such activity is perceived as defying authority or rejecting assistance, staff may respond to such behavior personally.

By understanding the *chronic nature* of addictions, which are progressive illnesses that must be addressed over a lifetime, the nurse is better able to work with the client to establish realistic treatment goals. It is important for the nursing student to understand the magnitude of efforts necessary to deal with an addiction, whether it is to food, to nicotine, to alcohol, or to other drugs. When alcohol or another drug becomes the *primary defense against painful feelings,* and a rewarding way to cope with stresses, attempts to abstain from use are associated with a sense of vulnerability and feelings of inadequacy. *Anxieties* that have long been tempered by the drug, and realizations from which the client has been retreating, are now inescapable and necessitate attention and resolution. Most individuals who have depended on drugs to cope lack basic, healthier coping skills, learned by experience and with the support of others. Often they have not developed decision-making or problem-solving skills that allay anxiety and allow them to proceed in confronting stresses and emotional conflicts.

The central and overriding dynamic of substance abuse illness is *denial.* This primary defense mechanism operates unconsciously to limit the individual's awareness of dependence on a drug and its increasing importance in life. In a conscious and consistent way, the individual denies to others that problems in life are the consequences of obtaining and self-administering drugs. The initial breakthrough in denial brings the person to treatment, but does not necessarily ensure an acceptance of the illness and the need to learn about and live a drug-free life-style. Resistance to recognizing these factors extends to the counseling or therapeutic relationship with nursing staff and others. Attempts to confront the client's denial compromise opportunities to build a trusting relationship. The gradual introduction of realistic facts can promote the client's trust and acceptance of the nurse's concern. Denial has been the primary mode of handling life stresses, feelings of isolation and inferiority, absence of self-respect, and conflicts about sexuality. Directly confronting the client's denial threatens the individual with the loss of a last support.

Some psychological conflicts and dysfunctional interpersonal patterns commonly arise as treatment issues with the substance-abusing individual. Conflicts over feelings of *dependence* and the desire and need for *independence* are commonly encountered. Adults who develop addictions have frequently been observed to have adopted a "pseudo-independence" early in life. Because of a variety of family circumstances, these persons as children took on adult responsibilities, so their needs for dependency and nurturing were not met. As a result, they may lack a solid sense of autonomy and independence, and may have many unmet dependency needs. In the therapeutic relationship, it is important to accept and acknowledge the client's dependency needs and to establish realistic expectations. This is done by supporting independent decision-making and assisting clients with problem-solving.

When persistent drug use is a retreat from active participation in social, occupational, and emotional spheres of the individual's life, it establishes a predominant pattern of withdrawal. Frustration in interpersonal relations, anxiety, and self-doubt become triggers to use of drugs. Because drugs effectively suppress anxiety and relieve psychological discomfort on a short-term basis, recovering individuals, freed of this buffer, experience threatening and disturbing emotions. Support is essential to their efforts to deal with feelings in a new way. *Anger*[52] is often central to these struggles. It has been postulated that anger is learned as a means of neutralizing the threat one experiences in the face of anxiety. The insecure and anxious individual, therefore, may rely heavily on anger as a means of coping with feelings of frustration and powerlessness. Persistent and disturbing feelings of anger and rage may provoke or support self-medicating to temper these emotions. At the same time, drugs impair cognitive capacities and weaken the individual's judgment. Expression of verbal or physical abuse may result. Control over the destructive expression of anger is a realistic goal more easily achieved in a sober state, but the client needs firm direction in ways to recognize angry feelings and find appropriate outlets for their expression.

The individual who becomes substance-dependent has failed to find fulfillment of self or personal needs in

NURSING CARE PLAN: AMY

Acute Withdrawal From Alcohol and Minor Tranquilizers (Diazepam)
DSM-III-R Diagnostic Category: Alcohol Withdrawal Delirium
                     Anxiolytic Withdrawal Delirium

ASSESSMENT	NURSING INTERVENTIONS	EVALUATION CRITERIA

NURSING DIAGNOSIS: Alterations in Defensive Human Response Patterns, Excess of or Deficit in Defenses (40.)
Impaired Functioning of Defenses (40.01)
Denial (40.01.01)

SUBJECTIVE DATA	Do not confront denial directly.	Client will be able to disclose drug use.
Client states, "I am a social drinker." "I take 30 mg of Valium a day—it helps me stay calm."		
OBJECTIVE DATA		
Client denies drug dependence.		

NURSING DIAGNOSIS: Alterations in Circulation: Biological Response Patterns (10.)
Alterations in Neurologic/Sensory Functioning (15.)

SUBJECTIVE DATA	Monitor vital signs.	Vital signs will return to normal range.
(No statement)	Observe for changing signs and symptoms.	CNS activity will be controlled by medication
OBJECTIVE DATA	Provide calm, well-lighted environment.	and environmental management.
Tremors, BP 170/80, P = 100, distortions of visual stimuli	Administer medication as prescribed.	

NURSING DIAGNOSIS: Alterations in Motor Behavior (22.01)
Restlessness (22.01.12)

SUBJECTIVE DATA	Observe signs and administer anti-convulsant and sedative medication as ordered.	Client will respond to sedation.
(No statement)	Reassure client.	Seizure threshold will be lowered.
OBJECTIVE DATA	Orient client to persons and place in clear, direct language.	Client responds to clear, direct messages.
Client manifests signs of alcoholic hallucinosis, is restless and agitated. Client manifests potential for self-injury.	Assess environment for risks to safety. Modify environment to reduce auditory and visual stimuli.	

NURSING DIAGNOSIS: Alterations in Nutrition/Metabolism (14.)

SUBJECTIVE DATA	Hydrate client: offer fluids frequently. If sedated, initiate I.V. therapy as indicated.	Adequate hydration and urinary output will be established.
(No statement)	Monitor client's electrolyte and fluid balance.	
OBJECTIVE DATA		
Temperature elevation—101°		

(Continued)

NURSING CARE PLAN: AMY (CONTINUED)

Acute Withdrawal From Alcohol and Minor Tranquilizers (Diazepam)
DSM-III-R Diagnostic Category: Alcohol Withdrawal Delirium
　　　　　　　　　　　　Anxiolytic Withdrawal Delirium

ASSESSMENT	NURSING INTERVENTIONS	EVALUATION CRITERIA
NURSING DIAGNOSIS: Alterations in Perception/Cognition (50.) Alterations in Perception (50.06) Hallucinations (50.06.02)		
SUBJECTIVE DATA Client states, "There are cats climbing in the window." OBJECTIVE DATA Client is agitated, distracted.	Reassure client of the unreality of those perceptions, but validate the experience as real for the client.	The client will become less fearful.
NURSING DIAGNOSIS: Excess of or Deficit in Dominant Emotions (30.) Impaired Emotional Experience (30.01) Hopelessness (30.01.10)		
SUBJECTIVE DATA Client states, "I can't manage my life or my illness." OBJECTIVE DATA Client feels dejected.	Assist client to assess self objectively. Encourage verbalization of cognitive problem-solving. Support emotional expression.	Client will demonstrate more active role in recovery. Client will consider future treatment.
NURSING DIAGNOSIS: Alteration in Role Performance (23.) Impaired Work Role (23.03) Lack of Direction (23.03.02)		
SUBJECTIVE DATA Client states, "I'll never be a nurse. I'll never be anything." OBJECTIVE DATA Inadequate problem-solving related to career.	Reassure client that drug dependence is a treatable disease and that sources of help are available. Refer client to recovering nurses' support group.	Client will joint a weekly support group.
NURSING DIAGNOSIS related to Amy's husband: Alteration in Role Performance (23.) Impaired Family Role (23.01) Dependence Excess (23.01.02)		
SUBJECTIVE DATA (No statement) OBJECTIVE DATA Husband reports distress over wife's illness and sick role behavior.	Teach husband about alcohol and prescription drug dependence. Refer husband to Al-Anon.	Husband will seek further counseling.

NURSING CARE PLAN: TONY

Intoxication Secondary to Inhalation of Phencyclidine (PCP)
DSM-III-R Diagnostic Category: Phencyclidine Intoxication (305.90)
On admission:

ASSESSMENT	NURSING INTERVENTIONS	EVALUATION CRITERIA

NURSING DIAGNOSIS: Alteration in Biological Human Response Pattern

SUBJECTIVE DATA (No statement)	Perform gastric lavage. Monitor input and output.	Client will attain normal biological response pattern.
OBJECTIVE DATA Inhalation of PCP	Give charcoal, Vitamin C, or cranberry juice to facilitate drug elimination. Obtain blood and urine samples. Monitor blood pH, gases/electrolytes.	

Four days later, Tony was still in the restraint room, but was becoming less agitated and more compliant with staff requests. His violent outbursts were inconsistent and often confusing and nonsensical. He would thrash around and struggle to break through the leather restraints. Staff maintained a strict one-to-one relationship with him 24 hours a day.

NURSING DIAGNOSIS: Alteration in Neurological/Sensory Functioning (15.)
Impaired Level of Consciousness (15.01)
Drug-Related Impairment (15.01.03)

SUBJECTIVE DATA Client states, "I can fly. My legs are flying."	Orient client to time, place, and person. Explain the need for the restraints. Reassure client about body integrity.	Client will remain safe while experiencing hazardous drug effects.
OBJECTIVE DATA Distorted perceptions of body due to drug use.		

NURSING DIAGNOSIS: Alteration in Circulation (10.)
Hypertensive (10.01.04)

SUBJECTIVE DATA (No statement)	Monitor vital signs. Administer antihypertensive medication as ordered.	Blood pressure and pulse rate will decrease.
OBJECTIVE DATA Blood pressure 170/100 Pulse = 110 Diaphoresis		

(Continued)

the external world; the use of a substance becomes a solution to a variety of dissatisfactions and disappointments. Often, the individual has been *unable to trust* or depend on others for basic emotional, social, or economic needs. Self-esteem is low for many reasons, including the absence of positive regard from parents and others during developmental years. A drug-using life-style and its associated withdrawal from relationships, self-care, and responsibilities, have consequences that result in feelings of guilt, low self-worth, and depression. Nurses must be aware of clients' attitudes and beliefs about themselves, and the fact that these will be expressed in relation to the care-giver. Some examples include a skepticism about the nurse's motives, self-deprecatory remarks, and the assumption of guilt for happenings and events over which the individual has no control.

Successful helping relationships with the substance-abusing individual require that the nurse understand the nature of addictions and the patterns that emerge in their development. Facilitating change in those patterns

NURSING CARE PLAN: TONY (CONTINUED)

Intoxication Secondary to Inhalation of Phencyclidine (PCP)
DSM-III-R Diagnostic Category: Phencyclidine Intoxication (305.90)
On admission

ASSESSMENT	NURSING INTERVENTIONS	EVALUATION CRITERIA
NURSING DIAGNOSIS: Excess of Dominant Emotion (30.) Impaired Emotional Experience (30.01) Anxiety (30.01.02)		
SUBJECTIVE DATA Client states, "I'm going crazy."	Place client in a non-stimulating environment.	Client will not repeat feelings of "going crazy."
OBJECTIVE DATA Client is restless, has dysarthria (poorly articulated speech).	Do not attempt to "talk the client down;" such an intervention may increase PCP agitation.	Client will be more coherent.

FOLLOW-UP

Institute comprehensive drug assessment as soon as crisis has passed. Client and/or family will participate in interview and provide history.

1. Obtain a comprehensive drug history, including:
   a. Type of drug used
   b. Route of administration
   c. Length of time using the drug
   d. Alcohol use
   e. Circumstances leading to the crisis
2. Obtain a psychosocial history, including:
   a. Previous treatment
   b. Attitudes and life-style related to drug use
   c. Willingness to change abusing habits
   d. Family or friends to assist client with treatment follow-up
   e. Community agencies or resources that can provide follow-up support, treatment

Refer client to a community agency substance-abuse treatment program, mental health clinic follow-up
Evaluation Criteria: Client will pursue further treatment.

means tolerating and working with old modes of expression and helping to resolve old feelings before a new sense of the individual's self is manifested.

The Family and Substance Abuse

In U.S. society, the family is the smallest and most influential unit of socialization. It is responsible for the development of basic attitudes, values, and beliefs for the individual, and the preparation and support of its members in the implementation of their social roles. In the Bowen theoretical framework, two forces within the family predict how members will function: the level of differentia-

tion of self achieved by its members, and the level of anxiety achieved.[10] These forces are interactional inasmuch as greater levels of anxiety limit the capacity of family members to differentiate separate selves. Because the family is a system, change in the functioning of one member is followed by change in other family members. Imbalance of forces within the system results in a dysfunctional family with characteristic dysfunctional patterns of behavior by all members.

Consequently, substance-abuse illness within the family system results in dysfunctional behavior patterns of all members, not only the alcoholic or drug addict. Bowen links the development of substance-abusing patterns, in particular excessive drinking, to high family anxiety, which then increases as a result of drinking. These illnesses limit the capacity of the family system to facilitate physical, intellectual, emotional, spiritual, and social growth in its members.

Theoretical observations about families have particular meaning for the development and continuation of substance-abuse illness in the family. These include the existence of generational patterns of interaction, and the tendency in families to replicate patterns over time. Family dynamics that maintain homeostasis even in the presence of dysfunction must be identified in order to delineate and interrupt such patterns. Common modes of dealing with conflict within the family, such as *emotional distancing* and triangulation, are basic to an understanding of the process within the substance-abusing family. *Triangulation* is the process by which emotional energies are directed away from the marital dyad and new bonds are formed with a person, substance, or behavior. While only one member may be alcoholic, the problem affects the entire system and modifies the extent to which the family can successfully fulfill its social tasks.

The study of processes within substance-abusing families has focused almost totally on the alcoholic family. Similarities in the process through which addiction develops, and the course of the illness, suggest, however, that the dysfunctions that affect family process probably occur when a parent is addicted to drugs other than alcohol. Factors that determine changes and predict certain patterns include characteristics of families in general, such as ethnicity, religious values, social class, sex roles, cross-cultural variation, and the family structure, *e.g.,* nuclear or extended, single-parent, and the like. Determinants that have added importance in families in which a parent is addicted included additional factors such as the sex and age of the children at the onset of parental addiction, the temperament of the children, the behaviors of the addicted parent and spouse, and patterns of parental drug use. Observation indicates that many varieties of relationships develop in families with an addicted parent, and that alcoholism *per se* is probably not a very good predictor of the quality of parent–child relationships. How the parent's illness influences the family depends on many factors that increase or counteract the negative effects. Similarly, children in the family develop attitudes that range from ambivalence to consistent distancing and rejection of the ill parent.

Normal family processes are changed by the presence and functions of the drug to which a parent is addicted. Basic issues must be addressed in all families, and remain consistent. The response to conflict by members is central to family dynamics. Conflict is an inevitable occurrence in a family, and its management and resolution are important parental activities and learning experiences for children. When conflict occurs in the marriage, for example, and one spouse or the other has difficulty in dealing with it, the response is often to move away emotionally from the other spouse or family members, using distance as a way of dealing with emotional and psychic strain. Within the Bowen framework, this distancing maneuver may result in the development of a triangle, that is, a relationship with work, a person, or a group that is external to the marital relationship and involves the formation of new emotional bonds. The alcoholic spouse who distances has, in fact, triangulated to a substance. His or her relationship to that substance serves the purpose of relieving stress and anxiety, but moves the individual out of the marital dyad. The distance that develops between the substance-addicted spouse and the nonaddicted spouse and family members may become a chronic characteristic of relationships, leading to the estrangement, anger and hostility, and lack of involvement described by members of alcoholic and other drug-abusing families.

Problems with role are commonly observed in substance-abusing families. The alcoholic parent cannot function as a healthy role model; consequently, role reversal and role confusion result. One or more children may be called on to perform parental duties such as household tasks or childcare. While the child accepts these responsibilities and often performs admirably as the little adult, the process by which the child assumes a parental role interferes with the successful completion of the developmental tasks of childhood. When children assume a role that takes precedence over normal growth and development, it is hard for them to develop a separate sense of self. Often, the disorganization and incapacity of an addicted parent force children to assume roles limiting their growth.

Work with children of alcoholic parents has delineated *role patterns* observed in addicted families. Black notes that the child may adopt one role or a combination of roles identified as the responsible one, the adjuster, or the placater.[7]

It is often the oldest or only child who becomes *the responsible one,* working to provide the structure and stability that are lacking in the home because of a parent's addiction. Bowen uses the term *parentification* when this phenomenon is observed in family process.[10] The *responsible* one often develops an organized style of work and study and is very goal-oriented. Self-worth may be enhanced as a function of this role. While positive aspects of this role are clear, problematic aspects include the development of rigid behavior and the failure to experience feelings and events appropriate to the child's age and developmental level.

Another child may develop a role as an *adjuster,* or simply adopt some of its characteristics. The adjuster easily follows directions and is flexible in ability to respond to changing demands and expectations of a situation. Because the behavior of the addicted parent and the spouse's response are often unpredictable and changing, the child learns to adjust in order to survive emotionally. This "reactive" style may include physical and emotional fluctuations, however, that are potentially problematic.

The child who becomes a *placater* deals with the dysfunctional family process by helping others to adjust and feel comfortable. By listening and being sensitive to others, this child develops certain social skills that facilitate relationships.

The adoption of roles within the substance-dependent family promotes emotional survival for children in situations in which emotional neglect is a frequent problem. While enacting these roles achieves for the child some level of adjustment, unconscious patterns of thinking and attitudes develop as part of the process. These patterns, as well as the roles that are enacted, are more rigid and reactive in nature than roles developed in normal families. The defenses that constitute the roles are never more than partially successful, and children often have difficulty developing a sense of self separate from the role that they play. It may also be difficult to initiate behaviors that reflect desires, and physical and psychological changes that derive from individual vs. role-related needs.

The mechanism of *denial,* central to the development and continuation of drug dependence, characterizes the family system as well as the thinking of the alcoholic or drug addict. Denial is evidenced in family patterns that range from avoidance of the issue and attempts to ignore the problem to efforts to limit the ill adult's access to drugs or alcohol by restricting finances, hiding the car keys, or disposing of all available alcohol. In both instances, denial functions at conscious or unconscious levels. The illusion that family members can control the adolescent, parent, or spouse's behavior is based on a failure to recognize that individuals must be responsible for accepting and treating their own disease. Denial results in a progression of the individual's disease and delays the seeking of assistance, because the family avoids admitting that the individual's condition is worsening.

Behaviors that frequently accompany denial are called *enabling* behaviors. These are activities that spouses and children may unwittingly engage in through attempts to change or protect the addicted individual. They may include reporting absences to employers, loaning money, and angrily attacking the drug-using individual. Angry criticism and rejection become the abuser's excuse to continue using alcohol or drugs to squelch the psychological pain induced by others' disdain. The enabling overfunctioning of the nonaddicted spouse often permits the addicted individual to pursue drug use, because the spouse compensates for the addicted person's failure to meet role-related responsibilities. While painful for all involved, family confrontation of the need to face the consequences of the individual's loss of competence is a necessary step to move the family member toward treatment.

Emotional patterns within the family system demonstrate the family's attempts to handle emotional needs of the system and its members. Sibling relationships take on added importance when both parents are preoccupied with an addiction or with attempts to counteract its effects. Brothers and sisters may become overly attached to one another or intensely competitive for limited emotional resources. Spouses become emotionally estranged and may become overly reliant on children to meet emotional needs and support feelings of self-worth. Bonds within the marital dyad are weakened by sexual dysfunction and the emotions generated by the spouse's withdrawal into a relationship with a drug and away from marital interaction. Alliances form between children and the

nonalcoholic spouse or between children who feel they must maintain the family alone because both parents are unavailable. The nonalcoholic spouse assumes the majority of the responsibility for generating income, solving problems, and meeting emotional needs. Patterns of behavior develop as a function of the family members' responses to the addicted individual. Known as *co-behaviors* or *co-dependency* behaviors, they may become fixed over time and decrease the individual's flexibility to form new ways of relating within and outside of the family.

Social isolation develops as a result of attempts to deal with changes in family life caused by the addiction of its member. Because it is often unpredictable when a parent may become high on drugs or intoxicated, children stop bringing friends home, couples do not entertain in the home, and the addicted individual withdraws from community activities. A parent's illness is perceived as a source of shame that increases when legal problems such as drug trafficking, driving while intoxicated, or assaults on others occur.

Communication patterns in these families are dysfunctional and shaped by the emotional climate. Often, problems are not discussed and a conspiracy of silence functions to forestall action and limit the freedom of the family to reach out to friends or relatives. The conspiracy of silence is reinforced by fears that talking about the problem or seeking help will be viewed as betrayal or disloyalty and will result in the loss of the family. The "family secret" of a child or parent's illness becomes a burden and distorts or inhibits communication patterns. Communication with the addicted individual may consist mainly of attempts to bring about change by inducing guilt, blaming, downgrading, or otherwise pleading for improvement. Drunkenness further complicates communication, leading to exasperation and angry withdrawal by other family members. Verbal communication is often fraught with tension that characterizes the emotional atmosphere. There is an anticipation that behavior could change at any moment, from a restless but steady state to chaos induced by a parent's loss of control. The potential for the expression of destructive impulses against a spouse, children, or property is an ever-present reality and often adds to underlying tensions.

Effects of Parental Substance Abuse on Children

Dysfunctional patterns are documented by observation of alcoholic families. There is little evidence to suggest, however, that these families suffer any more deeply than families with members who are chronically mentally ill or afflicted with a progressive disease that is both psychological and physical in nature.[8] Additionally, it is difficult to identify or predict the probability with which children from alcoholic families will develop particular kinds of problems. Research studies conducted on these populations are limited in their applicability because of problems with research methodology. Offspring of alcoholic parents do, however, appear to be at increased risk for the development of psychosocial problems, psychiatric illness, and alcoholism. Behavioral changes vary according to the forces within the family that offset the problems associated with substance abuse, the severity of the illness, and the ages of the children during periods of parental disturbance. Constitutional factors, such as heredity and the biological predisposition to drug dependence thought to be associated with alcoholism contribute to the effects, and interact with environmental factors frequently observed in these families. These include sensory deprivation in childhood, parental separation, rejection, and more subtle disturbances in parent–child interaction.

Specific symptoms observed in children of alcoholics include excessive fearfulness, temper tantrums, stuttering or stammering, and bed wetting. Other researchers have identified problems related to school performance such as problems with concentration and limited attention span. Aggressive behaviors may include fighting with peers, problems in the neighborhood or school, and antisocial behavior that comes to the attention of the law. Adolescent children of alcoholics, when compared with other adolescents, evidenced greater degrees of psychiatric disturbance of a more severe nature.

In summary, the family system in which one parent (or both) is emotionally disengaged because of addiction is a closed system, with many conflicts. Inconsistent role expectations and role performance characterize behaviors; communication patterns are disturbed; and members are generally inhibited in their progress through the usual developmental stages. Fears of family dissolution and a sense of vulnerable and fragile emotional networks tend to reinforce a conspiracy of silence and the denial of family illness. Treatment of the family is directed toward modifying family relationships within the system to decrease dysfunctional behavior in all members.

Primary Prevention

The nurse prepared at the generalist level implements a variety of roles that include interventions to prevent mental and emotional illness and to promote health in the client and family. Of particular importance for the generalist nurse in substance-abuse illness are the roles of health educator and counselor.

Education about the effects of drugs on the body and the consequences of both habitual use of alcohol and experimentation with and continued use of other drugs should begin at school age. Continued, age-appropriate educational efforts are essential in health education for the adolescent and young adult, because the development of drinking patterns and the initiation of drug use commonly occur during these periods. The nurse who conducts health screenings and counsels children and adolescents in school settings, prenatal clinics, psychiatric facilities, and collegiate health services must use interviewing and teaching skills. The manner in which these skills are used is determined by the setting in which

the nurse practices and the health care needs of the population served. Clients in all age groups need information about the physiological effects of alcohol and all drugs, including prescription medications, and need information about drug-related problems sufficient to recognize problems if they develop in themselves or others.

An increasing awareness of the relationship between habits and health has been an important factor in the development of wellness-oriented drug and alcohol education. In the educational setting, high school as well as college, students are organizing workshops, seminars, and campaigns to increase understanding and awareness of the health risks associated with drug use. These activities are appropriate modes of primary prevention for the nursing student, the graduate nurse, and the nurse specialist.

The psychiatric nurse and nurses employed in substance-abuse treatment centers address drug-related problems at both primary and secondary levels of prevention. Primary prevention is accomplished through educating the psychiatric client about drug interactions and potential development of addictions. Drug interaction, particularly the interaction of psychotropic drugs and alcohol, can result in serious cognitive and psychomotor impairment and life-threatening depression of the respiratory system. Minor tranquilizers, in particular the benzodiazepines, become addicting in prolonged use at high dosages.

In addition to broad areas addressed in general drug education, specific phases of the life cycle have associated health care needs related to drug use. One of these is the child-bearing phase. Nurses need to promote optimal wellness in the pregnant adolescent or woman during this period. In counseling the pregnant female, the nurse must understand the risks associated with drug use and its implications for fetal development, the neonate, and the developing child.

Addiction to heroin and the opiate drugs, including synthetic morphine-like medications, may result in addiction of the fetus and the onset of a withdrawal syndrome in the neonate. The same is true for the infant born to the alcoholically-intoxicated mother. Because the placenta functions as a direct conduit, blood alcohol and drug levels in the newborn reflect those of the mother. The newborn will manifest signs of irritability of the central nervous system, including restlessness, sleep disturbance, and frequent crying. The infant of the heroin-addicted mother often has a high-pitched cry and cold-like symptoms, including excessive tearing and nasal secretion. Nursing care includes the administration of decreasing doses of barbiturates or major tranquilizers to offset the symptoms of withdrawal.

Fetal Alcohol Syndrome

Primary prevention of withdrawal at birth, and later behavioral and developmental effects, is a key activity for the nurse whose client population includes female adolescents and women who desire pregnancy or are in its early stages. Research initiated in the early 1970s has clearly defined the effects of alcohol on infants and children.[2,22,45,46] While medical and literary sources have alluded to generalized effects for many years, it is only recently that systematic studies of children of heavily-drinking and alcoholic mothers have been undertaken. In addition, extensive animal studies have shown a clear relationship between alcohol ingestion and structural changes in the developing fetus. The effects of alcohol on the developing fetus vary along a continuum of severity ranging from mild or minimal fetal alcohol effects (FAE) to a more complete collection of clinical signs known as *fetal alcohol syndrome (FAS)*. In the infant, FAE may be manifested in a weak sucking reflex, a slow habitual response to stimuli, sleep disorders, and decreased alertness. The relationship between patterns and the amount of alcohol ingested is not clear, but alcohol is clearly a teratogen at certain phases of fetal development. For a diagnosis of FAS, the child must exhibit three main characteristics. These characteristics are listed in Table 20-8.

Dysfunctions that result from subtle neuroanatomical or neurochemical changes in the brain are less detectable than the characteristics listed above. They are inferred to be related to alcohol ingestion on the basis of a drinking history in conjunction with behavioral distur-

bance, primarily in learning/memory performance. Signs of such disturbance include attention deficit, distractibility, impulsiveness, disciplinary problems, and hyperactivity in children of normal intelligence. Fetal alcohol syndrome is believed to afflict children born in the U.S. at a rate ranging from 0.4/1,000 births to as high as 3/1,000, depending on the population groups studied and the criteria used to diagnose FAS and FAE.

Behavioral changes exhibited in FAS may also occur as results of other constitutional and behavioral characteristics of both parents. Therefore, careful assessment of parental histories is necessary to ascertain the existence of alcohol-related effects. In addition, a number of other factors affect the degree of severity of signs, as well as whether or not the signs occur. These factors include:

1. Differences in *in utero* blood alcohol exposure. Greater consumption of alcohol appears to decrease birth weight.
2. Exposure to alcohol. Daily exposure and "binge" drinking may have different effects.
3. Genetic sensitivity. Genetic factors influence the metabolism of alcohol and its concentration in the blood.
4. Developmental phase of gestation at the time of exposure.
5. The use of other drugs, and alcohol's interaction with them.
6. Nutritional status of the mother. Undernutrition and deficits in thiamine and folic acid may increase the effects of alcohol.

Counseling the Pregnant Client

Preventing fetal alcohol syndrome requires that the nurse recognize the implications of alcohol consumption for fetal development and use strategies for the identification of, and intervention with, pregnant women who drink heavily. The following areas of information have been identified as essential for the implementation of this role by the health care provider:

1. Self-assessment of attitudes on child-bearing and drug/alcohol use
2. Information about the effects of alcohol during pregnancy
3. Interviewing techniques for obtaining a comprehensive drinking history
4. Strategies in supportive counseling[49]

Health care providers, like the general population, have strong feelings about alcohol use and its social and economic consequences. Similarly, health care providers view child-bearing from a variety of perspectives that are greatly influenced by their views on sexuality and child-bearing and by personal family experiences. As the health care provider learns about fetal alcohol effects, strong attitudes may develop that influence counseling and health education of the pregnant woman and adolescent. Awareness of one's own attitudes helps the health care provider recognize the importance of an unemo-

TABLE 20-8.
DIAGNOSTIC CHARACTERISTICS OF FETAL ALCOHOL SYNDROME

I. Growth deficiencies (greater than two standard deviations for length and weight)
   A. Intrauterine growth retardation
   B. Postnatal growth retardation
II. Facial anomalies/characteristics
   A. Short palpebral fissures
   B. Indistinct philtrum (groove below the septum of the nose)
   C. Epicanthic folds (exaggerated skin folds extending from the eyelid to the inner canthus)
   D. Ptosis (drooping) of the eyelids
   E. Shortened nasal bridge/upturned nose
   F. Underdeveloped jaw
   G. High arched palate
   H. Cleft palate/lip
III. Evidence of central nervous system dysfunction
   A. Mental retardation
   B. Hyperactivity
   C. Fine motor dysfunctions
IV. Other characteristics of Fetal Alcohol Syndrome
   A. Microencephaly
   B. Limb and joint anomalies
      1. Abnormal palmar creases
      2. Abnormal finger structure
      3. Immature or underdeveloped nails
      4. Hip dislocation
   C. Cardiovascular defects
   D. Urogenital defects

(Adapted from Weiner L, Rosett H, Mason E: Training professionals to identify and treat pregnant women who drink heavily. Alc H Res World 48:32, 1985.)

tional, nonjudgmental, and supportive interviewing style. Building a relationship characterized by trust rather than critical appraisal facilitates communication and the maintenance of a health-oriented alliance between client and nurse.

A brief, screening drinking history should be included in the initial evaluation. When this is not possible, it should be done on first contact with the pregnant client. A ten-question drinking history should include the following questions about the frequency, quantity, and variability in pattern of beer, wine, and liquor consumption:

Beer: How many *times* per week do you drink beer?
         How *many cans* do you drink each time?
         Do you ever *drink more*?
Wine: How many *times* per week do you drink wine?
         How *many glasses* do you drink each time?
         Do you ever *drink more*?
Liquor: How many *times* per week do you drink liquor?
         How *many shots* (or drinks) do you have each time?
         Do you ever *drink more*?
Has your drinking pattern changed during the past year?

Problem drinking describes a pattern defined by frequency and amount of consumption, as well as by the function of alcohol in the individual's life. The woman who is a problem drinker places the developing infant at risk primarily because of the amount and frequency of her drinking. Modifying drinking patterns, however, requires that the nurse acknowledge certain psychological needs that drinking meets, and base counseling on those needs. If the drinker is not psychologically dependent on alcohol, abstinence or modification of alcohol intake can be initiated more readily.

Motivating the pregnant woman who drinks heavily is best accomplished in the framework of overall prenatal counseling. Efforts to engage the mother-to-be in health-related behaviors for the good of her child should result in modified behavioral change that may not be accomplished if she is referred to an alcoholism specialist early in the relationship. Such a referral may provoke defensive behaviors that interrupt a beginning relationship with the nurse, and result in a resistance to further counseling. While it is important to share information about the effects of alcohol on pregnancy, excessive information or elaboration on the possibilities of fetal damage may overwhelm the client with guilt or create a climate of self-criticism that provokes further drinking. An attitude of optimism and its communication to the client promotes self-esteem and the opportunity for the woman to act in ways to offset negative outcomes, thereby promoting some control over her own, and her infant's, health.

Secondary Prevention

Nurses who are knowledgeable about substance-abuse illness perform important nursing interventions in institutions and in the community. Early detection of illness, that is, case-finding and treatment of drug dependencies

and alcoholism, occurs in a variety of settings. Of all acute states treated in emergency rooms, the greatest number are drug overdoses or responses to combinations of drugs and alcohol.[38] It is generally known that more alcoholics go untreated than the number who receive appropriate care. At any given time, it is estimated that 20% to 30% of adults hospitalized in medical-surgical units have problems that range from heavy drinking to frank alcoholism.[39]

The nurse who encounters an individual in an acute state of illness, whether substance abuse is the primary or the secondary diagnosis, must be prepared to implement or participate in a comprehensive assessment that includes:

1. A complete physical examination
2. A brief form of the mental status examination
3. A drinking history
4. A recreational and prescription drug-use history
5. Assessment of social support systems, life-style factors, and occupation-related factors

The history and physical examination may reveal some of the signs and symptoms described in Table 20-9. Central components of the mental status exam, including observation and assessments of cognitive processes, affect, and alterations in consciousness, will indicate the presence of intoxication or sedation. Because denial is a key symptom of alcoholism and other drug dependencies, the client's self-report provided in a drinking history may not be valid for the amount consumed (which is generally minimized), but still provides

TABLE 20-9.
EFFECTS ON THE BODY OF DRUGS OTHER THAN ALCOHOL

GENERAL	MANIFESTATIONS
NEGLECT OF HEALTH CARE	
	Undernutrition or malnourishment
	Dental caries
	Poor muscle tone
	Digestive problems
	Trench mouth
SPECIFIC ROUTE OF ADMINISTRATION	
Inhalation	Destruction of internal nasal structure
	Irritation of nasal mucosa
	Depression of respiration
	Seizure activity
Intravenous	Contact dermatitis
	Scarring of veins
	Skin infections
	Abscesses, ulcerations
	Sepsis
	Hepatitis, jaundice
	Organ damage
	Autoimmune Deficiency Syndrome (AIDS)
	Aids-Related Complex (ARC)
	Thrombophlebitis
	Endocarditis

CLINICAL EXAMPLE: ELIZABETH

The nursing care plan for Elizabeth that follows details nursing interventions to address a longstanding problem wherein the client has sustained significant systems damage. A comprehensive approach to this client requires that the nurse view the client in the context of systems interaction, so that nursing interventions reflect the totality of Elizabeth's health.

Elizabeth is a 76-year-old native of Jamaica, in the West Indies. She emigrated to this country 20 years ago with her husband, Alvin, who was employed as a carpenter. When her husband, who was a heavy drinker, died last year, Elizabeth moved in with her sister, Grace. Her sister brought her to the mental health clinic because of behavioral changes, including the consumption of at least one pint of distilled spirits weekly. Grace expressed concern because her sister has withdrawn from her children and their families, and shows marked changes in mood after drinking. She has caused some disturbances in their apartment building because she has been loud, argumentative, and belligerent with the neighbors. Elizabeth and her sister are interviewed by a clinical nurse specialist.

an estimate of frequency and types of beverages consumed.

The role that alcohol and other drugs play in the life of the individual can be assessed by obtaining a description of family and social patterns: Does the client drink when alone? Has obtaining the drug or abuse of alcohol interfered with attendance at work? How many episodes of medical illness has the individual experienced in the last year? What psychological functions does drug use serve . . . to increase relaxation? . . . kill painful feelings?

Interview components, as part of the nursing assessment in the acute setting, are directed toward identifying the drugs ingested with the goal of decreasing the noxious effects of the drug itself or the uncomfortable symptoms of withdrawal from it. The two case examples presented earlier, of Amy and Tony, demonstrate assessment and intervention in secondary prevention.

Tertiary Prevention

Alcoholism and drug dependencies are diseases characterized by phases and observable progression in severity until the disease process is arrested.[33] They differ from periodic episodes of excessive or recreational use in that the body has developed a physiological tolerance and/or dependence. The user feels compelled to take the drug frequently, and in a pattern that is socially and/or physically damaging. Throughout the period of time the individual is actively using a drug, episodes of acute illness occur within a pattern of chronic use. Once the crisis period in acute episodes has passed (such as intentional or accidental overdose, endocarditis, or hemorrhage), there are opportunities to initiate tertiary intervention directed toward rehabilitation and restoration of health. In diseases of substance dependence, relapse can be a common occurrence but does not necessarily persist for indefinite periods. By recognizing this, the nurse can work with the client toward maximizing the health benefits of healthy and sober periods, rather than viewing the inability of the client to abstain as failure.[12]

The central components of rehabilitation and restoration of levels of wellness for the substance-dependent client include:

1. A comprehensive medical history and physical
2. Assessment and history of substance abuse
   A. Length of time used
   B. Associated social, legal, psychiatric, and physical problems
   C. Patterns and circumstances of use
      (1) Substances used
      (2) Social patterns associated with use
   D. Previous history of substance use and treatment
   E. Assessment of social support systems from which the client can obtain assistance, including family, friends, and social service agencies
3. Evaluation of the client's need for detoxification from the substance
   A. Assessment of the need for inpatient or ambulatory treatment
4. Initiation of long-term treatment
   A. Referral to a long-term therapeutic community or halfway house
   B. Referral to self-help groups such as Alcoholics Anonymous or Narcotics Anonymous
   C. Provision of or referral for:
      (1) Substance-abuse counseling
      (2) Psychotherapy
      (3) Education on health problems associated with substance abuse
      (4) Education on diseases resulting from substance abuse
5. Assessment of the need for vocational counseling or occupational assistance
6. Assessment of the need for referral to financial or social assistance agencies

Therapies

The acute and rehabilitative aspects of substance-abuse treatment require that the client have access to a variety of public and private care facilities. During the acute episodes, the resources of the general hospital, psychiatric

NURSING CARE PLAN: ELIZABETH

ASSESSMENT	NURSING INTERVENTIONS	EVALUATION CRITERIA
NURSING DIAGNOSIS: Alterations in Circulation (10.) Hypertension (10.01.04)		
SUBJECTIVE DATA Client states, "I have trouble with my pressure." OBJECTIVE DATA BP = 180/90 P = 82	Refer to general medical clinic or private practitioner for comprehensive evaluation.	Client will be assessed for medical problems.
NURSING DIAGNOSIS: Alterations in Nutrition/Metabolism (14.) Less than Body Requires (14.01)		
SUBJECTIVE DATA Client states, "I have no appetite." OBJECTIVE DATA Ht: 5 ft. 6 in. Wt: 103 lb.	Refer for nutritional evaluation.	Client's nutritional status and needs will be established.
NURSING DIAGNOSIS: Alterations in Sleep/Arousal (25.) Early Morning Awakening (25.01.02)		
SUBJECTIVE DATA Client states, "I'm not sleeping so good." OBJECTIVE DATA Sister reports sporadic sleeping patterns, early morning awakening.	Obtain drinking history. Evaluate for depressive symptoms.	Client will resume REM sleep.
NURSING DIAGNOSIS: Alterations in Conduct/Impulse Control (21.) Aggression/Violence Toward Self (21.03) Substance Abuse (21.03.03)		

(Continued)

unit, or substance-abuse treatment center are essential to treat the toxic effects of substances or drug withdrawal, which can be life-threatening. The components of successful rehabilitation derive from client characteristics, severity of illness, and availability of support systems.

Detoxification

Some facilities, public or private, specialize in medical support and nursing care for detoxification, or withdrawal from the drug. Nonmedical detoxification centers also exist in a number of large cities. These facilities are lim-ited in their capacity to treat acute and potentially dangerous syndromes associated with delirium tremens and withdrawal from benzodiazepines, but can act as entry points into more comprehensive treatment programs. Voluntary admission to detoxification programs is not necessarily the first step in recovery. These facilities are also used when individuals feel the need to stop drinking for a limited period, but do not plan to discontinue drug use. Emergency support that includes a safe environment, shelter, and nutrition may be the primary concern. The time required for the elimination of drug metabolites from the body differs, depending on the drug upon which individuals are dependent, their physiology, and

NURSING CARE PLAN: ELIZABETH (CONTINUED)

ASSESSMENT	NURSING INTERVENTIONS	EVALUATION CRITERIA
NURSING DIAGNOSIS: Alterations in Conduct/Impulse Control (21.) Aggression/Violence Toward Self (21.03) Substance Abuse (21.03.03)		
SUBJECTIVE DATA Client states, "I used to drink sometimes." OBJECTIVE DATA Sister reports sporadic drinking bouts.	Obtain drinking history. Identify alcohol-related problems. Do mental status exam and evaluation. Potential psychiatric referral, evaluation for medication.	Client will report drinking patterns. Client will acknowledge effects of alcohol consumption.
NURSING DIAGNOSIS: Alterations in Role Performance (23.) Impaired Social/Leisure Role (23.02) Withdrawal/Social Isolation (23.02.01)		
SUBJECTIVE DATA Client states she does not want to go out— even to church. OBJECTIVE DATA Client is not engaging interpersonally.	Counsel client on reasons for withdrawal, relationship of isolation to mood. Identify local Alcoholics Anonymous groups with elderly members.	Client will spend less time alone, more time in the community.
NURSING DIAGNOSIS: Excess of or Deficit in Dominant Emotions (30.) Impaired Emotional Experience (30.01) Grief (30.01.07)		
SUBJECTIVE DATA Client states, "It's just not the same since Al died." OBJECTIVE DATA Client is depressed when talking about Al.	Engage client in counseling/psychotherapy to explore feelings about spouse's death.	Client will engage in grieving process.
NURSING DIAGNOSIS related to Grace (sister): Alterations in Role Performance (23.) Impaired Family Role (23.01) Disengagement (23.01.04)		
SUBJECTIVE DATA Sister states, "I can't tell when she is in trouble."	Educate client and family about manifested physical and behavioral symptoms of alcohol ingestion. Refer sister to Al-Anon.	Family will articulate increased understanding of client's problem.

their pattern of drug use. The effects of some drugs on the central nervous system may persist for several weeks.

Residential Treatment

When addiction is of long duration, or is interrelated with other psychiatric diagnoses, hospitalization for periods of four months or more may be the treatment of choice.

Long-term treatment goals may be accomplished in private or public long-term psychiatric hospitals or in facilities specifically planned around the needs of the substance-abusing client. The components of rehabilitation described above are incorporated into care delivered by a multidisciplinary team. Nurses, social workers, physicians, and recreational and art therapists collaborate in planning care within the therapeutic milieu. Desired treatment outcomes may include direct return to the community or progression to a halfway house or day treatment program.

The Halfway House

Halfway houses, as adjuncts to private and public long-term programs, provide transitional settings that promote the client's growing independence from the structured treatment regimen while continuing involvement with newly-established relationships and therapeutic modalities. The client resides with other adults in a communal living situation and participates in the management of the household. The client eventually works outside the treatment center in the larger community while continuing to attend therapy sessions and group meetings. Gradually increasing the client's involvement with the larger community provides opportunities for the client and care providers to explore the potential conflicts and stresses that will be encountered on returning home.

Therapeutic Communities

Phoenix House and Daytop Village are two examples of residential settings that were founded in the 1960s for the treatment of addiction to drugs other than alcohol. Alcohol is addressed in these programs, however. The major therapeutic tool is the encounter group, designed to promote catharsis and facilitate understanding of self and others. Residents work in a variety of rehabilitative activities directed toward modifying behaviors associated with drug abuse and its negative social consequences. Drug and alcohol education, formal classes, and vocational counseling are also offered. Therapeutic communities are primarily run by former addicts, or "residents." They are supported by an interdisciplinary staff of physicians, nurses, teachers, psychologists, and social workers who provide consultation and resources. The individual who enters the therapeutic community must adopt the goal of a drug-free life and agree to the personal and so-

cial changes that accompany it. A commitment to remain within the community for periods in excess of a year is usually required.

Day and Evening Programs

Treatment programs are now available as alternatives to inpatient hospitalization and the limited support of outpatient therapy. These programs may be a full or part day in length, and include group meetings as well as individual sessions. For the unemployed client or the individual who is not ready to return to work, partial programs facilitate the transition from hospitalization to independent living. When medical and nursing services are available, it is possible to conduct detoxification from certain drugs in these settings. Evening programs meet the needs of recovering people who are able to return to work but who need daily attendance at self-help meetings, therapy sessions, vocational counseling, social services, and socialization. Day and evening programs have been developed in the community mental health centers (Fig. 20-1) and outpatient clinics, and in free-standing services such as employee assistance programs.

Therapeutic Modalities in the Treatment of Substance Abuse

Self-Help Groups

In 1935, two sober alcoholics organized the fellowship of Alcoholics Anonymous (AA). It is structured as a self-supporting, voluntary program, and has provided a model for other self-help groups, particularly those intended to help individuals who are coping with addictions and compulsive behaviors. Its philosophy is based on Twelve

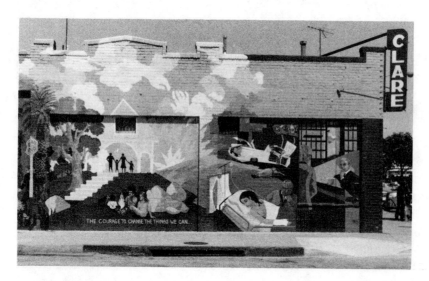

Figure 20-1. An alcoholism treatment center providing drop-in groups, referral information, and family support programs. The mural on the building was painted by clients at the center.

Steps and Twelve Traditions for Recovery, listed in Table 20-10. Important tenets of the program are confidentiality of meeting activities, protection of anonymity, and the 24-hour plan (keeping sober for the current 24 hours). The program is designed to help the individual achieve, to the greatest possible degree, a drug- and alcohol-free life. Through self-assessment, group support, humility, and positive thinking, participants develop perspectives on their disease and make restitution for past social transgressions. In large urban centers, AA meetings are available many hours of every day and are readily accessible. In smaller towns, finding a meeting may present problems for the individual in the shaky, early stages of sobriety. Most regions do have an AA resource, however, and AA has chapters in 110 countries in the world. Groups that have followed the AA model are described below.

Al-Ateen and Al-Anon are groups for family members, friends, and concerned associates of someone with a drinking problem. Through shared experiences, members help each other to cope with the stresses of these relationships and to keep the illness of others in perspective. These programs help teenagers, spouses, and others to detach themselves and to deal with shame, anger, guilt, and other emotions experienced in relation to the substance abuser.

Narcotics Anonymous (NA) is a program adapted from the AA model for narcotics addicts. Twelve Steps and Twelve Traditions provide guidelines for dealing with this addiction. Overeaters Anonymous and Gamblers Anonymous have also developed approaches and tenets of belief about recovery from these disorders.

Adult Children of Alcoholics, which also uses the Twelve Step Program, was developed in recognition that common problems and behaviors occur among children of alcoholic parents. Faced with the withdrawal, emotional neglect, inconsistent parenting, and climate of anxiety that characterize the alcoholic home, children develop ways of responding that are shaped by a parent's illness. Such adaptive behaviors can prove maladaptive

in later relationships. This group supports members in examining these issues and relearning patterns of relating.

Women for Sobriety is a recently organized program that seeks to address the needs of women drinkers for strong female support systems. Based on the belief that the problems women face in recovery are unique to their socialized role, this group has developed literature, guidelines, and group models that are contemporary and affirming of women's identity and emotional needs.

Professional Groups

With the recognition that occupational choice and professional membership bring special considerations to the lives of the active addict or recovering person, a number of groups have formed to provide support to professional colleagues. These include programs for pilots, dentists, women in religious orders, lawyers, physicians, nurses, and others. While a variety of approaches, such as support groups and peer assistance models, are used, their goals are the same—to identify the need for treatment and to support colleagues with a drug or alcohol problem. Information about these groups can be obtained from district branches of professional associations or organizations.

Counseling and Psychotherapy

Therapeutic approaches that use interviewing and verbal communication as predominant modes are also appropriate in the treatment of the substance-abusing individual. Theoretical frameworks that form the bases for these approaches derive from the education and experience of the clinician. Of primary importance to successful psychotherapy with the alcoholic or addict is a comprehensive base of knowledge about the addictions and the pharmacologic, psychodynamic, and social issues central

TABLE 20-10.
THE TWELVE STEPS OF ALCOHOLICS ANONYMOUS

1. We admitted we were powerless over alcohol—that our lives had become unmanageable.
2. We came to believe that a Power greater than ourselves could restore us to sanity.
3. We made a decision to turn our will and our lives over to the care of God as we understood Him.
4. We made a searching and fearless moral inventory of ourselves.
5. We admitted to God, to ourselves, and to another human being the exact nature of our wrongs.
6. We were entirely ready to have God remove all these defects of character.
7. We humbly asked Him to remove our shortcomings.
8. We made a list of all persons we had harmed, and became willing to make amends to them all.
9. We made direct amends to such people wherever possible, except when to do so would injure them or others.
10. We continued to take personal inventory and when we were wrong promptly admitted it.
11. We sought through prayer and meditation to improve our conscious contact with God as we understood Him, praying only for knowledge of His will for us and the power to carry that out.
12. Having had a spiritual awakening as the result of these steps, we tried to carry this message to alcoholics, and to practice these principles in all our affairs.

(Alcoholics Anonymous: The Twelve Steps of Alcoholics Anonymous. New York, Works Publishers, 1939.)

to their treatment. Individual, couples, family, and group psychotherapy techniques can be used successfully to address psychodynamic and interpersonal conflicts experienced by the substance-abusing client. These techniques are methods for learning new coping mechanisms.

Family therapy techniques are highly effective in assessing and intervening in the dysfunctional family system that developed as a result of substance-abuse illness. Because the total family system and patterns for relating are distorted by the drug use of one or more members, change in the behavior of all family members is necessary to address problems successfully. The psychotherapies are greatly enhanced in effectiveness when the client and/or family members are concurrently involved in self-help groups such as NA, AA, or Al-Anon. These are useful adjuncts to behavioral change because they address drug use specifically, and focus on the client's denial. The positive reinforcement provided by the group for the client's "clean" state and sobriety builds self-esteem and increases the client's accessibility and motivation for change.

Psychopharmacologic Approaches

The nurse must be aware of and knowledgeable about the various medications used in the treatment of acute and chronic phases of addiction. Because the addicted individual continues to be at risk for the abuse of drugs and intentional or accidental overdose, the nurse should be familiar with drug interactions and contraindications to use. The primary nursing activities include client teaching, administration, observation, and documentation.

Dolophine (methadone) maintenance is a treatment modality in which methadone hydrochloride, a synthetic and legal narcotic, is given to prevent a craving for heroin or other opioids. The client receives daily doses of the drug that are dispensed in a clinic setting. Methadone produces physical dependence but not sedation or narcosis. Although use is controversial, its greatest advantage has been to attract heroin addicts into treatment and toward the development of a structured life-style that includes work and family support.

Narcotic antagonists are given to prevent or reverse many of the pharmacologic effects of the opioid-like drugs, particularly respiratory depression. These drugs include naloxone, Narcan, and Lorfan. They may be used to inhibit self-administration of narcotics because they produce sudden and uncomfortable withdrawal symptoms in the opioid addict. Their most frequent use is in emergency situations to reverse respiratory depression induced by overdose.

Disulfiram (Antabuse) therapy is used exclusively as an adjunct to the treatment of alcoholism. It produces a severe hypersensitivity to alcohol by inhibiting the action of liver enzymes that usually act on alcohol. The resulting accumulation of acetaldehyde produces flushing, dizziness, dyspnea, anorexia, nausea, and vomiting. It should never be given when an individual is intoxicated, and

should be used with caution with narcotic addicts. The client must be aware of the role and consequences of Antabuse therapy, including the highly unpleasant effects that occur if alcohol is ingested in any form. Clients being treated with Antabuse should carry identification stating that they are in treatment and listing the symptoms of alcohol–disulfiram interaction.

The Nursing Role With the Substance-Abusing Client

Nurses encounter clients with alcohol and drug abuse and dependency problems in the general practice of nursing and in all specialty areas. The education of the nurse, the clinical setting, and the phase of the client's illness are all determinants of the implemented nursing role and the scope of the nurse's practice. Settings include inpatient detoxification units and residential treatment settings, long- and short-term psychiatric facilities, emergency rooms, and health maintenance organizations. In addition, nurses working in schools or community health agencies frequently encounter drug users and abusers with nursing needs. Nurses practicing in such settings use the nursing process in primary, secondary, and tertiary prevention. The key nursing skills used fall into the categories of functions of the nurse generalist and functions of the clinical nurse specialist.

The nurse generalist, educated in a baccalaureate, diploma, or associate degree program, is prepared to implement the nursing process in accord with client, family, and community needs. The broad areas of nursing education that are used most frequently and are required for competent practice with the alcohol- and drug-dependent client are:

1. Interpersonal skills in communication, counseling, and health education
2. A comprehensive base of knowledge about alcohol and other drugs: their use and abuse, and dependence on them

These categories of theoretical knowledge and clinical skill prepare the nurse to meet client needs in the following areas:

1. Prevention of substance-abuse illness through health education and intervention with individuals at risk
2. Identification and assessment of substance-abuse illnesses in early, middle, and late phases
3. Counseling of the client, family, and community about the implications and consequences of substance abuse on the human system, the community, and society
4. Initiation and maintenance of therapeutic relationships with individuals in various phases of substance-abuse illness

5. Referral of clients and families to appropriate treatment resources and personnel.

At the generalist level, the nurse is educated to perform these activities in all settings, and may choose to work exclusively in a setting where these skills are central to job performance—for example, in a rehabilitation unit. In this case, practice in the specialty is determined by clients' nursing needs and the treatment goals of the practice setting.

The clinical nurse specialist working with substance abuse is a nurse with a Master's degree in nursing or another discipline. The clinical nurse specialist in substance-abuse treatment settings usually holds an advanced degree in psychiatric/mental health or substance-abuse nursing, in addition to having completed continuing education. Education at the Master's degree level provides skills that enable the nurse to function as a psychotherapist with individuals, families, and groups; as a consultant and independent practitioner; and as a researcher and peer educator. The advanced level of function provides a new autonomy for the nurse working with substance-abuse clients, and facilitates the development of nursing roles in a variety of settings.

Advanced knowledge of the addictions, as well as the development of therapeutic interpersonal and management skills, expands the practitioner's assumption of responsibility for comprehensive client care. It also makes the nurse a valuable contributor of nursing expertise to the interdisciplinary team.

Like the nurse generalist, the clinical specialist utilizes interpersonal skills in the context of advanced knowledge of addiction. A data base is compiled and nursing diagnoses are formulated. Client education about the potential impact of alcohol and other drugs on body systems and the need for a balanced plan of nutrition and exercise is important. A major focus is the identification, with the client, of the problems consequent to the abuse of substances, and approaches to problem-solving.

The psychotherapeutic skills of the clinical nurse specialist are particularly important for the development of a trusting relationship with addicted individuals, whose denial and involvement with the drug(s) make them less than accessible to a therapeutic relationship. In long- and short-term contacts, the nurse directs the client's attention to the need to achieve sobriety, develop coping skills relating to current life problems, and become actively involved with support systems in treatment settings and in the structure of Twelve-Step programs in the AA model. The clinical nurse specialist who practices independently must recognize that the one-to-one relationship has limited potential for assisting the client to change. Self-help groups are important adjuncts to treatment that provide round-the-clock support in the form of the AA fellowship, structured steps for changing life patterns, and education on the impact of addiction on emotional, spiritual, and social life. Family involvement in treatment, when possible, is key, and the establishment or maintenance of employment provides a person-ally- and economically-rewarding structure. Prognosis is greatly improved when the client is connected in a meaningful therapeutic relationship, has social support from other caring individuals, and is able to utilize vocational and community resources.

Summary

1. Substance abuse is a serious global health problem. Alcoholism alone ranks among the four major health problems in the United States.

2. The idea that there is an "addictive personality type" has been set aside for a more complex model of the development and continuation of substance abuse. Today, psychological, medical (disease), sociopsychological, and interactional models are used to explain the complex phenomena of substance abuse.

3. Precipitating factors leading to substance abuse combine in a systems framework to promote substance abuse. Subsystem factors are environmental factors (such as peer pressure), family history, sex, age, and sociocultural factors (such as the high percentage of substance abuse among certain ethnic groups).

4. *Addiction* refers to the degree to which circumstances associated with procuring and administering a substance control the behavior of the individual. *Withdrawal* refers to a substance-specific set of symptoms following the cessation of, or reduction in, intake of a regularly-used substance.

5. Caffeine, nicotine, and alcohol are the drugs most frequently used in the United States. Other substances that are abused include phencyclidine, marijuana and hashish, stimulants, cocaine, inhalants, depressants, and opioids.

6. Health care providers are also susceptible to drug addiction. Health workers are around addicting substances in their practice, and they are susceptible to feeling society's misconception that health care workers are immune to substance-abuse problems. Today, many programs exist to help the impaired professional to avoid substance abuse.

7. Many clinicians working in the area of substance abuse view the illness as a "family disease." In one way or another, substance abuse in the family becomes a central concern around which family activity revolves. Children and spouses of substance-abusing individuals assume certain roles as a means of dealing with substance abuse in the family.

8. Substance abuse in a pregnant woman increases the likelihood of abnormalities in the child. Nurses can provide much-needed counseling in the care of mothers to prevent birth defects.

9. Nurses can provide valuable assistance in primary, secondary, and tertiary care in dealing with substance abuse. In some instances, nurses must deal with their own negative attitudes about substance abuse in caring for clients.

References

1. Ablon J: Family Behavior and Alcoholism. In Tabakoff B, Sutker P, Randall C (eds): Medical and Social Aspects of Alcohol Abuse. New York, Plenum Press, 1983

2. Alcoh H Res World: Alcohol-related birth defects. 10:4, 1985

3. American Nurses' Association: Taxonomy for the Classification of Human Responses of Concern for Psychiatric/Mental Health Nursing Practice. Kansas City, Missouri, American Nurses' Association, 1986

4. American Nurses' Association: Addictions and Psychological Dysfunctions: The Profession's Response to the Problem. Kansas City, Missouri, American Nurses' Association, 1984

5. American Psychiatric Association: Diagnostic and Statistical Manual of Mental Disorders, 3rd ed, revised (DSM-III-R). Washington, DC, American Psychiatric Association, 1987

6. Bissell L, Haberman P: Alcoholism in the Professions. New York, Oxford University Press, 1984

7. Black C: Children of alcoholics. Alcoh H Res World 4:23, 1979

8. Blane H: Psychotherapeutic Approach. In Kissin B, Begleiter H: Treatment and Rehabilitation of the Chronic Alcoholic. New York, Plenum Press, 1976

9. Bohman M, Sigardsson S, Cloniger C: Maternal inheritance of alcohol abuse. Arch Gen Psychiatry 38:965, 1984

10. Bowen M: Alcoholism as viewed through family systems theory and family psychotherapy. New York Acad Sci 223:115, 1974

11. Brodsley L: Avoiding a crisis: The assessment. Am J Nurs 83:1865, 1983

12. Burkhalter P: Nursing Care of the Alcohol and Drug Abuser. New York, Macmillan, 1975

13. Cahalan D, Cisin I, Crossley H: American Drinking Practices: A National Survey of Behavior and Attitudes. Monograph No 3. Washington, DC, George Washington University, Social Research Group, 1967

14. Clark W, Midanik L: Alcohol Use and Alcohol Problems Among U.S. Adults: Results of a 1979 National Survey. In Department of Health and Human Services: Alcohol Consumption and Related Problems, Pub. No. ADM 82-11990. Washington, DC, Department of Health and Human Services, 1982

15. Cohen S, Gallant D: Diagnosis of Drug and Alcohol Abuse. Monograph Series I (6). Brooklyn, New York, SUNY Downstate Medical Center Career Teacher Program, 1981

16. Cohn L: The hidden diagnosis. Am J Nurs 82:1862, 1982

17. Collins R, Marlatt G: Psychological Correlates and Explanations of Alcohol Use and Abuse. In Tabakoff B, Sutker P, Randall C (eds): Medical and Social Aspects of Alcohol Abuse. New York, Plenum Press, 1983

18. Cotton N: The familial incidences of alcoholism. J Stud Alcohol 40:80, 1979

19. Criteria Committee, National Council on Alcoholism: Criteria for the diagnosis of alcoholism. Am J Psychiatry 129:65, 1972

20. Donovan J: An etiological model of alcoholism. Am J Psychiatry 143:1, 1986

21. Dupont R, Goldstein A, O'Donnell J: Handbook on Drug Abuse. Washington, DC, National Institute on Drug Abuse, 1979

22. El-Guebaly N, Offord D: The offspring of alcoholics: A critical review. Am J Psychiatry 134:357, 1977

23. Estes N, Heinemann E: Alcoholism: Development, Consequences, and Interventions. St Louis, CV Mosby, 1982

24. Ewing J: Recognizing, confronting, and helping the alcoholic. Am Fam Physician 18:107, 1978

25. Goffman I: Stigma: Notes on the Management of a Spoiled Identity. Englewood Cliffs, New Jersey, Prentice-Hall, 1963

26. Gomberg E: Problems With Alcohol and Other Drugs. In Gomberg E, Franks V: Gender and Disordered Behavior: Sex Differences in Psychotherapy. New York, Brunner-Mazel, 1979

27. Goodwin D et al: Alcohol problems in adoptees raised apart from alcoholic biological parents. Arch Gen Psychiatry 31:164, 1973

28. Goodwin D, Schulsinger F, Knop J: Alcoholism and depression in daughters of alcoholics. Arch Gen Psychiatry 34:751, 1977

29. Hagland R, Schuckit M: The Epidemiology of Alcoholism. In Estes N, Heinemann E (eds): Alcoholism: Development, Consequences, and Interventions. St Louis, CV Mosby, 1982

30. Hanna J: Ethnic Groups, Human Variation, and Alcohol Use. In Everett M, Waddell J, Heath D (eds): Cross-Cultural Approaches to the Study of Alcohol. The Hague, Mouton, 1976

31. Jellinek EM: Phases of alcohol addiction. Q J Stud Alcohol 13:673, 1952

32. Johnston L, O'Malley P, Bachman J: Use of Licit and Illicit Drugs by America's High School Students. Pub. No. ADM 85-1394. Washington, DC, Department of Health and Human Services, 1985

33. Lewis D, Senay E: Treatment of Drugs and Alcohol Abuse. SUNY Brooklyn, New York, Downstate Medical Center Career Teacher Program, 1981

34. Macky R: Views of caregivers and mental health groups about alcoholics. Q J Stud Alcohol 30:655, 1969

35. National Commission on Marijuana and Drug Abuse: Problems in Perspective. Washington, DC, U.S. Government Printing Office, 1972

36. Naegle M: Creative management of impaired nursing practice. Nurs Admin Q 9:16, 1985

37. Oakley R: Drugs, Society, and Human Behavior. St Louis, CV Mosby, 1978

38. Pattison M: Selection of Treatment Modalities for the Alcoholic Patient. In Mendlesohn J, Mello N: The Diagnosis and Treatment of Alcoholism. New York, McGraw-Hill, 1979

39. Resnick H, Ruben H: Emergency Psychiatric Care: The Management of Mental Health Crises. Boston, Charles Press, 1975

40. Ryser P: Sex Differences in Substance Abuse. Int J Addict 18:1, 1983

41. Sanders J, David M, Williams R: Do women develop alcoholic liver disease more readily than men? Brit Med J 282:1140, 1981

42. Schuckit M, Pastor P: The elderly as a unique population: alcoholism. Alcohol Clin Exp Res 2:31, 1978

43. Sigell L, Kapp F, Fusaro G et al: Popping and snorting volatile nitrates: A current fad for a high. Am J Psychiatry 135:10, 1978

44. Smith D: Alcohol and Other Drugs of Abuse. In Gold H (ed): Comprehensive Textbook of Psychiatry. Chicago, Aldine, 1988

45. Stone M, Salerno L, Green M et al: Narcotic addiction in pregnancy. Am J Obstet Gynecol 109:716, 1971

46. Streissguth A, LaDue R: Psychological and Behavioral Effects in Children Prenatally Exposed to Alcohol. Alcoh H Res World 10:6, 1985

47. Vaillant G: The Natural History of Alcoholism. Cambridge, Massachusetts, Harvard University Press, 1983

48. Vourakis C, Bennett G: Angel dust: Not heaven-sent. Am J Nurs 79:649, 1979

49. Weiner L, Rosett H, Mason E: Training professionals to identify and treat pregnant women who drink heavily. Alcoh H Res World 10:32, 1985

50. Wilford B: Drug Abuse: A Guide for the Primary Care Physician. Chicago, American Medical Association, 1981

51. Whitfield C: The Patient With Alcoholism and Other Drug Problems. Chicago, Year Book Medical Publishers, 1981

52. Zamora L: Anger. In Haber J et al (eds): Comprehensive Psychiatric Nursing. New York, McGraw-Hill, 1982

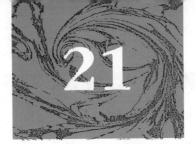

21

LORETTA M. BIRCKHEAD AND WILMA BRADLEY

FAMILY VIOLENCE

Learning Objectives

Upon completion of this chapter the student should be able to do the following:

1. List the factors that promote family violence.
2. Define major types of family violence.
3. Explain the family process whereby family violence becomes repetitive.
4. List frequent psychological problems of victims of family violence.
5. Define the nurse's role in intervening with victims of family violence.
6. Define legal aspects of the nurse's role in family violence.

Introduction

The fact that many homes are the scene of physical and sexual abuse, conflict, and even torture is sad. Home has always been considered the place where one should feel safe, loved, and refreshed. However, for some it is a place where they feel terrorized and are made to feel less than human. The idea of the home as a place where love reigns is being replaced in clinicians' minds by the reality that the home is often a place of suffering.

Barnhill, Squires, and Gidson[3] reported on what has been termed an epidemic of child and spouse abuse in the United States. They reported that 7% of one Detroit family service agency's cases involved violence. The authors also studied the occurrence of violence among clients in a small Midwestern town's community mental health center. The area had a population of 200,000, with a diversity of ages and income levels that ranged from average to poverty. Other differences included life-styles that varied from agrarian to university backgrounds.

CLINICAL EXAMPLES

JOHNNY

A community health nurse visits the home of the Barker family. Mr. and Ms. Barker have four children and two grandparents living in the home. The nurse is working on diabetic counseling with one of the grandparents who was recently released from the hospital.

The nurse notices that four-year-old Johnny has large bruises and burn marks on his hands. He is very anxious and does not speak.

JANE

A psychiatric nurse in a day treatment center is working with Jane, a 19-year-old incest survivor. While talking about the incest expe-

rience, Jane becomes anxious and has difficulty in speaking. When Jane speaks, she hesitates to discuss the incest.

PHYLLIS

A nurse working in a women's center talks with Phyllis, who arrived at the center in a distressed state. She describes a history of

abuse, but cannot decide what she should do about her husband, the perpetrator. She is worried that her husband will beat the children.

The researchers collected data using the Violence Needs Assessment, an instrument used to gather descriptive information about the violence occurring in the respondent's life. Data were collected on all routine and emergency admissions and discharges in a four-county area for a three-month period in the winter of 1978-1979.

Of 837 cases included in the study, 39.5% or 331 individuals reported a general concern about violence. Violence was a "current concern" in 24.5% or 205 cases, and was a past concern for an additional 15.0% or 126 cases. "Since this area of the country is not particularly characterized by a high degree of violence, the fact that a current concern about a problem of violence was expressed in one fourth of the cases appears to be strong evidence that the problem warrants serious concern."[3]

Of 173 cases that reported a current concern about violence and for whom complete ratings of the level of violence were obtained, 49.1% described a concern with a "low" level of violence. These incidents included threats, reported impulses to be violent, rare acts of violence, and verbal abuse. Also, 26.6% of the 173 cases reported violence at the next highest level, including repetitive minor violence (such as hitting), serious threats, or serious attacks on property (such as arson). Extreme violence, including fighting, was reported in 13.3% of the cases. Eleven percent of the cases reported experiences of the highest level of violence, including attempted injury with a weapon, attempted murder, and maiming.

The researchers emphasized that lower levels of violence should not be dismissed, but should be taken seriously. Even an occasional slap is still violence. Individuals may live in homes where more extreme incidents of violence may erupt. It is known that previous violence is the best predictor of "future (at times more extreme) violence."[3]

Four fifths (79.6%) of the assaulters were male. Females were the victim of assault in 67.2% of the cases. Victims' ages ranged from under 1 year to 67 years, and 29.1% of the assaulted individuals were under 18 years of age. Spouse abuse and child abuse were almost equivalent in number of cases, and combined they accounted for two thirds of all violence reported. Because this study did not include incest as a form of family violence, it is probable that violence in the home is occurring even more frequently than the figures above indicate.

Erlanger[13] also reported on current rates of violence, drawn from a study in New York City. The author noted that:

1. The typical chain of violence is no longer simply: "Husband beats wife, wife beats kids, kids beat dog." More often, one abuser abuses others in the family.
2. Between 20% and 40% of the homeless people in New York City are battered women (women who have been beaten by their spouse or a significant other).
3. Twenty percent of the women who enter hospital emergency rooms for injuries have been battered.
4. Forty-five percent of the mothers of abused or neglected children have been battered.
5. Twenty-five percent of all women who commit suicide have been battered.
6. Fifteen percent of all households in one Bronx precinct called the police for help with domestic disputes over the period of a year.

The Relevant Research box on page 467 demonstrates additional findings in the area of family violence.

Although cases of family strife provide sufficient cause to focus on incidents of family violence, the cost of medical care necessitated by intrafamily assault, violence, and homicide provides another reason to study this problem. Based on data from 1984, Straus[28] reported that approximately 1,453,437 medical visits per year were made by women who needed care for injuries resulting from assault by a spouse. Also, there were 1,695,897 medical visits made by children for injuries resulting from assault by a parent. Husbands had a total of 479,634 visits

---

RELEVANT RESEARCH

This study explored the connection between experiences of violence and psychiatric status. Three hypotheses were considered: (1) that a significant proportion of outpatients would report having experienced serious violence; (2) that sex differences would be observed in the reporting of experiences of violence; and (3) that several psychiatric diagnoses would be associated more frequently than others with experiences of violence.

The sample consisted of 105 women and 85 men. Most were single and between 20 and 40 years of age. Most were white and were employed. The data collected included psychiatric diagnoses, experiences of physical or sexual abuse, and demographic information, including age. The data were collected by a clinician/interviewer during the course of ordinary clinical evaluations. Written evaluations were then reviewed by the research team.

A variety of psychiatric diagnoses were reported. Results indicated that 22% of the clients had at least one experience in which they were victims of physical or sexual violence. Thirty-one clients, or 16%, had been physically or sexually abusive to others. Most offenders were male (81%), and most victims were female (81%).

Most of the abuse was intrafamilial. Child abuse was reported most frequently, followed by wife-beating. Twenty-three percent of the married women had been beaten by their husbands, and 20% of the men had assaulted their wives. Thirteen percent of the women in the study had experienced sexual abuse, while none of the men had experienced such abuse.

Among the women who had been victimized, the most common diagnoses were borderline personality disorder and substance abuse. Women with a history of having been victimized were four times more likely to be diagnosed as substance abusers than those who had not been victimized. These findings point to the devastating effects of family violence.

Substance abuse and psychosis were not associated with violence toward others among the men in the sample. However, all six of the women in the study who had been violent toward others had a diagnosis of some psychosis or substance abuse.

The researcher reported that the results of this study were minimum estimates because many clinicians may have been hesitant to question clients about experiences of violence. The researcher further reported that the topics of sexual and domestic violence have not yet been integrated into teaching or clinical practice. The researcher encouraged clinicians to assess for family violence, and to be aware of appropriate treatment procedures for family violence.

(Herman J: Histories of violence in an outpatient population: An exploratory study. Am J Orthopsychiatry 56:137, 1986.)

for medical care necessitated by injuries from a spouse. In total, intrafamily violence required about 1,234,000 office visits, 2,141,000 emergency-room visits, and 254,000 hospital admissions lasting a day or more. These figures are in addition to the care needed by those who were injured seriously enough to die, and those admitted for care who did not admit that their injury was a result of intrafamily violence. Incest is one type of violence included in the latter category.

As indicated by the above figures, understanding family violence is a necessary part of understanding the family in today's society. Clinicians must be able to assess for the presence of violence in the family as well as plan and intervene in the troubling patterns of abuse.

This chapter will cover three types of family violence:

1. *Incest,* including all forms of sexual contact, sexual exploitation (*e.g.,* pornography), and "sexual overtures initiated by anyone who is related to the child by family ties or through surrogate family ties (the adult shares a primary group relationship with the child)."[30] Molestation will not be considered in this chapter because the perpetrator of molestation is not a family or surrogate family member.
2. *Child abuse,* defined as nonaccidental physical injury, with resultant cognitive, psychological, and/or maturational damage inflicted upon a person under the age of 18 years by any family member or surrogate family member

3. *Conjugal violence,* or severe, deliberate, and repeated physical violence inflicted on one partner by another with whom the former has or has had an intimate relationship[8]

Other identified forms of family violence include violence against older adults, which is covered in Chapter 26. Rape, a form of violence that occurs in many types of relationships, including marriage, is discussed in Chapter 25.

Theories of Violence in the Family: A Systems Theory Perspective

The systems theory perspective, one of the important bodies of knowledge used in this text, helps in the understanding of why violence in the home occurs. The causes of family violence lie in the physical, psychological, societal, cultural, and environmental aspects of the family or its members. Each of these etiologies will be discussed.

Physical Factors

Physical factors in this section refers to the biological characteristics of the perpetrator. Campbell[9] divided this discussion into the "instinctivist" and the "neurophysiological" perspectives.

According to the *instinctivist* position, men and animals are aggressive by nature. This allows the transmission of the strongest genes to future generations. Campbell referred to this theory as simplistic. The authors of this theory have been strongly criticized for equating animal needs for aggression in hunting for food with examples of parents who need to increase their self-esteem by cruelly abusing defenseless children. It has also been found that in "nonhuman primates, male aggression . . . (is) a minute fraction of the total interactions." Indeed, many animals are "almost entirely passive."[9]

The *neurophysiological* theories include findings that indicate that "different kinds of aggression (predatory, competitive, defensive, irritative, territorial, maternal-protective, and sex-related) have been elicited by electrical stimulation in different neuroanatomical places."[9] Also, levels of certain endocrines in the blood seem "to affect selectively different kinds of aggression." Other substances in the blood, such as alcohol, can also facilitate "neural mechanisms for aggression."[9]

In critiquing the concept of a neurophysiological basis of aggression, one is led to the conclusion that this explanation must be viewed in conjunction with other system concepts (such as societal, cultural, psychological, and environmental). The evidence suggesting a hormonal etiology of aggression is not conclusive; therefore, the lower likelihood of female aggression necessitates an examination of social learning as a mediating factor of aggression. Also, it is known that even individuals with brain damage who live in passive cultures do not become violent.

Psychological Factors

The psychoanalytic framework explains aggression as a basic instinct in individuals. This instinct is influenced by other internal and external factors that foster or hinder its expression. Once aggression has been expressed, the individual's hostility and further aggression will decrease. However, studies have shown that "overt aggression does not inevitably lead to physiological tension-reduction or a reduction in subsequent aggression."[9] Indeed, some forms of aggression, such as verbal aggression or watching violent films or sports, increase rather than decrease later aggression. Another theory in the psychological perspective is that of an "over-controlled personality type." These individuals display extreme violence. They are "instilled with such excessive inhibitions against aggression in childhood that their hostile impulses build up."[9] However, scales developed to measure this personality type have not been validated.

A number of problems occur with this psychological perspective on violence.

1. Mothers have been blamed for their children who demonstrate violence, because they are typically the primary care-givers. However, it is known that violent men "have also frequently been exposed to abusive and alcoholic fathers," and not just violent mothers.

2. Studies concerning the violent personality typically have small samples, and rarely include women as subjects.

3. Violent prisoners are rarely given psychiatric diagnoses by the courts or by psychiatrists outside the legal system. Therefore, these cases are excluded from research studies because they are undiagnosed.

4. If violence and psychological abnormality are so interwoven, it is hard to explain why "former mental patients commit fewer crimes (including violent crimes) than the normal population."[9]

Other writers considering the psychological aspect of aggression have not based their ideas on the instinctivist position. Erich Fromm, for example, considered forms of aggression that are "adaptive and life-serving," such as self-assertion and defensive aggression. Fromm believed that harmful aggression comes from the "dishonest and unalive atmosphere characterizing many families and social situations."[9]

Another theorist, Rollo May, characterized aggression as arising from a sense of low self-esteem and powerlessness. Alfred Adler believed that individuals act violently out of a feeling of inadequacy and the need for power.[9]

Societal Factors

Theorists who feel that societal factors promote violence view aggression as being learned from others. Other individuals in the aggressive person's environment either role-model or involve the aggressive person in violence. For example, an abused child is involved in violence as a child, and may become violent as an adult. Research supports the idea that the more violence a child sees in the home, the more violent that child will be as an adult. Also, violent men are more likely to have been abused as children.

Another societal factor concerns society's sanctioning of violence on television. One study described by Campbell reported that "the single best predictor of boys' aggressive behavior at age 19 was how much violent television they were watching at age 19."[9]

Cultural Factors

Cultural factors include belief systems that foster violence. These belief systems include the value of using violence as a means of resolving conflict. Subjects in one research study, for example, justified police shootings for the purpose of social control, not just in situations involving self-defense or protection. Twenty to thirty percent would advise police to shoot to kill in such instances.[3]

Another cultural factor can be seen in society's acceptance of attaining material goods by exploiting others.

There is a need for "competition, and lust for power and control over other human beings." One feels good by knowing that in some way one is better than someone else. Our "society's rewards or power and prestige tend to go to the least compassionate members."[9] In many ways, our culture is violent.

In studies that look at violence across societal groups, some researchers have noted that there is a significant correlation between violence and rigid sex roles, post-marriage sexual restrictions on women, and an inferior status of women.[9] It has also been found that societies with high levels of class differences also have high levels of violence.

Environmental Factors

Poverty is accompanied by feelings of anger generated by racism and discrimination. Violence, in light of stressful environmental factors, is a "desperate message that a situation of inequality, frustration, and rage exists that badly needs correction."[9] The environment of the ghetto is itself violent and uncertain. The incidence of violence is far greater in ghetto environments than outside them.

It is clear, then, that no one single factor leads to family violence. Many factors combine to produce a pattern of family behavior that causes emotional and physical pain for many, and great losses in society. Figure 21-1 depicts the combination of factors that produce family violence.

Child Physical Abuse

Child physical abuse is not unique in today's society. Humanity has witnessed and participated in various forms of child physical abuse for more than 5,000 years.[7] The following section presents a brief history of child physical abuse, along with a definition and a discussion of the prevalence of child physical abuse. The nursing process is used as a framework for dealing with abusive families, and a care plan is presented.

Society's Historical Views of Child Abuse

Over the last 5,000 years, all societies and cultures have supported the practice of child physical abuse in one

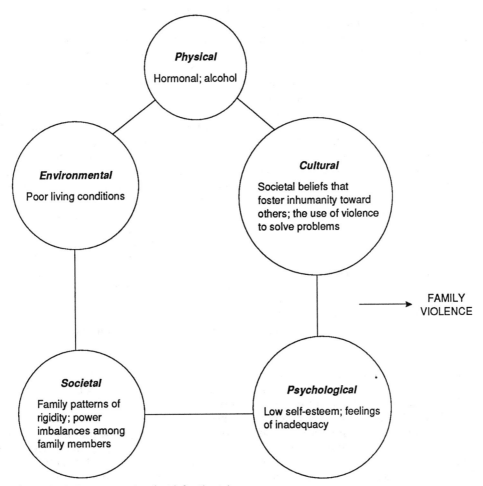

Figure 21-1. Factors associated with family violence.

form or another. Abuses of children were often willful and indiscreet. Ancient Sumerians employed men whose only purpose was to whip boys who did not behave. The Spartans abandoned weak and deformed children, or threw them into deep canyons to die. Some cultures offered young children as sacrifices to the gods for various reasons. From the advent of the industrial revolution until as late as the early 1900s, child labor was a common and socially acceptable custom. Although these examples are seldom seen now, except in the most primitive societies, child physical abuse continues to exist.

It was not until 1875 that children in the United States were protected from physical abuse by the legal system.[7] A young victim of child abuse was finally removed from her environment by the courts only after she had been granted status and protection equal to those of an animal, under the auspices of the Society for the Prevention of Cruelty to Animals. However, this case did not expedite the cause of physically-abused children. Further legal action did not ensue until 1968, when all 50 states had passed legislation mandating the reporting of child abuse. Not until 1974, almost 100 years after the case of 1875, was the Child Abuse Prevention and Treatment Act put into effect. As a result of this legislation, the National Center on Child Abuse and Neglect was established.[7] Although child physical abuse had finally come to the nation's attention, it still remains an unsolved problem.

The reasons for the reluctance of the judicial system, as well as of society in general, to recognize and act to prevent child physical abuse are founded largely in American tradition. Religious and legal customs gave men the right to discipline their wives and children as if they were property, thereby legitimizing physical abuse.

However, changes have occurred in the traditional family. With more women in the labor force and a greater variety of family structures, there is a greater sense of equality in the relationships between men and women. The traditional "man of the house" now is usually more responsible for the *well-being* of others in the home. Perpetrators of violence, however, do not view these changes positively. Unfortunately, there is still an increase of family violence in the United States.

The Definition of Child Abuse

In order to understand child abuse, a working definition is necessary. A review of the literature shows that there is not a universally accepted definition of child physical abuse. What some individuals consider abuse is viewed by others as acceptable and even prudent behavior. In 1961, C. Henry Kempe and Ray Helfer offered the term "battered child" to increase public awareness of a serious health problem.[23] In their definition, the term *battered* includes ". . . any child who suffered nonaccidental physical injury as a result of acts (or omissions) by his parents or guardian."[23] Although this definition began to delineate the circumstances and perpetrator of the battering of the child, it did not express the full impact of child physical abuse.

Brown[7] further defined child physical abuse by limiting the age to 18 years or younger, and by including other persons responsible for the child's welfare and care as perpetrators. Friedman[15] supported this broader definition of the family when she stated that a family is ". . . composed of people (two or more) who are emotionally involved with each other and live in close geographical proximity." This interpretation of family structure increases the number of potential perpetrators of child physical abuse. Further elaboration of the definition of child physical abuse included mention of the scope of the detrimental effects of abuse upon a family member. The staggering impact of the adverse effects of physical child abuse (*i.e.,* impairment of cognitive, psychological, and maturational development), in conjunction with the more obvious physical traumas, were completely detailed.

A combination of the previous definitions will be used in this chapter. Here, the definition of *child physical abuse* is: nonaccidental physical injury to any child under 18 years of age, with resultant cognitive, psychological, and/or maturational damage, inflicted by any family member (or surrogate family member). Friedman's definition of family will also be used.

Prevalence

The prevalence of child physical abuse is monumental. According to Brown,[7] at least seven children die each day from abuse. Keefe[23] reported that, in 1983, 26.9% of the total documented cases of child abuse in the U.S. were categorized as "major." In the state of California alone, 120,000 cases of child abuse are reported every year.[14] Brown[7] further stated that the highest number of physical abuse cases occur among boys six years of age or older. Keefe[23] cited very young children (under age four, and most commonly under age three) as the targets of major abuse-related physical injuries. A more detailed account of the victim of child physical abuse will be discussed under the assessment phase of the nursing process.

It is not difficult to understand the magnitude of the problem of child physical abuse in view of the large number of cases. Unfortunately, the psychological and cognitive impairments that result from child physical abuse are not as easy to document or count.

The Nursing Process

Assessment

All nurses who come in contact with the general population have roles in the assessment and diagnosis of child physical abuse. These nurses can work in hospitals, in community clinics, as school nurses, and/or as community health nurses. During home visits, nurses can provide initial assessment of child abuse.

Before nurses can begin to deal effectively with the problem of child physical abuse, they need to understand families at risk, individuals who commit child physical abuse, why perpetrators act as they do, who the victims are, and the effects of the physical mistreatments. It must be remembered that child physical abuse is a family-oriented problem. Therefore, singling out the perpetrator and/or the victim does not ensure the resolution of the family-centered problem. Nurses must recognize that any family experiencing developmental transitional crisis is at risk. "All families hold the potential for internalized destruction."[6]

Keefe[23] cited families in the early child-bearing and child-rearing stages of family development as the group at highest risk for child physical abuse. According to Friedman,[15] these stages continue from the birth of the first child (Stage II) to the middle years (Stage VII). This time-frame could conceivably cover a total of 30 years or more, with the parents in Stage VII (45–55 years of age). This is important for nurses to acknowledge, because children up to 18 years of age can be victims of child physical abuse.

The next family factor to be considered is the incidence of *family isolation*. Bolton and Bolton[6] describe the isolated family as one that is geographically and socially removed from assistance in times of distress. This family is generally characterized as a closed and rigid system. These families are particularly challenging to nurses because they shun outside assistance and interaction during times of distress (*e.g.,* marital disharmony and financial difficulty). Other contributing factors in the abusive family's dynamics include early, forced marriages and constant high levels of family stress.

Nurses must remember that families that fit these characteristics can be traditional families, single-parent families, and same-sex households. In fact, Keefe[23] indicated that 43% of the abusive families studied had a single female parent. Astute nurses must be aware of all these factors when assessing family systems.

The next focus of the nurse is to determine the perpetrator or adult abuser. Brown[7] stated that 90% of child physical abuse is committed by the parents. Men and women are perpetrators in equal numbers, but usually only one of the parents commits the act. Generally, the nonperpetrator is aware of the abusive parent's behavior, but is unwilling to act on behalf of the child for fear of retribution against the child and nonabusive parent, and/or family separation. Nurses must maintain a nonjudgmental posture toward both the perpetrator and the nonabusive parent if intervention and family treatment are the ultimate goals.

Certain personality characteristics are found in the abusive adult. Most authorities agree that abusive adults were usually abused children. The abusive pattern is modeled as an acceptable pattern of coping from generation to generation.[23]

Bolton and Bolton[6] presented a list of 11 characteristics commonly found in the perpetrator of child physical abuse. These characteristics focus on what the Boltons described as a flaw in the personality of perpetrators: "They are incapable of joining in a solidly-attached, reciprocal, and protective relationship with other family members."[6] The following is an adaptation of Bolton and Bolton's list, with brief definitions:

1. *Psychopathology.* The parents are neurotic. Their behavior may be ritualistic, with unpredictable assaults.

2. *Unresolved interpersonal conflict.* This occurs in perpetrators who have experienced early deprivation. Perpetrators have no complete sense of self, are immature, and are self-serving.

3. *Inappropriate and distorted dependencies.* These result in distorted relationships between perpetrators and their children. In other words, perpetrators are dependent on the children for fulfillment of their own needs.

4. *Immaturity.* Perpetrators exhibit a lack of impulse control, neediness, low frustration tolerance, and a need for instant gratification. Perpetrators with this characteristic are often termed "child parents."

5. *Low self-esteem.* Perpetrators view themselves as worthless and have a negative self-image. Perpetrators' judgments of themselves can relate to their own childhood traumas of hostility, rejection, and abandonment.

6. *Lack of preparation for the family role.* Perpetrators are both educationally and personally not prepared for the role of parent. They lack empathy for the child, and place unrealistic expectations upon the child relative to the child's capabilities. Perpetrators are driven to be perfect parents, an image that they believe is reflected in the actions and behaviors of their children. Misbehavior by the children is seen as purposeful by the perpetrators.

7. *Need for dominance and control.* Perpetrators demand strict and rigid obedience from children. Unfortunately for the children, the rules of the perpetrators are usually as changeable and unpredictable as the perpetrators' behavior.

8. *Approval of the use of violence.* Perpetrators come from a background of violent and abusive behavior learned early. They believe they have the right to punish children for misbehaving. This is especially the case if children's misbehavior is viewed by perpetrators as intentionally directed toward them.

9. *Lack of social and interpersonal skills.* Perpetrators are incapable of dealing with their children without the use of force and authority. Common feelings of warmth, kindness, and understanding are elusive or absent traits. Failures in interpersonal relationships of perpetrators are blamed on the children because of the perpetrators' inability to accept responsibility for their own actions.

10. *Denial and defensiveness.* Perpetrators believe that their abusive actions are rightful, and even rationalize and minimize the effects of the physical abuse. Perpetrators are convinced that they are the victims of their children's willful misconduct.

11. *Distorted view of the victim.* Perpetrators see children as different. Sometimes the differences include

premature birth, or mental or physical handicaps. Often the reason for the perceived difference results from the child's not fulfilling the expectations of the perpetrators, who feel they are not receiving the anticipated and demanded gratification they expect from the child.

As nurses become more familiar with these traits of perpetrators and comprehend the causes of the personality flaws, it will be easier to identify the warning signs of potential and actual situations of child physical abuse. This knowledge will also help nurses to prevent abused children from becoming abusive parents. What children learn, experience, and practice in childhood is brought with them into adulthood. Because abused children experience parental/perpetrator rejection, inconsistencies in behavior, and physical injury, they may emulate the same patterns with their own children. Therefore, it is essential for nurses to be able to assess victims of child physical abuse, not only by the physical signs, but also by being cognizant of the psychological, cognitive, and maturational developmental stunting that occurs in these children.

Victims of child physical abuse are confused, frightened, and emotionally deprived individuals. Many of the victims' personality flaws parallel those of the perpetrators. Victims experience low self-esteem, dependency, social isolation, difficulty in trusting, lack of self-control, impaired intellectual and cognitive functions, and a sense of feeling different from others.

Victims of child physical abuse are either overly compliant or overly aggressive toward adults. Aggression is usually uncontrollable and is the way the victims tend to solve problems. The social isolation usually corresponds with the forced demands of perpetrators and the children's own perceptions of being different and unacceptable to their peers. Often victims resort to antisocial behaviors (*e.g.,* delinquency, running away, prostitution, substance abuse, suicide attempts, or premature adulthood) in order to escape the physical abuse.

The overt symptoms of child physical abuse are obviously more apparent in the assessment and diagnosis of the problem. The presence of bruises, welts, lacerations, burns, and fractures may indicate child physical abuse. Nurses must clarify the circumstances surrounding questionable injuries and be alert to unsatisfactory answers or the direct avoidance of mention of such injuries. Nurses who are aware of the overt (physical) signs and symptoms and covert signs (deviance in behavior, abnormal maturational and developmental levels) are better prepared to make accurate assessments and diagnoses of victims of child physical abuse.

In the assessment phase of the nursing process, nurses must be aware of high-risk families, the personality flaws of perpetrators, the causes of such flaws, and the overt and covert signs and symptoms exhibited by the victims.

Diagnosis

While there are no nursing diagnoses specific to child abuse, it can result in a number of different problematic behavior patterns. It is important that, in making a diagnosis, the abuse remains a focus. Possible diagnoses may include the need to find a protective environment for the child. However, it is essential to assist abused children to deal with their history of abuse. See Chapter 22 for a description of how to work with children's psychological/societal issues.

Planning

Once the diagnosis of child physical abuse has been made, nurses begin planning interventions. According to Keefe,[23] nurses must accomplish two major tasks: (1) the formation of a cooperative relationship with the family, and (2) development of mutually agreed-upon goals. Both steps require excellent communication skills, as well as a nonjudgmental attitude and approach.

This stage of the nursing process can be very frustrating for nurses because of abusive families' characteristics of isolation. This family structure is dependent on the immediate members for support and guidance. Nurses are outside the family framework, and are most likely seen as uninvited intruders. In addition to the problem of isolation, the perpetrators' belief in their rightful conduct hampers the planning for interventions. These families typically do not listen to or want advice, especially when it involves a change in behavior patterns. Before any interventions can begin, nurses must establish trust with the family and with the perpetrator. Again, the importance of acutely refined communication skills and a nonjudgmental posture cannot be overly emphasized. By establishing trust among the family members and nurse, the pattern of isolation can be broken. Bolton and Bolton[6] summarized the impact of this breakthrough: "Isolation must be reduced before any hope for the elimination of the problem is realistic."

In order for the break from isolation to remain intact, the planning phase should include referrals to appropriate support systems within the health profession and community. This step is done gradually and without misinterpretation by the family that they are being abandoned by the initial nurse, with whom the trust and cooperative relationship have been developed.

Intervention

The nursing interventions applicable to the care of the abusive family and the victim concentrate on immediate and long-term needs. The immediate needs include providing the necessary physical care to the abused child and family, and continual reassessment of the family's situation and health needs.[23] Once these interventions are begun, nurses devote their efforts to long-term needs: establishment of trust and a cooperative relationship; coordination of family treatment activities; referral to necessary community resources; facilitation of direct problem-solving techniques through education and teaching; the provision of emotional support through nonjudgmental attitudes; and resocialization of the family. The child physical abuse situation must also be reported to the proper agencies. Families must be reassured that this is

NURSING CARE PLAN: JOHNNY

ASSESSMENT	NURSING INTERVENTIONS	EVALUATION CRITERIA

Aggression/violence toward others—family-focused (21.02)

NURSING DIAGNOSIS: Abuse—Physical (21.02.01)

SUBJECTIVE DATA		
Mother states, "Johnny is clumsy. He falls and hurts himself or he burns himself."	1. Assure safety of child by hospitalization, removal from home, removal of perpetrator from home. File abuse report.	Child will receive no further abuse.
OBJECTIVE DATA	2. Treat injuries.	
Old healing scars, burns on arms. Child is withdrawn, nervous, and acts more mature than age.	3. Begin to establish family trust by: phone contacts and home visits; work with family on treatment plan; provide information; remain nonjudgmental.	Child will obtain treatment for injuries. Family will maintain contact with nurse; will ask questions; will follow through with appointments.
	4. Refer family and individual members to counseling as needed. (See Chap. 12 and Chap. 22 for discussions of family- and child-focused interventions.)	Family members will begin collective or individual treatment plans as needed.

confidential and is not handled by the police. This is important in order to maintain the fragile interaction between the nurse and the family. A nursing care plan focusing on the family in which child abuse occurs is presented below.

Evaluation

Evaluation of the effectiveness of the plan and interventions occurs simultaneously with the reassessment of family needs. The more concrete and measurable the goals are, the less the possibility of recurrence of child physical abuse after the therapy and treatment have been terminated. Accessibility of the family through phone and mail contacts should be determined during planning, reassessment, and evaluation prior to termination of services. This is necessary in order to prevent reversion to isolation.

Levels of Prevention

Early case-finding is the most important concept in *primary prevention* of child abuse (Fig. 21-2). Children are actually or potentially susceptible to further abuse when they remain in the home for longer periods of time. There is no assurance that the family who abuses a child will spontaneously stop the abuse. There are indications that abuse continues unless an outside force interferes. Most states have mandatory reporting laws that require professionals, such as nurses, to report suspected cases of child abuse to authorities. Failure to report suspected

cases of child abuse can result in nurses' losing their licenses.

Secondary prevention includes immediate treatment for the victim of child abuse as well as treatment for the family. Such intervention can be life-saving, and may involve steps such as finding a temporary home for the abused child and the initiation of help for the perpetrator.

Tertiary care involves long-term care of the abused child and the family. This process can allow much growth in the family, giving them the sense that after therapy they are leading "new lives." Tertiary prevention is more difficult because it implies a failure in early case-finding. As the abuse continues, it frequently becomes worse, and feelings such as guilt, fear, terror, and aloneness intensify. However, treatment is certainly possible. In many cases, treatment includes counseling for individual family members, as well as for the family as a whole. Support groups, such as multiple family groups for families in which there has been incest, Al-Anon, Alcoholics Anonymous, Adult Children of Alcoholics, and others, offer long-term support for needed family changes.

Child Sexual Abuse

In a study of 50 adult survivors of child sexual abuse (specifically, incest), one theme was consistent among the survivors. They all stated that "there is no part of my life as an adult that has not been affected in a negative way by my incest as a child."[4] This comment documents the need for all health care providers to understand the phe-

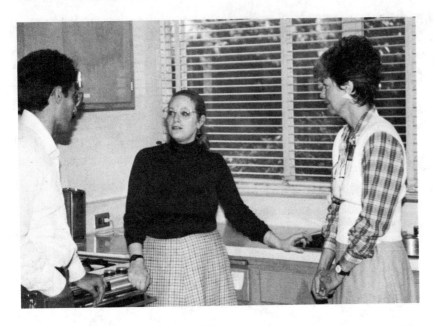

Figure 21-2. A psychiatric nurse meets with parents in their home to discuss parenting skills.

nomenon of incest—both how to assess the family environment for incest and how to intervene.[18]

Incest is still a "taboo" topic in our society, despite current media interest. Health care providers, including nurses, are not immune to wanting to avoid dealing with the topic of incest.[24] Yet incest behavior in a family is one area in which prompt and effective action on the part of the health care provider is most needed.

"It is estimated that one out of every four females is sexually abused before she reaches the age of 18."[22] Sexual abuse of children and adolescents (referred to in this section as "sexual abuse of children" in order to avoid repetition) may occur in families of any socioeconomic class. More cases are reported in lower economic classes, partially because those classes are overrepresented in research. Gelles reported that, in fact, sexually-abusive families may have an annual income "as much as 10% higher than physically-abusing families."[17]

The Family

Families in which incest occurs tend to be isolated, either socially or geographically. As members withdraw from others outside the home, relationships among members inside the home become overly important. Also, because there is little outside scrutiny of the family, an environment is provided in which abusive behavior can more easily occur. "Importantly, this is a pattern completely hidden from the outside world."[6]

"The sexually-abusive family may appear to others as being stable, financially competent, and with a male in the household who is respected in the community."[6] Family members are isolated psychologically from one another. Hence, incest occurs and is maintained as a behavior "through the cooperative acceptance of this family secret by family members." Murphy described an exception to the "secret" aspect of incest. In this case, the in-

cestuous behavior was done openly in the family and accepted by all members.[25]

In the sexually-abusive family, unresolved parental conflicts, within each parent and between the parents as a couple, serve as a starting point requiring a source for release of the tension in the parent(s). The child becomes the target of the abuse.

Summit reported that most mothers are not "aware of ongoing sexual abuse. Marriage demands considerable blind trust and denial for survival."[29] If the child does mention the abuse (which is rare), the mother finds herself in a bind. One person in the child–father dyad is lying. Both are individuals to whom the mother has deep attachments of trust and security. Typically, the mother does *not* comfort the child. At best, the mother asks why the child did not come to her sooner to talk about the incest. At worst, the mother denies the allegation or ignores it.

The Survivor

Frequently, incest victims are referred to as "survivors." This term is commonly applied to individuals who have endured abuse in an atmosphere of terror, from which there is no escape. The term also denotes the fact that many women seek help from other incest survivors and clinicians to avoid being the "victim" in the family and in society. They seek to attain and maintain a sense of personal power and assertiveness. In this chapter the term *survivor* is used to refer to incest victims because of the countless acts of personal courage shown by so many women in the face of repeated acts of personal violation and even threats of death. The term "victim" does not connote these acts of courage.

Summit has identified the *child sexual abuse accommodation syndrome.*[29] This syndrome describes the behavior expected of a normal child subjected to sexual assault. The five categories of the syndrome are: secrecy; helplessness; entrapment and accommodation; delayed, conflicted, and unconvincing disclosure; and retraction.

Secrecy. Perpetrators use various forms of threat to maintain the secrecy of the incest. In some instances, children are told that if they tell anyone about the incest the perpetrator ("Daddy") will get into trouble, or the family will fall apart, or "Mommy" will be upset, or "I'll hurt you." The perpetrator is trusted and/or feared, so the child maintains the secret. The secrecy "makes it clear to the child that there is something bad and dangerous"[29] occurring. Even in cases in which the child does inform the nonperpetrator parent about the incest, that parent may believe that the child is fabricating the incest. The child "feels stigmatized with a sense of badness and danger from the pervasive secrecy."[29]

To counteract the secrecy, the child must (1) find the "permission and power to share the secret," and (2) find the recipient of such information "engaging and nonpunitive." This combination of conditions is rare. "The child is likely to spend a lifetime in what comes to be a self-imposed exile from intimacy, trust, and self-validation."[29]

Helplessness. Society assumes that, while children should not "talk with strangers," they can relate with those in the home. Yet trusted family members (or those in similar relationship to the child, such as a step-father) often violate the child's trust. "A child is three times more likely to be molested by a recognized trusted adult than by a stranger."[29]

One incest survivor stated, "There is little, and there is big."[4] This simple phrase presents the difficulty of the small child faced with much larger adults. "No child has equal power to say no to a parental figure or to anticipate the consequences of sexual involvement with an adult care-giver."[29] Approximately 25% of the children treated for incest are five years of age or younger. The adult bears "sole responsibility for any clandestine sexual activity with a minor." The image of the seductive minor who approaches the family member is "an artifact of delayed disclosure and a prevailing adult wish to define sexual abuse within a model that is similar logically to adult behavior." Hence, blame can be attributed to the victim rather than to the perpetrator.[29]

Entrapment and Accommodation. The perpetrator finds the forbidden nature of the incest experience inviting, and the acts are accomplished with ease. "A compulsive, addictive pattern is established within the abuser. In many instances the abuse does not stop until the survivor is much older or leaves home. The child is trapped in the home."[29] The "healthy, normal, emotionally resilient child will learn to accommodate to the reality of continuing sexual abuse."[29]

The types of accommodations are varied. Survivors may mutilate themselves, avoid reality, or develop multiple personalities (see the discussion of Personality Disorders in Chap. 19). Children who are incest survivors may come to believe that *they* are to blame for the incest. The thought of having a trusted adult inflict pain is unbearable, and the children protect an image of the "good" parent by blaming themselves. They may come to hate the mother who does not protect them, or they may engage in antisocial behavior. The child may withdraw in school and feel a lack of a sense of self. Part of the sense of self is a feeling of personality boundaries, and the survivor's boundaries are continually violated.[4]

Delayed, Conflicted, and Unconvincing Disclosure. "Most cases of incest are unreported. Reported cases are the exception, not the norm."[29] Very often survivors who report the incest are adolescents. Yet adolescence is the time in which survivors are "least likely to find understanding and intervention."[29] Authorities tend to be alienated by the rebelliousness automatically attributed to adolescence. Many authorities believe that adolescents are simply trying to "get back at a controlling adult." The adolescent risks "disbelief by others and also humiliation and punishment."[29] In cases in which the adolescent is an obedient, seemingly adjusted child, the survivor also may not be believed because there is nothing obviously wrong with the child.

Retraction. Children frequently deny their accusations of sexual abuse. When the incest becomes known, the child is often abandoned by the accused father and typically is not supported by the mother, who may believe the child has "ruined the family." The child may be removed from the home. For the sake of peace, the child retracts what has been said. The secret is maintained.[29]

The Perpetrator

There is no indication that incest perpetrators are "mentally defective" or psychotic. Two cases studied by Birckhead[4] included the family physician as a perpetrator. The physician was subtly encouraged to abuse the child by the child's father. Another perpetrator was the male therapist of a female incest survivor.

Some researchers find in the perpetrator traits of "immaturity, inadequacy, vulnerability, helplessness, and isolation" rather than a specific psychiatric diagnosis. Because of these traits, perpetrators often find adult sexuality frightening or threatening, and therefore focus on children as sexual partners. Children are seen by perpetrators as "adults" who can relate to the "child" perpetrator. Hence, sexual contact with children is pleasing to perpetrators.

The perpetrator may expect his wife and children to be totally dependent on him and to see him as the "power" in the home. Yet the abuser also is dependent on his wife and may relate to her as if she is his mother. The perpetrator may idealize women, and therefore may not want his wife to participate in sexual behavior—something that the perpetrator would view as "dirty." "Sexual activity with children is not seen as dirty. Children are somehow different—less frightening to the perpetrator and easier to control." The abuser's abstinence from sex with his wife may be thought of by the perpetrator as demonstrating strength and control to his wife.[29]

Gelles[17] urged caution in assuming that perpetrators of sexual abuse were sexually abused during their childhood. An intergenerational transmission pattern of abuse indicates that abusers repeat abuse patterns they learned in their families. Generally, it appears that "the previously sexually-victimized individual may have some small likelihood of increased risk of perpetration. Due to incomplete research on the topic of generational transmission of the abuse pattern, only a 30% to 60% perpetration rate is suspected among males who themselves were victims of child sexual abuse."[17]

The perpetrator may or may not abuse alcohol. Gelles stated that clinicians can disregard the family's statements that the incest behavior occurred "because" of the alcohol.[17] The causes of the abuse lie beyond the abuse of alcohol, and a focus on substance abuse may serve as a way for the family to avoid the topic of incest.

The Nursing Process

Assessment

Every physical and psychiatric history taken of individuals—both adults and children—should ask incest-related questions. Renshaw[27] reported a number of factors that lead to suspicion of incest behavior in a family. These factors include: a disrupted marital sexual relationship; previous incest experiences in the childhood of the adult members of the family; substance abuse in the home; a value system that contains stronger negative injunctions against masturbation than against incest; extended periods of time spent alone together by the perpetrator and the child; and newly-admitted family members (such as step-fathers).

Typically, childhood incest is first discovered in one of two ways, in a crisis situation or incidentally. For example, a teenager may become pregnant, or a nurse may ask "How are things at home?" as part of an assessment. The response of the client may be an unfolding of the history of incest. The incest may also be discovered during the course of counseling (begun because of issues *other than* incest) or during participation of the survivor in a research project.

Assessment data gathered from a child suspected of being sexually abused would include:

Appearance (including the appearance of clothing)
Injuries (anatomical drawings can be used to locate injuries)
Fingernails
Pelvic exam (A vaginal opening of more than 4 mm [VO+] indicates child sexual abuse in girls under 13 years of age.)
Menstrual history
The nature of the assault (Describe the acts that occurred, whether ejaculation occurred, whether the client lost consciousness.)

What might the client have done that would affect evidence of incest (such as bathing)?
Laboratory tests (such as a gonorrhea culture)

Birckhead's[4] research identified other characteristics of children (or adolescents) that may predict incest. This assessment data may be identified in any child, not only those already suspected of having a history of incest. These characteristics include:

Behavior that is suddenly different from typical behavior (An active child may suddenly become withdrawn.)
Marked personality differences from one moment to the next (indicative of multiple personalities)
Not wanting to go home
Fear of adult men or women
Self-mutilation
Substance abuse
Sudden weight gain
Suicidal thoughts/actions
Episodes of running away from home
Hostility/aggression
Statements such as "something is going on at home"
Low self-esteem
Depression
Problems with authority
Shame
Pregnancy

Researchers[4,12] have described assessment data in adults that may predict a history of incest. Birckhead has also identified assessment data indicative of incest in research subjects. Such data are important because clients may not volunteer that they are incest survivors. Clients may never have told anyone about the incest, or they may begin to remember the experiences of incest after being prompted to do so by incest-related assessment questions from nurses. Many incest survivors in Birckhead's research study stated, "If the health care worker or school counselor had only asked," or "All the symptoms were there; why didn't anyone care enough to ask?" Data indicative of incest may include:

Troublesome dreams that suggest incest. Themes in the dreams may include violence, threats made to a child, and family turmoil.
Repetitive, disturbing thoughts
Repetitive client reports of "not being present," "leaving my body for a while," or "not being here"
Beliefs that stimuli in the environment are threatening (Shadowy figures in a doorway, for example, may cause anxiety.)[12]
Symptoms that symbolize incest (One client stated that she remembered being taken as a child to the emergency room with a foaming mouth. The client later remembered that this symptom occurred after she had been forced to engage in fellatio and that she could have been saved years of psychotherapy if her therapist had made the connection between this symptom and incest.)
Sexual difficulties

Concerns about sexual preference; questioning whether the individual is heterosexual, homosexual, or a lesbian

Self-mutilation
Suicidal thoughts or actions
Sudden changes in behavior (multiple personalities)
Sudden weight gain
Promiscuity
Provoking attacks by others

The family is another important area of assessment. Nurses are in an important position to help incest survivors. *The incest occurring in a family can be detected by careful observations and questioning by nurses.* As a result, survivor suffering can be greatly reduced. Areas of family assessment that may predict incest include:[4,19]

Family violence
An ill or disabled mother
A mother who is absent from the home for periods of time
Male baby sitters
Periods of time when the perpetrator is left alone with the incest survivor
Psychosis in family members (One research subject was sexually abused by her psychotic brother.)
Depression in family members
Periods of time when the incest survivor was placed in the care of others as a child
The presence of more than one child in the family
Adult responsibilities performed by the children
Parental conflict
Parental behavior that encourages children not to trust one another
Threats with guns or knives among family members
Attempts by the father to keep the incest survivor at home, or to direct the life of the survivor

Diagnosis

It is most important *to first identify that the individual is an incest survivor.* Current practice indicates that tortuous acts of incest against unsuspecting children are surrounded by threats and secrecy. Most cases of incest are not reported. Nurses come in contact with many individuals and families and can fulfill the important function of case-finding.

The diagnosis of incest is the most important step. The road to recovery is then set into motion. While the process of recovery in treatment is difficult, many incest survivors grieve, in part, for the amount of time they lost in fulfilling their lives. They have spent their lives in the aftermath of the incest with no assistance from professional care-givers to work through and understand the incest and how it has affected their lives.

Birckhead's[4] research involves studying incest survivors (N = 50) who participated in psychotherapy within the two months preceding the research interview. The purpose of the study is to determine the nature of the incest awareness process of the survivor in psychotherapy. When asked to respond to the statement, "The incest experiences were a continued trauma to me after their occurrence," all 40 of the survivors interviewed thus far answered "strongly agree." Most survivors stated that the incest experience affected "every part of my life."

Because of the degree to which incest survivors are affected by their incest experiences, and because the trauma involved a form of terrifying abuse or even torture, discussing the incest acts themselves *must* be a focus of the therapeutic work. However, there is no specific nursing diagnosis in the existing taxonomies that describes sexual abuse/torture. Such a diagnosis would lead to the necessary intervention of recounting the incest experiences and grieving for the self who was tortured.

Other sequelae of the incest could be covered by a variety of nursing diagnoses. Nursing diagnoses should be formulated on an individual basis, because some clients experience overwhelming depression while others experience low self-esteem.

Planning

The long-term goal of the work with incest survivors is to understand the effects of incest on the person's life and to work through the resulting issues surrounding the incest. Short-term goals may include providing safety for the survivor in support groups for incest survivors. The survivor may be removed from the home (in the case of a child or adolescent) and placed in a foster home or shelter. Often adult survivors take off time from work or school (in the case of college students) to deal with the incest trauma. Nurses may work with a number of other professionals while assisting with cases of incest. These professionals include child care workers, lawyers, police, other therapists, and clergy.

Most survivors of incest need therapy. Where the survivor has certain benefits (such as previous therapy experience, whether or not related to incest, education, financial resources, and social support), professional nurses can use individual relationship intervention to help clients discuss their incest experiences and understand the effects of the incest on their current lives. Unfortunately, many incest survivors do not have these benefits. In such cases, the individuals typically need individual psychotherapy with professionals such as psychiatric nurse clinical specialists, psychologists, and others who are prepared to work with the client on the incest and related issues. Unfortunately, it is naive to believe that, with current social policies leaning toward cutting social services, most incest survivors will have the benefit of (typically long-term) professional counseling.

Davanloo[11] stated that there is currently an unfortunate bias in U.S. psychiatry toward providing only supportive (superficial) psychotherapy for incest survivors. Many U.S. psychiatrists believe that incest survivors cannot benefit from intensive psychotherapy, even intensive psychotherapy modeled on Davanloo's model of short-term psychotherapy. The Diagnostic and Statistical Manual of Mental Disorders (DSM-III-R)[2] has no classification for abusive behavior. Davanloo has had much success in treating incest survivors with short-term psychotherapy. Nurses can and should serve as ombudspersons for clients by referring them to appropriate treatment sources. Psychotherapists must foster an open discussion of incest among the survivors, their families, and our society in which incest occurs.

Although it is not possible to elaborate on all aspects of planning, another area should be mentioned. Recent research reports that most incest survivors benefit from discussing the incest with the perpetrator.[4] This discussion takes place after much preparation and planning with the survivor. Contact with the perpetrator is discouraged until the survivor is sufficiently prepared not to be put in a position to be victimized again by the perpetrator. Once the acts of incest stop, there is no reason to assume that the perpetrator does not think like a perpetrator. The perpetrator can easily relapse and again abuse the incest survivor. The benefits of a discussion with the perpetrator include the survivor's witnessing the narcissistic behavior of the perpetrator, which counters the survivor's tendency toward self-blame while giving the survivor a sense of personal power in telling the perpetrator that the perpetrator has harmed the survivor.

Intervention

The history of treatment of incest survivors is replete with examples of how survivors have *not* been helped to deal with the incest trauma.[24] Some members of the therapeutic community who could assist incest survivors have instead: (1) dismissed survivors as individuals who describe incest trauma as a disguised childhood "wish" to have sex with "Daddy", (2) believed that the incest was unimportant, and misdiagnosed the individual as depressed or hysterical, (3) failed to ask about incest, or (4) continued the abuse of the client. One client who served as a research subject in Birckhead's[4] research reported that she had multiple personalities as a result of the incest (see Chap. 19). One personality was "angry," and protested against the incest. When the survivor would become angry in the therapeutic session, the therapist placed the client in a psychiatric hospital. The topic of incest was never addressed.

As stated previously, the top priority in working with incest survivors is to have the survivor describe the incest incidents to a caring, professional care-giver. This is essential for the successful recovery of the client. Other issues of concern during the therapeutic process include depression, low self-esteem, feeling low self-worth, and others.

One frequent problem of incest survivors is their anxiety-avoidance behaviors. While these behaviors have served the client well in past times of anxiety (such as during the incest), they limit the survivor's discussion of the incest. Anxiety-avoidance behaviors may include: dissociation (or a splitting of thoughts, feelings, or actions from the client's sense of will or purpose), withdrawal, silence, or mistrust. Dissociation is a frequent symptom of incest survivors.[5] Many research subjects report "going to a safe place in my mind" during the incest.[4] Survivors dissociate in this manner to avoid the overwhelming panic experienced during the incest. Some report going to a forest scene that is safe, or leaving their bodies and watching the scene from the ceiling to avoid what was occurring.

Many survivors also reported *experiencing the same dissociation during therapy*. While discussing the incest in therapy, the survivor became silent and "left my body," as one incest survivor reported. In these instances, the survivor relived the incest trauma so vividly that the same anxiety-decreasing defenses were used as were used during the incest. The client repeats the dissociation process learned during the incest trauma as a way to deal with the trauma.

While this defense is understandable, the therapist must be prepared to assist the client to progress beyond the use of the defense in order to discuss the incest trauma. The nursing care plan below discusses how nurses can work with clients who are dissociating. In the classification of nursing diagnoses,[1] *dissociation* is referred to as *inattention,* meaning that the client cannot focus consciously on the anxiety-laden material being discussed. A nursing care plan for Jane, introduced in the clinical examples at the beginning of this chapter, follows.

Evaluation

A successful treatment program for an incest survivor involves the client's understanding of the incest experience. Indications of this understanding include being able to freely discuss: the incest itself; how the client reacted to the incest while it was occurring (how the client's life was affected); how the family of origin fostered the incest behavior; how the client coped with the incest; and how the client is presently affected by the incest. Effectiveness of a treatment plan is also demonstrated by the client's statement of a present sense of well-being, supportive interpersonal relationships, and self-care.

It is obvious from these standards of effective treatment that working on the effects of the incest experience is *central* to any therapeutic endeavor between the client and the clinician. Increasingly, clinicians and the general public recognize that incest usually has disastrous effects on individuals. These effects cannot be avoided in treatment by minimizing their importance. Nor is it appropriate to focus on the ramifications of an incest history (such as depression) rather than to focus on the incest itself.

Effective treatment programs view incest as events that may still affect incest survivors deeply, even as adults. The adult survivor of incest is viewed as a courageous person who has survived frightening trauma, and who, as an adult, will take the responsibility along with the clinician of working through incest-related issues. The goal of the survivor and clinician is to heighten the client's sense of self-respect and ability to hold others accountable for their actions toward the survivor.

Levels of Prevention

At the *primary level of prevention,* it is critical for nurses to assess for the presence of incest, thereby allowing for

NURSING CARE PLAN: JANE

Alterations in perception/cognition (50.)
Alterations in attention (50.01)

ASSESSMENT	NURSING INTERVENTIONS	EVALUATION CRITERIA

NURSING DIAGNOSIS: Inattention (50.01.03)

SUBJECTIVE DATA
Client states, "Nothing really happened."

OBJECTIVE DATA
Client states that she believes she is an incest survivor, yet has difficulty discussing the topic.

1. Provide a caring, trusting response while maintaining incest trauma as focus of discussion.
2. Focus on any and all emotions brought up by the client.
3. Acknowledge and empathize with painful emotions, yet maintain a focus on discussing the incest.
4. Allow for and discuss "deeper" incest-related issues as they surface. Do not allow these issues to overwhelm the client and promote inattention. Deeper incest-related issues may include the pain, anger, fear, and sense of loss felt when the adult client was a child.

Client will place trust in the nurse and will indicate a willingness to consider the topic of incest.
Client will become comfortable discussing presently experienced emotions.
Client will be able to tolerate painful emotions while maintaining focus on incest.

Client will continue to discuss incest-related issues even when feelings associated with past incest trauma surface.

a safe environment in which children can thrive. Assessment for incest in the family must take place as a matter of course rather than exclusively when there are obvious signs of abuse. Without appropriate interventions, many families have the potential to become violent. Invasion of family privacy must be avoided, but significant safeguards should be taken to determine when violence is occurring, and to provide high-quality care once abuse has been detected.

Secondary prevention necessitates prompt intervention in cases of abuse. In many cases, the abuse is determined only when the violence has reached an extreme degree. Further delay in intervention can mean death of a family member.

In *tertiary care,* health care providers are beginning to learn ways to intervene effectively in order to restore the family to a more effective level of functioning. There is often much prejudice against the perpetrator. The health care system also further victimizes incest survivors with combative court testimony, with judgmental attitudes, and in a variety of other ways.

A positive finding in the area of incest is that, to some degree, reporting of cases of incest trauma are occurring. The secrecy surrounding incest is beginning to be broken. Some families and incest survivors are working through their incest experience and are coming to an understanding of how it has shaped their lives.

Conjugal Violence

Families in which conjugal violence takes place are typically isolated from others. These families may move frequently, thus keeping themselves and their patterns of violence from becoming known to others.

The couple is isolated at the community level, as well as at the individual level. The victim is cut off from all social supports, including her spouse.

The typical psychological profile of the batterer "is that he has a low sense of self-esteem and he compensates for his sense of inadequacy through the use of violence. Somehow, in his mind, the violent behaviors are interpreted as an indication of masculinity."[6] The batterer may be depressed and feel that he does not measure up to societal expectations of manhood. He does not know how to function in a relationship. He lacks "compassion, assertiveness, coping skills, and control over emotions."[6] He does not trust his partner, and experiences extreme jealousy. He believes his partner should understand him, and sees the world from a narcissistic perspective.

Violence between spouses occurs in approximately 50% to 60% of the general population. It is estimated that three to four million women are battered by a significant other each year in the United States. "One out of every four suicide attempts by women, and half of all suicide

RELEVANT RESEARCH

The purpose of this research was to describe the psychological adjustment of children who had witnessed parental violence, and who were temporarily living in shelters for battered women. The ages of the children and whether or not they had personally been physically abused were taken into account.

Children in the study ranged in age from 3 to 12 years. They were divided into two groups: those who had been physically abused in addition to having been exposed to violence, and those who had witnessed conjugal violence but had not been abused themselves.

Mothers and children living in the shelter were matched with mothers and children not living in a shelter to allow a comparison of distress between the two groups of children. The children not living in a shelter had neither been abused nor had been witnesses of conjugal violence. In the sample, 40 children had been witnesses of abuse but had not been abused; 55 children had been witnesses and had been abused; and 83 children were in the comparison group.

Mothers in the sheltered group were questioned about their histories of abuse. Children in the sample were assessed for behavioral problems, anxiety, and self-esteem.

Results of the study indicated that abused children received significantly higher problem behavior scores than did the other two groups. Anxiety scores of both groups of abused children were significantly higher than those of the comparison group. The scores of preschool children who had been witnesses of abuse and abused themselves were significantly higher in the intensity of behavioral problems than the older children's scores on behavior problem scales.

The comparison group children showed the highest levels of self-esteem, followed by children who had witnessed abuse, followed by children who had witnessed abuse and had been abused. These findings point out the devastating effects of family violence on children.

(Hughes H: Psychological and behavioral correlates of family violence in child witnesses and victims. Am J Orthopsychiatry 58:77, 1988.)

attempts by black women, are triggered by battering."[20] Although cases of women battering men do occur, they are much less common than women being beaten.

The effects of family violence on children, whether abused themselves or witnesses of conjugal violence, can be devastating. The above Relevant Research box explores the impact of family violence on children, and the possible resulting behavioral problems.

Lenore Walker,[31] one of the first researchers to focus on the problems of battered women, mentioned a number of myths surrounding spouse abuse. For example, the battery occurs in all socioeconomic classes. Batterers include physicians, attorneys, and college professors, as well as laborers, construction workers, and the unemployed. In the middle and upper classes, incidents of battery are more likely to be dealt with privately, whereas individuals from lower socioeconomic classes have no buffer between themselves and reporting agencies. Rather than being referred for couples' counseling, in the lower socioeconomic classes the man may be incarcerated and the woman ignored, or the entire situation may be ignored by clinicians and other authorities.

Walker[31] also stated that conjugal violence happens to both educated and uneducated women. Women with successful careers are often willing to sacrifice their career to meet their partner's demands. Also, many batterers are *not* violent in other areas of their lives.

The Battered Partner

Walker identified common characteristics among battered women. Typically, these women have low self-esteem. They believe they could not possibly be involved in a relationship in which battery occurs, because it happens to "desperate women in the lower class" (a myth). They may believe that it will stop once they are married to the batterer or once the children are older. The women typically believe "in family unity and the prescribed feminine sex-role stereotype."[31]

Battered women may also accept responsibility for the batterer's actions. The women may "suffer from guilt and also deny their terror and anger."[31] They may present a passive face to others, yet maintain the "strength to manipulate (their) environment sufficiently to avoid being killed."[31] Battered women may have severe stress reactions and psychophysiological complaints. While they may engage in sex with their partners as a way to be intimate, they may exclude other forms of intimacy. Also, these women feel alone. They feel that they are their only resources for help. According to Walker, most women who are battered have not been exposed to violence prior to their relationship with the batterer.[31]

Battered women are *not* masochistic: they do not experience pleasure from being hurt. Battered women do not "like it and deserve it," as has been stated in one belief system. The provocation occurs because of the actions of the batterer, not those of the woman. The woman's passivity is an attempt to ward off further attack.[31]

Walker discussed why women are battered from the standpoint of the woman. The situation of the woman can be compared to that of anyone who receives negative reinforcement that is not dependent on any specific behavior of the individual. These individuals come to believe that they have no control over their fate. Men can batter women without warning, so most women feel a lack of control over what happens to them. They become passive and powerless, and learn helplessness.

The Batterer

Bolton and Bolton reported that batterers frequently experience "an early exposure to a deprivational childhood environment that may have contained a paternal model who physically assaulted the mother." It appears that "violence in childhood need only be observed and not necessarily experienced for it to be duplicated."[6]

Walker also identified characteristics of the batterer. She stated that batterers maintain a "traditionalist belief in male supremacy and the stereotyped masculine sex role in the family."[31] They blame others for their actions and are pathologically jealous. They present a dual personality; on one hand, the batterer may violently attack the victim, and then in the next moment may soothe his partner's wounds. They experience severe stress, and beat their significant other or drink excessively in order to cope. They may be sexually aggressive with their partner to enhance their sense of power or self-esteem. Also, batterers do not believe that their violent acts can have any negative consequences.

The batterer may deny the battering or minimize it by not "really recalling what happened." He may report that "he did not mean to hurt her, just teach her a lesson."[6] As an example of the batterer's jealousy, he may not allow his partner to leave the home except for a few hours to do grocery shopping. He may not allow her to have keys to the car. He is suspicious of what his partner does, and in many cases he believes her to be having an affair. In one case reported by Walker, the husband "escorted his wife to the door of the ladies' room in any public facility they visited."[31]

The Cycle of Violence

Walker[31] identified a battering cycle consisting of three phases, which vary in intensity and time with each couple. The phases are: the tension-building phase, the explosion or acute battering incident, and the calm, loving respite. In the *tension-building phase,* minor battering incidents occur. The woman may try to stay away from the man, or soothe him. The woman does not believe that she should be abused. She believes she can prevent the attacks. In this manner, the batterer is not expected to take full responsibility for his behavior, and he does not see the need to take this responsibility. The woman denies the significance of the battering, and excuses the battering by believing that perhaps he is under some stress or that perhaps she really is not "doing things right for him anyway." She believes that, if she waits, things will improve.

The battering incidents usually escalate. The woman has no control over the man, and the "batterer, spurred on by her apparent passive acceptance of his abusing behavior, does not try to control himself."[31] He fears that she may become so disgusted with him that she will leave him. He becomes more suspicious of her. She tries harder to control what may upset him. She abandons all outside interests and directs the children to maintain quiet. She becomes exhausted from the constant stress, and withdraws from him more. He moves "oppressively towards her. . . . Tension between the two becomes unbearable."[31]

The *acute battering phase* is characterized by a lack of control of the batterer's impulses and their destructiveness. This stage of violence lasts from 2 to 24 hours. The batterer stops the violence only because he becomes "exhausted and emotionally depleted." During the acute phase, the "man cannot stop even if the woman is severely injured."[31]

During the attack, the woman feels physical pain and feels "psychologically trapped and unable to flee the situation. She believes that, if she resists, the violence will escalate."[31] Some women report a sense of dissociation; they feel themselves split from their bodies, as if the incident is not really happening to them.

After the attack, the woman has a sense of shock and

TABLE 21-1.

ASSESSMENT GUIDELINES TO DETERMINE ACTUAL OR POTENTIAL CONJUGAL VIOLENCE

BATTERED SPOUSE	PERPETRATOR	FAMILY
Delay in seeking medical treatment	Inappropriate responses to others' injuries	Poverty
Vague description of cause of injury	Ignoring seriousness of injuries	Social isolation
Going to emergency room with vague complaints of tension	History of physical or sexual abuse	Inadequate problem-solving skills
Substance abuse	History of perpetrator's mother having	Presence of other abuse in the home,
History of: depression, anxiety, feelings of powerlessness, low self-esteem, suicidal thoughts, spontaneous abortions, injuries during pregnancy, eating problems, shame	been abused	*e.g.,* child abuse
	Jealousy	Traditional beliefs about women's and
Anxiety in presence of perpetrator	Low self-esteem	men's roles in marriage
Poor grooming	Aggressiveness in sexual intimacy	
Physical injuries on: face, breasts, chest, upper arms, abdomen, genitalia, rectum	Display of machismo	
Neurologic signs of hyperactive reflex responses, numbness	Unemployment	
	Substance abuse	

(Adapted from Campbell J: Nursing Care of Abused Women. In Campbell J, Humphreys J (eds): Nursing Care of Victims of Family Violence. Reston, Virginia, Reston, 1984.)

disbelief. Both batterers and victims rationalize the seriousness of the attack. In a pattern similar to that of disaster victims, the women generally "suffer emotional collapse 22 to 48 hours after a catastrophe. Their symptoms include listlessness, depression, and feelings of helplessness."[31] They may wait several days before obtaining medical or psychiatric care.

Most women do not call the police. Walker stated that these women believe the police cannot deal with the tenacity of their partner's battering pattern. If neighbors call the police, it is not unusual for the woman to become abusive toward the police for fear of reprisals from her partner when the police leave.

In the *kindness and contrite loving behavior phase,* the batterer becomes kind. "It is during this phase that the battered woman's victimization becomes complete."[31] There is no tension. The batterer apologizes. The "battered woman is held responsible for the consequences of any punishment he receives."[31] Most battered women believe that they need to keep the family intact. They remain with the batterer. According to Walker, however, "the chances of the batterer's seeking help are minimal if she stays with him."[31]

"Battered women sense their men's desperation, loneliness, and alienation from the rest of society. They see themselves as the bridge to their men's emotional well-being."[31] Walker reported that some men told the victim that something terrible would happen to them if the victim left them. Ten percent of these batterers committed suicide after their victim left them.

The calm, loving behavior of phase three ends with the beginning of small battering incidents. The cycle of violence begins again.

The Nursing Process

Assessment

Homes in which conjugal violence occurs are "closed systems." The threat of violence, or actual acts of violence, in the home occurs in couples that are isolated from others. The couple does not deal with the topic, and thus the assessment must be done with certain points in mind.

Campbell[8] suggested that it is not enough to begin to intervene in conjugal violence when the woman comes to the emergency room with injuries. The "question, 'Does your husband or boyfriend ever hit you?' should be included in the history of *any woman who indicates a close relationship with a man. . . .* One can also ask, 'Have you ever been physically hurt by anyone?' while inquiring about past trauma or injuries." The nurse can ask about the use of physical aggression when asking about methods to resolve differences in the home.

Battered women typically are embarrassed about the incidents of violence and are afraid of their spouse. The nurse must reassure the client that what she says will be held in confidence, as required by law. Campbell[8] reported that women do want to talk about the violence.

They wish "somebody would come right out and ask" about the violence. In many instances, women want relief of the tension they endure in their day-to-day lives.

The nurse should not ask the woman to discuss the abuse in front of her children. Also, the spouse may not want the battered wife to have visitors, so the nurse may have to meet the woman at a local clinic or even at a restaurant if the woman fears retaliation from her spouse for going to a clinic.

Campbell[8] reported that gentleness is important in talking with the battered spouse. The nurse should ask direct questions and model a sense of strength in discussing the topic of family violence. The woman will probably deny or minimize the abuse at first. Even if the woman

TABLE 21-2.
SUGGESTED NURSING DIAGNOSES TO BE CONSIDERED IN CASES OF CONJUGAL VIOLENCE

THE VICTIM
20.02.03	Circumstantial
21.03.04	Suicidal
23.03.02	Lack of direction (impaired work role)
24.05	Impairment in solitude/social interaction
30.01	Impaired emotional experience
30.01.01	Anger/rage
30.01.02	Anxiety
30.01.06	Fear
30.01.08	Guilt
30.01.09	Helplessness
30.01.12	Loneliness
30.01.14	Shame/humiliation
40.01	Impaired functioning of defenses
40.01.01	Denial
40.01.07	Rationalization
50.01.02	Hyperalertness

THE PERPETRATOR
21.02.01	Abuse—physical
21.02.03	Abuse—verbal
21.02.04	Assaultive
21.03.04	Substance abuse
21.07.02	Regressed behavior
21.08	Unpredictable behavior
21.03.02	Lack of direction (impaired work role)
24.05	Impairment in solitude/social interaction
24.05	Impaired emotional experience
30.02	Impaired appropriateness of emotional expression
30.03	Impaired congruence of emotions, thoughts, behavior
40.01	Impaired functioning of defenses
50.03.07	Impaired judgment
50.07.05	Impaired self-esteem

THE FAMILY
21.01.02	Dependence excess
21.01.03	Enmeshment
21.02.01	Withdrawal/social isolation

(American Nurses' Association: Taxonomy for the Classification of Human Responses of Concern for Psychiatric/Mental Health Nursing Practice. Kansas City, Missouri, American Nurses' Association, 1986.)

NURSING CARE PLAN: PHYLLIS (CONJUGAL VIOLENCE)

Impaired emotional experience (30.01)

ASSESSMENT	NURSING INTERVENTIONS	EVALUATION CRITERIA
NURSING DIAGNOSIS: Anxiety (30.01.02)		
SUBJECTIVE DATA Client states, "I can't think what I should do next. I feel nervous. What if he finds me?" **OBJECTIVE DATA** Client's voice tone is pressured.	1. Focus on what can be clearly understood by the client. 2. Focus on concrete, specific tasks. 3. Tell client how to perform tasks. 4. Ask client to tell you what each family member is doing at the time. 5. Assess physical and emotional safety of each family member. 6. Provide reassurance that client is not alone and that she is meeting her family's needs. 7. Assist client to select a method of decreasing tension. 8. Instruct client to lock the room door and keep curtains closed. 9. Provide client with phone numbers to call in case of an emergency.	Client will state her planned behaviors correctly after they have been discussed with the nurse. Client will understand the required tasks. Client will perform needed tasks. Client will describe what each family member is doing. Client will describe each family member as safe from physical/emotional harm. Client will report decreased anxiety. Client will report increased relaxation. Client will provide for family's safety. Client will know numbers to call in an emergency.

does not wish to discuss the abuse, the offer of help is important, as is a nonjudgmental approach. Women may keep the business card of the nurse for months before they are ready to reach out for help.

It is important for nurses to examine their own reactions to the woman who is battered. Nurses may be frustrated that the battered woman remains with her husband. Nurses may also feel pity, anger, and helplessness. It is best if nurses remember the cycle of violence and how traumatic it is for the battered wife to be deeply in love with or dependent on someone who acts in unloving ways. Nurses can also meet regularly (*e.g.,* once a month) with other nurses who work with clients with difficult emotional problems in order to feel unburdened and refreshed in their work. Table 21-1 lists several assessment guidelines to use in determining actual or potential conjugal violence.

Diagnosis

In the process of forming the nursing diagnosis, Campbell[8] suggested emphasizing the strengths of the battered spouse. These women have shown courage in the face of terror and have attempted to perform heroic acts, such as protecting the children in an abusing household. A focus on strengths can increase the self-esteem of the woman

and foster a positive alliance between the nurse and the victim. The positive alliance is in contradiction to the ridicule that many abused women expect. Table 21-2 lists many of the psychosocial diagnoses that may be applied to conjugal violence.

Planning

The battered woman must be included in her care planning. It may seem most logical to remind the client that she is, indeed, in an abusing situation, and that she should leave the batterer. Such a statement, however, will make no impact if the client is not ready to hear this information. The client may deny the batterer's actions, and may not be able to imagine herself without her home, even if it is tension-filled. Campbell[8] recommended asking clients to develop their own goals rather than doing this step for them. In this manner, battered women begin to develop their own problem-solving skills.

Short-term goals should be specific and easily understood by the client. It is possible that long-term goals may *not* include ending the cycle of violence (such as leaving the batterer). This goal may be unimaginable to the woman. Long-term goals may include developing effective problem-solving skills, establishing a social support system, or other long-term goals that are more acceptable initially to the client. Campbell[8] stated that long-term goals may only be established later in the nurse–client relationship, once the woman can focus on a period of time beyond the present.

Intervention

Intervening with battered women requires flexibility, caring, and patience. Intervention is complex, in part because these women may have no social supports, no education, no job training, one or more children, no financial resources, no home, and a significant other (such as a spouse) who may be trying to find "his woman" to bring her back home.

Legal ramifications may exist as a result of the abusive situation. For example, the children may have been beaten by the perpetrator and removed from the home, or the woman may need assistance in filing a restraining order (a court order demanding that the batterer not bother the victim).[21]

In many cases, intervening with battered women involves more than one care-giver. Many women, for example, profit from the assistance of care-givers at women's shelters. Women and their children remain at these shelters until other arrangements can be made. Battered women gain many insights by being around other battered women who are also making different lives for themselves.

Crisis intervention may be an important aspect of care. While working with battered women in a women's center, one of the authors of this chapter assisted a woman in leaving her abusive situation. After an initial interview the woman, Phyllis, made the decision to take her children and leave the home. She refused to go to a shelter.

The author and client maintained phone contact (hourly at times) with each other on a periodic basis over a 24-hour period. Phyllis located a motel where she and her children could stay temporarily. However, she had to obtain funds from her bank, locate a motel that was not easily noticed, and hide her car. She feared that her husband would come to look for her and beat her and her children if he found them. Phyllis had to obtain provisions for her infant and three-year-old son. For a brief period of time, the victim was so anxious that she could only perform minimal functions. She had to be reminded how to care for herself and her children. However, she was able to maintain herself and her children until her mother arrived two days later. The care plan for this case appears on page 483.

Interventions for the perpetrator include group therapy in which several batterers discuss their common problems with violence and related issues. Referrals to substance-abuse treatment programs may also be needed, although the violent behavior should be treated in addition to the substance abuse. Stopping substance abuse is no guarantee that the violent behavior will cease. The occurrence of violence must not be minimized nor avoided as a focus of treatment.

Evaluation

In evaluating the nursing care of victims of conjugal violence, the nurse determines whether or not the goals established by the client and nurse have been achieved. The goals may not be achieved in a short period of time. Readjustment to a new life outside the violent home may take months or even years. Many areas of the client's life must be reestablished—areas that can easily be taken for granted by others. The client may need to find new housing, begin financial savings again, make new friends, assist her children to adjust to a new environment and a new school, attain a new perspective on herself as one who lives outside a violent relationship, and develop new relationship skills. The client may also have to cope with setbacks in life planning and maintain a sense of motivation to move forward again in her life.

TABLE 21-3.
INTERVENTIONS FOR PRIMARY, SECONDARY, AND TERTIARY PREVENTION OF CONJUGAL VIOLENCE

PRIMARY LEVEL OF PREVENTION

Work to change sexist attitudes toward women whereby they are seen as "objects" or something over which to maintain power.

Work to eliminate the economic, political, and social dependence of women.

Encourage full participation of men in parenting.

Encourage health promotion activities for men, including support groups for discussion of how to handle feelings without using aggression.

Assist in the establishment of support groups for women, for both those who are battered and those who are not.

SECONDARY LEVEL OF PREVENTION

Be alert to symptoms of abuse in all clinical areas (*e.g.*, psychiatry, medicine, substance abuse, emergency care, maternity, occupational health, etc.)

Assess clients and families for the presence of abusive behavior.

Assist clients to learn about conjugal violence.

Assist clients to leave the home if they are ready to take this step.

Engage clients in individual relationship intervention to discuss issues of self-esteem, assertiveness, and self-care.

Assist clients to obtain health care for physical problems.

Assist clients to obtain needed community resources such as help in filing a restraining order, entering a battered women's shelter, and obtaining financial assistance, social support, and educational loans.

Assist the family as they begin to examine the abusive situation.

Refer the family for family counseling.

Refer the perpetrator for counseling.

Provide respite and relief from exhaustion.

TERTIARY INTERVENTION

Assist battered women in rehabilitation shelters or mental health settings.

Provide care for the physical health/illness needs of battered women and their children.

Facilitate a group for battered women or locate groups for clients in which they can discuss abuse patterns and solve problems realistically.

Involve women in individual relationship intervention to work on feelings such as fear, anger, resentment, and guilt.

Maintain a focus on clients' strengths.

Levels of Prevention

Interventions occur across all levels of prevention. Much effort is needed to establish resources and to carry out research in each level of prevention. Table 21-3 describes a few of these interventions.

Summary

1. The factors that are thought to promote family violence include: little (or superficial) contact with others outside the family, emotional distance, rigid family rules and structure, low self-esteem, and beliefs supporting the limiting aspects of the traditional male/female family roles.
2. Family violence includes child physical and sexual abuse, conjugal violence, rape, and elder abuse.
3. Violence begins in a family, in part, because violence or abuse is seen as one way to deal with family or individual conflicts. The violence continues because the members cannot break out of the cycle of violence, or because the perpetrator experiences no force inside or outside the family requiring the perpetrator to stop the violence.
4. Victims of family violence experience lasting psychological/societal problems as a result of family violence. These problems include difficulties in forming and maintaining relationships, difficulties in concentrating, and low self-esteem.
5. The nurse's role in family violence includes early case-finding, prompt intervention or referral to treatment resources, and long-term intervention and follow-up to assist clients in achieving their potential.
6. Nurses are required by law to report instances of child physical and sexual abuse to authorities. Nurses can also assist victims of conjugal violence in obtaining restraining orders to prevent perpetrator/victim contact.

References

1. American Nurses' Association: Taxonomy for the Classification of Human Responses of Concern for Psychiatric/Mental Health Nursing. Kansas City, Missouri, American Nurses' Association, 1986
2. American Psychiatric Association: Diagnostic and Statistical Manual of Mental Disorders, 3rd ed, revised (DSM-III-R). Washington, DC, American Psychiatric Association, 1987
3. Barnhill L, Squires M, Gidson G: The Epidemiology of Violence in a Community Mental Health Center Setting: A Violence Epidemic? In Hansen J, Barnhill L (eds): Clinical Approaches to Family Violence. Rockville, Maryland, Aspen, 1982
4. Birckhead L: The Trauma Awareness Process in Survivors of Incest in Psychotherapy (research in progress)
5. Blake-White J, Kline C: Treating the dissociative process in adult victims of childhood incest. Soc Casework 66:394, 1985
6. Bolton F, Bolton S: Working with Violent Families. Beverly Hills, California, Sage, 1987
7. Brown W: Understanding Child Abuse and Neglect. York, Pennsylvania, William Gladden Foundation, 1985
8. Campbell J: Abuse of Female Partners. In Campbell J, Humphreys J (eds): Nursing Care of Victims of Violence. Reston, Virginia, Reston, 1984
9. Campbell J: Theories of Violence. In Campbell J, Humphreys J (eds): Nursing Care of Victims of Family Violence. Reston, Virginia, Reston, 1984
10. Cantwell H: Update on vaginal inspection as it relates to child sexual abuse in girls under thirteen. Child Abuse Negl 11:545, 1987
11. Davanloo H: Intensive Short-Term Dynamic Psychotherapy With Highly Resistive Patients: Personal Dialogue. Conference sponsored by the Department of Psychiatry, University of California at San Diego, February 6–7, 1988
12. Ellenson G: Detecting a history of incest: A predictive syndrome. Soc Casework 15:525, 1985
13. Erlanger S: A Widening Pattern of Abuse in New York Case. New York Times, Nov 1, 1987
14. Fisher R: Abused children, depressed children: They may be one and the same. Child Adolesc Ment Health Rev: Fall, 1985
15. Friedman M: Family Nursing: Theory and Assessment. Norwalk, Connecticut, Appleton-Lange, 1986
16. Gelinas D: The Persisting Negative Effects of Incest. Psychiatry 46:312, 1983
17. Gelles R: The Violent Home. Newberry Park, Sage Library of Social Research, 1987
18. Hansen J, Barnhill L (eds): Clinical Approaches to Family Violence. Rockville, Maryland, Aspen, 1982
19. Herman J, Hirschman L: Families at risk for father–daughter incest. Am J Psychiatry 138:967, 1981
20. Hirschmann M: Intervening With Newly Married Couples and Marital Violence. In Leahey M, Wright L: Families and Psychosocial Violence. Springhouse, Pennsylvania, Springhouse, 1987
21. Humphreys J: The Nurse and the Legal System: Dealing With Abused Women. In Campbell J, Humphreys J (eds): Nursing Care of Victims of Family Violence. Reston, Virginia, Reston, 1984
22. Joy S: Retrospective presentations of incest: Treatment strategies for use with adult women. J Counsel Dev 65:317, 1987
23. Keefe M: Intervening With Families of Infant and Child Abuse. In Leahey M, Wright L: Families and Psychosocial Problems. Springhouse, Pennsylvania, Springhouse, 1987
24. Miller A: Thou Shalt Not Be Aware. New York, New American Library, 1984
25. Murphy P: Searching for Spring. Tallahassee, Florida, NAIAD, 1987
26. Pascoe D: Management of Sexually Abused Children. Pediatr Ann 8:309, 1979
27. Renshaw D: Incest: Understanding and Treatment. Boston, Little, Brown & Co, 1982
28. Straus M: Medical Care Costs of Intrafamily Assault and Homicide. Bull N Y Acad Med 62:556, 1986
29. Summitt R: The Child Sexual Abuse Accommodation Syndrome. Child Abuse Negl 7:177, 1983
30. VanderMey B, Neff R: Incest as Child Abuse. New York, Praeger, 1986
31. Walker L: The Battered Woman. New York, Harper & Row, 1979

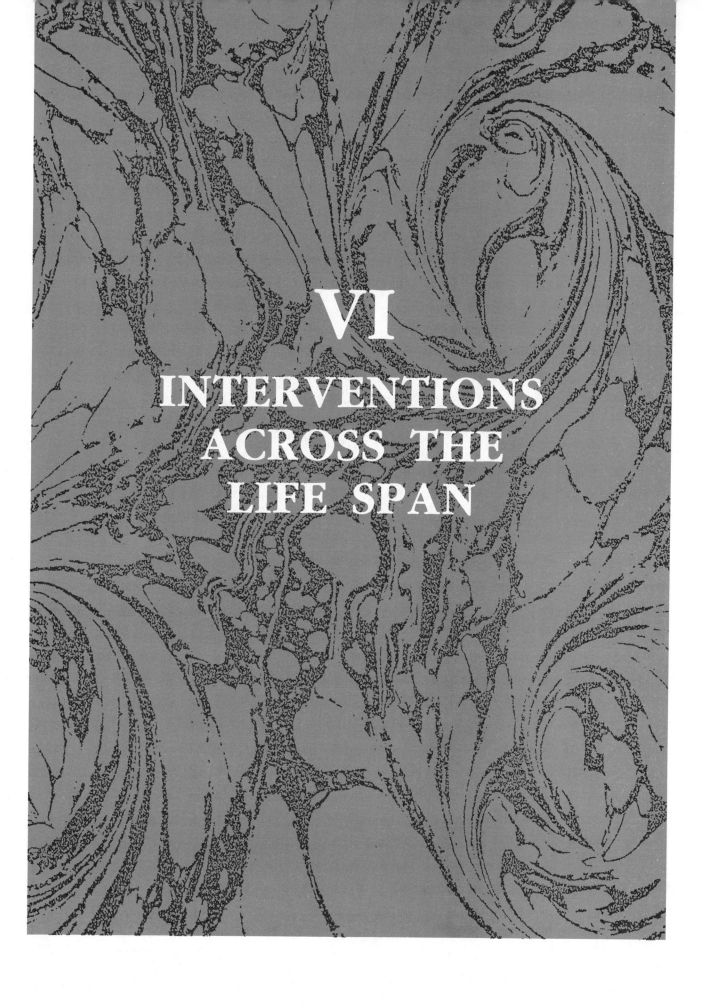

VI

INTERVENTIONS ACROSS THE LIFE SPAN

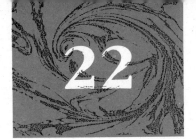

22

ELIZABETH C. POSTER AND KATHLEEN DELANEY

MENTAL HEALTH COUNSELING OF CHILDREN

Learning Objectives

Upon completion of this chapter the student should be able to do the following:

1. Explain how the three levels of prevention apply to child psychiatric nursing.
2. Recognize the impact of various factors (environmental, cultural, societal, psychological, and physical) on a child's experience and developmental progress.
3. Understand how a child uses a therapeutic relationship to change self-attitudes and attain a higher level of mental health.
4. Identify five ways the nurse can promote trust and decrease the child's anxiety during an interview.
5. Describe the key elements of a child's psychiatric assessment.
6. Discuss several of the more common child psychiatric disorders—their incidence, behavioral picture, and treatment.
7. State how the DSM-III-R is used in assigning a child's formal diagnosis.
8. Understand how children's play can represent their thoughts and concerns, and how children use play to gain mastery over conflicts.
9. Identify the general goals of mental health counseling with children.
10. Understand how therapeutic interventions are formulated to address the underlying dynamics of a child's behavior, and describe therapeutic responses to acting-out behavior, inadequate social skills, low self-esteem, and lack of trust.

Introduction

Growth of Child Psychiatry

Historians of the U.S. mental health system generally trace the beginnings of adult psychiatric care to the 1790s and the moral treatment movement, a philosophy that ushered in an era of humane treatment for the emotionally disturbed. Interestingly, child psychiatry and concern for the mental health of children only gained momentum in the 1890s, about 100 years after the start of the moral treatment movement. Even at this point, no classification system of childhood psychopathology existed, there was no definite body of knowledge covering behavior disorders, and there were no extensive theories of child development.[32]

Several factors account for this delay in the child psychiatric field. The first was the low status of childhood. Prior to the 20th century, parents thought that children were put in this world for their amusement and to work hard to support the family.[13] This attitude influenced mental health care because, as Cullinan points out, psychiatric treatment is usually tied to the beliefs, attitudes, and politics of society at large. Because they were undervalued by society, children were denied special treatment or status. A second factor that influenced the delay of treatment methods was the belief that children's problems were small versions of adult disorders.[32] As a result, children failed to receive treatment that was unique to their needs and in line with any development considerations. For example, delusional adults and delusional children were given the same type of care.

The field advanced at about the turn of the century. The societal and scholarly developments that supported child study included:

- *Compulsory Education.* Once all children were forced to go to school, previously unrecognized problems became apparent.[13] Troubled children, once kept at home, found themselves being evaluated by teachers. As the public school system grew, so did special classes to help disturbed pupils and "hard to manage" children.
- *Child Study Movement.* Cullinan cites several major advances in the 20th century that changed the way children and their problems were viewed. The first was the publication of child development studies that demonstrated the progressive and orderly unfolding of children's psychological make-up. Next came the development by Alfred Binet of the intelligence test. Through use of this test, children could be systematically evaluated and some gauge could be made of normalcy and deviance. Finally, the early 20th century saw the publication of the first longitudinal studies of children. Scholars such as Piaget and Gesell charted the course of children's behavior and began to identify characteristics that typified each age.[13]
- *National Committee for Mental Hygiene.* In 1908, Clifford Beers chronicled his mistreatment at a state

mental hospital in *A Mind That Found Itself.* This book so raised public awareness of the bad conditions in state hospitals that Beers, along with other mental health professionals, formed the National Committee for Mental Hygiene. This committee worked to promote better treatment and emphasized the need for prevention and research. The committee took special interest in the needs of children and established the first child guidance clinics which, in addition to providing treatment, led to the multidisciplinary approach in children's psychiatric care.[32]

At the same time, advances were being made in the practice of *inpatient* child psychiatry. These changes can be attributed partially to the popularity of Freudian thought. Freud originated the notion of unconscious motivation for feelings and behaviors. August Aichhorn carried this notion into the inpatient arena, and experimented in using psychoanalytic principles to rehabilitate children.

Since these early developments, child psychiatry has continued to grow. In 1944, Bruno Bettelheim founded the Orthogenic School for the treatment of severely disturbed children. He developed a program that emphasized staff relationships with the children and with each other.[8] His principles of unit and staff organization are evident in the current practice of milieu therapy.

Yet, in many aspects, child psychiatry remains in its infancy. As Rie points out, we are still striving to understand how children become mentally ill.[32] What role does environment play in a child's emotional problems? Is disturbed behavior hereditary or is it genetically determined? As evidenced in the Diagnostic and Statistical Manual of Mental Disorders, Third Edition, Revised (DSM-III-R),[3] professionals continue to reorder their thinking on classification and the interplay between the many factors that have an impact on psychopathology. In this chapter we will discuss these factors and review the current thinking on a number of childhood disorders.

Mental Health Services for Children

It is estimated that two million children have mental disorders that require immediate intervention, and that an additional 10 million would also benefit from some type of mental health care. Yet only a very small number (7%) receive any kind of treatment in the mental health care system.[2] The primary source of psychiatric care for troubled children and families is the community mental health center. The children served in these centers have both emotional and behavioral problems and usually live at home while attending school. The aim of the centers is to provide diagnostic services and treatment, while fostering family integrity and school attendance. However, most of the 671 approved centers are adult-centered, with limited services for children. Of these facilities, only 50 have inpatient units for children.[41]

Children who have severe mental illness and are not able to be cared for in the home and school require inpatient facilities. The cost of inpatient care is high, however, even with the use of third-party payments (e.g., insurance). An alternative is special education classes in the public school. As a result of legislation, schools are now required to meet the educational needs of all children.[13] Because of this requirement, schools must provide therapeutic services to disturbed children, along with special education. Even with the emergence of special education services, children with psychological problems are an underserved population. In this decade of cost trimming and cutbacks, children's mental health services have suffered.

Levels of Prevention: The Role of the Nurse

In 1978, the President's Commission on Mental Health reiterated the importance of childhood as a critical period for the development of mental health, and called for more research and services in the areas of primary and secondary prevention of children's mental disorders.[31] The President's Commission emphasized the need for *primary* prevention of mental illness in populations of children at risk of pathological development, as well as the need for *secondary* prevention, *i.e.,* early case-finding and intervention with children already exhibiting signs of disturbance.

Nurses have many opportunities for primary prevention with children. Nursing emphasizes concepts such as adaptation, effective coping, mastery, and competence. Feelings of self-esteem and self-worth are basic to mental health, and nurses working with children can intervene in ways that promote these positive attributes. Primary prevention occurs in the hospital setting with interventions aimed at prevention of psychological problems that can result from the stress of hospitalization, *e.g.,* helping a child deal with body-image changes following an accident or operation.

Nurses are also in a unique position among health professionals to provide secondary prevention. While working as public health nurses or in schools, nurses are able to make assessments of both children's behavior and constantly changing environmental factors. Because of their access to children's worlds, nurses are able to identify high-risk children. Children at high risk may have physical and/or intellectual handicaps, may be nutritionally and/or economically deprived, may be abused and neglected, or may have a disruptive family life. Examples of secondary nursing prevention include developmental counseling, anticipatory guidance, discussion of child-rearing practices with parents, support of children and families in crisis and under stress, and consultation with teachers and school personnel.

However important these two types of prevention are, the majority of psychiatric nurses focus their efforts on tertiary prevention. They work in settings with children already identified as having emotional distress and/or maladaptive behavior. The focus of this chapter is on working with these children, and on helping them move toward higher levels of mental health and functioning. Although the focus is on tertiary prevention, much of the chapter applies to primary and secondary prevention as well, because many of the interventions discussed can be used by nurses to promote children's mental health.

The Child as a System

During childhood, the first 12 years of life, each person undergoes numerous physical and biological changes. Accompanying these changes are psychological and sociocultural tasks that also present challenges to the child's development. The term *child development* reflects this complex process of change in all areas of life. In order to understand fully the dynamics of human growth and development, a number of theories need to be integrated: psychosexual, psychosocial, and cognitive. In addition, the influence of environment, society, and culture must be taken into consideration. As an open system, constantly exchanging information with the environment, the child grows and develops a sense of self.

The Physical System

The mind and body are in constant interaction and influence one another. For instance, how we perceive our bodies affects our self-concept. Physical illness tests our coping mechanisms. Children experience similar mind–body interactions, but generally express them through behavior. Children who perceive themselves as clumsy, for example, may become daredevils to prove their prowess. Children's reactions to physical changes or illness depend on the *meaning* of the event to the child. A six-year-old boy who is being teased because of wearing glasses may feel rejected and react by isolating himself. Another boy may see the teasing as a challenge and fight with the children who make fun of him.

With more serious physical problems comes the possibility of more serious emotional difficulties. For example, Tourette's syndrome (TS) is a movement disorder often accompanied by emotional turmoil. A child with TS suffers from recurrent involuntary tics affecting the head as well as other parts of the body. These children may blink, grimace, or stutter.[10] TS can be such an intrusion on a child's life that children with it may suffer social isolation and all of the attendant problems, including low self-esteem and poor social skills. Without adequate social interaction and peer identification, they can fail to reach developmental milestones. In these cases, a basically physical problem has spawned significant emotional complications.

Developmental and physical assessments are components of care for all children being considered for mental health counseling. For children who are not functioning at grade level and present a possible learning disability, a neurological exam or assessment may also be appropriate. Consideration of the interaction between

CLINICAL EXAMPLE

SEPARATION ANXIETY DISORDER

In the first grade, Marilyn missed 100 days of school. Her mother insisted that Marilyn was ill, but could not produce documentation of visits to a doctor. She refused to discuss the problem with Marilyn's teachers, so the school referred the family to a community mental health center. After a thorough evaluation, the team reported that Marilyn needed special education, individual therapy, and family treatment. They recommended that Marilyn be placed in a therapeutic day school.

At the school, Marilyn presented herself in a pseudo-mature manner. She was flip and confident with the interviewer, for example, rolling her eyes at a request to draw a picture of her family. She was like a "little mother" to her brother and sister, mindful of their actions and frequently correcting their behavior. When she was alone with the interviewer, however, she sat quietly and seemed fearful and apprehensive.

Marilyn's mother reported that her home life was chaotic and stressful. At this time there was no male figure in the home, and there were few friends or relatives. Mrs. M. was unemployed and the family lived on public aid. Mrs. M. viewed the world as a dangerous place and kept her children close to her at all times. They all slept in the same bed. This family lived an isolated and impoverished existence.

At school, Marilyn was quiet and appeared frightened. Her adult mannerisms masked inadequate social skills, an inability to play with peers, and learning disabilities. She had numerous somatic complaints, and frequently visited the school nurse. Her therapist found that she feared many things. While playing, she often repeated a scene in which a child was in grave danger with no adults to rescue her. Marilyn's diagnosis of separation anxiety disorder was based on her school avoidance, her excessive fears of long duration, and the family dynamics.

All children have fears. By three or four years of age, children are easily frightened by a scary T.V. show, and may be afraid of the dark. These fears are usually of short duration, specific to the situation, and cease as the child matures. Some children, however, develop intense fears centered on harm befalling themselves or their parents. They become very frightened at any separation from their parents, fearing a terrible occurrence like death or kidnapping. These fears are unrealistic, with little or no basis in reality, and cannot be reasoned away. These children are identified as suffering from a *separation anxiety disorder.*

The DSM-III-R[3] lists the essential features of this disorder as morbid fears that danger will befall either the child or someone close to the child. These children resist separation, and experience extreme discomfort when they are away from home. When hospitalized, these children often ask to call home because of a sense that something terrible is happening to their parents. In addition to separation fears, they may be phobic about large animals or feel threatened by imaginary monsters. The clinical picture includes problems with going to sleep at night or staying in a room alone. Their refusal to go to school is often centered on vague somatic complaints. Frequently, the mother believes the child and is at odds with the doctor who suggests that the complaints are psychosomatic.[17]

In separation anxiety disorders there is a pattern to the family dynamics. Gardner describes a close-knit family with an overprotective mother.[17] The mother often fears letting the child leave home alone either to play or to attend school. By her behavior, the mother delivers the message that "you are safe only with me." The child learns the message well, and separation fears become exacerbated. The standard treatment for separation disorders is psychotherapy for both the family and the child. It is important to address the problem when it arises, because the disorder will persist if untreated.

---

the child's physical health and mental health is essential for a comprehensive assessment and treatment plan.

The Psychological System

Adults mistakenly believe that a child's inner life parallels their own. Actually, children experience the world quite differently. Their perceptions of events and relationships vary with the level of their emotional development. Numerous developmental theories explain the orderly unfolding of a child's inner life. Two examples are *Piaget's cognitive theory* and *Erikson's developmental stages.*

It is important to understand how cognitive abilities affect children's behavior and their perceptions of experiences. For instance, an outgrowth of a seven-year-old's concern with order is the belief in strict equality in action. At seven, most children believe that everyone must be treated absolutely the same, *e.g.,* that every child in a group should receive the same amount of candy. It does little good to appeal to the child about changing the rules. The seven-year-old does not yet possess the cognitive abilities to understand why any person should receive special treatment.[14]

Children's behavior is also a reflection of their emotional development. Erikson[15] delineated development in eight psychosexual stages. Erikson's stages are helpful in understanding children's behavior because they provide clinicians with guideposts for a child's psychological life. By school age, children typically have had the opportunity to master three developmental challenges: developing a sense of trust, achieving a measure of control over bodily functions (autonomy), and controlling impulses without excessive guilt (initiative). School-age children now face the task of leaving behind more youthful ways of play and fantasy, and begin to apply themselves at school. The child's sense of enjoyment begins to rest on accomplishments—achievements earned through effort and persistence.

If children maneuver through this challenge, they emerge with a sense of industry. Conversely, failure at this task may result in feelings of inferiority. An example of failure at this task is illustrated in the clinical example below of Marilyn, who has a separation anxiety disorder.

Erikson's stages are only one way to view developmental changes in children's emotions, but they are invaluable to the professional struggling to understand how children's behavior reflects their emotions and inner turmoil. Piaget's theory of cognitive development serves a similar purpose. Piaget provided insight into how children perceive the physical world at various stages of their lives. From these sequential stages, clinicians have been able to observe patterns of children's responses to their social world, *e.g.,* role-taking skills, development of empathy, and emergence of a sense of justice. Most adults have forgotten their childhood experiences. Developmental and cognitive theories provide an entrée into the child's inner world.

The Societal System

Children's development takes place in the primary societal unit, the family. Families influence virtually every aspect of their children. Children's basic attitudes bear the imprint of familial norms and values. Similarly, much of children's behavior is a reflection of how they were parented. Considered here are two important by-products of the parenting process: *internal controls* and *self-esteem.*

As toddlers approach the age of two, the family is confronted by an impulsive (and often strong-willed) little person. From this point through the remainder of children's youth, an important parental task is to teach controls, that is, to help children curb to impulses and, later on, to call on judgment and reasoning to monitor their behavior. How parents teach controls depends on their parenting style.

We all have our own notions about what constitutes good parenting; however, researchers have demonstrated how particular parenting styles make a difference in children's impulse control. Three parenting styles have been described: the *authoritarian* style that values obedience and maintenance of tradition; the *authoritative* style that seeks to be rational and issue-oriented, and involve children in decision-making; and the *permissive* style that allows children to make decisions with little parental influence. Baumrind's longitudinal study of 134 children found that the authoritative parenting style was associated with the most competent children.[6] These children believed in themselves, felt responsible for their actions, and believed that what they did was important. Their parents gave firm controls, but were reasonable in their expectations and rules. These parents rarely used punishment to achieve control, and they considered their children's feelings when making decisions.

Parenting style also plays an important role in the development of children's self-esteem. During infancy, children's interactions with care-takers set up certain expectations about their competencies and abilities to affect others. Children's first impressions of what they are about are gathered from how significant adults respond to them. A father who consistently gives his daughter the message that "you are impossible" or that "dealing with you is a headache" leads the child to conclude that she is impossible; she then begins to carry these labels inside.[9] As Briggs underscores, "Words have power." Words can either build or erode self-esteem.[9] Thus, early on, parents deliver important messages to children by how they label behavior and respond to misbehavior. To build self-esteem, Briggs recommends that parents have realistic expectations of their children's capabilities, accept children for what they are, be empathetic with the child's experiences, and not be judgmental in correcting the child.[9]

A stable, loving, and supportive family fosters children's mental health, yet many families are so distressed that they are unable to provide an emotionally positive environment. The nurse's professional role is to identify these families and assess how support might raise the families' functional level and ability to meet their children's needs. As children become older and become involved with people outside the home, such as teachers and peers, they rely less on the family to meet their needs. However, the family continues to exert a strong influence throughout childhood and well into adulthood.

The Cultural System

As described in earlier chapters, culture is made up of the values, beliefs, and habits that shape experiences. Cultural biases have a tremendous impact on child-training practices. Parents' perceptions and beliefs about discipline are based, in part, on cultural norms and values. Their cultural beliefs influence how parents proceed with the task of child-rearing.

Waldron cites the following general areas that come under the influence of culture:

> The length of time a child is coddled, the degree of security and protection to which each child is entitled, the age at which serious learning and work begin, the very existence of adolescence as a transition period from childhood to adulthood, all are heavily influenced by culture and the stage of development of that culture.[37]

Waldron continues with examples of how child-rearing practices differ across cultures. For instance, the way that Chinese women approach infants as treasures, providing constant gratification and protection, is in direct contrast to the approach of U.S. mothers, who view children as separate from an early age, encourage independence, and encourage children to think for themselves. Parental differences in expectations of children's behavior result in variations later in children's behavior with peers and outside the home.[37]

Families also have cultural underpinnings for their perceptions of illness and treatment. Depending on cultural differences, parents may view psychiatric problems as a result of supernatural experiences, as physical problems with behavioral manifestations, or as results of internal conflict within the child.[37] An example is a family's reaction to their 12-year-old daughter's developing delusions, paranoia, and hallucinations. They believed she needed rest and quiet, not psychiatric treatment. In the father's view, his daughter was "strange," would probably remain so, and most of all needed the security and protection of home.

The nurse's role is to understand individuals' culture-specific values and beliefs. Professionals need to ascertain how parents define their children's problems, and to consider these perceptions when planning treatment. For instance, when drawing up a problem list of inappropriate behaviors, nurses need to recognize behaviors that the family considers troublesome. Behaviors that the nurse labels "depressed" and "blunted" may appear to the parent to be the child's quiet manner. A comprehensive treatment approach to troubled children demands that professionals consider parental beliefs, values, and perceptions.

The Environmental System

Space and family living arrangements are strong influences on children's worlds. For instance, *space* influences a child's privacy. A child living in a crowded apartment may not have even a small amount of territory for books and toys. This is especially problematic because it is important for children to have some control over their possessions. Beyond the issue of available space is the issue of how families use space. For example, it is not uncommon for parents of troubled children to become so overwhelmed by their children's misbehavior that they respond to misconduct by isolating the child. During the assessment interview of one 13-year-old boy, the family reported that they handled the boy's defiance by sending him to his room. It became clear that the boy spent almost every evening alone in his room. He failed to respond to limits, in part, because he never learned to negotiate controls at home.

Another important environmental factor is the *quality of the child's home life.* This encompasses not only the household economics, but also the closeness and support within the home. A child's environment is also affected by community support or, conversely, by the amount of neighborhood crime. Children's fears of harm are powerful emotions. Just how powerful is evident when children enact these fears during play. One six-year-old boy always set up his play situation so that another person was in terrible danger and he came to the rescue. In his play world he was powerful enough to fend off all "bad guys." This boy lived in a crime-ridden neighborhood, and his fears were grounded in reality. However, his fears so dominated his thoughts and play that they contributed to his inability to master more pressing developmental tasks.

Understanding a child requires having some knowledge of *the child's living environment.* When assessing the child's environment, the nurse explores areas such as the living arrangements, who else resides in the home, the surrounding neighborhood, and the proximity to en-

vironmental assets or pollutants. In a hierarchy of problems, these environmental factors may be the family's most pressing issue. The treatment team may need to address these problems before moving into the psychological issues. It is essential to understand the total system of the child and to fit all the elements of the system together when considering treatment planning and therapeutic interventions.

The Nursing Process

Assessment

Psychiatric assessment of a troubled child requires gathering information on the child's behavior at home, in school, and in the community. If indicated, a physical assessment may be conducted. If there is a possibility that the child's problem is the result of a specific disease of the nervous system or a lesion, a neurological exam must also be performed. Psychometric tests are administered and interpreted by psychologists to provide additional information about the child. Before any diagnosis or conclusion about a child's problem is reached, information from various sources is contrasted. How does the child behave at home compared to at school? Is the child violent and oppositional with the parents, but withdrawn at school?

The depth and breadth of the nursing assessment depends on the health care setting and the nurse's role there. As a child health nurse in a community clinic, the RN might document a child's current behaviors, and then refer the client to a community mental health center. In a general hospital, a nurse specialist might function as the intake worker, screening children who arrive at the emergency room. Here the nurse would gather a brief history, document the current problem, perform a mental status exam, and then decide on an appropriate referral. On a child psychiatric inpatient unit, the nurse typically gathers a history, does a short review of the child's health history and physical status, and concentrates on documenting the child's current behavior and initial reaction to the unit.

In the following section, the elements of a child psychiatric assessment will be explained. Various methods of gathering data, *e.g.,* play and observation, are outlined. Finally, there are general suggestions on talking with children and gaining their trust during the interview process.

Structuring the Assessment Interview

In addition to health and developmental history, there are three major questions about the child that should be answered as a result of the assessment process: (1) What is the child doing? (2) What is the child feeling? (3) What is the child thinking? These three questions are meant to organize data-gathering and the observation process.

What is the Child Doing?   With this first question, information about the child's behavior and the events surrounding the presenting problem is obtained. What brought the child to the hospital? What behaviors alarmed the parents or school personnel enough to persuade them to seek professional help? This information can usually be obtained from interviews with the family. It is useful to compare these data with school reports, because the information from the latter source may not agree with the parents' perceptions of the problem. For example, if the teacher reports that the child is becoming more aggressive in school, hitting other children and breaking objects, the nurse needs to determine if this behavior is evidenced in the home as well. For each maladaptive behavior reported, the nurse inquires where it happens (the *site*), how long it has been occurring (*duration*), and how much it interferes with the child's functioning and relationships (*intensity*).

What is the Child Thinking?   The child's perceptions of the reasons for being brought to the hospital or agency for mental health counseling need to be determined. Children under the age of 10 years have a limited awareness of their own mental health problems, and have difficulty identifying and expressing them verbally. Usually they do not express their difficulties in emotional terms because they do not have the words and because their thinking is concrete. They may express their problems in terms such as, "The other kids in school don't like me," "I get stomach-aches a lot," or "My parents yell at me all the time."

Despite the immaturity of the child's cognitive ability, the nurse still inquires about the child's perceptions or ideas about treatment. The nurse might ask, "What are you telling yourself about why your parents brought you here?" If this draws little response, the child can be asked directly, "Do you feel that you are being punished?" Often younger children (6–10 years) see treatment in this way.

What is the Child Feeling?   A psychological assessment includes information on the child's mood. Children feel and express emotions that fit the present situation; they have difficulty reporting past feelings. Although nurses might ask children 10 years old or older about their feelings, generally direct questioning about mood draws little information. Therefore, the assessment of mood is based on the child's behavior during the interview, supplemented by the parents' report.

In this context, things to observe about the child are:

- *Mood:* Is the child's mood sad or euphoric? Does the mood change as the interview progresses or in response to a question?
- *Posture:* How does the child sit: relaxed or tense? Does the child look at the interviewer or avert the gaze?

- *Speech pattern:* Is the speech pressured or rapid or does the child speak slowly? Do words flow, or is the speech pattern retarded?
- *Motor activity:* Does the child play with available toys during the interview? Does the child sit still in the chair or move about? Does the child fidget?
- *Facial expression:* Does the child smile? Does the child maintain a bland or blank expression? Does the expression change with the topic?

The Mental Status Exam

The mental status exam is a formalized and systematic probe into the child's thoughts. It is an important diagnostic tool used to determine the presence or absence of a thought disorder. While the nurse does not usually diagnose, RNs can perform a complete mental status exam if relevant to their role in the assessment process. The usual components of this evaluation include the following key areas:[12,20]

- *Appearance:* age-appropriate behavior, size, stature, mannerisms, dress, physical appearance, any handicaps
- *Mood and affect:* predominant feelings expressed either overtly or covertly. Are expressions of feelings consistent with content?
- *Orientation:* knowledge of place, time, and person
- *Coping ability:* method of dealing with anxiety and problem-solving, types of defenses
- *Thought processes and verbalizations:* flow of ideas, quality of associations. Are ideas presented in a logical order or are statements difficult to follow?
- *Fantasy–reality testing:* ability to distinguish fantasy from reality; nature of fantasy material
- *Superego functioning:* concepts of right and wrong, feelings of guilt or shame
- *Concept of self and relations with others:* relationships with family members and peers; expressions of self-image/self-concept in play, in drawings, and verbally; ability to relate to the interviewer
- *Suicidal/homicidal ideation:* thoughts of hurting self or others, incidents of suicidal acts in the past, any specific plans for suicide right now

Most children are anxious when confronted by a total stranger who is asking personal questions. To help children verbalize, the professional creates a comfortable and nonthreatening atmosphere. The interviewer should not sit behind a desk, because that may symbolize authority and power, intimidating the child. Positioning chairs so that the interviewer and the child are sitting near one another facilitates communication. Providing a physical outlet for the child's anxiety may be helpful. The interviewer might have a ball of clay and say to the child, "Sometimes children get nervous talking to strangers and it helps to hold something while we are talking."

An assessment interview is a slow exploration of children's inner worlds. The first part of the interview is an orientation period in which children and adults become acquainted. A good way to begin the interview is by ask-

CLINICAL EXAMPLE

CONDUCT DISORDER

Albert, a six-year-old, was referred for mental health counseling because of behavior problems at school. The parents were reluctant to see a therapist because they maintained that he was well-behaved at home. However, the teacher reported that Albert's disruptive and non-compliant behavior had increased over the past several months.

He refused to do projects and did not respond to direct questions. His withdrawal from peers had increased; he rarely played or talked to other children. In group activities he often pushed and hit other children without any apparent provocation. In addition, other children's missing possessions were frequently found in Albert's desk or locker, although Albert denied taking them.

While these changes were apparent in school, the parents had not noticed any behavioral problems in the home. Here, Albert continued to be the ideal child. They described him as "nice and quiet and polite." His mother stated that, although there had been increasing marital conflict over the past months, with the possibility of a divorce, Albert had not been informed of the problems and knew nothing of the parental strife.

During the initial interviews, Albert sat slumped in a chair. He frowned and, at times, clenched his teeth in response to questions about his home life. He told the nurse that he was not going to stay in the hospital, and that he had not done anything wrong. He said that he hated school and that the teacher picked on him. In Albert's case, it was ineffective to ask the parents about Albert's behavior. They seemed to have grown accustomed to his abrupt mood changes. To gain insight into Albert's home behavior, nurses probed indirectly about Albert's habits, daily activities, and responses to parental expectations.

After gathering the various assessment data, the team made the provisional diagnosis of conduct disorder, undifferentiated type. They did not rule out that Albert's recent rash behavior was a reaction to his home life and not really indicative of psychopathology.

A *conduct disorder* is a behavioral syndrome marked by a persistent pattern of antisocial behavior that violates the rights of others. The behaviors (*e.g.,* stealing, vandalism) are not just pranks, but are more in the realm of juvenile delinquency. These children consistently refuse to conform to societal rules. Associated features include aggression, oppositional behavior, destructiveness, meanness, and low self-esteem. The category is subdivided into group type or solitary aggressive type, depending on whether the conduct problems occur predominantly as a group activity or are initiated by the child alone. The solitary aggressive type is also marked by the presence of aggressive physical behavior.

It is not known what causes the disorder, although strongly associated are: family discord (divorce), heredity, temperament, and inconsistent or harsh parental discipline style.[24] A more general hypothesis is that conduct disorders are maladaptive strategies of adjustment by which children learn to cope with the demands of living.[21] For example, a child who lived through a chaotic upbringing and much rejection might have learned that it was less of a risk to rely on oneself. Although maladaptive, these children survive at home by insulating themselves; unfortunately, they become keyed on their own psychological survival.

The clinical picture is that of a dishonest child who doesn't know right from wrong. These children fail to think before they act, and lack self-control.[21] Because they are self-centered, they do not form social bonds. Boys and girls differ in the type of conduct problems they display; boys are more likely to be involved in antisocial acting-out and girls in precocious sexual behavior.[34]

Research shows that, in the extreme forms of conduct disorder, children do not outgrow their antisocial behaviors; rather, they mature into juvenile delinquents and adult criminal offenders.[21] Thus, children with conduct disorders pose a potentially serious threat to society, and need early diagnosis and treatment.

ing nonthreatening questions about special interests or daily activities. The interview should not begin by reviewing complaints about the child. The child may perceive that the interviewer already knows the situation, and that there is little point in adding the child's side of the story. Finally, the child should be allowed to ask questions. To encourage questions, the nurse might say, "Many children have questions when they come to the clinic, but they think they are not supposed to ask them. It is OK to ask whatever questions you want."

Children rarely ask for psychiatric treatment, so the nurse anticipates that the child may be resentful or angry. The nurse should be empathetic with angry feelings. This initial empathy with the child's experience sets the tone for the staff responses the child can expect. During the assessment, not only is the nurse observing the child but the child is learning about the professional staff. Thus, while gathering data, the nurse lays the groundwork for the relationships that will follow.

What follows is a clinical example of an assessment of a six-year-old boy, along with a theoretical explanation of his tentative diagnosis, conduct disorder.

In summary, the assessment interview initiates treatment. For the nursing assessment, information is gathered from both the parents and the child. The child's behavior and problem areas are documented, and developmental functioning is ascertained. In addition, the initial assessment interview provides an opportunity for the interviewer to develop a therapeutic alliance and convey interest and concern. Table 22-1 summarizes the type of information essential to a complete nursing assessment.

Diagnosis

The DSM-III-R

The completion of the health team's assessment yields a formal diagnosis, that is, a diagnosis that is placed in the

TABLE 22-1.
THE CHILD PSYCHOLOGICAL ASSESSMENT

WHAT IS THE CHILD DOING? (PROBLEM IDENTIFICATION)
Specific problem behaviors: duration, intensity, site
Typical behavioral responses: at home, in school, in the community
Relationships: with peers, with family
Interests, hobbies
Self-care
Hygiene
Elimination
Sleep and eating habits

WHAT IS THE CHILD FEELING? (MOOD ASSESSMENT)
Mood: quality, fluctuations
Posture, stature, quality of eye contact
Speech: rate, quality
Motor activity

WHAT IS THE CHILD THINKING?
Perception of hospitalization
Perception of treatment
Reaction to treatment
Perception of problems

MENTAL STATUS EXAM
Thought process
Orientation
Coping
Reality testing
Presence of hallucinations
Suicidal or homicidal ideation

child's clinical record. There are numerous ways to organize childhood problems and symptoms of psychopathology, but the most widely used classification scheme is found in the Diagnostic and Statistical Manual of Mental Disorder (DSM-III-R).[3] The DSM-III-R classifies psychiatric disorders of both children and adults, and specifies criteria for each diagnosis. This descriptive system tells clinicians specific behaviors a client has in common with others who have similar clinical syndromes. It does not, however, propose specific etiologies or modes of intervention. In fact, in child psychiatry there is little knowledge about the cause of disorders.

Childhood disorders are categorized according to problems that are usually first evident in infancy, childhood, or adolescence (see Table 22-2). They do not represent all diagnoses applicable to children. In addition to receiving a childhood disorder diagnosis, children can be given a diagnosis from the adult sections of the manual. For example, a child may be diagnosed as having an affective disorder, such as depression. Currently, the essential features of depression are considered to be the same in children and in adults, so the diagnosis of depression is given regardless of age as long as the individual meets the diagnostic criteria.

The DSM-III-R is a multiaxial system. The multiaxial approach enables clinicians to focus systematically not only on the predominant diagnosis but also on related factors that are significant in the client's problem. This is

particularly important for children, because developmental issues and familial involvement are usually significant components of the clinical picture.

Nursing Diagnosis

Nursing diagnoses are drawn from the nurse's assessment. These diagnoses differ from the medical diagnosis because they list specific behaviors that the nurse intends to monitor or intervene with. Nursing diagnoses serve as the basis for the initial problem list and care plan. To formulate nursing diagnoses, the nurse reviews the assessment material, and evaluates specific problem behaviors in terms of their intensity and the degree to which they interfere with functioning. The child's behavior must also be considered in terms of the child's present life situation. For instance, a five-year-old child experiencing an abrupt life change may return to bed-wetting. The concept of "normal" is difficult to define in adults, and even more so in children.

It is also important to assess behaviors within the context of expected developmental norms. Because children are in the process of developing, the same behavior may have different meaning at different stages.

In our clinical example of a conduct disorder, Albert did not respond to the interviewer's questions. However, the nurse would not immediately include poor communication skills in the problem list. Six-year-olds are not expected to articulate problems and analyze daily life experiences. However, the nurse can expect at least parallel play from a six-year-old, so Albert's withdrawal from peers is significant. The nursing problem list might include *poor peer relationships* or *social isolation*. Albert's affect and mood were markedly hostile, so the additional problems of anger/hostility would also be added. Note that these problems are behaviorally-based and, thus, appropriate for nursing interventions.

Table 22-3 illustrates how nursing diagnoses parallel similar categories in the DSM-III-R.

In summary, after the assessment, the process of assigning a diagnosis begins. All materials are reviewed, and the physician or admitting officer decides on an initial diagnosis. The childhood disorders found in the DSM-III-R are the classification scheme most widely used. The DSM-III-R is a multiaxial classification system. Information on development and familial stress is also defined in the diagnostic process. The nursing assessment data provide information on which to base nursing diagnoses. These diagnoses are behaviorally-based, and include problems in which the nurse intends to intervene.

Planning

Selection of a Treatment Modality

When the initial assessment process is completed and it is determined that mental health intervention is warranted, the specific treatment modality and level of treatment need to be determined. *Level of treatment* means

TABLE 22-2.
THE DSM-III-R CLASSIFICATION OF DISORDERS USUALLY FIRST EVIDENT IN INFANCY, CHILDHOOD, AND ADOLESCENCE

DEVELOPMENTAL DISORDERS

Mental Retardation

Mild mental retardation
Moderate mental retardation
Severe mental retardation
Profound mental retardation
Unspecified mental retardation

Pervasive Developmental Disorders

Autistic disorder
  Specify if childhood onset.
Pervasive developmental disorder NOS (not otherwise specified)

Specific Developmental Disorders

Academic skills disorders
  Developmental arithmetic disorder
  Developmental expressive writing disorder
  Developmental reading disorder
Language and speech disorders
  Developmental articulation disorder
  Developmental expressive language disorder
  Developmental receptive language disorder
Motor skills disorder
  Developmental coordination disorder

Disruptive Behavior Disorders

Attention-deficit hyperactivity disorder
Conduct disorder
  Group type
  Solitary aggressive type
  Undifferentiated type
Oppositional defiant disorder

Anxiety Disorders of Childhood or Adolescence

Separation anxiety disorder
Avoidant disorder of childhood or adolescence
Overanxious disorder

Eating Disorders

Anorexia nervosa
Bulimia nervosa
Pica
Rumination disorder of infancy
Eating disorder NOS

Gender Identity Disorders

Gender identity disorder of childhood
Transsexualism
  Specify sexual history: asexual, homosexual, heterosexual, unspecified.
Gender identity disorder of adolescence or adulthood, nontranssexual type
  Specify sexual history: asexual, homosexual, heterosexual, unspecified.
Gender identity disorder NOS

Tic Disorders

Tourette's disorder
Chronic motor or vocal tic disorder
Transient tic disorder
  Specify: single episode or recurrent.
Tic disorder NOS

Elimination Disorders

Functional encopresis
  Specify: primary or secondary type.
Functional enuresis
  Specify: primary or secondary type.
  Specify: nocturnal only, diurnal only, nocturnal and diurnal.

Speech Disorders Not Elsewhere Classified

Cluttering
Stuttering

Other Disorders of Infancy, Childhood, or Adolescence

Elective mutism
Identity disorder
Reactive attachment disorder of infancy or early childhood
Stereotypy/habit disorder
Undifferentiated attention deficit disorder

(American Psychiatric Association: Diagnostic and Statistical Manual of Mental Disorders, Third Edition, Revised. Washington, DC, American Psychiatric Association, 1987.)

---

where the child will receive therapy, *e.g.,* counseling at school, treatment at a community mental health center, hospitalization at an inpatient facility. The *mode of treatment* refers to the different types of therapy available—individual, group, family, or a combination. The modality and level are based on a number of factors:

1. Age and developmental level of the child
2. The role of the family in the child's disturbance
3. The clinical diagnosis
4. The severity of the disorder

For example, a four-year-old boy judged to be hyperactive, with the diagnosis of attention deficit disorder, might not be referred for immediate treatment. Rather, the parents might be put in contact with support groups,

the boy's behavior monitored at home, and a "wait and see" attitude taken until the boy enters school. Conversely, an extremely depressed 11-year-old boy who attempted to hang himself would be admitted immediately to a child inpatient unit, if for no other reason than self-protection.

The treatment team, in conjunction with the family, makes the decision on the level of treatment that is called for. The family plays a critical role because the child is the responsibility of the parents and, ideally, the parents are the child's advocate. Some treatment settings require that parents agree to be involved in treatment based on the rationale that the gains made by the child will not be sustained unless there are changes in the family as well. Regardless of the amount of their involvement in the

TABLE 22-3.
NURSING DIAGNOSES I (PNDI)

DSM-III-R*		PNDI†
DISRUPTIVE BEHAVIORAL DISORDERS		
Attention-deficit hyperactivity disorder	50.01	Alterations in attention
Conduct disorder	21.	Alterations in conduct/
Group type		impulse control
Solitary aggressive type		
Undifferentiated type		
EATING DISORDERS		
Anorexia nervosa	14.	Alterations in nutrition
		metabolism
Bulimia nervosa	14.01.01	Anorexia
Pica	14.02.02	Bulimia

*American Psychiatric Association: Diagnostic and Statistical Manual of Mental Disorders, Third Edition, Revised.
† Psychiatric Nursing Diagnoses I.

child's treatment, a therapeutic alliance with the family, in which family members feel supported by the therapist and communication is open, is important.

Nursing Function in Treatment Planning

Where a child goes for therapy is generally a decision made by the entire assessment team or, if the child is seen privately, by the child's psychiatrist. However, once the mode of therapy is clarified, the nurse may assume responsibility for planning therapy. This is especially true in outpatient facilities in which nurses with advanced degrees are primary therapists. A nurse functioning at a staff level also develops treatment goals, but these are usually suited to the milieu management of specific behaviors. For the purposes of this chapter, the RN's role will be discussed primarily in terms of therapeutic interventions with specific behaviors rather than "how to" methods for conducting therapy.

In planning treatment for specific behaviors, the nurse reviews the problem list and formulates long- and short-term goals. Broadly speaking, treatment goals encompass the following areas of desired change: attitude, behavior, self-understanding, relationships, and self-esteem. The following clinical example describes a depressed boy and his treatment planning. Note that, in treatment planning, goals are written in behavioral terms.

Intervention

Once a child's behavior is assessed, problems are identified, and therapy is planned, the treatment team moves into the *intervention phase*. For children, several modes of therapy are available: play, group, individual counseling, and family treatment. Who performs treatment depends on the setting (mental health center, school, inpatient facility) and the qualifications of the therapist. Thus, a clinical nurse specialist might be the individual therapist for a child seen weekly at a community mental health center. In the same facility, social workers might conduct play therapy groups.

What follows is a discussion of four modes of therapy: play, group, behavior modification, and art therapy. The emphasis then shifts from therapy to therapeutic intervention techniques used by nursing students and beginning nurses. Here we suggest interventions for dealing with specific problem behaviors.

Play Therapy

Play therapy is a major mode of intervention with young children. Therapy is based on the principle that play is a form of symbolic communication, *i.e.,* through the use of play materials children symbolically express themselves. The play materials they choose and the ways in which they use the materials give evidence of children's underlying thoughts, feelings, and needs.[4] This is especially true for young children whose speech is not yet their most effective mode of expression for feelings. As children become more skilled and comfortable with verbalizing (somewhere between the ages of 9 and 11), play becomes an adjunct to therapy.

How does a structured opportunity for play help children? The therapeutic benefit is accomplished through the play experience itself. Play provides children with an opportunity to elaborate their lives. Specific childhood experiences may be too complex for children to comprehend, *e.g.,* living with an abusive parent who both loves and hates. In play therapy, the child repeats these complicated experiences and, through repetition, psychologically assimilates the trauma. The concept is mastery through repetition.[36] Repeatedly playing out an ordeal is similar to an adult's need to verbally retell a traumatic event (*e.g.,* a car accident) until the incident "sinks in."

When children elaborate experiences in play therapy, they frequently switch roles in the event. For instance, a small child will become the mother trying to help a child in need. In this way the child is no longer the passive recipient of painful stimuli. Again, the child brings an excessive experience down to a level that can be dealt with and, through play repetition, starts to resolve the conflict.

The second important aspect of play therapy is the relationship between the therapist and the child. The therapist is a healthy adult role model. Because a major problem for many troubled children is developing and maintaining relationships, the continuity and stability of the therapeutic relationship is extremely important. Often, for children who have little trust, this relationship can be built slowly and the child can then reexperience the adult–child relationship in a positive light.[4]

Group Therapy

In the literature, group treatment of children with mental health problems is variously referred to as group therapy, play groups, and discussion groups. Generally these terms are used interchangeably. However, there are some basic differences in procedures and goals, depending upon the therapist's school of thought and the children's

CLINICAL EXAMPLE

CHILDHOOD DEPRESSION

David was a 12-year-old boy admitted to an inpatient facility because of depression and suicidal ideation. Two days prior to admission he had written a suicide note. David reported feeling sad, lonely, and worthless. David's parents were divorced, and recently his father had stopped visiting. David had made repeated attempts to contact his father, but was rejected each time. His mother stated that this was an important relationship for David and he was very upset over the rejection. She reported that David currently had problems sleeping at night and concentrating in school.

On the unit, David was quiet and compliant with the milieu program. He followed the rules and gained perfect points in the unit's behavior modification program. However, he avoided any discussion of his problems. He told staff that he was quiet and did not think talking helped him. When David did discuss his father's withdrawal, he reasoned that something about his looks or personality made his dad turn away; he blamed himself for his dad's behavior.

David's relationships with his fellow patients varied. In free play, he was congenial and cooperative. In competitive situations, however, he exploded in anger whenever he sensed he was losing a game. At that point he protested that the rules were unfair and that staff was biased. He became loud and abusive to peers.

The treatment plan focused on David's impairment in social interactions, his family's problems, his suicidal ideation, and his anger and rage. Table 22-4 is a sample of how the treatment goals were formulated for three of these problems.

Depression is a severe disturbance in mood. Depressed people feel sad and lack energy; they see themselves as failures or as worthless. It is now recognized that children also become depressed, although it may not be manifested in precisely the way that adult depression is manifested. The notion that children become depressed received serious consideration in the 1930s when Levy linked an eight-year-old girl's lack of emotional responsiveness and inability to form attachments to the child's disruption in mothering. In the 1950s and 60s many syndromes (e.g., object loss and separation anxiety problems) were linked to depression in children.[26]

Debate on the existence of childhood depression, and how it is manifested, raged through the 1970s. One school of thought was that depression in children was masked—that behavioral symptoms such as enuresis, school phobia, and delinquency were expressions of the child's depression.[35] A second group of clinicians maintained that there was no such syndrome as childhood depression—that all children experience some sadness and depressive feelings as they progress through normal development, but that they grow out of these feelings.[25]

A third group of clinicians concluded that childhood depression exists in a form similar to the adult phenomenon. In their report on 14 overtly depressed children, Poznanski and Zrull[30] describe the sadness, withdrawal, and negative self-image projected by the children they diagnosed as depressed. Research tools to measure symptoms of childhood depression are now being developed, and quantifiable support for the syndrome is emerging.[23] However, at this time the DSM-III-R does not have a diagnostic category of childhood depression, and thus clinicians use the adult classification of affective disorders.

Depressed children show changes in four major areas: affect, self-esteem, behavior, and somatic problems.[16] They are often sad children who maintain a flat tone of voice. Poznanski describes them as follows:

> A child with moderate to severe depression looks distinctly unhappy. It is not difficult to recognize these children as depressed. Any smiles are fleeting and quickly replaced by a bland, frozen look of depression.[29]

Because children often have a difficult time expressing sadness, noting their affect and facial expressions is important. Freeman notes that young children often confuse sadness and anger, or they may report a feeling of boredom.[16] The following Relevant Research box demonstrates the importance of and difficulty in assessing childhood depression.

Changes in self-esteem are part of the clinical picture. These children see themselves as unlikable, and they report that other children make fun of them and that nothing they do is good enough. Parents report that the children isolate themselves from friends, and that they no longer seem to have any fun. Finally, depressed children may experience changes in appetite or sleep. Although sleep disturbances are not as common as in adult depression, children do report difficulty in falling asleep and middle-of-the-night waking.[16]

When working with depressed children, nurses focus on the deficits in the child's self-image and low self-esteem. Often, depressed children have suicidal thoughts. If one suspects that a child is depressed, the child should be directly questioned about suicidal intent. Other forms of treatment include chemotherapy, social skills training, and behavior modification to increase activity level.[23]

In summary, *where* children are treated and *what* modality of therapy meets their needs are decisions of the assessment team or the child's psychiatrist. Nurses become involved in treatment planning when they function as primary therapists or when they draw up care plans for the milieu management of specific behaviors. Treatment planning involves conceptualizing problems and then developing long- and short-term goals for interventions. Goals should be behaviorally-based so that the nurse can evaluate whether or not they are met.

stage of development and individual needs. Play groups are usually most beneficial for young children, activity groups for latency-age children, and discussion groups for adolescents.

The aim of group therapy for children is to provide opportunities for socialization, to improve reality testing, and to provide ego support. During group sessions with other children and therapists, children learn to interact with others in healthy ways and develop social skills and a sense of competence. For shy and withdrawn children, the group experience helps them become more outgoing and develop feelings of belonging. Aggressive children can learn to control their impulses through group controls and peer pressure.

TABLE 22-4.
TREATMENT GOALS IN CLINICAL EXAMPLE: CHILDHOOD DEPRESSION

I. PNDI 24.05 IMPAIRMENT IN SOCIAL INTERACTION

GOAL	INTERVENTION
1. David will have daily contact with staff member.	a. Set a specific time each day for one-to-one attention from a staff member.
	b. Begin with short, frequent contacts.
	c. Staff should be warm and supportive during daily interactions.
2. David will view talking out problems as one avenue of dealing with depression.	a. Provide opportunities for structured discussion of David's problems.
	b. Encourage David to state possible ways of dealing with his problems.

II. PNDI 50.08 ALTERATIONS IN THOUGHT CONTENT
50.08.07 SUICIDAL/HOMICIDAL IDEATION

GOAL	INTERVENTION
1. David will be protected from himself—suicide attempts will be prevented.	a. Note any cues to possible suicidal behavior.
2. David will verbalize the relationship between life events and occasions of suicidal feelings.	a. Encourage verbalization of suicidal feelings and life events.

V. PNDI 50.07 ALTERATIONS IN SELF-CONCEPT
50.07.04 IMPAIRED SELF-ESTEEM

GOAL	INTERVENTIONS
1. David will accept staff feedback about his strengths.	a. Help David to identify his strengths.
	b. Foster successful experiences.
	c. Provide verbal praise for neat appearance, success in activities, and tasks well done.
2. David will verbalize his own strengths and how he might use them to form relationships in school, etc.	a. Have David identify his own strengths to staff during one-to-one interaction.
	b. Encourage discussion with David about how his strengths can be used in daily activities and in establishing peer relationships.

In therapeutic groups, children tend to replicate problem behaviors they display at home and at school. Children who have had difficulties in interacting with other children at school exhibit the same difficulties in the group setting. Here, these problem behaviors are confronted by other children and, with the therapist's intervention, problems can be worked through in positive ways.[19] For example, a child who bullies others and demands control of play things will be confronted by group members. The therapist can enforce fairness and point out to the child how the aggressive behavior affects others. Additionally, when children are ready to give up problem behaviors they can practice more adaptive ways of behaving, in an environment that is accepting and nurturing.

Most people have a need to be accepted and to be part of a group. Being accepted by a group promotes feelings of belonging and self-esteem. The longing for group acceptance motivates children to change their behavior and attitudes. The group leader is positive and accepting of children, and for many children being unconditionally accepted by an adult is a new experience. In many ways, group leaders become figures children identify with, and over time the leader's values are internalized into children's value systems.

Behavioral Therapies

Behavioral therapies focus on the child's present, observable behavior rather than on the psychodynamics of behavior or the influence of past experiences. The aim of these therapies is to change, modify, or control behavior. Although the focus is on behavior, emphasizing doing and action, the child's feelings are also taken into consideration. According to Wilson,[39] cognitive processes are currently receiving a greater emphasis in behavioral therapies. Two of the major forms of cognitive behavioral therapy are *coping-skills therapies* and *problem-solving therapies*. The goals of these approaches are to increase the client's coping skills and increase response options.

Much of the negativism toward behavior modification can be traced to the much publicized works of B. F. Skinner, who emphasized that individuals are "controlled" by manipulation of external rewards and punishments. Today's behavioral therapies have become more eclectic and modified, giving the decision-making and control to the client. Although the therapist takes a scientific view of human behavior, the relationship with the client is still important. A wide variety of techniques and procedures are used in contemporary behavioral therapies with children.

RELEVANT RESEARCH

Depression in children is often difficult to define and measure. In order to assess childhood depression accurately, pediatric nurses must rely on the information provided to them by the children and their parents. Nelms's study compares the assessments of depressive behaviors by parents and their chronically ill, school-age children. In the Study findings, Nelms attempts to identify the discrepancies in the parent–child assessments, and their important nursing implications.

Subjects for the study were recruited from camps, private physicians' offices, clinics, and health maintenance organizations. The sample included 80 chronically ill children (ages 9 to 11) and their parents. Of the 80 subjects, half were asthmatic and the other half were diabetics. Sex distribution was equal. The parents participated in the study with their children (79 mothers and 67 fathers). Each of the 80 children and 146 parents completed the Children's Depression Inventory (CDI). The children rated their own behaviors, and parents were asked to assess their children's behaviors. The CDI is a 27-item, self-rated depression symptom scale developed in 1978 by Kovac to assess depressive behavior in school-age children and adolescents.

The study results follow. With the exception of the asthmatic children's fathers, the parents had lower depression scales than the children. Of the 80 chronically ill children, 30 scored above 13 and could be classified as "depressed." When a repeated analysis of variance was done on the mean scores for the mothers, fathers, and children, the scores were found not to be significantly different. Although the mean scores were not different, the relationship between the parent and child scores was significant.

Parents are usually the primary information providers concerning their child's behavior, and therefore nurses must know whether children and parents agree on their behavioral assessments. This study found that parents agreed with each other on their assessment of the child, but that little agreement was found between the child and parents. Parents of the diabetic children tended to underestimate their child's depression.

Due to possible discrepancies in parent–child assessments, nurses should use multiple information sources to assess childhood depression. In addition to its assessment implications, this study also has implications for patient education. Nurses need to educate families regarding depression signs. The difference between illness symptoms and depression signs should be explained to parents. With such knowledge, parents and children can provide information on the child's emotional state so that the diagnosis of depression can be made accurately.

(Nelms BC: Assessing childhood depression: Do parents and children agree? Pediatr Nurs 12:23, 1986.)

The most common form of behavior therapy used with children is the *token economy*. In this system, specific target behaviors are identified for elimination or modification. The aim is to replace the targeted maladaptive behaviors with adaptive behaviors. These target behaviors are reinforced with tokens (*e.g.,* points, chips) that can be used to buy toys or special activities, *e.g.,* field trips. A key to the success of a token economy program is selection of reinforcers that have value and meaning to the child. It is also essential that staff work cooperatively; all staff members must be convinced of the value of the token economy and be knowledgeable about its implementation.[1]

Because the emphasis is on doing, behavioral techniques are particularly applicable to work with children. In addition, because children have specific behaviors to change and are rewarded for change, they feel a sense of competence, achievement, and increased self-esteem. It is important to start where the child is and to reinforce or reward for gradual approximation of the behavior expected as the final goal. A key to success is determining rewards or reinforcers that have meaning to the child.

Art Therapy

Art therapy with children is usually a supplement to other forms of therapeutic intervention. In some mental health facilities there are art therapists who plan, coordinate, and evaluate the art activities of children and staff. However, because many settings do not have trained art therapists on staff, nurses can develop a basic understanding of the use and evaluation of art as a therapeutic intervention. A number of resources on art therapy provide a guide.[33]

Art therapy supports the child's ego, fosters development and adaptive behavior, and, in addition, serves as a medium of expression and creativity. In the various forms of art therapy (painting, clay, crafts, and the like) children gain a sense of competence because they are able to accomplish an activity and use a variety of motor skills. In addition to serving as a vehicle for expression and activity, art therapy can also be used to promote the development of relationships between the child and the nurse and among children in a group.

Art therapy is a substitute for verbal communication, and is therefore one means by which children can sublimate aggressive or other socially unacceptable behaviors into acceptable channels. For example, the use of materials such as clay, which can be pounded and physically manipulated, allows children to express their anger and hostility. Nurses who are interested in art as a mode of therapeutic intervention can use their own creativity in planning and implementing specific activities with children. Becoming involved in art activities with children can be another means of establishing and maintaining a therapeutic alliance.

CLINICAL EXAMPLE

Sheila and Amy were both inpatients on a child psychiatric unit. They were both 12 years old, and they both presented excessive demands for staff attention. Yet, staff responded to these problem behaviors in two different ways.

Sheila was hospitalized for a conduct disorder. She had been aggressive with siblings and peers and expelled from three different schools for constant fighting. She was troubled with serious family problems and was plagued by anxiety about the possibility of placement in residential treatment. Sheila reacted to her anxiety by agitating other clients. She caused such conflict on the unit that intervening with her behavior meant constant one-to-one staff intervention. She perceived herself in constant crisis and demanded staff time to discuss these issues, yet staff attention failed to resolve anything. After one-to-one sessions, Sheila invariably appeared at the desk, needing to talk again.

Amy was admitted to the unit for a severe attention-deficit hyperactivity disorder. Amy also had a history of poor peer relationships; she only played with much younger children in the neighborhood. Her behavior at school had deteriorated to the point that the special education teacher could no longer contain her in the classroom. Amy also had a problem with being alone, especially during afternoon quiet times. She came out of her room constantly, asking staff to talk or play. During T.V. time she was unable to sit quietly, instead asking staff to play games or requesting one-to-one time.

In weekly conferences, staff discussed how to deal with these two girls' constant requests for attention and time. Amy and Sheila presented similar behaviors in their demands on staff time and their inability to tolerate aloneness, yet staff realized that entirely different dynamics motivated these behaviors.

Sheila was plagued by a sense of loneliness. She was unable to hold onto a sense of contentment or goodness about herself. She had little awareness of the causal relationships in her inner world, that is, how feelings affected her behavior. One theoretical explanation for Sheila's behavior (which her early history supported) was that failures in her early maternal relationship left Sheila with a predisposition to depression, anxiety, and abandonment fears.[27] Sheila never received the consistent nurturing she needed to develop a strong internal sense of goodness about herself. Once staff understood the underlying dynamics of Sheila's behavior, they no longer expected her to be calm or especially satiated with one-to-one staff time. They understood that

Sheila wanted a soothing person constantly, and once alone she collapsed into anxiety.

Staff members were aware, however, that they could not meet her unrealistic demands for attention, and that even if they could it would not be therapeutic. Instead, at the start of each shift they set up specific times for one-to-one time with staff. They tried to teach Sheila to look forward to these times, but otherwise follow the milieu program. Sheila still manipulated staff members to keep them in her room, but ultimately began to conform with the program. Staff confronted Sheila gently on how she acted out anxiety by agitating others, and tried to teach her to deal with anxiety by structuring herself into an activity.

Staff dealt with Amy's needs in a different way. They interpreted her inability to be alone in her room as secondary to boredom and her problems with organizing herself into an activity: problems related to her attention deficit. In addition, Amy had few hobbies or things she enjoyed doing. Thus, when faced with quiet time in her room, Amy occupied herself by thinking of constant little requests to engage staff and keep herself amused. In response to this, staff members sat with Amy prior to quiet time and planned out how she might spend her time alone. They tried to help her cultivate some interests in puzzles or card games. Staff checked on Amy frequently during quiet time, offering praise for her sticking with an activity.

The staff interpreted Amy's demanding behavior at T.V. time as her inability to understand the behavioral requirements of that situation (i.e., to sit quietly). In addition, Amy quickly became bored and distracted at T.V. because she often did not follow the plot of a show. The staff conceptualized her general problem as an inability to read cues of a social situation and mold her behavior accordingly. Thus, they would explain and reexplain the expected behaviors for a given activity. During T.V. time, they would check in and update Amy on what was going on in a show. With increased knowledge of behavioral expectations, Amy was quieter at T.V. time.

The clinical example shows how two clients who presented excessive demands for staff time were dealt with in two different ways: with Sheila the staff provided ways to control her anxiety and hold onto a feeling of support, and with Amy the staff structured and cultivated her interests. In this example, we see the necessity of formulating interventions based on the individual, underlying dynamics of behavior.

General Principles of Therapeutic Interventions

Therapeutic interventions with disturbed children demand that the nurse have a thorough knowledge of both the client's history and diagnostic formulation. In intervention with children, the nurse's behavior is purposeful, directed by a theoretical rationale for the intervention, and directed by the outcomes the nurse hopes to achieve. In addition, interventions should address the *underlying dynamics* of a child's behavior. The nurse does not just respond to the surface behavior (*e.g.,* provoking peers),

but before intervening asks *why* the child displays such behavior. What sets the negative behavior off? Does the behavior serve a need for the child? The following clinical example demonstrates how staff considered underlying dynamics of behavior when responding to the excessive demands of two clients.

Interventions Specific to a Diagnosis

In addition to recognizing the underlying dynamics of behavior, interventions are also formulated based on diagnosis-specific behaviors. For example, depressed chil-

CLINICAL EXAMPLE

ATTENTION DEFICIT DISORDER WITH HYPERACTIVITY

Jane, an 11-year-old, was admitted to a short-term psychiatric unit due to her hyperactive behavior. Her parents reported that she was unable to control her constant motion, and asked questions incessantly. Jane had fierce temper tantrums over seemingly minor incidents. She hit her sister and became violent with peers. She was socially withdrawn and spent most of her time alone in fantasy play. Her parents sought admission because they were at "wit's end" in dealing with Jane's behavior, especially her rage outbursts.

School reports corroborated the parents' data. Jane attended a special learning disability classroom. Even in this controlled setting, her behavior was difficult to manage. In class, Jane stood about and did not get down to her work. She was easily distractable, and often seemed lost in a daydream. She demanded almost constant individual instruction, and even then became easily frustrated. During the assessment interview, Jane was extremely restless. She constantly touched items on the interviewer's desk. She voiced her dislike for school and the other children there—"Those kids are just jerks."

Jane was admitted to the unit for a complete evaluation including neuropsychiatric testing, a trial of Ritalin, and being placed on a behavioral program. The parents agreed to family therapy and attended the unit's parents' group.

On the unit, Jane had difficulty in complying with the milieu program. She could not understand the behavioral expectations for given situations. For example, in occupational therapy, instead of sitting she wandered about the room touching things she shouldn't. At meals, she talked constantly, and usually it was 30 minutes before she began eating. She played with the younger children on the unit, often bullying them and taking their toys without permission. Verbal limits were ineffective with Jane. When staff verbally corrected Jane's inappropriate behavior, she would continue as if she didn't hear. When pressed to conform to limits, Jane would stomp away, crying about the staff's unfairness.

The nursing management of Jane's behavior focused on her poor impulse control and lack of social skills. The staff reacted to Jane's inappropriate behavior immediately. If verbal intervention failed, she was placed on a two-minute time out (sitting on a chair in a quiet area of the hallway). The staff's goal was to teach Jane to *listen* and then follow through on adults' requests. Limit setting was always accompanied by empathetic statements indicating staff's awareness of Jane's poor impulse control. The staff wanted Jane to know that they understood how difficult it was to stop herself from certain action, *e.g.*, running down the hall, coming out of her room at quiet times.

To help Jane in social situations, staff engineered her environment to limit stimulation. In occupational therapy and at meals, Jane was placed with quiet children away from the flow of activity. Staff emphasized what was expected in particular situations, attempting to teach Jane how to read a situation and its inherent expectations.

Finally, staff's efforts focused on increasing the range of Jane's play style. Jane was extremely restricted in her play—she basically liked run and chase games.

The staff learned Jane's strengths and built on them to teach her new skills. She had good fine motor coordination, and thus did well at games requiring fine manipulation. They taught her how to play simple card games. Staff monitored her in play to help her with taking turns and following rules. The above interventions were devised for Jane because her interpersonal and behavioral problems were tied to the ADDH syndrome of poor concentration, distractibility, and poor impulse control.

Attention-deficit hyperactivity disorder (ADDH) is a syndrome marked by a short attention span and poor concentration. It occurs in an estimated 3% to 10% of the school-age population, and it is 10 times more common in boys.[5,18] The hyperactive syndrome was first described in 1845 by Heinrich Hoffman. Since then, the behavioral problems of hyperactivity, impulsivity, and distractibility have been categorized under various labels: hyperkinetic syndrome, hyperactive child syndrome, minimal brain dysfunction, and minimal cerebral dysfunction.[11] Because there is such variation in terminology and symptom identification, comparison of research findings across studies has been difficult and, although ADDH is a widely-studied disorder, there is a lack of consensus on the syndrome.

ADDH children are usually referred from school, where the demands for concentration and organization bring their attention problems to the fore. However, when parents are questioned, they may report that by two to three years of age the child displayed symptoms of hyperactivity: high energy level, little need for sleep, always climbing.[11] Once in school, teachers report that the child can't sit still, fidgets, daydreams, and is easily distracted. Cantwell notes that the activity of these children is haphazard and poorly organized, and that their impulsivity often takes the form of dangerous behavior, *e.g.*, jumping in front of cars or climbing out on high roofs.[11]

The cause of ADDH has not been determined, and there is no known cure. Treatment includes the use of stimulant drugs, the most popular being Ritalin, which increases the child's attention span and decreases non-goal-directed activity. The following Relevant Research box cites recent findings on the use of Ritalin to improve social functioning. ADDH children have specific learning disabilities and generally have low academic achievement.[11] Thus, treatment usually involves an academic component, special education classrooms, and specific approaches to help the child learn. The child can be drawn into counseling secondary to emotional problems of low self-esteem and depression.

dren often have cognitive distortions in which they see themselves as worthless. Nurses intervening with these thoughts realize that the lack of esteem and negative self-image are rooted in cognitive changes. Thus, the interventions might be aimed at reality testing (since their negative self-definitions are often groundless) and also at empathetic statements recognizing how bad the children feel about themselves. Conversely, the negative self-image of children with attention-deficit disorder might be rooted in an awareness of their deficits and their realization that they are different from other children. Here, interventions are more aimed at skill acquisition and com-

RELEVANT RESEARCH

The most common intervention for children with attention deficit disorder with hyperactivity (ADDH) is stimulant medication. The poor social functioning of ADDH children is well-documented, so it was seen as valuable to investigate the effects of stimulant medication on these children's social behavior. The main objective of this study was to answer the following question: what is the effect of stimulant medication on the interaction patterns of ADDH children with peers and teachers in the classroom?

Twenty-eight children (20 boys and 8 girls) ages 6 to 12 were chosen as subjects for the study. Fifteen of the subjects were on an inpatient evaluation and placement unit; the remainder were from an outpatient pediatric neuropharmacological clinic. All of the children were found by a psychiatrist and pediatrician to meet the DSM-III-R criteria for the diagnosis of ADDH, and to score two standard deviations above the mean for sex and age on both the hyperactivity and distractibility factors of the Conner's Teacher Rating Scale. None of these children had ever taken stimulant medication prior to the study. Based on a double-blind crossover design, subjects received a placebo, 0.3 mg/kg of methylphenidate (low-dose), or 0.6 mg/kg of methylphenidate (high dose).

Classroom observations were conducted one to two hours after administration of the drug. The subjects were observed while participating in group activities in their regular classrooms (outpatients) or in the hospital-based classroom (inpatients). The tool used for the observations was a modified version of the Ecobehavioral Assessment System (ECO). The ECO consists of 24 categories that account for the behaviors displayed by the children and those directed toward the children by peers and teaching staff. Fifty (10-second) intervals were scored during each 16½-minute observation session.

Results of the observations yielded the following information. Compared to the placebo group, the children who were medicated showed improvements in oppositional (verbal or physical assault), off-task (inappropriate actions), and on-task (sustained attention towards people, appropriate activities) behaviors. Significant effects on peer interaction were seen only in the outpatient children. With more on-task behaviors occurring in the medicated children, peers were able to reinforce this positive behavior in these children. There was a low rate of social behavior from the ADDH children toward adults and vice versa. This behavior did not significantly change due to medication use.

The authors suggest that further research is needed in this area before broad generalizations can be made about the results. Stimulant medication has been found to decrease behavioral excess. However, it does not by itself increase appropriate social interactions. Interventions must also focus on improving the social acceptance of ADDH children.

Nursing can make a contribution in this area by helping to improve the social skills deficits of ADDH children, and thus improving their social acceptance.

(Wallander JL, Schroeder SR, Michelli JA et al: Classroom social interactions of attention deficit disorder with hyperactivity children as a function of stimulant medication. J Psychol 12:61, 1987.)

petence to improve self-esteem. The following clinical example further illustrates interventions specific to a diagnosis.

General Intervention Techniques With Disturbed Children

In a children's milieu, whether inpatient setting, special classroom, or therapeutic day program, children suffer from a variety of childhood disorders, *e.g.,* attention-deficit disorder, anxiety disorders, conduct disorders, and depression. Each diagnosis carries its own symptoms and behaviors. However, there are basic problem areas that are common to many children found in treatment. Four of these areas are outlined below, with examples of possible staff intervention. These areas include: acting-out behaviors, poor peer relationships, self-esteem issues, and lack of trust.

Acting-Out Behaviors

Many disturbed children experience a great deal of inner turmoil because of anger, anxiety, or depression. At times, children express these feelings behaviorally and project their inner conflicts onto staff and peers.[7] Examples of acting-out behaviors include unprovoked aggression, stealing, smuggling contraband, sexual acts, and excessive manipulation of staff. The following intervention addresses acting-out behaviors.

1. *Set firm limits.* It is common wisdom that children may be acting out because they feel unsafe, and if they are allowed to continue their inappropriate behavior they will increase the amount of acting out to provoke adults to set limits. Setting limits is a logical response to acting-out behaviors. For safety reasons alone, one cannot have children being aggressive with staff or other children. Give children clear messages about expectations and the consequences of their behavior. When acting out occurs, staff members enforce these consequences quickly, firmly, and consistently.

2. *Process acting-out behavior with the child.* Disturbed children frequently act out conflicts. Staff members should move the child toward the use of words, not actions, to express problems. Once a child is in a calmer state, a staff member sits with the child and examines the acting-out behavior, the events that led up to it, and what the child was thinking. The staff then explores alternate ways the child could have dealt with the problem.

3. *Encourage verbalizations of feelings.* Parallel with the use of action to express conflicts, disturbed children use action to express feelings. Disturbed children often lack contact with their inner world; feelings are in a jumble, are mislabeled, or go unrecognized. For example, what a child may call anger is really the feeling of sadness. The staff urges the identification of feelings, and has the child sort feelings out and then learn how to label them correctly.

Poor Peer Relationships

Disturbed children often have few friends. They involve themselves with peers by fighting and provoking. Often these children crave friends but do not know how to approach peers or do not have the skills to maintain friendships.

The staff can intervene in this problem in the following ways:

1. *Point out how their behavior affects others.* Troubled children often do not see how their behavior affects peers. A child with low self-esteem may cope by putting peers down, without seeing how it erodes chances for friendships. When the occasion arises, point out to these children how their behavior affected a peer, and help them become more attuned to social situations and relationships with peers.

2. *Clarify a child's perception of a peer conflict.* As Wineman pointed out, troubled children "don't get the hang of" social interaction unless someone explores the situation and puts it together for them.[40] Moreover, these children may operate on a set perception of how things happen. For instance, children may feel that peers are always out to embarrass them, and may apply this preconception to any peer conflict. Thus, when working through a peer conflict with a child, be sure to ascertain the child's perception of the event, and then point out how negative beliefs entered into the child's reaction in the situation.

3. *Help the child during group games.* Some children have particular problems with competitive group games. If you know that this is a child's weakness, stay near during the game. Be encouraging when the child seems to be losing confidence, supportive when the child seems to be losing face, and empathetic when the child takes a loss badly. With your presence, help the child stay in the game, within the bounds of appropriate behavior, if possible. When the child has made it through, be sure to point out progress in cooperating with rules and the norms of group play.

Self-Esteem Issues

Disturbed children sense that they are different from peers. Perhaps they have been ridiculed, or they have learned to see themselves as inadequate. Sometimes, this is realistic and the child has a limited repertoire of skills and abilities. At times, however, a negative self-image is a cognitive distortion; the children feel so bad that they see themselves as useless, ignoring obvious strengths. The following interventions are aimed at helping children with self-esteem issues.

1. *Help the child develop skills.* As Hobbs states, "Competence makes a difference." A sense of competence increases children's confidence and self-regard, and earns them a degree of acceptance from peers.[22] In helping a child develop skills, staff builds on the child's strengths and interests. Teach the child quietly, not exposing the child to an audience of peers. Demonstrate confidence that the child can learn, and give positive feedback on any signs of progress.

2. *Emphasize strengths.* Learn a child's strengths and point them out frequently. Be concrete when giving feedback on strengths. Avoid general statements such as "You're nice." Say instead, "When other kids are feeling bad, I've noticed you reach out and try to make them feel better. Caring about others is an important quality." Have the child write down a list of strengths. This can be difficult; to help the child get started, list some of your own strengths to show the child how to name strengths.

3. *Learn to like a child.* Often, troubled children are unlikeable. Their mannerisms may be annoying and their interactions hostile. Sometimes they are mean and manipulative. It is necessary to move beyond these behaviors and pay attention to more subtle qualities. Perhaps the child has a sense of humor or an enthusiasm for a hobby. By learning what is likeable about children, the staff can teach children to begin to like themselves.

Lack of Trust

Some children have learned that adults are not to be trusted and are not a source of help in the problems of growing up. As Hobbs explains:

> The disturbed child is conspicuously impaired in his ability to learn from adults. The mediation process is blocked or distorted by the child's experience-based hypothesis that adults are deceptive, that they are an unpredictable source of hurt and help. He faces each adult with a predominant anticipation of punishment, rejection, derision, or withdrawal of love. He is acutely impaired in the very process by which more mature ways of living may be acquired.[22]

Thus, to help these children it is necessary first to establish a bond of trust. Some useful techniques to accomplish this include the following:

1. *Be consistent in behavior.* Children who have grown accustomed to unreliable adults need to reexperience the adult–child relationship in a different way. To provide a corrective emotional experience, staff members need to be consistent in their behavior, to be on time, and to keep promises. Being consistent also means showing children a consistent level of involvement. A staff member is not "on" one day and

distant the next. Children should be able to count on a certain degree of interest from a particular staff member.

2. *Establish an empathetic bond with children.* Children learn to trust adults who understand their world, yet children are not always able to verbalize their feelings, thoughts, conflicts, and worries. Learn to read when a child is distressed. Pay attention to facial expressions and body language. Be sensitive to how children express themselves in play, fantasy, and art work. When the staff member senses that a child is troubled, make contact with the child. It doesn't always have to be a verbal intervention—sometimes a reassuring and caring arm around the shoulder is what children need.

3. *Develop a degree of closeness.* Certain children keep adults at a distance by hostility, and others maintain distance by their own withdrawal. Whatever the mechanism, these children remain aloof, not revealing their thoughts and feelings. Nurturing closeness is a slow process. First, display expressions of caring to children. Note subtle things about them. Show interest in their interests. Distant children often feel awkward in face-to-face interactions, so find times and situations in which the child can feel comfortable—over a board game, on a walk, or at bedtime when the room is darkened. Remember that interaction with an adult may be a new experience or a threatening one, and that the child needs time.

In summary, while formulating interventions with troubled children, staff members are cognizant of the underlying dynamics of the children's behavior. They respond to children in a way that indicates their understanding. In intervening, staff members should also consider how a behavior is indicative of the child's particular psychopathology. Many disturbed children have similar problems with self-esteem, trust, acting out, and peer relationships. For this reason a psychiatric nurse needs to cultivate certain skills in working with troubled children: how to care and display caring, how to read the subtle messages of a child's behavior, and how to be of support to a child who may not always accept what is offered. Again, in dealing with children, so much depends on the adult's attitude and ability to empathetically enter the world of the child.

Evaluation

Children are intensely involved with their environment and the relationships they hold. In child treatment centers, there is constant interaction between staff and children. In the quiet moments of a shift, it is common to find staff discussing behavior changes in particular children and evaluating their responses to these changes. This ongoing evaluation process is a vital way in which child psychiatric nursing staff remain attuned to the children they treat.

Along with evaluating behavioral changes, nurses also refine children's psychodynamic formulations. The psychodynamic formulation is a theoretical view of a person's behavior. For example, one five-year-old boy entered treatment because of rage attacks. These outbursts were seemingly unprovoked by any person or environmental factor. However, after two weeks in treatment, the interplay between the mother and child emerged and the staff noted the subtle ways tension built between them until the boy exploded into a rage. Staff observations prompted an increased focus on the maternal relationship. As new observational data mounted, the staff began to suspect flaws in the maternal–child attachment. It became clear that the rage attacks were tied to this flawed attachment. Thus, the evaluation process increased understanding of the child's behavior and also served as a basis for refining the psychodynamic formulation. Note that in this evaluation process the data base was also expanded.

The evaluation process also requires nurses to review goals and time frames. In the initial stages of treatment, staff members pinpoint behavioral problems, set goals for changes they hope to see, and estimate the time required for these changes. However, only in the process of treatment do staff members learn a child's ability to change or, conversely, how tenaciously a child will hold on to maladaptive behaviors. One eight-year-old girl displayed severe defects in her interpersonal relationships when admitted to the unit. She had been so abused and neglected as a child that, initially, staff doubted that she could change her manner of relating to adults. After seven months of treatment, however, she began to negotiate control with staff and respond calmly to limits. She developed close relationships with her doctor and primary nurse. This girl utilized her cognitive strengths to gather new information about how adults behave, and then trusted enough to test out relationships. She surprised staff with her adaptability and, happily, treatment goals were evaluated and revised.

During the evaluation process, the texture of the nurse–client relationship is scrutinized. The way in which children relate to adults is particularly pertinent because the therapeutic relationship is often a reenactment of the primary parental relationship. For example, abused children who are adept at sending staff into a rage are, in a sense, replaying the role they learned growing up. As treatment progresses, staff members examine how the relationship is evolving. Is a sense of warmth developing? Do the staff feel they know the child, or does distance remain? Countertransference issues are particularly important. "Countertransference" refers to the feelings children evoke in adults. Does the child infuriate the staff? Do the staff fantasize about rescuing the child? Supervision provides an excellent opportunity to examine countertransference issues.

For the nurse clinician, the evaluation process holds great research potential. In advanced practice, research opportunities arise from a critical review of both client and staff behaviors. It is here in the clinical arena that nurses will discover ways to solve clinical problems through research inquiries. With a research-based practice, the field of child psychiatric nursing will surely advance.

The Therapeutic Use of Self

Establishing relationships with children means gaining their trust. Children come to know adults through their actions, and trust adults whom they view as fair, consistent, and caring. Developing trust means demonstrating these qualities to children. For instance, rather than telling children that they will be consistent, adults should behave in a predictable manner by keeping their promises, being on time, and being consistent in their responses to children's behavior.

To work with children, one must basically like them. Not all children are easy to like. There are hostile children who use anger to express hurt and may be cruel to other children. The nurse must move beyond this negative presentation of self and find qualities to like. Because these children have learned a negative way of relating, the nurse's task is to discover their positive aspects and, in turn, help them recognize their strengths.

Within the context of the relationship, nurses strive to promote children's sense of self-worth. Children need to experience success. A number of recent authors have supported the view that interacting effectively and mastering situations lead to a sense of competence, whereas being helpless leads to a negative self-image and a diminished sense of competence. When working with children, professionals pay close attention to how they progress in tasks or operate in group situations. The nurse then supports the child over rough spots, and verbally confirms any successes.

The general goal of relationships with children is that they begin to see themselves as accomplished, likeable, and having strengths. For troubled children, such a relationship is a corrective emotional experience. They begin to see adults as trustworthy. They also begin to understand how their behavior affects others, and the motivations for their behavior. Drawing upon the relationship, the children are not such strangers to themselves but begin to make some sense of their internal world.

Summary

1. Nurses utilize their understanding of the child as a system to assess, plan, intervene, and finally evaluate their interventions. The foundation on which the nursing process rests is the nurse's therapeutic use of self.

2. Utilization of all phases of the nursing process is based on an understanding of the child's growth and development and on knowledge of the influences on the child of culture, society, environment, and physical and psychological development.

3. Assessment of children's mental health is based on three questions: what is the child doing, what is the child feeling, and what is the child thinking?

4. The nurse uses a number of tools to assess the child: verbal techniques, child mental status exam, drawings, and play. In the assessment process, the nurse's attitude and manner lay the groundwork for the relationship to follow.

5. Treatment planning incorporates parents' perception of the problem, treatment goals, and beliefs about therapeutic interventions. In treatment planning, five general areas of change are attitude, behavior, self-understanding, self-regard, and relationships.

6. Interventions are based on the results of the assessment process. Modes of intervention include play therapy, group therapy, behavior therapy, and art therapy.

7. When planning interventions with children, the nurse uses diagnostic information and the child's history and assessment data to individualize interventions in order to address the underlying dynamics of the child's behavior.

8. If children are allowed to continue acting-out behaviors, they will intensify their inappropriate actions to provoke adults to set limits. Cultivating controls in children includes teaching them to use words instead of actions, and to express anxiety and conflicts.

9. To work with troubled children, nurses need to develop interpersonal skills such as empathy, caring, and how to convey support.

10. The evaluation of the nursing process (assessment, diagnosis, planning, and intervention) occurs throughout treatment. This ongoing evaluation is especially important with children whose responses to staff and the treatment environment often reveal significant aspects of their psychodynamics.

References

1. Agras WS: The Token Economy. In Agras WS (ed): Behavior Modification: Principles and Clinical Applications, 2nd ed. Boston, Little, Brown and Co, 1978

2. American Journal of Psychiatry: Mental disorders of childhood and adolescence: Research progress on special populations. Am J Psychiatry 142(Suppl):25, 1985

3. American Psychiatric Association: Diagnostic and Statistical Manual of Mental Disorders, 3rd ed (revised). Washington, DC, American Psychiatric Association, 1987

4. Axline V: Play Therapy. New York, Ballantine Books, 1983

5. Barkley R: Hyperactivity. In Morris RJ, Kratochwill TR (eds): The Practice of Child Therapy. New York, Pergamon Press, 1983

6. Baumrind D: Parents as Leaders: The Role of Control and Discipline. In Corfman E (ed): Facilities Today, Vol 1. National Institute of Mental Health, Cat. No. 79-66916, DHEN Pub. No. (ADM) 79-815, 1979

7. Berlin IN: Developmental issues in the psychiatric hospitalization of children. Am J Psychiatry 135:1044, 1978

8. Bettelheim B, Sanders J: Milieu Therapy: The Orthogenic School Model. In Marrison S (ed): Basic Handbook of Child Psychiatry, Vol 3. New York, Basic Books, 1979

9. Briggs DC: Your Child's Self-Esteem. New York, Dolphin Books, 1979

10. Bruun RD: Gilles de la Tourette's syndrome: An overview of clinical experience. J Am Acad Child Psychiatry 23:126, 1984

11. Cantwell D: The Hyperactive Child. New York, Spectrum Books, 1975

12. Critchley D: Mental status examinations with children and adolescents. Nurs Clin North Am 14:429, 1979

13. Cullinan D, Epstein MH, Lloyd JW: Behavior Disorders of Children and Adolescents. Englewood Cliffs, New Jersey, Prentice-Hall, 1983

14. Elkind D: Children and Adolescents: Interpretive Essays on Jean Piaget. New York, Oxford University Press, 1974

15. Erikson EH: Childhood and Society. New York, WW Norton, 1950

16. Freeman LN: Depression in children: How it differs from adult depression. Med Aspects Hum Sexuality 18:206, 1984

17. Gardner RA: Separation Anxiety Disorder: Psychodynamics and Psychotherapy. Cresskill, New York, Creative Therapeutics, 1985

18. Garfinkel BD: Recent developments in attention deficit disorders. Psychiatr Annals 16:11, 1986

19. Ginott HG: Group Therapy With Children. In Gazda GM (ed): Basic Approaches to Group Psychotherapy and Group Counseling. Springfield, Illinois, Charles C Thomas, 1975

20. Goodman J, Sours J: The Child Mental Health Status Exam. New York, Basic Books, 1967

21. Herbert M: Conduct Disorders of Childhood and Adolescence. Chichester, England, John Wiley & Sons, 1978

22. Hobbs N: Helping disturbed children: Psychological and ecological strategies. Am Psychol 21:1105, 1966

23. Kaslow NJ, Rehm LP: Childhood Depression. In Morris RJ, Kratochwill TR (eds): The Practice of Child Therapy. New York, Pergamon Press, 1983

24. Kazdin AE, Frame C: Aggressive Behavior and Conduct Disorder. In Morris RJ, Kratochwill TR (eds): The Practice of Child Therapy. New York, Pergamon Press, 1983

25. Lefkowitz MM, Burton N: Childhood depression: A critique of the concept. Psychol Bull 85:716, 1978

26. Malmquist CP: Childhood Depression: A Clinical and Behavioral Perspective. In Schulterbrandt JG, Raskin A (eds): Depression in Childhood: Diagnosis, Treatment, and Conceptual Models. New York, Raven Press, 1977

27. Masterson JF: Treatment of the Borderline Adolescent: A Developmental Approach. New York, Brunner-Mazel, 1985

28. Nelms BC: Assessing childhood depression: Do parents and children agree? Pediatr News 12:23, 1986

29. Poznanski EO: The clinical phenomenology of childhood depression. Am J Orthopsychiatry 52:308, 1982

30. Poznanski EO, Zrull JP: Childhood depression: Clinical characteristic of overtly depressed children. Arch Gen Psychiatry 23:8, 1970

31. President's Commission on Mental Health: Vol 1. Mental Health in America, 1978. Washington, DC, U.S. Government Printing Office, 1978

32. Rie H (ed): Historical Perspective on Concepts of Child Psychopathology. In Rie H (ed): Perspectives in Child Psychopathology. Chicago, Aldine-Atherton, 1971

33. Rubin J: Child Art Therapy. New York, Van Nostrand-Reinhold, 1978

34. Stewart MA, DeBlois CS, Meardon J et al: Aggressive conduct disorder of children. J Nerv Ment Dis 168:602, 1980

35. Toolan JM: Depression in Children and Adolescents. In Kaplan G, Lebovici S: Adolescence: Psychosocial Perspectives. New York, Basic Books, 1969

36. Walder R: The psychoanalytic theory of play. Psychoanal Quart 2:208, 1933

37. Waldron J, McDermott JF: Transcultural Considerations. In Harrison SI (ed): Basic Handbook of Child Psychiatry, Vol 3. New York, Basic Books, 1979

38. Wallander JL, Schroeder SR, Michelli JA et al: Classroom social interactions of attention deficit disorder with hyperactivity children as a function of stimulant medication. J Psychol 12:61, 1987

39. Wilson T: Cognitive Behavioral Therapy: Paradigm Shift or Passing Phase? In Foreyt JP, Rathjens DP (eds): Cognitive Behavioral Therapy: Research and Applications. New York, Plenum Press, 1978

40. Wineman D: The life-space interview. Soc Work 4:3, 1959

41. Wolfe J: Community mental health center and runaway programs working together. In Gorden J, Beyer M (eds): Reaching Troubled Youth: Runaways and Community Mental Health. Rockville, Maryland, U.S. Department of Health and Human Services, 1981

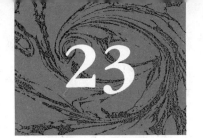

23

RONDA MINTZ

MENTAL HEALTH COUNSELING OF ADOLESCENTS

Learning Objectives

Upon completion of this chapter the student should be able to do the following:

1. Name at least one reason that treating the adolescent client is so challenging.
2. Discuss the physiological changes that occur in female and male adolescents.
3. Discuss the environmental, cultural, and societal systems as they apply to adolescent development.
4. Name at least four of Havighurst's developmental tasks of adolescents.
5. Describe Mahler's theoretical framework, with specific attention to its application to adolescents.
6. Name at least one of the traumas described by Rinsley that the adolescent client expects the adult to repeat while in the hospital.
7. Give one example of a technique that an adolescent client might employ to defeat psychiatric treatment.
8. Name three goals for hospital treatment of adolescents.
9. Name and describe at least two theories of adolescent drug-taking behavior.
10. Describe the relationship between depression, social role failure, illness behavior, and the use of drugs by high-risk adolescents.
11. Describe at least one etiological factor of anorexia nervosa.
12. Name at least three diagnostic criteria for anorexia nervosa.
13. Detail appropriate nursing goals and interventions for the following nursing diagnoses as they apply to the treatment of anorexia nervosa: inappropriate food intake, increase in feeling expression, altered body image, excessive exercise, and staff splitting.

14. Detail appropriate nursing goals and interventions for two nursing diagnoses of bulimia nervosa.
15. Name at least three ways that staff members can better relate and work with adolescent clients.

Introduction

Engaging in therapeutic treatment with an adolescent client can be an exciting and challenging experience for a psychiatric nurse. Teenagers are struggling with many deeply-rooted emotions and issues as they leave the dependent years of childhood and move into the more autonomous and independent phase of adolescence. If this transition is stressful, the confusion and struggling build to a point at which the adolescent may seek activities to relieve this pressure by socially-unacceptable means such as drug abuse, delinquency, suicidal gestures, and/or eating disorders. However, with appropriate nursing interventions in the form of guidance, teaching, support, and interpretation of their actions in relation to their emotions adolescents can find more healthy ways to cope. One challenge in working with adolescents consists of building a good therapeutic alliance with adolescents who are attempting to extricate themselves from adult figures. Hesitation on the part of the client must be overcome to build rapport with adolescents. Psychiatric nurses who specialize in the treatment of adolescents cite two other challenges that face the care-giver on a personal level:

1. As growth into adulthood continues, memories of adolescence tend to become more remote. However, when working with teens, nurses may find that past struggles, turmoil, pain, and/or excitement can easily be recreated, or can resurface. Nurses may find themselves stating phrases that parents or other authority figures said to them when attempting to set limits on inappropriate behaviors. Nurses may see themselves as if their parents were with them, or perhaps how they wish their parents might have been.

2. Adolescents are remarkably gifted at projecting their intense feelings onto nurses, especially in inpatient settings. These feelings of pain, helplessness, despair, confusion, anxiety, and rage are uncomfortable for anyone to feel, so nurses attempt to avoid feeling the depths of these experiences whenever possible. Yet it is almost inevitable that nursing staff members will experience these feelings when working with struggling teens. One reason may be that, developmentally, adolescents are physiologically and emotionally experiencing a spectrum of feelings in a very heightened and stimulating way that is then transmitted to others in their environment.[23,29]

The following box lists only a few of the many and varied psychiatric nursing diagnoses adolescent clients may have.

In understanding these phenomena of adolescence, it becomes quite clear why adolescent clients can be so emotionally challenging, producing uncomfortable feelings within the therapeutic care-giver. Recognizing these feelings within themselves is a very important first step for nurses. To listen truly and offer support effectively, it is essential to remember and understand past experiences and feelings, but in a nonjudgmental and nonbiased way. If a staff member had a very rough or difficult adolescent developmental period, and experiences a barrage of intense emotions, the staff member should seek supervision and/or individual psychotherapy to understand better how these inner emotions may be affecting the level of nursing care and empathy delivered to clients. Rather than avoid working with teens altogether, the staff member may gain newly derived insight from self-exploration that could, in fact, facilitate becoming a very gifted clinician with adolescents.

The Adolescent as a System

To obtain a clear picture of the intrapsychic world of the adolescent client, a systems theoretical approach can be applied. As defined in previous chapters of this text, general systems theory is a useful construct in analyzing the dimensions of the ever changing adolescent's body, mind, and emotions in relation to the world at large. Aside from the first year of human life, probably no other period of development involves such a surge of hormonal, emotional, physiological, familial, societal, cultural, and psychological experiences as does the period of adolescence.

In the following sections, the systems components of the adolescent will be discussed. It is understood that the adolescent period covers the ages from 12 to 18 years.

The Physical System

The developmental phase of adolescence begins with the emergence of the secondary sexual characteristics, also known as puberty. These physiological changes appear to be the result of rapid level rises of two hormones,

PSYCHIATRIC NURSING DIAGNOSES FOR ADOLESCENTS

11. Alterations in Elimination
    11.99 Alterations in elimination NOS (not otherwise specified)
14. Alterations in Nutrition/Metabolism
    14.01 Less than body requires
        14.01.01 Anorexia
    14.02 More than body requires
        14.02.01 Bulimia
17. Alterations in Reproductive/Sexual Functioning
        17.01.01 Amenorrhea
        17.01.07 Unwanted pregnancy
21. Alterations in Conduct/Impulse Control
    21.03 Aggression/violence toward self
        21.03.03 Substance abuse
        21.03.04 Suicidal
    21.07 Age-inappropriate behavior
        21.07.01 Pseudomature behavior
        21.07.02 Regressed behavior
23. Alterations in Role Performance
    23.01 Impaired family role
        23.01.01 Dependence deficit
        23.01.02 Dependence excess
        23.01.03 Enmeshment
        23.01.04 Role loss/disengagement
        23.01.05 Role reversal
    23.02 Impaired social/leisure role
        23.02.01 Withdrawal/social isolation
    23.03 Impaired work role (play/academic/occupational)
        23.03.01 Dependence
        23.03.02 Lack of direction
        23.03.03 Overachievement
        23.03.04 Truancy
        23.03.05 Underachievement
24. Alterations in Self-Care
    24.05 Impairment in solitude/social interaction
30. Excess of or Deficit in Dominant Emotions
    30.01 Impaired emotional experience
        30.01.09 Helplessness
        30.01.14 Shame/humiliation
50. Alterations in Perception/Cognition
    50.06 Alterations in perception
        50.06.05 Impaired self-awareness
    50.07 Alterations in self-concept
        50.07.01 Impaired body image

(American Nurses' Association: Taxonomy for the Classification of Human Responses of Concern for Psychiatric/Mental Health Nursing Practice. Kansas City, Missouri, American Nurses' Association, 1986.)

follicle-stimulating hormone (FSH) and luteinizing hormone (LH), along with increasing levels of 17 ketosteroids.[38] In males, a higher level of androgen hormones including testosterone, is produced, while in females, estrogen hormones, including estrogen and progesterone, are produced at higher levels. As a result of increased production of these hormones, the following physiological changes occur:

In males: (a) increase in the size of testicles and penis; (b) growth of pubic hair, along with underarm, chest, and facial hair; (c) active production of spermatozoa leading to the first experience of ejaculation through masturbation or wet dreams; (d) increased muscle growth and height; (e) change in the larynx, leading to gradual deepening of the voice

In females: (a) increase in size of breasts, uterus, and external genitalia; (b) growth of pubic hair, with a minimal amount of underarm and facial hair; (c) beginning of vaginal secretions; (d) onset of the menstrual period, which tends to be very irregular at first but slowly regulates to a 25- to 30-day cycle; (e) muscle growth, along with weight gain and height increases

Sexual preoccupation, acne, concerns about body appearance, first infatuation, and, with some adolescents, first sexual experience are all common events before the teen years have ended. Some uncommon physical problems that can occur are severe weight-related issues, such as obesity or self-starvation (called *anorexia nervosa*), hormonal imbalances that can cause delayed growth, painful ejaculation and/or menstruation, urinary tract infections, vaginal infections, mononucleosis, anemia, and, with intercourse experimentation, venereal disease and pregnancy.

The Psychological System

In briefly describing the physiological changes occurring in the adolescent, it is easy to feel overwhelmed in remembering adolescent times, and wonder how we made it to where we are now. The processing of all the conflicts and turmoil of each part of the system falls ultimately on the psychological system within the adolescent. More specifically, the *ego* acts as a moderator of all stress and conflict.

Havighurst[22] summarizes the eight major developmental tasks that the adolescent must complete during this maturational time period:

1. Emotional independence of parents
2. Acceptance of one's physique, thereby effectively using the body
3. Achievement of mature peer relationships
4. Achievement of socially responsible behavior
5. Acquisition of a set of values
6. Preparation for an economic career
7. Preparation for marriage and family life
8. Achievement of feminine/masculine social roles

In Chapter 6, Sullivan's five stages of development are presented. His stages focus on the interpersonal struggle of adolescence, that of achieving intimacy with the peers of both the same and the opposite sex. However, what Sullivan does not expand upon fully is the need for intimacy and role modeling on the part of the family, as well as the incorporation of a successful separation and individuation. To understand fully the psychological conflicts and turmoil that the adolescent faces, an object-relations view of familial dynamics must be employed. Of all the object-relations theories, Mahler's detailed psychological theory of separation–individuation, published in 1968,[33] is still a highly-regarded classic. To understand how Mahler's theory can be applied to adolescents, a quick review will be presented.

In 1968, psychoanalyst Margaret S. Mahler published a psychological theory of separation–individuation that specifically outlined a developmental sequence of phases through which infants and children progress.[33] In essence, the theory describes the process by which a person learns to differentiate experiences related to a sense of self from those related to a sense of another.

Adolescent theorists propose that, if this original separation–individuation process is not fully completed, similar difficulties will occur at the time of adolescence. In particular, children who suffered a *major loss* or trauma during their first years of life tend to have marked disturbances at the adolescent development level.

Mahler's theory of child development was based on recorded observations of emotionally disturbed and normal infants and children, and their mothers. The central theme of Mahler's theory revolved around the hypothesis that an individual's current psychological functioning has its origin within the original interpersonal relationship between the mother and the child.[33,34]

Mahler's separation–individuation process takes place between the ages of 4 months and 36 months. *Separation* refers to the child's movement out of a symbiotic (oneness) fusion with the mother. *Individuation* consists of the child's development of unique and special characteristics.[33] Mahler views separation and individuation as two complementary, but not identical, developmental intrapsychic processes that reverberate through the lifecycle. Her theory suggests that this process always remains active, and that derivatives of this first separation–individuation attempt are noted in all new phases of the lifecycle.[33]

During adolescence, a second phase of ego maturation occurs, similar in degree to the maturation of the ego described during earlier childhood. *Regression,* a coping mechanism whereby a person reverts to an earlier pattern of behavior, occurs naturally at this developmental time.[33] The growing adolescent once again comes into contact with the earlier infantile emotional experience of separation–individuation. At this time, the individual who has successfully completed the previous growth process can successfully alter the irrationalities of the child mentality in the achievement of a higher, more developed ego. In essence, the previously powerful and dependent child–parent dyad, essential for child growth and development, dies to enable the teenager to meet the tasks and conflicts of this new developmental period.[3]

Even in optimal circumstances, this is a very difficult time period of tension, struggling, and confusion for adolescents as well as for parents. Ultimately however, the child–parent dyad changes toward a more mutually satisfying and symmetrically equivalent adult–adult relationship.

In adolescents who were unable to resolve the first separation–individuation process adaptively, this developmental time period becomes an overwhelming and taxing stressor. In general, adolescents who have experienced little satisfaction from their childhood, who have become isolative and lack meaningful relationships, as well as those who function ineffectively with environmental or intrinsic stress, are unable to cope with the pressure to separate from parents.[37] Their inner conflicts and struggles may be expressed through behavior that is problematic enough to direct them to inpatient residential facilities for help.

The disturbed adolescent presents in one of two impaired developmental ways on the inpatient adolescent service. These are general psychological categories based on separation–individuation difficulty with parents and/or fixations (an overfocus on early developmental tasks) that surfaces prior to admission.

The first category encompasses the child who was never able to experience a satisfactory symbiosis, and thus has had very little psychic or emotional integration.[23] The original psychological mechanisms are presumed to have gone awry. The early history usually contains faulty or traumatic interpersonal contact that ultimately led to some form of withdrawal, fragmentation, or decompensation by the infant. With the pressures of adolescence, these teenagers experience a severe breakdown of their mental state leading to some form of psychotic, schizophrenic, or otherwise mentally incongruent functioning.

The second category accounts for situations during the early symbiotic relationship when the child never had the opportunity to become completely independent from the mother. If a mother was unable to allow for the separation–individuation of the toddler, chances for an adolescent to complete the task are minimal. The adolescent experiences the separation as a loss of a part of the self, an abandonment of the magnitude of death.[37] Initially, a clinging to the lost object, in the expression of a reunion, helps defend against the overwhelming feelings. Ultimately, the clinging fails to provide a strong enough defense and a major depression ensues. The onslaught of rage, despair, and hopelessness are of such an intense nature that these teenagers attempt to defend themselves further by acting out (drug use, sexual promiscuity, aggression, truancy) or by manifesting other maladaptive defenses (obsessive–compulsive or schizoid behaviors) that protect them from the despair and abandonment experience.[37] These adolescents are generally classified as manifesting the criteria for Borderline Personality Disorder (see Chap. 19).[9,35,37]

The Societal System

Based on the importance of peer relationships during adolescence, the societal system of the teen is quite large. It exerts substantial pressure that can be positive, facilitating growth into young adulthood, or negative, fostering maladaptive coping skills and unhealthy relationships.

Erikson's psychosocial theory of personality development was previously described in Chapter 7. To summarize, the developmental task of adolescence is the struggle between identity and role confusion. *Identity* can be defined as the integration of past identifications with significant role models and authority figures,[17] and the acquisition of a set of values and, therefore, a personal ideology.[22] Both of these help adolescents decide who they are and what they believe. *Role* can be defined as "the structurally given demands, including norms, expectations, responsibility, and taboos, associated with a given social position."[12]

The majority of adolescents, faced with stress surrounding the psychological and social conflicts of this developmental period, do cope appropriately and formulate a socially acceptable role as they enter young adulthood. However, many adolescents do not tolerate the stress of this developmental period, and choose alternative means of decreasing stress. Rather than engaging in socially acceptable behaviors, some adolescents move toward a negative peer group and engage in socially inappropriate behaviors such as vandalism, theft, aggression, and drug abuse.[28] In doing so, these adolescents do not complete their psychological tasks and, therefore, acquire what Erikson calls a "negative identity" in society, a sign of social failure. Erikson[17] further elaborates by stating that "young people, driven into the extreme of their condition, may find a greater sense of identity in being withdrawn or delinquent than in anything society has to offer." From a sociological perspective, troubled adolescents put energy into becoming what the careless community expects them to be. An example of this concept is the presence of "punk rocker" and "heavy metalist" lookalikes in our adolescent population today. Burr[7] coined the phrase "ideologies of despair," and hypothesized that the two adolescent groups he studied in England, the punks and the skinheads, use very self-destructive drugs (barbiturates) along with their clothing and violent outbreaks to express their inculcated negative values in the form of outlandish social protest.

In understanding the societal factors, we must not underestimate the importance of the family as a major social pressure. Although the attachment to peers is a very prominent force for teens, the attitudes, limit-setting capabilities, and understanding that parents can maintain are also crucial to the formation of an identity and a role in society. Family theorists agree that families must change their definition of themselves and their roles toward adolescents to allow for the process of separation and individuation to occur fully. Although the process may be turbulent, stressful, and at times painful, the majority of families with adolescents can allow a successful separation to occur, and a new and more mature relationship with their growing and maturing adolescent ensues. However, in some cases, a maladaptive separation–individuation begins and is never fully completed. This can cause pain and anger, and can continue indefinitely. It is not surprising that the majority of drugs abused by adolescents are pain killers (marijuana, alcohol, barbiturates, and cocaine), and that those who use them have the least ability to tolerate pain and/or anxiety.[47] It is also not surprising that the accelerating divorce rate in the United States,[36] has closely paralleled the rise in drug use among adolescents.[42]

The Cultural System

Similar to environmental factors, cultural aspects also appear to be in the background during adolescence. Values imposed upon growing adolescents by their parents may or may not have a significant effect on their growth. Adolescents who agree with their home life and cultural values may seek similar racial and religious same-sex and opposite-sex friends, while adolescents who need to rebel dramatically against their families may purposefully seek different racial and/or religious friends to flaunt in front of their families in order to anger or hurt them.

Most attitudes that growing adolescents adopt reflect their own personal experiences with members of differing cultures and religions in their association either with peers in school or with teachers and administrators who make up the culture of their communities.

The Environmental System

Although some adolescents choose to become interested in their environment on political and/or societal levels, to the majority the state of the environment is of little importance compared to the other impending stressors that need confrontation and resolution. One obvious area of environmental impact on the growing teen is the effect of the condition of the immediate area surrounding the adolescent's home and school. Using this assumption, the presence or absence of factors such as gangs, graffiti, drugs, delinquency, and environmental attitudes will have strong effects on the development of the adolescent. If there is a permissive atmosphere, drug and gang activities in the form of delinquent acts will be highly visible. If there is a strong negative atmosphere regarding drugs, gangs, and delinquency, the adolescent most likely will subscribe to those negative values.

Another major environmental concern that appears to be affecting teens is the threat of nuclear war. Adults need to be careful not to express apathy to adolescents. Adolescents are quick to absorb apathetic attitudes, and can become withdrawn and angry. They may look for chemical means to feel better in the form of legal and illegal drugs.

Hospitalization

Why is treating adolescent clients so demanding, frustrating, and difficult? Rinsley[49] describes what he terms the *adolescent position,* which treatment team members need to understand in order to be able to break down the known defense mechanisms and resistances. Included in the adolescent position are various formed expectations and behaviors that confront the treatment team during the early phases of treatment. These are:

1. When adolescents are psychiatrically hospitalized, they must confront the reason for hospitalization. In doing so, they need to consider whether they are, in fact, "mentally sick," a horrible and frightening thought.

2. Because the treatment team is composed entirely of adults, adolescents must overcome the fantasy, and for some the past proven reality, that adults *cannot* understand them.

3. It can be assumed that the traumas in the lives of hospitalized adolescents were caused by adult figures. Adolescents fear that new adult treatment team figures will repeat these traumas. The three major traumas identified by Rinsley[49] are:

   "a. The adult will retaliate punitively and hurt him/her

   b. The adult will reject and/or abandon him/her

   c. The adult will prove that s/he is not perfect, blameless, omnipotent, or omniscient, qualities which adolescents desperately want to believe, yet protest against. . . ."

4. When these traumas did occur, it is most likely that they were inflicted by the adolescents' parents. These adolescents can be expected to project these features onto the treatment team members in the form of a heightened transference that needs to be understood and analyzed.[49]

5. Adolescents will struggle to prevent these traumas from occurring again. The major way to protect themselves is through refusing to engage in the treatment and/or therapeutic relationships. Rinsley calls this resistance the adolescent's attempt to "defeat the structure of the hospital."[49]

Of the many ways of defeating the hospital structure that Rinsley summarizes, a few are very apparent, and worth mentioning here. They are the classic mechanisms that the majority of adolescents will employ:

1. *Leveling:* Adolescents will attempt to diminish the importance of therapeutic adults by minimizing their position and approaching the staff as peers rather than as authority figures.

2. *Scapegoating:* Adolescents will subtly or covertly provoke a more disorganized or impulsive peer to act out and divert the staff's attention from the resistant adolescent onto the peer who is acting out. The adolescent thus avoids therapeutic contact, and forces staff attention to be diverted.

3. *Seductive behavior* or *flirtatiousness:* In confronting their own sexual urges and feelings, which are often frightening, teens will become very flirtatious with staff of the opposite sex. They may sometimes make very blunt sexual statements and advances. This is most common with teens who have a history of having been sexually abused as children or early adolescents.

For teenagers who are frightened of becoming individuated and separated, hospitalization poses a major threat to their psychological being. Hospitalization enforces a major and sudden separation from their families, school system, peer group, and society. The issues and conflicts regarding separation–individuation must be recognized, addressed, and allowed to be resolved throughout the entire management of treatment. It is suggested that, although individual psychotherapy is the most powerful change agent, the milieu setting provides the basis for meaningful therapy.[43] The staff members supply the many ego functions that the adolescents are unable to provide for themselves. Ultimately, as the teenagers begin to grow and change, these functions are reclaimed by the clients and incorporated into their personality structure. To encourage this type of internalization effectively, it is essential that staff show empathetic and positive interactions while setting limits and providing external boundaries that are crucial for this age group.[32]

The Therapeutic Use of Self

It is crucial in therapeutic interactions with adolescent clients that staff members appear real and authentic. Adolescents who are fearful and hesitant in interactions with adults can accurately assess a staff member's interest, concern, and/or honesty quite quickly. In attempting to nurture clients and move them to uncover themselves, it is important for staff members to know their own selves, including their shortcomings. Adolescents are incredibly gifted at pointing out adults' shortcomings to them. If staff members react with concern or are offended, adolescent clients remember the weak point and continue to use it to defeat the power of the therapy and the relationship with the adult.

Given the issues of separation and individuation with which the adolescent client now struggles, it is essential that staff members maintain and enforce the therapeutic boundary between the client as Self and the staff as Other. Staff must role model the importance of maintaining boundaries of personal space and emotional attachment to avoid enmeshment and fusion. This is not easy, since it certainly did not occur in these clients' earlier development. Yet, to truly experience attachment and intimacy, as described in Chapter 7, it is crucial that boundaries of differentiation be maintained for a healthy therapeutic relationship to ensue. With the maintenance of the boundary, trust and respect will develop between client and staff, thereby promoting the working phase of treatment in which growth and more adaptive coping mechanisms can be fostered and incorporated into the client's life.

Goals of Hospitalization

The need to individualize nursing care has been repeated throughout this textbook. However, with disturbed adolescents in the inpatient system, certain basic ego functions that are immature or nonexistent can become the focus of general goals of treatment for most teens. These include:

1. To teach the importance of talking rather than acting out the conflict, problem, or dilemma at hand
2. To increase self-control within the adolescent to avoid explosive verbal and/or physical acts
3. To increase impulse control so that the client does not immediately act without cognitively processing the situation at hand
4. To increase the delay-of-gratification mechanism so that the client will not constantly expect his/her needs to be met immediately and then become frustrated and angry if it does not occur this way. In doing so, patience is increased.
5. To increase the number of autonomous and individuated relationships to which the adolescent is exposed
6. To aid the adolescent in the development of appropriate boundaries between the Self and Others in order to experience attachment and intimacy to their fullest

Drug Abuse and Depression in Adolescent Clients

The most common symptom shared by adolescents in psychiatric hospitals is their drug use history. Illegal drug use has become a monumental social, familial, and personal problem for families of adolescents and their communities. Once detoxified, a majority of teens show clear clinical signs of a preexisting biochemical depression that can usually be traced back to a period just before the adolescent turned to pain killers and/or illegal drugs.

One of the major causes of clinical depression in children and adolescents is the loss of a parent, either through death or, more likely, through parental divorce. Especially in early childhood, parental separation or divorce is an overwhelming stressor to the offspring, eliciting feelings such as helplessness, abandonment, and anger.[18]

Researchers are just beginning to investigate statistically whether the occurrence of clinical depression precedes drug abuse behavior.[8] Of the published research thus far, longitudinal studies by Kaplan and colleagues[27] and by Kandel[25,26] have found depressive symptomatology and self-derogation to precede drug use, which im-

plies causality. In a study of the correlation between adverse health behaviors and depressive symptomatology, Kaplan[28] reported that adolescents who scored high on an Adverse Behavior tool also scored high on a Depressive Inventory tool. Aside from these studies, drug abuse research has reported a wide spectrum of possible etiological factors, numbering more than 30.[52]

Review of the Literature

The majority of published drug abuse research and/or theory construction focuses on: disturbances within the adolescent's family, self-development, school conflict, and peer relationships (summarized in Table 23-1), and/or prevention (summarized in Table 23-2).

Most of the hypothesized etiologies of drug abuse focus on attitudes and personality traits within the adolescent drug abuser. Recent studies have uncovered a broad range of personal and social factors that have been found to contribute to adolescent experimentation with drugs (Kandel,[25,26] and Cook[11]). Byram and Fly[8] reported the following findings related to family structure, race, and adolescent alcohol consumption: (1) as family closeness decreases, the adolescent's investment in a peer group increases; (2) alcohol abuse was greater in family configurations other than that of both natural parents living together; (3) for nonwhites, there was less drug or alcohol use in families with one or both natural parents missing compared to use in white adolescents and their families; (4) overall, adolescents' alcohol use increased as friends' use of alcohol increased, family closeness diminished, and adults' use in the family increased. The adolescent usually models appropriate (and inappropriate) behaviors of the parents.

Along similar lines, Reeves and Draper[48] found that adolescents refrain from drug or alcohol consumption for the following reasons: (1) concern about health, (2) fear of losing control, and (3) parental disapproval. They point to evidence that adolescents identify and imitate parents who are nurturant and involved in their lives in a constructive, yet nonintrusive, way.

A third study presented longitudinal data collected to test a model that uses four broad constructs rooted in sociological and psychological theory in understanding drug usage. Kaplan, Martin, and Robbins[27] selected the following four complementary constructs: (1) self-derogation, (2) peer influence, (3) social control, and (4) early substance use, and reported the effects and influences of these four groups of predictors on adolescent drug use. Of the four, the three that were shown to be predictive of later drug use included self-derogation, peer influence, and social control. All four initiated indirect influences on later drug use. Of particular significance is the reported *adolescent rejection experience.* This begins with rejection by one peer group, which leads to increased feelings of rejection by family and school, as well as by peers. This could account for the movement of these adolescents toward a new, possibly drug-taking peer group, for reasons of enhancing self-esteem and support to counter the earlier experiences of rejection.

A fourth article of particular interest compares substance abuse in Israel and France with abuse in the United States. Kandel[26] substantiated a cumulative sequence of drug use that begins with beer and/or wine and then progresses to cigarettes and/or hard liquor, and then to marijuana, and finally to more serious illicit drugs. Of equal significance is her hypothesis concerning greater prevalence of drugs in a culture based on the following four social processes: (1) greater involvement in drugs, (2) greater persistence of drug use as reflected in the proportion of adolescents who remain current users among those who have ever used a drug, (3) the earlier age of initiation into drug abuse, and (4) a spread phenomenon throughout all groups in society so that group differences in drug experience are decreased. This process is widened by decreased sex and age differences in drug use patterns in adolescents in France as compared to those in Israel. The U.S. adolescents had much higher rates of illicit drug use than did adolescents in either of the other two countries.

A large portion of the current drug abuse literature focuses on new prevention techniques rather than on critiques of previously unsuccessful campaigns. To highlight a few articles of particular relevance to this chapter: Durell and Bukowski[15] suggest creating a climate of nondrug use, not only within the media but also among parents, teachers, and community agencies. Peele[47] takes an even stronger approach aimed directly at parents, who he feels must "arm our children with a set of values that will inoculate them against the dangers of exposure to drugs and alcohol." He details five specific values that must be inculcated: (1) a sense of healthfulness or concern for health, (2) a belief that it is worthwhile to problem-solve to resolve a conflict, (3) an appreciation of achievement and involvement in a positive enterprise, (4) a sense of community and obligation to others, and (5) a sense of one's own value. Bruns and Geist[6] appeal to school counselors and administrators to incorporate a prevention program in their schools based on the following approach: (1) educate students about drug use as one alternative to stress. Teach coping mechanisms for life that reduce stress, rather than increasing stress as drug-taking does; (2) have counseling options available within the school

TABLE 23-1.
THEORIES OF DRUG ABUSE

FAMILY CONFLICT
Dissension in home[56]
Breakdown in communication between parents and youth[56]
Alienation from parents[15]
Parental involvement in smoking/drinking and/or drugs[42]
Decreased positive parental involvement in adolescent's life[48]
Perceived lack of close relationship with parents[27]
Increased time away from home[42]
Questionable genetic link—generational predisposition[31]
Parental rejection[28]

SELF-DEROGATION/DEPRESSION
Sensitivity to peer and family attitudes[28]
Personality deficiency and/or decreased coping[52]
Low self-esteem and/or loss[28,52]
Interpersonal skill deficits[15]
Poor self-concept[48]
Poor self-control[48]
Loss of motivation to achieve[28]
Boredom and/or curiosity[56]
Previous behavioral disorders/psychiatric problems[52]
Suicidal and/or depressed feelings[27]

SCHOOL DIFFICULTIES
Low academic performance[52]
School failure[15]
Problems with authority figures, i.e., teachers, principals[52]
Increased delinquency—truancy, theft[52]
Loss of commitment to school[27]
Loss of motivation to achieve[27]

REJECTION BY SOCIALLY-APPROPRIATE PEER GROUP
Side-effect of clinical depression, i.e., withdrawal[28]
Increased aggression[52]
Increased rebelliousness[52]
Decreased concern about appearance[28]
Problems with authority figures[52]
Increased alienation from society[15]

ACCEPTANCE BY SOCIALLY-UNACCEPTABLE PEER GROUP
Friends incompatible with values of parents[42]
Seeking out of friends who feel the same way[42]
Alliance with new support group increases self-esteem[27]
Substitute for parent and school and previous peer rejection[27]

TABLE 23-2.
PREVENTION TECHNIQUES

MACRO
Climate of Non-drug Use[15]
Media
Schools
Parents
Community agencies
Prevention Programs in Schools[6]
Stress reduction in schools
Availability of counseling
Prevention Programs in Schools[11]
Improve interpersonal skills
Improve self-esteem, power, and problem-solving
Improve number and variety of positive behaviors
Prevent alcohol and drug abuse

Family Value Inculcation[47]
Sense of healthfulness
Problem-solving
Achievement appreciation
Sense of community/obligations to others
Sense of one's own value

or on a consultant basis to deal with drug abusers; and (3) do not neglect abstainers who, like drug abusers, are considered deviant by "normal" peers. They stress that drug experimentation is normal, but it can and does lead to abusive and addictive tendencies. Cook[11] reports the results of implementing an alternatives-oriented, school-based drug abuse prevention program over a two-year period for junior and high school students in Milwaukee, Wisconsin. The premise underlying this program was originated by Dohner,[14] who suggested that the way to prevent drug abuse is to provide adolescents with ways of gaining the desired rewards and pleasures through healthy and nonchemical activities. The goals were: (1) to improve interpersonal skills, (2) to improve self-esteem, feelings of power, and problem-solving abilities, (3) to improve the number and variety of positive behaviors, and (4) to prevent alcohol and drug abuse. Findings indicated that students who actively participated in the alternatives program moved toward a more future-oriented attitude, viewed drug use more negatively and healthful activities more favorably, and exhibited a more responsible attitude toward the use of drugs and alcohol.

Illness Behavior—Legitimizing Failure

When an individual experiences pain or discomfort and chooses to seek a means of relief, the individual is engaging in illness behavior. Clearly, the goal is to provide a means of symptom relief. As long as the person searches for a cure, or seeks a diagnosis for the presenting symptoms, the person is considered to be engaging in illness behavior (Wu[57]). The ultimate illness behavior is to call on a physician, who legitimizes and validates the presence of a disease and details the course to regain health.

Two studies indicate that people can engage in illness behavior as a means of coping with the presence of failure. Shuval[50] states: "Failure to obtain certain desired goals can also be coped with through illness. . . . Feelings of failure represent a subjective state that can arise from different situations. . . . Inadequate role performance as measured by one's expectations or against the performance of others can bring about this feeling." Her basic premise questions how the medical profession can legitimize an illegitimate claim of illness. Cole and Lejeune[10] make a similar point in discussing how a status of illness can excuse people from socially prescribed roles.

Drug Abuse and Illness Behavior

Based on the above theories of the etiology of drug abuse, role theory, and illness behavior, the following model presents a new means of viewing adolescent drug abuse—that of illness behavior as a means of dealing with an underlying depression, concomitant with social role failures. Figure 23-1 demonstrates the process whereby a sense of social role failure leads to drug abuse.

To begin, many adolescents experience family conflict, often including parental divorce or similar adult-focused crisis. During such crises, adolescents' needs are not met because the conflict in the home receives the majority of attention. There occurs a perceived lack of positive attention, along with a parental role model engaging in increased drug-taking behaviors due to the impending stress in the home. The adolescent experiences severe perceived parental rejection. This particular adolescent is sensitive to feelings of abandonment and rejection by the parents, and the adolescent becomes overwhelmed with the stress, pressures, and loss, and manifests clinical signs of a depression. The adolescent also struggles with

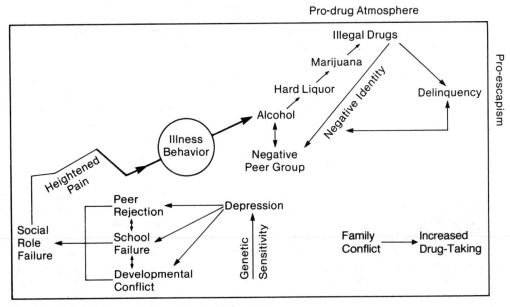

Figure 23-1. Role failure and drug-taking in adolescence.

his/her own stress of the adolescent developmental period, during which gaining emotional independence of parents is one of the major tasks.

At this point, the adolescent should seek symptom relief by consulting a health care worker. However, most adolescents do not want to engage in illness behavior and, based on their developmental level, are struggling to dissociate from adults, including physicians and nurses. Although psychological disorders are more commonly accepted and understood today, most families and their offspring choose to deny symptoms that indicate a possible clinical disorder, especially depression.

As the depression continues, however, the adolescent find it harder and harder to study in school and/or engage in achievement-oriented tasks. The inability to attend class affects school-related activities, and over the course of a few months the adolescent's grades decline. The adolescent's positive peer groups, who notice the significant change in their classmate, are also affected. They are unable to help him or her, or to offer suggestions. The peer groups, organized around group similarities, slowly pull away from the affected adolescent, and engage in their normal social activities, excluding the depressed and conflicted adolescent. This is experienced as a major rejection; when coupled with school problems and family disinterest, it helps to perpetuate depressed feelings and causes an escalation in psychic pain.

At this point, the adolescent can no longer deny the pain, and engages in illness behavior for symptom relief. Because of feelings of distrust of adults stemming from familial experience, concomitant with school difficulties (also considered authoritarian), the affected adolescent moves toward new peer groups, filled with other adolescents who are anti-authority and share the same feelings of depression. This new peer group may engage in drug use to temporarily remove the heavy feelings of sadness and produce a euphoric experience. Depressed adolescents are drawn to "socially unacceptable" negative peer groups, and maintain membership for the following reasons: (1) need for symptom relief, (2) need for peer acceptance, (3) heightened feelings of role and societal failure exacerbated by experiencing rejection from family, peers, and school, (4) new peer group identification correlated with inner feelings of societal failure, and (5) incorporation of a negative identity that is congruent with negative peer group stigma.

Discussion

This model helps to explain the motive behind seeking a negative peer group in a society that applauds only success and achievement. Second, this model accounts for the presence of depressive symptomatology in adolescents who engage in adverse health behaviors. Finally, it provides a means of intervening that can: (a) provide legal symptom relief in the form of psychotherapy and/or antidepressants, (b) target high-risk adolescents and provide alternatives to new "negative peer identification," (c) parallel concurrently employed anti-drug and prevention programs, and (d) acknowledge the struggles

and stressors that adolescents are faced with, yet provide a measure of relief that maintains self-esteem.

The model is based on the hope that these adolescents, who are medicating themselves with harmful and destructive drugs, will opt for a legal alternative. This alternative seeks to alleviate the overwhelming feelings of uncontrollable depression, return their self-control, and aid in their school behaviors by helping them concentrate again. These goals can be achieved with the use of antidepressants. Rather than allowing these adolescents to build up a psychological and physical dependence on illegal drugs that only perpetuate delinquency and self-destruction, antidepressants can aid in maintaining a stable and positive feeling, but not euphoria, for a period of three to five months. Antidepressants help adolescents to achieve "positive" and acceptable health behaviors while boosting their self-esteem. If psychotherapy is also instituted, adolescents can fill deficits in their previous nurturing experiences, relieving the stress and anxiety of their family situation, and once again turn toward resolving the developmental tasks of adolescents.

As seen in Figure 23-2, the school system, as well as the family, plays an essential role in aiding adolescents to channel their efforts appropriately into seeking symptom relief through adaptive means. If the environment maintains an anti-drug, pro-support stance, the option to engage in antisocial, illegal behaviors can be drastically reduced.

To substantiate the validity of the model depicted in Figure 23-2, research needs to be directed toward finding the etiology and prevalence of clinical depression in adolescents, and its direct effects on peer withdrawal, school difficulties, and developmental conflicts; and toward finding the patterns of drug abuse in a large population of students. Because it appears that junior high school students are engaging in drug-taking behaviors at an earlier age, perhaps this type of study should begin in third or fourth grade and be traced for five to seven years. The study should also attempt to discover the extent of learning disabilities in students who engage in drug-taking. With a higher incidence of learning problems being detected in children and adolescents, it might be useful to measure whether or not the onset of a learning disorder affects students' decisions to choose drugs because of "failing" in their role in society, namely, that of achieving in school. Students' degrees of role success and/or failure should also be studied as a means of determining if role perception has a causal impact on the decision to seek drugs.

Studies on the motivations of students to seek drugs as a means of coping with societal stress and/or depression are in their early phases; theoretical frameworks are being proposed to encourage research in this area. Kandel[25] calls for greater integration and sharing of complementary frameworks because each perspective emphasizes a unique part of the process that affects drug involvement. The research review in this chapter appears to call for an integration of nursing, social work, public health, psychology, and psychiatry to conceptualize fully the extent of the variables involved in the complicated

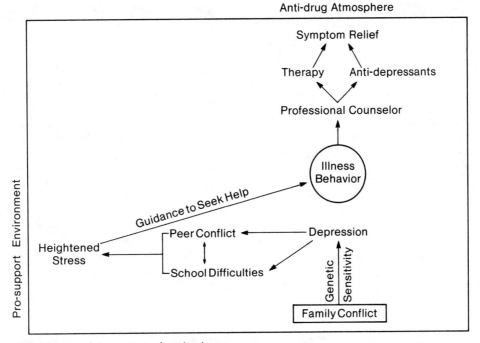

Figure 23-2. Early intervention by school system.

process of drug-taking behaviors. Before successful prevention programs can be designed, it is necessary to understand fully the elements involved in drug-taking choices. Ultimately, the best prevention is better control of drug availability in society. Miller[38] makes an excellent point: "Society fails to protect its youth and may be colluding in its own destruction. . . . The nuclear threat and provision of pathological escape mechanisms are a lethal combination." With respect to the family, Peele[47] directs parents and school teachers to orient adolescents toward something stronger and more valuable than drugs. He gives examples of good parenting, presenting healthy life-styles, teaching ways to develop constructive lives, and aiding in the growth toward adult developmental processes. Kaplan and colleagues[28] address the need for a fourth category of health behaviors, which they call *adverse health behaviors,* to cover those who purposely engage in adverse, self-destructive behaviors (see the Relevant Research box below, concerning adolescent suicide). This group includes drug abusers, among others. If this could guide us to better interventions, then a fourth category could be useful. However, a means to eradicate the need for such a category would make better use of our time and research skills. Clearly, adolescents need help coping with overwhelming stressors that face them in their growth process. In light of their failure to accomplish their developmental tasks of gaining a flexible identity and role status, coupled with family conflict and break-ups, it is understandable that adolescent suicide rates continue to grow.[38] Drugs continue to be a major avenue toward suicidal attempts. Clearly, in their nonassertive, anti-adult way, adolescents are asking for adult control and limit-setting regarding their engagement in negative behaviors.

The Nursing Process Applied to Adolescent Clients: Anorexia Nervosa

The nursing process can be applied to adolescent psychiatric care in the same way it has been applied throughout this textbook. To exemplify further, *anorexia nervosa,* a psychiatric disorder that appears to have its etiology in adolescence, will be addressed through the use of the nursing process and a nursing care plan.

Assessment

The most prominent (or obvious) feature of clients with anorexia nervosa is their physical appearance, consisting of muscle wasting and a bony skeletal look with protruding clavicles and hip regions, resulting from self-imposed starvation without the presence of a medical disorder. These clients have an unrealistic body image; they think that they are fat and, therefore, must continue to lose weight. This disorder is reported to occur in females 95% of the time at a prevalence of 1 in 250 between the ages of 12 and 18 years.[2] Age of onset is predominantly during adolescence, yet cases have been reported during prepubescence as well as in adults. Cases of male clients have been published at a much lower rate, with the age of onset more frequently in early adulthood, before the age of 25.[30] The severe and consistent weight loss, usually greater than 25% of the original body weight, mandates hospitalization to prevent death by starvation. Due to the persistent and consistent drive to lose weight, the mortal-

RELEVANT RESEARCH

This research replicates a previously published study that examined the effects of television movies with suicidal themes on the recorded number of adolescent suicides during the two-week period after the airing date. The initial study focused on the effects in New York City. This study examined records during the same time period as the first study, but looked at records in California and Pennsylvania. Three movies, fictionalizing the effects of suicide, were aired from October 1984 to March 1985.

Data from New York City demonstrated an increase in suicides following the broadcast of each movie; a decrease in suicides followed each movie showing in California and Pennsylvania. The researchers then looked at three large metropolitan cities in California and found, again, that the number of suicides was not higher after the broadcasts.

The second question focused on why suicides appear to increase after a true suicide has occurred, as compared to a fictional movie suicide. The authors question the extent of media coverage of a true suicide, which is headlined in the newspapers and on the television news and probably discussed by the media for many days. The authors speculate that perhaps in New York City the airing of the movies coincided with a publicized true suicide, which then caused a higher rate of suicide.

Given the California and Pennsylvania results, the authors conclude that in their study fictional portrayals of suicide did not increase the number of recorded suicides in two states. The authors encourage testing with larger populations.

(Phillips D, Paight D: The impact of televised movies about suicide: A replicative study. N Engl J Med 317:809, 1987.)

RELEVANT RESEARCH

Twenty-four female adolescents who met the DSM-III-R criteria for anorexia nervosa and were inpatients of the Eating Disorders Program of the Children's Hospital at Stanford, California, were separated into two groups: 16 females were vigorous exercisers, having engaged in running and school team sports before admission to the program; 8 were considered sedentary, because their history lacked athletic participation. The clients were followed for an average of three years. The average age for the athletic group was 14.7 years, while the average age for the sedentary group was 15.6. Data obtained consisted of menstrual history, demographic characteristics, and hormone levels of luteinizing hormone (LH), follicle-stimulating hormone (FSH), and prolactin. Radioimmunoassay testing was performed on samples collected in the early morning, indicative of fasting levels.

Results indicated that both groups with anorexia nervosa had low body weights, low gonadotropin levels, and cessation of menses. LH levels were more suppressed than FSH levels. The athletic group had greater disruption of the menstrual process (due to an earlier cessation), with subsequent return of menses, as well as lower levels of gonadotropins.

These findings appear to dispel the current hypothesis that menses cessation in anorectic clients is due to excessive exercise, because the sedentary population studied also had amenorrhea. The authors suggest, however, that there may be an additive effect of combined starvation and strenuous physical activity on the menstrual function of these adolescents, since the athletic group had more serious menstrual disruptions than did the sedentary group.

(Litt I, Glader L: Anorexia nervosa, athletics, and amenorrhea. J Pediatr 109:150, 1986.)

ity rate is between 15% and 21%.[2] The following Relevant Research box describes one study of amenorrhea in female anorexics.

A specific etiology for anorexia nervosa is unknown. The current treatment under investigation is aimed at lowering excessive secretions of the hormone cortisol, which is found in anorectic patients. Psychiatrists Parsons and Sapse[46] state that, once high cortisol levels are reduced, anorectic patients begin to eat normally, gain weight, and then respond to a combined psychotherapy, nutritional, and food reeducation protocol.

A second possible etiologic factor is linked to theories of development that propose that anorexia nervosa is manifested due to pubertal changes that emphasize deficits in autonomy and self-regard and underscore weight phobias.[54,55] The onset of adolescence can be a crisis period for normal and healthy children. In the anorectic client, the newly emerging adolescent is unable to meet the challenges of adolescence due to unresolved earlier developmental tasks. Maturation is viewed as painful and disruptive, and therefore unwanted. With the onset of the symptoms of anorexia nervosa, maturation is stopped, which then decreases the complexities faced by the adolescent.[13]

A third possible etiologic theory utilizes family development theory to explain the anorectic adolescent.[5,40] More specifically, treatment is focused on familial issues, such as the adolescent's need to separate from the family, which has been avoided or unsuccessfully attempted.[39] To enhance this important task, therapists do marital ther-

TABLE 23-3.
DSM-III-R CRITERIA AND NURSING DIAGNOSES FOR ANOREXIA NERVOSA

DSM-III-R	NURSING DIAGNOSIS

A. Refusal to maintain body weight over a minimal normal weight for age and height, *e.g.,* weight loss leading to maintenance of body weight 15% below that expected; or failure to make expected weight gain during period of growth, leading to body weight 15% below expected	Alterations in nutrition
	  Less than body requires
	    Anorexia

B. Intense fear of gaining weight or becoming fat, even if underweight	Alterations in perception Impaired self-awareness
C. Disturbance in the way in which one's body weight, size, or shape is experienced, *e.g.,* the person claims to "feel fat" even if emaciated, believes that one area of the body is "too fat" even when obviously underweight	Alterations in self-concept Body image
D. In females, absence of at least three consecutive menstrual cycles when otherwise expected to occur (primary or secondary amenorrhea)	Alterations in reproductive/sexual functioning Amenorrhea

apy with the parents to strengthen the parental coalition, individual therapy with the anorectic client, and family therapy.

Currently, all of the above theories are used in combination to treat anorectic clients, along with the sociocultural and familial variables that interact in unique patterns that predispose adolescents to anorexia nervosa.

Diagnosis

The DSM-III-R[2] specifies four diagnostic criteria for anorexia nervosa. Table 23-3 compares the DSM-III-R criteria with the appropriate nursing diagnoses.[1]

In depressive disorders and certain physical disorders, weight loss can occur. However, the major difference is the presence of an intense fear of weight gain that is inappropriate in light of the emaciation in the anorectic patient. In bulimia (discussed later in this chapter) there is never a 25% loss of body weight. There is a disorder called bulimorexia that meets the criteria for both anorexia nervosa and bulimia.

Anorexia nervosa is a psychiatric disorder and, therefore, is predominantly treated with intensive milieu and individual psychotherapy. The following psychological issues are frequently found in anorexic clients:[19]

1. Difficulty in feeling in control of their lives as manifested by the appearance of their bodies, poor recognition of inner bodily states, and revulsion at physical bodily functions and regulations

2. Difficulty in emotional and/or psychological separation from the family and/or particular people, along with difficulty in autonomous living

3. A high degree of personal mistrust. Rather than trust their bodies and their mental processes, anorectics fear them

4. Confusion of personal identity and personal goals, as well as the presence of externally dictated feelings

of worth rather than internally developed feelings of self-worth

5. Starvation perpetuates many of these psychological symptoms, along with the will to diet, by increasing the self-focused concerns of esteem and control.

Research is currently focused on delineating subgroups within the diagnosis of anorexia nervosa. Strober describes three separate anorectic subtypes based on individual responses to a variety of scales and tools.[53] Type 1 is the dominant group; these clients resemble traditional stereotypes of the described personality and familial characteristics. Clinically, these clients exhibited a greater remission of symptoms, as well as achieved a more rapid weight gain, than did clients in other subtypes. Type 2 demonstrates a more neurotic personality, with high levels of anxiety, self-doubt, and social inhibitions. These clients exhibited higher levels of premorbid social avoidance, obsessionality, and intra-familial ten-

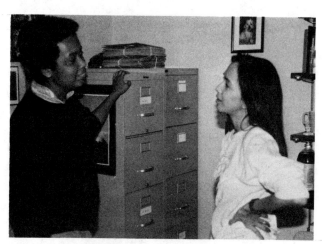

Figure 23-3. A psychiatric nurse on an adolescent unit communicates with a troubled adolescent.

NURSING CARE PLAN

Alteration in Nutrition: Less Than Body Requires (14.01)

ASSESSMENT	NURSING INTERVENTIONS	EVALUATION CRITERIA

NURSING DIAGNOSIS: Anorexia (14.01.01)

SUBJECTIVE DATA
Client states, "I know I just don't eat."
OBJECTIVE DATA
Low body weight. Client looks emaciated.

A daily caloric requirement, prescribed by the client's physician, is to be ingested either in solid food or by liquid replacement (Ensure or Sustacal), as follows:

1. A pre-selected meal of the appropriate calories is checked by a dietician, as well as by the nurse. All warm foods are warmed, and expiration dates on milk cartons are checked.
2. The tray is set in front of the client. The client has 30 minutes to consume as much (or as little) as the client chooses.
3. After 30 minutes, the tray is removed from the client and the calories of the intake are counted. The balance of the food left on the tray is then presented to the client in the form of a liquid supplement. The client has another 15 minutes in which to drink the liquid. At the end of 15 minutes, if any liquid is left, it is given in the form of tube feeding.
4. To ensure that clients will retain the caloric intake, they are usually placed on a close observation status for 1 to 24 hours; decision is based on initial assessment, dietary history, and/or the engaging in regurgitation after meals. If clients need to use the bathroom, they are accompanied by a staff member and observed.

The client will gain weight consistently at about two pounds a week until the pre-selected target weight is reached.

(Continued)

sion, and were more symptomatic of anorexia nervosa at follow-up. Type 3 presents a profile of low ego strength, impulsivity, proneness to addictive behaviors, and increased turbulent interpersonal dynamics. These clients are given a poorer prognosis based on high levels of family psychopathology, along with greater overall degree of anorectic symptomatology.

Planning and Intervention

Implementation of the nursing process for clients with anorexia nervosa requires a firm and consistent, but em-

pathetic, approach (Fig. 23-3). Nurses must focus on building therapeutic relationships with the clients while ensuring that their self-destructive behavior is carefully monitored. The nursing care plans detailed below provide appropriate nursing interventions, along with evaluation criteria, for key nursing diagnoses.

Evaluation

Evaluation of nursing care for clients with anorexia nervosa focuses on both psychological and physical problems. Clients must become aware of misperceptions re-

NURSING CARE PLANS (CONTINUED)

Alteration in Nutrition: Less Than Body Requires (14.01)

ASSESSMENT	NURSING INTERVENTIONS	EVALUATION CRITERIA
	5. Should vomiting occur, or if the client leaves the eyesight of staff when on close observation, all of the calories required for the previous meal are replaced by the liquid supplement. The client is again alloted 15 minutes to ingest the supplement, or tube feeding is instituted.	
	6. After every meal, the amount and type of caloric intake is recorded on a dietary intake form that is part of the client's medical record.	
	7. Clients are monitored at mealtime, as well as directly after food ingestion, until there is a decrease in rigidity, food and eating rituals, and overall anxiety and discomfort. Usually, this occurs after the client has met and stayed at the target weight for 1–3 weeks.	
	8. Clients are weighed in hospital gowns no more than twice a week, prior to breakfast and after voiding. For clients who are maintaining a rigid anorectic stance and appear to be gaining weight at an unbelievable rate, or who are maintaining a weight on little food intake after mealtime supervision has ceased, unexpected weighing is done to check the weight gain when the client is off guard.	

garding body weight as well as the issues of self-concept and body image. As clients begin to gain an understanding of the nature of these problems, nursing interventions are increasingly directed toward weight gain and other physical problems.

Bulimia Nervosa

The predominant manifestations of bulimia are episodes of binge eating that are accompanied by an awareness that the eating pattern is abnormal, a fear of being unable to stop the uncontrollable eating, and a depressed mood that demonstrates signs of self-deprecation and negative thoughts and feelings toward the self. The binge eating episode is most likely terminated by self-induced vomiting, sleep, and/or abdominal pain. In many cases, indi-

viduals use laxatives or excessively reduced diets following an overeating episode to attempt to control their weight and neutralize the effects of the binge episode. It is not uncommon for some individuals to consume 20,000 calories over a four- or five-hour period during a bulimic binge. It is also not uncommon for some individuals to take 15 to 20 laxatives to induce diarrhea and intestinal emptying after a binge. Table 23-4 lists DSM-III-R criteria and nursing diagnoses.

The results of a recent study of college freshmen, cited by the DSM-III-R, showed that 4.5% of the females and 0.4% of the males met the criteria for a diagnosis of bulimia nervosa.[24] Most often bulimia begins in adolescence or early adulthood, when a normal or slightly overweight girl becomes obsessed with food and diets. Frequently, the parents of these adolescents are obese, and the DSM-III-R[2] reports that recent published studies indi-

NURSING CARE PLAN

Excess of or Deficit in Dominant Emotions (30.)

ASSESSMENT	NURSING INTERVENTIONS	EVALUATION CRITERIA

NURSING DIAGNOSIS: Impaired Range of Expression (30.04)

ASSESSMENT	NURSING INTERVENTIONS	EVALUATION CRITERIA
SUBJECTIVE DATA Client states, "I should be allowed to eat like I want." **OBJECTIVE DATA** Client overfocuses on eating.	1. Allow and encourage ventilation of any feelings *except* those that directly involve fear of eating, weight gain, and/or fat. When client attempts to engage the nurse in anorectic fears, the client is to be redirected toward other accompanying feelings such as loss of control, anger, anxiety, and/or interpersonal feelings.	Client will begin initiating interactions with staff members that focus on inner feelings that are *not* related to fears of fat, eating, and the like.
	2. Encourage a trusting and accepting therapeutic relationship by validating the client's feeling expressions and facilitating a beginning self-exploration of the client's attitudes, values, and feelings that are age-appropriate. Role model-appropriate communication skills, feedback, and toleration of negative and positive affect will be important.	Clients will focus on a variety of feelings, predominantly positive at first, that they experience during the course of the hospitalization.
	3. With a developing therapeutic alliance, clients often become angry and jealous if the nurse is interacting with other clients or staff members. They usually have extreme difficulty in confronting and expressing these feelings, but instead express acceptance, flattery, and understanding, which are incongruent feelings. The nurse must repeatedly state that negative feelings are a normal part of relationships and lead to better understanding and trust between nurse and client.	Client will begin verbalizing fears of loss of love, engulfment, and abandonment related to the nurse, beginning in the third or fourth month of hospitalization. Client will experience a therapeutic alliance that accepts negative feelings. Once secure in this trusting atmosphere, client will begin exploring elements of the self that are frightening and new.

cate a higher frequency of a major depression in the nuclear family surrounding the client afflicted with bulimia nervosa.

Psychotherapists tend to view bulimia nervosa as a psychological disorder that occurs in females who have difficulty controlling their emotions—in particular, anger, depression, loneliness, and boredom.[16] They use food as a means of medicating themselves to allay these feelings, or, more appropriately, to "eat away the feelings." Food is viewed as something over which these clients feel they have total control, and that will never reject them as people, parents, friends, and significant others do. Inevitably, these clients eat compulsively, to the extent that they lose control over their eating and the emotional emptiness inside becomes bigger and bigger, forcing them to eat more and more.

Edmands[16] reported on a pattern of bulimia that becomes continuous and addictive, especially when the client feels tense with feelings of guilt, shame, or disgust that lead to cravings for food to help release the boredom and loneliness. The cycle becomes repetitious, leading into a continual pattern of binge eating and vomiting.

Clients with bulimia nervosa appear to be more psychologically impaired than do clients with Anorexia Nervosa. In an important comparative study, Strober[55] looked at etiologic factors for anorectic and bulimic adolescents and concluded that the bulimic adolescents appeared to have more emotional instability and a higher frequency

NURSING CARE PLAN

Alterations in Motor Behavior (22.)

ASSESSMENT	NURSING INTERVENTIONS	EVALUATION CRITERIA

NURSING DIAGNOSIS: Hyperactivity (22.01.07)

SUBJECTIVE DATA
Client states, "Exercise is good for me."

OBJECTIVE DATA
Client overexercises to detriment of physical health.

1. The nurse must set limits on nonscheduled client exercising. This can include reinforcing why inappropriate exercising is maladaptive, and attempting to aid the client in exploring what feelings were occurring when the client began extra exercising.
2. If extra exercising is not decreased, client can be placed on 24-hour close observation to consistently set limits on the overwhelming need to exercise, until client regains control over compulsion.
3. During recreational therapy, staff needs to involve client in the scheduled activity and set limits on extra jogging, pool laps, and continuous walking or running.

Client will begin to find and initiate a conversation with staff when client feels the urge to exercise, thereby appropriately seeking therapeutic help at a time of feeling loss of control and anxiety.

Client will gradually decrease the amount of extra exercising, when confronted with limit-setting and restrictions.

Client will use recreational therapy appropriately as a means of increasing interpersonal and group skills, rather than as a means of expending extra calories.

NURSING CARE PLAN

Excess of or Deficit in Defenses (40.)
Impaired Appropriateness of Defenses (40.02)

ASSESSMENT	NURSING INTERVENTIONS	EVALUATION CRITERIA

NURSING DIAGNOSIS: Staff Splitting

SUBJECTIVE DATA
Client states, "You all are idiots. Only Dr. Allen understands me."

Client is attempting to arouse tension among staff members.

1. All members of nursing staff will participate in weekly treatment conferences to discuss feelings elicited by these clients, as well as to discuss treatment goals and rationale for interventions.
2. The nurse will point out to the client the dynamics of the split, and aid the client in exploring the meaning of and need to engage in this type of defense mechanism.

Nursing staff will remain in touch with their feelings and thoughts regarding the treatment of this client and will be able to discuss perceptions with others.

The client will view the treatment team as a unified whole, and will then be forced to look inward and understand the need to split off feelings, ultimately leading to an integration of feelings toward others and those toward the self.

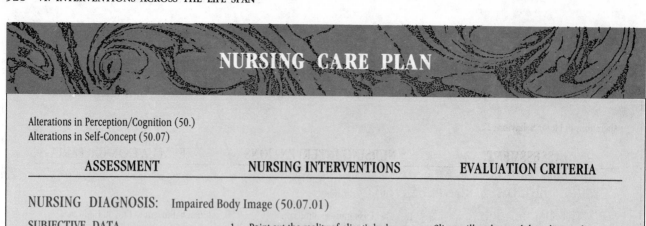

NURSING CARE PLAN

Alterations in Perception/Cognition (50.)
Alterations in Self-Concept (50.07)

ASSESSMENT	NURSING INTERVENTIONS	EVALUATION CRITERIA
NURSING DIAGNOSIS: Impaired Body Image (50.07.01)		
SUBJECTIVE DATA Client states, "I'm too fat." **OBJECTIVE DATA** Client distorts the reality of client's body size.	1. Point out the reality of client's body weight and expected weight. 2. Discuss fears and anxieties with client, such as client's concerns that others will reject client if client is at a normal weight.	Client will understand that client is distorting body weight. Client will label and discuss feelings about body.

of behavioral abnormality in their childhoods. In another comparative study, Sights and Richards[51] examined the parents of bulimic and nonbulimic college women. Their research indicated that mothers of bulimic women showed traits of dominance and controlling, while holding higher expectations of their daughters to achieve and succeed; fathers of bulimic women appeared to be emotionally close to their daughters in early childhood but distanced during their adolescence.

Outlined on the next few pages is a nursing care plan for clients with bulimia nervosa. Therapeutic work with bulimic clients focuses on improving the client's ability to verbalize feelings, seek support, and maintain proper nutrition. Evaluation criteria are also included.

Effective Treatment—What Really Works?

To work effectively with adolescent clients, it is essential to know, understand, and empathize with their struggles, conflicts, and turmoil. This means that care-givers must remember that turmoil and moderate levels of anxiety are normal, although unpleasant, components of development that must be experienced before adaptation to adulthood is possible.[45] Psychiatric nurses must be aware of the difference between normal rebellious attitudes and psychiatric disturbance. In two recent epidemiologic studies of adolescents in different communities,[41,44] results indicated that only 20% of the surveyed adolescents appeared to be psychiatrically disturbed, with severe and disruptive behaviors. Although a relatively small percentage, this translates into an estimated 3.4 million adolescents in the United States who need some type of mental health intervention.[44]

With this relatively large number of estimated adolescents needing mental health intervention, why are professionals so reticent to treat this population? It is most likely because confusion and fear surface in everyone's mind when troubled adolescents are discussed or observed. There is much confusion regarding what to say or do, and fear about the aftermath of a confrontation or limit-setting with an angry and potentially aggressive teenager. However, it is essential to understand that an-

TABLE 23-4.
DSM-III-R CRITERIA AND NURSING DIAGNOSES FOR BULIMIA NERVOSA

DSM-III-R	NURSING DIAGNOSES
A. Recurrent episodes of binge eating: rapid consumption of a large amount of food in a discrete period of time	Alterations in nutrition/metabolism More than body requirements Bulimia
B. A feeling of lack of control over eating behavior during the eating binges	Impaired emotional experience Helplessness Shame/humiliation
C. Regularly engaging in self-induced vomiting, use of laxatives or diuretics, strict dieting or fasting, or vigorous exercise in order to prevent weight gain	Bowel excess Diarrhea Alterations in elimination Not otherwise specified
D. A minimum average of two binge eating episodes a week for at least three months	Alterations in nutrition/metabolism More than body requirements Bulimia
E. Persistent overconcern with body shape and weight	Alterations in self-concept Body image

ger and aggression are deterrents that adolescents often use to prevent adults from seeing their more vulnerable and needy parts, the parts that have been mistreated, misunderstood, and deeply and painfully hurt. To break through their very powerful defenses slowly and delicately is the goal for building a healthy therapeutic relationship. Nurses must then attempt to heal adolescents' deep pain through interventions aimed at doing what their parents might not have been able to achieve; providing a consistent and safe environment in which they can understand right from wrong, acceptable from unacceptable, and ultimately who, and what, they are.

Adolescents are not children any more. Children are dependent on their environment and their parents because they are not fully developed physically or intellectually. Adolescents are physically maturing into adults and intellectually reaching the formal operations phase of thinking, equal to that of adults. Therefore, they are striving to be and feel respected for their thoughts, their actions, and their performance. They are striving to be noticed, to be commended, and to be a part of something: a family, a peer group, or a team. If parents and teachers don't supply them with the positive regard they desperately need, they will search elsewhere, whether in a cult, in a gang, or in a drug-abusing culture. If this fails as well, most likely the adolescent will attempt suicide in a despair of aloneness. According to a recent survey of contemporary threats to adolescent health,[4] the three leading causes of death for adolescents are (1) accidental injuries, including automobile accidents, drownings, poisonings, firearms, burns, and falls; (2) homicides and assaults; and (3) suicide. Results of a study that explored youths' perceptions of life stressors in an adolescent's world indicated that school-related problems ranked first, followed by parental conflict and family issues.[21] These studies support the importance to the adolescent of success in school and family systems. If adolescents sense or feel impending failure, aggressive or violent behaviors may result.

Adults are easily able to nurture and support children, but seem to struggle with giving the same amount of positive emotion to adolescents. Perhaps the difficulty is in knowing how. Adolescents make it known when they sense they are being treated like children, and yet will appear uncomfortable and confused if spoken to like an adult. Appropriate interventions, therefore, include those that support their autonomy and acknowledge their thoughts. Interventions should also address their more needy emotional side in a noncondescending, warm, playful way that demonstrates respect for their achievements yet offers them a chance to ask questions and to learn without experiencing embarrassment or intimidation. This necessitates being available to provide emotional support and intervention, education, and exploration of thoughts and values, while maintaining consistent, yet appropriate, limits and personal boundaries. It means allowing adolescents to make decisions, such as the subject of discussion during one-to-one sessions, or which recreational activity to play. However, if the choice is to withdraw rather than talk about a pending

hospital discharge, a compromise is appropriate. The adolescent could agree to withdraw for five minutes, after which discharge issues will be addressed for the next 10 minutes. This demonstrates respect for the adolescent's decision, yet sets a limit on the appropriateness of the subject.

When an adolescent is angry and begins yelling, rather than yelling back or setting down one limit after another terminating with a room restriction for days, the staff should try to appeal to the hurt and pain and humiliation that the adolescent is experiencing and discharging through acting out the anger to avoid the deeper hurts. Instead of recreating the family interactions of power and control through yelling, the nurse should gently and compassionately appeal to the "wounded child" part of the adolescent. Very often staff accidently exacerbate angry adolescents' behavior by immediately setting limits rather than diffusing the anger through verbal intervention. Staff members frequently tell adolescents to "Talk it out, don't act it out"—yet, when adolescents begin to act out, instead of role modeling appropriate verbal interventions, the staff person acts out by yelling back, by setting a variety of limits, or by prematurely preparing for physical restraint. All of this might have been avoided through talking instead of acting. If staff members act out, adolescents have no alternative but to act out further, in order to demonstrate power and authority, defending themselves against humiliation, submissiveness, and the child-dependent position.

Being reminded of uncomfortable childhood feelings like helplessness and dependency evokes pain and despair in these adolescents. Those feelings, the root of acting-out and aggressive behaviors, should be elicited through therapeutic relationships when trust and safety have been secured, not through a power struggle in which the adolescent is placed in a predicament that recreates the situation the therapeutic staff are struggling to repair. To heal painful emotional wounds, adolescents must experience consistent and therapeutic empathy to then show the vulnerabilities of their inner emotional world. Through understanding, care, and appropriate interpretations of what is occurring, the adolescent heals intrapsychically. Focusing attention on inappropriate behaviors only ignores the roots of the symptoms.

In an article addressing room restrictions as a method of limit-setting for adolescents, Gentilin[20] describes three behaviors that result in a room restriction in a program for substance-abuse treatment: (1) running away, (2) drug use, and (3) violent behavior. Gentilin describes how a plan is developed with the client, and how a mutually acceptable program is then enforced. The adolescent is given some control and is respected, even while being disciplined. Often in behavioral programs for adolescents, limits in the form of time-outs, room restrictions, and/or activity restrictions are designed without any input from the adolescent. Therefore, the adolescent will not submit, and a power struggle ensues, ultimately resulting in compounded limits and more restrictions. The adolescent then feels more alienated from the staff and withdraws further. Too often, treatment

NURSING CARE PLAN

Excess of or Deficit in Dominant Emotions (30.)

ASSESSMENT	NURSING INTERVENTIONS	EVALUATION CRITERIA

NURSING DIAGNOSIS: Impaired Range of Expression (30.04)

SUBJECTIVE DATA Client states, "Food doesn't really matter." OBJECTIVE DATA Client cannot express feelings about food.	Encourage client to write down what feelings surface before, during, and after eating. Client should also write down any feelings regarding individual foods. Feelings to focus on should include: boredom, loneliness, anger, depression, guilt, and shame.	Client will identify and discuss feelings regarding food.

Alterations in Self-Care (24.)

NURSING DIAGNOSIS: Impairment in Solitude (Social Interaction) (24.05)

SUBJECTIVE DATA Client states, "My life is empty." OBJECTIVE DATA Client experiences boredom, inability to comfort self when emotionally upset.	1. Help client make a list of things to do (write, call a friend, listen to music). Make a list of resource people who are available to call and talk to. 2. Encourage soothing, nurturing self-thoughts rather than negative, critical self-thoughts.	Client will identify realistic ways to occupy self. Client will understand self-critical thoughts and identify positive self-thoughts.

Alteration in Nutrition/Metabolism (14.)

NURSING DIAGNOSIS: Post-Meal Vomiting

SUBJECTIVE DATA Client states, "I just feel a little nauseous after a meal. Maybe it's the food."	1. A staff member must remain with the client for two hours after meals, including trips to the bathroom and	Client will not vomit after a meal.

(Continued)

teams feel successful when adolescents comply with the design of the unit. The question at this time is whether the team was truly effective or the adolescent chose to be compliant solely to be discharged out of the "prison" hospital without really dealing with the true emotions and roots of the noncompliance. Often adolescents learn, and then manipulate, a treatment team only to be discharged without learning about emotions and behavior. They then return to their families and communities to engage, once again, in inappropriate outbursts and rebelliousness. This is the hazard of enforcing and providing only a behavioral treatment framework with adolescents. It teaches submissiveness to someone else's structure without respecting or encouraging shared responsibility or commitment. Once again, a repetition of the messages from the adolescent's disturbed home is reinforced rather than encouraging dignity and self-esteem through emotional expression and gaining insight.

To see a disturbed, emotionally troubled, angry adolescent slowly transformed into a friendly, emotionally relieved, verbal adolescent is exciting therapeutic work. To be tested and then to be accepted by an adolescent is an amazing and fulfilling accomplishment. Finally, to be there when the anger melts and the pain of childhood is tearfully shed can be a powerful, mutually shared experience of trust and safety, giving the staff the greatest compliment an adolescent can give: being appreciated, accepted, and heard.

Summary

1. Aside from the first year of life, probably no other period of development involves such a surge of hormonal, emotional, physiological, familial, societal,

NURSING CARE PLAN (CONTINUED)

Alteration in Nutrition/Metabolism (14.)

ASSESSMENT	NURSING INTERVENTIONS	EVALUATION CRITERIA
OBJECTIVE DATA Client vomits after meals. Teeth are eroded.	while in the bedroom. 2. Encourage client to ventilate feelings about observation and the desire to vomit.	Client will discuss the need to vomit and the treatment plan to prohibit vomiting.

Excess of or Deficit in Dominant Emotions (30.)

NURSING DIAGNOSIS: Impaired Range of Expression (30.04)

SUBJECTIVE DATA Client states, "I don't know how the food got into my locker. Maybe another client left it there." OBJECTIVE DATA Client is sneaking in and hoarding extra food.	Staff members will monitor visits with client's family and friends. Instruct the client, family, and friends to not bring extra food to the client.	Client will tolerate three meals a day.

Alterations in Conduct/Impulse Control (21.)

NURSING DIAGNOSIS: Aggression/Violence Toward Self (21.03)

SUBJECTIVE DATA Client states, "So what if I hold my pocketbook." OBJECTIVE DATA Client is guarding pocketbook, which may contain laxatives or diuretics.	Search room and personal belongings before hospitalization for any such medications. If there is reasonable cause for suspicion, a room search may be performed per patient rights and hospital procedure.	Client will have normal elimination.

cultural, and psychological experiences as does the period of adolescence.

2. Mahler, a psychoanalyst, proposed that if the separation–individuation growth and development phase of infancy and childhood is not successfully mastered, disturbances may occur in adolescence.

3. Hospitalization can cause a number of difficult concerns for adolescents: they may fear that adult hospital staff members may inflict the same emotional pain as have other adults in their lives.

4. Staff members who work with adolescent clients must maintain the ability to appear real and authentic as individuals, yet maintain appropriate boundaries of personal space and emotional attachment.

5. Drug abuse is common among adolescents with psychiatric/mental health concerns.

6. Anorexia nervosa most frequently appears in adolescence, and may require hospitalization to provide treatment and prevent death by starvation.

7. Bulimia most frequently begins in adolescence and includes an obsession with food and diets as a way to deal with emotions.

8. When working with adolescents, staff members should remember that anxiety and turmoil are natural parts of adolescence, and that staff can best respond by remembering to focus on the vulnerable, previously mistreated, and misunderstood aspects of the clients.

References

1. American Nurses' Association: Taxonomy for the Classification of Human Responses of Concern for Psychiatric/Mental Health Nursing Practice. Kansas City, Missouri, American Nurses' Association, 1986

2. American Psychiatric Association: Diagnostic and Statistical Manual of Mental Disorders, 3rd ed, Revised (DSM-III-R). Washington, DC, American Psychiatric Association, 1987

3. Bloom M: Adolescent–Parental Separation. New York, Gardner Press, 1980

4. Blum R: Contemporary threats to adolescent health in the United States. JAMA 257:3390, 1987

5. Bruch H: The Golden Cage: The Enigma of Anorexia Nervosa. Cambridge, Massachusetts, Harvard University Press, 1978

6. Bruns C, Geist C: Stressful life events and drug use among adolescents. J Hum Stress 10:135, 1984

7. Burr A: The ideologies of despair: A symbolic interpretation of punks and skinheads' usage of barbiturates. Soc Sci Med 19: 929, 1984

8. Byram O, Fly J: Family structure, race, and adolescents' alcohol use. Am J Alc Abuse 10:467, 1984

9. Carser D: The defense mechanisms of splitting. J Psychosoc Nurs Ment Health Care 17:21, 1979

10. Cole S, Lejeune R: Illness and the legitimation of failure. Am Soc Rev 37:347, 1972

11. Cook R: An evaluation of the alternatives to drug abuse prevention. Int J Addict 19:767, 1984

12. Coser L: Sociological Theory—A Book of Readings. New York, Macmillan, 1976

13. Crisp A: Anorexia Nervosa: Let Me Be Me. New York, Macmillan, 1980

14. Dohner V: Alternatives to drugs—A new approach to drug education. J Drug Educ 2:3, 1972

15. Durell J, Bukowski W: Preventing substance abuse: The state of the art. Public Health Rep 99:23, 1984

16. Edmands M: Overcoming eating disorders: A group experience. J Psychosoc Nurs Ment Health Serv 24:19, 1986

17. Erikson E: Identity, Youth, and Crisis. New York, WW Norton, 1968

18. Gardner R: Psychotherapy With Children of Divorce. New York, Jason Aronson, 1976

19. Garfinkel P, Garner D: Anorexia Nervosa: A Multidimensional Perspective. New York, Brunner-Mazel, 1982

20. Gentilin J: Room restrictions: A therapeutic prescription. J Psychosoc Nurs Ment Health Serv 25:12, 1987

21. Green J: Stressful life events and somatic complaints in adolescents. Pediatrics 102:456, 1985

22. Havinghurst R: Developmental Tasks and Education. New York, David McKay, 1972

23. Hedges L: Listening Perspectives in Psychotherapy. New York, Jason Aronson, 1983

24. Johnson C: Bulimia: A descriptive survey of 316 cases. Int J Eating Disorders 2:3, 1982

25. Kandel D: Epidemiological and psychosocial perspective on adolescent drug usage. J Child Psychiatry 21:328, 1982

26. Kandel D: Substance abuse by adolescents in Israel and France. Public Health Rep 99:277, 1984

27. Kaplan H, Martin S, Robbins C: Pathways to adolescent drug use, self-derogation, peer influence, weakening of social controls, and early substance use. J Health Soc Behav 25:270, 1984

28. Kaplan S, Landa B, Weinhold C, Shenker I: Adverse health behaviors and depressive symptomatology in adolescents. J Child Psychiatry 23:595, 1984

29. Keith C: The Aggressive Adolescent. New York, Free Press, 1984

30. Kielcott-Glaser J, Dixon K: Postadolescent-onset male anorexia. J Psychosoc Nurse Ment Health Serv 22:10, 1984

31. Lewis C: Alcoholism, antisocial personality, and narcotic addiction. Psychiatr Dev 3:223, 1984

32. Linnell Z: Authority as a treatment modality with adolescents in a psychiatric hospital. J Hillside Hosp 9:48, 1960

33. Mahler M: On Human Symbiosis and the Vicissitudes of Individuation. New York, International Universities Press, 1968

34. Mahler M, Pine F, Bergman A: The Psychological Birth of the Human Infant. New York, Basic Books, 1975

35. Marks B: Hospital treatment of borderline patients: Toward a better understanding of problematic issues. J Psychosoc Nurs Ment Health Serv 18:25, 1980

36. Marriage and Divorce Newsletter. New York, Ed Brown, 9/10/84

37. Masterson J: Treatment of the Borderline Adolescent: A Developmental Approach. New York, John Wiley & Sons, 1972

38. Miller D: The Age Between: Adolescents and Therapy. New York, Jason Aronson, 1983

39. Minuchin S, Rosman B, Baker L: Psychosomatic Families: Anorexia Nervosa in Context. Cambridge, Massachusetts, Harvard University Press, 1978

40. Mushatt C: Anorexia nervosa: A psychoanalytic commentary. Int J Psychoanal Psychother 9:257, 1982–1983

41. Myers J, Weissman M, Tischler G et al: Six-month prevalence of psychiatric disorders in three communities. Arch Gen Psychiatry 41:959, 1984

42. Nicoli A: Drugs: The extraordinary epidemic. World Health Forum 5:138, 1984

43. Offer D, Marohn R, Ostrov E: The Psychological World of the Juvenile Delinquent. New York, Basic Books, 1979

44. Offer D: The Epidemiology of Mental Health and Mental Illness Among Urban Adolescents. In Call J (ed): Significant Advances in Child Psychiatry. New York, Basic Books, 1987

45. Offer D: In defense of adolescents. JAMA 257:3407, 1987

46. Parsons J, Sapse A: Anorexia treatment—100% success reported. J Psychosoc Nurs Ment Health Serv 22:30, 1984

47. Peele S: Influencing children's use of drugs. Focus on Family 1:5, 1984

48. Reeves D, Draper T: Abstinence or decreasing consumption among adolescents. Int J Addict 19:819, 1984

49. Rinsley D: Treatment of the Severely Disturbed Adolescent. New York, Jason Aronson, 1980

50. Shuval S, Antonovsky A, Davies A: Illness: A mechanism for coping with failure. Soc Sci Med 7:259, 1973

51. Sights J, Richards H: Parents of bulimic women. Int J Eating Disorders 3:3, 1984

52. Sommer B: The troubled teen: Suicide, drug use, and running away. Women Health 9:128, 1984

53. Strober M: An Empirically Derived Typology of Anorexia Nervosa. In: Anexoria Nervosa: Recent Developments in Research, pp. 185–196. New York, Alan R. Liss.

54. Strober M, Yager J: The Treatment of Anorexia Nervosa in Adolescents—Theoretical Foundations and Clinical Strategies. In Garner D, Garfinkel P: Handbook of Psychotherapy for Anorexia Nervosa and Bulimia. New York, Guilford Press, 1984

55. Strober M: The significance of bulimia in juvenile anorexia nervosa: An exploration of possible etiological factors. Int J Eating Disorders 1:28, 1981

56. Wright J: The psychology and personality of addicts. Adolescence 12:399, 1977

57. Wu R: Behavior and Illness. Englewoods Cliffs, New Jersey, Prentice Hall, 1973

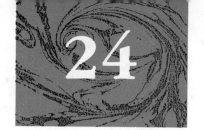

JEAN MOORE

MENTAL HEALTH COUNSELING OF ADULTS

Learning Objectives

Upon completion of this chapter the student should be able to do the following:

1. Identify the three developmental stages of adulthood.
2. Describe the major developmental crises of adulthood identified by Erikson.
3. Identify at least three developmental tasks associated with each of the following stages: early adulthood, adulthood, and middle age.
4. Describe the significant biological event of middle age.
5. Give an example of a life event that is a positive experience and yet is potentially stressful.
6. Identify at least two personality traits that are indicative of adaptive coping behavior.
7. Define cultural bias and give an example of how it can interfere with treatment planning.

8. Identify the two psychiatric disorders for which significant sex differences have been found in diagnosis rates.
9. Identify three behaviors or attitudes that reflect the nurse's therapeutic use of self.

Introduction

Adults who, at different stages of adulthood, cannot cope effectively with current stressful events may manifest a broad range of psychiatric symptoms for which they may seek psychiatric treatment. The failure to cope effectively may be related to a specific life event or trauma for which the individual lacks sufficient emotional resources to manage effectively. Some people demonstrate lifelong patterns of maladaptive coping with the developmental or situational crises experienced throughout the course of adulthood. In order to assess and treat clients effectively in the practice of psychiatric nursing, nurses must be aware of the influence that developmental stages of adulthood may have on the manifestation of psychiatric symptoms.

Early Work on Developmental Stages

Freud was once asked to identify the behaviors he attributed to a mentally healthy adult. He replied, "To work and to love." Freud, like many other early theorists of human development, presented a framework that identified stages of emotional development that begin in infancy and end in adolescence. Major theorists adhered to the belief that adult personality was shaped in infancy and childhood. Psychiatric symptoms arising in adulthood were seen within the context of an individual's childhood experiences. Positive experiences during this critical developmental period enhance the likelihood of an individual's ability to work and love effectively.

Little attention was paid to developmental issues that might arise after adolescence. Erikson is regarded as a pioneer in advancing developmental theory into adulthood.[11] His work strongly reflects Freudian thinking. Freud's psychosexual stages of development were translated by Erikson into psychosocial stages. However, Erikson added adult developmental stages, proposing that these stages emerge throughout the course of a lifetime. Erikson defined these psychosocial stages of development as *maturational crises,* that is, normal processes of growth and development involving the occurrence of potentially stressful events. The maturational crises of adulthood identified by Erikson include the following:

1. *Intimacy vs. isolation* is the developmental crisis that occurs in young adulthood. *Intimacy* is the ability to establish a positive and satisfying relationship with another person, although such a commitment could be made to a cause or a creative effort, as well.[27] *Isolation,* the failure to achieve intimacy, is usually seen as self-absorption and the tendency to avoid intimate contact with others, or to make goal-directed commitments.

2. *Generativity vs. stagnation* is the developmental crisis of adulthood. *Generativity,* a concern for the needs of others, may take the form of using one's skills and abilities to plan for the future in order to guide the next generation. *Stagnation,* the lack of concern for others, is typically characterized by self-preoccupation.

3. *Ego integrity vs. despair* is the developmental crisis of middle age and late adulthood. *Ego integrity* is characterized by emotional integration, evidenced by satisfaction with one's life accomplishments. *Despair,* a sense of unhappiness with one's life events, is characterized by a sense of failure and fear of aging and death.

Erikson's psychosocial developmental crises of adulthood were supported by Havinghurst,[18] who identified tasks of adulthood. Havinghurst identified three chronological periods: early adulthood, middle adulthood, and later maturity, and described behaviors associated with each of these periods. Table 24-1 compares Erikson's developmental crises with Havinghurst's tasks of adulthood.

Current Work on Developmental Stages of Adulthood

Theorists such as Erikson and Havighurst laid the groundwork for research into the developmental stages of adulthood. Since the publication of their works, there have been many empirical studies that not only verify their theories, but also elaborate on the issues of adulthood, especially the influence of changing family roles on developmental stages.

In examining current research on this topic, it is interesting to note that there is little agreement on the age definitions for early adulthood, adulthood, and middle age.[16,27,33] However, the descriptions of issues associated with these stages are very consistent with each other. Neugarten[28] summarized the critical issues of adulthood as follows:

. . . it might be said that they are issues which relate to the individual's use of experience; his structuring of the social

TABLE 24-1.

A COMPARISON OF THE DEVELOPMENTAL CRISES IN ADULTHOOD IDENTIFIED BY ERIKSON AND DEVELOPMENTAL TASKS IDENTIFIED BY HAVINGHURST

ERIKSON		
Intimacy vs. isolation	Generativity vs. stagnation	Ego integrity vs. despair
HAVIGHURST		
• Start a career. • Select a mate. • Find a congenial social group. • Start a family. • Manage a home.	• Achieve adult civic and social responsibility. • Rear children. • Establish and maintain an acceptable economic standard of living. • Raise children to teens.	• Raise teens to adults. • Adjust to children leaving home. • Relate to spouse in the absence of children. • Adjust to physiological changes associated with aging. • Adjust to aging parents.

Ages	18	20	30	40	50	60

world in which he lives; his perspectives of time; the ways in which he deals with the major life themes of work, love, time, and death; the changes in self-concept and changes in identity as he faces the successive contingencies of marriage, parenthood, career advancement and decline, retirement, widowhood, illness, and personal death.

Differences in the age definitions may result from a number of variables that include: (1) increasing longevity of human life span, thus extending the age definitions for the stages beyond their earlier definitions, and (2) social and cultural variations in movement through adult developmental stages.[29]

Each of the three developmental stages of adulthood will be examined separately, and the significant issues that fall within each will be identified.

Systems Theory

One can determine from the above quote by Neugarten that the adult is easily thought of as *not* separate from others, but a part of a system of persons with whom the adult interacts. System interactions are expected: withdrawal from other adults is seen as potentially problematic.

Parenthood, work, marriage, illness, and death are all phenomena in which the adult has a role, and the role involves others as system members. Even in illness, the adult can dramatically affect others in the member's family system—for example, who must provide care for the ill member—and alter roles accordingly. In death, the system is still a concern—even if in its disintegration, as in the example of a spouse losing a mate.

Early Adulthood

Early adulthood is the developmental stage that follows adolescence and, for the purpose of this discussion, be-

gins at age 18 and concludes at age 30. Many theorists agree that the most significant accomplishment of this stage is the development of a stable self-concept based on adult identity.[11,16,17,35] Frequently, this adult identity evolves as an individual proceeds toward emotional and financial independence from the family of origin.[27] This process is significantly affected by the response of the family of origin to bids for independence on the part of the offspring. Optimally, the family of origin must be able to accept and support their offspring in the development of a separate and distinct adult identity. This requires a reorganization of the family system in response to the loss of offspring.[38] The young adult's relationship with the family of origin usually manifests itself in one of four ways: overinvolvement; superficial, impersonal contact; no contact at all; or adult-to-adult personal relationship.[15]

A descriptive study of young adults at ages 18 to 21 indicated that getting away from parents was a major concern of that age group, while young adults at ages 22 to 28 were more concerned with becoming autonomous and established.[17] This finding was substantiated by a second study, which found that 18- to 21-year-olds identified separation from their families of origin as a major concern, and 22- to 28-year-olds showed an increasing interest in marriage and career development.[35]

The young adult may manifest a bid for independence through the pursuit of higher education, by initiating a career, or through marriage. A variety of factors influence the course that is chosen, the most significant of which are mobility and cultural considerations, which play critical roles in movement through all adult developmental stages.[38]

While the development of adult identity once tended to follow rather stereotypic, sexually defined roles, recent trends indicate significant changes in these patterns. More women are pursuing careers in young adulthood and, as a result, are postponing marriage and children to a later point in the life cycle. As a result of this, women and men are more often competitors in the pursuit of career achievement, and there is more general acceptance of diversity in lifestyles and relationships of young adults.

There are more single young adults who proceed with the development of an intimate bond with another but are not pressured to make an immediate commitment to marriage. This choice is most likely influenced by relaxed sexual mores that make such behavior widely accepted, as well as by a high divorce rate that may discourage young adults from rushing into marriage too soon. Homosexual relationships are also more widely accepted than they were in the past, and people inclined toward homosexuality are freer to pursue such relationships openly.

Despite these significantly changing attitudes, the general trend suggests that young adults often choose the most culturally acceptable option of developing a heterosexual relationship and marrying prior to age 30. Young adults who marry face the tasks of (1) developing an identity as a couple, (2) reestablishing relationships with both families of origin to incorporate the new spouse, and (3) deciding on parenthood.

Marriage requires the establishment of a strong bond that draws the couple to each other and can, at the same time, create a healthy emotional distance from families of origin. The types of relationships that develop with families of origin after marriage are strongly influenced by the relationships that existed prior to the marriage.

In addition to establishing a primary relationship with another, if that happens, the young adult must also develop a secondary network, usually consisting of friends and family. The involvement of family in such a support system usually depends on emotional and physical proximity.

As indicated earlier, choosing a vocation or career is another developmental task of young adulthood. The choice of a career can be as critical as the choice of a marital partner in shaping the life of an individual. Career choice may be influenced by a number of factors, including: educational opportunities; parental expectations; personal abilities, interests, and aspirations; and generally accepted sex roles and the tendency toward sex-role stereotyping. The most successful career choice is one that results in the individual's finding the work meaningful, experiencing personal satisfaction from productivity, and achieving financial security.[27]

In summary, the young adult strives to separate from the family of origin in order to achieve an adult identity. Establishment of a primary intimate relationship and a stable support group usually also emerge during this time. The completion of education signals the beginning of the pursuit of a career by the young adult.

The Nursing Process With Young Adults

Assessment

It is important for nurses to be able to assess the young adult's progress in completing these developmental tasks. Nurses must use investigative interviewing techniques to gather these data. Table 24-2 lists the specific topics and suggested approaches nurses may use in such an assessment.

Diagnosis and Intervention

It is clear that these forgotten experiences (refer to Clinical Example on p. 537) play a significant role in Debbie's present symptomatic behavior. As the client attempted to move toward the development of an intimate relationship with someone of the opposite sex, the unresolved feelings from repressed childhood experiences provoked tremendous anxiety. Her encounters with the opposite sex could only take place when she was under the uninhibiting influence of alcohol. The contact was superficial, and limited mainly to brief sexual encounters that reflected both her need for intimacy and her fear of it, based on the previous repressed experience.

Nursing interventions in this case must be aimed at the identification of underlying thoughts and feelings that the client has about herself and her relationships

TABLE 24-2.
NURSING ASSESSMENT OF THE YOUNG ADULT

AREA OF ASSESSMENT	INVESTIGATIVE QUESTIONS
Relationship with family of origin	• Tell me about your parents. • How often do you see your parents? • Tell me about your brothers and sisters. • How would you describe your relationship with your family? • With whom are you closest? With whom are you least involved? • With whom are you most likely to discuss your problems?
Relationships with others outside your family	• Who is the most important person in your life right now? • How long have you known each other? • How often do you see each other? • What do your parents think about this relationship? • What problems are you able to discuss with each other? Give me an example. • Tell me about your friends. • How often do you see them? • If you had a serious problem, with whom would you be most likely to discuss it?
Career	• Tell me about your job. • What do you think about this sort of work? • How did you come to get this job? • Tell me about your future career plans. What other job would you like to be doing? What plans have you made to achieve this?

CLINICAL EXAMPLE

Debbie, a 23-year-old college student, seeks psychiatric counseling. She indicates that recently she has had episodes of drinking to the point of blackouts. She has no memory of what she did while intoxicated and worries that she is promiscuous during these times. She describes herself as quiet and studious until the recent onset of this behavior. She has no idea what precipitates this behavior.

The case of Debbie illustrates how a young adult can have difficulty in accomplishing the developmental tasks of young adulthood. Using an investigative interviewing approach, the nurse determines that the client has little recall of childhood experiences, and what she does remember indicates serious problems with her family of origin. Her father had a history of alcohol abuse and her mother tended to be passive and withdrawn. The client remembers fights between her parents in which her father was both verbally and physically abusive to her mother, who did not attempt to defend herself against these attacks.

Over the course of individual sessions with this client, the repressed memories slowly emerge into consciousness. She recalls being "forgotten" by her parents, who were too preoccupied with their own problems to care for her. She remembers the angry feelings she had toward her parents for abandoning her. She remembers being sexually molested by an older brother when she was eight years old, and being too frightened to tell anyone about this experience.

with others. The client's avoidance of intimacy must be addressed. The therapeutic relationship with the nurse may serve as a corrective experience in the establishment of an intimate relationship with another person. The issue of alcohol abuse must also be dealt with directly. The family history of alcoholism must be examined carefully, since the client may be at high risk for similar problems as an adult. Table 24-3 identifies the appropriate diagnoses, goals, and interventions to be used in working with this client. Nursing diagnoses related to Debbie should concern past traumatic issues that are unresolved as well as current coping behaviors. An introduction of the client to Alcoholics Anonymous would be an important aspect of treatment.

Evaluation

This case demonstrates that unresolved issues of previous developmental stages clearly impinge on the successful negotiation of future developmental stages. It is important to collect all necessary data in order to assess the impact of past experiences on present behaviors.

The evaluation of treatment would incorporate both short-term goals and long-term goals. Short-term goal evaluation would involve determining the degree to which Debbie can recognize her feelings and cope better with them. Long-term goal evaluation would include determining sobriety, and the degree to which Debbie's early family history currently affects her.

TABLE 24-3.

DSM-III-R Diagnosis: Adjustment disorder with mixed disturbance of emotions and conduct

NURSING DIAGNOSES: Ineffectual Individual Coping; Anxiety

GOALS	INTERVENTIONS
1. Client will become aware of the unresolved issues that lead to self-destructive behavior, such as episodic drinking and promiscuity.	a. Assist client in understanding the influence of traumatic childhood experiences on symptomatic behavior. b. Encourage client to identify and describe feelings associated with her traumatic childhood experiences. c. Recognize and accept client's feelings about these experiences. d. Encourage client to attend Alcoholics Anonymous.
2. Client will begin to develop more appropriate relationships with people, especially members of the opposite sex.	a. Assist client in developing relationships that will promote intimacy without inducing anxiety. b. Help client to learn the necessary communication skills to reduce her anxiety in intimate relationships.
3. Client will learn to recognize her anxious feelings in interpersonal situations and find more adaptive ways of coping.	a. Help client to understand that her family's history of alcohol abuse places her at great risk for developing a similiar problem. b. Help client to identify the stressful situations in which she is most likely to use alcohol as a means of coping. c. Explore with client other behavioral and/or verbal alternatives she could use in these stressful situations.

Adulthood

The developmental stage of adulthood follows early adulthood and, for the purpose of this discussion, begins at age 30 and concludes at age 45. If the adult lifetime were to be characterized by a period of ascent leading to a period of decline, then awareness of the decline becomes apparent in this period.

Descriptive studies indicate that, at approximately age 30, individuals begin to look inward and pose existential questions regarding the direction of life goals and values.[17,35] One study identified and ranked the major concerns of individuals in the age group of 29 to 36 as follows: self, children, marriage, and career.[35] This trend continues from ages 36 to 45, with concern for parents also emerging as a major issue. It is generally believed that *interiority*, the tendency toward introspection, increases with age,[17,28,35] and descriptive studies indicate that interiority is first noticeable in early adulthood, with an increasing tendency toward interiority in the late 30s and early 40s. This is attributed to the increasing, and perhaps more desperate, awareness of time as it begins to be measured in "time left to live," instead of "time-from-birth."[28] One descriptive study found that adults aged 35 to 43 felt an increasing disparity between "what I want" and "what I've got," and dissatisfaction with their marriage and career was found to be highest in this age group.[17] This period of dissatisfaction is occasionally referred to as *mid-life crisis.* The term is confusing, because mid-life is generally thought to occur from ages 45 to 60. It is more important to recognize the individual's tendency to experience such feelings at this time, and the behaviors that may result from these feelings.

Erikson's description of the developmental stage of generativity vs. stagnation indicates that emotionally healthy adults sublimate their concerns about their own individual mortality into a more universal concern for the greater good of future generations. Thus, generativity may be successfully channeled into guiding one's own children.[10]

Families in this age group commonly have children. As indicated earlier in this chapter, child-bearing is often postponed by women who are establishing careers during young adulthood. The developmental task of becoming parents leads to fairly significant changes for the couple, and especially so for the woman bearing the child. The internal and external changes in a woman as a result of motherhood include the following:

- *Social*—there are changes in the way that a woman relates to her husband, family of origin, and social network.
- *Biological*—there are changes in a woman's body as a result of pregnancy, lactation, and the symbiotic bond that develops with the fetus during pregnancy.
- *Emotional*—there are changes evidenced by the development of a normative symbiotic bond with the infant.
- *Cognitive*—there are changes in the way that a woman views her responsibilities to herself and to her child.[34]

In addition to the impact of motherhood on a woman, the introduction of children into a family system also results in the need for adjustments to the changing needs of growing children. These changes are summarized as follows:

Families with infants must:

- Integrate the new member into the family.
- Accept and integrate the new roles that accompany parenting.
- Maintain intimacy in the marital dyad while accommodating the presence of a new family member.

Families with preschoolers must:

- Encourage socialization of children.
- Allow for physical and emotional separation.

Families with school-age children must:

- Encourage their children to be involved with a peer group.
- Accept the influence of school and peers on children.

Families with teenagers must:

- Accept the increasing need for autonomy by teenagers.
- Adjust their degree of marital intimacy to accommodate increasing absence of adolescent children.
- Begin to shift concern toward aging parents and grandparents.[38]

The Nursing Process With Adults

Assessment

Nurses must be able to use their skills in investigative interviewing to identify an individual's ability to negotiate successfully the developmental stage of adulthood. Table 24-4 lists specific areas of assessment and suggested approaches that nurses may use to collect data. A genogram may also be helpful, since diagramming a family can provide nurses with valuable information on intergenerational relationships.

Diagnosis and Intervention

The case in the Clinical Example on page 540 illustrates an instance in which the situational crisis of divorce, coupled with the failure to address issues related to the developmental stage of adulthood, affected the client's emotional well-being. In planning for Barbara's treatment, the nurse must not only aim to help her recover from the loss of a significant relationship, but also help her identify the developmental issues that must be considered.

TABLE 24-4.
NURSING ASSESSMENT OF INDIVIDUALS IN ADULTHOOD

AREA OF ASSESSMENT	INVESTIGATIVE QUESTIONS
Relationship to nuclear family system	• Tell me about your family. • To whom are you closest? With whom are you least involved? • Whom do you usually talk to about problems? • What sort of help do you usually get? • How do you show your anger in your family? With whom? • How do you show your sadness? With whom? • What would you like to change about your family?
Career	• Tell me about your job. • What do you like about your job? • What do you dislike about your job? • If you could, what would you like to change about your job? • What sort of career had you hoped to achieve? (If there is dissatisfaction with career) • Where do you see your career going over the next ten years?
General satisfaction with current life situations	• How would you describe yourself? • What would you say are your biggest concerns right now? • What do you think you can do about them? • If you could change anything in your life right now, what would it be?

Evaluation

The treatment program for Barbara is successful if the client can deal with her intra*psychic and inter*personal issues. She would be expected to understand the impact of her husband's leaving on her life and to express her emotions about his absence (intrapsychic tasks).

The client should also accomplish interpersonal tasks. She should become more open to support from others outside her home, and make realistic plans for her future through career or educational opportunities.

Middle Age

Middle age is the developmental stage that follows adulthood and, for the purpose of this discussion, begins at age 45 and ends at age 60. Unlike the other developmental stages described, middle age is a time of significant biological change.

The major biological event of this period is known as the *climacteric.* During this time, women undergo long-

term physiological changes caused by ovarian involution,[6] including cessation of menstruation. Men more often experience a decline in sexual activity.[27] Hormonal production declines, resulting in symptoms that women are more prone to experience. The most common symptoms include:

• Musculoskeletal symptoms, including back or shoulder pain, muscle cramps, numbness in fingers and toes
• Vasomotor symptoms, including hot flashes, headaches, perspiration, chills, dizziness
• Sexual symptoms, including increase or decrease in libido
• Psychological symptoms, including depression, anxiety, irritability, fatigability, insomnia[6,27]

At the same time, the middle-aged family undergoes a significant transition as children in the family proceed to early adulthood. Developmental tasks of the middle-aged family include:

• Allowing children to develop separate and independent identities as young adults
• Reinvesting in the couple's relationship as children leave home
• Incorporating in-laws and grandchildren into relationships with children
• Accepting disabilities and death of the older generation[38]

Attitudinal studies of this stage of development found that people aged 44 to 50 reported increasing marital satisfaction, and people aged 51 to 60 seemed generally accepting of their current life circumstances while beginning a review of their life's accomplishments.[17,35] People in this age group indicated an increasing concern with aging parents and, at the same time, indicated less concern for grown children. Middle-aged adults show an increasing tendency toward interiority, and this is believed to be a forerunner of the detachment process thought to accompany aging.[28] Middle-aged adults also demonstrate an increasing awareness of their own physical vulnerability. The term *body monitoring* is used to describe protective strategies employed to maintain one's body at a given level of performance.[28] All of these behaviors indicate that middle age is a time when an individual comes to terms, in very concrete ways, with his or her own mortality. This resembles Erikson's description of ego integrity, which involves an acceptance of one's life in order to prepare for the approach of aging and, ultimately, death.[10]

Another significant area of study in this age group is the impact of aging on cognitive abilities. Longitudinal studies of cognitive functioning indicate that there is no decline in mental ability during adulthood, including middle age. Generally, any significant changes in cognitive abilities occur after age 60.[7,32]

Individuals in this developmental stage, especially women, undergo significant, and potentially stressful, physical and interpersonal changes that have been referred to as "exit events," involving the loss of important

CLINICAL EXAMPLE

Barbara, a 33-year-old woman, is admitted to a psychiatric unit of a hospital. She is tearful and complains that life has no meaning for her, and that she has accomplished nothing. She admits to thoughts of killing herself by jumping from a bridge. She recently separated from her husband; she and her eight-year-old son and five-year-old daughter now reside with her mother, a widow.

The case of Barbara is that of an individual experiencing difficulty during the developmental stage of adulthood. In obtaining a history, the nurse learns that the client had lived at home with her widowed mother until age 23, when she married. The client graduated from high school and held a number of clerical jobs prior to her marriage, when she immediately became pregnant with her first child. She has not held a job since then. The client described her marriage as "okay." Her husband, a construction worker, was described as "distant" and "un-communicative," but a steady worker. The client spent much of her time at home with her children. She had few friends and socialized rarely with anyone except her mother. Her husband left her six months ago, when he moved in with another woman, and is filing for divorce.

After a number of individual sessions with this client, it becomes clear that she is extremely dependent on others for her sense of self-esteem. Her only significant relationships are now limited to those with her mother and her children. She appears to be overinvested in these relationships and extremely overattached to her children.

The client describes herself as someone concerned with "doing the right thing." She recalls her childhood as a happy time, when she acted like "a little lady," as her mother wanted her to do. At her mother's insistence, her pursuit of a career was limited to the study of clerical courses in high school. Her mother's rationale was that Barbara should be more concerned with "finding a husband" than pursuing a career. The client recalls that her only aspiration was to be married and have children.

This client's socialization to the limited sex-role expectations identified by her mother placed serious restrictions on her capacity to assume adult roles. The failure of her marriage precipitated a crisis for her because of her limited expectations of herself. Her role as "wife" was one of her few sources of self-esteem.

Nursing interventions in this case must be aimed at helping the client identify the source of her low self-esteem, which is contributing to feelings of depression. The client must examine her feelings regarding her lack of productivity, and identify strategies for involving herself in relationships and activities that could enhance her self-esteem and provide opportunities for feeling successful.

The development of a therapeutic relationship with the nurse can help this client to learn the importance of mutuality in a relationship. Table 24-5 identifies the appropriate diagnoses, goals, and interventions that would be used in working with this client.

TABLE 24-5.
DIAGNOSES, GOALS AND INTERVENTIONS: BARBARA

DSM-III-R Diagnosis: Major Depression, Single Episode

NURSING DIAGNOSES: Dysfunctional Grieving; Disturbance in Self-Concept

GOALS	INTERVENTIONS
1. Client will grieve about the loss of a significant relationship (her husband) as well as a significant role in her life (being a wife).	a. Encourage client to identify and describe her feelings about these losses.
	b. Help client learn to verbalize her feelings (sadness, anger) instead of acting on them.
	c. Recognize and acknowledge client's feelings (sadness, anger) about these losses.
2. Client will develop and utilize more supportive relationships with others.	a. Assist client to understand the effect her over-dependence on family relationships has on her self-esteem.
	b. Help client increase contacts with friends, extended family, church groups, clubs.
	c. Refer client to a support group for divorced women.
3. Client will participate in activities that will build self-esteem and create opportunities for success.	a. Encourage client to make realistic plans for herself that may include career counseling and/or educational opportunities.
	b. Support client in developing plans that foster increasing self-sufficiency.

relationships and important body functions.[6] Consequently men, and more often women, during this period may be at risk for psychological symptoms resulting from these stressors. This age group has been studied in an effort to identify predictors of high risk for the development of psychological symptoms.

A study of women's attitudes toward menopause found that, while most women view menopause as an unpleasant event, middle-aged women did not, however, view the psychosocial events of middle age negatively.[30] Other studies have examined a number of psychosocial variables of middle-aged women, and have identified the following factors that predict the likelihood of psychological symptoms: loss of mother before age 11, unemployment, and few emotionally intimate relationships.[6] A study of stressors that result in psychosis or depression in middle age found that the loss of a significant relationship was the predominant stressor for persons in these two diagnostic categories.[3]

It is thought that a woman is less vulnerable to an adverse response to losses during this time period when her roles extend beyond those of wife and mother. A woman who has a career or is involved consistently in a similar type of meaningful activity is less likely to be threatened by "the empty nest syndrome."[8] Men, on the other hand, are thought to need more experience with feelings of relatedness, both with spouses and families.[8] The emotional isolation characteristic of many men is thought to leave them more vulnerable to the stress of middle-age events.

The Nursing Process With Middle-Aged Adults

Assessment

Middle age is a developmental period involving both physiological and psychosocial changes that have significant potential for emotional disturbance. In view of this, it is critical for nurses to assess the significant variables in the life of a middle-aged client in order to predict the client's ability to cope effectively with these changes. Table 24-6 identifies important areas for assessment and suggested questions that can be used to obtain these data.

Diagnosis and Intervention

The nursing diagnoses in the Clinical Example on page 542 would be focused on issues related to the family's ability to cope with common stressors, including separation of children and family relationships. Treatment in this case should involve working with the family, and ultimately with Adam and Jane. Helping the elder child achieve independence from this family, while attempting

TABLE 24-6.
NURSING ASSESSMENT OF MIDDLE-AGED INDIVIDUALS

AREA OF ASSESSMENT	INVESTIGATIVE QUESTIONS
Biological changes	• What changes have you noticed in the way you feel? • To what do you attribute the changes? • How does this make you feel? • What do you think you can do about it?
Relationship with family of origin	• Name the person in your family with whom you feel closest. • How would you describe your marriage? • What is it like for you as your children leave home? • How have you and your spouse adjusted to the children's leaving?
General satisfaction with current life situations	• How would you describe yourself? • Name the things you do that are important. • What do you find most troubling right now? • Name one thing you do that you enjoy doing. • Name something you wish you could have accomplished, but just weren't able to.

to support the marital dyad in dealing with this loss, is an important therapeutic goal. If the nurse can successfully help the couple cope effectively with this transition, they may be receptive to addressing other unresolved issues in their relationship. Table 24-7 identifies the appropriate diagnoses, goals, and interventions to be used in working with this client and his family.

The clinical example also demonstrates that, while the manifestation of psychiatric symptoms may be seen in only one family member, nursing interventions may include working with other family members to address problems within the system. It is crucial that nursing assessments of a client's psychiatric symptoms always include an assessment of that client's support systems. Psychiatric symptoms can, at times, be more readily understood when viewed within the context of the client's system of relationships.

Systems theory interprets an individual's behavior as an adjustment between social demands and personal needs. Developmental and situational crises often require adjustment.[36] Thus, Adam's recent episode of drinking can be seen as a reaction to his son's decision to leave home. Disequilibrium within the system leads to specific reactive behaviors on the part of each member of the family. Adam's behavior is the most problematic and, as a result, he becomes the identified client. When planning treatment for Adam, it is important to recognize the needs of other family members as well.

The nurse who works with this family is promoting mental health at all three levels of prevention.[36] Supporting the younger son's participation in Alateen illustrates primary prevention: health promotion through educa-

CLINICAL EXAMPLE

Adam, a 49-year-old man, is brought to the emergency room of a general hospital. He is acutely intoxicated, and admits to having beaten his wife. He claims to be an alcoholic and asks for help to "get off the booze so I can take care of my family again."

The case of Adam is that of a middle-aged man who lacks the coping skills to successfully address the developmental tasks of middle age. The nurse determines that Adam has a history of alcohol abuse, and that he and his family have periodically sought counseling to deal with this, and other, family problems.

In discussions with a nurse therapist who has treated this family in the past, it becomes clear that the current situation reflects long-standing unresolved issues within the family. Adam and his wife have two children, both in their late teens. He has had numerous blue-collar jobs, which usually ended in termination because he came to work intoxicated. His wife has been employed as a secretary for the past 20 years, and her income has been the main source of support for the family. Both children have been involved in an Alateen program for many years. The current episode of acute intoxication was precipitated

when the older son told his parents he planned to move into his own apartment, continue to work part-time, and enroll in night school. Adam's wife, Jane, became upset, saying her son was too young to make such a move. Adam was outraged, claiming that it was irresponsible of the son to leave and not continue to contribute to the family. The son refused to reconsider. Jane, who was very overattached to this son, became apathetic and withdrawn. Adam continued drinking heavily and became increasingly abusive to his wife and sons, both verbally and physically, until the police were called and he was taken to the hospital.

The family dynamics make it very difficult for this family to progress through the developmental stages of family life. Jane has coped with her husband's alcohol abuse through an overattachment to her children. The marital dyad is weak, and the presence of children in this family keeps pressure off that relationship. The nurse can predict that the younger son will have just as much difficulty with separation from this family.

tion. The nurse's work with the marital dyad to help them adjust to the impending departure of their son illustrates secondary prevention: interventions directed at relieving immediate stress. Encouraging Adam's participation in a group such as Alcoholics Anonymous is an example of the rehabilitative approach used in tertiary prevention.

This case is an example of a couple at high risk for

developing psychological symptoms in response to the stressful life events of middle age. Neither person appears to possess enough inner and outer supports to deal effectively with these experiences. A nurse who has a good understanding of the developmental tasks of middle age can use this information to plan treatment for this family.

TABLE 24-7.
DIAGNOSES, GOALS AND INTERVENTIONS: ADAM

DSM-III-R Diagnosis: Alcohol Dependence (Alcoholism)

NURSING DIAGNOSES: Potential for Violence; Ineffective Family Coping

GOALS	INTERVENTIONS
1. Client will express his thoughts and feelings to family members verbally, not physically, and in an appropriate manner.	a. Work with the family to identify "trigger events" that lead to client's verbal or physical abuse of other family members.
	b. Assist all family members to find more adaptive ways of dealing with "trigger events" to avoid confrontation.
	c. Help client to understand the connection between his ingestion of alcohol and his potential for verbally and/or physically abusing family members.
	d. Support all efforts of client and family members to cope with client's alcoholism (e.g., participation in AA, Al-Anon, Alateen).
2. The marital dyad (Adam and Jane) will develop a stronger, more positive bond between them.	a. Work with the couple to promote increased communication and discussion of their feelings about the impending loss of their elder son.
	b. Encourage the marital dyad to work together to identify problem-solving strategies to help them deal with impending changes in their family.

Evaluation

The treatment plan evaluation would involve looking at the family system. Has Adam begun a recovery program for both his alcoholism and his violent behavior? Have other family members examined their role in the alcoholism? Are they involved in their own recovery program to decrease the negative effects of the substance abuse in the home?

Also of concern in the evaluation of the treatment of this family is the family conflict concerning the plans of the older son to leave the home. Have the family's members coped effectively with its altered membership? Have the parents regained their alliance with each other, and do they offer support for each other?

Variables Influencing the Manifestations of Emotional Distress in Adulthood

Adult developmental stages and the tasks associated with these stages strongly influence the behavior of adults. When nurses are aware of this, they can use the information to predict as well as interpret behavior. There are a number of other variables that can also help nurses assess problematic behavior and use this to plan treatment effectively. The variables that will be examined include: stressful life events, personality traits that influence adjustment to aging, cultural differences that affect behavior, and sex differences in the diagnosis of psychiatric disorders.

Stressful Life Events

Much research has been conducted to identify the life events that people find most stressful. One of the most important findings to date is that stressful life events are not necessarily negative events, but rather events that signify change in the life of the individual.[36] The most widely acknowledged research on stressful life events was conducted by Holmes and Rahe, who developed a "Social Readjustment Rating Scale."[20] The scale identified the most stressful life events by the amount of coping behavior needed to adjust to the event. The ten most stressful life events listed on this scale include the following:

- Death of spouse
- Divorce
- Marital separation
- Jail term
- Death of close family member
- Personal injury or illness
- Marriage
- Being fired at work

- Marital reconciliation
- Retirement[20]

If change is one key to understanding the degree of stress caused by life events, then it is critical for nurses to determine the amount of change an individual has experienced, that is, the number of stressful life events experienced over a specific time period. Clearly, the more stressful life events that are experienced over a short time period, the more potential exists for emotional distress.

While the concept of stressful life events is useful in predicting and interpreting behavior, it must be considered in conjunction with other factors, such as personality traits that influence the individual's ability to cope with stressful life events.

Personality Traits

It is generally agreed that personality development occurs early in life and lays the basis for adjustment throughout the adult years. However, certain personality traits can significantly enhance an individual's ability to cope with both developmental and situational life events. The following traits have been identified as most adaptive for individuals, particularly as they experience aging throughout the adult years. They include:

- The ability to channel energy into the development of new relationships or activities
- The ability to use previous experience in solving new problems
- The ability to enjoy and find meaning in a variety of roles
- The ability to accept changing sexual needs and desires throughout adulthood
- The ability to accept bodily changes occurring throughout adulthood without loss of self-esteem[31]

Individuals who manifest these traits are more able to adjust to the psychological, social, and biological changes occurring throughout adulthood. These traits can help prepare them for the aging process and the acceptance of death. As mentioned previously, the basis for personality originates in early developmental experiences, and consequently individuals have the potential to exhibit traits shaped by these experiences throughout the course of their adult lifetimes. Nurses may assess clients for the presence of these traits, or the potential for the development of these traits, at any point at which emotional distress is experienced.

Cultural Considerations

Another important factor for nurses to consider is cultural differences, and the impact of these differences on an individual's behavior. Each individual's attitudes, beliefs, and mores must be considered within a cultural context. An individual's cultural background can shape the definitions of health, mental health, and illness, as well as identify the parameters of a family system and the boundaries of a social network. This can vary greatly from culture to culture, for any of the following reasons:

- Differences in the identification of stressors, including stressful life events
- Differences in the range of acceptable emotional expression
- Differences in expectations of social group cohesion
- Differences in definition of and tolerance for deviant behavior
- Differences in progression through adult developmental tasks[24,36]

The client with a different ethnic background may have communication difficulties related either to fluency in English or to differences in the meanings of words or phrases.[24] The nurse who conducts a mental status examination on such a client must consider the impact of such communication barriers and attitudinal differences on the client's affect, basic cognitive level, reasoning, and ability to abstract.[24]

A final consideration in evaluating cultural differences is the nurse's own cultural biases. The tendency to stereotype the behaviors of different cultural groups has serious implications for therapeutic effectiveness.

To summarize, cultural differences affect a client's belief system, and the nurse must evaluate a client within a cultural context in order to gain a better understanding of this influence on the client's inner resources, social support system, and behavior.

Sex Differences in Rates of Psychiatric Disorders

The final factor to be considered is the sex differences noted in the diagnosis of psychiatric disorders. There is evidence to indicate that the number of women seeking psychiatric treatment has increased significantly since the early 1960s.[4] Another significant and consistently documented trend is that of sex differences in rates of certain diagnoses: women more often receive a diagnosis of a depressive disorder and men more often receive a diagnosis of a personality disorder.[2,4,5,9]

Much research has been done in an effort to identify the variables contributing to these trends, but no conclusive findings have been obtained. However, two theories are consistently cited regarding the tendency to diagnose women more frequently as having depressive disorders. The first theory emphasizes biological differences, specifically the changes in hormonal output during the menstrual cycle, during the postpartum period, and during menopause.[5,22] The second theory emphasizes the sex-role differences between men and women, especially the fact that women tend to assume socially expected roles (such as wife and mother), and incorporate socially expected values (such as youth, beauty, and passivity), that result in a decreased capacity to influence their environments. This, coupled with the tendency toward social, le-

gal, and economic discrimination, may leave women more prone to depression. A recent survey of attitudes of the general population toward the mentally ill found that the participants clearly differentiated attributes of a "normal" man and a "mentally ill" man. However, attributes of a "normal" woman were not as clearly distinguishable from the attributes of a "mentally ill" woman. Men were perceived as being closer to the norm of psychological health than women.[21] More research is required before any firm conclusions can be drawn about the sex differences in the rates of psychiatric diagnosis.

AIDS

The AIDS (acquired immune deficiency syndrome) virus was first reported in the United States in 1981. The virus attacks the body's immune system, and the person with AIDS is then susceptible to other illnesses such as infections. AIDS usually occurs in the following groups: sexually active homosexual and bisexual men; users of illegal intravenous drugs; persons who have had transfusions of blood or of blood products; sex partners of individuals with AIDS; and infants born to mothers with AIDS.[14]

Flaskerud stated that the client with AIDS has many of the same characteristics as the medically ill client. In brief, the nurse should assess the client with AIDS according to the following areas in which the client can have particular strengths or vulnerabilities to psychosocial stressors:[14]

Interpersonal relationships
Education
Career
Substance abuse
Degree of coping skills in dealing with stress prior to the illness
Degree of crisis experienced after the diagnosis of AIDS
Social supports available
Life cycle phase and comfort of clients with that phase (if 40 to 50 years of age, the client may be less stressed if, prior to diagnosis, the client believed that his/her life choices of mate, career, and so on were satisfying)
Degree of comfort with existential issues (is the client comfortable with the idea of death, the meaning found in life, and so on?)
The degree of loss experienced in the illness (the client with large medical bills as a result of the illness who has to sell his/her home to pay for the costs of care may experience more stress than someone who does not have financial concerns)

Psychosocial Stressors

Flaskerud described AIDS as generating immense psychosocial stress for clients, "their lovers/spouses and family members, and health care professionals."[14] Psychosocial stressors that may occur include the following.

Psychosocial Stressors of Clients with AIDS

Disbelief upon hearing one's diagnosis, followed by numbness, denial, anger, and acute turmoil

Knowledge that they have a lethal illness

Anxiety, fear, depression

Suicidal ideation

Physical weakness

Social isolation, hypochondriasis

Demanding behavior, overdependence

Hopelessness, low self-esteem

Cognitive impairment (because of central nervous system involvement in the disease)

The degree of a sense of resolution (during the terminal stages of the illness)

Psychosocial Stressors of the Lover/Spouse of the AIDS Client

Possible guilt about transmitting the illness to the client

Shock, denial, anxiety, depression, fear

Fear of getting AIDS from the client

Physical and/or emotional suffering from adjusting to the altered level of activity of the client in the relationship and in participating in activities in the home. The lover/spouse may also feel drained from providing physical care for the client.

Anticipatory grief over the loss of the client

Psychosocial Stressors of Nurses of AIDS Clients

Concerns about getting the illness from the client

Possible belief/value conflicts accompanying providing care for an IV drug abuser or a homosexual individual

Fatigue from the provision of care to a client with complicated physical and emotional needs

Fears accompanying caring for clients with AIDS, many of whom are the same age as the nurse

Conflicts arising when the client who is dying from AIDS is given multiple treatments that have little effect. The professional identity of "nurses as persons who improve clients' lives is called into question."[14]

Interventions

Psychiatric/mental health nursing principles are an important adjunct to the care of clients with AIDS. As stated by Flaskerud, "therapy skills needed are those that nurses have always used to help their clients face catastrophic illness."[13] Listed below are several interventions which the nurse may use in dealing with psychosocial concerns of the AIDS client.

The AIDS Client

Crisis intervention

Individual therapy to deal with feelings of extreme anxiety, fear, anger, impulsivity, suicidal ideation, guilt

The provision of an opportunity for the client to express feelings and to go through the grieving process

The provision of psychopharmacology to deal with anxiety, insomnia, depression

The facilitation of the client's entrance into support groups for AIDS clients

The provision of education about the illness and its treatment, stress management, practice in problem solving

The facilitation of helpful interactions of family and friends with the AIDS client

The Lover/Spouse of the Client

Individual therapy for the lover/spouse of an AIDS client to deal with his/her crises and sadness

The facilitation of the person's entrance into a support group for lovers/spouses of AIDS clients

Discussions with the lover/spouse concerning ways to minimize stress

The Nurse

Because of the stress involved in caring for the AIDS client, Flaskerud proposed a "multifaceted program of institutional support" for the nurse.[14] This support should include the following:

Regularly scheduled educational updates about AIDS (including instruction on transmission, homosexuality and bisexuality, assessment of mental status and delirium, assessment of cognitive capabilities to follow prescribed procedures, hospital and community resources)

Clear policies about infection control adhered to by all staff

Regularly held staff conferences (including all disciplines) about goals for care

Support groups for staff

Easy access to mental health consultants to help in planning care

Support of administration in the form of adequate personnel to prevent the staff from becoming overtaxed

It should also be noted that nurses in all areas of nursing practice face the challenge of assisting clients with AIDS to focus on their psychosocial concerns. Community health nurses, for example, have an opportunity to educate members of the community about fears related to AIDS. Nurses on inpatient psychiatric units have the opportunity, at times, to facilitate the AIDS client admitted for psychiatric problems to become part of the therapeutic milieu.

Women's Health

The current women's health movement is an example of the work being done now in the developmental stage of adulthood. The women's health movement is the con-

RELEVANT RESEARCH

This study examined the extent to which life changes after the birth of a baby and instrumental support of parenting predict the occurrence of illness in mothers. It is known that the birth of an infant causes major alterations in the mother's patterns of living, as well as a decreased sense of well-being and increased stress. Prior to this study, no studies were performed regarding the association of major life events and social support to physical illness in mothers following birth.

The sample for the study included 155 women selected from urban university hospital and suburban community hospital records. All infants of mothers in the sample were six months old. The mothers ranged in age from 15 to 39 years; 53% were white and 47% were nonwhite; they had a seventh-grade or higher education; they were single (42%), married (55%), or divorced/separated (3%). Most respondents were primiparas (57%), and unemployed (78%).

Life-change events were measured by counting events occurring in the six-month period between the infant's birth and data collection. Instruments used included the Social Readjustment Rating Scale and an instrument to measure events affecting the health of preschool children.

Instrumental support was described as the provision of material assistance (such as shelter or income) and parent-assisting resources (such as babysitting). This support was measured by a structured interview.

Illness was *defined* as the number of illnesses reported by the mothers within the month before the interview. The instrument used was a structured interview. The number of illnesses during the previous year were also measured for comparison with the number of illnesses reported during the six-month period postpartum. Data were collected in the mothers' homes.

Results indicated that demographic variables (socioeconomic level, age, race) were not related to illness. Life change was positively related to illness, allowing for prior illness. Support network size was negatively related to illness. Taking into account demographic characteristics, prior illness, and life changes, the following findings were reported:

1. Increased support network size is associated with a decrease in reported illness.

2. Neither composition of the network (such as maternal kin) nor the helpfulness of the support was associated with illness.

Life-change events predicted illness, but less strongly than did prior illness.

The researchers stated that nurses can assess the extent to which life changes occur, and can identify mothers who may be at higher risk of illness. The study contributes to what is known about variables that can be adjusted (such as the mothers' support network) to promote women's health.

(Lenz E, Parks P, Jenkins L et al: Life change and instrumental support as predictors of illness in mothers of 6-month-olds. Res Nurs Health 9:17, 1986.)

certed effort by lay people and health care workers to provide women with health care or education at each level of prevention (Fig. 24-1). The study in the following Relevant Research box supports the idea that women's health is affected by the special experiences of women (such as pregnancy).

The inadequacies of health care tailored to the needs or health status of women were addressed in 1980 by a committee of women doctors. The committee asked the American Medical Association to examine:

1. The high number of hysterectomies and radical breast cancer surgeries being done each year
2. The unnecessary prescription of tranquilizers and antidepressant drugs to women
3. The lack of attention to medical research on menstrual and menopausal problems
4. The lack of attention to dietary, nutritional, and exercise needs of women
5. The lack of respect of male physicians for the needs of female clients

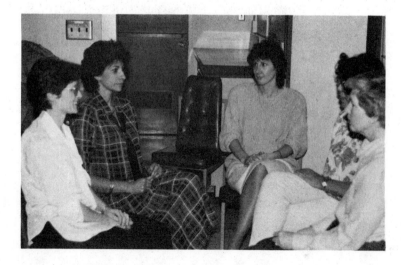

Figure 24-1. Women participating in a support group to discuss issues they have in common.

6. The inadequacies of explanations of diagnoses and treatments given to women[37]

Weiss reported that women have "historically been regarded by medical science as neurotic"[37] or as mentally ill in some way just because they are female. A review of medical texts reveals certain patterns in health care provided by male physicians for female clients: women's physical diseases are often not taken seriously by physicians; women undergo more unnecessary surgical removal of sex organs than do men; and women receive more prescriptions for sex hormones for the treatment of common problems than do men. Medical texts tend to foster sex-role stereotypes.

Weiss[37] reported that in the last 15 years "the women's movement has succeeded in changing many of the historical medical attitudes toward women that have resulted in inappropriate and poor treatment. Yet the medical care offered women during their life stages is still characterized by a lack of effectiveness, safety, and consideration."[37]

The Female AIDS Client

A new concern in women's health is the presence of AIDS in women. Evans reported that, in 1985, more than 12,000 cases of AIDS were diagnosed; this number was expected to double by 1986, and to continue increasing thereafter. "One hundred and eighteen of these cases are women whose only risk factor was that of heterosexual contact with a risk-group member or an AIDS client."[12]

The effect on adult women diagnosed with AIDS is particularly tragic because many of them must cope, not only with their own possible death due to the illness, but with the risk of death to their children if they give birth. Pregnant women with AIDS also have a higher risk of complications during pregnancy.

Evans, in reporting on one case of a 34-year-old female client with AIDS, stated that this client was difficult for the female nurses to deal with, although they had become accustomed to caring for AIDS clients. "The fact that she is a young woman with a previously normal history and lifestyle has made the disease even more frightening." "You realize it could happen to you,"[12] said one nurse working with this client.

Evans emphasized the need for AIDS education for both adolescent and adult women concerning heterosexual transmission of the virus. "Too many women believe they are inherently safe from the disease."[12]

Evans also emphasized the need for the nurse to "learn to deal with her feelings of identification and empathy" with female AIDS clients. Even experienced nurses can be overwhelmed with caring for "a young, heterosexual woman dying from what she previously considered an 'abnormal disease'."[12]

The Therapeutic Use of Self

The nurse who understands the developmental stages of adulthood can apply this knowledge to the assessment of individuals who seek psychiatric care. Effective planning, as well as implementation, of treatment is influenced by the nurse's behaviors and attitudes, which can have a significant impact on treatment outcomes.

The three clinical examples presented earlier clearly illustrate the need for nurses to promote change in individuals and families through communication. Nurses' communication with clients is deliberate and planned, in order to achieve specific goals (for example, reduce anxiety, increase self-esteem, or foster trust). Therapeutic communication occurs over a period of time, and key to its success are nurses' abilities to establish therapeutic alliances with clients.

When establishing these alliances with clients, nurses must carefully consider each of the following principles:

- Nurses must accept clients for who they are, and convey this acceptance to the clients.
- Nurses must possess self-awareness and an understanding of motives and needs (*e.g.*, cultural bias).
- Nurses must demonstrate emotional involvement and, at the same time, maintain objectivity.
- Nurses must convey feelings of empathy to clients.
- Nurses must demonstrate and role model open and honest communication.

The most effective therapeutic alliances develop when nurses convey genuineness, acceptance, honesty, and respect for clients. Nurses' ability to manifest these attitudes and traits with clients exemplifies the therapeutic use of self in the nursing process.

Summary

1. Adulthood includes individuals whose ages range from 18 to 60 years. It is composed of three stages: early adulthood, adulthood, and middle age.
2. Erikson described the maturational crises of adulthood as: intimacy vs. isolation, generativity vs. stagnation, and ego integrity vs. despair.
3. Important events occurring in early adulthood include developing a stable sense of identity and independence, while establishing a primary relationship with another person.
4. Individuals in the adult stage, or the mid-phase of adulthood, work on the task of establishing a career, a family, and a sense of self.
5. During middle age, individuals work to maintain physical health, separate from children, and adapt to losses, such as the death of peers.
6. By being aware of the tasks and problems of adulthood, nurses can more effectively offer care tailored to the developmental needs of adult clients.
7. There are differences in the progression through adult development stages within various cultures.

8. Differences in mental health care needs among adults of different genders are evidenced by variations between the sexes in the rates of mental illness diagnoses.

9. The women's health movement advocates the study and provision of appropriate health care for women.

References

1. Balswick J, Peels C: The Inexpressive Male: A Tragedy of American Society. In Sze W (ed): Human Life Cycle. New York, Jason Aronson, 1975
2. Belle D, Goldman N: Patterns of Diagnoses Received by Men and Women. In Guttentag M (ed): The Mental Health of Women. New York, Academic Press, 1980
3. Bowers M: Psychoses and depression arising in the mid-life period. J New Ment Dis 169:12, 1981
4. Chesler P: Women and Madness. New York, Doubleday, 1972
5. Cochrane R: The Social Creation of Mental Illness. New York, Longman, 1983
6. Cooke D: A Psychological Study of the Climacteric. In Broome A, Wallace L (eds): Psychology and Gynecological Problems. New York, Tavistock, 1984
7. Cunningham W, Owens W: Iowa State Study of the Adult Development of Intellectual Abilities. In Schail K (ed): Studies of Adult Psychological Development. New York, Guilford Press, 1983
8. Davidson L: Preventive attitudes towards mid-life crisis. Am J Psychoanal 39:165, 1985
9. Dohrenwald B, Dohrenwald B: Sex Differences in Psychiatric Disorders. In Grusky O, Pollner M (eds): The Sociology of Mental Illness. New York, Holt, Rinehart, & Winston, 1981
10. Erikson E: Generativity and Ego Integrity. In Neugarten B (ed): Middle Age and Aging. Chicago, University of Chicago Press, 1968
11. Erikson E: Growth and Crisis of the Healthy Personality. In Kludsolm C, Murray H: Personality in Nature, Society, and Culture. New York, Knopf, 1959
12. Evans K: The female AIDS patient. Health Care for Women Int 8:1, 1987
13. Flaskerud J: AIDS: Implications for Nurses. Journal of Psychosocial Nursing and Mental Health Sciences 25:4, 1987
14. Flaskerud J: AIDS: Psychosocial Aspects. Journal of Psychosocial Nursing and Mental Health Sciences 25:8, 1987
15. Framo J: Family of origin as a therapeutic resource for adults in marital and family therapy: You can and should go home again. Fam Process 15:193, 1976
16. Frenkel-Brunswik E: Adjustments and Reorientation in the Course of the Life Span. In Neugarten B (ed): Middle Age and Aging. Chicago, University of Chicago Press, 1968
17. Gould R: The Phases of Adult Life: A Study in Developmental Psychology. Am J Psychiatry 129:33, 1972
18. Havinghurst R: Human Development and Education. New York, Longmans, Green & Co, 1953
19. Hobfoll S, Leiberman J: Personality and social resources in immediate and continued stress resistance among women. J Counsel Consult Psychol 52:18, 1987
20. Holmes T, Rahe R: The social readjustment rating scale. J Psychosom Per 11:213, 1967
21. Jones L, Cochrane R: Stereotypes of mental illness: A test of the labeling hypothesis. Int J Soc Psychiatry 27:99, 1981
22. Klerman G, Weissman M: Depressions Among Women: Their Nature and Causes. In Guttentag M (ed): The Mental Health of Women. New York, Academic Press, 1980
23. Lenz E, Parks L, Jenkins L et al: Life change and instrumental support as predictors of illness in mothers of 6-month-olds. Res Nurs Health 9:17 1986
24. Louie K: Cultural Issues in Psychiatric Nursing. In Lego S (ed): The American Handbook of Psychiatric Nursing. Philadelphia, JB Lippincott, 1984
25. Lewinsohn P: Age at first onset for nonbipolar depression. J Abnorm Psychol 95:378, 1986
26. Menninger K: Work as Sublimation. In Sze W (ed): Human Life Cycle. New York, Jason Aronson, 1978
27. Murray R, Zentner J: Nursing Assessment and Health Promotion Throughout the Life Span. Englewood Cliffs, New Jersey, Prentice-Hall, 1975
28. Neugarten B: Adult Personality: Toward a Psychology of the Life Cycle. In Sze W (ed): Human Life Cycle. New York, Jason Aronson, 1978
29. Neugarten B, Moore J: The Changing Age-Status System. In Neugarten B (ed): Middle Age and Aging. Chicago, University of Chicago Press, 1968
30. Neugarten B: Women's Attitudes Toward Menopause. In Neugarten B (ed): Middle Age and Aging. Chicago, University of Chicago Press, 1968
31. Peck R, Berkowitz H: Personality and Adjustment in Middle Life. In Neugarten B (ed): Personality in Middle and Late Life. New York, Arno Press, 1980
32. Schaie K: The Seattle Longitudinal Study: A 21-Year Exploration of Psychometric Intelligence in Adulthood. In Schaie K (ed): Longitudinal Studies of Adult Psychological Development. New York, Guilford Press, 1983
33. Shanan J, Kedor H: Phenomenological Structuring of the Adult Lifespan as a Function of Age and Sex. Int J Aging Hum Dev 10: 343, 1979–80
34. Shectman K: Motherhood as an Adult Developmental Stage. Am J Psychoanal 40:273, 1980
35. Stein S: Mid-Adult Development and Psychopathology. Am J Psychiatry 35:676, 1978
36. Stuart G, Sundeen S: Principles and Practice of Psychiatric Nursing. St Louis, CV Mosby, 1987
37. Weiss K: Women's Health Care. Reston, Virginia, Reston, 1984
38. Wright L, Leahey M: Nurses and Families: A Guide to Family Assessment and Intervention. Philadelphia, FA Davis, 1984

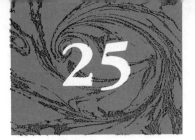

JUDITH F. KARSHMER

HUMAN SEXUALITY

Learning Objectives

Upon completion of this chapter the student should be able to do the following:

1. Define and discuss the nature of human sexuality.
2. From a systems perspective, identify the components that form an individual's sexuality.
3. Identify and define the dimensions of sexual identity.
4. Describe sexuality across the life span.
5. Discuss historical trends and emerging scientific knowledge of sexuality and sexual behavior.
6. Identify and describe common sexual dysfunctions and sexual disorders.
7. Describe nurses' responsibilities in primary, secondary, and tertiary levels of prevention of sexual dysfunctions.
8. Discuss the importance of nurses' understanding and feeling comfortable with their own sexuality as a prerequisite for therapeutic interventions.
9. Identify common nursing interventions used to treat sexual dysfunctions.

Introduction

Mention of the topic of the nurse's role in sexuality sends faculty members hurrying through reference materials, students into a frantic, secretive study of illustrated sex manuals, and nurses deciding that clients "really don't want to talk about THAT anyway." While it is acknowl-edged that sexuality, sexual development, and sexual behavior are important considerations in client care, there remains a basic discomfort in dealing with sexual issues in health care.

In a poll of a group of senior nursing students, 96% agreed that "dealing with patients' sexual issues is a nurs-ing responsibility." However, only 31% of the students felt comfortable doing so. In a review of the nursing care plans of these students, only 3% documented nursing interventions related to sexual issues.[17] Both students and faculty appear to have difficulty dealing with sexual issues. Fontaine[9] reported that faculty were less able to discuss sex with clients than their self-identified level of knowledge would indicate. These findings are inconsistent with the direction that the topic of sexuality took initially. In September of 1982, *Nursing Clinics of North America*[34] addressed the issue of incorporating the topic of sexuality into nursing literature and practice. In 1978, Mims and Swenson[26] suggested that human sexuality had become an accepted part of nursing care of clients. However, nurses' comfort with, and integration of, topics related to sexuality have not dramatically increased.

There is little doubt about the importance of dealing with sexual issues in client care. Sexuality is a key concept because so much of human interaction is directly or indirectly related to sexual affirmation and communication. The lack of comfort, rather than the lack of knowledge, often prevents nurses from dealing with sexual issues with clients. This chapter will provide students with the necessary knowledge base and background for nursing interventions based on the therapeutic use of self. It will also stress the development of personal comfort with sexual issues and the development of a knowledge of one's own sexuality. These topics will be addressed within a systems perspective, and will include sexuality across the life span, sexual variations, dysfunctions and disorders, and nursing interventions for the three levels of prevention.

Sexuality: A Systems Perspective

Sexuality is not limited to the reproductive organs. It is far more complex, and affects all aspects of individuals' lives and their interactions with others. Sexuality is more than the sum of individual experiences, emotions, or anatomical parts. It is an ever-changing, dynamic aspect of the human system that is in constant interaction: when one portion of an individual's sexuality is altered, all other aspects are changed. It is difficult to separate "normal" sexuality from problematic sexuality. Individuals are constantly bombarded with input about how, with what, and when they are supposed to react or respond sexually, resulting in a clouding of individuals' understanding of how they experience or identify sexuality. While this problem occurs in adults, it is also seen during the development of sexual identity.

Systems Dimensions of Sexual Identity

Sexual identity is a key concept of human sexuality. The common use of the term "opposite sex" implies a distinction between men and women. However, only the different responsibilities during conception make such a clear distinction. There are few distinct differences between male and female hormones, and fewer physical and behavioral distinctions. There are probably more physical differences between individuals of the same sex than there are between the two sexes. The overall development of sexual identity involves a complex interaction among four areas: (1) biological identity, (2) gender identity, (3) social sex roles, and (4) sexual orientation.[39]

Biological Identity

Biological sexual identity is determined at the moment of conception by chromosomal typing. This genetic determination establishes the development of sex organs, and determines the sex label given at birth.[39]

Gender Identity

Gender identity is the child's conviction or understanding of his or her own sex. A child's understanding of gender identity usually takes place between the ages of 18 months (the initiation of language acquisition) and three to four years.[27] During this period, children tend to identify with members of the same sex and begin to feel pride in their own genitals. This development is a result of the interaction of chromosomal and hormonal factors, as well as internal cues and, most significantly, cultural and social cues.

Social Sex Roles

An individual's *social sex role* is determined by the cultural and social behavioral expectations of members of each sex. Sex role is largely determined by the culture in which individuals live, and is usually assimilated between the ages of three and seven years.[7] Immediately after birth, sex roles begin to be reinforced; boys are usually dressed in blue, and are handled more roughly than girls, who are dressed in pink. Baby girls are treated more delicately, and are cooed to sweetly.[37] A 1974 study by Rubin, Provenzano, and Luria[33] found that parents' perceptions 24 hours after birth differentiated between male and female babies. Girls were identified as softer, finer, and more delicate; boys were labeled stronger, hardier, and better coordinated. In spite of changing sex stereotypes, a 1980 replication of this study[39] indicates that this form of sex typing continues.

By the age of two to three years, these sex-linked behaviors are established within individuals, and provide individuals with a sense of being either male or female. Sex-role expectations from significant others, especially parents, teachers, babysitters, and friends, continue the differentiation between the sexes. Rodgers[32] describes girls' early childhood years as a "honeymoon period." Girls have greater verbal, perceptual, and cognitive skills, all of which please adults. Therefore, from an early age girls become dependent on adults for approval. Boys, on the other hand, are more likely to be scolded, and learn to become individuals and self-sufficient. The following Relevant Research box shows that, while changes are taking place in traditional sex-role stereotyping, these changes continue to be slow.

RELEVANT RESEARCH

The author of this study used a longitudinal design employing surveying techniques to assess change in a measure of traditional sex roles. In 1975, the author surveyed three independent groups of university graduates from the classes of 1954, 1964, and 1974. The same study was repeated with the same groups in 1980. Subjects completed five-item Likert scales portraying conceptions of appropriate behaviors for men and women. Data showed that the overall change during the five-year period indicated a decrease in traditionalism. This, however, varied importantly for subgroups in the study: women changed more than men, and subjects that graduated more recently changed more than those from the earlier years.

(McBroom WH: Changes in sex-role orientations: A five-year longitudinal comparison. Sex Roles 11:583, 1984.)

Sexual Orientation

Sexual orientation is determined by individuals' physical and emotional sex preferences. There is considerable controversy regarding when sexual orientation becomes established. Kinsey and colleagues[21] first demonstrated that sexual orientation was defined by the sources that provide erotic stimulation, rather than by a fixed, immutable self-identity. Previous theories explained normal sexual preference as static and exclusively heterosexual. Today, sexual orientation is much less clearly defined, and a range of variations exists.

Throughout history, sexual functions and behavior have been surrounded by secrecy, myths, prohibitions, and misinformation. Higgins and Hawkins[13] identified four reasons for this: (1) the human race depends on sexual drives and reproduction for continuity; (2) sexual responses are strong emotions that involve individuals in intimate relationships; (3) sexual interaction affects the establishment and preservation of families (including property rights) as well as the security and psychological growth of members; and (4) human sexuality induces fear because of a lack of knowledge about reproduction and sexual function. Individuals have sought control of the powerful and mysterious forces of sexual attraction and behavior. These controls have come from families, churches, the state, individuals themselves, and, until recently, the scientific community.

From childhood through old age, societies have had expectations about how members should feel about their bodies, seek sexual pleasures, and establish sexual patterns. Society has also dictated the ages and conditions under which sex is allowed. Healthy sexual development includes learning how to differentiate between expected and actual behaviors.

Sexuality Across the Life Span

Infancy

Infants are sensual human beings whose gratification comes from feeding, warmth, closeness, and caressing. Infants whose needs are met tend to develop higher levels of self-esteem and feelings of security. They respond to verbal and (even more significantly) to nonverbal reactions of their parents to their actions. Infants engage in random genital play. Nondramatic, accepting responses of parents to their activities increase infants' development of self-trust.

Early Childhood

Genital play during early childhood is less random and more purposeful than that during infancy. During toilet training, parents and children focus more attention on the genitals. While the approach and severity of the training have an impact on the psychosocial development of the child, the training has a greater impact on the child's acceptance of basic sexual functioning. It is common for young children to engage in sexual exploration and masturbation. Less aversion shown by parents results in greater acceptance by children of the appropriateness of the time and place for these activities.[22,30]

Late Childhood

As children grow and develop, their involvement with sexuality also grows and develops. In contrast to the view of late childhood as one of sexual latency,[10] this period is clearly one in which children begin to engage actively in sexual behavior. These activities include masturbation, genital manipulation with peers (same-sex and opposite-sex), and genital exhibition.[21] During this period, children concentrate on playing with friends of the same sex in school, and delight in telling dirty jokes.[13]

Adolescence

The time period from puberty to adulthood is marked with many developmental tasks. Physically, the individual is growing and changing rapidly. (For a complete discussion of the physiology of sexual maturation, see Higgins and Hawkins, 1984.[13]) Sexual development is a major part of these changes. "The blossoming of sexuality in each generation of adolescents is as fascinating a sight as the unfolding of spring each year: predictable and repetitive, yet nonetheless enchanting."[18] The increased production of hormones and the spontaneity of physical arousal establish sexual response and behavior as a major adaptation mechanism of adolescents for coping and interacting with their world.

Sexual activity fills adolescents' needs for the entire range of intense feelings, including dominance, submission, belonging, exploration, competence, and love. Adolescents who experience healthy sexual activity and sexual growth increase their self-esteem; increased self-esteem enhances healthy sexuality. Unhealthy, exploitative sex increases guilt and lowers adolescents' self-esteem; low self-esteem potentiates an unhealthy sense of sexuality.

Faced with many decisions concerning sexuality and sexual behavior, adolescents frequently question the normalcy of their behavior. During this developmental phase, it is common for the self to be a focus of sexual pleasure. Sorenson[35] found that 58% of all male adolescents and 39% of all female adolescents masturbated. However, many individuals believe that masturbation is not acceptable and is a dangerously immoral act. It is not unusual for adolescents to worry about being homosexual; Jensen[16] found that 25% of all adolescents have had sexual experiences with others of the same sex.

Changing norms and expectations of teenagers have emphasized sexual activity and have reduced societal constraints. Sexual activity among teenagers has increased by more than 60% since 1970.[38] Of 29 million adolescents between the ages of 13 and 19, 12 million have experienced sexual intercourse. There are more than 1 million teenage pregnancies in the United States each year.[13] Births to adolescents have reached epidemic proportions. Increased sexual activity has not been accompanied by related knowledge and understanding on the part of adolescents, their parents, or society. Therefore, problems related to sexuality have multiplied.

Adulthood

Adolescence, in part, prepares individuals for adult life. Because sexuality is physical, cognitive, affective, and behavioral, participation in healthy sexuality is a benefit of adulthood. Knowledge and understanding of sexual responsiveness enable us to explore more clearly the nature of adult sexuality. Kinsey and associates[20,21] provided details about sexual behavior. Hite[14,15] focused on what men and women think, feel, and like about sex. Masters and Johnson[23,24] established a whole new field of scientific inquiry into the physiology of sexual functioning, and created an approach to the treatment of sexual dysfunction and enhancement of sexual enjoyment. As our understanding of sexuality grows, so does our comfort with exploring, experiencing, and responding.

Older Adulthood

Sex among the elderly has only recently become a focus of study for professionals. However, older individuals have been interested all along. It is significant that older adults continue to participate in sex and experience their sexuality in direct relation to their interest and sexuality in earlier years. In other words, sexual behavior patterns continue into older adulthood. However, the effects of aging do have an impact on individuals. A number of factors, including alcoholism, the side-effects of drugs, eating disorders, and declining health all directly affect sexual activity and ability. Stereotypes, however, are more influential in affecting the sexual patterns of the elderly. There seems to be a continual effort to convince both the young and the elderly that old people either "can't do it" or "aren't interested" in sex or sexuality.

Understanding Sexuality

Although reproductive anatomy has long been understood, until recently the nature of sex physiology has not been explored. Medical study of sexuality was largely restricted by societal and religious morality, which condemned all forms of nonreproductive sex.

In the late 19th century, theorists, not experimentalists, established criteria for what was considered "normal." In contrast to those that perceived any form of sexual behavior (other than for procreation) to be perversion, these theorists had a more "enlightened" view. They differed from theorists such as Freud, who considered any variation from the "norm" as indicative of pathology or arrested development.

By comparison with other bio-psycho-social aspects, study of human sexuality did not evolve until relatively recently. In 1948 and 1953, Kinsey[20,21] conducted surveys that raised the sexual consciousness of the entire country. He documented that, while men were more sexually active than women of all age groups, their sexual behavior peaked in the early 20s; women seemed to reach a peak between the ages of 30 and 45. He found that both men and women masturbated frequently, and that married couples reported women experiencing multiple orgasms, an notion that was unheard of prior to this time. Kinsey also found that homosexuality was more prevalent than had earlier been thought, with 10% of the men and 2% to 6% of the women identified relatively exclusively as homosexuals. Perhaps even more significant was the fact that more than 25% of the men reported having had homosexual experiences at one time. Kinsey's work sparked research in an area in which little was known and documented.

In 1966, Masters and Johnson published their first work, which documented the nature of human sexual response. They outlined the responsive nature of the entire body and, through observation, validated Kinsey's finding that women were able to have multiple orgasms. Masters and Johnson[23] outlined the four phases of the *sexual response cycle* as: excitement, plateau, orgasm, and resolution. The initial, or *excitement phase,* can result from any reflexogenic or psychogenic stimulation. Different individuals respond to different stimuli. During this phase, the body prepares for continuation of the stimulation until orgasm. If the stimulation from the excitement phase continues, the individual will pass into the second, or *plateau phase*. If, however, the stimulus or drive is removed, there will be decreased sexual tension and movement into a prolonged resolution phase, without orgasmic relief.

If stimulation continues, the person experiences an *orgasm,* which usually lasts from a few seconds to several minutes.[18] During orgasm, the vasoconstriction and muscle tension developed during stimulation are released. Orgasm is an involuntary climax that represents a release of the maximum sexual tension attained. Orgasms are focused in the pelvic region; for women they are usually centered on the clitoris, vagina, and uterus, while for men they are usually centered on the penis, the prostate, and the seminal vesicles. Women seem to have greater variation in duration and intensity of orgasm than do men.

The fourth phase is the *resolution phase.* This is an involuntary period of tension loss in which individuals move, in reverse order, through the plateau and excitement phases. During the resolution phase, women may quickly reach second and third orgasms. For men, the resolution phase also includes a *refractory period,* a time of nonresponse to further stimulation. Effective restimulation is not possible until refraction is over.

Sexual Orientation

The Hite survey of women[15] and a 1982 study[31] documented a wide range of sexual behavior, practices, and attitudes. Sexual expressions can be placed on a continuum according to the relative frequency of homosexual or heterosexual ideation, affect, and behavior.

Most individuals are aware of their sexual orientation from early childhood.[12] This is different from the notion that one event or a series of experiences can cause an individual to become either heterosexual or homosexual.[39] Often, individuals are confused and feel pressured to decide whether they are homosexual, heterosexual, or lesbian. In general, sexual orientation has little or nothing to do with an individual's desire to be one sex or the other. The determination of hetero- or homosexuality depends on whether an individual becomes erotically aroused by people of the opposite or the same sex, and/or whether that person engages in sexual activities with individuals of the same or opposite sex.[4,29] Of key interest is the *arousal,* or feeling of sexual interest in the same or the opposite sex, not necessarily acting on the feelings. Bisexual individuals respond equally, although in different ways, to a variety of people regardless of sex. In spite of the fact that few differences have been found between heterosexual and homosexual individuals, homosexuals have been victims of blatant discrimination in Western society.

Homosexuality

Weinberg[39] found that male homosexuality is more threatening than female, because of the special power position and benefits afforded to men in society. It is perceived as far worse for a man to act like a woman (who is thought of in prejudicial fashion as being weak and inferior to a man) than it is for a woman to act like a man. It is beyond comprehension for many that a man would choose to give up his "male status." On the other hand, women strive for power and status, and therefore it "makes sense" that they would want to become more masculine.

As indicated earlier, medical views and attitudes toward sex grew from religious sexual morality. Because the church condemned any form of nonprocreative sex, masturbation and homosexuality were seen as particularly immoral, and were viewed by the medical community as harmful to health. In the mid-19th century, medical professionals split from the church in their beliefs about homosexuality. In an effort to view the homosexual as a variant rather than a deviant, doctors sought to reduce pressure by removing responsibility for homosexuality from the individual. One theory[18] proposed that homosexuals' development was arrested at an early age. This view suggested that homosexuals were not responsible for their behavior and, therefore, should not be punished.

During the first three-fourths of the 20th century, homosexuality was considered an illness. The American Psychiatric Association defined homosexuality as a psychiatric disorder. In 1974, the Association removed homosexuality as a diagnostic category. Unfortunately, the new knowledge and understanding of the medical community has not removed the social stigma attached to homosexuality.

Homosexuality is currently defined as the erotic arousal of an individual by people of the same sex, and/or sexual behavior between individuals of the same sex.[4,29] Although homosexuality is no longer considered pathological, some individuals still seek to change homosexuals to heterosexuals. The most common approaches include *systematic desensitization* and *aversive techniques.* These approaches seek to recondition the individual's sexual responses to homosexual behavior. Psychotherapy is sometimes used as an implicit or explicit tool to "eliminate" a client's homosexuality. On occasion, clients seek therapy to reduce homosexual feelings. More frequently, however, individuals seek therapy for a range of emotional difficulties that the therapist ascribes to the homosexuality. When this occurs, therapists confound the treatment regimen, and seek resolution by "helping" individuals change their sexual orientation. Interestingly, therapeutic treatment of homosexual individuals is no different than treatment of heterosexuals. Both experience a range of interpersonal difficulties, sexual and nonsexual. However, just as heterosexuals' problems cannot be viewed as having been caused by heterosexuality, neither can homosexuals' problems be attributed to their homosexuality.

The Nurse and the Homosexual

Although homosexuality is no longer viewed as a psychiatric disorder, it is still risky for homosexuals to disclose their lifestyle choices to others. This is also true in nurs-

RELEVANT RESEARCH

In a large, urban teaching hospital having many clients with AIDS, 37 medical house officers and 91 RNs completed a questionnaire designed to measure attitudes about homosexuality. Mean scores for both physicians and nurses indicated fewer negative feelings toward homosexuality than historical mean scores for non-health professionals. The women in the study were significantly more "homophobic" than the men. However, the most alarming finding was that nearly 10% of all respondents agreed with the statement that homosexuals who get AIDS were "getting what they deserve." The authors concluded that this may indicate that homophobia is actually higher than the mean attitude scores may indicate, and very much higher than is desirable in a group of health professionals.

(Douglas CJ, Kalman CM, Kalman TP: Homophobia among physicians and nurses: An empirical study. Hosp Community Psychiatry 36:1309, 1985.)

ing. If clients share this information, they risk having all of their feelings reinterpreted in the light of their homosexuality, and face possible prejudicial care by nurses.

Homosexuals who have AIDS are a particularly vulnerable population. Douglas, Kalman, and Kalman[8] found that health care professionals demonstrated homophobic attitudes toward AIDS clients, as is shown in the above Relevant Research box.

Nursing Interventions in Human Sexuality

The Therapeutic Use of Self

Nurses must have a clear understanding and appreciation of their own sexuality in order to work with issues related to clients' sexuality. This is not a static comprehension, but an ongoing affirmation of nurses' views of themselves. As with all nurses' special backgrounds, skills, knowledge, and motivations, sexuality is a unique part of their sense of themselves. Sexuality is a key aspect of all interpersonal relations, and has the potential to become therapeutic in nurses' working relationships with clients who have sexual problems as well as with those who don't.

Primary Prevention

Nursing interventions are directed toward promoting health and preventing illness. Developing healthy sexuality involves a variety of factors, including psychological, cultural, societal, environmental, and physical. Understanding sexuality from a systems perspective guides nursing assessment and intervention by helping nurses to consider all facets of clients' lives. Often the most basic but necessary intervention to promote sexual development is the explicit discussion with clients of their views toward and understanding of their sexuality. While this may seem superficial and obvious, it is the intervention least frequently used.

The most important intervention in the area of sexuality is the explicit identification of sexuality as an issue, followed by a discussion of clients' views of their personal sexuality. The social norms that inhibit open discussion of sexuality have taught clients to avoid dealing with their perceptions of sexual development and behavior. Only when nurses identify sexuality as an area of importance are clients free to bring up areas of concern or confusion. Through conscientious interviewing, nurses allow clients to explore and consolidate their views and understanding of their sexuality. By directing clients to consider all systems aspects, nurses help clients to understand the effects of each part of the system on their sexuality. This aspect of primary prevention is dependent on nurses' comfort with their own sexuality, which serves as a model for clients. This form of intervention is appropriate for clients of all ages, and is an essential part of nursing care for all clients, even those being treated for problems that are not sexually related.

Secondary Prevention

The early case-finding and treatment of potential and actual sexual problems fall into two major categories: *predictible developmental events and situations* and *unexpected crises*. A number of predictible events can directly influence an individual's sexuality. Anticipation of possible difficulties allows nurses to intervene and avert negative outcomes. Developmental events that can potentially cause sexual problems include: pregnancy, the birthing process, the postpartum period, menopause, dysmenorrhea, premenstrual syndrome, contraceptive choices, abortion, and sexually transmitted diseases.

Each of these events forces individuals to recognize and analyze their personal sexuality and sexual behavior. Nurses must anticipate this and, when possible, initiate interventions before the event occurs. Nursing interventions should include: (1) identifying with clients the possibility that sexuality may be affected by the experience; (2) exploring the impact of the experience or event before it occurs, when possible; (3) using the basis of trust developed in the nurse–client relationship, encouraging clients to identify and understand the impact of the event on their sexuality; and (4) facilitating clients' recovery after the experience by synthesizing the events and clients' response patterns, while helping clients learn about personal sexuality.

Sexual disruptions following crises may also force clients to reevaluate their sexuality. Whether or not crises are sexually related, nurses must help clients return to, or attain, peak levels of sexual functioning and healthy sexuality. The impact of the crisis on sexuality should be considered for all health problems, whether a broken leg or an acute psychotic episode.

Rape

One of the most devastating forms of sexual crisis is sexual assault, or *rape*. The National Institute of Mental Health defines rape as "intercourse, cunnilingus, fellatio, anal intercourse, or any intrusion of any part of another's body, or any object manipulated by another into the genital or anal opening of the victim's body, or intentional touching of the victim's sexual parts by another when this is accompanied by force or threat of force, or against the victim's will."[39] Rape is not a sexual act, but an act of violence in which sex is used as a weapon. In accord with this definition, using force to induce individuals to perform acts against their will cannot rationally be seen as anything but a severe danger.[39] Nurses are usually the first health care providers that rape victims encounter. It is essential that nurses know the proper protocols for treatment, including legal ramifications and the need for teaching and counseling. Nurses must also be prepared to provide anticipatory guidance to rape victims.

It is believed that fewer than 10% of all rapes are ever reported. Of these, only about 1% get to trial, where 30% result in convictions.[36] There are a number of reasons why rapes are not reported. These include fear and guilt, the worry that the victim might not be believed, and the victim's desire to forget the experience.

Rape trauma syndrome, first described by Burgess,[6] delineates two phases an adult victim undergoes as a result of forceable rape. The *acute phase* is marked by either an expressive or a masked style. The *expressive style* is characterized by fear, anger, sobbing, restlessness, and tension. Its opposite, the *masked style,* is calm, subdued, and hidden. Victims suffer from a variety of somatic difficulties, and demonstrate extreme fear of violence and death. The acute phase usually lasts for less than one month.

The length of the *recovery phase* depends on a number of factors, such as the degree of physical injury and the victim's self-esteem. Burgess' research[5] has documented that 37% of all rape victims are "back to normal" within several months. Another 37% of the victims recover within a year, but 30% are still recovering four to six years after the experience. Those who recovered quickly had high self-esteem, and evaluated their parts in the episodes as appropriate. These victims worked to ascribe some "meaning" to the experience, and defined behaviors that would enable them to prevent such attacks in the future.

The nursing diagnosis and clinical approaches related to the rape trauma syndrome indicate that the primary responsibilities of nurses are: (1) dealing with clients in a relaxed, sympathetic, nonjudgmental manner; (2) providing emergency health care; (3) performing a nursing assessment and collecting evidentiary material and documentation; (4) preventing unwanted pregnancy and venereal disease; and (5) arranging for follow-up. The immediate kindness and support shown by nurses to rape victims may be the single most important aspect of nursing care provided to these victims.[28]

Rapists are also of concern to nurses. Rape can be categorized by three different motivations: anger, power, and sadism. Rape is never a result of sexual arousal, but, rather, is an expression of power over another person.[39] For most rapists, the act results from a specific fear of and feeling of hostility toward women.[11] Most rapists believe that the act will be sexually rewarding, but find that it is not. Weinberg[39] indicated that rapists suffer from either temporary or chronic psychiatric dysfunction, and are unable to deal with the stresses of life. Emotionally weak and immature, they lack close interpersonal relationships.[11] More than half of the offenders in this study were found to have been victims of sexual assault when they were children, half had been drinking at the time of the assault, and more than one third experienced sexual dysfunction during the rape.

Nurses must work with offenders to facilitate their search for and securing of treatment. It is essential to view offenders as individuals, and avoid making judgmental and prejudicial comments. Nurses' therapeutic interpersonal relationships can have a positive impact on offenders. The factors and experiences that led offenders to commit such violent acts, as well as their reasons for seeking treatment, are appropriate topics to explore during the nursing interview.

Nurses have varying attitudes toward the victims of rape, as is shown in the following Relevant Research box. This research calls into question the degree to which nurses maintain the perspective of placing blame for rape where it belongs—on the rapist. Nurses must initiate secondary prevention in relation to rape. Each act of sexual aggression forces individual victims to focus on sexual behavior or function. As a result, their views regarding sexuality are reassessed and potentially enhanced or negatively affected. Nurses must anticipate this, and raise the issue with clients before they become overwhelmed by the experience and lose their ability to cope, or attempt to avoid sexual issues. The following clinical example presents a nursing care plan for a rape victim.

Nursing Interventions

When working with clients who are experiencing events that have potential impact on their views toward and understanding of their sexuality, nurses should initiate discussion of clients' fears and hopes as well as the nature of the influence on them. Nurses should encourage clients to explore what occurred during the sexual aggres-

RELEVANT RESEARCH

One hundred eighty senior baccalaureate nursing students read six different accounts of a rape victim who drove to a drugstore on a legitimate errand. In the different versions, the rape victim either locked or failed to lock her car door and was traveling at either 5 p.m., 9 p.m., or midnight. Students who read the versions in which the car door was unlocked viewed the victim as predisposed to being raped. They also viewed her less sympathetically, and felt that she was more careless and responsible for having been raped. The versions of the account that placed the victim running the errand at midnight were also viewed less favorably by these students.

(Damrosch S: How perceived carelessness and time of attack affect nursing students' attributions about rape victims. Psychol Rep 56:531, 1985.)

---

sion, as well as the significance of the experience for their sexuality and their sexual behavior.

It is essential for nurses to anticipate the potential impact of such assaultive experiences on clients. Often, individuals become so enmeshed with the specifics of their physical condition that they do not consider the sexual issues. Conversely, some clients may focus extensively on their sexuality, think that their focus is "out of proportion," and hesitate to discuss it. In either case, nurses must label the potential issues and encourage clients to consider and work with them. When these interventions are timely, clients have the opportunity to integrate the experiences with a new level of understanding of their sexuality.

Tertiary Prevention

The goal of providing nursing care for clients who have sexual difficulties is to help them attain an optimum level of functioning. The two major categories of sexual problems are *sexual dysfunction* (or disturbed sexual response) and *sexual disorders* (such as pedophilia). While these are disparate problems, nurses' goals in tertiary prevention are similar.

Sexual Dysfunction

Formerly, sexual dysfunction was thought to be caused by underlying psychological problems or neuroses. It was believed that once the underlying problem was resolved the sexual problem would also be solved.[3] Masters and Johnson[24] rejected these ideas. They documented a treatment approach based on the premise that sexual response is a natural function, and that it is influenced by physiological *and* psychosocial factors such as depression, anxiety, and stress. The Masters and Johnson approach focuses on education and communication.

Impotence

The major form of sexual dysfunction for males is primary or secondary impotence. Individuals who suffer from *primary impotence* have never been able to achieve or maintain an erection sufficient to perform coitus. Approximately 15% of all impotent men suffer from some sort of physiological or metabolic problem. The remaining 85% have no physiological reason. Clinical treatment focuses on exploration of traumatic first attempts at intercourse and basic fears of an inability to perform sexually. Men who suffer from *secondary impotence* have successfully had intercourse on one or more occasions, but later developed difficulty in achieving and maintaining an erection. For a large portion of men, performance fears are the cause of the problem. However, alcoholism is the second leading cause of secondary impotence.[25] Treatment centers on explaining and removing the so-called "spectator role" during sexual activity.[39] This difficulty arises when individuals sacrifice spontaneity and become detached spectators during sex, usually because of a fear of inadequacy. Treatment focuses on communication techniques and removing pressure for performance during intercourse. Individuals are encouraged to *sensate focus* (experience comfortable sexual feelings while gently caressing their partner's body and desisting from intercourse and orgasm).

Disorders of Ejaculation

Whether individuals have problems with premature ejaculation (ejaculation before the individual's partner is satisfied), ejaculation incompetence (the inability to ejaculate), or retrograde ejaculation (the absence of semen as an ejaculate due to emptying of the ejaculate into the bladder), nurses have several responsibilities in working with these clients. Initially, nurses must gather assessment data to rule out physical causes for ejaculation disorders. At the same time, nurses must work with clients to allow them to express their fears and concerns and encourage them to discuss the impact the problems have on their sense of self and interpersonal relations.

Anorgasm

The major sexual dysfunction in women is *anorgasm*, or lack of orgasm, which may be caused by organic or psychological factors. Once the cause is determined and physiological conditions are remedied, treatment focuses on removing performance pressure. This is done to assist clients to explore, define, and communicate erotic foci, needs, and preferences to their partners.

CLINICAL EXAMPLE

Police found Elaine wandering around the neighborhood near the university in total disarray, with several superficial cuts and bruises. She seemed to be dazed and confused, and was unable to explain where she had been or what had happened. The police took Elaine to the hospital's emergency room. During the initial nursing assessment, Elaine cried, and told the nurse that she had gone to a party with friends and had met "some guy." Although she knew his first name, that is all she knew about him. After the party, he had offered to take her home. On the way, he had driven to a deserted road and raped her.

Elaine told the nurse that all she wanted to do was to make sure she wasn't pregnant, and then "forget" the whole awful experience. She hadn't said anything to the police because she didn't want to press charges, and particularly didn't want any of her friends to find out what had happened.

NURSING CARE PLAN: ELAINE

ASSESSMENT	NURSING INTERVENTIONS	EVALUATION CRITERIA

NURSING DIAGNOSIS: Rape Trauma Syndrome—Acute Phase

SUBJECTIVE DATA
Client states, "I was raped."

OBJECTIVE DATA
Client was brought to the ER by police. She was found wandering the streets in disarray, with superficial cuts and bruises.

1. Provide a private area in the ER where the nurse and the client can talk.
2. Stay with client; do not leave her alone.
3. Give client choices.
4. Encourage client to relate details in her own words.
5. Reassure client that forgetting details is normal.
6. Elicit essential data: when; where; was there a threat of or actual violence; did client see a weapon or was it referred to; was there physical abuse; was a foreign object inserted into the rectum or vagina; were restraints used; did the client lose consciousness at any time?
7. Remain accepting and nonjudgmental.
8. Inform client that she may permit or refuse the collection of physical evidence. If she is unsure or thinks she might change her mind about pressing charges, the hospital can collect evidence and hold it for seven days, releasing it only with her permission.
9. Prepare client for the medical examination. In addition to treating cuts and bruises, the physician will conduct a pelvic exam and provide prophylaxis against unwanted pregnancy and sexually transmitted diseases. This may be traumatic, reminding the client of the attack. The nurse must remain with the client and provide emotional support.

By the end of the interview, client will appear more relaxed and be able to talk freely about what has occurred.
Client will appear to have gained self-esteem and self-control.
Client will tell the nurse, in her own words, what happened and how she feels about the assault.

Client will provide sufficient details regarding the assault.

Client will state that she understands her rights regarding the collection of evidentiary material.

Client will be able to cooperate with the physician during the exam, and make her wishes known regarding treatment.

(Continued)

NURSING CARE PLAN: ELAINE (CONTINUED)

ASSESSMENT	NURSING INTERVENTIONS	EVALUATION CRITERIA

NURSING DIAGNOSIS: Rape Trauma Syndrome—Potential for long-term difficulties
30.   Excess of or deficit in dominant emotions
30.01   Impaired emotional experience
30.01.08   Impaired emotional experience

SUBJECTIVE DATA
Client states, "I never should have let him take me home. I shouldn't have gone to the party in the first place. Why me? What did I do? I don't want anyone to know. . . . I only want to forget the whole thing."

OBJECTIVE DATA
Client is crying and has difficulty in talking between sobs.

1. Assure client that she is not to blame, and that her attack was violent and potentially life-threatening. Remind client that she was a victim of a sick person who wanted to disgrace and humiliate her, *not because of her,* but because she represented something to him.
2. Work with client to help her regain a sense of control over her life. She must come to the conclusion that she can prevent such experiences in the future.
3. Explore with client her decision not to press charges. Explain that she has time to change her mind.
4. Contact any person client may want to help her during discharge and at home.
5. Provide client with an opportunity to bathe and change into clean clothing and leave the hospital in a dignified manner.
6. Initiate provision for follow-up care: contact client the following day and at intervals for the next month; explain availability of rape counselor and refer client to community resources. Long-term care focuses on victim's feelings of control and self-esteem.

Short-term: Client will verbalize that she was not to blame, but was a victim.
Long-term: When contacted over the next few weeks by the nurse, client will be able to discuss the assault and her ability to survive. She will place the blame for the attack on the rapist.

Short-term: The client will discuss how her actions could be modified to reduce the chances of such violence occurring again.
Long-term: Client will demonstrate behaviors that reduce the risk for potential assault. Client will verbalize that she understands the implications of her decision, and that she knows that she can change her mind.
Client will supply the name of a person to assist her during discharge and at home.

Client will bathe and change clothes.

Client will utilize available resources.

Vaginismus

Vaginismus is the involuntary constriction of pelvic musculature. It is a reflex stimulated by imagined, anticipated, or real attempts at vaginal penetration. The severity varies from making penetration impossible to mild dyspareunia with stinging on penetration. The most frequent causes are psychogenic in nature, and include severe psychosocial conditioning against intercourse; religious orthodoxy; rape or sexual assault; trauma associated with a first pelvic examination; and repeated male sexual dysfunction, causing pelvic congestion.[39]

Initial treatment for vaginismus establishes and demonstrates to the women that the spasm is involuntary. The use of increasingly large dilators can be helpful. Nurses must encourage these women to discuss their perceptions of the causes of the problem, and their beliefs about its resolution. It is imperative that the women be encouraged to discuss the significance of the difficulty for their involvement in sexual behavior, the impact it has on sexual partners, and their overall sexuality.

Dyspareunia

A common reason for decreased sexual activity in women is *dyspareunia,* or painful intercourse. The causes vary,

CLINICAL EXAMPLE

Richard was admitted to the hospital for overnight observation after having received a head injury following a motorcycle accident. Shortly after Richard was admitted, his wife was seen by a nurse leaving his room crying. Soon thereafter, the nurse entered the room, and asked Richard if there was anything upsetting him. Richard hesitated, and then began to dismiss the nurse's inquiry. The nurse then explained to Richard that she was really interested in him, and was concerned because she had seen his wife leaving in tears. She explained the nature of the nurse–client relationship, and assured him that everything he said was confidential. She told him that she hoped that he would trust her enough to let her help him deal with whatever was troubling him.

Richard explained that he had recently been laid off from his job, and was having difficulty in finding a new one. He said that "relations with his wife were strained" (a phrase he used at least four times). After Richard outlined his perceptions of the problem, the nurse asked if "strained relations with his wife" meant that he was having some sexual difficulty. Richard appeared relieved to have the topic made explicit and labeled.

and include vaginal infections, frequent douching, allergic responses, torn tissues, and lack of lubrication. After the cause is established, nurses should initiate discussion of the implications of the problem for the women and their sexual partners. To achieve effective treatment, it is important that any feelings of failure or guilt be explored and allayed. The work of Masters and Johnson has been instrumental in disproving the myths that sexual behavior comes naturally, that only vaginal orgasms should be experienced, and that men are responsible for women's orgasms. Nurses must provide clients with such information.

Nursing Interventions

Nurses must establish for clients the importance of discussing sexual issues. This is done by asking explicitly about: the nature of the problem; the client's perceptions of the cause of the problem; and the impact of the problem, and potentially the treatment, on the client and the client's sexual partner(s) and on the client's significant others.

People of all walks of life, men and women, the experienced and the inexperienced, the young and the old, periodically experience some degree of interruption in ideal sexual response patterns. Employing the therapeutic use of self, nurses are in a unique position to identify sexual problems and intervene with clients to facilitate their movement toward positive sexual growth. The following clinical example presents a nursing care plan for a client with a sexual dysfunction.

Sexual Disorders

The American Psychiatric Association's *Diagnostic and Statistical Manual of Mental Disorders* (DSM-III-R)[2] identifies and defines a variety of sexual disorders having different degrees of frequency and severity. The major disorders will be presented below, followed by a discussion of nursing interventions.

Gender Identity Disorders

Gender identity disorders are characterized by individuals' feelings of discomfort and inappropriateness about their anatomic sex, and their persistent abnormal behaviors associated with the opposite sex. These disorders are rare, and should not be confused with the common phenomenon of feeling inadequate in fulfilling the expectations of one's gender identity role.

Transsexualism

Transsexualism is a disorder found in individuals who are genetically of one sex but psychologically and emotionally of another. They have a persistent sense of discomfort and inappropriateness about their anatomic sex, a desire to be rid of their own genitals, and a desire to live as members of the opposite sex.

Paraphilia

Paraphilia is the use of unusual imaging or acts for sexual excitement. Acts tend to be involuntarily repetitive (or compulsive), and generally involve a preference for nonhuman objects for sexual arousal, repetitive sexual activity with humans involving real or simulated suffering, or repetitive sexual activity with nonconsenting partners.

Fetishism

The use of an object for sexual arousal is called *fetishism*. The fetish object may be used to increase sexual excitation, and often becomes the preferred sexual partner or object. *Partialism* is a fetish for a particular body part. There is a fine line between normal arousal and partialism, since certain body parts initiate arousal in most people. *Object fetishism* occurs when an inanimate object, of any form, becomes sexually revered. Most often the object is a piece of women's apparel. The fetishist often masturbates in the presence of the object, and frequently involves it in the sexual act.

NURSING CARE PLAN: RICHARD

ASSESSMENT	NURSING INTERVENTIONS	EVALUATION CRITERIA

NURSING DIAGNOSIS: 26. Alterations in sexuality
26.01.06 Impaired sexual desire

SUBJECTIVE DATA

Client states, "Relations with my wife are strained. Ever since I was laid off things have been terrible. My wife and I seem to argue all the time—we don't ever seem to get along. I feel she thinks I'm a failure, even though she hasn't ever said it. I can't even seem to make love any more."

OBJECTIVE DATA

The client's wife left the room crying. He appeared tense and seemed to want to talk about his relationship with his wife and his sexual difficulties.

1. Nurse must form a contract with client, explicitly defining confidentiality as well as her interest in helping and ability to help him deal with his interpersonal difficulties.
2. The nurse must listen and respond appropriately to the information shared by client about sexual difficulties, and label it, making it explicit.
3. The nurse must elicit answers to questions that enable client to explore the nature of the dysfunction in order for the nurse to arrive at specific nursing diagnoses.

Client will feel comfortable in discussing his sexual difficulties.

Client will explain the specific nature of his sexual difficulty, *e.g.*, his inability to maintain an erection.

NURSING DIAGNOSIS: 26. Alterations in sexuality
26.01.05 Impaired sexual activity

SUBJECTIVE DATA

Client states, ". . . I seem to be watching myself . . . always worried whether or not I will get an erection, but mostly if I will be able to keep it. . . . I feel like such a failure."

1. The nurse must explore with client his perception of the problem—what he believes to be the cause, how things have changed, when he noticed difficulty in achieving and maintaining a erection.
2. During the interview, the nurse must

Client will be able to share with the nurse what he perceives to be the nature of his problem.

Client will be able to explain the negative

(Continued)

Transvestism

Achievement of sexual gratification by dressing in the clothing of the opposite sex is called *transvestism*. Contrary to popular opinion, those who receive gratification from cross-dressing are usually heterosexual.

Zoophilia

Zoophilia is the use of animals as the exclusive or repeated and preferred method of achieving sexual excitement. Most often the animal is one with which the individual has had contact during childhood.[18]

Pedophilia

The act or fantasy of engaging in sexual activity using prepubertal children as the repeated and preferred object of sexual excitement is termed *pedophilia*. The sexual orientation of the individual may be either heterosexual or homosexual.

Exhibitionism

Exhibitionism is the exposure of one's genitals to unsuspecting individuals in order to achieve sexual arousal. This disorder occurs only in males, and is the most common sexual offense in the United States.

Voyeurism

Observing people undressing or engaging in sexual behavior, without their permission, for the purpose of sexual gratification is termed *voyeurism*. The observer does not seek sexual activity with those who are being observed. Taking pleasure in watching a partner undress as part of a sexual act is different from being obsessed with watching a stranger in secret. The former is not diagnostic of a disorder.

Sadism

Inflicting pain, whether psychological or physical, to achieve sexual arousal is termed *sadism*.

NURSING CARE PLAN: RICHARD (CONTINUED)

ASSESSMENT	NURSING INTERVENTIONS	EVALUATION CRITERIA
OBJECTIVE DATA Client displays concern and worry about his sexual performance. Client views overall ability in terms of his sexual abilities.	explore client's performance fears as well as establish whether alcohol is a significant factor. 3. Facilitate reducing client's "spectator role" during intercourse, thus reducing performance fears. 4. Encourage client to discuss his performance fears with the nurse and his wife. 5. As the therapeutic relationship evolves, the nurse may encourage client and his wife to discuss their relationship jointly with her. 6. Reassure client and his wife that sexual difficulties and fears are normal, occur in most people from time to time, and should not be considered pathological. 7. Treatment for secondary impotence is based on education and communication. Behavioral prescriptions include: removal of pressure for actual coitus; focusing on comfortable sexual feelings during mutual stimulation; verbal feedback from one partner to the other regarding the impact of particular contacts; regular use of relaxation techniques before sexual contact; participation in self-arousal; and verbalization of thoughts and fantasies during sexual arousal. These techniques are suggested by the nurse and explored with client and his wife. They form the basis for behavioral prescriptions.	impact alcohol has had on maintaining an erection. Client will be able to explain the cyclic nature of performance fears. Client will be able to discuss the difficulty with his wife by _____ (date). Client and his wife will explore the problem with the nurse by _____ (date). Client will state that the difficulties he is experiencing are normal and not an indictment of his entire personality. Over the next two months, client and his wife will follow the behavioral prescriptions and report their impact to appropriate follow-up person. Client will experience decreased anxiety related to the sexual dysfunction prior to discharge from the hospital. Within the next four months, client will experience fewer episodes of secondary impotence.

Masochism

Masochism is the opposite of sadism. It is the need to experience physical pain or humiliation in order to achieve sexual arousal. Although some degree of sadism and masochism are found in normal sexual behavior, extremes are deemed pathological.

Nursing Interventions

Nurses work as part of a treatment team when assisting clients with sexual problems. They utilize the nursing process to assess client needs, plan and implement appropriate strategies, and evaluate their impact on improving the mental health status of clients. Working with clients who have primary diagnoses of sexual pathology can be extremely challenging for nurses. Not only are these individuals experiencing emotional problems, but they must face the stigma attached to socially inappropriate sexual behavior and often face legal problems as well. While nurses are required to explore the nature of the difficulty, they must demonstrate nonjudgmental acceptance of these clients at the same time. This is often difficult for nurses because they may find it distasteful to deal with clients who have broken taboos that are strongly ingrained in their value systems. If nurses are unaware of the impact such biases may have on nurse–client relationships, the therapeutic effect of the relationships may be in jeopardy. Nurses must explore their views of personal sexuality and work to understand the impact that value systems have on therapeutic outcomes.

Nurses must first understand their own sexuality,

value systems, and evaluative judgments of certain sexual acts before they can have a positive impact on the treatment of clients with sexual pathology. Work with these clients should be based on a direct and unconditional positive regard, which is fundamental to therapeutic relationships.

The key to establishing unconditional positive regard toward clients is nurses' understanding of how their own sexuality influences others, and how others' sexuality influences their own. The metacommunication that takes place in interpersonal relationships is primarily sexual. When nurses understand this dynamic, they are able to sort through the messages that are sent and received, and maximize the positive impact of therapeutic relationships.

Application of the Nursing Process in Human Sexuality

There are a number of barriers, actual and perceived, that can prevent nurses from providing comprehensive nursing care for clients with sexual problems. Many nurses feel that sex is the client's private business, or that, although it is reasonable for others to explore sexual issues, it is inappropriate for nurses. Nurses may worry that clients will think they are promiscuous, or may believe that certain individuals are "not sexual." Whether or not individuals are sexually active, we are all sexual beings.

There are four levels of nurses' ability to promote sexual health. At the first level, nurses may utilize life experiences to guide interventions. These experiences may be either intuitively helpful or destructive. The second level of ability is the assessment phase of the nursing process. This level is dependent upon nurses' awareness and knowledge of sexual issues, and facilitates data-gathering. The third level is based on nurses' ability to implement and evaluate nursing care based on nursing diagnoses. All professional nurses should be able to function at this level. The fourth level of ability is that of sex therapist or counselor, and requires advanced academic preparation.

Assessment

A sexual history is basic to the assessment phase of the nursing process. An outline for a sexual history is included in Table 25-1. It is essential to prepare clients for discussions of sexual issues by explaining the reasons for, and the importance of, dealing with sexual issues. With this foundation, nurses should be explicit about the discussion, which will facilitate the establishment of trust.

As with other assessments, the sexual data base is composed of subjective and objective information. A complete physical examination may be indicated after completion of the sexual history. This includes a Pap test and pelvic and breast examinations for women, and a genitourinary examination for men. The physical examination provides an opportunity for client teaching as well as emotional support.

Nursing Diagnosis

Based on the findings of the nursing assessment, including sexual history, subjective and objective data, and a physical exam, nurses formulate nursing diagnoses. Only two nursing diagnoses approved by the North American Nursing Diagnosis Association (NANDA)[19] relate specifically to sexual problems; these include the broad categories of "sexual dysfunction" and "rape trauma syndrome." The American Nurses' Association includes the following diagnoses in its Taxonomy for the Classification of Human Responses of Concern for Psychiatric/ Mental Health Nursing Practice (PND-I)[1]:

26.   Alterations in sexuality
26.01.01 Excess in masturbation
26.01.02 Excess seductiveness
26.01.03 Excess sex play/talk/activity
26.01.04 Exhibitionism
26.01.05 Impaired sexual activity
26.01.06 Impaired sexual desire
26.01.07 Impaired sexual objects

PND-I also includes diagnoses related to perpetrators of sexual aggression, including:

21.   Alterations in conduct/impulse control
21.02   Aggression/violence toward others
21.02.02 Abuse—sexual

Additional diagnoses that may pertain to clients with sexual problems include diagnoses in every major diagnostic category of PND-I. These include physiological problems (such as headaches or nausea in response to sexual activity) and emotional problems (such as guilt).

Planning

Nursing diagnoses are derived from the assessment data, and establish the short- and long-term goals for nursing interventions. Based on the goals, a nursing care plan is developed that guides the nursing interventions used to deal with sexual problems. The care plan also establishes the resources that will be necessary for implementation of the care plan.

Intervention

Depending on the nursing diagnosis, goals, and care plan, nurses may engage in direct treatment of clients with sexual problems. However, nurses usually work in collaboration with the entire health care team in designing and providing care for clients. The objective of sex therapy is to assist clients in resolving personal and

TABLE 25-1.
PSYCHOSEXUAL HISTORY

The following psychosexual history is best completed in a face-to-face interview, with the nurse conducting the discussion. A psychosexual assessment form should not be left for clients to complete by themselves with no discussion. Because many individuals have difficulty discussing sexuality, a face-to-face interview best obtains needed information.

This approach allows the nurse to assess the client's ease in talking about these topics during the interview. If the assessment is done with a couple the nurse can also assess the couple's interaction during the interview.

Initially the nurse states the purpose of the interview by saying, "This aspect of the assessment procedure concerns your psychosexual history. Begin by telling me about your early experiences with affection." The nurse then begins to cover the topics listed below. The nurse may also include the psychosexual history as part of the psychiatric assessment (see Chapter 4). In this case the nurse simply asks questions to prompt a discussion of psychosexual history and behavior rather than announcing it as a separate part of the interview.

I. Early childhood background
  A. Family background
    1. Birthplace
    2. Parents' occupations
    3. Were one or both parents emotionally distant, close, warm, affectionate, seductive, clinging?
  B. Attitudes and belief systems
    1. Were there early attitudes in the home of trust, closeness, egalitarian male–female relationships, a sense that sex was normal and comfortable?
    2. Religious influences on attitudes about sexuality
    3. Was affection demonstrated between the parents? Under what circumstances? What does the client know about the parents' sex lives? What was the parents' attitude about sex between themselves and about the client's developing sexuality?
    4. Was the client allowed to ask questions about sexuality? Was sexuality (and related topics such as venereal disease) discussed?
    5. What were the rules about nudity in the home?
    6. What were the client's ideas about sex, pregnancy, and the functioning of body parts as a child?
  C. What were the client's early sexual experiences?
    1. Experiences of incest in which members of the family or close friends of the family (or neighbors) touched the client inappropriately? (See Chapter 21 for a more thorough discussion of the assessment of incest.)
    2. Did the client play any sex games? Was the client caught?
  D. Emerging sexuality
    1. At what age does the client recall having pleasurable genital sensations? How does the client describe the circumstances?
    2. At what age did the client first experiment with masturbation (or any other solitary activity that produced genital feelings and pleasures)? Describe how and where the client did this. How did the client feel about this? Was the client discovered; if so, what happened?
II. Puberty and adolescence
  A. Did the client receive sex education? From whom?
  B. Females
    1. Was menstruation explained in advance? By whom?
    2. Did the client discuss it with her friends?
    3. How did the client feel in anticipation of menstruation?
    4. How did the client feel when menstruation started? At what age did menstruation occur?
    5. Were there any problems with menstruation?
    6. Did the client ever have sex during her period? How did the client feel about that?
  C. Males
    1. Age of first wet dream
    2. Had the client been told about this?
    3. What was the client's reaction?
  D. Dating behavior
    1. Age of the initiation of dating:
      a. In groups?
      b. On single dates?
    2. What were the parents' rules about dating?
    3. Did the client date several people or one person at a time?
    4. How attractive did the client feel? How popular?
  E. Petting behavior
    1. What kind of petting took place (clothes on, skin to skin, breasts touched, genitals touched)?
    2. Under what circumstances did petting occur?
    3. What influence did peer pressure have on the client?
    4. What kind of emotional relationship did the client have with someone they became involved in petting with?
    5. How did the client respond or feel about engaging in these behaviors?
    6. What would the client's parents have thought?

(Continued)

TABLE 25-1. (CONTINUED)
PSYCHOSEXUAL HISTORY

F. Coital experiences
   1. When did the client first engage in intercourse? (If client is female, was it her choice?)
   2. What were the circumstances of the first time?
   3. How did the client respond (orgasmic, premature ejaculation, erectile difficulty)?
   4. What emotional conditions did the client need to engage in intercourse?
   5. What feelings usually accompanied intercourse (satisfaction, guilt, pleasure, embarrassment, anxiety)?
   6. Method of contraception?
   7. Did the client ever become pregnant or have an abortion?
G. Other experiences
   1. Has the client ever had any homosexual or lesbian experiences?
III. Adulthood
   A. When did the client leave home?
      1. What was it like being free?
   B. How many partners has the client had during adulthood, and under what circumstances?
   C. Past marriages and relationships
      1. What was the emotional quality of the relationships?
      2. What was the quality of the sexual relationship?
      3. How did these relationships end?
      4. Does the client have any children from previous relationships?
IV. Current experiences
   A. What relationships does the client currently have?
   B. What sexual relationships does the client currently have?
   C. What attracted the client to the present partner?
   D. What was the relationship like in the beginning?
   E. Historically, what has happened in the relationship (emotionally and sexually)?
   G. Are there any present (emotional or sexual) problems in the relationship?
      1. When did the problem(s) begin?
      2. What does the client describe as the precipitant of the problem?
      3. What has been done to assist with the problem?
      4. Does the problem occur at some times and not at others?
      5. Describe any physical problems that may affect sexual behavior.
      6. What medications does the client take that may affect sexual behavior?
   H. Has the client ever had extramarital affairs?

(Lemon M: Psychosexual History, 1988. [Used in private practice in counseling for sexual functioning.])

interpersonal problems related to sexuality. Nursing interventions may involve sexual counseling, including educating and advising clients about the biological, psychological, developmental, behavioral, and social aspects of sexuality. Education, as part of both treatment and prevention, is the most common nursing intervention. Client advocacy is another key role for nurses, and often involves protecting clients' privacy and modesty. Table 25-2 provides several hints for establishing a nurse–client relationship that is conducive to therapeutic intervention.

Evaluation

Evaluation criteria should include clients' perceptions of success as well as some comparison of clients' sexual behavior or attitudes to normative bases provided by the lit-

erature. Because much information is reported to nurses by clients, a trusting nurse–client relationship is essential. Clients should be involved in both the establishment of goals and the determination of whether and when the goals have been met. The ultimate evaluation of nursing interventions merges the client's subjective report and objective data.

Summary

1. Sexuality is concerned with more than individuals' reproductive organs. It encompasses all sensual thoughts, feelings, and actions.

2. Sexual identity includes individuals' biological make-up; their understanding of themselves as either male or female; their social role according to

TABLE 25-2.
THERAPEUTIC INTERVENTION HINTS

- Don't assume that clients are knowledgeable about human sexuality.
- Strive to establish a trusting nurse–client relationship.
- When clients resist discussing human sexuality, focus on the process of the discussion.
- If you believe that the client is reluctant to discuss sexuality, you can ask, "Do you wonder why you are silent?"
- Clearly state common misperceptions and biases that others may hold in order to remove fear and guilt from the client and open the channel of communication.
- Make all implicit or suggestive remarks explicit and available for discussion.
- Be aware of and sensitive to cultural variations in client comfort with sexuality and sexual issues.
- Allow sufficient time for clients to divulge information at their own pace.

their femaleness or maleness; and their emotional and physical sexual preferences.

3. Sexuality differs at each level of growth and development, and is shaped by each. For example, many alterations of the physiology of sexual maturity occur in adolescence.

4. There are definitive stages or phases of human sexual response in males and females.

5. Nurses use the nursing process to intervene with clients' sexual problems at each level of prevention.

6. Rape victims work through phases of recovery, known as the rape trauma syndrome, while recovering from the experience of sexual aggression.

7. Sexual dysfunctions, such as impotence, include varying levels of sexual performance, based on physiological and psychological concerns.

8. Sexual disorders, as outlined by the American Psychiatric Association, are rare, and are accompanied by feelings of discomfort related to sexuality.

9. Nurses must work to understand their own sexuality and their attitudes toward sexuality in order to provide professional care to clients with all types of problems related to sexuality.

References

1. American Nurses' Association: Taxonomy for the Classification of Human Responses of Concern for Psychiatric/Mental Health Nursing Practice. Kansas City, Missouri, American Nurses' Association, 1986
2. American Psychiatric Association: Diagnostic and Statistical Manual of Mental Disorders, 3rd ed, revised (DSM-III-R). Washington, DC, American Psychiatric Association, 1987
3. Barbach L: For Yourself: The Fulfillment of Female Sexuality. New York, Signet, 1975
4. Bell AP, Weinberg MS: Homosexualities: A Study of Diversity Among Men and Women. New York, Simon & Schuster, 1978
5. Burgess AW, Holstrom LL: Rape Crisis and Recovery. Bowie, Maryland, Robert J Brady, 1979
6. Burgess AW, Holstrom LL: Rape: Victims of Crisis. Bowie, Maryland, Robert J Brady, 1974
7. DeCecco JP, Shively MG: Children's development: Social sex-role and the hetero-homosexual orientation. In Oremland EK, Oremland JD (eds): The Sexual and Gender Development of Young Children: The Role of the Educator. Cambridge, Massachusetts, Ballinger, 1977
8. Douglas CJ, Kalman CM, Kalman TP: Homophobia among physicians and nurses: An empirical study. Hosp Community Psychiatry 36:1309, 1985
9. Fontaine KL: Human sexuality: Faculty knowledge and attitudes. Nurs Outlook 24:174, 1976
10. Freud S: Three Essays on Sexuality. In Strachey J (ed): The Standard Edition of the Complete Psychological Works. London, Hogarth, 1953
11. Groth AN, Burgess AW: Motivational intent in the sexual assault of children. Crim Just Behavior 4:253, 1977
12. Gochros H, Gochros J: The Sexually Oppressed. New York, Association Press, 1977
13. Higgins LP, Hawkins JW: Human Sexuality Across the Life Span: Implications for Nursing Practice. Monterey, California, Wadsworth, 1984
14. Hite S: The Hite Report on Male Sexuality. New York, Ballantine, 1982
15. Hite S: The Hite Report: A Nationwide Study of Female Sexuality. New York, Dell, 1976
16. Jensen GD: Teenagers' fears that they are homosexual. Med Aspects Hum Sexuality 15:47, 1981
17. Karshmer J: Nursing students' attitudes toward dealing with clients' sexual issues (informal survey), 1985
18. Katchadourian H, Lunde D: Fundamentals of Human Sexuality, 4th ed. Philadelphia, WB Saunders, 1980
19. Kim MJ, McFarland GK, McLane AM: Classification of Nursing Diagnoses: Proceedings of the Fifth National Conference. St Louis, CV Mosby, 1984
20. Kinsey AC, Pomeroy WB, Martin CE: Sexual Behavior in the Human Male. Philadelphia, WB Saunders, 1948
21. Kinsey AC, Pomeroy WB, Martin CE et al: Sexual Behavior in the Human Female. Philadelphia, WB Saunders, 1953
22. Martinson FM: Eroticism in Childhood: A Sociological Perspective. In Oremland EK, Oremland JD (eds): The Sexual and Gender Development of Young Children: The Role of the Educator. Cambridge, Massachusetts, Ballinger, 1977
23. Masters WH, Johnson VE: Human Sexual Response. Boston, Little, Brown and Co, 1966
24. Masters WH, Johnson VE: Principles of new sex therapy. Am J Psychiatry 133:5, 1976
25. Masters WH: Sex therapy: Concepts and format. Paper presented at seminar on human sexuality at Masters & Johnson Institute, St Louis, Missouri, Nov 6–7, 1978
26. Mims FH, Swenson M: A model to promote sexual health care. Nurs Outlook 26:121, 1978
27. Money J, Ehrhardt AA: Man and Woman: Boy and Girl. Baltimore, Johns Hopkins University Press, 1972
28. NAACOG: Rape. Washington, DC, Nurses' Association of the American College of Obstetricians and Gynecologists, 1979

29. O'Leary V: Lesbianism. Nurs Dimensions 7:78, 1979

30. Peltz M: Sexual and gender development in the latency years. In Oremland EK, Oremland JD (eds): The Sexual and Gender Development of Young Children: The Role of the Educator. Cambridge, Massachusetts, Ballinger, 1977

31. The Playboy Readers' Sex Survey, Part I. Playboy 1: 1983

32. Rodgers JA: Struggling out of the feminine pluperfect. Am J Nurs 75:1655, 1975

33. Rubin JZ, Provenzano FJ, Luria Z: The eye of the beholder: Parents' views on sex of newborns. Am J Orthopsychiatry 44:4, 1974

34. Schuster E: Sexuality and nursing practice. Nurs Clin North Am 17:3, 1982

35. Sorenson RC: Adolescent Sexuality in Contemporary America. New York, World Publishing, 1973

36. Sredl DR, Klenke C, Rojkind M: Offering the rape victim real help. Nursing '79 9:38, 1979

37. Walum LR: The Dynamics of Sex and Gender: A Sociological Perspective. Chicago, Rand-McNally, 1978

38. Wallis C: Children having children: Teen pregnancies are corroding America's social fabric. Time 26:78, 1985

39. Weinberg JS: Sexuality: Human Needs and Nursing Practice. Philadelphia, WB Saunders, 1982

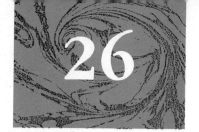

26

LORNA MILL BARRELL AND JEAN F. WYMAN

PSYCHOSOCIAL NURSING WITH OLDER ADULTS

Learning Objectives

Upon completion of this chapter the student should be able to do the following:

1. Describe the process of normal aging, including biological and psychological changes.
2. Recognize and categorize systems components of the older adult, including physical, psychological, societal, cultural, and environmental components.
3. Identify three types of common stressors affecting older adults.
4. Identify and differentiate among the major psychological alterations affecting older adults.
5. Identify the unique aspects of each step of the nursing process that are used in interactions with older adults.
6. Identify intervention strategies in primary, secondary, and tertiary levels of prevention.
7. Articulate examples of the therapeutic use of self in interaction with older adults.

Introduction

The dramatic growth in the number and proportion of people over the age of 65 years is directing attention toward the mental health needs of older adults. Aging is associated with unique, and often multiple, losses. The losses that occur, in combination with increased demands from physical illness and decreased coping resources, place the aged at high risk for mental health problems. Estimates of the prevalence rate of mental disorders in the elderly population range from 15% to 25%, far exceeding the prevalence rate of 10% in the general population.[63,64] Although older adults need mental health services, they underutilize available outpatient services. Older adults constitute only 3% to 5% of client loads in community mental health services, hospital clinics, and private psychiatric practice.[26] In addition, the mental health care that is provided is often deficient in quality, reflecting biased societal attitudes toward the aged as well as the lack of training of mental health professionals in care of older people.[42]

This chapter will provide a systems perspective on the older adult that describes normal aging processes in the context of the complex interactions among the biological, psychological, sociological, cultural, and environmental subsystems. It will also discuss the special problems of the aged and the common high-risk alterations in mental health functioning that occur with aging. Specific techniques in mental health assessment, and interventions appropriate for selected nursing diagnoses, will be presented.

Characteristics of Older Adults

When does a person become "old"? This is a difficult question to answer because "old age" does not begin on a specific date. Technically, each of us ages from the moment of conception. Because of considerable variations in the aging process among individuals, use of chronological age to define old age presents a biased and limited view of a person's actual functional status. Some elderly individuals retain a remarkable youthfulness of spirit and excellent physical condition, while some younger people show behavioral and functional limitations commonly associated with old age. It is important to recognize that older adults are an extremely heterogeneous group, with individuals aging in different ways and at different rates.

Traditionally, the definition of old age was arbitrarily set at age 65. This age was adopted as the mandatory retirement age in the United States with passage of the social security laws in 1935. Thus, for social purposes, this age has been adhered to as a means of determining the point of retirement or eligibility for various services available to older citizens. Gerontologists, recognizing the great differences in health status and functional abilities in the 20 to 30 years of post-retirement, have divided the older population into four age categories: the young-old, 55 to 64 years; the middle-old, 65 to 74 years; the old-old, 75 to 84 years; and the very old, 85 years and over. Several authors cite the age of 75 as a more accurate marker of when old age begins.

Recent demographics indicate that 29.2 million (or 12.1%) of the U.S. population is over the age of 65. This percentage is expected to increase to 21% of the population by the year 2030.[2] The fastest-growing segment of the total population is in the age group of 75 years and over, and this group is expected to increase from 38% to 47% of those over the age of 65 years by the year 2003.[15] This has significance because, after the age of 75, morbidity and mortality rates increase sharply, chronic diseases affect functional abilities, and there is an increased likelihood that organic brain disorders, such as senile dementia of the Alzheimer's type (SDAT), will appear.

The significant differences in life expectancy that exist between men and women are attributed to lifestyle differences, higher incidence among men of mortality from disease and accidents, and differing rates of suicide. The role of genetic factors in longevity has not yet been determined. The average 65-year-old male can now expect to live for 79 years, and the average 65-year-old female for 83 years.[2] This longer life expectancy in women means that women outnumber men by increasing proportions, so that by age 85 there are slightly more than twice as many women as men.[15]

White persons constitute the majority of the elderly population. However, the elderly nonwhite population is growing faster than the elderly white majority. In 1980, 10% of those over 65 were nonwhite; by 2025, this figure is expected to be 15%.[2] In general, minorities tend to require greater social, health, and income supports than do the majority of white elderly people.

Most elderly people live in families that consist of an elderly married couple with no children or other relatives residing in their homes. The most striking difference in living arrangements, regardless of age or ethnicity, reflects marital status differences. A higher proportion of men (78%) are married and living with spouses, whereas only 37% of elderly women live with their husbands. Slightly more than half the women (52%) are widowed, whereas only a small percentage of the men (14%) are widowed.[15]

According to the 1985 National Nursing Home Survey, approximately 5% of the elderly population were residents of institutions (*e.g.,* nursing homes).[55] The majority of those institutionalized were over the age of 75 (78%). More than 50% of those in nursing homes had psychiatric diagnoses. Estimates indicate that approximately 20% of all people over age 65 will be institutionalized in a nursing home at some time.[15]

Many older people live in poverty. However, based on income alone, the number of poor elderly persons actually declined slightly, from 15.3% in 1981 to 12.4% in 1984. Another 9% of the aged are classified as "near-poor." In total, more than one fifth (21%) of the older population are poor or near-poor. Women, minorities, and those living alone are overrepresented in the group of poor elderly. Retirement is associated with a one-half to two-thirds cut in income. This means that many aged become poor, or must restrict their standard of living, when they retire. Social security benefits are the sole source of income for one fifth of all elderly persons in the U.S.[2]

Definitions of Mental Health in Old Age

What is mental health in later life? This question is difficult to answer, not only because there are no well-accepted criteria for mental health in any age group, but also because the professional's knowledge of the inner world of older people tends to be stereotypical.[17] Health, either physical or mental, has commonly been defined as the absence of illness. Therefore, we sometimes define individuals as mentally healthy if they do not exhibit any signs or symptoms of a psychiatric disorder.

Jahoda[34] provided several criteria of mental health that reflect optimal psychological functioning in people of any age. These include:

1. Positive self-attitudes
2. Growth and actualization
3. Integration of the personality
4. Autonomy
5. Reality perception
6. Environmental mastery

Individuals vary in their level of attainment of each of these criteria, and no one reaches the ideal on all criteria. However, through mental health intervention, each person can approach the ideal, and thereby improve his or her quality of life and life satisfaction. According to these criteria, the mentally healthy older adult possesses a sense of identity and self-acceptance that will help negotiate the future with a sense of security and optimism. If people cannot accept their lives as meaningful, the result may be depression, bitterness, remorse, and fear of death.

Ebersole and Hess[23] define mental health as the capacity to interact with others and negotiate the environment in a manner enriching to self and others. In addition, mental health might be measured as satisfactory adjustment to one's life stage and situation. Thus, using these criteria, a contented institutionalized older adult might be considered mentally healthy.

The mentally healthy person at any age adapts to changing external requirements and internal needs. Individuals with poor mental health fail to adapt, or adapt in ways that limit their optimal functioning or place them in danger of harming themselves or others.

A Systems View of the Older Adult

Aging is a complex phenomenon that involves interaction among biological, psychological, sociological, environmental, and cultural subsystems. These subsystems and their associated components are illustrated in Figure 26-1. The mental health of the elderly can not be sepa-

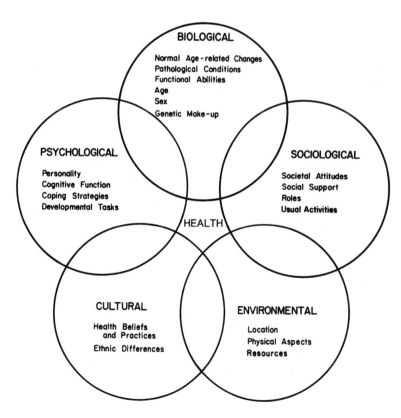

Figure 26-1. A systems perspective on the older adult.

rated as a single factor, but can only be understood in relationship to all of these subsystems. Physical and psychological well-being are intimately intertwined. Many acute physical illnesses often present atypically in elders, usually with cognitive or behavioral changes rather than classic signs and symptoms of disease. Daily coping with the effects of chronic conditions can significantly affect mood and morale. Mental well-being of the individual is closely tied to environmental considerations, such as living in unsafe neighborhoods where fear of being a crime victim leads to social isolation. In addition, the environment can exert a powerful influence over physical health either by supporting optimal function or by placing an individual at risk for the development of illness.

The Biological System

Biological components include: age, sex, genetic constitution, normal age-related changes, pathological changes associated with acute and chronic physical disease, and functional abilities. Increasing age is associated with increased vulnerability to physical and psychological illnesses and with a greater decrease in functional abilities as a result of such illness.

Aging is considered a normal, inevitable, and relatively benign process. Although it is a universal phenomenon, individuals vary considerably in their rates of aging. Rather than becoming homogeneous, older adults tend to become more heterogeneous in their responses to aging because of differences in genetic background, environments, lifestyles, and nutritional patterns. In general, there is a physiologic age-related decline in organ function beginning at age 40. Most older adults are able to adapt well to age-related changes that affect physical structure and function of cells, tissues, organs, and organ systems. Many of the physical problems associated with aging occur when acute or chronic disease is superimposed upon normal aging changes.

Normal Changes

Changes in physical appearance are a hallmark of aging. The skin of the older adult gets wrinkled due to changes in elasticity and loss of subcutaneous fat. Changes occur in hair texture, color, amount, and distribution. Hair loss occurs in both sexes; for men, hereditary baldness may result. Women may develop skin whiskers as a result of hormonal changes. Gray or white hair that becomes thin or fine is common.

Changes in body composition result in an overall increase in body fat. Although subcutaneous fat is lost, fat around the body's organs increases. Fat redistributes from the extremities to the trunk of the body, changing body shape.

All five senses show a decline in function, and each has the potential for having a major impact on psychosocial functioning. Visual acuity decreases. Presbyopia (far-sightedness) results from changes in the lens and ciliary muscle, so that by age 40 to 45 years most people need corrective glasses for close work and reading. The extent of the visual field declines; adaptation to the dark is impaired. Cataract formation is common. Hearing ability also declines with age, with high-frequency tones being lost first. Presbycusis (hearing loss in old age) begins to affect individuals at age 60. Taste sensitivity declines after age 50, particularly the ability to taste sweets. This decline is related to a decrease in function of taste buds and also to a decline in the sense of smell.

Changes in the musculoskeletal, cardiovascular, and central nervous systems contribute to decreased mobility in later life. Joint stiffness, loss of muscle fiber, decreased muscle strength, and decline in flexibility can limit functional abilities. However, research has shown that many of these changes are due to a lack of use rather than true aging. Regular exercise can often help to reduce the effects of aging and to maintain good muscle and joint function. Loss of bone tissue through osteoporosis is common, and can predispose individuals to fracture, particularly of the hip, shoulder, wrist, and spine. Women are especially prone to bone loss. Hip fracture, the most serious consequence of osteoporosis, leads to immobilization and a greater risk of mortality. Intervertebral discs lose water, thus contributing to loss of height.

Cardiovascular changes include a thickening and stiffening of heart valves, with some hypertrophy of the myocardium. Although the resting heart rate remains unchanged, maximum cardiac rate and stroke volume are decreased. The ability of the heart rate to return to normal after stress is prolonged. Blood vessels become thicker and less elastic, resulting in a rise in the systolic blood pressure and widening pulse pressure.

The nervous system shows a number of changes. If lost, postmitotic nerve cells are not replaced. Studies indicate that there is a significant loss of brain cells, resulting in a decrease in brain weight and possibly affecting some brain functions. There is an increase in lipofuscin deposits, senile plaques, and neurofibrillary tangles in brain cells. Whether this is part of normal aging or a disease process is unclear. Cerebral blood flow is decreased. Nerve conduction velocity is slowed, which affects psychomotor reaction times. Several of the neurotransmitters are affected. Monoamine oxidase (MAO) and serotonin increase with age, whereas norepinephrine, the active precursor of epinephrine, and dopamine decrease. Depression and Parkinson's disease have both been linked to changes in the neurotransmitters.

Loss of cells in the liver and kidney alters their function, especially under stress. This loss of function helps to explain why the elderly are at higher risk for iatrogenic effects from drug therapy. They are less able to metabolize and excrete drugs from the body, and thus maintain higher drug levels in their blood, leading to increased drug effect.

The respiratory system shows alterations in both structure and function with age. The anteroposterior diameter of the chest increases with age. Chest-wall compliance is reduced, with decreased strength in the expiratory muscles and increased rigidity in the thoracic wall. Alveoli are lost, with rigidity in the lung occurring.

Changes in various lung volumes balance each other so that there is no significant change in total lung capacity or ability to manage stress. A reduced cough efficiency, decreased ciliary activity of the bronchial lining, and increased lung dead-space enhance the potential for respiratory complications, particularly with immobilized individuals.

The gastrointestinal system shows few changes in function. Although motility changes are commonly assumed to occur, especially given the frequent complaint of constipation in the elderly, few studies have documented age-related changes. Secretion of saliva, gastric juices, and pancreatic enzymes does occur, but does not appear to affect digestion significantly. Absorption may be affected, however.

Endocrine-system changes include loss of receptor sites in target cells and decreased secretion of several hormones. However, the significance of these alterations is not known. The immune system also shows decline with age. These changes, which are not yet clearly understood, are associated with reduced survival.

Functional Abilities

Chronic disease, in combination with normal aging changes, can significantly affect functional abilities, yet there is no predictable relationship between the morbidity associated with a chronic disease and functional ability. One individual may have three chronic diseases, such as hypertension, arthritis, and heart disease, and have no activity impairment, whereas another person could have only one chronic disease, diabetes mellitus, and have serious activity restriction due to complications that have resulted from the disease process itself, such as blindness, lower-leg amputation, and kidney disease requiring dialysis therapy.

In general, the majority of elderly persons, even in the oldest age groups, do not suffer from functional limitations or require assistance. A recent survey conducted on functional abilities of community-dwelling older Americans indicated that more than three fourths of the elderly did not have functional limitations.[53] The risk of functional limitations does significantly increase with advancing age. The percentage of individuals with functional limitations ranges from 13% of people aged 65 to 74 years, to 25% of those aged 75 to 84 years, to 46% of those over age 85 years. As would be expected, older adults residing independently in the community are less impaired than those residing in nursing homes.

The Psychological System

The psychological system includes the following factors: personality, cognitive abilities, coping strategies, developmental tasks, and future perspectives. Psychological adaptation is closely intertwined with physical health status. Alterations in physical health can produce changes in mental functioning. Acute illness, such as myocardial infarction, pneumonia, and other systemic infections, is often manifested in older adults as changes in cognition or behavior. Sensory impairments, particularly hearing deficits, can lead to personality changes such as suspiciousness and paranoia.

Personality

Older people show great diversity in their personalities and abilities to cope with stress. Personality traits remain consistent from middle age through old age. Behavioral responses tend to become more exaggerated. Individuals who were opinionated, rigid, and difficult to get along with as younger people are usually only more opinionated and inflexible and harder to live with as older people. If someone was flexible and actively involved in life with many friends and social activities, those characteristics will continue into old age.

From a series of cross-sectional and longitudinal studies, Neugarten, Havinghurst, and Tobin[56] identified four personality patterns associated with aging: integrated, defended, passive-dependent, and unintegrated. Those with *integrated* personalities are mature, happy individuals who vary in their amounts of activity. They may be reorganizers, who maintain active lives and substitute new activities for lost ones. They may be focused individuals, who maintain a medium level of activities that are highly satisfying, or persons disengaged and content to move away from role commitments and activities. The second personality pattern, *defended,* is striving, ambitious, and achievement-oriented. These individuals may either continue to hold on to the roles of middle age and be content, or they may become discontent and preoccupied with their losses. The third pattern, *passive-dependent,* may be either help-seeking individuals with strong dependency needs, or apathetic persons who are passive and unhappy, withdrawing from contact with others. The last pattern is composed of *unintegrated* personalities, who show a disorganized pattern of aging and suffer mental health impairment. Havighurst and his colleagues found that, in general, as one moved from the integrated to the unintegrated personalities, life satisfaction and morale decreased.

Most older people adapt to changes in their physical function and to the presence of chronic disease. However, these physical changes lead to a change in self-concept, because self-image is related to body image. Although the majority of people can accept and cope with these changes, the potential for a decrease in self-esteem is possible.

Cognitive Abilities

Except for a decline in perceptual motor skills, intellectual abilities remain relatively stable in later life, even in the presence of major illness. *Verbal* or *crystallized intelligence* shows little or no decline up to age 70. After age 70, there is some decline, although without major impairment. Reasoning and perceptual-integrative abilities, or *fluid intelligence,* do show decline with age. Speed of response decreases on almost all performance measures.

This slowed response may affect other cognitive abilities, such as problem-solving and information retrieval.

Memory is affected by the aging process. Research indicates a minimal impairment in ability to recall the distant or remote past, but less accuracy in recall of recently-learned information. The capacity to store information in short-term memory is altered. Only items that have considerable meaning to the person are remembered. Older people also have difficulty in transferring information from short-term to long-term memory.

Learning may be affected by changes in memory. Motivation can significantly affect learning; older learners show less motivation to learn materials not directly related to an immediate need. Anxiety can also interfere with the learning process: higher levels of performance anxiety have been demonstrated to occur in elderly than in younger subjects, altering the amount of information learned. Older learners are also more cautious in test situations and tend to do less well on tests involving timed performance.

Developmental Tasks

Erik Erikson's[24] stage theory is one of the earliest and most accepted models of personality development across the life span. He divided life into eight stages. At each of these stages, individuals must resolve a psychological issue or conflict before they can progress to the next higher stage of development. The first five stages are similar to Freud's stages of psychosexual development, and cover infancy through adolescence. The last three stages deal with early, middle, and later adulthood. The last stage, *integrity vs. despair and disgust,* has the most significance for older adults. Individuals who successfully achieve integrity feel satisfied and happy with their life experiences, and accept full responsibility for their lives. Life changes are viewed positively and accepted, without the wish to change them. In contrast, individuals who have a negative resolution of this stage feel depressed and unhappy about life, emphasizing failures and fears of getting older. Life changes are viewed negatively, with the wish that they could have been different. Despair results because the individual realizes that there is not enough time to start over. Disgust may be substituted for despair, and is manifested as displeasure with particular people or institutions.

Erikson's theory has been criticized as being too broad to cover the tasks involved in late adulthood. Later theorists, such as Peck and Havinghurst, have identified additional tasks associated with later life.

Havinghurst[29] lists six tasks:

1. Adjusting to declining physical strength and health
2. Adjusting to retirement and its reduced income
3. Adjusting to changes in the health of one's spouse
4. Establishing an explicit affiliation with one's age group
5. Adopting and adapting social roles in a flexible way
6. Establishing satisfactory physical living arrangements

With increasing age, individuals begin to experience social, physical, and psychological losses. Role loss is associated with retirement, widowhood, death of friends, moves to new neighborhoods, and the completion of the parental role. New roles must occur for life satisfaction to be maintained. Proximity of age-appropriate people is a critical factor in maintaining a social network.[31] A close confidant has been demonstrated to be more important to satisfaction than degree of social interaction.[47]

Peck[58] identified the following developmental tasks of old age:

1. Ego differentiation vs. work-role preoccupation
2. Body transcendence vs. body preoccupation
3. Ego transcendence vs. ego preoccupation

The final task of old age is coming to terms with one's mortality and accepting the reality of death. This adaptation requires an active effort of the individual, and should not be seen as passive resignation or denial. The need to leave a legacy, ensure the welfare of one's family, and gain closure on and acceptance of one's life are included in this task.

Aging poses a great challenge in terms of adaptation to many life changes, including changes in physical health, lifestyle, financial status, living arrangements, and role losses. Coming to terms with one's past life, dealing with the present, and preparing for an uncertain future can significantly affect the mental health of older adults. Coping with these events is made more difficult in light of the declining health and loss of social supports and resources that are common for the elderly.

The Sociological System

The societal system involves the following: societal attitudes toward the elderly, social support and networks, social roles, and usual activities. Social theories of aging attempt to describe and predict how an individual will respond or adapt to old age. Four theories have been proposed: disengagement theory by Cumming and Henry,[21] activity theory by Havinghurst and Albrecht,[30] exchange theory by Dowd,[22] and continuity theory by Atchley.[7]

Theories of Aging

Disengagement theory, an early theory that has received considerable criticism, contends that it is normal and inevitable for people to decrease their activity and seek more passive roles as they age. Disengagement is viewed as a positive and necessary process that enables the individual to achieve optimal functioning. Research support for this theory is inconsistent. Several studies contradict disengagement, and support the conclusion that "engaged" people are more likely than "unengaged" people to express life satisfaction.

The theory most widely used, *activity theory,* proposes that individuals must retain adequate levels of social activity if they are to age successfully. Individuals who maintain their social activities and roles of middle age, or are able to replace them with new ones, are predicted to have higher self-esteem and life satisfaction. People who are unable to replace lost roles and activities with new ones will have a less positive self-concept and less life satisfaction. Research support for activity theory has also been inconsistent. Basic assumptions of the theory have been criticized for disregarding the effects of the aging process and its associated changes, such as health problems, reduced income due to retirement, and inadequate transportation, which may alter ability to participate in activities. In addition, the theory does not take into consideration that the meaningful activities of middle age, such as vocational or professional activities, may not be so easily replaced by the leisure activities available to older people.

Activity and disengagement theories describe a decrease in social interaction in old age. *Exchange theory*, which has not been tested, postulates that patterns of interaction exist among individuals and groups because they are rewarding. In seeking rewards, however, there are costs. According to the theory, the participant in the relationship who values the reward more highly loses power; the other participant gains power. In exchanges between the aged and their social environment, the aged gradually lose power. This is inevitable because of losses in friends, family, health, and income. Thus, society holds a distinct advantage in the exchange relationship between the aged and society. The elderly can rebalance the relationship by voluntary withdrawal (disengagement), extension of the power network (development of alternative relationships that are more rewarding), emergence of status (recognition of a critical skill possessed by the elder), and coalition formation (banding together of the elderly to exert sufficient power to achieve rewards).

Continuity theory, a newer theory that appears promising, contends that successful adjustment to old age is based on continuity of life patterns. The more people can do what they have always done, the higher their morale and life satisfaction will be. As individuals grow older, they are predisposed to maintain stability in coping strategies, habits, preferences, and associations. These predispositions constantly evolve from interactions among personal preferences, biological and psychological capabilities, situational opportunities, and experience. Change is viewed as an adaptive process involving interaction among all these components.

Societal Attitudes

The term *ageism* was coined by Butler[16] to describe the discrimination that often accompanies old age. Society often acts to discredit older people in a variety of ways. The basis for this lies in the many myths and stereotypes regarding old age that influence our attitudes and behavior toward the elderly. These attitudes, often shared by the aged themselves, influence the delivery and utilization of mental health services. Some of these myths include:[23]

1. The majority of old people are senile or demented.
2. Old people feel miserable most of the time.
3. Most older people cannot work as effectively as can younger people.
4. Most older people are unhealthy, and need assistance with activities of daily living.
5. Most older people are set in their ways and unable to change.
6. Most old people are alike.
7. Most old people are socially isolated.

These stereotypes have the potential for shaping the pattern of aging for people who believe them. They can turn into self-fulfilling prophecies in which aging individuals believe they should behave in certain ways, and therefore act out their beliefs. Kermis[38] pointed out that old people who believe senility is inevitable may label normal memory changes as signs of senility. If this concern is shared with a family member, then that person also may begin to evaluate the older relative's behavior in light of this statement. Gradually, the older person's self-esteem may erode and he or she may lose importance in the family's functioning. In this way, a normal older adult becomes vulnerable to the risk of social isolation, loneliness, and depression.

Health care professionals' perceptions of the aged are also influenced by these myths and stereotypes. Research has indicated that mental alterations in older people are often assumed to be normal expected consequences of the aging process or damage to the central nervous system. Often, the conclusion is drawn that the mental condition is irreversible, with a prognosis of further deterioration. Negative attitudes toward the elderly on the part of health workers contribute to the neglect of mental health problems of the aged, in terms of case-finding and active treatment of identified problems.

Nurses are no exception to the prevailing societal attitudes toward the elderly. Until recently, most schools of nursing failed to provide content in gerontologic/geriatric nursing. Studies on nurses' attitudes have consistently documented negative attitudes. They have also demonstrated that these same attitudes influence nurses' behaviors. For example, nurses may choose not to work with the elderly or have a custodial rather than a rehabilitative philosophy about delivery of care to the elderly.

Social Support and Networks

Social support and networks play a critical role in the maintenance of health and well-being in later life. *Social networks* are the structural interrelationships of family, friends, neighbors, coworkers, and others who provide support. *Social support* refers to the psychosocial and tangible aid provided by social networks.[67]

Family members are major providers of support for older people. The majority of the elderly population who reside at home live near children or other relatives and have frequent contact with them. Across several ethnic groups, older adults typically turn to their families in times of need.[68] Contrary to the myth of family alienation (that is, that families do not care for their elders), the majority of home care today is provided by adult children. Elderly individuals who are childless tend to be more socially isolated than those with children. However, the well-being of older women appears to be less influenced by contact with their own children than by contacts with other relatives, friends, and associates.[10]

Research indicates that social support is a significant buffer of stressful life events and moderator of psychological and physical well-being. Elderly individuals, particularly those with chronic health problems resulting in functional limitations, require social support to manage daily living needs. Studies have demonstrated positive benefits of social support in reducing mortality rates and in the rate and completeness of recovery from injuries, myocardial infarctions, cancer, and other physical illnesses. In addition, the adequacy of a social network and the quality and type of support provided can help alleviate the stressors associated with aging, so that mental health problems are minimized.

Social Roles

Aging is associated with a loss of and change in social roles. Middle-age roles associated with raising children and work are changed with children's leaving home, retirement, and widowhood. New roles, such as grandparenting, may be assumed. Relationships with children are changed, particularly if a parent becomes physically or mentally dependent. Marital roles may be altered, with a redistribution of household responsibilities when one spouse or both retire. Adjustment is necessary for spouses who have never worked outside the home and spouses who suddenly find themselves at home all day with no planned activities. Death of a spouse requires the surviving spouse to take over household responsibilities and tasks that he or she may never have done. For example, if one spouse took care of financial matters such as paying bills while the other took care of household matters such as shopping, cooking, and cleaning, each may have difficulty in assuming the new responsibilities in the event of the other's serious illness or death. In addition, assuming the role of a no-longer-married person, after years of marriage, is difficult.

Usual Activities

Activity patterns also change with aging because of changing roles, health problems, and reduced income. New or changed roles require different types of activities. Retirement brings added hours in the day that need to be filled with activities. Many older people report that they have more new activities than they can find the time to do. Others, whose only activities in younger years centered around work, find the time difficult to fill. Declining health influences whether a person can continue to do certain preferred activities such as physical recreation. For example, activity intolerance associated with cardiovascular or pulmonary problems may limit a person's participation in tennis, golf, or swimming. A reduced income that decreases the amount of discretionary money available may alter the type and amount of preferred activities in which individuals can engage. Vacations, restaurant meals, sports events, and cultural events may become luxury items.

The key factor in life satisfaction in the later years appears to be the maintenance of meaningful activities. Bingo games, television, and bird watching, although activities that could be enjoyed even by people in declining health and on limited incomes, may not carry the same value as activities enjoyed in younger years. Lost activities need to be replaced with those that have value and meaning to the individual, so that enjoyment and quality of life can be maintained.

The Cultural System

Cultural differences in coping patterns, perceptions, manifestations of illness, and attitudes toward utilization of health care services all influence the health and well-being of older adults. However, relatively few studies have addressed the differing effects of aging in different cultural groups, including racial and ethnic minorities. Research is needed to identify the variations in health perceptions, beliefs, and practices among various cultural groups of the elderly.

Butler and Lewis[17] point out two major issues regarding minority age groups: (1) the unique cultural elements found in each minority group that have affected people's lives, and (2) the effects imposed on older people of living in a majority culture, particularly the direct effects of racial and ethnic prejudice. Black persons especially face the double jeopardy of ageism and racism as they grow older.[17]

Socioeconomic status, including income and education, has significant impact on physical and mental health. Research among different minority groups in the United States indicates that social networks of family, friends, and neighbors are among the most important mechanisms to assist elderly individuals to cope effectively with health-related problems. Each cultural group uses the network in a slightly different manner. Neighbors and church members often assist elderly blacks and Hispanics with problems that involve illness or physical disability. Most minority elderly, even those with severe physical and psychological impairments, remain in the community and are cared for by family, relatives, and friends. White elderly, however, are more likely to rely on formal sources of support and services. They also have higher rates of institutionalization.

Death rates and disease prevalence vary among different racial and ethnic minority groups in the United States. One reason for this variation is the influence of socioeconomic factors (*i.e.,* low income and the other factors associated with poverty). For example, mortality of Mexican Americans, blacks, native Americans, and native Alaskans is significantly higher than the rate of death among whites. Suicide rates show dramatic age-related "cross-over" differences. During early adulthood, blacks, native Americans, native Alaskans, and Mexican Americans commit suicide more frequently than do whites. This reverses after age 60, when white males show the highest suicide rate. Some studies indicate that certain psychiatric disorders are more prevalent among older blacks, American Indians, and Alaskan Indians.

Folk remedies and practices may be important therapies for some ethnic groups. For example, elderly persons in some ethnic groups tend to consult folk healers and others outside the traditional health care system. Persons in some groups may attribute their health status to good or evil forces, and in some groups spiritual ritual and homemade drugs may be used to treat disease.

Patterns of health service utilization also differ by cultural background. Many minority groups, such as blacks and native Americans, view the formal health care system with caution and distrust. Other ethnic groups, such as Jewish Americans, are encouraged to use health services; however, rabbinical consultation may be desired for decisions involving organ transplantation or life-sustaining measures.

The Environmental System

The impact of environment on health, psychological well-being, and human behavior has long been recognized. As one ages, the environment becomes increasingly important as it affects independent living and contributes to the quality of life. The interrelationships among biological, psychological, and social factors and the environment are complex, especially with respect to the elderly population.

Living arrangements are an important consideration, particularly when an individual develops physical or mental health problems and is in need of a care-giver. Most older adults reside independently in their own homes (house, apartment, hotel room), either with a spouse or alone. Alternative independent living arrangements may include the provision of homemaker/chore services and personal care services within an individual's home, or licensed adult boarding homes, or other congregate housing in which there are common dining, recreational, and medical facilities. Only a small percentage (5%) of older adults reside in nursing homes.

Relocation to another living accommodation, either as a voluntary and planned move or as an unexpected and involuntary move, can affect significantly the health and well-being of older people. Relocation involves several categories of moves: residential (home to another home), inter-institutional (transferring from one institution to another, *e.g.,* hospital to nursing home or the reverse), intra-institutional (transferring from one room or unit to another within the same institution), and residential-institutional (transferring from a residence to an institution, or the reverse). All of these relocations are potentially stressful. For the elderly individual, relocation is often accompanied by declining health, financial problems, death of a spouse, and/or urban renewal, placing the person at higher risk for alterations in both physical and psychological health status.[65]

Findings from relocation studies are inconsistent. In general, they indicate that, although stressful, most relocations are not necessarily detrimental in terms of increasing mortality rates. Some relocations may be beneficial. The crucial factor in how well people adapt to relocation is based on both their perceptions of their own control over the events related to the move, and the differences in controllability between pre- and post-location environments.[66] Thus, inter-institutional relocation is more stressful than residential relocation. Intra-institutional relocation, if managed properly, has little negative effect on the older person. A caution in relocation decisions involves inappropriate placement of older people in more restrictive environments when their functional abilities do not warrant the change. In these situations, increased depression and more rapid physical deterioration can occur.[51]

Location

Location of the home environment is important because of accessibility to essential services such as medical care, pharmacies, banking, grocery stores, and shopping centers. Also important is accessibility of social services that provide both health and recreational programs, such as those found in senior centers, and nutritional programs, such as Meals on Wheels and the governmental hot lunch programs. Availability of transportation is another significant characteristic that will influence health-seeking behavior and treatment follow-up. Obtaining needed health services, particularly home care, is often more difficult for rural elderly people than for those who reside in cities with easy access and good transportation.

Personal safety is another relevant feature of location. Although older adults are commonly assumed to be frequent victims of crime, they are not at higher risk when compared to people in other age groups. However, older adults are more afraid of crime than of ill health, loneliness, or inadequate income.[28]

Physical Aspects

The design aspects of the environment can directly affect the physical and psychological functioning of older adults. Architectural features such as stairs, arrangement of rooms or facilities, lighting, and available equipment are key aspects. Accident hazards such as uneven flooring, cluttered living space, and frayed and loose rugs can lead to falls. Poorly-insulated housing without adequate heating systems can lead to accidental hypothermia. Toilet facilities and the doorway leading to the toilet are of special importance for older persons using mobility aids such as walkers or wheelchairs.

Psychological functioning can be affected in several ways. The lack of privacy in communal living situations and institutional environments can lead to psychological stress. Too little or too much sensory stimulation within the environment can contribute to depression and confusion. Personal possessions are important in the environment, particularly in an institutional environment where depersonalization and disorientation can occur.

Resources

The availability of community resources to assist older adults in daily living is a key factor in maintaining independence. This is critical for elderly people with physical and psychological impairments who do not have family care-givers available to help them meet basic living and health needs. Major contributing factors in institutionalization are the lack of available and adequate community resources to meet health needs and inadequate financial means to obtain required community resources.

Common Stressors Associated With Aging

Aging is associated with several events and conditions that can stress the adaptive mechanisms of older adults, placing them at risk for alteration in health status. These events are considered part of normal aging, but they have the potential of taxing people's coping abilities and leading to impaired physical and psychological functioning. For people with impaired functioning, the events may trigger serious mental health consequences. Three common stressors are loss, change, and health alterations. The nurse should be aware of these common stressors in order to provide optimal care to aging individuals.

Common stressors of aging reflecting loss, change, and health alterations include:

Changes in physical appearance and function
Loss of physical stamina and energy
Onset and complications of chronic illness
Retirement
Decreased income
Death of a spouse, adult children, siblings, and friends
Relocation, involving loss of home and friends

Loss

The common denominator of stressors is loss. Losses in mid- and late life are common. For some people, losses are predictable with aging; for others, losses are not anticipated and are severely disruptive. Losses are usual across the life span. Losses experienced in childhood and early and mid-adulthood may differ in type and number but, as a rule, do not differ in intensity. What is different is the reserve of physical and emotional energy and resilience needed to make peace with the loss and move on. Examples are a young person's not being accepted in the college of choice, not winning an honor, or not receiving membership in an organization. Another loss faced by young adults and their children is divorce; with time and effort, most adults and children are able to make peace

with the failed marriage and the failed expectations of a family life with all members living together harmoniously.

For the older adult, losses require substantial efforts, in both physical and emotional energy, in grieving and in resolution. Older people often face multiple losses that occur simultaneously. The death of a spouse may set in motion a number of confounding losses, such as the loss of companionship, loss of usual roles, losses in financial and social resources, and, perhaps, losses surrounding a move to a new residence. For example, an elderly minister, who continued to serve a church congregation, moved with his wife to a retirement community in which they shared a two-room apartment and joined other residents for meals in a common dining room. Shortly after the move, his wife died and he was told he was no longer eligible for the two-room space and must move into a single room. His losses were many: his spouse of many years, their expectations of life in the retirement community, home and possessions that were sold prior to the move, neighborhood and friendships with neighbors and a neighborhood dog, and loss of his previous lifestyle. Even with his advanced age, his assets of having an occupational purpose, a religious belief system, mobility with his car, supportive adult children, and substantial financial resources were sufficient to give his life meaning until his health began to fail and he experienced multiple illnesses and died. For many older people, the resources needed to deal with losses are insufficient in quality and quantity for positive outcomes, even for a time.

While loss of one's spouse may be severely disruptive, loss of an adult child is a more threatening and disorganizing event. Older people do not expect to survive their children; recovery is difficult because the lost object is irreplaceable.

The impulse to preserve the thread of continuity in life is critical for survival and for making sense of life.[49] Losses must be accepted somehow and understood to capture the thread of continuity and restore meaning. That understanding and making sense is as important to children and young adults as it is to mid- and late-life adults whose losses are more numerous and, for the most part, are losses of irreplaceable objects. In all losses, there is rupture of attachment.[18] The strength of the attachment that is broken may be comfort, security, esteem, predictability, roles, or lifestyles. Losses are usually threatening, leading to disorientation of purpose and undermining the structure of meaning on which new learning and adaptation depend.

Losses must be acknowledged and grieved over to restore meaning and continuity to life. Unless losses can be understood and meaning assigned, people cannot go on. Coming to terms with loss, balancing and making peace with what was and what is, helps put the loss into manageable perspective. Working through losses requires both time and emotional energy. When losses are multiple, disrupt strong attachments, and occur in close proximity, loss overload and crisis may occur.

Grieving follows no certain pattern and no predictable timetable. Resolution of grief probably is never completed. The work of grief, as described by Lindemann,[46] includes emotionally separating from the lost object, be it a person or a job or a long-time family home. This work includes considering positive and negative features of the object and developing a balanced memory that is comfortable to live with. Grieving includes adjusting to the environment with the lost object missing, that is, making the changes necessary to living alone, to no longer leaving the house to go to work each day, or to living in a smaller space. Finally, grief work includes trying to establish additional ties with people, to involve oneself in new roles, or to revive former relationships and roles. Grief work must be accomplished for the resumption of a reasonably whole and meaningful life. Major psychosocial alterations may occur in the absence of this sense of closure from the loss.

Change

Change, like loss, is a stressor in the lives of older people. Change and loss are related concepts because loss accompanies every change. Change is so much a part of life that it is talked about as if there is universal agreement about its meaning. Furthermore, change is a value-laden concept that triggers feelings and reactions that are negative (disruptive) or positive (energizing). Change may be planned, developmental, spontaneous, unplanned, or haphazard. Whether change is sought or resisted or whether it happens by chance or design, people usually respond with mixed emotions.[49] The will to change has to overcome the impulse to continue or restore the past. Resistance to change is a fact of life.[49]

As with loss, the impulse to preserve the thread of continuity is crucial. People's lives and comfort are dependent on the ability to predict events and to anticipate what is ahead. New experiences are more comfortably incorporated when they can be filtered through the screen of what is known and what has been experienced before. Change is understandable in terms of the balance between continuity, growth, and loss.[49] Many changes are incremental or substitutional; patterns of expectations are uninterrupted. An example of incremental change is an older couple's plan for retirement, when they would move from a large family home to a home in a retirement community. While the move itself may be disruptive, the meaning of their lives together is not disturbed. The move is part of their shared developmental shift to life as a retired couple. A second group of changes represent growth, in which familiar purposes are incorporated and elaborated, as with the previously described couple. For them, the continuity of their lives is unbroken. They move on to another developmental period in their relationship in a new setting. The third kind of change may involve the loss of a person or of assumptions about life, which may result in a crisis of discontinuity. An example is a couple who planned throughout their lives to move to a retirement community when they retire. One of them becomes seriously ill, which necessitates a change of plans and the decision to stay where they are, where med-

ical care is available and where existing support systems are in place. As they come to terms with the loss of their life-long goals, the structure of the meaning of the illness and the resultant shift in plans may result in despair. With time, it may result in innovation, as they incorporate the changes into the continuity of their lives.

One critical change is the transition from the role of wife to the role of widow. The success of the transition, as reported by widows, is congruent with their previous lifestyles.[9] Older people undergo numerous changes in all domains of their daily lives. For some, the changes lead to crisis, despair, and major psychosocial alterations. For others, the change is incorporated, understood, and accepted; life continues with new meaning.

Health Alterations

Normal aging is a relatively benign process, yet as people grow older they have increasing risk of developing physical and psychological health alterations. By age 60, most individuals have at least one chronic disease. Because the incidence of chronic disease increases with age, people at age 75 years and older are likely to have an average of three or more chronic diseases. The impact of these health conditions may range from relatively minor impairment to severe functional limitation. In most cases, only relatively minor changes in lifestyle are necessary. In other cases, increasing amounts of care and health services are required.

Older people tend to experience multiple health problems at the same time, which makes diagnosis and management extremely difficult. Problems in one organ system can affect the functioning of another system. Physical health problems can lead to mental health difficulties, and the reverse is also true. Drug therapy may induce new problems, such as depression, dizziness, and palpitations.

Acute or chronic conditions in interaction with normal aging changes may mask clinical diagnoses. Often, older adults will present with atypical disease signs and symptoms. Rather than show well-defined symptoms, as observed in younger people, the aged will present with vague and nonspecific complaints. Elderly people are more likely to show mental manifestations of their physical problems. In many instances, they will demonstrate functional changes such as confusion, incontinence, and falls. All of these problems may be symptomatic of a wide range of different illnesses, ranging from infection to cardiac problems to iatrogenic (drug-induced) complications. For example, a previously alert and oriented 78-year-old woman becomes confused and incontinent. Although she is afebrile, on closer examination it is discovered that she has a systemic bacterial infection. Once treated appropriately with antibiotics, she returns to her normal alert, oriented, and continent status.

In spite of having several chronic conditions, most older people are healthy and able to function independently in the community. The majority of the elderly rate their health as good or excellent when compared to that of others in their own age group. As nurses, we need to be aware that a disease process may underlie any acute change in physical or mental functioning. If treated properly, many individuals will revert back to their normal baselines of functioning.

Physical Alterations

Older adults, in comparison to younger adults, are less likely to experience acute illnesses such as infections. Instead, they are more likely to experience an acute problem related to their chronic disease conditions. Once an acute illness does occur, elderly individuals usually have a longer recovery period. This longer time for recovery is due to a decreased organ system reserve capacity that leads to a decreased ability to respond to stress.

Chronic conditions reported most frequently by older adults include arthritis, hypertension, heart disease, hearing impairment, orthopedic impairment, cataracts, chronic sinusitis, visual impairment (other than cataracts), diabetes mellitus, and varicose veins.[54] Other disease processes that increase in incidence with aging include neurological disorders such as cerebrovascular accident and Parkinson's disease; musculoskeletal disorders such as osteoporosis, with potential for fractures of the spine, wrist, and hip; nutritional anemias such as iron, folate, and Vitamin B_{12} deficiencies; respiratory disorders such as chronic obstructive lung disease; and genitourinary disorders such as urinary incontinence and severe prostatic enlargement. Malignant neoplasms such as breast and lung cancers also increase in incidence with age.

Psychological Alterations

The prevalence of psychiatric disorders in the elderly has not been well-documented. Personality disorders and neurotic or psychotic conditions that were present early in life may persist for many years. These disorders do not shorten the life span of the person. However, recent studies conducted in populations of community-dwelling elders indicate that, for most psychiatric conditions, the incidence declines with age. The major exceptions are a high prevalence of depression in the elderly, and the suicide rate for white males age 75 to 84 years, which is higher than for all other age and racial groups.[61] In the noninstitutionalized elderly male population, severe cognitive impairment was the most common psychiatric disorder, followed by phobia and alcohol abuse or dependence. For elderly women, the most common disorder was phobia, followed by severe cognitive impairment.[52]

Cognitive impairment increases with advancing age. Estimates indicate that 20% of individuals over age 65 suffer from mild cognitive impairment. It has been predicted that 20% of those over age 80 and 30% of those age 85 and over will develop senile dementia of the Alzheimer's type (SDAT).[26,61] These predictions are important because these individuals require extensive monitoring and care, whether it be at home or within an institution. This places heavy burdens on care-givers, especially family members who are unable to obtain mental health services for their relatives. Mental disorders, including the loss of cognitive functioning, are a leading cause of institutionalization. While it is not necessarily the primary reason for admission, a high proportion of the nursing home population has a senile dementia.[12]

Major Psychosocial Alterations

Older adults face challenges in their lives that are similar to those of younger persons. However, they face the challenges at a time when their adaptive skills and resources, as well as their physical, social, and psychological resources, may be limited. Older adults are faced by losses in both quantity and quality that exceed the usual and predictable losses of younger individuals. From a systems perspective, older adults may face systems overload, with physical changes, illness, and care needs complicated by losses of former health status and abilities, by the need to change residence or other activity patterns, by losses in support systems, and by other threats to the person's definition of self as a self-sufficient person. Vulnerability increases with advancing age and predictable concomitant changes.

Depression

The incidence of depressive disorders and symptoms of depression is notable in people age 65 and older. Readily-recognizable signs of depression range from sadness and despondency to immobility and dejectedness. Persons experiencing clinical depression demonstrate alterations in affect, thinking, physiological responses, and social behaviors. The usual symptoms include: depressed mood; weight loss, resulting from diminished interest in food and the process of eating; sleep disturbances, such as early awakening and difficulty in falling asleep; psychomotor changes, such as severe slowing of activities and responses or agitation; loss of interest; inner distress; diminished self-esteem; and feelings of hopelessness and helplessness. While some people may experience symptoms of depression, others experience primary affective disorders. The clearest agreement to date on differentiating depression from other disorders may be found in the Diagnostic and Statistical Manual of Mental Disorders, third edition, revised (DSM-III-R).[6] (See Chap. 15 for DSM-III-R criteria for depression.)

While knowledge is growing, there is no agreed-upon cause for depression. Depression results from the mix of stressful personal and environmental events, genetic endowment, and personality development and structure. The regular challenges faced by elderly individuals contribute to their risk of depression. The challenges include: alterations in physical health status, with chronic diseases and resultant reactions to illness; reductions in mobility and fewer opportunities for interaction;

losses of significant people in their lives; social isolation; and loss of financial resources.

Depression resulting from these changes may be difficult to differentiate in older adults. Klerman[40] identified three major problems that confound the diagnosis of depression. One is *pseudodementia,* in which the depressed older adult shows cognitive impairment, memory and orientation impairment, and delusions. The depression in pseudodementia can be treated and reversed; *senile dementia,* with more mental deterioration, is not reversible. A second condition confounding the diagnosis of depression is that of somatic manifestation in endocrine disorders and electrolyte disturbances. Somatic and organic complaints of older adults may be signals of depression. Finally, drug-induced reactions confound the diagnosis of depression. The medications for typical chronic illnesses may yield depressive side-effects, as may polypharmacy, or multiple use of drugs; both drug interaction and toxicity provide important cues.

Mood disorders, with the exception of organic disorders, are classified in the major group of affective disorders in which depressed mood is the predominant feature. Depression is the most relevant psychosocial condition for older adults. The major affective or mood disorders are classified in two groups: bipolar disorders and major depression. The essential feature of *bipolar disorder* is a distinct period of elevated mood, increased activity, and poor judgment that lasts from one to two weeks. Most people with bipolar disorder subsequently develop depression. A *major depressive* episode lasts for at least two weeks, and clients experience loss of energy, loss of interest, disordered eating and sleeping, difficulty in concentrating, psychomotor agitation or retardation, self-reproach, and thoughts of suicide and death. The symptoms occur in the absence of other disorders and persist, impairing the person's ability to function.

In the last three decades, there have been major advances in understanding and treating depression and related mood disorders.[40] However, many critical issues involved in depression and treatment in older people have not been addressed: (1) Is depression one or several disorders? (2) Is the process of depression in late life similar to the process of affective disorders in earlier stages of life? (3) Should the treatment be the same as at earlier ages? (4) How does a diagnosis of clinical depression relate to feelings of loneliness and depression reported by elderly people? (5) What are the roles of biological correlates and psychosocial stresses found in depression in the elderly?

It has been estimated that the manic type of bipolar disorder occurs in only 10% of elderly people with affective disorders. The characteristic elation seen in younger clients is not usual with older clients. Elderly persons are more often aggressive and surly. They may show suspiciousness and paranoid thinking. Grandiose ideas and unwise conduct are usually present, as they are in younger clients. Awareness and cognitive functions may be impaired. There may be bursts of tears and sadness followed by resumption of grandiosity. Single attacks of mania in the elderly are exceptional; the more usual pattern is for early recurrence of both manic and depressive symptoms.

Major depression is the most common and recurring affective disorder experienced by older people. The characteristic picture of depression occurs: melancholy mood, low self-esteem, feelings of unworthiness, hopelessness, and self-doubt, and tearfulness or inability to cry; behavioral changes such as decreasing activity and social interaction; and biological difficulties, including somatic complaints, sleep disturbances, gastrointestinal complaints, weight loss, tachycardia, and chest pain.

In all instances, depressive symptomatology in older adults warrants careful medical assessment, including extensive family history data, mental status data, physical examination and laboratory data, and psychological testing, in addition to data on the history and present physical and social status of the person. The key to an accurate diagnosis is the client's past and present history of symptoms and the family's history of affective disorders. Given the scope of depression, the complexity involved in determining an accurate diagnosis cannot be overemphasized. The continuum for depression begins with depression as a normal emotion, an expected part of the human condition; continues with depression as a symptom experienced by people with various medical, neurological, and psychiatric disorders, as well as by individuals making transitions caused by losses and changes in their lives; and concludes with depression as a clinical condition classified as mood or affective disorder.

Grief, reacting to the loss of a loved person, is classified as Uncomplicated Bereavement in the DMS-III-R. It is not classified as a mental disorder unless there is severe impairment or an extended bereavement episode or an adjustment disorder. Grieving individuals experience depressionlike symptoms of sadness, sighing, loss of interest in the environment, and crying, as well as physical symptoms that follow the death of a loved individual. Following a period of mourning, those symptoms usually subside as the loss is accepted, the environment with the lost person gone is accepted, and new people are added to the lifestyle and life space.

Dementia

Dementia is characterized by losses of brain functioning that result in impaired intellectual functioning, memory, judgment, and orientation. Shallow, labile affect may also result. The changes may have an insidious onset, but usually result in the older adult's inability to function in social and occupational spheres. Personality changes occur concomitantly. For some, the changes exaggerate long-standing personality characteristics and coping styles. For others, the changes result in the person's withdrawal from previous patterns. In any case, the losses to the self are severe and, for the most part, irreversible.

The individual with dementia in advanced states is "in the world" but not "of the world" in terms of physical and mental functioning, appearance, and behavior. While the physical person remains, the self that was known to the person and to significant others is no longer present. The age of the person, combined with the nature of the brain changes, influences life expectancy for the individual with dementia.

Multi-infarct dementia is a vascular disease affecting vessels of the brain. It often accompanies other signs of heart disease. Causes often include hypertension and arteriosclerosis. Unlike senile dementia, multi-infarct dementias often have sudden onset, with rapid changes in intellectual functions due to small strokes. Other impairments follow, including changes in memory, judgment, and orientation, along with emotional lability, and neurological and personality changes.

A thorough physical examination will aid in the diagnosis. Treatment includes both medical and surgical interventions focusing on the impaired circulatory system. The prognosis is dependent upon a combination of factors, including lesion sites, progression of the illness, age of the client, and the number of risk factors involved.[71]

Pseudodementia

Pseudodementia is a common condition in the older adult population. The constellation of depressive symptoms closely parallels the symptom-picture of dementia. The distinguishing features can be assessed on the basis of history, appearance, affect, and cognitive functioning.

In a true dementia, the depression follows the loss of cognitive functioning, while in pseudodementia the depression precedes cognitive impairment. Assessment of the depressed older adult will likely reveal a history of recent, significant losses, and depressive symptoms such as helplessness, hopelessness, undue focus on physical conditions and functions, and eating and sleeping difficulties. A history of previous depressions is not unusual. In the older adult with a true organic dementia, the history of recent losses and previous depressive episodes is not likely. To mislabel a depressed person as senile is a costly error. Depressions are responsive to treatment and are reversible. Table 26-1 shows characteristic differences between pseudodementia (depression) and dementia.[70]

Suicide

Taking one's life by suicide is a type of coping behavior. Common sense suggests that, when faced with problems that are challenging or difficult and for which obvious solutions are not evident, individuals may consider fleeing the problem by taking their own lives. Suicide is one coping mechanism; the person removes himself or herself from the problem. With older adults, whose coping repertoire may be insufficient for the challenges being faced in a long life, suicide is one solution. As with any crisis, it is not an event, but the person's reaction or definition of the situation, that leads to suicide.[8] How well-developed and useful the coping abilities are is the crucial factor.[50]

TABLE 26-1.
A COMPARISON OF PSEUDODEMENTIA AND DEMENTIA

PSEUDODEMENTIA	DEMENTIA
1. Symptoms of short duration suggest pseudodementia.	1. Symptoms of long duration suggest dementia.
2. Clients usually complain much of cognitive loss.	2. Clients usually complain little of cognitive loss.
3. Clients' complaints of cognitive dysfunction are usually detailed.	3. Clients' complaints of cognitive dysfunction are usually imprecise.
4. Clients usually communicate a strong sense of distress.	4. Clients often appear unconcerned.
5. Memory losses for recent and remote events are usually equally severe.	5. Memory loss for recent events is more severe than that for remote events.
6. Memory gaps for specific periods or events are common.	6. Memory gaps for specific periods are unusual (except when due to delirium, trauma, or seizures).
7. Attention and concentration are often well-preserved.	7. Attention and concentration are usually faulty.
8. "Don't know" answers are typical.	8. "Near miss" answers are typical.
9. Clients emphasize their disability.	9. Clients conceal their disability.
10. Clients make little effort to perform even simple tasks.	10. Clients struggle to perform tasks.
11. Clients highlight failures.	11. Clients delight in accomplishments, however trivial.
12. Clients do not try to keep up.	12. Clients rely on notes, calendars, and the like to keep up.
13. There is marked variability in performing tasks of similar difficulty.	13. There is consistently poor performance on tasks of similar difficulty.
14. Affective change is often pervasive.	14. Affect is labile and shallow.
15. Loss of social skills is often early and prominent.	15. Clients often retain social skills.
16. On tests of orientation, clients often give "don't know" answers.	16. On tests of orientation, clients mistake unusual for usual.
17. Behavior is often incongruent with severity of cognitive dysfunction.	17. Behavior is usually compatible with severity of cognitive dysfunction.
18. Nocturnal accentuation of dysfunction is uncommon.	18. Nocturnal accentuation of dysfunction is common.
19. History of previous psychiatric dysfunction is common.	19. History of previous psychiatric dysfunction is unusual.

(Modified from Wells CE, Duncan GW: Neurology for Psychiatrists. Philadelphia, FA Davis, 1980.)

CLINICAL EXAMPLE

PERSON AT RISK FOR SUICIDE

Ms. Gordon retired at age 70 from a long career in nursing administrative roles. She moved back to her hometown, where she had not lived for 50 years. Within the space of five years, she experienced the deaths of her only siblings, two brothers, an aunt, and a cousin. Her physical health was sufficient for her to attend Mass weekly and to shop for groceries in a nearby center. Within the next five years, her housemate of 35 years died suddenly of a ruptured aneurysm. Other cousins died.

Now, at age 85, Ms. Gordon lives alone. She does not leave her house for months at a time. She has been declared legally blind. A woman helper shops and writes checks for her, as needed.

She has exhausted her coping repertoire and continues to exist in an environment that is substantially devoid of human contact. She rejects a move because she fears depletion of her funds. She also does not have sufficient physical or emotional energy to accomplish a move, or to undertake the process of change.

All outside indicators suggest her life is over. She is a passive participant in living each day, eating a mid-day meal and little else.

Older adults are at high risk for losses in all domains of their lives. While many can absorb losses and continue, others do not have the resilience and strength to meet the challenge. Loss overload may be the critical factor. When losses occur with both frequency and intensity, grief work and problem-solving are not completed before another loss occurs.

Older adults at risk for suicide are those who: have experienced loss of family and social ties; have physical illnesses; have made suicidal gestures; have psychiatric disorders; have organic mental disorders; abuse alcohol; or have heightened physical complaints. Osgood[57] expands the list of those at risk for suicide by including those who have had disorderly occupational lives, are retired, are unemployed, are living alone, have had recent change of residence, have poor health or a terminal illness, are lonely, or are from a broken home of family origin. The distinction is made between quality of life and quantity of life. Miller[50] suggests that within each person there is a subconscious line of unbearability. When people find themselves in an intolerable situation, one for which coping skills are insufficient or absent, the line of unbearability comes into awareness. When the situation is defined as intolerable, and the will to live is insufficient, the person may choose to die.

While there is rarely a single reason for a person's decision to commit suicide, the patterns of suicide in older adults provide categories of major threats to people who reach the line of unbearability. In reality, patterns overlap and reflect salient motivations for dying. These patterns include reaction to:[50]

1. Severe physical illness
2. Mental illness
3. The threat of extreme dependency and/or institutionalization
4. The death of a spouse
5. Retirement
6. Pathological personal relationships
7. Alcoholism and drug abuse
8. Multiple factors

Suicide is more prevalent among the elderly than among other segments of the population. Unmarried white males in lower socioeconomic classes and low-status occupations, the lonely, and those who are isolated in urban areas are at higher risk. The above clinical example depicts an older adult at risk for suicide.

Elder Abuse

Elder abuse is a family systems issue. While it is not a new problem, it has received increased attention recently. As with child and spouse abuse, definitional issues abound. A useful, encompassing definition has not been established. Most agree that abuse includes physical and psychological abuse and neglect. Material abuse and violation of individual rights are also included.

Reporting of abuse in the elderly is inadequate. Estimates by some are that one elderly person in ten is abused;[43] others[13] estimate that elder abuse occurs in one of every two households. Victims rarely report abuse. They may be physically or mentally unable to report, they may be embarrassed about reporting, or they may fear abandonment or other reprisals. Perceived physical and psychological costs of reporting may exceed the costs of being abused.

To understand why abuse occurs, one needs to look at the total family system, including family roles and needs. The usual elderly abused person is a Caucasian woman, over the age of 75, who is dependent because of a physical or cognitive impairment.[14] In many instances, the individual has troublesome behavior such as incontinence, confusion, and disorientation. Abusers may be spouses, daughters or sons, or other family members. Abusers have often been mistreated themselves, and view abuse as a means of problem-solving.[35] Abusers are categorized as pathological abusers and stressed care-givers. *Pathological abusers* include those who are mentally or physically disabled themselves, and those who are substance abusers. *Stressed care-givers* may be individuals who function normally, but who are stressed because of the physical and emotional demands of providing care for a dependent elderly person.

Human interest stories in the popular press describe care provided by spouses and daughters for years without

RELEVANT RESEARCH

The purpose of this study was to estimate the economic costs of Alzheimer's disease (AD) to the individual and society. This is the first study measuring the economic toll of this fatal degenerative disease.

The authors used published reviews of research related to Alzheimer's disease as the data source. Specifically, epidemiological projections and cost information for the 1983 United States population were used. Autopsy samples and data from foreign studies were also included. The estimated costs of AD were measured by assessing diagnostic costs, "nursing home care, long-term mental hospital care, short-term acute hospital care, physician services," and so on. Costs were also estimated for "home care provided by the family, and travel time."

The estimated diagnostic costs were $874. Nursing home care for one year was $5,326. Other findings related to costs included: long-term mental hospital care, $322; home care, $1,744; short-term acute hospital care, $434; physicians' services, $418; drugs and medical supplies, $244; and family-provided home care, $8,684. Including other totals, the net annual expected total cost for the first year was $18,517. For the second and later years, the cost was $17,643.

The annual cost in the United States for AD was found to be between $27 and $31 billion; this will increase dramatically as the size of the aged population increases. The authors state that, "given the magnitude of potential savings—if AD could be prevented or arrested at an early age—a substantially increased federal commitment to AD research is clearly warranted."

(Hay J, Ernst R: The economic costs of Alzheimer's disease. Am J Pub Health 77:1169, 1987.)

relief. The story will then report an act of violence that is identified as elder abuse. These instances reflect family systems tension and strain, and are somehow understandable in light of family systems issues such as inadequate communication, problem-solving, and coping. Further, the family system may be strained because of depleted financial and personal resources. In some instances, the abuse is reciprocal, with the frail elderly individual being abusive to the care-giver.

Primary Degenerative Dementia

Senile Dementia of the Alzheimer's Type (SDAT)

SDAT is characterized by changes within the brain: senile plaques, neurofibrillary tangles, granulovacuolar structures, and loss of neurons.[73] Causes are hypothesized to be genetic, viral, biochemical, immunological, or toxic. In the DSM-III-R,[6] SDAT consists of three components: (1) memory and other cognitive impairment, (2) functional and structural brain impairment, and (3) behavioral manifestations that affect the person's capacity for self-care, interpersonal relationships, and adjustment in the community. Because definitive diagnosis can be made only at autopsy, in clinical practice the diagnosis is made by ruling out other known causes of cognitive and memory impairment. Diagnostic tools include: history and physical examination; mental status, neurological, and psychological evaluations; laboratory studies of blood and urine; and computerized axial tomography.[1] In the last decade, attention to this disease process has had positive and negative effects. The positive effects include increased public understanding and research. The negative effect has been indiscriminate labeling of older individuals who do not have dementia.

SDAT involves gradual deterioration in functioning. There are considerable variations in symptoms from client to client, as well as in longevity following the onset of symptoms. One prototypic pattern of progression is: initial memory impairment, reduction in spontaneity, progressive intellectual deterioration, and changes in behavior. Symptom constellations vary in degree and in their combinations; included, in varying degrees, are disorientation, memory impairment, emotional lability, and changes in concrete thinking and concrete language and word use.

SDAT is more common in women than men. Clustering of cases of the disease has been found in some families, but no consistent pattern of genetic transmissibility has been established. It is the fourth or fifth leading cause of death for people over age 65. Risk factors have not been associated with SDAT, except for advancing chronological age. SDAT is irreversible; it involves progressive loss of cognitive ability, self-care skills, and adaptation. Prevalence of the disease increases steadily with age. Alzheimer's disease accounts for 50% to 70% of the diagnoses of dementia in elderly people; 15% to 25% of the dementias can be accounted for with multi-infarct dementias, and the remaining 5% to 35% are due to the reversible pseudodementia.[20]

Present knowledge about the clinical course of SDAT is limited, particularly in relation to early phases. Initially, individuals may complain of forgetting names and objects but show no other deficits in social and employment situations. At that point, it is difficult to identify the meaning of the symptoms. With SDAT, the memory loss continues, with failing recall of contexts and events. The person may become lost when traveling to an unfamiliar place, and experience mild to moderate anxiety.

With further declines, the individual experiences additional memory losses; difficulty with complex tasks; social withdrawal; flattened affect; and loss of initiative, judgment, and tact. Denial is frequently used as a de-

RELEVANT RESEARCH

This study explored experiences of families from the first recognition of symptoms of SDAT throughout the course of the dementia. The research questionnaire, developed at the University of Michigan Institute of Gerontology, was sent to a random sample of 413 families on the mailing list of the Minnesota Chapter of Alzheimer's Disease and Related Disorders Association. Most of the 289 respondents were the primary care-givers for their relatives. Care in the home was being provided by 130 respondents (45%), and 159 (55%) respondents had relatives in nursing homes and other institutions. More than half (55%) of the respondents were spouses. Individuals with AD ranged in age from 42 to 82 years of age; 61% were men and 39% were women.

Study findings were consistent with those of other care-giving studies. Initially, families struggled with the changes in their relative's behaviors. The insidious onset of the changes caused families to mistrust their perceptions. Early symptoms were experienced as unrelated, until the symptoms increased and they could no longer be ignored.

Diagnoses for some took years and visits to several physicians. Physicians' explanations of the progressive, irreversible deterioration of the family member were most helpful when they extended over several visits and allowed family members time to process the information and to absorb the advice and suggestions for care. Physicians' availability by phone during the course of the illness was seen as particularly helpful. Support of family and friends made coping with problems less stressful for care-givers. Unexpectedly, for some, the care-giving experience drew families and friends closer together.

The fact that care-givers could not continue to provide 24-hour care was the most common reason for institutionalizing the family member with dementia. Even when care-givers went beyond their capabilities to provide care for their family members with AD, the care-giver required the support and urging of family members and physicians to make the decision for institutionalization. From the insidious onset throughout the course of the disease, families of clients with AD adapt and adjust to new problems and challenges with courage and determination. Appropriate professional care can assist them to adapt to the different stresses along the way.

This research, conducted by a gerontologic nurse specialist and a social worker, demonstrates the need for a family systems approach in providing nursing care to SDAT clients and their family care-givers. It underscores the importance of making a careful nursing assessment of, not only the client's physical and psychosocial needs, but the family care-giver's knowledge of the disease and coping resources. Further, the research supports the need for nurses, when teaching family members about the disease, to present only as much as the care-giver can take in at one time, and to reassess and repeat as needed. The need for the nurse to have knowledge of supportive community resources is demonstrated in this study.

(Chenoweth B, Spencer B: Dementia: The experience of family caregivers. Gerontologist 26:267, 1986.)

fense. Progressively, the person is unable to remember relevant facts, and needs assistance with activities of daily living. The combinations of symptoms that follow include personality and emotional changes, obsessive symptomatology, and anxiety, agitation, and abusive behavior. Individuals may no longer recognize their spouses or care-givers. Ultimately, they lose verbal ability, and require assistance to eat and use the toilet.

The client is not the sole victim of SDAT. Families and family systems are affected by the disease and disease process. Care-giver stress, in the case of people maintaining family members at home, is enormous. Stresses arise both from the total care-taking functions and from the role realignments and boundary ambiguity with the SDAT person physically present but psychologically absent. The care family members must provide often takes all of their time and emotional energy.

In working with SDAT clients and their families, there are two important tasks for the nurse. The nurse must assess both the client's problems and the care-giver's reactions to the problems, in order to determine the help the care-giver needs. The nurse must also assess the care-giver's coping skills and social supports in order to identify specific sources of burdens on the care-giver.[73] Care-giver stress is not directly correlated with the behavioral and cognitive symptoms of the client. How the care-giver manages the client's memory loss and behavioral problems has a great impact on the care-giver's stress. The social support systems available to the care-giver and the quality of the dyadic relationship prior to the SDAT diagnosis are also important influencing factors. For the most part, families seeking help are not aware of the resources that are available for them and for the person with SDAT. Nurses working with clients and their families should be certain that they are aware of the variety of alternatives available. Nurses should take into consideration the needs and preferences of the clients and their families.

Nurses are likely to encounter people with SDAT in hospitals or other institutional settings. Within these settings, it is important to have a systems view of the SDAT client. All elements of the five-systems model need to be considered within the institutional system: the biological, psychological, sociological, environmental, and cultural subsystems. It is expected that the move to an institutional setting will be stressful and disruptive for clients. Being in an unfamiliar setting with many more unfamiliar people can be disorganizing and disturbing. For a time, clients may regress, not maintaining their prior levels of functioning. Typical behavior seen in hospital settings may include: withdrawal, confusion, disorientation, wandering, broken sleep patterns, inability to eat without assistance, incontinence, ritualized behavior, agitation, and, at times, angry outbursts and violent behavior.

Recent work by Hall,[27] a nurse, has moved care of clients with SDAT from trial-and-error, generically-implemented nursing practice to theory-based practice. The model developed by Hall is the progressively lowered stress threshold model (PLST). Conceptually, the model considers symptom clusters in three groups of losses (cognitive, affective, and functional loss). Hall's model adds PLST as the fourth cluster of symptoms, which are stress-related. Three types of behaviors are exhibited by SDAT patients. *Baseline* or normative behavior is exhibited by persons who are functioning within the limits of their neurological deficits; they are socially and cognitively accessible. *Anxious* behavior is seen when the patient is stressed; care-givers may still be able to be in contact with the person. *Dysfunctional* behavior occurs if stress continues or increases. As the label suggests, the person's behavior becomes dysfunctional, and cognitive and social contact with care-givers is lost. The person cannot communicate effectively and cannot use the environment appropriately. These behaviors include: agitation, withdrawal, panic, fearfulness, purposeful wandering, and combativeness. Together, these symptoms represent Hall's fourth symptom cluster.

States of stress occur when people do not have mastery of internal and external stimuli and cannot cope with the environment. As the disease progresses, SDAT patients are less able to receive and process stimuli and information. As abilities decline, challenges for maintenance increase, and frustration, anxiety, and fatigue result. Hall's PLST model seeks to support maximum functional levels and to anticipate and control for potentially stress-related factors in the environment. Anxiety is used as the barometer to determine what the patient can tolerate, and when environmental stimuli need to be modified and simplified. The principles of providing care to a person with progressive cortical degeneration using Hall's PLST model are presented in Table 26-2.

It is important that care planned for persons with SDAT be individually planned and evaluated frequently in light of their changing cognitive and intellectual abili-

TABLE 26-2.
PLST PRINCIPLES OF CARE FOR PERSONS WITH PROGRESSIVE CORTICAL DEGENERATION

1. Maximize the level of safe function by supporting all areas of loss in a prosthetic manner.
2. Provide the patient with unconditional positive regard.
3. Use behaviors indicating anxiety and avoidance to determine limits of levels of anxiety and stimuli.
4. Teach care-givers to "listen" to the patient, evaluating verbal and nonverbal responses.
5. Modify environment to support losses and enhance safety.
6. Provide ongoing education, support, care and problem-solving for care-givers.

(Hall GR, Buckwalter KC: Progressively lowered stress threshold: A conceptual model for care of adults with Alzheimer's disease. Arch Psychiatr Nurs 1:404, 1987.)

ties. An active rehabilitation program with reality-orientation activities may be a serious stressor when clients are not oriented in the environment, when they misperceive an action or event, or when the judgments are inappropriate.

In the PLST model,[27] a client's losses are considered in establishing a routine and providing rest periods. Clients' orientation is assisted by environmental cues for dates and time and by presentation of reality as needed for security, comfort, and safety. Therapies that do not contribute to added stress are suggested, such as: music therapy, reminiscence groups, and therapeutic recreation. As part of the model, families, care-givers, and staff are taught the PLST principles. When care is implemented using this plan, patients remain at their highest level of functioning and their behavior remains normative.

The Nursing Process

The nursing process enables the nurse to assess, diagnose, plan, implement, and evaluate care directed toward meeting mental health needs of older adults. Consideration of the physical, psychological, social, environmental, and cultural subsystems is critical in this process.

Assessment

The key to an accurate nursing diagnosis is a careful and thorough assessment that gathers pertinent information on the older adult's presenting problem and associated symptoms, cognitive skills, functional abilities, medication history, relevant past health history, social history, family history, activity patterns, and environment. It is important to identify the older adult's normal behavior and functional abilities prior to the onset of the presenting problem. In addition, a physical examination is necessary to screen for treatable physical conditions that may be presenting as psychological symptoms. Components of the psychosocial assessment of the older adult are summarized in Table 26-3.

The nurse needs to be especially sensitive to the possibility of atypical presentation of acute medical illnesses, appearing as confusion or behavioral changes. In addition, the nurse should keep in mind as the client proceeds through the initial description of the problem that older adults may somatize their complaints rather than identify that they are depressed. Reports of sleep problems, loss of appetite, and constipation may be symptoms of depression. However, reports of changes in bowel habits, nausea, vomiting, weight loss, heart palpitations, fatigue, headaches, and shortness of breath may be indicative of a physical illness and warrant referral for a medical evaluation. If cognitive abilities appear significantly impaired, a comprehensive medical and psychological examination should be conducted. A variety of standardized instruments to assess mental status, affect, and func-

CLINICAL EXAMPLE

Ms. Martin was admitted to a psychiatric unit of a general hospital when she became unmanageable in her home environment. She was brought to the hospital by her husband and daughter. They reported that her behavior had changed gradually over the previous five years. Recently, she had become increasingly restless, on some days showing belligerence and hatefulness and on other days being lethargic. She had become more confused about elimination—sometimes soiling herself, at other times using the bathtub for a toilet, and only occasionally using the toilet. She needed help with bathing and dressing. She needed cues about how to eat, and no longer remembered how to use a knife and fork. Her sleep was sporadic. She reported disturbing dreams and nightmares that made her agitated and anxious.

In view of the recent symptoms, she was admitted to the hospital for a complete work-up by a geropsychiatrist and neurologist. Her husband, Mr. Martin, had been her full-time care-giver for the past three years. He reported that he sleeps for only one or two hours at a time and often sits outside his wife's room when she is unable to sleep. For reasons of personal safety, she has not been able to stay alone even for short periods of time for more than a year.

He said that the family first noticed changes in Ms. Martin's behavior five years earlier, when she was 60 years old. She became less and less able to manage in her secretarial position, and was asked by her supervisor to seek medical help for her confusion and forgetfulness at work. She was seen at a nearby medical center, but no definitive diagnosis was made. She and her husband decided that she would resign her position and stay home. One morning, after her resignation,

Mr. Martin found her in her car at 5 a.m., stating that she was leaving for work. On two other occasions she went out during the day and could not remember where she had left her car. With help from the police, the car was located. Mr. Martin decided she was no longer capable of being alone, and he applied for early retirement to be with her. He stated, "We've been married 39 years. She gave me 35 good years—now it's my turn."

It is apparent that the family cares about Ms. Martin and wants her to be with them. However, this stay in the hospital for assessment and evaluation is transitional, prior to placement to a long-term care facility because of the gravity of her symptoms. The goals for her hospital stay are to evaluate her physical health and functional status, as well as to begin nursing care planning for the future based on her strengths as well as her deficits. Mr. Martin and their daughter will be included in planning her care and in helping the staff know Ms. Martin as the person she was before her SDAT.

Ms. Martin will be assigned a primary nurse for her stay in the unit. The primary objective for nursing care during this hospitalization is to maintain her mental and physical functional status in the unit, to provide a low-stress environment that does not evoke undue anxiety, and to prepare her, to the extent possible, for the move to the long-term care facility. Her husband and daughter will be encouraged to visit for short periods several times each day to help them, as well as Ms. Martin, with the transition from roles as direct care-givers to more indirect, consultative, advocacy roles in her future care.

tional abilities have been developed for use with elderly clients. These tools can be easily administered and scored, and provide good baseline data with which to assess health status as well as to monitor changes resulting from nursing intervention. These instruments, described in a following section, are recommended as a useful adjunct to the nursing history and assessment process.

Interviewing the Older Adult

Nurses may have to adapt their usual interviewing techniques when completing psychosocial assessments of older clients. Several factors may influence the accuracy and completeness of information collected from elderly individuals. These include: (1) the attitudes toward and beliefs of nurses about elderly people, (2) the setting in which the assessment is conducted, (3) the trust and rapport established with the clients, (4) consideration of the special needs of adults with sensory or cognitive impairments, and (5) the pace and timing of the interview itself.

Nurses' stereotypes about older people can often bias data collection and data interpretation. Often, we are unaware that our personal views influence the communication process. Younger nurses may feel that, because of the large age discrepancy, older people will be uncom-

fortable in answering certain questions. When nurses receive responses such as, "You're too young to understand" or "It's none of your business," they may become more cautious in the questions they ask. In general, most older adults are interested in relating to others and will talk about their problems and feelings, particularly if they sense that the interviewer is genuinely interested in them. Sometimes, assumptions about older individuals interfere with obtaining data. We may not ask certain questions because we assume that the person cannot answer. For example, a nurse may fail to ask a question on the sexual history if the older adult is a widow or widower. A common mistake of interviewers is to interview the client and family together, believing that the family member will provide more accurate information. The older adult, even if confused, should always be interviewed alone. A later interview can be conducted with the family.

Providing comfortable and conducive settings in which to interview clients is important for all age groups, but is particularly important for elderly individuals, who often have sensory impairments. If at all possible, the interview should be conducted in a quiet, private area and not in the middle of the hall or in an activity or recreational area of a health care setting. Because of hearing

TABLE 26-3.
PSYCHOSOCIAL ASSESSMENT OF THE OLDER ADULT

DEMOGRAPHIC INFORMATION

(What are the person's strengths and problems at the time of assessment?)
Description of presenting problem
Current health status
Current medications and treatments
Functional abilities
Description of current social system
Psychological/cognitive functioning
Economic status
Environmental assessment

PAST HISTORY

(What has preceded the current status?)
Physical health/medical history
Medication/drug-use history
Cognitive abilities
Developmental history
Usual coping styles
Social history (education, occupation, people resources, belief system)
Family history
Functional abilities across time
Past environmental factors (housing, transportation)

PHYSICAL EXAMINATION

and vision deficits, modification of the environment may be necessary. An individual's lack of response to a question may reflect, not an unwillingness to answer, but that the question was not heard clearly. To overcome hearing deficits, the interviewer should sit close to, and directly in front of, the client. Talk slowly, using a low-pitched voice. Raising the voice or shouting, which involves higher-pitched tones, actually interferes with hearing. A well-lighted room may help to compensate for vision deficits.

The timing of the interview can influence the accuracy of the data collected. Mental alertness is often best earlier in the day for older adults. Therefore, the morning is the most appropriate time to schedule an interview and to test mental status.

The flow of the interview may need to be adjusted for an older adult. Reminiscence is common in the elderly, and one question may lead to a chain of thoughts, making it difficult to keep the client on the topic. Although the process of life review can yield valuable data in the psychosocial assessment, it is often helpful to set a time limit at the beginning of the interview. This helps to orient the client to the purpose of the interview. The time limit should be shorter than for younger age groups, and may depend on the level of cognitive impairment. The length of the interview should avoid exceeding the client's attention span and tolerance, or errors in communication may occur. Usually, healthy aging clients tend to show fatigue after 45 to 60 minutes. Clients with cognitive impairments may not attend to the interviewer for longer than 5 to 10 minutes. Therefore, it may be necessary for

the nurse to see the client several times until sufficient information is obtained. The interviewer needs to allow sufficient time for elderly clients to respond to questions. Often response time is greatly lengthened. If the nurse rushes a client through an interview, valuable information may be lost.

Establishing trust and rapport with the older adult is essential before an adequate assessment can be completed. It may be necessary to spend several short sessions of 5 to 15 minutes in social discussion about the client's family, friends, or hobbies in order to establish the necessary rapport. Once rapport is gained, questions assessing the client's impairments should be spaced throughout the interview. These should only be raised after the individual has relaxed. This is of particular importance for the mental status examination, which can only be done accurately if there is good rapport between the interviewer and the client.

Standardized Assessment Instruments

Mental Status. A variety of tests have been developed to evaluate cognitive function in the elderly. The instruments most widely used in geriatric research and practice to assess mental status are short-item, standardized questionnaires: the Mental Status Questionnaire (MSQ),[36] the Mini-Mental State Examination,[25] and the Short Portable Mental Status Questionnaire (SPMSQ).[60] Each instrument is designed to screen for cognitive impairment and changes in cognitive function, and is not intended to diagnose specific organic disease. All have high reliability, and good validity when compared with other indicators of cognitive impairment.

The MSQ provides a good example of the types of items included on mental status questionnaires. It consists of ten questions:

1. Where are you now?
2. What is this place?
3. What day is this?
4. What month is this?
5. What year is this?
6. How old are you?
7. When is your birthday?
8. In what year (or where) were you born?
9. Who is the president of the United States?
10. Who was the president before him?

Individuals who score 0 to 2 errors on this test are presumed to have no, or mild, cognitive impairment; 3 to 8 errors indicate moderate impairment; and 9 to 10 errors indicate severe impairment. If a person scores in the range of moderate to severe cognitive impairment, additional testing by a psychiatrist or psychologist should be done.

In addition to the mental status questionnaires, several other instruments are useful in the assessment of cognitive impairment due to depression or other psychological disorder. They include the Set Test,[32] the Face–Hand Test,[36] and the FROMAJE.[45]

The *Set Test* is a simple, quantitative verbal test that can easily be used by nurses to screen for mental status changes in older adults. The client is asked to name as many items as he or she can recall in each of four categories or sets: fruits, animals, colors, and towns. No time limit is given. One point is awarded for each correct item. No points are given or deducted if items are repeated. The total maximum score is 40. Isaacs and Kennie[33] found that clients with total scores under 15 had a clinical diagnosis of dementia; scores between 15 and 24 were questionable, and clients with scores of 25 or higher were not demented.

The *Face–Hand Test* is a useful examination to distinguish clients with brain damage from those who are psychotic without an organic cause. The test requires that the individual recognize tactile stimulation on the cheek and palm of the hand. The individual is touched simultaneously on one cheek and the dorsum of one hand, in a specified order. The test is administered twice, once with the person's eyes closed and then repeated with eyes open. The attention span must be sufficient to follow instructions. Persons with hallucinations who might perform poorly on the MSQ tests generally will not make errors on tactile stimulation.

The FROMAJE is a brief and easily-administered instrument designed to evaluate mental, emotional, and physical functioning. FROMAJE is the acronym for the areas that are assessed: functional status, reasoning, orientation, memory, arithmetic, judgment, and emotional state. It is helpful as an initial screen for distinguishing depression from dementia.

Caution must be exercised in interpreting the results of any of the mental status tests. One abnormal mental status test is not indicative of dementia. The results obtained on this test can be affected significantly by the individual's anxiety, fear, or fatigue, as well as by how the test is administered and the time of day it is administered.

Affective Status. Assessment of mood is essential in the evaluation of psychological functioning, and is especially important with older adults because of the high prevalence of depression. Several instruments are recommended to assess for the presence of depression: the Geriatric Depression Scale,[72] the Center for Epidemiological Studies-Depression (CES-D) Scale,[62] and the Zung Self-Rating Depression Scale.[74] Each is a brief questionnaire that can be self-administered or used in an interview format. All have high reliability, and good validity when compared with other indicators of depression.

In contrast to the other scales that were developed to assess depression in the general population, the Geriatric Depression Scale was designed specifically to assess affect in older adults. One advantage of this scale is the response format, which asks for a yes or no answer. The other scales incorporate a four-item response format that is difficult for older adults with alterations in cognitive function to use.

Functional Status. Psychosocial assessment of the older adult should include an evaluation of functional abilities. Alterations in affective and cognitive functioning in later life are closely related to impairments in physical function. Two categories of functional abilities have been used to assess the needs of the elderly population. *Activities of daily living (ADL)* refers to self-care functions such as bathing, dressing, eating, walking, and toileting. *Instrumental activities of daily living (IADL)* refers to functions other than self-care activities that are required for living independently, such as grocery-shopping, meal preparation, laundry, housework, managing money, using the telephone, taking medications, and arranging transportation.

The Katz Index of ADL Functioning,[37] Barthel Index,[48] and Physical Self-Maintenance Scale[44] can be used to assess ADL function. All are short instruments, easy to score, and useful to measure changes in function over time. The Scale for Instrumental Activities of Daily Living[44] was designed to measure IADL function in community-dwelling elderly persons. In contrast to these scales, which rely on self-reports of the client, reports of other care-givers, or the rater's impression of the client's ability to perform items, the Performance Test of Activities of Daily Living[41] is based on actual observed behavior on specific tasks, and includes both ADL and IADL items. It was designed for use with psychogeriatric patients.

Carefully gathered, integrated, and analyzed data about older adults' presenting problems and past histories are critical in identifying problems, determining nursing diagnoses, and planning appropriate interventions. Assessment is a dynamic process, and assessment data are gathered throughout the entire nursing process. As new data are identified, modifications are made in diagnoses and in interventions. In the following section, selected nursing diagnoses typically made with older adults are identified.

Diagnosis

Nursing diagnoses are the basis for specific interventions by nurses. Unlike medical diagnoses, which describe pathology and diseases, nursing diagnoses describe an individual's response to a health state or altered interaction pattern. This orientation follows from the 1980 *ANA Social Policy Statement,*[3] which defines nursing as the diagnosis and treatment of human response to actual or potential health problems. Numerous diagnostic categories, agreed upon by the North American Nursing Diagnosis Association (NANDA),[39] are applicable to the nursing care of older persons with psychosocial alterations. The list is extensive because of the wide range of potential symptomatology in older adults. Among the present diagnoses used with older adults are:

Bowel elimination, altered incontinence
Communication, impaired verbal
Coping, ineffective individual
Coping, ineffective family: compromised
Coping, ineffective family: disabled
Family process, altered

Grieving, dysfunctional
Hopelessness
Injury: potential for
Powerlessness
Role performance, altered
Self-care deficit: feeding, bathing/hygiene, dressing/
grooming, toileting
Self-concept, disturbance in: body image, self-esteem,
personal identity
Sleep pattern disturbance
Social interaction, impaired
Social isolation
Thought processes, altered
Urinary elimination, altered patterns
Violence, potential for: self-directed or directed at others

It is important that nursing diagnoses be explicit and meaningful.[11] Broad labels are not useful because they are not concrete and descriptive enough to use in identifying etiology and prescribing the intervention needed. To give greater specificity to the nursing diagnosis: altered thought process, Berry[11] suggests using more concrete diagnoses: potential for violence to others related to suspiciousness; fluid-volume deficit related to suspiciousness of oral fluids; or impaired social interaction related to auditory hallucinations and suspiciousness. With these examples of specification, the interventions are evident and can be accomplished by nursing to affect problems in the daily life of the person. Powerlessness is another diagnosis that can be further specified to use with older patients experiencing significant losses: powerlessness, related to progressive loss of function or progressive loss of memory.

Intervention

Levels of Prevention

Nursing interventions with older adults and their families occur within the primary, secondary, and tertiary levels of prevention. The following box describes interventions commonly used with elderly clients at each level of prevention.

The levels of prevention describe the points of intervention used to prevent development of crises or maladaptive behaviors. The objective in *primary* prevention is the elimination of factors that may lead to the development of disease. In primary prevention and intervention, the nurse anticipates further problems that may become maladaptive. For example, because of the demographic realities of married women outliving their husbands, a program of study focusing on grief work for all losses would help women anticipate what they will experience as widows and would potentially offset a prolonged or dysfunctional grief reaction. *Secondary* prevention is the early detection and treatment of disease. The use of medications in the treatment of the affective disorders in older adults is an example of secondary prevention. The

---

LEVELS OF PREVENTION USED WITH ELDERLY CLIENTS

PRIMARY

Anticipatory socialization for late life—retirement planning, grief counseling
Reminiscence groups
Life review groups
Respite care
Seniors groups
Family support groups

SECONDARY

Individual therapy/counseling
Group therapy/counseling
Family therapy/counseling
Electroconvulsive therapy
Medications

TERTIARY

Sensory stimulation
Reality orientation
Pet therapy
Activity therapy
Milieu therapy
Day treatment programs

---

objective is to intervene to prevent further disability. *Tertiary* prevention is the elimination or reduction of residual disabilities following a disease process. Day treatment programs help people with SDAT to remain in a community setting reflective of patterns of their work lives, and help to retain functional abilities by providing necessary structure for their days and weeks. For their care-givers, day care for SDAT clients provides primary prevention, that is, prevention of burnout from the caregiving burden. The objectives of tertiary prevention are to help the person maintain functional activities at the highest possible level and to reduce further disability.

In the above list of common interventions some, such as sensory stimulation, pet therapy, and activity therapy, might also be classified as primary prevention for use by older clients prior to the onset of a disability. Individuals involved with activities or a pet may find life engaging and satisfying and thereby maintain mental and physical well-being. Reminiscence groups and life review groups may be used at the secondary level of prevention, too.

Common Interventions

Activity therapy takes various forms, depending on the target group of clients. Activity therapy is a generic label for specialized programs for groups of clients in both inpatient and day treatment environments. Usual group activities include music, art, dance/movement, dramatics, horticulture, creative writing, poetry, oral history/reminiscence, and sports and games. Objectives include both interaction among group members and stimulation of personal interests, involvement, and creativity in individuals in the group.

Pet therapy, one type of activity therapy, is a generic label for a variety of activities involving the use of animals. With the previously-described losses in late life, pets may be used to fill the role of a substitutional object. Pets may have permanent residence in some settings; in other settings they may be brought in on a regular schedule, usually weekly. Pet therapy may be particularly useful with people who are withdrawn. Pets may facilitate communication between clients and staff and among clients.

Sensory stimulation or *sensory training*[69] is another type of activity therapy. It is used most often with individuals who are regressed and withdrawn. The objective is to facilitate individual–environment interaction, in order to provide experiences that stimulate the five senses. The groups typically consist of five to seven clients who are at approximately the same functional levels. The leader's creativity in challenging the group's interest and enthusiasm is the key variable. The technique of sensory training includes use of a four-phase model: orientation, body awareness exercises, stimulation of the senses, and conclusion.[69] Reinforcement in the environment is important for stimulation/training.

Evaluation

Like assessment, evaluation is a part of the nursing process that takes place throughout the process. As nursing care plans are implemented, it is important to provide opportunities for the interventions to be evaluated objectively and subjectively. Objectively, nurses look for affective, behavioral, and cognitive changes in the older adult as a result of the planned interventions. Nursing staff and multidisciplinary staff meet regularly to assess clients' progress. Subjectively, clients and family members may report changes as they are experienced and observed. In a systems approach, evaluation data are part of the feedback loop that leads to reassessment, diagnosing, planning, and intervening. In open systems, feedback data on the outcomes of the nursing process take into account data from all subsystems of the older adult clients and enable use of the data in reformulating diagnoses and interventions.

Application of the Nursing Process: Elder Abuse

The *nursing assessment* of the dysfunctional family system includes a variety of factors. Within the family, nurses should try to identify strengths, family roles, family ties,
the family's sense of role responsibilities, family supports, and financial resources. In assessing the family's weaknesses, nurses should investigate role conflict, role expectations, and communication patterns. For the care-giver, nurses should assess care-giving skills, usual problem-solving skills, and lifestyle, as well as family and personality characteristics. Signs of neglect and abuse are sought in the appearance and behavioral indicators of the elderly individual. History-taking will reveal injuries and repeated encounters with health care providers. Neglect may be evident in the individual's appearance. Wariness, defensiveness, withdrawal, and aggression need to be noted.

The two most probable *nursing diagnoses* that follow from the nursing assessment are:

Coping, ineffective family: compromised
Coping, ineffective family: disabled

Planning and *intervention* have four points of contact: the elderly abused person, the care-giver, the family system, and the community. For the abused individual, the short-term goal is to attend to physical and psychological deficits, with attention given to the safety of the person. The nurse's therapeutic use of self in this instance includes establishing a trusting relationship with the abuse victim and the care-giver; it is important to be aware of judgmental attitudes and personal feelings in this situation. It is also important to enlist the abused person and the care-giver, as well as the family, in a partnership to correct the system's problems.

Nurses can intervene at each level of prevention in elder abuse. The *primary* prevention-level objective is to prevent abuse by reducing the risk that elderly individuals will be abused. Primary prevention can be accomplished by acknowledging the potential for care-giver strain and by providing services to teach, support, and relieve care-givers at the community level. Care-givers can be taught how to mobilize and use their social networks (family, church, neighbors, community), how to ask for help, and how to use help that is offered. They can join with other care-givers in organized care-giver support networks, and they can seek and use relief from care-giving through use of formally- or informally-arranged respite care.

Secondary prevention can be accomplished by early case-finding and identification of the instance of elder abuse. Care-giver strain and elder abuse may both be identified by family and community members, community health nurses, and health care professionals. Investigation and interventions at the point of identification are critical.

Tertiary prevention may involve separation of the elder from the abuser through temporary or permanent change of living arrangements, or through introduction of different or additional care-givers. Interventions require multidisciplinary planning that addresses the needs of the total family system, including homemaker and home health services, adult day care, home-delivered meals, transportation, respite care, and counseling services.

The long-term goals are to support family strengths and to engage in problem-solving activities to correct the deficits in relationships and in the family environment. Counseling may be individual- or family-oriented. It is directed toward increasing self-esteem and increasing feelings of mastery and competence in the care-giver–care receiver dyad. Teaching and practicing concrete problem-solving may help to increase the repertoire of possible solutions. The relationship with the nurse is important to both client and care-giver as a symbolic statement of concern, hope, and understanding. The nurse may role model interventions that may expand the care-giver's skills.

The family system may profit from family counseling to explore existing and potential role allocations and role assumptions and to establish norms for greater openness in communication and for further sharing in provision of care. Societal interventions include increasing awareness for case-finding, and teaching to expand knowledge of elderly people in general and of those at risk for abuse in particular.

Evaluation of nursing interventions in elder abuse begins with the implementation phase of the nursing process. Each intervention is monitored to ensure that it supports the immediate goal of cessation of the abuse and the long-term goal of improving family relationships. Frequently, new interventions may be used to alleviate family stress and improve coping skills.

The Therapeutic Use of Self in Providing Psychosocial Nursing Care for Older Adults

Nurses employ the therapeutic use of self to provide care and to facilitate the learning by clients of more positive and effective behaviors. This includes the application of theoretical knowledge in the process of nursing. The nursing process is educational and therapeutic when the client and the nurse can come to know and respect each other as people who are alike, and yet different, and as people who share in solving problems.[59]

In optimal interactions with older adults, nurses are aware of theories of aging. They must also be aware of how their reactions to older people are influenced by personally-held myths and stereotypes about older people and the aging process. Nurses are aware that older adults' life experiences exceed their own in both numbers and kinds. Care-givers and care recipients are members of different generations and are influenced by different social worlds. Each belongs to a different, dynamic, heterogeneous group. From this perspective, they influence, and are influenced, by one another.

Openness, acceptance, trust, honesty, and respect characterize the role behaviors of participants in therapeutic interactions. The objective of the relationship is to maximize health through primary, secondary, and tertiary prevention. The primary ways in which nurses relate to older adults are through advocacy, assessing, and intervening. In each instance, the nurse empathetically takes the role of the client, to work in tandem with the older adult toward a higher level of health and satisfaction.

Roles and Functions of Nurses Providing Psychosocial Nursing Care for Older Adults

The subspecialty of geropsychiatric or psychogeriatric nursing is relatively new in nursing, although nurses have provided psychosocial nursing care to older adults throughout the history of nursing. Psychosocial nursing care for the aged may be provided by baccalaureate-prepared nurses who are generalists or by masters-prepared nurses who are clinical specialists.

Nurse generalists may function as primary nurses, as nursing team leaders, and as members of multi- or interdisciplinary teams. They function from the broad knowledge bases of nursing, psychiatric mental health nursing, and gerontological nursing. Theoretical knowledge from the physical and behavioral sciences, including the biology, psychology, and sociology of aging, contributes directly to their practice. They may practice in homes, general hospitals, psychiatric hospitals, clinics, and units, nursing homes, and adult day care centers.

Specialist practice in psychosocial nursing care for older adults may be grounded either in advanced gerontological nursing or in advanced psychiatric mental health nursing. Preparation in geropsychiatric nursing is available in a number of schools at both master's and doctoral levels.

Nursing practice for both generalists and specialists is based on theory and on the ANA Standards of Practice in gerontological nursing[4] and in psychiatric mental health nursing.[5] Both sets of standards provide the structure for achieving excellence of care. The organizing framework of the standards is the nursing process, including assessment of the older adult, identification of nursing diagnoses, planning and implementation of care, and evaluation of the individual's response to the care.

The ANA Standards of Gerontological Nursing[4] address the systematic collection and communication of data about the health status of older adults, deriving nursing diagnoses from knowledge of normal responses to aging and the collected data, and initiating plans of care with older adults and/or their significant others from the goals following the nursing diagnosis. Further, the plans of care include establishing priorities and nursing interventions to meet the goals. Plans are implemented using appropriate nursing actions. The older adult, together with the nurse, determines the progress attained in goal achievement as well as the continuation of nursing care. The standards reflect the nursing profession's concern for providing responsible, high quality services to the public, and for involving older adults to the fullest extent possible in decision-making and implementing care.

Both gerontological nurse generalists and specialists apply the Standards in providing care to older adults. The nurse specialist has additional diagnostic and management skills, and functions at an advanced level in meeting the needs of older adults.

The ANA Standards of Psychiatric and Mental Health Nursing Practice[5] also address the systematic collection and communication of data about the health status of individuals, the derivation of nursing diagnoses, the initiation of plans of care, and the evaluation of goal achievement. In the psychiatric nursing standards, interventions are identified in terms of psychotherapeutic interventions, health teaching, activities of daily living, somatic therapies, and therapeutic environment. Both nurse generalists and specialists intervene in these areas. Specialists, using advanced knowledge and skills, function as individual, group, and family therapists with older clients. They also participate in community health systems that affect services for primary, secondary, and tertiary prevention of mental illness. Participation in research is another important standard of practice implemented by nurse specialists.

Geropsychiatric nursing, as a subspecialty of both gerontological and psychiatric nursing, includes implementation of specialized nursing knowledge and skills with older adults. Meeting the psychosocial needs and problems of older adults is within the domain of both clinical specialities.

The need for nurses to provide psychosocial care for older adults is evident by the demographic trends outlined earlier in this chapter. The population of older adults is projected to continue to grow steadily well into the 21st century. The mental health needs of the growing population fall within the identified subsystem domains: biological, psychological, sociological, cultural, and environmental. These needs vary with the heterogeneity of the older adult population. While a portion of the population maintains a high level of functional abilities and good physical and mental health, another portion experiences substantial physical and emotional losses and, subsequently, develops psychiatric impairments requiring intervention. Issues of depression, dementia, suicidal behavior, and abuse require knowledgeable intervention.

Opportunities for nurses in geropsychiatric nursing are limitless. The rewards and challenges of providing psychosocial nursing care to individuals in institutions and in the community continue to grow, as does knowledge development in the therapeutic use of self in the delivery of humanistic nursing care.

Summary

1. The growth in the number and proportion of people over the age of 65 years is dramatic. The elderly population is at risk for mental health problems because of the losses that come with aging in combination with decreased coping resources and physical health status.

2. There is no single definition of or set of criteria for mental health in older adults. In general, mental health is chacterized by the capacity to interact with others and negotiate the environment in ways that are enriching to self and others.

3. The health of older adults is viewed from a systems perspective that takes into account complex interactions among biological, psychological, sociological, cultural, and environmental subsystems.

4. Common stressors associated with aging are loss, change, and health alterations. The common denominator for all stressors is loss. Losses are to the self. They may be losses of people, of physical functioning, of roles, or of other resources. In every case, losses must be grieved over if a person is to restore meaning to life and go on. When losses are unresolved, individuals may experience major psychosocial alterations.

5. Major psychosocial alterations include depression and dementia. The difference between pseudodementia (depression) and dementia were identified. Suicide and elder abuse were described as two areas of special concern with older adults.

6. The nursing process enables the nurse to assess, diagnose, plan, implement, and evaluate psychosocial care for older adults. Consideration of the biological, psychological, sociological, cultural, and environmental subsystems is critical throughout the nursing process.

7. Assessment is a key component in the nursing process. Assessment is particularly critical with older adults. It is important to identify normal or baseline behavior and functional abilities, to gather pertinent information on the presenting problem and symptoms, and to determine relevant past history. Standardized assessment instruments are useful in determining mental status, affective status, and functional status.

8. Accurate nursing diagnoses can be determined only after carefully gathering, integrating, and analyzing assessment data. Diagnoses are the bases for specific nursing interventions. The more explicit and meaningful the diagnoses are, the clearer the prescribed interventions can be.

9. Nursing interventions are developed at primary, secondary, and tertiary levels of prevention. At each level, the objectives are to maintain the highest possible levels of mental health and functional abilities, to prevent further disability, and to reduce residual disabilities.

10. Evaluation is a necessary component of the nursing process. By completing the feedback loop, behavioral, affective, and functional changes are measured and reassessment begins.

11. Elder abuse is a psychosocial problem in which interventions are planned at each level of prevention and take into account the older adult's total system.

12. The subspecialty of geropsychiatric nursing is relatively new. Specialist practice in psychosocial care for older adults may be grounded in advanced gerontological nursing or in advanced psychiatric mental health nursing. Psychosocial practice with older adults is based on ANA Standards of Practice and is structured by the nursing process.

References

1. Alzheimer's Disease Report of the Secretary's Task Force on Alzheimer's Disease (DHHS Publication No. [ADM] 84-1323). Washington, DC, U.S. Government Printing Office, 1984

2. American Association of Retired Persons and Administration on Aging, U.S. Department of Health and Human Services: A Profile of Older Americans. Washington, DC, American Association of Retired Persons, 1987

3. American Nurses' Association: Nursing: A Social Policy Statement. Kansas City, Missouri, American Nurses' Association, 1980

4. American Nurses' Association: Standards of Gerontological Nursing Practice. Kansas City, Missouri, American Nurses' Association, 1988

5. American Nurses' Association: Standards of Psychiatric and Mental Health Nursing Practice. Kansas City, Missouri, American Nurses' Association, 1982

6. American Psychiatric Association: Diagnostic and Statistical Manual of Mental Disorders, 3rd ed, revised (DSM-III-R). Washington, DC, American Psychiatric Association, 1987

7. Atchley RC: The Social Forces in Later Life. Belmont, California, Wadsworth, 1977

8. Barrell LM: Crisis intervention—partnership in problem-solving. Nurs Clin North Am 9:5, 1974

9. Barrell LM: From wife to widow: The transitional process. Diss Abstr Int 41(10):4509-A, 1981

10. Beckman LJ: Effects of social interaction and children's relative inputs on older women's psychological well-being. J Per Soc Psychol 41:1075, 1981

11. Berry KN: Let's create diagnoses psych nurses can use. Am J Nurs 87:707, 1987

12. Blazer D: The Epidemiology of Mental Illness in Later Life. In Busse E, Blazer D (eds): Handbook of Geriatric Psychiatry. New York, Van Nostrand-Reinhold, 1980

13. Bloch M: Symposium on abuse of the elderly. JAMA 243:1221, 1980

14. Block MR, Sinnott JD: The Battered Elder Syndrome: An Exploratory Study. College Park, Maryland, Center on Aging of the University of Maryland, 1979

15. Brody JA, Brock DB: Epidemiologic and Statistical Characteristics of the United States Elderly Population. In Finch CE, Schneider EL (eds): Handbook of the Biology of Aging, 2nd ed. New York, Van Nostrand-Reinhold, 1985

16. Butler R: Age-ism: Another form of bigotry. Gerontologist 9:243, 1969

17. Butler RN, Lewis MI: Aging and Mental Health—Positive Psychosocial and Biomedical Approaches, 3rd ed. St Louis, CV Mosby, 1982

18. Cassem NH: Bereavement as Indispensable for Growth. In Schoenberg B, Gerber I, Wiener A et al (eds): Bereavement: Its Psychosocial Aspects. New York, Columbia University Press, 1975

19. Chenoweth B, Spencer B: Dementia: The experience of family care-givers. Gerontologist 26:267, 1986

20. Cohen D, Dunner D: The Assessment of Cognitive Dysfunction in Dementing Illness. In Cole JO, Barrett JE (eds): Psychopathology in the Aged. New York, Raven Press, 1980

21. Cumming E, Henry WE: Growing Old. New York, Basic Books, 1961

22. Dowd JJ: Aging as exchange: A preface to theory. J Gerontol 30:584, 1975

23. Ebersole P, Hess P: Toward Healthy Aging: Human Needs and Nursing Response, 2nd ed. St Louis, CV Mosby, 1985

24. Erikson EH: Childhood and Society, 2nd ed. New York, WW Norton, 1963

25. Folstein MF, Folstein SE, McHugh PR: Mini-mental state—a practical method for grading the cognitive state of patients for the clinician. J Psychiatr Res 12:189, 1975

26. Gurland BJ, Cross PS: Epidemiology of psychopathology in old age: Some implications for clinical services. Psychiatr Clin North Am 5:11, 1982

27. Hall GR, Buckwalter KC: Progressively lowered stress threshold: A conceptual model for care of adults with Alzheimer's disease. Arch Psychiatr Nurs 1:404, 1987

28. Harris L: The Myth and Reality of Aging in America. Washington, DC, National Council on the Aging, 1975

29. Havighurst RJ: Developmental Tasks and Education. New York, David McKay, 1972

30. Havighurst RJ, Albrecht R: Older People. New York, Longmans, Green & Co, 1953

31. Hess B: Friendship. In Riley M et al (eds): Aging and Society. New York, Russell Sage Foundation, 1972

32. Isaacs B, Akhtar AJ: The set test: A rapid test of mental function in old people. Age Ageing 1:222, 1972

33. Isaacs B, Kennie AT: The set test as an aid to the detection of dementia in old people. Br J Psychiatry 123:467, 1973

34. Jahoda M: Current Concepts of Positive Mental Health. New York, Basic Books, 1958

35. Johnson DG: Abuse and neglect: Not for children only. J Gerontol Nurs 5:11, 1979

36. Kahn RL, Goldfarb AI, Pollack M et al: Brief objective measures for determination of mental status in the aged. Am J Psychiatry 117:326, 1960

37. Katz S, Ford AB, Moskowitz RW et al: Studies of illness in the aged. The index of ADL: A standardized measure of biological and psychosocial function. JAMA 185:94, 1963

38. Kermis MD: Mental Health in Later Life—The Adaptive Process. Boston, Jones & Bartlett, 1986

39. Kim MJ, McFarland GK, McLane AM: Pocket Guide to Nursing Diagnoses. St Louis, CV Mosby, 1987

40. Klerman GL: The Treatment of Depression. In Perspectives on Depressive Disorders: A Review of Recent Research. U.S. Department of Health and Human Services, PHS, ADAMHA. Rockville, Maryland, National Institute of Mental Health, 1987

41. Kuriansky T, Gurland B: The performance test of activities of daily living. Int J Aging Hum Dev 7:343, 1976

42. Lasoski MC: Reasons for Low Utilization of Mental Health Services by the Elderly. In Brink TL (ed): Clinical Geronotology: A Guide to Assessment and Intervention. New York, Haworth Press, 1986

43. Lau E, Kosberg J: Abuse of the aged by informal care providers. Aging 10:299–300, 1979

44. Lawton MP: The functional assessment of elderly people. J Am Geriatr Soc 19:465, 1971

45. Libow LS: A Rapidly Administered, Easily Remembered Mental Status Examination: FROMAJE. In Libow LS, Shuman FT (eds): The Core of Geriatric Medicine: A Guide for Students and Practitioners. St Louis, CV Mosby, 1981

46. Lindemann E: Symptomatology and Management of Acute Grief. In Parad HJ (ed): Crisis Intervention: Selected Readings. New York, Family Service Association of America, 1965

47. Lowenthal M: Interpersonal Relations. In Loether H (ed): Problems of Aging. Belmont, California, Dickenson, 1967

48. Mahoney FI, Barthel DW: Functional evaluation: The Barthel index. Md Med J 14:61, 1965

49. Marris P: Loss and Change. New York, Pantheon Books, 1974

50. Miller M: Suicide After Sixty: The Final Alternative. New York, Springer Publishing, 1979

51. Morris J: Changes in morale experienced by elderly institutional applicants along the institutional path. Gerontologist 15: 345, 1975

52. Myers JK, Weismann MM, Tischler GL et al: Six-month prevalence of psychiatric disorders in three communities, 1980–1982. Arch Gen Psychiatry 41:959, 1984

53. National Center for Health Statistics: Aging in the Eighties: Functional Limitations of Individuals Age 65 Years and Over. Advance Data from Vital Health Statistics, No 133. DHHS No. (PHS) 87-1250. Hyattsville, Maryland, U.S. Government Printing Office, 1987a

54. National Center for Health Statistics: Current Estimates From the National Health Interview Survey. DHHS No. 86-1588. Hyattsville, Maryland, U.S. Government Printing Office, 1986

55. National Center for Health Statistics: Health Statistics on Older Persons—United States, 1986 (Series 3, Analytical and Epidemiological Study, No. 25). DHHS No. (PHS) 87-1409. Hyattsville, Maryland, U.S. Government Printing Office, 1987b

56. Neugarten BL, Havinghurst RJ, Tobin SS: Personality and Patterns of Aging. In Neugarten BL (ed): Middle Age and Aging. Chicago, University of Chicago Press, 1968

57. Osgood NJ: Suicide in the Elderly. Rockville, Maryland, Aspen Systems, 1985

58. Peck RC: Psychological Developments in the Second Half of Life. In Neugarten BL (ed): Middle Age and Aging. Chicago, University of Chicago Press, 1968

59. Peplau HE: Interpersonal Relations in Nursing. New York, GP Putnam, 1952

60. Pfeiffer E: A short portable mental status questionnaire for the assessment of organic brain deficit in elderly patients. J Am Geriatr Soc 23:433, 1975

61. Rabin DL, Stockton P: Long-Term Care for the Elderly: A Factbook. New York, Oxford University Press, 1987

62. Radloff L: CES-D scale: A self-report depression scale for research in the general population. Appl Psychol Measurement 1:385, 1977

63. Redick R, Taube C: Demography and mental health care of the aged. In Birren JE, Sloane RB (eds): Handbook of Mental Health and Aging. Englewood Cliffs, New Jersey, Prentice-Hall, 1980

64. Romaniuk M, McAuley W, Arling G: An examination of the prevalence of mental disorders among the elderly in the community. J Abnorm Psychol 92:458, 1983

65. Rosswurm MA: Relocation and the elderly. J Gerontol Nurs 9: 632, 1983

66. Schultz R, Brenner G: Relocation of the aged: A review and theoretical analysis. J Gerontology 32:323, 1977

67. Tilden VP, Weinert C: Social support and the chronically ill individual. Nurs Clin North Am 22:613, 1987

68. Weeks JR, Cuellar JP: The role of family members in helping networks of older people. Gerontologist 21:388, 1981

69. Weiner MB, Brok AJ, Snadowsky AM: Working with the Aged, 2nd ed. Norwalk, Connecticut, Appleton-Century-Crofts, 1987

70. Wells CE, Duncan GW: Neurology for Psychiatrists. Philadelphia, FA Davis, 1980

71. Whanger AD, Myers AC: Mental Health Assessment and Therapeutic Intervention With Older Adults. Rockville, Maryland, Aspen Systems, 1984

72. Yesavage J, Brink TL: Development and validation of a geriatric depression screening scale: A preliminary report. J Psychiatr Res 17:37, 1983

73. Zarit SH, Orr NK, Zarit JM: The Hidden Victims of Alzheimer's Disease: Families Under Stress. New York, New York University Press, 1985

74. Zung W: A self-rating depression scale. Arch Gen Psychiatry 12: 63, 1965

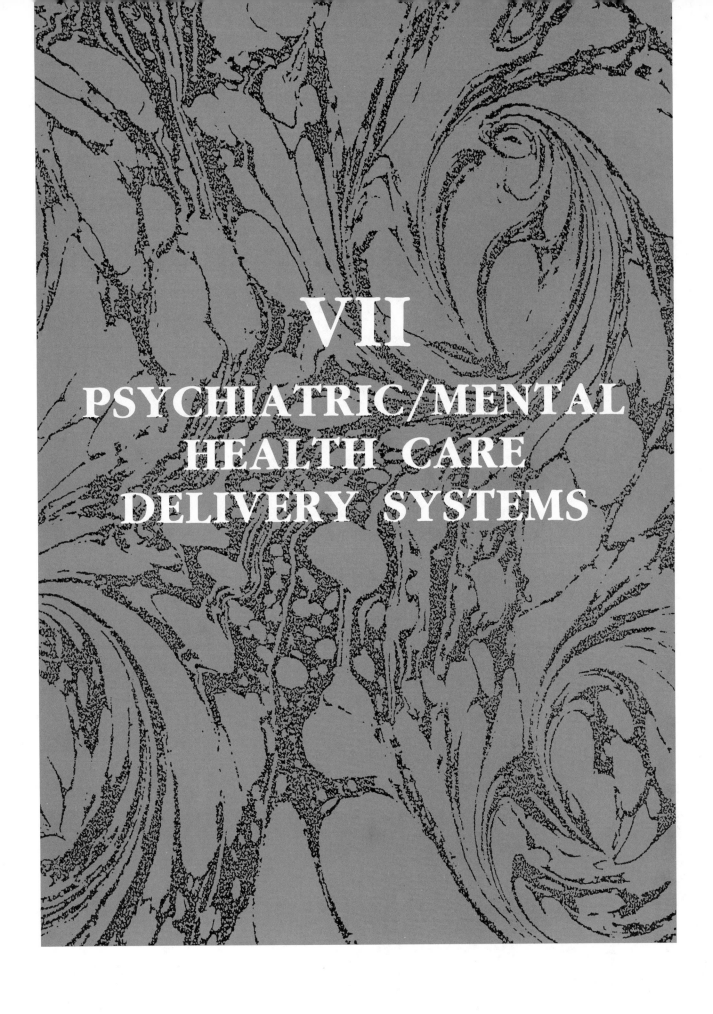

VII
PSYCHIATRIC/MENTAL HEALTH CARE DELIVERY SYSTEMS

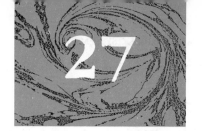

MARYANN H. OGONOWSKI

NURSING ADMINISTRATION IN A PSYCHIATRIC SETTING

Learning Objectives

Upon completion of this chapter the student should be able to do the following:

1. Describe the systems nature of nursing service in terms of supra- and subsystems components.
2. List four adjustments that nursing administrators have to make according to whether clients are in or out of control of their behavior.
3. Explain the parallel nature of the steps of the nursing process and those of the management process.
4. Differentiate between a problem orientation to nursing management and a developmental orientation.
5. List four functions of the nursing administrator that demonstrate an understanding of the therapeutic use of self.

The Organization as an Open System

The purpose of an organization is to complete some form of work, that is, to produce a product or deliver a service. Any health care facility, such as a hospital or a community mental health clinic, is a type of organization in which a group of people come together for the specific cause, purpose, goal, or mission of delivering health care. It is through people (employees) that the specific work of the organization gets done; the relationship between the people and the organization is very direct, interdependent, and integral, and represents an open system. Figure 27-1 illustrates some of the forces, societal and individual, that interact and influence the formation and character of an organization. Reciprocally, the organization, as a whole or as a particular experience, influences each individual. Constant interaction and influence among the people inside and outside the organization are further compounded by the fact that the focus of health care institutions is also people (clients). In mental health facili-

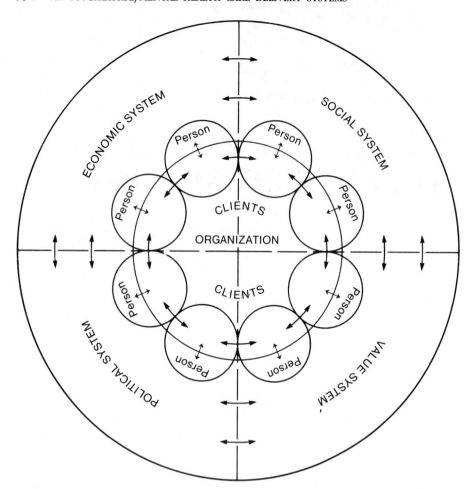

Figure 27-1. An organization is an open system and has a direct, interdependent, and integral relationship with people and society.

ties, attention is intensely focused on people, their behavior, and their relationships. Therefore, the maintenance of healthy relationships is paramount, is complex, and needs to be the focus of skilled nursing management practices.

Each organization has its own personality, goals, rules, values, and unique identity by which it is known or identified. This individualized culture reflects the totality of the overall system and is the environment in which the employees work. "Culture refers to the customs, habits, and shared beliefs which bind and bond people within an organizational framework. This interpersonal fabric is not passive, but a living, working element that permeates the aspects of the health care environment."[13] The continuous interaction among the elements of the organization and the people who work there creates a dynamic atmosphere with constant change in the work, the environment, and the people.

Internal and External Organizational Environments

An organization's external and internal environments influence and interact with each other and create a situation that is unique and dynamic. The *external environment* consists of such things as laws, economics, the politics of the community, the type of population, and the resources available. In a hospital or a community program for clients, the external environment includes such things as standards of practice, the availability of health care professionals, community or consumer groups, unions, politics, local or state laws, professional organizations, and the economic climate. The *internal environment* of the organization is created by the philosophy and mission, the internal rules and regulations, the organizational structure, the physical environment, and the individuals who constitute the organization—their philosophy, interests, and needs.

The internal and external environments interact continuously to make organizations entities that change constantly, although they have identifiable cultures and characters. External forces that affect the health care system demand continuous adjustment and readjustment to maintain a balance (or steady state) between the internal and external environments and to enable ongoing productivity and survival. The continuous need for change in a health care organization creates stress in the system and among health care workers. The nursing administrator's role, which is discussed later in this chapter, addresses this issue.

People are the major component of the internal organizational environment, and greatly influence the personality, culture, and productivity of an organization. A health care facility is people-oriented rather than product-oriented, and is subject to complex influences from clients and employees. The internal environment in a psychiatric/mental health care facility is influenced by the type of clients being cared for. Internal environments differ greatly, depending on whether the predominant population consists of clients with short-term, acute care needs or consists primarily of chronically ill, aggressive, or violent clients. The needs and behaviors of these two populations create very different physical, emotional, and social environments. The needs and behaviors of the clients influence the attitudes, skills, and type of personnel employed in the facility. Clients in a maximum security forensic unit need high levels of security services, and the environment has a predominant feeling of control and close observation. Clients in a community preparation unit have less need for a closed, secured, controlled environment; this type of unit has a more trusting, open, and developmental atmosphere. Therefore, in one organization there may be various services with different social, emotional, physical, and political characteristics brought about by the interrelationship between clients' needs and the services provided.

Each employee comes to the organization with a unique set of values, needs, skills, and expectations about the organization, its clients, the other employees, the work, and the services the institution offers. All employees bring their own education, experiences, values, and skills to the work environment, which all influence the work climate. Individuals also bring their own needs, liabilities, problems, and complexities to the work environment. The philosophy, mission, policies, attitudes, culture, and personality of the organization are formulated by the people who work in it through many complex interactions among individuals. Recognizing and respecting the human strengths and liabilities in personnel give nursing administrators an important key to developing management strategies and practices that enable people to accomplish work. The knowledge and skill of each individual and his or her place in the hierarchy of the organization determine how much influence each person can have on the culture of the organization.

Nurses' work is usually done within the organizational structure, and is subject to many influences in the organization's or agency's work environment. As employees rather than private entrepreneurs, nurses are subject to these influences and their effects on nursing practice. Because the organization is an open system, nurses and nursing administrators can influence the conditions under which nursing is practiced. As long as the system is perceived as one in which nurses can have some influence and autonomy, nurses' attitudes are more hopeful and positive. If nurses perceive that the system's administration listens and responds with respect and honest concern about issues, nurses will experience the positive force of having input into the system. Nurses in organizations in which nurses have an active role in the determination of the practice environment generally remain in their jobs longer and have greater satisfaction about their work.[10] If the system is not perceived as open, or if the system gives messages of being nonresponsive to input from employees, nurses may become apathetic, accepting of the status quo, frustrated, or rebellious.

Of the many types of organizations, hospitals are the most complex, with numerous systems, subsystems, and sub-subsystems. Personnel may be organized by function, discipline, service, team, or project. Many kinds and types of personnel, with many levels and types of education, experience, and interest, must come together to coordinate their activities to provide health care to clients. On an inpatient unit, the major components of a multidisciplinary team are a nurse, a psychologist, a social worker, a psychiatrist, and an occupational, recreational, and/or physical therapist. The work of this treatment team is complex, and the need for sound group dynamics that foster cooperation, communication, and collaboration among these very different disciplines is paramount. The goal of maintaining high-quality client care is sometimes diverted by struggles over practice domains, power, esteem, or image. Group dynamics among team members are complex, to say the least. In a psychiatric facility, sound, productive, cooperative relationships need to be fostered as an organizational value by administrators and practitioners alike in order to meet the organization's goal or mission: the delivery of high-quality client care.

Health care facilities are labor-intensive because the nature of the work or service requires people, rather than technology, to do the work. Machines have replaced people in many industries or businesses but, in health care, technology has often increased the need for people to deliver services. The nature of human services precludes automation. Nursing care, by its nature and purpose, necessitates intense and sustained human interaction. The more acute the needs of clients, the more intensive are their needs for nurses. There is a direct relationship between clients' needs and the importance of having nurses that cannot be substituted for by technology or automation.

The psychiatric hospital or mental health service is labor-intensive because of the special nature of the service or treatment needed in the therapeutic relationship. Human interaction and observation are the major components of treatment. Therefore, the need for therapeutic interactions as a treatment modality necessitates the presence of high numbers of nurses in the mental health system. It is also relevant that nursing care is needed 24 hours a day, every day, rather than only periodically.

Nursing administrators or managers must tend to a multitude of needs and problems in order to facilitate the practice of nursing for nurses and for clients. Through knowledge about and skill in management and strength in leadership, nurse administrators can develop and maintain effective and efficient nursing practice.[10]

As one service in a complex system, nursing practice is influenced by, and can influence, a multitude of external and internal forces. The ability of the nurse administrator is paramount in determining the scope of nursing practice, the general quality of work life for nurses, and the overall contribution nurses can make to clients' experiences and levels of wellness.

The Management Process in Nursing Administration

The management process is focused on getting work done (to produce a product or deliver a service) through others. The work, or content, of nursing is focused on delivering nursing care to selected groups of clients, and requires the use of the nursing process to formulate and complete the activities of client care. Getting work done by many people, as in a department of nursing in which as many as 100, 400, or 1000 employees need to be mobilized, is complex, and requires a process to formulate and complete those activities: the management process. The ultimate purpose of both the nursing process and the management process is to complete work in an efficient and effective manner. Orderliness in arranging work activities facilitates both the quality of the outcome (effectiveness) and the quantity of the outcome (efficiency). Each process gives order or sequence to the approach needed to complete the specified work, and each uses its specific, defined knowledge base.

The components of the management process—planning, organizing, staffing, directing, and controlling—are similar to the components of the nursing process. Each management function incorporates other common concepts or skills, such as communication, delegation, or prioritization. Managing people is a complex process. The way in which it is done has great bearing on the satisfaction of employees and the quality of their work to deliver health care. This relationship is illustrated in Figure 27-2. The ability and skill of the management team are reflected in measurements of productivity. Quality assurance (QA) reports, client length of stay (LOS) data, financial reports, turnover and absenteeism data, and

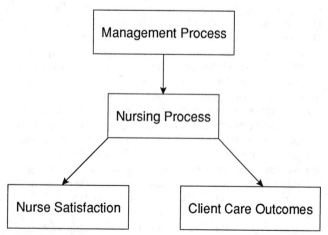

Figure 27-2. The management process influences the job satisfaction of employees and the quality of client care outcomes.

employee and client satisfaction information are indicators of the effectiveness and efficiency of the management process in a health care facility.

Similar indicators are used in a psychiatric/mental health care facility or service. Specific client indicators include clients' length of stay (LOS), medication compliance, or readmission data. The work of the treatment team is greatly influenced by the total atmosphere created by the administration, including the amount of professional and general support services given to the clinical team.

Planning

Although planning is the first management function, it is based on assessing and collecting data about a situation or condition. As in the assessment of a client, organizational situations need to be observed, evaluated, and diagnosed. As with clients, the more data that are gathered about the situation, the more clear and successful a plan can be. However, it is impossible to have all the information regarding any particular client or situation; decisions about a plan are usually made with less than all of the potentially available information.

There are two very different foci for the planning process, depending on the situation, the philosophy, and the perspective of the manager. A *problem orientation* responds only to a defined problem, and results in a narrow response to the difficulty encountered or in removing an obstacle or an impediment to a goal. This focus simply needs problem-solving skill. A *developmental orientation* responds to a situation by searching for ways to create a better solution, a better system, or a better product or goal. It focuses on redefining a goal or creating a new one, and demands keen thinking and problem-solving skill, coupled with vision and a futuristic perspective. This creative process brings "what is" to a new level of "what can be," and is energizing to the organization and its participants. In the same way that people strive for self-actualization, organizations have the potential to strive toward their collective, cumulative, or organizational actualization. The process of helping clients, through the use of therapeutic sessions and the environment, to move from their presenting state to a new (and hopefully better) state of self involves a developmental orientation. Helping a client to solve only a presenting problem may be very limiting and may serve to prevent the client's exploration and expansion of potential. Similarly, an organization is denied growth and dynamism when planning is done without vision, creativity, or an openness that invites ideas. Developmental planning has the underlying philosophy that, not only do things need to be fixed or problems solved, but everything has the potential to be better or improved.

When plans are developed by a nurse administrator, they most often have a client focus. Concern for client outcome (and nursing effectiveness) relates to almost any subject of planning, no matter how seemingly remote: planning a new facility relates to client care, financial planning relates to client care, human resource (personnel) planning relates to client care, and material resources (supplies and equipment) planning relates to client care. The nurse administrator, as an advocate for client care, spends an extraordinary amount of time in planning to enable and evaluate support systems on behalf of nurses and client care delivery. The planning function is done in collaboration and coordination with the two other major administrative groups: the hospital administration, which includes departments such as personnel, accounting, and support services; and the medical administration, which includes the physician staff and sometimes other professional staff. How well these three major administrative groups function together determines the efficiency and effectiveness of all support systems that provide client care services, and ultimately to the client care outcomes. Figure 27-3 illustrates the relationship of the management process and the nursing process to organizational function, structure, and purpose. The underpinning of clients' outcomes is sound, thoughtful, client-oriented administrative planning. Planning is essentially a cognitive activity that takes the nurse, manager, or administrator from a present situation to one in the future. In the same way, planning activities for a client's whole day at the beginning of the day or shift, or planning for a client's discharge from the unit the following week, requires thinking into the future and deciding what needs to happen. Without this function, results of activities for clients are not predictable, and any outcome, behavior, or activity (wanted or unwanted) may be the result. Concentrating on the planning function, therefore, can lead to greater predictability of activities, behavior, and other outcomes.

The nursing administrator in a psychiatric hospital needs to invest much time in planning, and may ask the following questions about the future of the department of nursing and the nursing personnel in the facility:

- Should nurses become primary therapists for clients?
- How will nurses do so if there is a strong resistance from other disciplines?

- How much education and supervision will the nurses need?
- Which model of nursing care delivery would be best for clients in this facility?
- How many and which types of nursing personnel are needed for each model?
- What other support systems (*e.g.,* activities therapy, psychology, housekeeping) will be needed?
- What will be the effect of each on client outcomes? Length of stay? Recidivism?
- Which model will most effectively decrease absenteeism, increase nurses' satisfaction, morale, and retention, and promote better recruitment?

These are just a few of the considerations involved in planning, but all of the questions relate to the future and need to be considered in that time context. The planning function demands creative and visionary thought, linked with the realities and constraints of any given institution. Planning by either a clinical or an administrative nurse pushes reality into the future in order to actualize the fullest potential for clients and the nursing staff. Planning is not an easy function, nor a reflex action; it demands concentrated cerebral effort. However, the product of such work enables nurses to determine their own and their clients' destinies, and to have some knowledge of and control over the direction of future activities, situations, events, and their related outcomes.

Organizing

Bringing order to ideas, thoughts, or plans for implementation requires that the various parts or specifics need to be identified and put in the proper sequence. Just as the total nursing care for a client needs to be broken down into parts that are placed in some relationship to each other before implementation, a management plan is broken down into specifics and given order and sequence. Attempting to jump from the plan directly into activity, without an organizing function, can result in unwanted

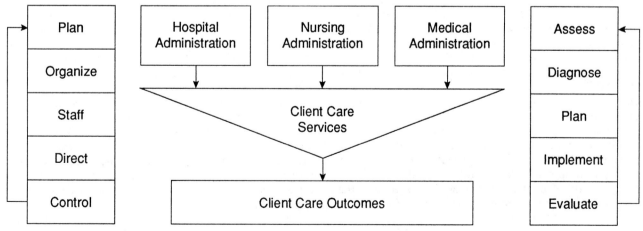

Figure 27-3. The management process and the nursing process are similar and, when done well, have a positive effect on client care outcomes.

outcomes or chaos in which there is much activity but nothing is truly accomplished.

For any plan to become action, there should be structure and form for the people, events, and activities. The form of the organizational structure fundamentally reflects the mission and goals of the organization as a whole, and its long-range or strategic plan. In the complex health care facility, there are many opportunities for diversion from a systematic flow of activities. Each employee has at least a hypothetical relationship with all other employees in an organization. The organizational chart delineates the formal structure, hierarchy, reporting relationships, and channels of communication and authority among employees. This is the formal organization.

There is also an informal structure that bypasses formal lines in the structure. It is a people-oriented, person-to-person process that overrides formality. It functions in spite of, and differently from, the organizational chart. For example, if it is very hot and clients could suffer hyperthermia, and the air conditioner is broken, the nurse may know the proper approach to getting things repaired: fill out a requisition and submit it to the head nurse. The formal process may take days before the air conditioner is repaired. However, the nurse may call the assigned unit mechanic directly and have the problem resolved in a short time. While this produces the needed outcome (the air conditioner gets repaired), it may have caused the mechanic to be unavailable for another critical situation.

Although informal mechanisms can sometimes facilitate action, they are potentially hazardous when total organizational needs are considered. From a management perspective, following formal lines in the organization promotes order and direction among the many people, events, and activities in a hospital, although it may hinder efficiency.

In a similar fashion, organizational structure in the nursing department strongly relates to the general plans for the future. Organizing nursing personnel and their work in a way that meets the overall plan is imperative. For instance, the formal committee structure is designed to relate today's work to intended future outcomes in the department. The Policy and Procedure Committee is formed with the knowledge that the organization is an open system with constant need for change. This is a mechanism to update the guidelines used to maintain orderliness and standardization in work, while assuring that certain external and internal standards of practice are met. An Ethics Committee may be developed because there are many conflicting values in delivering client care. In order to bring some uniformity and unanimity to client care dilemmas, this group is formed to explore and balance approaches to care that may be in conflict. Because ethical dilemmas are prevalent in health care, by having a group available for and knowledgeable about work on ethical matters, crises can be prevented, the rights of clients can be protected, and integrity in nursing practice can be promoted.

Thus, the plans set forth by the nursing administrator can begin to become reality when structure or form is developed. Making a plan operational necessitates coordination of many specific parts, with the development of structure and strategy. To develop primary nursing on a psychiatric unit, or to initiate a mental health nurse specialist role with surgical clients and staff, or to decrease non-nursing functions of nursing staff, forces thorough analysis and coordination of activities and events. These are combined with insight to envision and formulate plans to overcome unexpected problems. The ability to structure the work of many people for future goals is truly complex, and demands considerable talent, foresight, and wisdom.

Staffing

As mentioned earlier, health care is a labor-intensive industry, and nursing is the core in most facilities. All the planning and organizing of a nursing administrator are futile if personnel are not available to carry out the activities. The problem most discussed in nursing today is the shortage of nurses to take care of clients. It has taken years to create the problem, and years and concentrated planning and action will be required to resolve it. The shortage is a symptom of other major issues in the nursing profession such as status, economics, and general work content and conditions. There is an ongoing, concentrated effort on the part of nursing administrators to broaden recruitment efforts to increase the number of new nurses in their organizations. Without a unified, clear effort to resolve or improve the basic issues depleting the supply of nurses (such as public image, autonomy of practice, and economic and work conditions), no amount of recruiting will increase the numbers of working nurses and retain them in the work force. Other techniques need to be implemented to increase retention.[5,6]

A vital aspect of this shortage is that it belongs, not only to the administrators, but to all nurses. If all nurses work together to influence the system on many fronts, with collaboration, coordination, cooperation, and communication, this situation could change.

An ongoing problem in staffing for nursing administrators is the quantification of staffing needs. Since the number of clients and their conditions are variable and not truly predictable, it is difficult to predict from one day to the next, one shift to the next, and sometimes one hour to the next what the staffing needs on a unit will be. Great strides have been made in developing acuity or classification systems to evaluate, delineate, and quantify clients' needs for nursing care. These are then calculated and translated into the staffing needs for a given shift or day. However, psychiatric/mental health nursing care has been slower to develop these systems because of its interpersonal, rather than task activity, emphasis. The process of developing and validating psychiatric classification systems is progressing and an effective measurement tool is emerging.[4,11,12]

There is now a very objective and accurate method to determine the number and kinds of nursing personnel needed on a unit. As seen in Figure 27-4, client acuity

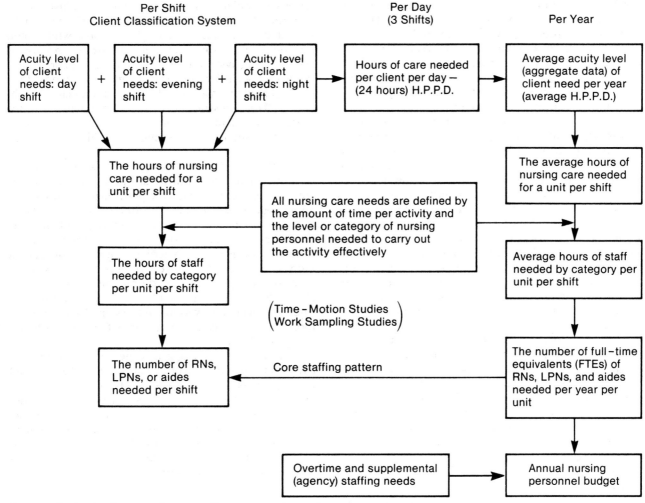

Figure 27-4. The development of a core staffing pattern and annual nursing personnel budget flows from direct client acuity data.

data, collected over a period of time, can be used to project the general staffing pattern and the annual nursing personnel budget required.

Staffing relates to the general number and kinds of personnel needed to meet the nursing needs of clients. Scheduling, another aspect of staffing, refers specifically to the days and shifts on which personnel are assigned to work. There are variations in the amount of care needed by clients on different shifts. Because acuity data are collected primarily by shift, they show the variation in the numbers and kinds of personnel needed on each shift, and also the variation in personnel needed for weekends or holidays if census and acuity levels differ on those days. Therefore, schedules determining when personnel work are also developed from the client acuity data.

A scheduling concern of nursing administrators is to allow personnel the needed time away from clients to recuperate from the intensity and stress of nursing work. Great care needs to be taken in schedule development to enable personnel to rest and relax from their work. Body rhythms influence nurses' productivity and general effectiveness. In designing a schedule for nursing staff on

a unit, individual preferences should be considered in relation to general productivity in order to assure high-quality care and to promote morale. The key to caring for clients rests with the quantity and quality of the nurses providing the care.

Directing

When the staffing plan and the schedules are complete, the next major management function is directing. Personnel may show up for their shift but, unless there is effort to clarify roles and responsibilities, personnel are likely to fall short of maximizing their potential on behalf of clients. Policies, procedures, and job descriptions give guidance for the activities of nursing personnel. Employees need to know what has to be done, when, how, how often, and by whom.

Managing a large work force involved in the complex activities of client care demands considerable attention, evaluation, and supervision on the part of those in charge.

It is the responsibility of those in authority, in supervisory or management roles, to give the necessary guidance to employees in order to get work completed.

The core of the directing function is communication. The style and approach the manager uses in giving directions or assigning activities can influence the outcome in terms of both efficiency and effectiveness. Communication ability is critical to productivity.[14]

The process of delegation of responsibilities or activities is important. To delegate a task to someone with trust and explanation, but without rejection or hostility, can be crucial to the outcome. Awareness of others' abilities and sense of commitment relates to the quality of the work done. The ultimate accountability, however, is vested in the person who originally was responsible for the task or activity. Delegating work to others does not negate the originator's accountability and need to check on progress or the final product. For example, the primary nurse on a unit may ask another nurse to give a p.r.n. medication to an agitated client. The primary nurse is still accountable for the proper completion of the task, or the consequences of its not being done or being done improperly.

Another aspect of directing involves disciplining, counseling, or assisting others. The nurse administrator, manager, or head nurse has a responsibility to take action when employees are not following directions about their work, behavior, or actions. If an employee does not stay within given parameters of expected behavior and performance, disciplinary action may be taken. In many circumstances, explaining, counseling, coaching, and generally helping the employee to do better may be effective. However, if performance does not improve, more firm, punitive, disciplinary action may be indicated.

Delegating, communicating, and disciplining all assist in guiding employees to complete the needed work. When people are involved, it is imperative to be thoughtful in determining the approach to use. A haphazard approach in directing others may lead to interpersonal disasters and decline in productivity. A developmental approach, whenever it is possible, usually yields long-lasting results. The developmental approach centers, not on problem-solving, but rather on making situations better. The developmental approach fosters a group's potential, and is preferable to an authoritarian, disciplinarian style.

Controlling

The last of the management functions is control. This term is used, not in the psychological sense, but to mean a process of examining results and feeding back information in order to bring something within the limits, standards, or parameters set for an activity, behavior, or outcome.

A quality assurance program is a control function because it reports outcomes measured against established standards in order to provide feedback for improvement. For example, evaluating the conditions or criteria used as rationale for placing a client in a quiet or seclusion room may reveal a lack of consistency. Some clients may be secluded for minimal behavioral symptoms, while others may be secluded only after demonstrating considerable assaultive behavior. If there are parameters or criteria for the use of seclusion, compliance with the standard can be evaluated by analyzing clients' documentation in the record. If the assessment reveals noncompliance with the criteria, action may be taken to correct the situation through in-service classes, meetings, films, or memoranda.

In the case of peer review, standards are established for performance and individuals' performance is evaluated against them. Again, if the performance is not within an acceptable, defined range, corrective action is taken.

The nursing administrator's role frequently involves the control function in order to assure that activities, performance, decisions, or outcomes are within acceptable ranges for the proper delivery of nursing care. Management reports give data regarding items such as budget, absenteeism, turnover, use of overtime, or supply costs. They are many and varied, and essentially are used as tools to assist in controlling events that are not within acceptable limits.

In summary, the major management functions have a relationship with each other and are, therefore, considered a process. They are not mutually exclusive, but overlap, and cannot be done in total isolation from each other. The process of management requires skill, knowledge, and sensitivity to the uniqueness of people. The nursing administrator needs to be flexible and thoughtful with people, while being knowledgeable and futuristic about the organization as a totality.

The Use of Self and the Role of the Nursing Administrator

The scope of the nursing administrator's responsibility encompasses both the context and the content of nursing practice: the environment where nurses practice and the breadth of their role and responsibilities.

> The primary goal of organized nursing services is the delivery of effective care to individuals. To meet the new demands placed on organized nursing services, nurse administrators must be knowledgeable, skilled, and competent in directing clinical practice, in data analysis, in business management, and in resource management. Nurse administrators are responsible for the provision of safe, efficient, cost-effective care to recipients served by organized nursing services.[2]

Clinical vs. Management Knowledge and Skills

Nurses are frequently promoted into management positions primarily because of their clinical expertise, efficiency, and effectiveness. Often, these nurses have had little formal management education or training, and encounter great frustration and even failure. Education for the nurse administrator usually includes coursework in organizational theory, health care finance, health care law, and the general management of people. As shown in Figure 27-5, different cores of knowledge and skill are used by management nurses and by clinical nurses. The shaded area in the figure represents the commonalities, or overlapping, of knowledge and skill between the clinical nursing and management processes.

If nurses bring only clinical nursing knowledge and experience to a management role, they will manage by commonsense, trial and error, intuition, or just plain luck. Not having a knowledge base in management limits the nurse administrator's effectiveness. Broad knowledge of and experience in clinical nursing are not substitutes for knowledge of and experience in management. Knowledge about one is not knowledge about the other; however, knowledge and skill in one area enhance knowledge and skill in the other area.

The knowledge base for administration is different and separate from the knowledge base used in clinical practice. However, basic principles used in psychiatric nursing, such as communication, understanding of Self and Other, and understanding of behavior, relationships, values, needs, and trust are applicable, needed, and helpful in managing people. The use of human relations skills and group dynamics approaches and the therapeutic use of self contribute greatly to the style and effectiveness of the nurse administrator. The administrator's skills in us-

ing the self in the management process, coupled with understanding of and insight into others and their dynamics in the organization, determine the administrator's ultimate effectiveness in the organization. At the organizational level, this knowledge of self enables the nursing administrator to create the culture in which nurses work. Silber and Tubbesing[13] translate the word *culture* into seven functions:

Create a bonding-linking climate.
Understand yourself.
Lead effectively.
Trust.
Utilize the cultural values.
Recognize rights and rituals.
Encourage excellence.

Creating an organizational climate in a complex organization such as a health care facility while being subjected to numerous external and internal influences is not an easy task. Many skills must be mastered and many roles are needed to effect change and create the desired culture.

Roles of the Nursing Administrator

At the individual level, the nursing administrator may need to be many things to many people in the organization, as shown in the following box. Understanding the self gives the nursing administrator the core ingredient of the flexibility needed for the many roles. Self-under-

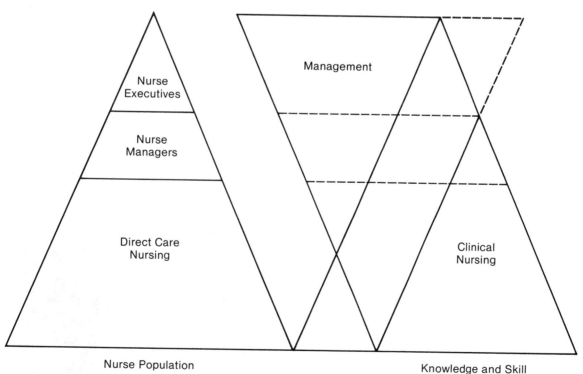

Figure 27-5. Use of management and clinical nursing knowledge and skill by direct care nurses, nurse managers, and nurse executives.

standing gives balance, direction, and stability during unsteady times and prevents confusion during times of organizational disorder or discord. The responsibility for high-quality nursing practice and for high-quality client care outcomes is enormous, and the role stress produced in this type of administrative position can be overpowering[9] if the person is not cognizant of the Self in its many and complex aspects. Mental, moral, and emotional insight and stamina produce the vision and wisdom needed for the many dimensions of the role and responsibility of the nursing administrator.

The tone and direction of the nursing department are set by the philosophy of the nursing administrator: the values and beliefs of that individual about human beings, work, health care, nursing, and the environment permeate the organization and become part of the culture of the department. The experience, personality, vision, philosophy, and wisdom of the administrator can enrich the operation, the climate, and the morale. The person's fundamental beliefs about the essence of nursing can permeate the nursing department.

As in the therapeutic relationship, the nursing administrator engages in, and promotes, healthy relationships with nursing staff and other employees. Within this climate, the chance is great that there is a clear client focus, with much energy available for caring. Essentially, the breadth of human experience of the administrator's Self will be reflected in the Relationships with Others in the department. It follows that, if the administrator fosters an environment of mental health among staff, then the staff can be more effective in fostering mental health with clients.

The nurse administrator may need to function as a healer for the nursing staff and in the organization. Many employees need, at one time or another, to be heard, listened to, comforted, or nurtured as individual human beings. The tragedies, stress, anxiety, and pain of life are not selective, and no one is immune. As care-givers, nurses also need to be cared for, and their wounds healed. Nurses undergo emotional wounds as part of their daily routine. They are not impervious to the pain, confusion, fear, turmoil, aggression, anxiety, or agitation of clients or the organization. If the emotional wounds of nurses are allowed to go unaddressed, they can deplete the energy and the therapeutic ability of nurses with clients. The nurse administrator cannot heal all wounds, but has a responsibility to acknowledge the humanness of the staff and provide mechanisms for renewal, support, nurturance, and healing. Developing support groups, educational programs, outside social or sports activities, or rap groups can be rejuvenating and energy-producing for staff. A moment of an administrator's listening ear offered to a nurse can generate respect, loyalty, and support (Fig. 27-6). An atmosphere that promotes health and wellness among staff will, in turn, be reflected in an atmosphere that promotes health and wellness among clients. The general health and harmony of the staff determine the quality of health and harmony in the client care environment.

The role of the nursing administrator as advocate for clients and personnel is important. With the business focus of health care institutions, "total absorption in nonhumanistic perspectives in the care of patients can critically jeopardize nursing's future as central in the health care delivery process."[7] The effective nursing administrator maintains a balance between business and humanitarianism.

In the mental health care setting, the nurse functions as an advocate to ensure rights and facilitate the coordina-

ROLES OF THE NURSING ADMINISTRATOR

Philosopher
Decision-maker
Communicator
Healer
Leader
Follower
Facilitator
Mentor
Care-giver
Supporter
Representative
Counsellor
Confessor
Priest
Judge
Disciplinarian
Futurist
Politician
Advocate
Risk-taker
Ethicist

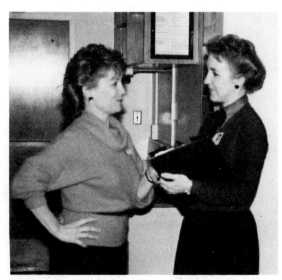

Figure 27-6. A nursing administrator confers with a psychiatric nurse staff member.

tion of care by a multidisciplinary team. The client can readily be shuffled from one person to another without defined purpose, and become lost in the complexity of the large system. The nurse's role is to help; advocacy in the system epitomizes this true professional purpose.

The nurse administrator empowers the clinicians through decentralizing decision-making and increasing autonomy and accountability. This decreases unhealthy needs to foster dependence of or hold power over clients. If the nurse is given the authority and autonomy to make clinical decisions, the search for health will be promoted and achieved at a faster rate for each client.

The organization's attitudes toward, and respect for, nurses and their contribution to clients' well-being are a concern for the nursing administrator. Advocacy on behalf of respect for and participation of the nursing staff not only improves self-esteem, but also enables nurses to maximize their contribution to client care. The success of nurses' participation in decision-making activities depends on the organizational structure and culture of the institution, and the established power of the nurse administrator within the executive management team. Frequently, the political role is prevalent, and risks must be taken to promote gains in professional authority and autonomy in nursing practice. A basic philosophy of respect for the practice domains of other disciplines frequently creates a reciprocal respect for nursing practice.

The nurse administrator brings concerns and information from the nursing staff to the other executive-level administrators. This role of representative requires a confident and assertive person who articulates the needs and issues of nurses. The nurse administrator, being a nurse, understands the issues and needs of clients and nurses, and can translate and articulate them to others on the executive team. Although it is difficult to quantify subjective information and make it meaningful to those who make organizational decisions affecting nurses and nursing practice, it must be done. In the data collection and analysis process, nursing administrators are able to quantify the needs of clients through the use of acuity or classification systems, and translate clients' need into staffing patterns. Because psychiatric clients' needs are more interactive and observational than task-oriented, quantification is significantly more difficult than with other clients.

With so much needed for clients, nurses need the nursing administrator to be a *leader*. This may take many forms: as advocate for both clients and nurses, as futurist in planning for change, and as visionary in defining new ways of caring. The nursing administrator must ask for and allow followers. Without followers, the nurse administrator is only a figurehead in the organization, and maintains the organization rather than creating its destiny. The role of leader demands the highest skill of interaction with all personnel, and true excellence in understanding the truth of Self and Other. The efforts put forth in developing truth in the relationships with Others can bear the many fruits of loyalty, productivity, effectiveness, and efficiency in the care environment.

The nursing administrator needs *followers*. There is often a subtle reluctance of administrators to seek the support of the staff, and a reciprocal reluctance on the part of staff to be supportive to managers. There seems to be an automatic, unwritten tendency in organizations to create distance between management and staff, with an innate organizational need to develop a we–they attitude between management and staff. With the current nursing shortage, there is a great force that negates nursing management. Now, more than ever, there is a need for unity among all nurses. The dynamic of the we–they separation, with no trust or strong relationship between the Self and the Other, disperses unity among nurses in the health care system and diminishes the maximization of nursing talent with clients. The astute staff recognizes the potential demise of this dynamic, and works toward fostering support for the nursing leader.

Ethical practice of nursing is monitored by the nursing administrator. Many questions, concerns, and dilemmas exist in the complexities of caring for human beings, but decisions must be made. The need for care does not cease when difficult ethical questions arise. Knowledge of ethical principles and biomedical ethics is vital to facilitating decisions and avoiding conflict and confusion for clients, families, and nursing staff. The ANA Code for Nurses[1] is a guide for ethical and professional practice in nursing. The nurse practice act of each state sets the legal parameters of practice and assists in some decisions regarding nursing practice. Also, there may be legislation guiding and guarding the human rights of the mentally ill and mentally retarded that can be used to clarify clients' rights.

Some nurses want and seek the nursing administrator to be a *mentor* to them. This is a role that is vital to the growth and development of staff. Some administrators have had broad experience that they are pleased to share. They are usually pleased that someone is interested in learning from them. The role of mentor is not necessarily easy, nor totally career-oriented. A mentor may not have similar clinical interests, but has experience and insight in life and in the ways of human beings that are helpful to the mentoree. In the mental health arena, having a mentor can help to bridge some of the gaps of life experience, both in the Self and the Truth of the Other.

The health care system, including the mental health care system, has not yet balanced the needs of people for a decent minimum level of care with the free enterprise aspects of the health care industry and the self-actualization needs of health care providers. The financial crisis in health care has occurred because there is not a clearly defined public policy regarding health care services in this country. Most efforts have surrounded cost containment issues rather than defining a decent universal minimum. Fear of potential rationing of services supersedes development of potential equity in distribution. With no limits or parameters, a system quickly gets out of control and behaves irrationally.

According to Peplau, "Although deinstitutionalization of psychiatric patients arose in part for humane reasons, such as providing the least restrictive environment, and with the introduction of psychotropic drugs, the greatest impetus to this movement came with efforts to contain health care costs."[8] The shift in care from institution to community has come about in a way that ultimately has not always been in the client's best interest. Humanizing care was, and remains, essential in institutions; however, one must be somewhat suspect of the true motivation to decrease the numbers of hospitalized chronically ill persons in state facilities. The tax burden of caring for the mentally ill in institutions is high, and the motivation to support mental health services is not so high. It is through the vigilance of nurses in the mental health system that changes will be made. Attentive and strong nursing administrators can make a difference in creating an environment that promotes excellence in psychiatric/mental health nursing and in leading other nurses in a challenge to make services better and more readily available to all clients.

> Nurses can and do control the environment of the institution, and nurses can institute progressive and humanizing changes if they so desire. Explanations and working together with a patient are not extras that nurses may choose to do, they are the essence of nursing, the essence of the nurse–patient relationship.[3]

Summary

1. Nursing administration in a psychiatric facility is an open system. It is affected by other systems, including the hospital administration, societal policy and culture, clients, and other professional groups.

2. The internal environment of a psychiatric facility is influenced by the specific client population. Clients in a geriatric unit of a psychiatric facility require different nursing administration behavior than do aggressive adults on a psychiatric unit.

3. Each individual employee comes to the nursing organization with unique personality, talents, and needs, and affects the nursing organization in correspondingly unique ways.

4. The management process is focused on getting work done through others to deliver a service. The components of the management process include planning, organizing, staffing, directing, and controlling.

5. Nursing management effectiveness is measured by quality assurance reports, client behaviors and improvement, and staff turnover and satisfaction.

6. A nursing administrator's ultimate effectiveness is based on the administrator's own therapeutic use of self in conjunction with an understanding of others.

7. The nursing administrator makes use of mental, moral, and emotional insight and stamina in working with nursing staff.

References

1. American Nurses' Association: Code for Nurses. Kansas City, Missouri, American Nurses' Association, 1985
2. American Nurses' Association: Standards for Organized Nursing Services and Responsibilities of Nurse Administrators Across All Settings. Kansas City, Missouri, American Nurses' Association, 1988
3. Curtin L: The nurse as advocate: A philosophical foundation for nursing. ANS 1:1, 1979
4. Eklof M, Qu W: Validating a psychiatric patient classification system. JONA 16:10, 1986
5. Huey FL, Hartley S: What keeps nurses in nursing: 3,500 nurses tell their stories. Am J Nurs 88:181, 1988
6. Loveridge C: Contingency theory: Explaining staff nurse retention. JONA 18:22, 1988
7. Miller K: The human care perspective in nursing administration. JONA 17:10, 1987
8. Peplau H: Tomorrow's world. Nurs Times 83:29, 1987
9. Scalzi C: Role stress and coping strategies of nurse executives. JONA 18:34, 1988
10. Scherer P: Hospitals that attract (and keep) nurses. Am J Nurs 88:34, 1988
11. Schroder PJ, Washington WP: Administrative decision-making: Staff–patient ratios (a patient classification system for a psychiatric setting). Perspect Psychiatr Care 20:111, 1982
12. Schroder PJ, Washington WP, Deering CD et al: Testing validity and reliability in a psychiatric patient classification system. Nurs Man 17:49, 1986
13. Silber M, Tubbesing B: Nursing director: Creator of culture. Nurs Man 19:64T, 1986
14. Wolf GA: Communication: Key contributor to effectiveness—a nurse executive responds. JONA 16:9, 1986

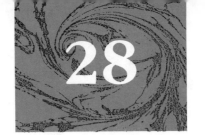

28

RONDA MINTZ

THE INPATIENT SYSTEM

Learning Objectives

Upon completion of this chapter the student should be able to do the following:

1. Describe feelings generated in clients when confronted with admission to a psychiatric facility.
2. Describe reactions of clients' families to clients' needs for psychiatric hospitalization.
3. Detail the components of a psychiatric facility, including: the physical environment, types of activities and programs available for clients; and members of adjunctive services, including RT, OT, and others.
4. Discuss the function of the interdisciplinary treatment team in relation to client care, and name one potential conflict that can occur among members of the team.
5. Describe the therapeutic use of self as an aspect of nursing care.
6. Give examples of two conflicts that can occur among members of a nursing team, and how the conflicts can be resolved.
7. Give an example of a conflict that can occur among members of two different nursing shifts, and how the conflict can be resolved.
8. Discuss the defense mechanism of splitting and how it can cause conflict among nursing team members.
9. Detail the importance of good and consistent communication among nursing staff members, and list ways to facilitate communication.
10. Name five of the major goals that inpatient clients should achieve during hospitalization.
11. Discuss the impact of discharge of clients on the clients' families.
12. Name at least four of the treatment ingredients that were present in the detailed clinical example that made positive contributions to the success of the treatment.
13. Name two cultural considerations that can influence a client's hospitalization.

Introduction

The world of inpatient psychiatry is still unknown to most of society. In addition to feelings of fear and confusion, common questions arise about what really occurs behind the "locked doors," who the clients are, who compose the staff, and how staff and clients interface. In movies such as "One Flew Over the Cuckoo's Nest," "I Never Promised You a Rose Garden," and "Sybil," the psychiatric hospital is presented as a frightening, controlling, and dehumanizing place. Clients are portrayed as helpless and defenseless individuals who inevitably yield to the administration of sedating medications or, in more severe cases, restraints, electrical shock therapy, and/or surgery.

Given these common stereotypes, it may be surprising to find that clients and staff members are not as they are portrayed, that units are often cheerful and colorfully decorated, and that there is an aura of calm and tranquility, rather than anxiety and fear. The psychiatric hospital, rather than being a frightening and dehumanizing experience, is, in fact, what Gralnick defined as a "remedial society to which we turn to undo what the environment has wrought upon the patient . . . and should be filled with healing, humanizing resources."[7] Therefore, to provide an optimal environment for emotional healing, staff members do not wear uniforms but wear ordinary street clothes and a badge or namepin. Visiting students usually find it difficult to discern who are clients and who are staff. Medications, restraints, and other invasive treatments are only ordered when deemed necessary by the psychiatrist coordinating the case, in conjunction with legally-sanctioned hospital policies.

Previously, Chapter 14 detailed the components of the milieu, including the nurse–client relationship, levels of communication, and the power of the milieu as treatment tools for clients in the form of therapy and group dynamics. This chapter explores the inpatient psychiatric system on a more concrete, organizational level, focusing primarily on the composition of the staff and interdisciplinary team members and the roles they play as clients progress from admission to discharge.

Admission

Before a person is considered for admission to a psychiatric facility, certain criteria must be met, including the following: (1) a completed assessment by a psychiatrist or other licensed clinical therapist, indicating the present need for hospitalization; (2) proof of health insurance coverage or other source of payment; (3) a psychiatric diagnosis that includes the severity of the problem(s), past and present functioning levels, and degree of affliction (*i.e.,* DSM-III-R diagnostic analysis); (4) signed consents for voluntary admission, signed by the client if over the age of 15 years, or by the legal guardian if the client

is under the age of 15, or legal documents indicating conditions for involuntary admission status, signed by the case coordinator if specific criteria are met (see Chap. 34 for more specific legal implications).

Many hospitalized psychiatric clients voluntarily agree to enter an inpatient facility for relief of their current emotional and psychological experiences. As difficult and, at times, demoralizing as it may be to acknowledge the need for hospitalization, the immediate sense of safety and security provided in a nurturing environment tends to be soothing, and alleviates pressure and tension before they build to an unbearable level. Once security and safety are felt, clients then must confront feelings of failure and inadequacy at being unable to cope with daily life without the structure of a psychiatric hospital. Nurses play extremely important roles in aiding clients to express these deep and painful feelings. This expression helps to build the foundation of support and concern in an honest and accepting environment. When these feelings remain unexpressed and out of the client's awareness, the therapeutic process is hindered and the relationship with the nursing staff stays superficial.

For the family and/or immediate support system(s) of the hospitalized client, the removal of the client from the home into the hospital can also be overwhelming, frightening, and confusing. For some, feelings of guilt or the anticipation of blame for the client's decompensation may surface, while for others the hospitalization may provide a feeling of relief and hope that the client will receive the necessary help and support.[8] What most families do not realize is that the client and family members will change or grow from the hospital experience. Mutual change and growth are based on systems theory, which has been discussed previously. Current research demonstrates the impact families have on the therapeutic outcomes of clients. For instance, Leavitt[9] detailed how the lack of family involvement in the inpatient treatment program leads to a stronger possibility of treatment failure, concomitant with a crisis at the time of discharge. Along these same lines, researchers are attempting to validate statistically the connection between repeated hospitalizations (influenced by unrealistic expectations of the client and the family), denial of the severity of the emotional problems, and lack of empathy toward the identified client.[4,12]

The Inpatient Hospital as a System

The psychiatric hospital can be considered a system, with all the activities, disciplines, and staff being viewed collectively as parts of the whole. Each separate unit can also be considered a distinct system (especially locked units, where only a select group of people enter and leave the unit). All the units together can be a part of the general system of the hospital in its entirety.

Unit Structure

The inpatient psychiatric hospital is most often subdivided into distinct, separate units, each with a capacity of 15 to 40 beds. Usually, the units are classified by age groups, as follows: (1) children, ages 3 to 11; (2) adolescents, ages 12 to 17; (3) adults, ages 18 to 55; and (4) geriatrics, ages 55 and over. Some hospitals have special units for developmentally delayed children and adolescents. Others differentiate by diagnosis. Some units are considered open units, indicating that there is no locked door restricting the movement of clients into and out of the hospital. Most psychiatric units are locked, restricting clients' movements into and out of the unit for their safety and protection.

Figure 28-1 shows the floor plan of an adult inpatient unit. It includes a glass-enclosed nurse's station; a social or day room equipped with a T.V. and ping-pong table; a dining room; a laundry room; a music room; and two separate hallways, one for female client bedrooms and one for male client bedrooms. This unit has a locked front entrance, and therefore is considered a locked unit. All staff members have a special key to the entrance. An intercom system at the entrance is connected to the nursing station so that the staff can be alerted when others request admission.

The term *structure* also refers to the recommended schedule of activities available to the clients. A usual day may include the hourly events listed in Figure 28-2. Contrary to the popular opinion that psychiatric hospitals provide a place for rest and relaxation, the opposite is more realistic. Clients are expected to participate actively in the different groups and special programs, as well as in recreational and occupational therapies. Each of these is intended to provide services to strengthen skills that are rarely used or are underdeveloped in individual clients, yet could help to reduce stress or assertiveness outside the hospital. The therapists who organize and lead the

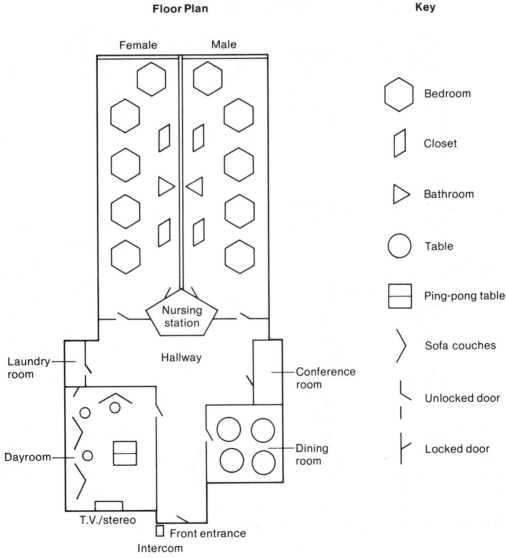

Figure 28-1. An adult inpatient closed/locked unit.

PSYCHIATRIC HOSPITAL

Closed Unit Daily Schedule

Adults

(Patients With Off-Unit Activities)

	MONDAY	TUESDAY	WEDNESDAY	THURSDAY	FRIDAY
7:00–7:30 AM	Wake-Up	Wake-Up	Wake-Up	Wake-Up	Wake-Up
7:30–8:00	Grooming	Grooming	Grooming	Grooming	Grooming
8:00–8:30	Breakfast*	Breakfast*	Breakfast*	Breakfast*	Breakfast*
8:30–9:00	Medications	Medications	Medications	Medications	Medications
9:00–9:30	Milieu Grp.	Milieu Grp.	Milieu Grp.	Milieu Grp.	Milieu Grp.
9:30–10:20	Free Time	Free Time	Free Time	Free Time	Free Time
10:20–11:10	O.T./Small Grp.	O.T./Small Grp.	O.T./Small Grp.	O.T./Small Grp.	O.T.
11:10–11:50	Small Grp.	Small Grp.	Small Grp.	Small Grp.	Small Grp.
11:50–12:30 PM	Free Time	Free Time	Free Time	Free Time	Free Time
12:30–1:00	Lunch*	Lunch*	Lunch*	Lunch*	Lunch*
1:00–1:15	Medications	Medications	Medications	Medications	Medications
1:15–2:15	O.T./Small Grp.	O.T./Small Grp.	O.T./Small Grp.	O.T./Small Grp.	O.T.
2:15–3:00	R.T.	R.T.	R.T.	R.T.	R.T.
3:00–3:15	Free Time	Free Time	Free Time	Free Time	Free Time
3:15–4:00	Milieu Time	Milieu Time	Milieu Time	Milieu Time	Milieu Time
4:00–4:30	Free Time	Milieu Grp.	Free Time	Free Time	Milieu Grp.
4:30–5:00	Medications	Medications	Medications	Medications	Medications
5:00–5:15	Free Time	Free Time	Free Time	Free Time	Free Time
5:15–5:45	Dinner*	Dinner*	Dinner*	Dinner*	Dinner*
5:45–6:30	Free Time	Free Time	Free Time	Free Time	Free Time
6:30–7:30	O.T.	O.T.	O.T.	O.T.	O.T.
7:00–8:30	Visiting	Visiting	Visiting	Visiting	Visiting
8:00–8:30	R.T.	R.T.	R.T.	R.T.	R.T.
8:30–9:00	Snacks/Meds.	Snacks/Meds.	Snacks/Meds.	Snacks/Meds.	Snacks/Meds.
9:00–10:00	Free Time	Free Time	Free Time	Free Time	Free Time
10:00–10:30	T.V.	T.V.	T.V.	T.V.	T.V.
10:30–11:30	Bedtime	Bedtime	Bedtime	Bedtime	Bedtime

WEEKEND SCHEDULE

	SATURDAY	SUNDAY		SATURDAY	SUNDAY
7:00–7:30 AM	Wake-Up	Wake-Up	1:00–3:00	Free Time	Free Time
7:30–8:00	Grooming	Grooming	3:00–3:45	R.T.	R.T.
8:00–8:30	Breakfast*	Breakfast*	3:45–5:00	Free Time	Free Time
8:30–9:30	Medications	Medications	5:00–5:15	Meds.	Meds.
9:30–10:00	R.T.	R.T.	5:15–5:45	Dinner	Dinner
10:00–10:30	Free Time	Free Time	5:45–6:30	Free Time	Free Time
10:30–11:00	Milieu Grp.	Milieu Grp.	6:30–7:30	O.T.	Free Time
11:00–12:30 PM	Free Time	Free Time	7:00–9:00	Movie	Movie
12:30–1:00	Lunch*	Lunch*	9:00–9:30	Snacks/Meds.	Snacks/Meds.
1:00–1:15	Medications	Medications	9:30–10:30	Free Time	Free Time
1:15–2:30	O.T.	O.T.	10:30–11:30	Bedtime	Bedtime
			11:00 AM–8:30 PM	Visiting	Visiting

* = Cafeteria

Figure 28-2. Client activities available Monday–Sunday. (Del Amo Psychiatric Hospital, Torrance, CA)

activities are specialists in their fields. For better understanding of the usefulness of each service, the following section describes the treatment modalities that are separate from, but closely interface with, the nursing staff.

Adjunctive Services

Recreational Therapy

Recreational therapy focuses on strengthening individual and group skills during physical activity and exercise. Individual skills include eye–hand coordination, familiarity with the rules of different sports, gaining expertise in participating in athletic activities, and generally building a repertoire of physical activities that are enjoyable and stress-reducing. Group skills involve learning the responsibilities of being a team member, including communication, sharing equally among members, learning how to be gracious winners and losers, and learning the boundaries of competitiveness. Also included are the organizing of and participating in field trips to museums, movies, or concerts, as well as hospital-based parties. These activities are presented to show alternate ways to have fun, relate to friends, and feel good.

Occupational Therapy

Occupational therapy is designed to provide activities that encourage the use of art materials such as paints, clay, pottery, woodwork, and the like. The objective is to produce products that are meaningful, and representative of clients' artistic abilities. Cooking and baking are also taught and encouraged, as is participation in making holiday decorations. Clients learn how to share materials, and how to join together in large projects.

Social Services

Social services are predominantly composed of licensed clinical social workers who are actively involved with the families of hospitalized clients, coordinate and lead family therapy, and help in discharge planning. In some facilities, members of the social services department also lead "small groups" for the inpatient clients. In these groups, clients intensely share and relate with each other in a confidential setting, and in a trusting and supportive group that is separate from the milieu. In some facilities, social services staff hold groups for the parents of hospitalized children and adolescents, during which more appropriate ways of parenting are taught.

Alcohol- and Substance-Abuse Programs

In some facilities, the effects of drug abuse are taught by specialists in the area of drug addiction. Preventive measures are also taught to individuals at high risk for assuming a drug lifestyle. Addicted clients are encouraged to express their underlying needs and feelings in small groups led by counselors. In some facilities, Alcoholics Anonymous, Narcotics Anonymous, and Cocaine Anonymous meetings are held daily, with emphasis on the 12-step program of breaking addictions.

School

In the majority of psychiatric hospitals, educational programs through 12th grade are available for hospitalized children and adolescents, as well as for some adult clients who did not complete high school. School credits are directly transferrable back into the previous school system. Inpatient school is quite unique because the courses are individualized to each student, based on the student's current levels of functioning. The teacher–student ratio is surprisingly low, averaging around 1:4 in most facilities. With such intense individualized attention and programming, students can quickly make up lost credits or failed courses.

The Interdisciplinary Treatment Team

In a hospital setting, it is essential that all staff members who interact therapeutically with clients have the opportunity to share their assessments and plans for intervention with each other on a regular basis. In this way, a consistent and unified treatment program can be maintained for clients. To expedite this process, an *interdisciplinary team* is created, consisting of one representative from each discipline that has direct client contact. The members of the interdisciplinary team include representatives from the adjunctive services listed above, usually one nursing staff member from each nursing shift, and the unit psychiatrist, the unit psychologist, the nursing unit manager/clinical coordinator, and the clinical nurse specialist.

The functions of the interdisciplinary team were summarized by Norman Brill, who stated that a team is "a group of people each of whom possess particular expertise; each of whom is responsible for making individual decisions; who together hold a common purpose; who meet together to communicate, collaborate, and consolidate knowledge, from which plans are made, actions determined and future decisions influenced."[3] Unfortunately, teams do not always function as effectively and smoothly as this definition implies. In the field of psychiatry, conflicts and struggles ensue quite often.

In a somewhat negative critique of the interdisciplinary team functioning observed by Ruch,[15] he stated that "establishing clear discipline boundaries is an important part of team function and should proceed based on areas of individual expertise." Ruch went on to comment specifically about the extent and intensity of the therapeutic relationships established between the client and team members who are not designated as the primary psychotherapist. His concern, via direct observations, was that, when a client has a number of close and therapeutically intimate relationships with numerous staff members, "it will be less likely that he or she will develop an effica-cious therapeutic alliance (with the assigned psychotherapist)."[15] The issue Ruch addressed is important for all members of treatment teams, and nursing staff in particular, because it is an issue that is raised repeatedly in psychiatric settings. In contrast to Ruch, Romoff and Kane[14] encouraged nursing staff members to utilize psychotherapeutic techniques (such as encouraging the exploration of past, traumatic, or painful events to aid in understanding the client's current emotional difficulties) when these techniques are thought to be therapeutically appropriate.

While nursing continues to define the scope of its practice, and until other mental health professionals adjust to this transition, the conflict will continue. As long as nursing staff members have strong therapeutic rationales for interventions, complete with short- and long-term goals, and as long as interventions are shared openly with members of other disciplines, the nurse is acting under the guidelines of the state Nurse Practice Act and is, therefore, legally supported.

Unsettled role confusion on the part of one or more interdisciplinary team members can have destructive repercussions in the overall treatment of the client from admission through discharge. Confusion can affect the daily milieu activities and involvement, and also raises issues concerning who should do what, with whom, and when (*e.g.,* family therapy, discharge planning, and the like). Benfer[2] summarized this conflict when stating that it is naive to expect that a group of interdisciplinary members will easily be able to design a comprehensive treatment program, especially a team "that deals with the stress of pathology and crises as well as the problems of team members learning to work together."

Given the above, frequent, regular meetings are needed to facilitate a clear and satisfactory work relationship among all interdisciplinary team members. Team meetings should provide an environment in which to question and confront, as well as support, each other's clinical assessments. Program activities and therapeutic interventions should be discussed so that they are as consistent as possible throughout all disciplines. The types and numbers of meetings vary with each facility, but it is essential for interdisciplinary team members to meet weekly for at least an hour, to work on their conflicts and concerns with each other as professionals. Other meetings, lasting from 15 minutes to half an hour, should be scheduled weekly to focus specifically on the client's progress and treatment.

Figure 28-3 is an example of the agenda for a weekly interdisciplinary treatment team meeting to be held on an inpatient adolescent unit. The major issue to be discussed is the goals of treatment for an aggressive and at times combative 15-year-old male PCP user who has been hospitalized for three days. Input from all disciplines is strongly encouraged. In this case, the major concern will be the views of the nursing staff, who are behaviorally intervening with the use of restraints.

The Nursing Treatment Team

The composition and number of staff of the nursing treatment team differ in every hospital. For example, some hospitals hire only licensed registered nurses and psychiatric technicians, while others hire fewer licensed personnel but add unlicensed psychiatric assistants who have majored in psychology in college. In some university hospitals, registered nurses are hired exclusively. To determine the required number of staff on each shift, many hospitals correlate the number of staff to the severity of the illness of the clients. This correlation is measured by behavioral rating scales similar to that in Figure 28-4, or it may be measured in terms of the expressed concerns and feelings of the staff members who interact

---

Week of: 1/15/89
Unit: Adolescent I

Members in attendance: _____
_____
_____

Agenda Items

1. 15 YO male PCP user hospitalized 3 days ago; behavior: aggressive and combative; in 5-point restraints almost the entire stay thus far; treatment goals and recommendations:

    a.

    b.

    c.

2. Vacation schedules—please write down dates you will be available and, if taking a vacation, please indicate dates and who will be covering.
3. Special Recreational and Occupational Therapy scheduling during the weeks of 1/22 to 1/28. Please note the changes.
4. New Business

Figure 28-3. Interdisciplinary team meeting agenda.

UCLA NEUROPSYCHIATRIC INSTITUTE
HOSPITAL & CLINICS

Nursing Service

Patient Classification Rating Form
Children's Service

Date: _____
Shift: ___ Night
    ___ Day
    ___ Evening
Unit: 6–West

Nursing Care Hour (NCH) Factors

	I	II	III	IV
NOC	1.0	2.0	4.0	8.0
Days	2.0	3.0	5.0	8.0
PMS	2.0	4.0	6.0	8.0
24°	5.0	9.0	15.0	24.0

Patient Name (Last name, Initial)	M	F	Ingestive	Eliminative	Affiliative	Dependency	Sexual	Aggressive–Protective	Achievement	Restorative	Overall Patient Category	Adaptive/ Appropriate	Inconsistent/ Needs Limits	Severe/Acute Problems	Very Severe/ Strict 1:1
1. JOHN	X		I	I	II	III	I	III	II	III	II		X		
2. HAROLD	X		I	I	III	III	II	III	II	II	II		X		
3. MAX	X		I	I	III	IV	IV	IV	III	III	IV				X
4. LEE	X		I	I	II	I	I	I	II	I	I	X			
5. LORENZO	X		II	II	III	III	II	III	II	III	III			X	
6. JIMMY	X		I	I	III	III	II	III	III	III	III			X	
7. ALLYN	X		II	I	II	III	II	III	II	II	II		X		
8. ERIC	X		III	II	III	III	I	II	III	III	III			X	
9. KIM		X	III	II	III	II	I	II	II	III	II		X		
10. LINDA		X	II	I	III	III	II	III	III	III	III			X	
11. FRANCES		X	I	I	I	I	I	I	I	II	I	X			
12. NANCY		X	I	I	II	II	I	I	II	I	I	X			
13. CATHY		X	I	I	II	II	II	II	II	III	II		X		
14. DIANE		X	II	II	II	III	I	III	III	III	III			X	
15. CHERYL		X	II	I	II	III	I	II	II	III	II		X		

Total # patients in each required Level of Care 1.   **3**   **6**   **5**   **1**

Enter Nursing Care Hours Factors for shift 2.   **2**   **3**   **5**   **8**

Multiply #1 by #2. Add across for total NCH . . . . 3.   **6** + **18** + **25** + **8** = **57**

Total NCH [**57**] ÷ 8 = [**7**]   Number of Staff required on duty   Total NCH

Lesley Wilbur   R.N.
Signature of Shift Coordinator

Figure 28-4. Acuity rating scale.

with the clients. In general, staff-to-client ratios range from 1:3 on a locked crisis unit to 1:7 on an unlocked, less structured treatment unit.

In most facilities, a "charge nurse" oversees the other nursing staff members and their interactions with clients (Fig. 28-5). The charge nurse also negotiates conflicts or concerns with client case coordinators, signs off on doctors' treatment orders, and organizes the overall operation of the unit. This staff member is usually responsible for completing staff–client assignment lists, coordinating staff lunch and coffee breaks, giving daily reports of clients' progress to other interdisciplinary team members, and assuring that charting has been completed by nursing staff members. The charge nurse should facilitate good working relationships among all staff members on all shifts, as well as encourage staff participation in treatment team meetings, in nursing meetings, and in one-to-one supervision.

Levels of Prevention

While the inpatient unit serves mainly as a secondary- and tertiary-level treatment-related facility, additional mention can be made of primary and secondary levels of prevention.

Primary prevention, or early case-finding, can occur on an inpatient unit. When an adult is admitted, a family assessment may reveal a substance-abuse problem in the adult's spouse or child. A family meeting can be called to discuss "total family" issues/problems. Physical problems occasionally are first assessed on psychiatric inpatient units.

When properly structured, an inpatient unit, operating at the secondary level of prevention, can serve as a mechanism for providing rapid, intense treatment of a client's problems. This is especially needed, for example, in cases of admissions related to crisis events, or first episodes of a language and thought disorder.

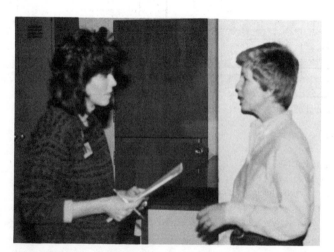

Figure 28-5. A psychiatric nurse confers with a client about the client's treatment plan.

The Therapeutic Use of Self

As discussed throughout the text, nursing team members need to offer a therapeutic self to clients, as well as to other nursing team members and interdisciplinary treatment team members. Staff members need to be aware of their own selves in all interactions while on duty. Staff members who can stay in touch with themselves tend to have better and more effective working relationships with fellow team members, and are highly respected by interdisciplinary team members. It is also imperative for psychiatric nurses to remain nondefensive and open to suggestions. To grow and mature in psychiatric nursing, nurses must always be open to constructive feedback, analysis of countertransference and transference issues, and awareness of staff conflicts. Although this kind of feedback may be painful, avoiding or denying it is more hazardous.

Nursing Team Conflicts

Conflicts within the nursing staff can have very severe effects on the milieu, client care, and coordination of treatment goals, for two reasons:

1. Conflicts within the nursing staff can affect the functioning of the interdisciplinary treatment team, and thus spread through all disciplines;
2. Once nursing becomes fragmented, the environment of the milieu is affected, which has repercussions for all clients.

Within nursing, the two major types of conflict are either between nursing staff members on one shift (*intrashift*) or between nursing staff members on separate shifts (*intershift*) e.g., days vs. evenings. When either occurs, the tension, anxiety, and emotional climate that exist can be felt by clients, visitors, and others on the unit.

Intrashift Conflicts

Examples of intrashift conflicts include:

1. A staff member does not agree with a decision made by the charge nurse and, rather than confronting the issue, talks negatively about the charge nurse to other staff members or to clients, or proceeds in direct opposition to the charge nurse.
2. A staff member becomes emotionally involved in a relationship with a hospitalized client, but does not feel able to discuss the feelings with other staff. Other staff members may become critical or angry at the amount of time the staff member is spending with the client. If the feelings of the staff are not expressed, the staff may then take out their angry feelings on the client by avoiding the client or making inappropriate comments regarding the relationship.

3. Conflict can arise if a relatively new and inexperienced registered nurse assumes the position of charge nurse on a weekend shift. Other staff members may either resent this acquisition of power or not trust the judgment of the new nurse. In this case, the staff, as a whole, may veto decisions made by the designated charge nurse, and carry out their assignments in ways they choose, showing no support or respect for the new leader.

These examples demonstrate lack of communication, inability to confront treatment or staff issues, and the results of ineffectual leadership.

Intershift Conflicts

Similar situations can occur among staff on different shifts, and can cause confusion and havoc for other staff members and clients. The following are examples of intershift conflicts:

1. A recently admitted client is on strict suicide observation. This entails removal of any sharp or potentially dangerous objects from the client's room, constant one-to-one sessions with a nurse, and careful and consistent monitoring. At 3:30 p.m., the evening shift assumes control of the unit and the incoming staff member assigned to this client finds that the room has not been thoroughly searched, potentially dangerous objects are within the client's reach, and the client is wearing clothes with long drawstrings. The staff member reports this directly to the charge nurse. When the same events occur the next day, the staff member who feels that appropriate action(s) were not taken writes in the client's chart a narrative of what was found, rather than again confronting the day shift and/or charge nurse.

2. A client enjoys working with a particular staff member on the evening shift, yet has difficulty in working with the assigned day-shift staff members. Hoping that the day-shift staff member will assume the same qualities, the client talks actively about the evening staff member in a very positive and enthusiastic way. The day-shift member becomes angry and, unable to accept the client's feedback or talk directly to the other staff member, projects the angry and hurt feelings onto the client. This angers and disappoints the client, and increases the client's positive feelings about the evening staff member.

3. Using example 2, a conflict could arise if the day-shift member responded with competitive feelings toward the evening staff member, and attempted to "win over" the client by awarding special favors, encouraging lengthy sessions, and/or talking negatively about the evening staff member.

Splitting

In the majority of these examples, a developmentally inappropriate defense mechanism called *splitting* has been utilized successfully. Usually, clients entering the hospital are already quite effective in splitting those around them. Therefore, staff members become prime targets to be split by these clients. From a developmental standpoint, these individuals have been unable to integrate and accept the notion that one can feel both positively and negatively toward a person. Because of poor ego development, they can only see people and events as either all good or all bad, with no compromise in between. Carser nicely summarized the effects of a client's splitting: "The patient externalizes the internal conflict and manipulates the staff to act out the patient's internal conflict."[5] Therefore, some of the staff members become "good" and are seen positively as nurturing and caring individuals who are liked and trusted by the client. Others are seen as "bad," and are viewed negatively as excessive limit-setters, unfair and inhumane.

If staff members do not have a forum in which to analyze the client's splitting tactics, or feel unsafe in bringing up the presence of a split in the nursing staff, the split will continue to mount. This leads to an environment that is unsafe, inconsistent, and, in most cases, an exact replica of the client's family life, in which faulty communication and splitting occurred. To rectify this struggle for the client, the unit must provide the consistency and stability that the family couldn't. Therefore, confrontation of this defense should be the treatment goal, rather than having the staff act out the conflict. There is a correlation between the acting out by a client of the good–bad staff split and an inherent, covert presence of nursing staff conflict that has been unsuccessfully addressed. These observations lend support to the call for regular nursing staff meetings within and between each shift, so that brewing conflicts can be resolved before the client's treatment is affected.

Effective Communication

For effective communication to occur on a unit, confrontation and questioning among staff members must be encouraged and facilitated. Staff members must be able to talk openly and honestly about issues with each other in a nonjudgmental and respectful manner. As professionals, it is essential that staff members realize that questions concerning an intervention are not personal insults or attacks, but rather questions of clinical judgment and/or therapeutic interpretation. These questions and confrontations can provide a forum for education. Therefore, to become defensive or closed-minded defeats the purpose of the team, and indirectly leads to stored feelings of frustration, anger, or competition that can be transmitted to clients. Once an open atmosphere exists and the goals of team meetings are explicitly discussed, constructive and nondefensive conflict resolution can begin. According to Thurkettle and Jones,[16] three basic elements must exist to facilitate conflict expression and resolution:

1. Open communication involves readiness on the part of team members to listen, talk, and feel heard by

others without rejecting comments. Team members should feel positive support and reinforcement for initiating the discussion of a concern.

2. Focusing on issues of task orientation, rather than person orientation, is used. This type of focus provides a safe and accepting environment rather than a critical one. At times, if a sensitive or anxiety-producing topic is addressed, a team member may change the focus of the meeting to a less threatening subject.

3. Mutual sharing of responsibility decreases the need for competition among team members, and eliminates dominance/subservience roles that inhibit conflict resolution.

Consistent team meetings are necessary because conflict among team members will always be present. It is essential that team members acknowledge its presence and learn strategies to resolve conflicts. Mallory[10] highlighted positive and negative differences in conflict-resolution approaches. She advocated the use of a "win–win" approach, in which an active role is maintained by both parties and a mutual decision is made, on which both parties agree. In contrast, she presented a "win–lose" situation, in which a solution to a conflict has been attained but one party feels frustrated and negative about the decision. A third approach is "lose–lose," in which the conflict is not resolved, neither party is satisfied, and both parties feel frustrated and angry.

Needless to say, consistent and honest communication among nursing staff members is essential in the treatment of all hospitalized clients to avoid unnecessary errors of judgment or partiality toward one or more clients. Even beyond client care, good communication among nursing staff members can help alleviate the potential for "burnout," a condition described by Alexander as "a condition of severe exhaustion found primarily among individuals who work in helping professions . . . characterized by physical and emotional fatigue, disillusionment, cynicism, depression, and a sense of total futility."[1] Of the five major factors that appear to foster burnout, faulty communication and work environment are both within nurses' control to correct.

The Inpatient Experience

With health insurance companies drastically cutting psychiatric benefits, the average length of hospitalization has been reduced to 2 to 5 weeks. This has begun to alter the focus of psychiatric treatment, from a long-term developmental approach to a more realistic crisis-intervention approach. Staff members have changed from use of interventions with long-term personality-change goals to use of interventions with short-term goals, in the hope that long-term change can still be achieved. However, need for work on the long-term goals will appear when clients are functioning on an outpatient basis without the consistent help of nursing staff and the safety and security that a hospital unit provides. In extreme and unfortunate

cases, repeated hospitalizations of one client have been known to occur two to seven times in one year.

Goals

The goals of short-term hospitalization vary, depending on the presenting mental status of the client and the initial psychiatric diagnosis. In a general sense, the following goals are realistic for most clients being hospitalized for the first time:

1. To stabilize the presenting conflicts and stressors/feelings that have risen to a level necessitating psychiatric hospitalization. Once these are stabilized, the client can slowly gain some clarity and insight into the conflicts and, hopefully, begin to learn stress/anxiety-reduction skills, as well as ways to avoid having feelings collect to such an immobilizing level.

2. To encourage verbalization of feelings and thoughts to members of the interdisciplinary team. This will help the client to validate or alter perceptions of reality, feel support from other adults, and gain a sense that people care for the client and want to help.

3. To provide a 24-hour-a-day medically-monitored environment for medication trials (if considered appropriate by the attending physician/psychiatrist). This is important for clients who cannot tolerate normal dosages of regularly prescribed medications.

4. To teach new coping skills that can be applied to a variety of life experiences that in the past have been frightening, overwhelming, or stressful. In some cases, trigger events in the environment repeatedly elicit maladaptive reactions or behaviors. New and more appropriate reactions can be rehearsed by the client in group therapy and in sessions with nursing staff while in the hospital, and can then be applied after discharge.

5. To encourage the client to continue psychological growth on an outpatient basis, either within the facility with the same case coordinator or in another mental health agency or private practice. The need for readmission is substantially reduced if the client can accept the need for psychological help and can actively and consistently take part in individual and/or group psychotherapy after discharge.

During hospitalization, all five goals are worked on simultaneously. Some can be achieved very quickly, while others may be achieved only partially. The focus of nursing care is to aid the client in meeting as many of these goals as possible during hospitalization.

The actual hospital stay has three distinct components or phases:

1. First, the client is in an *adjustment* or beginning phase of treatment while acclimating to the unit and becoming familiar with rules and time schedules. Even if the client believes that hospitalization is not

needed, the client begins to accept the reality of it. Usually the first three to six days are termed the "honeymoon" phase, because during them the client is often on his/her best behavior and does not appear to need psychiatric hospitalization. Immediately following the honeymoon, the client usually displays the maladaptive or inappropriate behaviors that caused hospitalization.

2. Second, the *working phase* emerges, in which trust begins to form and the client slowly opens up emotionally to the staff and other clients. The client becomes more receptive to the staff's input regarding life situations, conflicts, and how the client's inappropriate behaviors seldom elicit the responses the client really wants. The client's needs are slowly expressed, and adaptive ways of meeting those needs are shared. The client is encouraged to try out new behaviors in the milieu.

3. Third, the *termination phase* approaches once a discharge date is set. The client begins the painful process of separating from the safety and consistency of the hospital while attempting to integrate newly learned behaviors and insight into daily life.

Discharge Issues

Although clients constantly talk about how they wish they could be discharged and how they will never behave the way they did before hospitalization, clients do have difficulty in leaving the hospital, regardless of the length of their stay. For many, the caring and support they received from the interdisciplinary staff was stronger and more meaningful than what they felt at home or from their families. Saying goodbye and experiencing the feelings of loss as relationships with staff members end stir up unresolved feelings of past losses that were also painful. Therefore, clients are given the opportunity to complete a good and healthy termination, which can then serve as a model of a successful termination for future experiences.

The Family

For family members, the client's discharge stirs up many feelings as well. Prehospital anxieties surface again as the family begins to wonder if the client will be able to live outside the hospital and if the family will be able to give the support and guidance that the hospital staff has provided. Families also fear finding out whether the client really is "better," or if previously exhibited inappropriate behaviors will return. With this concern about the client's change comes the question of whether the family has changed. In most situations, family therapy throughout the hospital stay gives staff a sense of whether the client and family are compatible, and what issues need further psychological work. In many cases, family therapy is continued after discharge to provide a forum for continued exploration into conflicts occurring as the client readjusts to the home, the community, and the family.

Observing the Nursing Process

To comprehend fully the experience of an inpatient environment, it is necessary to spend time learning about the program, watching the different disciplines interacting with the clients, and, most important, talking with the clients and their families if possible.

The following clinical example summarizes the concepts presented so far in this chapter by utilizing the client's exhibited behavior as an indicator of the success of the individualized programs as well as the success of the communication among interdisciplinary and nursing team members. The three phases of treatment will be addressed, along with how nursing care plans were designed and implemented during the different phases to aid the client in working through the issues and conflicts that surfaced.

Cultural Considerations

Cultural considerations within the inpatient hospital structure include issues related to: (1) the client's cultural beliefs about family expectations, values, and home environment; and (2) the nurse's cultural background, including the same elements.

Situations have occurred in which these factors have played a major role. For example, a hospitalized black client refused to talk with anyone who was not black. Fortunately, a black staff member was able to begin the one-to-one sessions, and after this relationship was established the client slowly began to trust staff members who were not black. When a Filipino female nurse joined an adolescent nursing staff and had difficulty in pronouncing certain words, she was repeatedly mimicked by the adolescent clients. Slowly, as she adapted to the unit and became clearer in her conversation, the mimicking stopped and she was easily accepted and trusted. These are two concrete examples of how cultural considerations can affect inpatient treatment.

Many covert issues can exist, as well. Some can be resolved during hospitalization, while others may involve long-term prejudices and values. For instance, a wealthy Caucasian inpatient female was raised in a home environment with strong prejudices against Hispanics and blacks. This woman believed the stereotypes, and had never had an opportunity to change or even validate whether or not these perceptions were accurate. While in the hospital being treated for anorexia nervosa, she was shocked to see how concerned and caring Hispanic peers and staff were toward her, and that her preconceived notions were false.

Cultural variables should also be considered in the quality and type of communication expected from, and elicited by, clients and staff members. Nurses often expect clients to discuss or disclose things about themselves in certain ways that are based on the nurses' own standards. In many other cultures, however, discussing feelings is a sign of weakness and vulnerability, espe-

(*Text continues on p. 622.*)

CLINICAL EXAMPLE

Sandy was admitted to a 17-bed locked coed unit, structured around a token-economy behavioral system based on social learning principles.[13] In brief, clients were expected to earn up to 400 points per shift, based on the division of points outlined in each client's nursing care plan. At the end of each shift, the number of points earned was entered in each client's bank book. With the points, clients could buy numerous "reinforcers," which varied from special outings to extra snacks to one-to-one walks off the unit and other privileges. Each client had a regularly-assigned staff member for each shift for five of seven days a week. Staff members were responsible for continual assessment, diagnosis, intervention, and evaluation of their clients through alterations in specialized nursing care plans. In this way, consistency and continuity were provided, and growth was recognized and encouraged. On the remaining two days a week, other staff members worked with the clients by following the care plans. Therefore, clients received the same type of intervention from all shifts every day of the week.

Sandy, a 14-year-old, sullen, casually dressed, small-statured, Caucasian male was admitted for inpatient treatment to a university-based adolescent treatment unit for a three-month hospitalization. Seven months earlier, Sandy had been on a different adolescent treatment unit after making a suicide attempt. Due to a dispute with the case coordinator, however, his mother had prematurely removed him after one month, against medical advice. His mother chose to rehospitalize him, with a different case coordinator, when his inappropriate behaviors and communication problems with his family escalated sharply.

Sandy's problems upon admission were: increasingly aggressive outbursts leading to a fractured hand, deteriorating school performance, truancy, soliciting drugs, stealing, and drug experimentation (marijuana, cocaine, and LSD). Sandy had been enrolled at four different junior high schools. His mother, age 29, reported that she too had had numerous problems with drug abuse. She had had a history of numerous suicide attempts (two of which had resulted in comas), which had begun after she had been raped two years previously. Sandy's father resided in Europe, and had had no contact with Sandy since he was one year old. Sandy's upbringing was shared between his mother and his maternal grandmother, who lived separately. They had very different parenting styles. Sandy never knew who he would be staying with, or for how long. He viewed his mother as unstable, and, although he knew she had difficulty in caring for herself, he needed her nurturing and love so intensely that he had begun engaging in behaviors to attract her attention. During his development, Sandy had been hospitalized many times for pneumonia and gastrointestinal complications, along with numerous emergency visits for acute attacks of asthma.

During this second admission, Sandy presented as a withdrawn, regressed, teary-eyed adolescent with quiet ambivalence about this unexpected separation from his mother. Sandy allowed his mother to answer all the questions, even those addressed specifically to him. Occasionally, he began a sentence that his mother would interrupt and finish for him.

From the history detailed by his mother, she had been inconsistently overprotective, allowing him to do neighborhood activities for varying lengths of time, yet demanding emotional dependence from him. She seemed very attached and dependent on him, relying on him to do many household chores and make decisions that were inappropri-ate for his age and maturity level. Given this information and an assessment of their communication style, the two appeared enmeshed, with severe boundary problems stemming from the mother's inability to allow Sandy to confront adolescent individuation issues appropriately. This was further validated by the mother's expressed and demonstrated difficulty in leaving the unit, and expressions of guilt, ambivalence, clinginess, and tearfulness. Sandy, on the other hand, was excited to meet the other clients and was eager to learn about the unit's philosophy, expressing little fear or sadness about reentering the hospital or leaving his family temporarily.

While Sandy was in the *beginning phase* of the hospitalization, a standard care plan was implemented; it included encouraging Sandy to learn the names of staff and peers, and documenting any signs of aggressive threats or outbursts or self-destructive activities. A data base was collected over the next two weeks, which would supply the information necessary to create a more complex and individualized care plan. Behaviors were recorded while Sandy was engaging with peers and adults, as were defense and coping mechanisms utilized in stressful situations or during limit-setting, and the extent of ego regression.

Sandy's first two weeks were characterized by somatic complaints of headaches and muscle tension, and self-inflicted bruises, scratches, and scrapes. He initiated requests to enter the seclusion room to calm himself down. He experienced four acute asthma attacks while in self-requested isolation, three of which required subcutaneous injections of epinephrine. Clinginess, excessive demands, testing and rejecting of limits, and excessive attention-seeking were also noted. These behaviors indicated a level of ego regression and psychological development similar to that in borderline adolescents described by Masterson.[11]

To aid in the transition into the *working phase* of treatment, a second nursing care plan was formulated that targeted Sandy's inappropriate attention-seeking, display of aggression, limited social skills, and self-destructive acts. Sandy received a specific number of points for following staff instructions, use of effective ways to cope with anger, absence of self-abuse behaviors, and effective communication with others. Although initially overwhelmed by the complexity of the care plan, Sandy later expressed feelings of pride and motivation to achieve in these targeted areas. However, his inability to adapt to these expectations and developmental demands was evident with his first AWOL (absence without leave). A week later, he initiated a closed-door seclusion that resulted in banging and pounding, causing soft-tissue damage to his legs and hands. It was decided at this time that he would no longer have access to the seclusion room, but would be placed in four-point leather restraints at any sign of self-destructive behavior or aggressive acting out. Restraints were used once when he refused to stop hitting a wall.

A second AWOL occurred when he disagreed with a set limit. His difficulties with psychological growth and trust in adult role models were evident with intensified attempts to test limits, achieve autonomy, and feel comfortable and/or safe with care-taking adults. Interpretation and some confrontation were utilized in sessions to help Sandy connect with how difficult it was to follow specific limits, although they were set in his best interest and out of caring and concern for him as a person.

(Continued)

CLINICAL EXAMPLE (CONTINUED)

During the weekly interdisciplinary treatment planning, Sandy's skill in and love for recreational therapy were discussed, and the decision was made to use extra RT sessions as reinforcers for his appropriate unit behaviors. A recreational therapy participation criterion was implemented at the beginning of his second month of hospitalization. The criterion for RT participation was based on inappropriate behaviors exhibited in the milieu. Regular RT occurred at 10 a.m. for all unit clients. Two additional RTs were added to a client's program, based on skill level and emotional maturity demonstrated on the unit and during the recreational activities. Sandy responded well to this RT participation criterion, and his behavior settled down on the unit, which allowed him to take part in an average of two RTs a day.

As Sandy's behavior on the unit began to improve, day passes to home were added to his scheduled activities on Saturdays. These were also based on the effects of family therapy with his mother and grandmother. (See Chap. 12 for a discussion of family therapy.) However, with this surge of autonomy, acting out on the unit began to increase. He returned from one pass in an altered state of consciousness. In a suicide attempt, he was discovered with a pillow over his face and a bathrobe tied around his neck. He admitted to attention-seeking and testing to see if staff really cared, even if he was gaining maturity and independence. To help channel his anxiety and excessive amounts of energy, a supervised calisthenics program was instituted. He exercised whenever he felt anxious, and this promoted a sense of accomplishment as he increased his repertoire of exercises. This intervention had two benefits. He now had a healthy and adaptive activity to employ to release overwhelming feelings, and the activity nurtured his developing physique and aided in enhancing his body image and self-esteem.

Toward the end of his second month on the unit, Sandy asked to earn a higher responsibility level, a self-pass to activities, which allows the client to leave the unit unaccompanied by staff to attend an off-unit activity within the hospital. The criteria for advancement in responsibility level are outlined in Table 28-1. His initiation of this request was viewed by the interdisciplinary staff as a major step toward self-motivated autonomy; he was encouraged to meet the criteria established for him in the nursing care plan. These criteria specifically focused on self-control, impulse control, and development of appropriate and mature autonomy within socially-appropriate boundaries. On his second try, Sandy earned this privilege. He viewed this achievement as a major accomplishment, especially because there was only one other adolescent who had this privilege at this time. Two-day overnight weekend passes to home were instituted at this time as well, which Sandy tolerated well. Members of all disciplines agreed that Sandy was reformulating his self-esteem and self-concept around his new-found abilities. His success in the treatment program was also being maintained at home. His self-control improved as he showed signs of impulse control by not maladaptively acting out on the unit. Decreases in clinginess, somatic complaints, and verbal arguing were observed and documented. Sandy was definitely resolving feelings about adolescent independence and was receiving support and encouragement for each autonomous move.

During his third month, Sandy continued to try newly-formed self-controls, autonomy, and frustration tolerance. He continued demonstrating appropriate behaviors, and was becoming a more stable, less anxious, very approachable adolescent. Relationships with peers improved, and he became very outgoing, friendly, and warm. He earned the next responsibility level, an accompanied self-pass, which allowed him to go off the unit with another peer at the same responsibility level, for up to 1/2 hour at a time per shift.

Another care plan was instituted as the time for discharge approached. Sandy began showing slight behavioral regressions as he entered into the *termination phase* of treatment. This new care plan was designed to strengthen his autonomy, ego functioning, and delay of gratification, and counteract potential use of the maladaptive defense of splitting. Sandy was encouraged to be independent, and received reinforcement for appropriate moves toward individuation and autonomy. The care plan also focused on sessions in which he was encouraged to talk about surfacing feelings and fears as he approached discharge. These included anxiety and fears of abandonment and loss. Using this care plan, he attained the highest responsibility level, that of an unaccompanied self-pass, which allowed him to leave the unit unaccompanied for 1/2 hour. No other client had that status at the time, and this accomplishment was considered a major achievement by staff and peers.

Sandy continued to build his self-esteem, express his feelings, and take pride in his achievements and developing personal qualities. He was seen as a leader by staff and peers, and began initiating introductions and welcomes to the newer clients on the unit. He became less prone to taking part in activities that jeopardized his success. He tolerated and accepted delays before his needs were met, and enjoyed finding out why his needs were not met immediately. The occupational therapy staff reported that his ability to take part in long-term projects had improved, again illustrating a lengthened delay of gratification. Recreational therapy staff members reported an increase in positive peer relationships and abilities in team play. Episodes of disappointment and anger when on a losing team decreased. Finally, he was observed encouraging other peers to talk about their feelings and also attempt to gain self-control and a sense of self-worth. Previously-documented behaviors of self-destruction and somatizing had stopped, and his appearance changed into that of a mature, calm young man.

The week of discharge was difficult, with a surge of separation anxiety, self-doubt, and repeated fear of rejection and abandonment. However, he was able to express his concerns and fears verbally, and allowed the staff to reassure and nurture him. The staff encouraged him to spend time alone and then to discuss the experience, as well as to come up with ways that he could spend his time when he was at home, without engaging in drug use or other socially inappropriate behaviors. Staff members continued praising him for his accomplishments and his new-found maturity and self-control. With lots of hugs and expressions of sadness and loss, Sandy left with his mother and all of his belongings.

In summary, Sandy's treatment focused on altering self-injurious, impulsive, clingy, isolative, and anxious behaviors characteristic of impaired personality development. Utilizing social learning principles, more adaptive behaviors, and coping structures such as positive self-care, delay of gratification, increased impulse control, stable and positive interactions with peers and adults, increased tolerance of staying alone without signs of anxiety, and positive acceptance of earned free-

(Continued)

CLINICAL EXAMPLE (CONTINUED)

dom were rewarded with positive attention and encouragement. Freedom and independence seemed to be the most rewarding experiences for Sandy; when they were actualized, the negative attention-seeking activities decreased. Thus, he demonstrated that taking part in socially positive and adaptive activities felt better than having to experience the guilt and shame associated with involvement in socially maladaptive behaviors.

In analyzing the success of this case, the following variables are worth mentioning because they contributed positively to this boy's treatment:

1. Sandy's unique psychodynamic composition, along with his strong desire to grow and change, allowed the various interventions to be effective.
2. The milieu at the time of his admission was composed of predominantly nonaggressive, minimally obstinate adolescents.

3. The intricate and complicated attachments between Sandy and his therapist, assigned staff members, and interdisciplinary team therapists contributed to his improvement.
4. The extensive communication network among all members of the interdisciplinary treatment team facilitated their willingness to attempt new and different interventions, such as the detailed RT involvement.
5. Accurate assessment of Sandy's struggles and conflicts predicted when a new care plan needed to be instituted, and which variables should be included.
6. The establishment of a trusting, safe, and stable attachment with Sandy taught and role modeled adaptive and socially appropriate behaviors.
7. The staff-to-patient ratio of 1:3 allowed the time and energy to be invested in the development and follow-through of this individualized treatment program.

cially when clients have been raised by families that constantly reinforced this. If clients or staff members are unable to share, give, and accept honesty and deep emotional experiences, they are thought of as different from others. Staff and clients of other cultures can change, but it takes time, teaching, and role playing by staff members. Some individuals may decide to change some of their cultural patterns and not others. Staff can assist clients and other staff with these decisions.

Finally, the role of the family is crucial in the acceptance and understanding of the psychiatric difficulties of

the client during hospitalization. In some cultures, individuals who need psychiatric hospitalization are seen as truly ill because they are unable to cope with everyday pressures. In other cultures such ill individuals are kept at home. Flaskerud[6] has summarized many findings about cultural aspects of inpatient care and implications for nursing.

Summary

TABLE 28-1.
CRITERIA FOR ADVANCEMENT IN RESPONSIBILITY LEVEL

(for three consecutive days)
A. *Self-Pass to Activities:* Attained January 16, 1989
   1. Earning 300 points a shift based on the care plan
   2. Remaining on the unit or within eyesight of staff when off the unit
   3. Attending all of the scheduled recreational programs
B. *Accompanied Self-Pass:* Attained January 29, 1989
   1. Earning 350 points per shift based on the care plan
   2. Adherence to the rules of the Self-Pass to Activities, and remaining on the unit when not involved in off-the-unit activities
   3. Compliance at bedtime without need of further nursing intervention (*e.g.,* foot treatment for warts to be completed before 10 p.m., settling appropriately)
C. *Unaccompanied Self-Pass:* Attained February 16, 1989
   1. Earning 400 points per shift based on the care plan
   2. Adherence to the rules of the Accompanied Self-Pass and remaining on the unit when not involved in off-the-unit activities
   3. Adherence to milieu rules
   4. Remaining within eyesight of staff when in a group off the unit
   5. Compliance at bedtime, as described in B.3. above

1. Upon admission to a psychiatric unit, clients may feel a sense of safety and security as well as demoralized. Families of clients may feel overwhelmed, guilty, and frightened.
2. When the inpatient hospital is viewed as a system, the subunits of this system include the unit structure (physical environment) and the various adjunctive services, such as the nursing staff, management, and recreational and occupational therapy.
3. The interdisciplinary treatment team functions to assure high quality care. While the treatment team works to assure a high level of unit functioning, role confusion and other types of conflict can develop.
4. The therapeutic use of self by nurses includes a willingness to understand and work on the nurse's conflicts with clients, personal issues, and the interdisciplinary team.
5. Intrashift and intershift conflicts may affect the nursing team. These conflicts are resolved by frequent meetings and discussions among nursing staff.
6. Splitting occurs when clients project their own concerns about having a "good" self and a "bad" self onto staff. Clients then think of particular staff or

treatment programs as all good or all bad. Splitting is dealt with by recognition of clients' behaviors and remaining consistent in the treatment approach.

7. Effective communication among treatment team members includes honest and open discussion of problem treatment-related issues.

8. Clients on an inpatient unit achieve particular goals as a result of their hospitalization. These include learning new coping skills and adjustment to treatment regimens such as medications.

9. Family responses to a member's hospital discharge include anxieties about whether or not the client is truly better. Family discussions with staff can assist in smoothing the discharge transition.

10. Cultural considerations, such as clients' and staffs' belief systems, affect client care.

References

1. Alexander C: Counteracting burnout. AORN J 32:597, 1980
2. Benfer B: Defining the role and function of the psychiatric nurse as a member of the team. Perspect Psychiatr Care 18:166, 1980
3. Brill N: Teamwork: Working Together in the Human Services. Philadelphia, JB Lippincott, 1976
4. Brown G, Birley J, Wing J: Influence of family life on the courses of schizophrenic disorders: A replication. Br J Psychiatry 121:241, 1972
5. Carser D: The defense mechanism of splitting: Developmental origins, effects on staff, recommendations for nursing care. J Psychosoc Nurs Ment Health Serv 17:21, 1979
6. Flaskerud J: Community mental health nursing: Its unique role in the delivery of services to ethnic minorities. Perspect Psychiatr Care 20:37, 1982
7. Gralnick A: The nature of the psychiatric hospital: An exploration into the development of one such. Psychiatr Hosp 14:29, 1983
8. Harbin H: The Psychiatric Hospital and the Family. New York, SP Medical and Scientific Books, 1981
9. Leavitt M: The discharge crisis: The experience of families of psychiatric patients. Nurs Res 24:33, 1975
10. Mallory G: Turn conflict into cooperation. Nurs 85 15:81, 1985
11. Masterson J: Treatment of the Borderline Adolescent: A Developmental Approach. New York, Brunner/Mazel, 1985
12. Minuchin S: Families and Family Therapy. Cambridge, Massachusetts, Harvard University Press, 1974
13. Rimm D, Masters J: Behavior Therapy: Techniques and Empirical Findings. New York, Academic Press, 1974
14. Romoff V, Kane I: Primary nursing in psychiatry: An effective and functional model. Perspect Psychiatr Care 20:73, 1982
15. Ruch M: The multidisciplinary team: When too many is too much. J Psychosoc Nurs Ment Health Serv 22:18, 1984
16. Thurkettle M, Jones S: Conflict as a systems process: Theory and management. J Nurs Admin 8:39, 1978

SALLY KNORR-NEWMAN

AFTERCARE AND EXTENDED CARE SERVICES

Learning Objectives

Upon completion of this chapter the student should be able to do the following:

1. Define aftercare and discuss the historical roots of aftercare and extended care services.
2. Apply Caplan's concepts of prevention to aftercare and extended care.
3. Compare and contrast four types of residential care available to psychiatric clients as part of the mental health aftercare delivery system.
4. Describe the following: aftercare clinics, transitional care, partial hospitalization, vocational rehabilitation services, and self-help groups.
5. Describe the role and functions of the psychiatric nurse in aftercare and extended care services.

Introduction

"But it is so very hard to be an on-your-own, take-care-of-yourself-'cause-there-is-no-one-else-to-do-it-for-you grown-up."[42]

In the past 150 years, ideas about the care and treatment of the mentally ill have come full circle. Public pol-

icy has moved from an emphasis on care of the psychiatrically impaired in the local community, to one of housing them in state institutions, only to return to the recent trend toward shorter hospital stays and discharge back into the community. This trend began with the Community Mental Health movement in the early 1960s. With this shift in treatment philosophy, aftercare, once the stepchild of mental health services, is now an important focus in psychiatric care.

Historical Roots of Aftercare

Adolf Meyer, a Swiss psychiatrist and one of the most influential psychiatrists of the 20th century, served as director of the psychiatric clinic at Johns Hopkins University in the early 1900s. He advocated the therapeutic function of aftercare programs for the released mental patient. He developed the idea of using social workers, in conjunction with clients' families, to help clients return to the community.[22] Aftercare services were viewed, not only as a continuing treatment mechanism, but also as a social control mechanism for supervising former mental patients living in the community. The terminology, adopted from the penal system, reveals societal attitudes toward aftercare at the time; in the early days of aftercare, clients discharged from the hospital to community care were said to be "on parole."

Impact of Federal Programs

Prior to World War II, the federal government played a very small role in the mental health care delivery system. In the 1950s, however, a series of scientific, social, and political developments culminated in the movement toward community-based care for the mentally ill. Advances in psychopharmacology allowed many patients requiring long-term care to be hospitalized for shorter periods and discharged into the community. Paralleling the development of psychopharmacology were both the introduction of new psychosocial treatment modalities and the increasing availability of mental health facilities in the community that offered alternatives to lengthy hospital stays.

The Mental Health Study Act (Public Law 84-182) was enacted in 1955 as the U.S. Congress responded to the growing pressure for reassessment of the mental health care program in the United States. The Joint Commission on Mental Illness and Health was formed to carry out this congressional mandate. In 1961 its final report, *Action for Mental Health,*[8] was delivered. President Kennedy was receptive to the recommendations of the Joint Commission, and in a message to Congress proposed the establishment of a national mental health program. This was the first time in U.S. history that a president addressed the topic of mental illness and health. The Community Mental Health Centers Act (Public Law 88-164) was passed and signed into law in October 1963, less than a month before Kennedy's death.

This act provided funds for the construction of community centers that were to provide at least five essential services: inpatient care, outpatient care, partial (day and night) hospitalization, 24-hour emergency service, and community services (consultation and education). While

the Joint Commission had strongly recommended a detailed community aftercare program, legislators who drew up Public Law 88-164 did not include aftercare among these five essential services. Aftercare and rehabilitation were categorized as optional services. However, in the years following the passage of the Community Mental Health Centers Act, the U.S. Congress has extended or amended the act on several occasions. Public Law 94-63, enacted in 1975, gave new guidelines for the five essential services, and mandated provision of aftercare service.

Since the "Golden Age" of the community mental health movement in the 1960s and early 1970s, aftercare and extended care have received more attention and government support. Deinstitutionalization, however, an outcome of the community mental health movement, has had its share of problems. While advances in psychopharmacology, Medicare and Medicaid, and federal aid to the mentally disabled through Supplemental Security Income (SSI) have made the move to community care possible, the increasing number of "revolving door patients" and the presence of "psychiatric ghettos" in the community give evidence that much more funding is needed for community rehabilitative programming.

Aftercare and Extended Care Ideology

As described earlier, psychiatrist Adolf Meyer was an early proponent of aftercare and extended care. More than 70 years ago, Meyer expressed some of the basic tenets of this movement. He felt that chronic mental illness was not handled by "merely patching up" the patient. He advocated "straightening out the environment" and preparing the patient to meet the difficulties that might be encountered following discharge. Rejecting the earlier English model of aftercare that focused primarily on providing a few months of lodging for ex-patients in need of housing, Meyer described aftercare in broader terms and related it to prophylaxis:

> " 'Aftercare' . . . consists of finding an occupation for patients who are leaving the institution and trying to live again in the community, and helping make the reentrance into the community easy and safe against relapses."[17]

His comments highlight the need for aftercare, and his emphasis on community care remains valid today.

Definition

Aftercare and *extended care* are the terms used in psychiatric literature to describe the total treatment program for psychiatric clients after their discharge from the hospital. It includes pre-discharge planning, post-hospital residential living arrangements, medication follow-up, individual and/or group therapy, family education, partial hospitalization (day or night hospitals), vocational rehabilitation, and resocialization services such as self-help groups. It encompasses all clients discharged from mental hospitals, regardless of diagnosis.

Levels of Prevention

Caplan distinguished among three types of preventive efforts: *primary prevention* (the elimination of factors that cause or contribute to the incidence of mental disorders), *secondary prevention* (the early detection and prompt treatment of disorders that have already occurred), and *tertiary prevention* (the elimination or reduction of disability associated with a particular mental disorder).[4] Neither secondary nor tertiary prevention is prevention in the usual sense, so it may be less confusing to use the terms *treatment* and *rehabilitation* when addressing the subjects of aftercare and extended care.

Early detection and prompt treatment of mental disorders are the foci of secondary prevention efforts. Effective treatment includes aftercare planning, and should begin with the initial diagnosis of mental illness when hospitalization is required. Short-term hospitalization and discharge to a community care system may be the treatment of choice for both acute and chronic mental health clients.

In tertiary prevention, the focus is on the client who has suffered from a mental disorder and is attempting to readjust to community life. Aftercare and extended care services that enable clients to function with maximum effectiveness as soon as possible following discharge are *major* components of the tertiary prevention program. Rehabilitation is the primary goal, with the prevention of further deterioration or recurrence of a psychiatric disability as the ultimate desired outcome.

Community Support Systems Model

The rise of community mental health services and the parallel decreases in state mental hospital systems have led to the return of great numbers of chronically mentally ill persons to their communities. Community support systems have emerged as a new conceptual model to improve the quality of life of the chronically mentally ill who live in community settings. As adapted by the Community Support Program (CSP) of the National Institute of Mental Health, the model specifies essential guidelines for comprehensive care. These components are listed in Table 29-1. As defined, these components extend beyond the boundaries of the mental health system and require coordination with other health and human service agencies.[27]

The intent of the community support program is to make available a broad array of services to chronically mentally ill individuals, each of whom has needs that are unique and change over time. These services and opportunities can be clustered under the following general categories:

- Basic life needs
- Health and mental health treatment services
- Rehabilitation services
- Social support services
- Integrative services

These services are further defined in Table 29-2.

Planning for Aftercare

For most clients, the major function of psychiatric hospitalization should be preparation for aftercare. Unfortunately, it is easy for staff to overlook this perspective, focusing instead on specific treatments while attempting to help clients adjust to life inside (rather than outside) the hospital. The ultimate goal of hospitalization is to reintegrate clients into the community, restoring them to the fullest possible normal living within the limitations of their emotional handicaps.

Hospitalization produces unique problems that may foster dependency and regression. Hospitalized clients develop dependence on the hospital and staff and the sense of security associated with the hospital setting.[31] An

TABLE 29-1.
GUIDELINES FOR THE PROVISION OF A COMMUNITY SUPPORT SYSTEM

1. *Identify the population at risk* through outreach programs or case-finding, and assure access to needed services.
2. *Help disabled individuals apply for entitlement benefits* such as income assistance, SSI, and Medicaid.
3. *Provide 24-hour crisis assistance,* aimed at improving community ties by offering a rapid response to the disabled in the community, perhaps avoiding hospitalization.
4. *Provide psychosocial rehabilitation services,* including programs that train clients in community living skills, develop social skills, and improve clients' ability to secure employment.
5. *Provide supportive services of indefinite duration,* such as special housing options and sheltered employment.
6. *Provide adequate medical and mental health care,* including diagnostic evaluation, medication management, and community-based psychiatric services.
7. *Offer back-up support, assistance, and consultation* to families and significant others, to maximize benefits and minimize problems associated with mentally disabled individuals living in the community.
8. *Provide natural support systems* by involving concerned community members in planning community support systems.
9. *Protect client rights* by providing clients with education concerning their legal rights, mental health advocacy, and establishment of grievance procedures.
10. *Provide case management* to facilitate the movement of clients through the system and assist them in securing needed services.

(Adapted from NIMH Definitions and Guidelines for Community Support Systems, NIMH, July 29, 1977.)

TABLE 29-2.
COMPREHENSIVE SERVICES AND OPPORTUNITIES
FOR THE CHRONIC MENTALLY ILL

BASIC NEEDS/OPPORTUNITIES	SPECIAL NEEDS/OPPORTUNITIES
SHELTER *Protected* (services on site) • Hospital • Intermediate-care facility • Semi-independent (linked to services) • Family-care home • Board-and-care home • Cooperative apartments	**TREATMENT SERVICES** *Medical Services* • Physician assessment and care • Nursing assessment and care • Dentist assessment and care • Physical/Occupational therapy • Medication counseling • Home health services
FOOD, CLOTHING, AND HOUSEHOLD MANAGEMENT • Fully-provided meals • Access to food stamps • Homemaker services	*Mental Health Services* • Acute treatment services • Assessment and diagnosis • Medication monitoring • Psychotherapies • Hospitalization: acute and long-term care • Crisis intervention • Self-medication training
INCOME/FINANCIAL SUPPORT • Access to entitlements • Employment	**REHABILITATION SERVICES** • Social/recreational skills development • Life skills development • Leisure time activities
MEANINGFUL ACTIVITIES • Work opportunities • Recreation • Education • Religious/spiritual activities	**VOCATIONAL SERVICES** • Pre-vocational assessment and counseling • Sheltered work • Transitional employment • Job placement
MOBILITY/TRANSPORTATION • Special discounts for public transportation	**SOCIAL SERVICES** • Family support • Community support • Legal services • Entitlement assistance • Housing management
INTEGRATIVE SERVICES • Outreach • Case management • Advocacy • Community information • Education and support	

important step in planning for aftercare is to undo this dependency and regression as clients prepare to return to the community. Clients need help in developing positive attitudes toward rehabilitation.

The Nurse and the Therapeutic Use of Self

The role of the nurse is crucial in assuring post-discharge adjustment. Through their interactions with clients, nurses can use interpersonal relationships to enhance clients' learning of new skills. Clients can be helped to learn to trust others, to acquire self-confidence and self-esteem, and to progress from dependence to independence. Pre-discharge planning should begin at the time of admission and should involve both clients and their families. Nurses are the professionals that are most intimately associated with hospitalized clients, and are frequently the persons most keenly aware of their problems and needs. Nursing input to other members of the treatment team is vital in the formulation of a comprehensive aftercare treatment plan.

Discharge planning begins by addressing four questions:

1. Where will the client go, and with whom will the client live following hospitalization?
2. How will the client be supported?
3. How will the client's time be structured?
4. What kind of psychiatric follow-up will the client require?

The transition from hospital to community should involve preplanning and discussion. Schwartz and Schwartz discuss the importance of grading stress and tailoring aftercare to the individual's needs.[24] Through grading of stress (providing opportunities for the gradual assumption of responsibility), clients are enabled to resume social functioning and their vulnerability to incidents that could produce crises is decreased. Examples of grading stress in preparation for discharge include use of overnight passes and weekend visits that allow clients to readjust gradually to community living and family life.

The Client as a System

In planning for aftercare, nurses must assess each component of the client as a system. Specific concerns in planning for aftercare include five systems elements, as follows.

1. *The environment.* In what type of environment is the client presently? Will this environment provide the necessary support for this client after hospitalization? For example, the withdrawn and socially isolated schizophrenic client who lives alone may do better in a family-care placement than in a large board-and-care home where it is possible to "fade into the woodwork."
2. *Cultural aspects.* How is mental illness viewed in the client's culture? What impact will this have on psychiatric follow-up? For example, a Roman Catholic Latino client may be reluctant to attend an aftercare medication group held in the community mental health satellite clinic housed in a Baptist church in the neighborhood. The client might be more likely to utilize the medication group at the main clinic in the county psychiatric hospital where the client received inpatient care.
3. *Societal aspects.* Does the government provide adequate community supports for the client after hospitalization? Will new board-and-care homes be accepted by the local community? What does the community offer in the form of aid to the homeless chronically mentally ill? Often homeless mentally ill clients move to urban locations where there are shelters and meal programs, but are reluctant to apply for government aid due to the complexity of the application process. Clients may need to have social workers help them with the application process prior to discharge.
4. *Physical aspects.* What is the health status of the client? Are there any physical limitations that would interfere with the client's ability to manage medications or to provide self-care? The depressed older client with a hearing problem may not do well with a referral to a transitional care group because of difficulty in hearing group interactions. This client might do better with follow-up from a supportive individual therapist.
5. *Psychological aspects.* How does the client view the mental illness? What are the client's present coping skills? How does the client respond to stress? Will long-term follow-up be required? For example, the paranoid client may not do well in a short-term day treatment program with many students rotating

through it. This client may do better in a weekly supportive outpatient group with consistent co-leaders.

The Nursing Process

Assessment

Nurses working with clients in aftercare use the nursing process to provide care. Nurses assess clients according to the clients' cultural, psychological, social, physical, and environmental characteristics. Frequent concerns that appear with chronically mentally ill clients are:

Poor impulse control
Low self-esteem
Noncompliance with prescribed medication regimens
Lack of independent living skills
Social isolation
Poor time-structuring
Difficulty in making decisions
Inattention to grooming and personal hygiene
Lack of social skills
Few support systems
Limited ability to deal with stress

Nursing Diagnoses

Based on a thorough assessment, the nurse formulates nursing diagnoses. Common diagnoses that occur with the chronic psychiatric patient in need of aftercare are:

1. Noncompliance with medication regimens, related to:
   Recurrence of psychiatric symptoms
   Resistance to psychiatric treatment
   Lack of medication education
   Limited financial resources and ability to acquire medications
2. Low self-esteem, related to:
   Lack of social skills
   Ineffective interpersonal relationships
3. Poor time-structuring, related to:
   Lack of independent living skills
   Limited financial resources
   Recurrence of psychiatric symptoms

Treatment Goals

Nurses formulate treatment goals based on the assessment and nursing diagnoses. Specific treatment goals for clients with chronic mental health problems include:

Establishing interpersonal relationships in the community
Developing basic independent living skills
Decreasing social isolation and improving time-structuring through involvement in day treatment programs, three days per week
Developing or increasing feelings of self-worth

Expressing anger or hostility outwardly in a safe manner
Demonstrating an increased ability to cope with anxiety and stress

Nursing Interventions

Nurses carry out interventions based on assessment, nursing diagnoses, and goals of treatment. Some interventions used in providing aftercare follow:

1. *Help clients comply with prescribed medication regimens.* Explore clients' reasons for noncompliance. Can they afford the medicine? Do they forget to take it? Are they afraid of side-effects? If clients cannot remember to take medicine, set up a system with them to check off medication times or encourage use of a pill box with separate compartments for each dose.
2. *Help clients develop leisure skills, plans for unstructured time, and increased socialization skills.* Help clients make specific plans for unstructured time. Role play social interactions with clients. Encourage involvement in past hobbies. Assist clients in locating community resources, such as social clubs and community recreation centers.
3. *Promote clients' self-esteem.* Help clients increase self-esteem by demonstrating an honest interest and concern. Provide opportunities for clients to succeed at activities, tasks, and interactions. Give positive feedback and point out clients' demonstrated abilities and strengths. Support clients' positive actions in viewing themselves and their abilities realistically. Encourage clients to explore options for volunteer work.

Evaluation

Nurses should constantly evaluate treatment plans. If interventions are not successful, new ones should be tried. If interventions appear to be helpful but treatment goals have not been met, the interventions may need to be revised or expanded. The evaluation of the treatment plan for clients in aftercare is frequently carried out in the form of an interdisciplinary team meeting.

Transitional Care

Continuity of care is an important part of the aftercare delivery system. Transition group meetings can act as a link from hospital to community for many clients. Some types of transition groups begin while clients are still hospitalized, but help staff and clients to anticipate discharge in the near future. The group, frequently co-led by a nurse and an occupational therapist, deals with issues involving transition back into the community. It allows members to express their feelings about returning to the community and helps them deal with their separation from the hospital.

Transition groups are not strictly therapy groups, because they may also include the teaching of basic daily

living skills and education concerning medications and follow-up care. Often this type of transition group encourages former inpatients to continue to attend the group for the first two to three weeks after discharge. This allows role-modeling for clients newer to the group and provides support for former inpatients in their first weeks in the community.

Another type of transitional care group begins upon discharge. This transitional care program lasts for 10 to 12 weeks, and consists of a three-hour weekly meeting, usually held in the evening. Nursing staff members act as primary therapists and lead a team meeting in which clients review their treatment plans and progress. Group discussion ensures social reinforcement for adaptive change and assists in the development of problem-solving skills. Interactions among clients outside of the group are encouraged, and social support networks are formed. This system helps clients to see themselves as responsible and capable of assisting one another, rather than always looking for help from the staff.

A community meeting follows the team meeting, and is a time when issues related to the entire program are addressed. These issues may include absenteeism, lateness, and group structure as well as acknowledgement of a client's successful termination from the program. These meetings are member-led, with staff acting as consultants.

Transitional care programs have the potential to shorten hospitalization, decrease readmission rates, and maintain newly acquired behaviors after discharge.[9] Utilizing nursing staff who have worked with clients in the hospital to co-lead transition groups not only assures continuity of care for clients, but also provides a chance for inpatient nursing staff to see the fruits of their labor. The time-limited nature of these programs decreases the likelihood of fostering maladaptive dependency on the hospital as well as clients' unhealthy identification with the patient role.

Aftercare and Extended Care Services

Residential Care

In Belgium in the 15th century, the colony of Gheel was formed; it has offered sheltered community care to the mentally ill ever since then. Clients are placed with local families who provide foster home care. Gheel is an agricultural community, and almost two thirds of the clients live on farms. It is the philosophy of the colony that this rural setting offers a variety of activities and that a job can be found for everybody. The tradition of caring for the mentally ill in a family setting is still being practiced successfully today, not only in Gheel but also in many other countries. In the United States, family foster care is one of the variety of options available to mentally ill clients who require community-based sheltered placement.

Placement Considerations

Three possible community settings are available to psychiatric clients upon discharge from the hospital: they may live with their families, live alone, or live in a residential aftercare facility. The hospital has provided a highly structured, well-regulated, and tightly organized institutional shelter in which responsibility for clients' care has been largely assumed by others. The transition from this environment to the community, where individuals are expected to assume full responsibility for their conduct, often proves too stressful for former inpatients.

Residential aftercare facilities serve as "a bridge back to the community." Some provide less structured care with an emphasis on gradual increases in clients' control over their activities and interests. Others offer permanent residences for chronically mentally ill clients. Facilities vary in size, philosophy of care, and type of management. Small residences or family-care homes offer lodging for one to six former inpatients. They are run family-style, with shared meals and activities supervised by the family-care operator, who assumes a parental role in the facility. Board-and-care homes house larger numbers of clients and are more like apartments. They provide room and board, as well as varying degrees of supervision, recreation, and rehabilitation. Halfway houses, intermediate in size, provide a temporary residence, acting as a transitional environment for clients following discharge from the hospital.

Community-based sheltered care serves three basic functions:

1. A temporary, transitional facility for clients who are unable to live independently in the community
2. A permanent placement for clients with chronic mental illness problems
3. An alternative to hospitalization

Despite the diverse environmental settings of various sheltered care facilities, they all share a common goal: to integrate clients into the internal system of the facility and the external activities of the community.

Placement in sheltered care is usually the responsibility of two organizations, state mental hospitals and the bureau of social work (now referred to in some states as the community care services section of the Department of Health). Other agencies also involved in placement include county mental hospitals, county community mental health services, and private mental hospitals. The goal of successful placement is to match potential residents to the facilities that will best meet their needs.

Continuity of care is important in the transition from hospital to community. Pre-discharge planning is crucial. Medicaid and SSI are usually necessary to assure sufficient funds to cover residential care and follow-up psychiatric services and medications. If possible, clients should visit potential placement sites in the community, prior to discharge. The involvement of clients and their families in aftercare plans increases the likelihood of positive post-hospital adjustment for them. Ignoring clients' input diminishes their integrity at a time when their self-concept is already impaired. Frequently, clients know

better than the staff what type of placement would best suit their needs.

Several considerations are important in determining the best residential care placement for a given client:

1. What are the client's treatment needs?
2. At what level can the client be expected to function?
3. How will the client's personality match the personalities of the staff and other residents at a given facility?
4. What are the client's financial resources?
5. What residential care options are available in the local community?

By assessing the client's treatment needs and level of function, the facility best suited to the client can be chosen. Does the client need the closeness and nurturing environment that a family-care setting may offer? Is a locked facility with 24-hour supervision necessary to help the client regain a sense of security and control? Does the client's need for distance from others dictate placement in a large board-and-care facility? Is a transitional setting indicated by the client's need for greater freedom and a higher level of independent functioning?

Personality is another placement determinant. One must take into consideration, not only the personality of the client to be placed, but also the personality of the staff and fellow residents living in the facility. A mothering care-taker and passive, dependent fellow residents would cause conflict for an active, independent client. Likewise, a regressed or passive client would not do well in a facility where staff expect independent functioning and quick treatment successes.

Financial resources are a critical part of the placement process. Most clients who require community-based residential care depend on SSI to meet these costs. While residential care costs much less than hospitalization, there is little spending money left to cover living expenses after the SSI check pays for room and board. If the client is not already on SSI, the cost of placement must be assumed by either the client or the family until SSI is obtained. Private health insurance and Medicaid are necessary to cover treatment and medication costs.

After these issues are addressed, placement may still be a problem. Choices are often limited due to an inadequate variety of residential-care alternatives in the local community. Availability is also affected by timing. There may be appropriate facilities in the area, but they might not have a vacancy at the time placement is needed for a given client. This sometimes results in longer hospital stays or, more commonly, discharge to the client's home as an intermediate step in the placement process.

Another important factor in the consideration of residential treatment is the extent to which residents are *enveloped* by their housing facility.[14] The more care-taking a facility provides, the fewer life choices the residents are required to make for themselves, which provides a greater degree of envelopment. An example of a high-envelopment facility is the therapeutic residential center that provides 24-hour care in a highly structured and protected environment. Mid-range-envelopment facilities include board-and-care and family-care homes, where nonintensive interaction and some supervision are provided. Low-envelopment resources include satellite housing and cooperative apartments. In these facilities, groups of clients live and work together, managing their own activities of daily living with minimal professional assistance or supervision. A guiding principle in community placement is that the chosen facility should offer the least envelopment possible while still meeting the client's treatment needs. Treatment should also be geared toward moving the client toward lower levels of envelopment.

Types of Residential Care

Family-Care Homes

The family-care home is one of the oldest forms of community-based sheltered care for the mentally ill. Family-care homes have existed in the United States since the late 1800s, and have traditionally been a form of placement for the chronically mentally ill. These programs place mentally ill clients in the community with foster families, and are sometimes referred to as *family foster care.*

Family-care facilities are small (one to six beds), and qualify under state zoning laws as single-family units. They are usually located in suburban and single-family areas. Clients are supervised by a family-care operator who is provided with professional support, usually from a social worker. Many family-care homes are sponsored by social-service organizations and have their service needs brokered by a social worker from the organization.[25] The family-care operator relies on the social worker to obtain medical and social services when needed by clients.

While family-care programs have been in existence for many years, the overall growth of such programs has been limited. Morrissey reports that in 1963 there were 13,000 mentally ill people in family-care homes in the United States, plus about 4,000 in similar programs operated by the Veterans Administration.[19] The resident population in mental institutions at that time exceeded one half million.

The slow growth of family-care programs appears to be related to a number of factors: public anxiety about the return of mentally ill clients to the community; legislative resistance to appropriation of sufficient funds to support such programs; and the apathy and resistance to the idea of family-care placement on the part of some psychiatrists, especially those affiliated with state hospital systems. However, the concept of family care has been accepted for economic reasons: family-care homes are less expensive than hospitalization for clients and free beds for acutely ill clients.

Despite limited growth, family-care programs have made an important contribution to the establishment of community-based care for the mentally ill. They have provided chronically ill clients with sheltered care in the community, and have enabled segments of the public to become accustomed to the treatment of and care for the mentally ill in their own neighborhoods. Family-care programs have also moved mental health personnel out of hospitals and into communities, giving them experience in the placement and supervision of clients in sheltered-care settings. This experience proved especially valuable during the 1960s, when additional resources became available and a large community placement program was undertaken.

Halfway Houses

The name *halfway house* implies the transitional nature of these residential-care facilities. In the late 1800s, Britain provided the earliest model of halfway-house placement of the mentally ill, offering *hostels* as an intermediate form of care for discharged mentally ill clients; later hostels were used as an alternative to hospitalization for some emotionally disturbed individuals living in the community.[13] The formal development of halfway houses in the United States came much later, beginning in the 1950s.

Glasscote and colleagues defined a halfway house as follows:

> . . . a non-medical residential facility specifically intended to enhance the capabilities of people who are mentally ill, or who are impaired by residual deficits from mental illness, to remain in the community, participating to the fullest possible extent in community life.[10]

While the major aim of the halfway house is to provide a temporary residence, a permanent residence may be necessary for people who are unable to live independently, and some halfway houses also meet this need.

As transitional placements, halfway houses attempt to strike the proper balance between rehabilitation measures and the need to provide a homelike environment. These facilities are often started by professionals and community-sponsored. They are frequently viewed as models of care for the mentally ill residing in the community, and are more likely than other forms of sheltered care to have access to community funding.

Potential halfway-house residents may be referred by a therapist, a social worker, a vocational rehabilitation counselor, or their family. There is usually a screening process in which the application for residence is reviewed by the halfway-house staff and the applicant is interviewed. Each halfway house has specific admission criteria. While these may vary from house to house, conditions that usually disqualify an applicant for admission include: destructive impulses toward self or others; poor impulse control; drug or alcohol abuse; uncontrolled sexual promiscuity; and characterological problems. Careful screening of applicants is important because it helps the staff to assess clients' strengths and weaknesses and to evaluate whether or not this would be an appropriate community placement for them.

Once applicants are accepted, they are notified and, in many cases, move in following discharge from the hospital. Residents usually share a room, and an attempt is made to match roommates who are likely to be compatible and to develop a friendship. The roommate system helps to facilitate socialization and creates an internal support system for residents. It can also provide checks and balances for the house's clinical program and its behavioral codes, helping to prevent illicit drinking, sex, drugs, and antisocial behavior.[3] The clinical program of halfway houses focuses on helping residents to develop life skills. This may include learning how to manage money, becoming oriented to the local community and its resources, or even more basic tasks such as doing laundry, handling self-care needs, and maintaining clients' rooms. There is a strong emphasis on teaching the skills of daily living that allow residents to function more independently.

Social integration is another focus of the halfway-house program. Recreational and leisure groups are offered, and residents are encouraged to participate in these social activities. House meetings, usually held once a week, provide an additional source of social interaction. These meetings are sometimes resident-led, and topics include issues ranging from announcements and administrative changes to in-depth discussion of individual and group concerns.

Most halfway houses expect their residents to have some form of meaningful involvement during the day. Initially, this may take the form of participation in structured activities and treatment programs such as group therapy, which is offered at the facility. Because this is a transitional setting, however, residents are encouraged to expand their involvement to include community resources such as school, work, and recreational programs. The goal of treatment is to return residents to the community when they are able to function independently.

Board-and-Care Homes

The board-and-care type of community-based sheltered facility is the largest placement resource for long-term clients. Board-and-care homes are usually privately owned and operated, and usually offer the least therapeutic milieu.[14] While the size of the facility may vary, the majority of these homes serve 50 or more residents, who may be housed in converted apartment buildings. In California, board-and-care homes service 82% of the population living in sheltered-care settings.[25]

Most board-and-care facilities share certain common characteristics, including: (1) they are usually unlocked facilities; (2) shared rooms are provided; (3) three meals are offered a day; (4) administration of medications is supervised; and (5) staff supervision is minimal. The length of stay for a resident may vary from six months to an indefinite period for more chronically ill clients. The primary services offered are supervision and socialization. Unlike halfway houses, there is no emphasis on active rehabilitation. Perhaps this is the reason that critics of the board-and-care home programs refer to them as "mini-mental institutions in the community" and see the care provided as simply "warehousing" of chronically ill clients.

General health and medical supervision are often lacking. This may be due to the lack of coordination of services between involved agencies and the board-and-care home. Other factors include the reluctance of some physicians to treat this chronically ill population, the difficulty of chronically ill clients in recognizing problems and seeking help, and the lack of trained staff to provide care.

Given these problems, it is clear that an effort is needed to make board-and-care homes more therapeutic. Consultation to board-and-care operators and their staff by nurses is one way to upgrade the treatment programs. Educational training programs for residential-care administrators offer support and information that facilitate the process of involving these administrators in helping their residents make the transition to community life.

Cooperative Apartments

Perhaps the newest type of community-based sheltered care for the mentally ill is the cooperative apartment program. In this setting, adults labeled as mentally disabled can have their own apartments and live independently without on-site professional supervision, yet with an available agency support system. The movement toward this type of community residence can be traced back to the late 1950s, when Fountain House initiated some of the first cooperative apartments in order to help clients stay out of hospitals and hold jobs.[11] Since then, cooperative apartment programs, sometimes referred to as *satellite housing,* have spread, and are often part of transitional residential services provided by mental health agencies involved in community-based residential care programs.

The cooperative apartment program has the following basic characteristics: (1) a mental health-related agency may act as lessee of an apartment for two or more clients for a period of time; (2) the agency screens and selects the clients who are to live together; and (3) a mental health professional or paraprofessional acts as consultant and may call or visit at regular intervals. This type of program offers several advantages over traditional community residences, including decreased cost and normalizing community involvement.

One model of this type of program is the landlord-supervised apartment that provides a landlord, living on the premises, who serves a supportive and rehabilitative function, helping formerly hospitalized clients to learn daily living skills and community survival. Residents are responsible for their own cooking, cleaning, shopping, and laundry. They are expected to manage their own affairs, including budgeting and compliance with medication regimens.

For many clients who need to be maintained on medication, a long-acting phenothiazine (fluphenazine decanoate) is prescribed. Because the medication is given by injection, the client is expected to keep outpatient clinic appointments on scheduled dates. If the client does not show up within 48 hours, the staff nurse involved with the cooperative apartment program goes to the client's apartment to administer the medication.[6]

Cooperative apartment programs often interface with other residential care programs providing a stepping stone to community living. For some formerly hospitalized clients, gradual entry into the community may begin with a halfway house, followed by a landlord-supervised cooperative apartment with visiting staff from an affiliated mental health facility. This community group living situation can be either an endpoint for those who require a semi-sheltered setting, or the last part of a bridge to independent living in the community. This bridge is crossed when the client moves into a permanent housing arrangement.

Community Reactions to Residential Care

Residential-care facilities are a means of providing shelter to the mentally ill who have no available social networks and who are unable to live independently. The fact that these facilities are located in the community has naturally had an impact, and public response has not always been positive. Community reactions seem to be based on several factors: (1) a perceived threat to the community posed by former mental health clients; (2) a stereotypical fear of the mentally ill; (3) odd or bizarre behavior exhibited by some mentally ill persons in the community; (4) a concern about the effect of a residential-care facility on property values in the local community.

While the concern about a physical threat posed by former inpatients residing in the community is not without some basis in fact, a careful evaluation of studies in this area helps to clarify the issue. Most research on the threat that discharged mental hospital clients represent to the public does indicate a higher incidence of violent crime among these clients,[33] but does *not* distinguish between clients who return to their families or relatives or more transient lifestyles and those who are living in residential-care settings. The impression, based on available studies, is that the involvement in violent crimes of released clients residing in sheltered-care settings is overestimated by the public. Perhaps this is due, in part, to the publicity given to such crimes when they do occur.

Fear of having mentally ill persons reside in the community is largely the result of stereotypical concepts of mental illness. The image of the "lunatic" or the "raving maniac" does little to foster community acceptance of discharged clients living in the local area. While bumperstickers reading "Support mental health or I'll kill you" may appear amusing, they say much about the persistence of the stereotypical response to the mentally ill.

An "odd-looking" young man, somewhat disheveled, wandering the streets, talking loudly to himself about his mission from God, is going to receive public comment. This norm-violating behavior is often the stimulus for storekeepers or homeowners to call local police, who have to investigate and evaluate this complaint of "disturbing the peace." Critics of community-based sheltered care point out that police involvement with this population takes up valuable time and lessens the amount of protection given to the community. This "dis-

turbing the police" philosophy is another evidence of unwillingness to accept the mentally ill in the community.

Homeowners' concerns about decreases in property values because a residential-care facility is located in their neighborhood have led to some zoning regulations that attempt to restrict the presence of facilities in some communities. Strict definition of what should be considered a "family" for zoning purposes has successfully limited residential-care facilities in some areas.

These negative community reactions have great impact on the location of newly developing community-based sheltered-care facilities for the mentally ill. Unless these reactions are challenged and the public is educated to the realities of community treatment, mentally ill people will be forced to live in "ghetto"-type environments rather than returning to the healthy environments of their local communities.

Partial Hospitalization

Partial hospitalization dates back to 1933, when the first psychiatric day hospital was organized in Moscow, Russia. It was characterized as a "day infirmary for the mentally ill," and was created to relieve the acute shortage of hospital beds.[15] Thus, the main reason for the development of partial hospitalization was economic rather than theoretical or philosophical.

The first organized program of partial hospitalization in the North American continent did not occur until 1946, when a "day hospital" was established in Montreal, Canada. This program was seen as the extension of and supplement to full-time hospitalization, rather than as a substitute or alternative to hospitalization, as in the Russian model. By 1948, day treatment programs were in operation in the United States at Yale University Clinic and the Menninger Clinic. The former contained both day and night components, and both programs were designed as transitional treatment facilities.[15]

Partial hospitalization programs were slow to develop in the United States before the passage of the Community Mental Health Centers Act in 1963. As one of the five essential services to be provided by community mental health centers, partial hospitalization programs have increased in number since the 1960s, and have changed the complexion of psychiatric treatment. As an alternative to hospitalization, they play a role in secondary prevention, and as a transition from full-time hospitalization, they play a tertiary preventive role.

Washburn defined a psychiatric partial hospital as:

> . . . an organization designed to produce a therapeutic program more complex than the traditional outpatient services, yet without the 24-hour residence requirements, locked doors, quiet rooms, privileges or sanctions used by inpatient units.[29]

Partial hospitalization programs may be based in a hospital, in a mental health center, or in a free-standing location in the community. Given the nature of the programs and the population served, they require personnel that are trained and organized to deliver interventive, supportive, and rehabilitative services in an open system.

While objectives may vary from program to program, the three most common are:

1. To provide an alternative to 24-hour hospitalization
2. To provide transitional care to facilitate reentry into the community for previously hospitalized clients
3. To provide treatment and rehabilitation for chronically disturbed clients

Night Hospitals

One variety of partial hospitalization is the night hospital. This arrangement meets the needs of clients who are able to cope with school or work but are not yet able to deal with family or other home situations at night. The night hospital provides support and security for clients who are still too emotionally fragile to bridge completely the gap between the hospital and the community. Each morning, after breakfast, transitional clients leave for school or work. They return to the hospital in the evening and take part in ward activities such as group therapy, spending the night hours at the hospital.

Morgan and Moreno described the "evening–weekend" hospital, which uses the same space and facilities as the day program, providing a program for clients who have terminated in the day program in order to return to school or work, or for those whose illness does not disrupt their daytime activities.[18] Because of the availability of evening and weekend programs, clients are able to maintain important community involvement while receiving therapy and supportive treatment on two evenings a week, and a full day on Saturday.

Day Care/Day Treatment

The terms "day care," "day hospital," "day treatment," and "partial hospitalization" are often used interchangeably in the literature, but for this discussion the term "day treatment" will be used to describe such programs.

Day treatment programs serve a diverse population, from children and adolescents to adults and the elderly. Clients with a wide variety of diagnoses have been treated in these settings. The largest single category of clients reported in the day treatment literature, however, is the schizophrenic. Both acute and chronic schizophrenic adults have been treated successfully in day treatment programs.

There are limitations of the day treatment milieu. Therefore, certain admission criteria define the breadth of clients' disabilities with which day treatment programs can cope. Some programs exclude clients who are actively suicidal or actively destructive. Others require clients to have involved "significant others" who are available to work with the treatment team and provide support to the clients if they become disorganized, suicidal, or unable to cope. Many programs exclude clients with problems of alcoholism, drug addiction, mental defi-

ciency, or chronic brain syndrome. Because clients return to the community in the evening, a requirement for most programs is a stable living situation within commuting distance of the day treatment center.

Day treatment programs provide a wide range of therapeutic activities that reflect the philosophy of treatment and the needs of the client population. Many day treatment programs develop some variation of a "therapeutic community," as described by Maxwell Jones in the 1950s. In these programs, activities are conducted in a group setting with the premise that the experiences and group activities in a treatment day can be used by individuals to strengthen ego functions and/or modify maladaptive behavior patterns.

According to the standards set up by the American Association of Partial Hospitalization, day treatment programs must address at least four areas of dysfunction: psychological, interpersonal, primary role, and occupational.[5] Program components include group therapy, community meetings, goal-oriented social groups, recreational therapy, family evaluation/counseling, medication education groups, social skills training, creative expressive therapies (art, music, poetry, drama), and groups offering training in community living skills (Fig. 29-1).

Treatment goals vary, depending on the needs of the client population. For those who require resolution or stabilization of short-term problems, the goal of day treatment is to offer an intensive therapeutic experience that helps to eliminate or relieve dysfunction and allows the

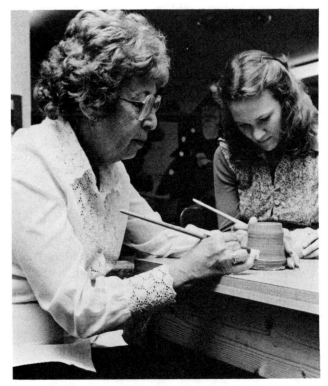

Figure 29-1. A client in day care (*left*) works on a project with a student nurse.

individual to return to a premorbid level of functioning in the community. The ambulatory setting of day treatment lessens the disruption of family, social, and community ties, making the idea of treatment in a mental health facility more palatable to both the client and the family. In this way, day treatment programs play a role in secondary prevention.

For mentally disabled individuals with long-standing social or vocational deficits, day treatment program goals are to reduce mental and functional disability and to maintain clients in the community by using supportive and rehabilitative services designed to improve their quality of life. In this respect, the day treatment program plays a tertiary preventive role.

Given the range of services needed in a day treatment program, staffing requires a mix of disciplines working together as a team to deliver adequate therapeutic care. The multidisciplinary staff most often involves psychiatrists, nurses, social workers, occupational therapists, recreation therapists, and psychologists. The staff–patient ratio varies, depending on the type of program and population served, but the suggested minimum ratio is 1:4 for programs with goals of resolution or stabilization of short-term problems, and 1:6 for programs with functions of rehabilitation of long-term problems.

Day treatment programs may be developed as an extension of an inpatient treatment setting, to offer specialized aftercare opportunities to specific client populations. The growth in day treatment has been accompanied by a concurrent expansion in the types of clients treated in these aftercare and extended care settings. Special populations currently being treated in the day treatment system include children, adolescents, the developmentally disabled, individuals with eating disorders, and the elderly.

Day programs specializing in the treatment of geriatric populations were first developed in England in the early 1950s. In the United States, geriatric day treatment programs have been created as a cost-effective way to meet many of the long-term psychiatric needs of older adults with chronic disabilities. These programs also serve a rehabilitative function, providing transition from hospital to community for older adults recovering from acute psychiatric illnesses who no longer require full-time hospitalization.

Among the candidates for geriatric day treatment are older adults who live alone and cannot completely care for themselves, those living with family or significant others who need relief from the total responsibility of their care, and older adults discharged from institutional settings. Services are oriented to prevention of illness; maintenance, rehabilitation, and restoration of health; and increasing social contacts to overcome isolation associated with illness and disability.[29] Geriatric day treatment as a component of aftercare services is a long-term care alternative to nursing homes or other institutional placements. It is a means of providing a comprehensive network of services for elderly persons who are psychiatrically impaired, thereby improving their quality of life.

There are many advantages of day treatment. These programs provide comprehensive treatment at a significantly lower cost than inpatient care. Day treatment avoids the regressive features associated with full-time hospitalization. The treatment setting does not completely disrupt the individual's existing social system; day treatment clients have more opportunities to maintain healthy areas of function in the community and with their significant others. Finally, there is less social stigma attached to this form of psychiatric treatment. There are indications that day treatment is more readily accepted by clients and their families as a treatment alternative.[32] This positive attitude may mean that clients will be more amenable to therapeutic intervention. Family support also favors a more successful treatment outcome.

The Role of the Nurse in Day Treatment Programs. There are two major functions that are essential parts of health care in a day treatment setting. The first is the provision of direct nursing care: the nurse is directly involved with health problems of individuals and groups of individuals. The second function is nursing coordination, which involves the nurse as a part of a multidisciplinary health care team that shares responsibility for implementing the broader goals of day treatment.

Both functions require nurses to have expertise in psychiatric nursing and the ability to engage in interdisciplinary communications. Nurses are involved in a diverse array of interactions with day treatment clients, their families, and other day treatment staff. Competent performance of these functions is essential for effective health care delivery. While these functions are described separately, it is important to keep in mind that direct nursing care and nursing coordination may be performed independent of one another or concurrently.

Direct Nursing Care. Direct nursing care involves assessment, problem identification, development of an appropriate plan, intervention or implementation of the proposed plan, and continuous evaluation. The objective of service is to restore functions or maintain them at the level of independence commensurate with clients' capabilities. The services required to produce this kind of functional outcome are interdisciplinary, and it is imperative that professionals from all involved disciplines plan jointly to meet the needs of the day treatment client.

Often, the most important members of the planning team—the clients and their families—are overlooked. Their goals, resources, desires, and limitations are important components of treatment planning. By including the client and family in all levels of problem identification and planning, there is an increased assurance of cooperation and compliance in carrying out the plan.

The first step in the provision of direct nursing care is *assessment*. Assessment is a "continuous, systematic, critical, orderly, and precise method of collecting, validating, analyzing, and interpreting information about the physical, psychological, and social needs of a patient and his family, the nature of the patient's self-care deficits, and other factors influencing his condition and care."[30]

CLINICAL EXAMPLE: ALBERT

Albert, a 28-year-old male, was referred to day treatment following hospitalization for a schizophrenic episode. It was his third hospitalization in the previous four years. At the time of admission, he lived in a board-and-care home and received SSI. He had a history of poor medication-regimen compliance, and was being maintained on fluphenazine decanoate, 25 mg IM every two weeks. He had a supportive family who provided some financial assistance and with whom he visited on weekends.

On admission, Albert was both socially and cognitively impaired, exhibiting extreme anxiety and poor eye contact. He defined his goals as wanting to be less socially isolated and better able to structure his time. He was encouraged to attend the day treatment program on Monday, Wednesday, and Friday, and to participate in the various group modalities.

The socialization effect of small-group therapy and communication skills groups led to his being less frightened of people. The groups provided a chance for him to listen to and share with other members, and brought a recognition that others have similar feelings and problems. The group format offered a controlled milieu in which he could practice social interactions. As Albert became more comfortable in groups, he began taking an active role by acting as a "buddy" to new group members.

Through leisure counseling and occupational therapy groups, he explored his leisure interests and vocational abilities. With encouragement from day treatment staff, he joined a self-help group that met once a week at a church near his residence. Following an occupational history and functional evaluation, he was given a referral to vocational rehabilitation for further assessment and possible sheltered-workshop training.

This culminated in Albert's graduation from the 12-week day treatment program to a sheltered-workshop placement. He continued to attend, one afternoon a week, an aftercare group run by the day treatment staff that provided him with ongoing support and medication management. He hoped to complete the job training program and eventually move into a paying job, doing factory work. He was actively involved in the self-help group, and began to take a leadership role there. He looked forward to moving into a satellite housing project where he would receive help and supervision while living more independently.

Initial assessment of a day treatment participant should be done at intake to establish a data base on which to plan care. It should emphasize functional abilities and limitations, based on data from many sources. Direct observation and interviewing clients and their families are the methods most frequently used by nurses. Other methods include obtaining information from a referral source, the acquisition and study of past records, and discussion with other personnel who know the client and have been involved with the client's care.

Drug therapy is an important aspect of treatment for many clients. Nurses are involved in monitoring clients' medication regimens, observing for possible side-effects, and providing medication education to clients and their families. Medication compliance is a key factor in the prevention of relapse; client noncompliance is one of the main reasons for rehospitalization. Often psychiatric clients fail to understand the reason they take the medication and the importance of adhering to the regimen even when they are without symptoms. They may not have been informed of possible side-effects, and can become frightened or annoyed if these occur, and therefore, stop taking the medication.

Nurses assume a major responsibility in medication education for day treatment clients. Frequently they co-lead groups with a psychiatrist or pharmacist that teach clients about their medications. According to Smith, the objectives of a medication education group are:

1. To provide client education on the primary action and side-effects of medications
2. To provide an opportunity for clients to verbalize their concerns regarding drug treatment
3. To provide clients with a positive attitude toward compliance with the drug regimen.[26]

Client education helps to improve medication compliance and fosters an increased sense of responsibility for self-monitoring of medications.

Formulation of care plans is another important nursing responsibility. Care plans must include specific short-term and long-term treatment goals. To be evaluated most easily, goals should be stated in terms of expected client behaviors. If goals are stated behaviorally, there will be no problem in measuring whether or not they are met. If a treatment goal is not met, it is necessary to review each of the steps in the process to determine possible causes. Was the assessment correct? Was the problem identified correctly? Were plans and approaches appropriate? How was the plan implemented? Client care planning is not effective unless it is an ongoing process. Reassessment and regular revision of the care plan are important components of the provision of comprehensive, individualized nursing care.

Nursing Coordination. The nurse in day treatment is a member of a multidisciplinary team that shares the responsibility for client care. The nurse coordinator has administrative responsibility to assure that the expertise and collaboration of the treatment team are utilized to assist in resolving the client's health problems. Developing, updating, and maintaining orderly recordkeeping systems is another function of the nurse coordinator.

Guiding the planning process is an important nursing role. The scheduling of regular treatment planning team meetings and case conferences allows representa-

CLINICAL EXAMPLE: MARIA

Maria, a 76-year-old Italian-American widow, was hospitalized for a second depressive episode with suicidal ideation. She had been living with her eldest daughter, Theresa, and Theresa's family since her husband died two years previously. During the hospitalization, family sessions were held to discuss aftercare plans. The client and her three children, Theresa, age 46, Rosa, age 40, and Anthony, age 38, were included in the sessions. Meetings with the children alone were helpful in allowing Theresa to express her feelings that her brother and sister did not share in the responsibility for care of their mother. She complained that she and her husband had had no real privacy since her mother had moved in. Neither Rosa nor Anthony had known that their sister felt this way. Because they both worked and Theresa was a homemaker, they had felt that Theresa was the logical family member to take care of their mother. When they recognized how overburdened their sister felt, they were able to discuss ways they could help relieve this stress, such as having their mother visit on weekends and assisting in providing transportation to doctors' appointments.

Medication education was needed because neither the client nor her family clearly understood the need for continuation of antidepressant therapy. Theresa agreed to monitor the medications because there was concern that her mother might sometimes forget to take them on schedule. It was made clear to Maria and her family that this was a temporary measure, and that eventually Maria would be able to manage her own medications.

Following discharge from the hospital, Maria began a two-day-a-week geropsychiatric day treatment program located near her home. This allowed free time for Theresa because her mother was able to take the bus to the program. Soon Maria began to explore community resources, including the local senior center and a church social club. Within six months, she was participating actively in these community groups and attending the day treatment aftercare program once a month for medication follow-up.

tives from the various disciplines involved to share their input. The nurse assumes a role in case coordination, making sure that all assessments, such as home visits, occupational history, and functional evaluation, have been completed prior to the case conference. The focus of the case conference is on both diagnosis and revision of the treatment plan.

Community outreach is another function of the nurse coordinator. Establishing community linkages with other agencies, while representing the day treatment center to the community, is an ongoing process for the nurse in day treatment.

Aftercare Clinics

One type of aftercare service frequently utilized for more chronically ill clients is the *aftercare clinic*. Aftercare clinics may be sponsored by the mental hospital or by a local community mental health center. Referral to the clinic is made at the time of hospital discharge. At this time, the client is provided with contact information and is instructed to call for an appointment following discharge.

Aftercare clinics typically provide medication follow-up and some form of supportive therapy. Some offer programs that combine individual supportive therapy with a period of informal socialization in a waiting room milieu. Schwab and Smith found it necessary to offer group therapy to facilitate social interaction and to enhance communication skills, because the "waiting room experience" did not offer the type of therapeutic interactions described by previous studies of aftercare clinics.[23] For the most chronically ill clients, this group therapy usually takes the form of a problem-solving or support

group, with a focus on teaching communication and social skills.

Nurses' roles in these clinics vary from primary therapist to co-leader of groups. They are available to administer medications, including injections of fluphenazine, and may also provide medication education to clients and their families. Family education is an important component of most aftercare clinics; counseling by aftercare nurses is aimed at upgrading families' coping skills and understanding of clients' illnesses.

Research on these clinics has shown that clients who attend are less apt to become rehospitalized, but it is not clear why this is so.[28] The one type of treatment consistently offered is medication, but to explain the reduction in recidivism on the basis of drug treatment alone ignores the factor of client motivation. Keeping aftercare clinic appointments may be clients' expression of their desire to become or stay healthy. This characteristic could be a more important factor than the type of treatment received.

Vocational Rehabilitation Services

A major objective of tertiary prevention is to increase the formerly hospitalized client's capacity to contribute to the occupational life of the community. However, the problems involved in rehabilitating psychiatrically disabled clients sufficiently to be able to function in a work environment are numerous. While studies of employment success rates show that approximately 30% to 50% of discharged clients obtain employment, they also point out that fewer than 25% maintain full-time employment.[1] Many lose jobs, not because of an inability to perform job tasks, but because of skill deficits in interpersonal functioning. Often discharged clients who lose jobs do not possess the skills necessary to find a new job, and are unaware of the vocational rehabilitation services available to assist them.

The process of preparing formerly hospitalized clients for work begins during hospitalization. Part of the client's therapy program should include involvement with an occupational therapist who reviews the client's prior work and functional history. An occupational history and functional assessment address such areas of concern as degree of autonomy or deficit in performing daily living activities, ability to problem-solve, level of socialization skills, and assessment of how the client's pathology affects occupational skills. The recommendations of the occupational therapist concerning the need for vocational rehabilitation services begin some client's return to work.

Vocational rehabilitation is composed of three basic interventions: work evaluation and work training, career counseling, and career placement. Vocational testing is usually offered to help the discharged client identify areas of aptitude and ability. If, by evaluation and testing, the client shows evidence of impairment in basic work and social skills needed to maintain a job, the client is referred to a work adjustment training program. This program attempts to re-shape work and social attitudes and behaviors in a work environment. Training settings may include hospital workshops, community-based workshops, or sheltered placements in industrial settings.

Career counseling is the second intervention in vocational rehabilitation. Its purpose is to assist psychiatrically disabled individuals to choose a career goal and to develop plans to meet their career objectives. Career counseling may begin at any point in the treatment process; beginning it in the hospital setting can provide an opportunity for psychiatrically disabled individuals to obtain career planning skills in a protected environment. If more skill training is required, a referral is often made to the local state office of vocational rehabilitation.

Career placement involves helping discharged clients find the best possible job available that is suited to their personal assets and qualifications. The steps involved in this process may include helping psychiatrically disabled individuals explore their assets, learn how to identify possible job openings, and how to take action to get a job. Support during this period may be in the form of role-playing job interviews, assistance in preparing a resume, or help in filling out a job application.

The need for vocational rehabilitation varies from client to client. Clients with more chronic illnesses may require a sheltered workshop placement because they are unable to withstand the pressures and competition of most jobs. These workshops pay slightly less than would be paid for the same position in general industry, but less pressure is placed on the worker and some guidance and supervision are offered. Volunteer work is another option for discharged clients who are not yet ready to return to salaried employment. It offers a flexible schedule, with less pressure, and provides an opportunity to explore new interest areas. Organizations such as Voluntary Action offer transitional volunteer opportunities to which psychiatrically disabled persons can be referred by the mental health agency, in which they will receive special support and help in the volunteer placement setting.

Alternative Mental Health Treatment System

Help for the emotionally disturbed comes from a variety of sources. Many groups of people from professions such as psychiatry, general medicine, psychology, psychiatric nursing, and social work offer treatment to this population. They practice within the official treatment system. There is also an alternative treatment system that was developed to fill some of the gaps in the official system and to offer alternative models of treatment. (See Table 29-3.)

There are certain characteristics that unite these diverse alternative care services. They offer care to all in need, and not just to those who are able to pay. The various groups are staffed primarily by volunteers and paraprofessionals. Alternative treatment system centers tend to be located "where the action is," usually in storefront operations in makeshift quarters. A typical feature of al-

TABLE 29-3.
AFTERCARE TREATMENT SYSTEMS

PROFESSIONAL AFTERCARE HELPING NETWORKS		NATURAL AFTERCARE HELPING NETWORKS	
(OFFICIAL TREATMENT SYSTEM)		(ALTERNATE TREATMENT SYSTEM)	
Residential care	Mental health centers	Family	Voluntary organizations
Aftercare clinics	Night hospitals	Friends/neighbors	Social clubs
Crisis/emergency services	Day care/day treatment	Free clinics	Neighborhood organizations
		→ Client movement between systems	
Neighborhood		Neighborhood	
		←	
Individual/group therapy	Transitional care services	Self-help groups	Natural helpers
Vocational rehabilitation services			

ternative services is a dislike for recordkeeping and program evaluation. Usually alternative programs focus on single problems such as alcoholism or drug addiction. Volunteers or paraprofessionals who become involved may have experienced the problem themselves or may closely identify with clients, often sharing clients' lifestyle.

Since the mid-1960s, the alternative treatment system has grown and expanded, mainly in response to the spread of drug use among young people. Alternative services for this population include runaway houses, drop-in counseling centers, free medical clinics, and telephone hotlines. Self-help groups such as Neurotics Anonymous and Recovery, Inc., can have a more direct impact on the needs of the aftercare and extended care population.

Self-Help Groups

Bean[2] divided self-help groups into various categories, including:

1. *Groups that help people with a permanent, fixed, stigmatized condition,* which help individuals deal with the stigma and improve their self-image. These groups may also fight prejudice and try to improve the public image of the condition. Members continue to use the group as long-term support. Examples of these groups include Recovery, Inc., and other groups for former mental patients.

2. *Groups that help people who are trapped in an addiction or a self-destructive way of life* offer a wide variety of techniques and assistance to help individuals change their behavior. They focus on helping people reorganize their lives, how they spend their time, relationships with others, and their personality structure and defenses. Examples of these include Alcoholics Anonymous, Weight Watchers, and Synanon.

"Self-help groups" and "mutual help groups" are terms that are used interchangeably in the literature. For discharged clients, these groups provide a peer-oriented helping network, and may serve as a transitional bridge from the hospital to the community. For those without family supports, the group may offer a substitute community support system. For some groups, the goal is to create a social and cultural environment that will help motivate and activate discharged clients to return to normal community life. For chronically mentally ill clients who see themselves as deviant and stigmatized, self-help groups assist in counteracting the isolation and alienation that result from being seen as different. The group creates a place where clients can belong and feel accepted; it assists clients in coping with long-term deficits.

The therapeutic value of these groups for aftercare clients cannot be overstated. Riesman termed it the "helper therapy principle."[21] He emphasized that giving help is often as beneficial to the helper as it is to the person being helped. Doing something worthwhile tends to improve one's self-image; the effective helper often feels an increased level of competence as a result of helping a peer.

Self-help groups such as Recovery, Inc., Project Return, and Emotional Health Anonymous offer opportunities for discharged clients to identify with others who have successfully dealt with similar problems. Mutual help and support, as well as positive role models, provide the impetus to change that is fostered by the group. While part of the alternative treatment system, these groups can be a valuable adjunct to more formal aftercare received through the official treatment system. The differences between traditional psychotherapy and self-help group therapy are detailed in Table 29-4.

Nurses have a dual role in self-help groups. They should be familiar with the various types of self-help organizations available and act as resources, providing information about these groups and helping discharged clients make initial contacts. They can also act as advocates, offering approval and support, not only to group members, but also to the group itself. Recognition and approval from a member of the official treatment system can do much to bolster the group's self-image, and may also lead to increased group membership.[16]

TABLE 29-4.
THE DIFFERENCES BETWEEN PSYCHOTHERAPY AND SELF-HELP GROUPS

	PSYCHOTHERAPY	SELF-HELP GROUP THERAPY
Group Leader	Professional therapist	Nonprofessional leaders
Cost	Fee	Free
Milieu	Therapy-oriented milieu (*e.g.,* psychiatrist's office)	Non-therapy-oriented milieu (*e.g.,* church, community center)
Therapist/Client/Member Relationship	Therapist is presumed to be normal. There is no identification between the therapist and the group.	Peers are similarly afflicted and identify with each other.
Emphasis of Therapy	Emphasis is on etiology, insight.	Emphasis is on faith, will-power, self-control.
Participant Title	Group members are referred to as patients or clients.	Participants are referred to as members.
Outside Contact Among Members/ Clients	Contact among clients outside of the group is discouraged.	Continuing support and outside socialization are encouraged.
Support	Clients expect only to receive support.	Members receive and must give support.

The Population Served by Aftercare

The aftercare population cannot readily be identified. The single factor its members share is a psychiatric hospitalization. Discharged clients who have successfully become reintegrated into the community tend to disappear from sight, and it is difficult to estimate their numbers. Chronically ill clients are much more visible, and are the type of clients most often referred to in the aftercare literature.

Chronically (long-term) mentally ill clients are frequently defined by diagnosis (predominantly organic, schizophrenic, or recurrent affective and active psychosis), degree of disability (with eligibility for SSI a common determinant), and duration of care (more than three months of hospital care). Using this definition, researchers have found that in the United States there are approximately 3 million individuals each year who suffer from serious mental illness, 2.4 million who continue to have some moderate to severe disability, and 1.7 million who suffer from prolonged severe mental disability. Of those with severe disability, it is estimated that about half reside in institutions (nursing homes account for approximately 44%), while half live in the community.[20]

Variables that determine the type of aftercare utilized by chronically ill clients include age, sex, education, length of illness, available social supports, and financial resources. The elderly often have no real family supports to return to, or their families may be unwilling to accept them because of the perceived burden. Nursing homes become a common "dumping ground" for these clients. Women are more likely to return to their home and family than are men. Families in lower socioeconomic classes are more likely to distance themselves from discharged clients following each successive rehospitalization. Black families are often more accepting than white, but may be less skilled at seeking and utilizing community placement.

In less than 30 years, the deinstitutionalization movement has lowered the population in public mental hospitals to one third of its former size. Unfortunately, this achievement has been offset by high readmission rates, and has resulted in the growth of a new type of chronically psychiatrically disabled client. Chronically ill young adult clients, sometimes referred to as "the new drifters," are usually between the ages of 18 and 35, and are frequently male. They are characterized by the fact that they have lived in the era of deinstitutionalization and have had the benefit of noninstitutional and nonrestrictive care. They are a heterogeneous group, which can be divided into three specific subpopulations described in Table 29-5.

Other subpopulations of chronically mentally ill clients include the elderly who suffer from organic brain syndromes, the developmentally disabled who also suffer from mental illness, children and adolescents with chronic psychiatric disorders, substance abusers, and criminal offenders.

TABLE 29-5.
COMMON CHARACTERISTICS OF THE AFTERCARE POPULATION

LOW-ENERGY, LOW-DEMAND GROUP

Passive, apathetic, poorly motivated individuals
Extremely dependent on the psychiatric service system
Have adapted to the "patient" role
Usually enter the mental health system in early adolescence
Appear "burned out"
May come from backgrounds of social deprivation

HIGH-ENERGY, HIGH-DEMAND GROUP

Aggressive, noncompliant individuals
Have a low frustration tolerance
May have had many encounters with the law
Often classified as "revolving door" clients because of their mobility within a single psychiatric service system
Frequently evicted, and when housing options are exhausted may become homeless "street" people

HIGH-FUNCTIONING GROUP

Highly motivated individuals who function while in remission, but who are seriously disabled by their psychiatric disorder
Often isolated, with few social supports
Are usually better educated and from higher socioeconomic levels
Desire to "blend" into the general population

Aftercare Referrals and Compliance

Continuity of care is a key concept in the provision of aftercare and extended care services. While studies show that organized aftercare programs can reduce recidivism rates by as much as 50%, aftercare is predicated on the fact that clients keep initially scheduled appointments.[7] The referral procedure plays an important role in assuring aftercare compliance.

Client failure to follow through with aftercare planning is considered one factor that predisposes clients to relapse and subsequent rehospitalization. For most clients, aftercare referrals are given at discharge, which is a time of high stress and anxiety. It is easy to understand why discharged clients, during the transitional period, may have difficulty in following up on aftercare services.

Nurses can facilitate the transition from hospital care to community aftercare by assuming an active role in the referral process. Helping clients to schedule specific appointment times with aftercare services and, if possible, establishing a contact with aftercare staff prior to discharge, can significantly increase aftercare compliance. Other factors that influence compliance include family involvement and aggressive follow-up on the part of the aftercare service to which the client has been referred.

Family members should be involved early and informed of the need for continued treatment, the need for medication follow-up, and the risk of relapse. The aftercare service should schedule an appointment as soon as possible following the client's discharge. If the client does not keep the appointment, outreach services may be necessary. Every effort should be made to reach the client and/or family by phone. If there is no response, a letter or home visit may be advisable. These active interventions are necessary for a wide variety of clients: schizophrenics who require maintenance medication but decide that they are feeling better and don't need it; manic-depressives who took lithium while hospitalized but prefer being "high" to taking medication; and housebound neurotics whose phobias prevent them from going to the aftercare service for follow-up.

Many factors affect successful continuity of aftercare, including the client's diagnosis, employment history, support systems, economic stability, educational level, and intellectual functioning, as well as the quality of the aftercare service. By increasing the follow-up compliance through good referral procedures, the chances of helping aftercare clients become functional members of the community and avoid relapse, are heightened.

Future Directions

The objective of modern treatment of persons with major mental illness is to enable the patient to maintain himself in the community in a normal manner. . . . Therefore, aftercare and rehabilitation are essential parts of all service to mental patients. . . .[8]

This statement on the need for aftercare made by the Joint Commission on Mental Illness and Health is as relevant now as it was in 1961. The need for improved aftercare services has become even more urgent because the number of clients residing in the community has increased as a consequence of deinstitutionalization policies and shorter hospital stays for acutely ill patients. Several factors must be addressed in planning for future aftercare services. These include:

1. *Funding of aftercare services* is crucial to their survival. While the government advocates the need for more and better aftercare and extended care programs, financial support has been slow in coming. Increased funding of aftercare programs, at both state and federal levels, is needed to ensure the provision of a high-quality, comprehensive network of services. Another source of financial support is through third-party insurance funding of aftercare programs. At this time, most health insurance programs, while providing some coverage for aftercare services (such as partial hospitalization), provide more comprehensive coverage for inpatient services. Aftercare programs have proven cost-effective, and it is time for increased reimbursement to reflect this.

2. *Training* is another vital factor in aftercare programming. Mental health professionals need education that includes an emphasis on aftercare and extended care services. Health care professionals require basic and continuing education in the provision of community care, including principles of rehabilitation,

supportive treatment, use of psychotropic drugs, referral procedures, and orientation to community resources. Nurses in both baccalaureate- and master's-level programs should have training in community care as it applies to both acutely and chronically ill psychiatric clients.

3. *The amount and type of aftercare services* available to discharged clients residing in the community must be improved. More residential care options are needed, as well as consultation and education services for existing facilities to help them upgrade the quality of care. Partial hospitalization and aftercare clinic programs should be developed as part of a coordinated network of community-based aftercare services.

As aftercare programs develop and expand their services, there is an increased need for *research* in this field. Program evaluation (*i.e.,* measuring the degree to which existing programs achieve stated program goals, judging the outcomes, and documenting the rationale for program changes) is a necessary component of aftercare services. Ongoing evaluation is closely integrated with the clinical and administrative aspects of program operation. The underutilization of aftercare services also requires further study. Additional areas of concern include questions such as:

What factors are predictive of complete utilization of aftercare services?
What kinds of clients require particular types of aftercare intervention?
What are the best means of coordinating aftercare services?

A more intensive and extensive research effort is necessary to provide answers to these and many other questions that have served as barriers to the expansion of aftercare services.

Finally, *advocacy,* the process of pleading the cause for another, is essential in the field of aftercare. Nurses can play an important role in protecting the rights of mentally ill clients. Discharged clients, struggling with the stresses of community living, often need a specific person to serve as an advocate while they become oriented to the community system. Nursing interventions may take the form of assisting clients to make phone calls to public agencies or actually accompanying clients to the particular organization involved. Indirect help may be given in the form of advocating the development of comprehensive community services such as housing and employment opportunities for the mentally ill. By assuring access to appropriate and adequate services, clients' rights are upheld and the best provision of aftercare services is guaranteed.

Summary

1. Aftercare and extended care services are a major component of the tertiary prevention system.

2. By utilizing the inpatient nursing staff, transitional programs help to assure continuity of care and offer a linkage from the hospital to the community for discharged clients.

3. Residential aftercare treatment facilities offer a "stepping stone back to the community" for clients. They provide structure and supervised transitional living for those who are unable to live independently in the community upon discharge from the hospital.

4. Partial hospitalization and aftercare clinics provide supportive treatment, medication follow-up, and rehabilitative service for discharged clients living in the community.

5. Vocational rehabilitation services increase the aftercare client's capacity for employment by offering work evaluation, career counseling, and job placement.

6. The alternative treatment system fills some of the gaps in the services provided by the official system. It offers alternative models of aftercare, such as self-help groups, that can provide discharged clients with positive role models and a sense of acceptance.

7. Nurses have many roles in aftercare and extended care. These roles include providing direct nursing care, coordinating treatment planning and intervention, community outreach, and client advocacy.

References

1. Anthony WA, Cohen MR, Vitalo R: The measurement of rehabilitation outcomes. Schizophr Bull 4(3):310–318, 1978
2. Bean M: Alcoholics Anonymous, Part II. Psychiatr Ann 5(3):8, 1975
3. Budson RD: The Psychiatric Halfway House. Pittsburgh, University of Pittsburgh Press, 1978
4. Caplan G, Killilea M (eds): Support Systems and Mutual Help: Multidisciplinary Explorations. New York, Grune & Stratton, 1976
5. Casarino JP, Wilner M, Maxey JT: American Association for Partial Hospitalization Standards and Guidelines for Partial Hospitalization. International Journal of Partial Hospitalization 1(1): 5–21, 1982
6. Chien C, Cole JO: Landlord-supervised cooperative apartments: A new modality for community-based treatment. Am J Psychiatry 130:156–159, 1973
7. Donion PT, Rada RT: Issues in developing quality aftercare clinics for the chronically mentally ill. Comm Ment Health J 2: 29, 1976
8. Final Report of the Joint Commission on Mental Illness and Health: Action for Mental Health. New York, Basic Books, 1961
9. Furdey R, Crowder M, Silvers P: Transitional care: A new approach to aftercare. Hosp Comm Psychiatry 28(2):122, 1977
10. Glasscote RM, Gudeman JE, Elpers JR: Halfway houses for the mentally ill: A study of programs and problems. Washington, DC, American Psychiatric Association, 1971
11. Goldmeier J et al (eds): New Directions in Mental Health Care: Cooperative Apartments. Adelphi, Maryland, Mental Health Study Center, National Institute of Mental Health, 1978
12. Kopp SB: If You Meet Buddha on the Road, Kill Him, p 224. Toronto, Canada, Bantam Books, 1976
13. Jones K: A History of Mental Health Services. London, Routledge & Kegan Paul, 1972
14. Lamb HR et al: Community Survival for Long-Term Patients. San Francisco, Jossey-Bass, 1976
15. Luber RF (ed): Partial Hospitalization: A Current Perspective. New York, Plenum Press, 1979
16. Marram G: The Group Approach in Nursing Practice. St. Louis, CV Mosby, 1978
17. Meyer A: Aftercare and Prophylaxis. In Lief A (ed): The Commonsense Psychiatry of Dr. Adolf Meyer. New York, McGraw-Hill, 1948
18. Morgan AJ, Moreno JW: The Practice of Mental Health Nursing: A Community Approach. Philadelphia, JB Lippincott, 1973
19. Morrissey JR: The Case for Family Care of the Mentally Ill. Community Mental Health Journal Monograph No. 2. New York, Behavioral Publications, 1967
20. Nielsen AC et al: Encouraging psychiatrists to work with chronic patients: Opportunities and limitations of residency education. Hosp Comm Psychiatry 32(11):767–775, 1981
21. Riesman F: The "helper" therapy principle. Soc Work 10:27–32, 1965
22. Rossi AM: Some Pre-World War II Antecedents of Community Mental Health Theory and Practice. In Bindman AJ, Spiegel AD (eds): Perspectives in Community Mental Health. Chicago, Aldine, 1969
23. Schwab PJ, Smith BH: A supportive clinic: Who comes, how often, and for what? Compr Psychiatry 18(5):503–509, 1977
24. Schwartz M, Schwartz CG: Social Approaches to Mental Patient Care. New York, Columbia University Press, 1964
25. Siegel SP, Aviram U: The Mentally Ill in Community-Based Sheltered Care. New York, John Wiley & Sons, 1978
26. Smith JE: Improving drug knowledge in psychiatric patients. J Psychosoc Nurs Ment Health Serv 4:16–18, 1981
27. Turner JC, Tenhoor WJ: The NIMH community support program: Pilot approach to needed social reform. Schizophr Bull 4(3):319–348, 1978
28. Vitale JH, Steinbach M: The prevention of relapse of chronic mental patients. Int J Soc Psychiatry 11:85–95, 1965
29. Washburn SI: Partial Hospitalization—Day, Evening, and Night—in the Changing Mental Health Scene. In Hirschowitz RG, Levy B (eds): The Changing Mental Health Scene. New York, Spectrum, 1976
30. Weiler PG, Rathbone-McCuan E: Adult Day Care: Community Work With the Elderly. New York, Springer Publishing, 1978
31. Wolman B (ed): International Encyclopedia of Psychiatry, Psychology, Psychoanalysis, and Neurology, vol 1. New York, Aesculapius Publishers, 1975
32. Zwerling I, Wilder JF: An evaluation of the applicability of the day hospital in treatment of acutely disturbed patients. Isr Ann Psychiatry Relat Disciplines 2(2):162–185, 1964
33. Zitrin A, Hardesty AS, Burdock EI et al: Crime and violence among mental patients. Am J Psychiatry 133(2):142–149, 1976

KATHLEEN L. PATUSKY

PSYCHIATRIC HOME CARE

Learning Objectives

Upon completion of this chapter the student should be able to do the following:

1. Identify key elements in the historical development of psychiatric home care.
2. Identify two qualifiers of the nursing process as it applies to home care.
3. Describe how psychiatric home care operates as a means of primary, secondary, and tertiary prevention.
4. Identify and discuss three models of psychiatric home care.
5. Discuss two potentially problematic issues regarding the therapeutic relationship that are specific to home care.
6. Discuss the preparation of the psychiatric home care nurse for effective psychiatric nursing practice in the home setting.
7. Summarize research findings regarding psychiatric home care nursing.

Introduction

History abounds with examples of ideas and practices that come full circle, returning like a pendulum. Health care is seeing this return with its recent reemphasis on medical treatment in the home. Psychiatric services are a logical and necessary component of this new model of home care. Their inclusion is just beginning to take hold, but not without precedent or supporting theory.

This chapter offers a speculative look at an area of health care that is in its infancy. Psychiatric home care has been implemented successfully in a number of settings outside of the United States, while its development has been all but ignored in this country. Cost-effectiveness issues force reconsideration of alternatives to hospitalization and fragmented services. Recognition of holistic and self-care concepts leads to rethinking of attitudes toward the client–health professional relationship. The nursing profession is in an ideal position to have a profound impact on the direction of this neonate. Psychiatric/mental health nurses can truly be pioneers in an area that expands the present hospital–outpatient continuum of psychiatric care.

Nursing's contribution will depend to a great extent on an understanding of the system that supports psychiatric home care, fundamental concepts that influence its implementation, and models of home care that have already been initiated. This chapter will address the background, theoretical considerations, and potential of psychiatric care delivered in the client's own environment.

Historical Development of Psychiatric Home Care

The earliest precedents for home care date back as far as does human existence. Cave dwellers, fresh from their latest battle with the saber-toothed tiger, returned to their cave to recuperate. Only in recent times have hospitals been considered superior to home care. Initially, sanitariums and hospitals became necessary to treat large numbers of clients with communicable diseases and chronic ailments. Such places were reserved for the poor, the homeless, or the dying. Clients were often admitted in a state of terror, because hospitals were perceived as the place to die.

Medical treatment in the home was standard for those who could afford it, with physicians supervising care provided by family members. In 1796, the first organized home care program, initiated at the Boston Dispensary, extended physician visits to the poor. Nursing services were considered unnecessary, an idea consistent with nursing's negative image at that time. In England after 1837, the work of William Rathbone and Florence Nightingale demonstrated that nursing could contribute a great deal in terms of treatment, instruction, and prevention in home care. By the late 1800s, lay-administered nursing services were organized in the United States. The first use of a graduate nurse in 1877 started a trend that later emerged as the Visiting Nurses' Associations.[7,21]

By the early 1900s, life insurance companies began to offer home care to policyholders, emphasizing health promotion rather than curative services. This trend continued until the 1940s, when long-term problems replaced communicable illnesses as the primary focus of health care. Hospitals became overcrowded and initiated programs of medical home care to shorten hospital stays. The National Organization of Public Health Nursing was founded in 1912 to promote professional standards and communication. In 1946, the organization recommended a health department pattern of preventive and curative nursing services. Their recommendation was largely unheeded.[7,21]

The prototype for today's concept of home care was initiated at the Montefiore Hospital, New York, in 1947. Services were extended to all clients and were viewed as a continuation of hospitalization. These included 24-hour medical service, social service, nursing service, housekeeping, transportation to the hospital, medications and restorative equipment, occupational therapy, and physical therapy. Inherent in this program was an acknowledgement of clients as a part of their own environments.[21]

A Public Health Service conference in 1958 responded to growing professional support for home care. It promoted the discussion of standards, funding, a wide range of services, and recommendations for research. By 1961, legislation was in place to provide grant funding for special projects in health care outside of hospitals. It was the passage of Medicare laws in 1965, however, that gave the greatest boost to home care, providing the federal funding and regulations that have been both the boon and the curse of the industry. Home care was declared mandatory for Medicaid programs in 1970.[21] At the present time, acceptance of home care is again becoming part of private insurance coverage, increasing the lucrative nature and, therefore, the growth potential of the home health field.

As can be seen from the preceding chronology, the nursing component of home care finds its roots in public health, with an emphasis on community-based services, teaching, and prevention. However, the state and federal support of home health care created a new system of agencies that split off from the public health arena. Initially, nurses who wanted to deliver care in the home could choose positions either with public health departments or with nonprofit home health agencies. Before long, nonprofit agencies, such as the Visiting Nurses' Associations, were outnumbered by for-profit or proprietary agencies. Additionally, hospital-based intervention programs, hospital-based home care agencies, health maintenance organization (HMO) home care services, and hospice programs have been added to the list. Services, regulations, restrictions, and funding vary with each type of organization. Home care is not the same in all settings. In short, the present state of home care services can be characterized as diverse, expanding, and generally confusing to care providers and recipients alike. However, chaos often provides the medium for change that can result in a higher level of organization.

Against this backdrop, psychiatric home care makes its appearance today. Actually, the history of psychiatric home care might begin with the first home exorcism attempted by a shaman on a deranged individual, or one could look to Freud's use of medical personnel living with one of his patients, the "Wolf-Man," to support the analytic process.[2] For our purposes, the research section of this chapter will cover studies back to the 1960s. These studies discussed the use of visiting nurses for psychiatric clients, predominantly in England, Canada, New Zealand, Israel, Finland, and India. Despite the positive results of such services in these countries, and supportive articles in American journals, there has not been an overwhelming movement to implement psychiatric home care on a wide scale in the United States. There is still a long way to go.

Theoretical Overview

The Person as a System

When clients enter the hospital or the outpatient setting, they bring a complex configuration of hopes, fears, and expectations into an artificial environment. As described in the chapter on milieu therapy (Chap. 14), the effectiveness of treatment relies to a great extent on the setting's ability either to recreate portions of the clients' natural environment or at least to anticipate the environmental impact on the client. Home care, on the other hand, goes directly to the natural environment. Clients are experienced in the process of dealing first-hand with their daily resources, limitations, and difficulties. Because this is the reality with which clients must live, intervention in the home is extremely relevant and potentially more effective in the long run.

There is a classic story of a therapist who had been seeing a client as an outpatient for some time, but who was distressed at the lack of progress being made. Of particular concern was the client's continued insistence that change was not possible, given the circumstances of his life. The therapist concluded that the client was resistant, noncompliant with treatment, and prone to externalizing his responsibility. One day, the client left the therapist's office without receiving a prescription that was to begin immediately. Because the therapist was to be in the client's vicinity that afternoon, he decided to deliver the prescription personally. One picture was worth a thousand words. Seeing the environment in which the client lived, and meeting the people who had a large impact on the client's existence, the therapist came away with a new understanding of the dynamics contributing to the client's position. The therapist developed a new respect for the client's strengths and persistence in dealing with that environment on a daily basis. Therapy was able to proceed once more, but this time with consideration for the client's reality. Denial of that reality, of the system that constituted the person, had compromised the therapeutic process.

System Components of the Person

Home care offers an opportunity to view the client in much greater depth than any other modality. Physical attributes and difficulties are noted on an outpatient basis, and dealt with briefly in the milieu. In the home, the key word is adaptation. The concern is not limited to "How does the client feel about limping?" or "Can the client ambulate around the unit?" Rather, home care asks, "Can the client function, let alone cope, on a daily basis?" "Can the client perform self-care?" If the answer is no, then, "What needs to be done with the environment, or what additional skills must be taught, in order for the client to live optimally outside of the hospital setting?" The safety of the environment is closely linked to the areas of physi-

cal and psychological limitation. Assessment of living conditions and potential hazards goes hand in hand with an evaluation of the client's ability to perform activities of daily living and exist in an independent setting without self-harm.

The psychological make-up of the person is seen intimately as it relates and reacts to its surroundings. Its threads are interwoven with all other components, influencing every facet of the client's lifestyle. In fact, much information can be deduced about how clients see themselves and their world simply by taking a look at how they combine the system components in their homes. The social component of the individual is truly seen as an interactive system. All significant others, including extended family, neighbors, and community supports, are assessed for their positive and negative contributions. The cultural influences apparent in the environment and the evidence of spiritual practices also play a major role in understanding clients' priorities. In combination, these system elements offer clues to effective interventions relevant to clients' actual circumstances.

The Therapeutic Use of Self

The therapeutic use of self, as described throughout this text, is similarly applicable in the home setting. However, something unique transpires when meeting with clients on their own ground—a difference that is both rewarding and problematic. Upon entering the home to provide treatment, nurses most closely approximate the role of the old family physician who made house calls. They are generally accepted as individuals who provide expert assistance, but who do so in an arena where the client is in total control. Hence, the relationship is more equal than one in which the client enters the therapist's domain (Fig. 30-1). As a result, the nurse is viewed in a more human light, which facilitates the therapeutic use of self. For therapists who delight in exercising their own humanity as a tool of treatment, the setting promotes a sense of challenge and reward. For therapists who are uncomfortable with such closeness, home care can be most threatening.

This closeness can also create some difficulty with issues of dependency and transference. Nurses walk a fine line. They must provide assistance in a very human and personal context, while intervening in such a way that the goals of treatment are not lost in the client's wish for a social companion. Therapists' ability to maintain awareness of this factor is crucial in ensuring effective treatment.

The Nursing Process

The nursing process is an integral part of psychiatric home care. However, it has two important qualifiers. First, elderly clients make up a large portion of the most appropriate clientele, because they may not have the mobility for outpatient treatment. Medical difficulties are

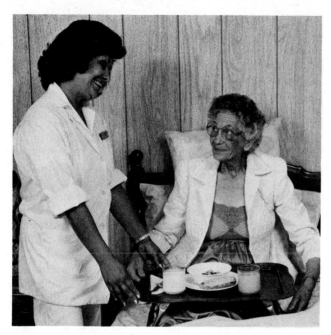

Figure 30-1. A psychiatric nurse doing home care establishes her relationship with a homebound client. (Courtesy of Allied Home Health Association, San Diego, CA)

common in this age group. Hence, it is particularly important that assessment and intervention emphasize the wide range of concurrent health problems possible. Particular attention is required for the special circumstances of the elderly. Included in this area are potential problems with medication effects and interactions. A strong medical nursing background is a real asset in providing psychiatric home care. Geropsychiatry also requires a different perspective in the areas of cognitive-perceptual, role-relationship, and coping-stress tolerance patterns. Nursing diagnoses in these categories involve an understanding that elderly clients may experience problems of a different nature and in a different manner than younger clients.

The second qualifier of the nursing process in home care relates to the case management nature of this type of service. It is potentially the most holistic kind of nursing, having an impact on the entire health care continuum. Home health nurses act as a liaison between physician, hospital, outpatient setting, community agency, and the entire ecological system of the client. All problem areas are addressed, with a full range of medical therapy services initiated as needed. Once a treatment plan is completed, contact is often maintained with the client to ensure early recognition of further difficulties. A case management perspective means that the nursing process is still in action, even when the visit or the case is concluded.

Levels of Prevention

Psychiatric home care operates at all three levels of prevention. This is not to say that it makes hospitalization

unnecessary, but it can influence the frequency and inevitability of hospitalization. The traditional public health role of nursing has already proven its efficacy in the promotion of health and prevention of illness through public education, *i.e., primary prevention.* The educative model also applies in the field of mental health. Educating clients is a skill employed by all public health and home care nurses, even without formal psychiatric experience.

Secondary prevention, which involves early case-finding and treatment, is generally initiated by referral from nonpsychiatric sources, such as physicians, community agencies, and families. In these instances, home care identifies the most appropriate level of intervention and assists clients in obtaining care. Entry into the mental health care system can often be frustrating and time-consuming, depending upon the financial status of the client. Home care facilitates the process.

When home care is carried out at its most sophisticated level, it is in essence an application of appropriate milieu concepts in the home setting. It becomes a rehabilitative program, operating as *tertiary prevention.* The entire knowledge base of psychiatric nursing is brought to bear to help clients attain an optimal level of function in the community.

Models of Psychiatric Home Care

The following models of psychiatric home care have been included in this chapter because they demonstrate formal, consistent programs of intervention that take place in the home environment. By rights, these programs are generally considered the province of community mental health. This discussion represents an extension of that section of this text, rather than an alternative to it. After briefly exploring these types of home care, we will take a closer look at one particular model that is gaining favor under the aegis of home health agencies.

The format of psychiatric care in the home setting can vary according to focus of treatment, base of operations, and time allotment. The following examples have been categorized to correspond with these variables, but the theoretical underpinnings are shared by all, and will be discussed separately.

Focus of Treatment: Crisis/Outreach Orientation

Home visit programs may be geared toward providing a very narrow and specific range of services with far-reaching effects. This has been the finding of the Geropsychiatric Outreach Team at the Illinois State Psychiatric Institute. They utilized a multidisciplinary team (psychiatric nurse, social worker, and psychiatrist) to conduct a one- or two-visit comprehensive evaluation of homebound elderly clients (Fig. 30-2). This team was then able to link the clients with necessary medical, mental health, and social services. Interventions included recommendations

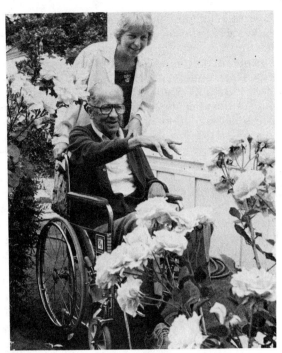

Figure 30-2. A psychiatric nurse doing home care meets with a client. (Courtesy of Allied Home Health Association, San Diego, CA)

for direct psychiatric services such as psychotherapy or medication, recommendations for increased medical or social services, and consultations with significant others and involved professionals. Follow-up evaluation interviews were conducted three months after the initial contact. The study concluded that an outreach program "can be instrumental in alleviating suffering and in providing a viable alternative to hospitalization and long-term institutionalization."[23]

The experiences of crisis teams in New York[4] and Philadelphia[24] support the effectiveness of emergency in-home services. The latter group provided the results of a four-year study detailing crisis-team operations. Staffed by an intake evaluator/social worker, psychiatric nurse,

and psychiatrist, the team functioned as part of a hospital-based 24-hour emergency service. They responded to calls concerning real or potential physical threat. The team evaluated clients and their situations, provided crisis intervention, and facilitated further treatment when necessary. The team was successful in defusing violent situations and effecting hospitalization in many cases. Follow-up treatment was often limited to the team's visits, since clients and families often refused any other services.

Base of Operation: Hospital Programs With Community Focus

Several hospitals and mental health centers have included home visits in their aftercare programs, deriving benefit from cooperation with, and utilization of, community resources (Fig. 30-3).[5,15,16] The most comprehensive plan described was undertaken in Israel.[17] It defined a specific geographical population, and then proceeded to work with the community in planning the types of services necessary, to be delivered in the most appropriate setting. While inpatient and outpatient components were available, a strong community emphasis included home visits by a coordinating nurse, social worker, public health nurse, and psychiatrist. Additionally, community members were called upon to assist with the formation of support systems and individual rehabilitation programs. These community members included the local rabbi, policeman, school nurse, and/or municipal authorities. With total coordination of all treatment systems and significant others, continuity of care was experienced to its best advantage.

Time Allotment: Home Health Model vs. In-Home Treatment

Home care nursing may be implemented either on a shift basis or on an intermittent visit schedule. While the latter is more common in home health agencies, it is possible

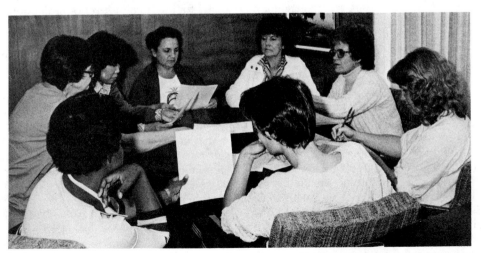

Figure 30-3. Psychiatric nurses in home care plan treatment with hospital staff. (Courtesy of Allied Home Health Care, San Diego, CA)

to assign in-home nurses for up to 24 hours a day. One author detailed this adjunct to psychoanalysis, specifying the need for close communication between the nurse and the primary therapist to ensure understanding of the dynamics, therapeutic plan, and countertransference issues.[2]

The home health model emphasizes treatment and rehabilitative services along with case management as aftercare[8,22] or in lieu of hospitalization.[3,12,18,19] Studies cite effective application with schizophrenics[11,12,13] and neurotics[14] and in family issues.[20] Psychiatric or public health nurses, as well as social workers, work closely with psychiatrists in support of mutual treatment plans. Nursing visits are made anywhere from twice a month to several times a week, depending upon clients' needs. Interventions center around medication therapy and compliance, psychotherapy, health care instruction, and family assistance. In the United States, these services are generally offered by a home health agency. This provides the additional advantage that medical treatment as well as physical, speech, or occupational therapy can be implemented as needed.

One such program at the Allied Home Health Association in San Diego was initiated in 1985 under a Public Health Service grant. Based on a full client assessment by clinical nurse specialists, intermittent skilled nursing visits are provided by clinical specialists and psychiatric nurses. Referrals to social workers, physical, occupational, and speech therapists, or home health aides are made, as needed. The inclusion of a rehabilitation clinical specialist provides further basis for a neuropsychiatric program dealing with stroke or head-injury clients. Referrals are initiated from a variety of sources, including physicians, hospital discharge planners, community agencies, and family members. A surprisingly large percentage of elderly clients are also referred from within the agency. The medical nurses benefit from staff consultation to identify depression or coping difficulties in their clients.

The program focuses on rehabilitation, evaluation, medication monitoring, client and family instruction, and counseling or psychotherapy. A strong case management system is also built in, with ongoing liaison between the agency and physicians. In fact, the system is often involved with encouraging and facilitating communication among several physicians providing care for the same client. Referral and liaison are also effected with a variety of community resources who deliver individually-tailored services to clients and are at risk of duplicating or fragmenting services.

A wide variety of clients have participated in the program so far. These include some with strictly psychiatric diagnoses and others whose medical problems combine with or result in emotional difficulties. Treatment has been initiated following and in lieu of hospitalization, with staff occasionally facilitating hospitalization. In one instance, a client was unable to be hospitalized because he did not meet the ambulatory criteria of the institution. Brief psychotherapeutic intervention addressed the client's lethargy while physical therapy was implemented

to increase endurance and ambulation. As a result, the client was able to be admitted and take full advantage of milieu treatment. The program has identified a number of possible subspecialties to be explored. It has also encouraged the development of policies and procedures to facilitate its smooth operation. However, it is just the beginning of a treatment option that will undoubtedly undergo further modification and growth. In the process, concepts basic to home care will be applied to the psychiatric arena.

Theoretical Considerations

Psychiatric home care nursing involves a good deal more than merely moving a nurse from the hospital setting to the community. The transition includes changes in treatment style prompted by three variables: the nature of home care itself, the population being served, and the differences in dynamics observed in the home setting. The necessary changes in treatment style lead to some guidelines for the preparation of nurses going into psychiatric home care.

The Nature of Psychiatric Home Care

Nurses who work in home health care give similar feedback about their field. The average length of employment in home care is either less than two years or forever. Nurses either love it or hate it, depending upon their ability to adjust from hospital nursing. Home health nurses operate with a degree of accountability and independence not required of hospital staff nurses. On the surface, the situation seems ideal. Nurses generally manage their own case loads, working with physicians to determine how many visits are appropriate for each client's needs. They then negotiate with clients to determine when these visits will be made. Nurses operate on their own in carrying out the nursing process and communicating results or problems to the physicians. The potential exists for the highest level of professionalism in providing care.

On the other hand, visit schedules are also influenced by the payer source and by agency policies regarding minimum daily visits. In home care, nurses learn firsthand that they are part of the business world. Their idealism in providing care cannot ignore financial reality. If costs are too high, or if the client's insurance coverage will not pay for the ideal treatment plan, the agency loses money and is not guaranteed to stay in business. As a result, nurses must have a greater familiarity with documentation requirements, insurance coverage guidelines, and other administrative parameters of health care delivery. Treatment regimens must be properly set up and put into operation without the "safety net" of 24-hour staffing or in-house physician coverage. Not all nurses are comfortable with what amounts to a mobile private practice. Nor are all nurses comfortable meeting clients on their own ground. The settings may be less than optimal or downright dangerous. Home care nursing offers many rewards for a special kind of nurse, but the decision to become a home care nurse must be considered carefully.

Home Care Clientele

The increasing use of home care services is leading to a well-known trend in hospitals—specialization. However, home health agencies are still more general in nature. Even in psychiatric home care, nurses will see a variety of clients from all age groups, with a diversity of diagnoses.

Age Groups

At the present time, elderly clients make up the largest percentage of home care clients. Psychiatric/mental health nurses must be willing and able to meet a strong need for geropsychiatric skills. As private insurance carriers increase mental health and home care benefits for their adult policyholders, this age group will be better represented. Insurance companies are already intrigued by the potential for psychiatric home care with children, particularly those who are receiving expensive care in residential treatment centers. While increased use of psychiatric home care and larger case loads will eventually make specialization more cost-effective, nurses in this field can expect to work with any age group, and must be flexible enough to adapt to each group's different needs.

Diagnostic Categories

A wide range of disorders will certainly challenge psychiatric home care nurses to exercise their skills. A certain percentage of clients will have strictly psychiatric problems. However, it is more likely, particularly with the elderly, that many complex issues will emerge. Depression may be difficult to separate from very real organic changes. Physical well-being may be compromised by medication effects or interactions. Otherwise normal recovery from health problems may be complicated by grief reactions due to the loss of a spouse or a friend. At any time, the impact of a dysfunctional family may require intervention.

Certain diagnostic configurations will also limit treatment goals. Home care treatment plans at present are formulated on a short-term basis, with the goal of returning clients' functional abilities. The assessment process includes an evaluation of clients' highest possible level of function. In some cases, nurses must be able to accept the fact that they are dealing with psychiatric symptoms that will not be resolved during the term of the treatment plan. The goals must then focus on improving function and adaptation, not on resolving issues that require long-term psychotherapy.

Dynamics in Home Care

Two of the interpersonal dynamics that undergo change in the home care setting are control and dependency. While both are issues in any therapeutic relationship, they take on a different character when the client is treated at home.

Home health care nurses know that control is in the hands of clients. Actually, this is true in all areas of health care, but nurses generally convince themselves otherwise. By recognizing this reality, nurses can address client noncompliance that is not directly attributable to a lack of knowledge. Home care clients make the final determination, directly or indirectly, regarding whether nurses will even be allowed in the front door. The professional role changes drastically. Clients are not going out of their way to appear at an office or hospital at the convenience of the health care provider. Rather, clients tell nurses what time to arrive, and have full control over what will happen once the nurse is there. Nurses who have difficulty in dealing with this role reversal find that their clients cancel appointments, or call another agency for service. Obviously, health care often involves telling clients things they may not want to hear, and prescribing changes in their lifestyles or daily routines that they may not wish to implement. The "reversal" of control does not mean that nurses should practice a lower standard of nursing in order to gain clients' approval. It does mean that nurses cannot afford arrogance in dealing with clients. Nurses must earn clients' trust and strive to understand their positions if they are to cooperate with treatment. Nurses must also avoid believing the fallacy that they have absolute control of clients' health care. Clients determine the parameters and the success. Nurses are expert collaborators and, once this is established as a part of the therapeutic contract, it is amazing how responsible and cooperative clients can become.

Upon entering clients' homes, nurses walk a fine line between maintaining their professional identity and being welcomed as pseudo-members of the family. A close transference can develop rapidly. Nurses must monitor its progress and intervene appropriately to avoid being perceived as nothing more than a social companion. This is particularly true in psychiatric home care. Hands-on nursing, such as dressing changes or drawing blood, is not a routine reinforcement of the psychiatric nurse's professional role. Isolated psychiatric clients are particularly vulnerable to using even the most distant clinicians as social contacts. This type of transference can happen in any setting, but is more intense in the home because there are fewer resources to dilute it.

A related question is raised for home care agencies: should psychiatric nursing services be delivered separately from or in conjunction with health care treatments? The answer may be provided by payer sources who insist that a nurse is a nurse, specialty or no, and that separate visits will not be paid for. It might be considered helpful in some cases for both types of care to be delivered by the same person, thereby reinforcing the nursing role. However, this short-sighted position fails to consider that the transference itself may be the very leverage necessary for progress. Combining the roles may actually dilute the therapeutic process—not to mention be more time-consuming and exploitive of the nurse. In fact, psychotic clients experiencing distortions of reality or of ego boundaries may not tolerate physical or invasive procedures being performed by the same nurse with whom they discuss conflictual issues. Until payer sources become more adaptable in this area, nurses will have to exercise their professional judgment regarding the appropriateness of combining roles.

Although the dynamics of psychiatric home care differ from those in any other setting, the therapeutic process can still be effective. It is a particular challenge, however, for nurses to consider the impact of these dynamics throughout the course of the treatment plan. Preparation in some pertinent areas of intervention is especially helpful.

Preparation of the Psychiatric Home Care Nurse

The effectiveness of psychiatric nursing care in the home setting depends upon identifying the specific skill components necessary. Professional care-givers must either have the required background or augment their current skill level to include new components. On-the-job psychiatric nursing experience is appropriate for certain levels of care. However, many clients require the advanced intervention capability learned at the graduate level. A high degree of accountability and independence is prerequisite, along with a sound medical background and a willingness to adapt to the administrative demands of the field. Certain characteristics of psychiatric home care dictate training in other areas as well.

Inpatient nursing care operates with an awareness that 24-hour follow-up of interventions is provided by skilled, complementary staff. This is not the case in home health care. This difference necessitates changes in the therapeutic approach as well as in the attitudes and awareness of nurses. Emphasis must shift from continuous care to intermittent care. There is an increased need for clarity and brevity of approach, greater awareness of safety issues and options, and resourceful use of the environment. Clients' strengths and resources must be utilized to the fullest. Maximum involvement of clients and their families in care planning is imperative to ensure follow-through. In short, psychiatric/mental health home care nurses must learn to use all available resources in order to guide therapy. They must then stand back and provide gentle guidance as interventions begin to work.

Familiarity with short-term treatment modalities and a strong ability to structure the interview process are necessary basic skills. However, brief intervention is not a cookbook approach to therapy. Its effectiveness depends on a solid theory base and an awareness of its limitations. Nurses must be able to recognize when referral for long-term treatment or hospitalization is necessary.

The presence or absence of the family is always an issue in home care. Certainly, the influence and interplay of family and significant others is important in effecting

behavioral change. With many inpatient populations, nurses participate only indirectly in this area. Additional training and supervision will assist nurses to better assess and utilize family dynamics in a therapeutic manner.

Each of the areas listed—intermittent treatment, short-term intervention, and family therapy—constitutes a set of skills that must be a part of the psychiatric home care nurse's repertoire. If these skills do not already exist, they must be developed in training and supervision. Experiences that increase nurses' abilities in these areas include: inpatient units with a short-term or strategic focus, outpatient treatment, crisis intervention, liaison psychiatry, and independent practice. Special training in geropsychiatric and child/adolescent psychiatric nursing are also helpful. Nurses interested in psychiatric home care can learn a great deal during these experiences.

Research

A number of studies explore the use of psychiatric home care with acute and chronic schizophrenic populations, the elderly, and medical clients with psychological difficulties. Home treatment is looked at following, and in lieu of, hospitalization. Some initial observations are offered concerning specific indications for home care.

The past 20 years have seen drastic changes in mental health care systems, both here and abroad. Public outcry over inadequate state mental hospitals, institutionalization, and inhumane treatment of clients led to the community mental health movement. Almost overnight, clients who had spent most of their lives in institutions were being released into the community, where mental health centers were supposed to supply their treatment needs. However, within a short period of time, questions were raised concerning the effectiveness of this "humane" move.

An English study addressed the status of 120 schizophrenic clients discharged from a mental hospital over a five-year period. This follow-up took place with individuals who had been out of the hospital for between five and nine years. Of the 120 clients identified, 105 were traced, 94 were alive, 66 were living at home and willing to be interviewed, and another 11 were hospitalized. Mental status and social situation were assessed by interview with both the clients and significant others. Of the 66 who lived at home, 18% showed no symptoms of psychiatric disturbance, while more than 50% demonstrated definite psychotic features. Despite this last number, no clients and few relatives wished a return to hospital care; 27% of clients had no contact with medical or social services; 24% saw only their general practitioner; and 14% saw only community nurses.[9]

The significance of these findings lies in the fact that, although severe emotional, social, and financial difficulties were identified in the majority of cases, the individuals and families were not seeking available help. The authors of the study believed this was due in part to the nature of psychiatric symptoms that lead to impaired judgment and poor cooperation. They also felt that it was partially due to the relatives' difficulty in dealing with the prognosis of the illness and comprehending the need for follow-up. Ultimately, while clients can be released from institutions, it cannot be assumed that this move has been successful simply because the client is not hospitalized elsewhere. The mental health system must consider alternatives for chronically ill clients with unmet needs who will not use the community center system.

An important consideration exists in reference to hospitalization of the elderly and hospitalization of the mentally ill. Society has determined that it is more humane to release the chronically mentally ill into the community than to limit their rights to freedom. Until recently, however, there has been an emphasis on placing the elderly population in convalescent or skilled nursing facilities rather than supporting their desires to live independently. Geropsychiatric needs are becoming increasingly recognized as an important component in maintaining independence for the elderly. Home visits are necessary, not only because of clients' homebound status, but also because they provide important relevant information regarding clients' living conditions and resources. The most idealistic treatment plans become meaningless if they are not applicable to clients' individual situations. Frequently, a part of that situation is the inability or reluctance to seek resources, in which case outreach programs become essential.[6,16,25]

The previously-cited model of a geropsychiatric outreach team was utilized in a study of 83 clients. They were referred by home health professionals for a variety of problems including depression, confusion, and bizarre behavior. At the three-month follow-up, information was available on 66 of these clients. It revealed that 73% of them had improved or stabilized. Of particular note, 50% of the clients with a primary or secondary diagnosis of dementia showed improvement in mood, level of confusion, or interpersonal tensions. While most clients experienced considerable physical, emotional, and psychiatric problems, 86% of them had been able to remain at home. Placement in a nursing home generally followed a hospitalization and was attributed to excessive dependency, anxiety, or physical disability in connection with inadequate social supports. On the whole, the outreach team demonstrated its potential as an alternative to hospitalization or long-term institutionalization.[23]

Whatever the age group, emergency response may become an issue at any time. The Emergency Psychiatric Home Visiting Team, a model that was described earlier, reported its findings on 624 visits made to 443 clients over a four-year period. The team anticipated a greater involvement in suicide prevention than actually occurred. However, its intervention was useful to facilitate hospitalization in emergency situations, and to difuse violent situations without physical harm to staff or family. Other findings of the study support the research previously discussed, since the team's case-load dealt with a large number of the chronically mentally ill requiring services. Many of these clients were seen for multiple episodes, but were unlikely to seek follow-up treatment and either did not qualify for, or refused, hospitalization. In such cases, team visits served as the clients' primary link with psychiatric care.[24]

While this discussion has mostly centered around care for clients with primary psychiatric diagnoses, attention has also been given to the need for psychological services among medical clients. Certainly the body of research supporting psychiatric liaison programs indicates that these services are effective with a wide range of medical disorders. The need increases when dealing with an elderly population who have multiple needs and problems. Programs utilizing psychiatric community nurses with the medical client population have been implemented successfully in England.[1] As psychiatric nurses become more involved with the home health teams in the United States, their role as consultants and therapists will potentially become as important for medical cases as for psychiatric clients.

Where does home care fit in with the existing treatment alternatives, specifically hospitalization and outpatient care? Research indicates that home care is effective both as follow-up and in lieu of hospitalization.

One study from Finland proposed to assess clinical recovery, adjustment into the community, rehabilitation, and expense associated with home care. A group of 102 schizophrenic and paranoid psychotic clients were compared with a control group of the same number of similar clients treated in a traditional hospital setting. During the follow-up period of four years, the home care clients received treatment in the home 44% of the time and were hospitalized 7% of the four-year period. By comparison, the control group was hospitalized 28% of the time. Outpatient contacts for the home group averaged once a week, while the hospital group had outpatient contact about once in four months. Only two of the home group clients, and none of the hospital clients, were attending a rehabilitation center. With regard to the parameters studied, 63% of the home treatment clients and 30% of the hospital clients had recovered clinically at the end of four years. Relapse and hospital readmission occurred more frequently in the hospital group. By the end of the study, 40% of the home care clients and 30% of the hospital clients were employed—not a significant difference. Overall, hospital clients cost the community approximately three times as much as the home care patients. This was calculated by comparing 413 hospital days for the control group against 108 hospital days and 638 home care days for the home treatment group. The authors concluded that psychiatric home care had a definite positive influence on clinical recovery, insignificant results regarding rehabilitation, positive results in minimizing hospitalization, and all at less expense than that of hospital care.[10]

Other studies with smaller populations and more limited parameters support the effectiveness of psychiatric home care in preventing hospitalization.* One study also compared home treatment with outpatient therapy for neurotic clients. The sample of 36 outpatients and 35

---

* References 3, 11, 12, 13, 18, and 19.

home care clients were assessed every six months for 18 months. While no significant differences were found between the two groups with regard to symptoms, social adjustment, or family burden, the home care clients reported greater satisfaction with treatment. At the same time, the home care group demonstrated a reduction in outpatient contacts and more discharges. The home treatment group was slightly more expensive during the first six months, but significantly cheaper over the total 18 months.[14]

None of these studies that investigate psychiatric home care as an alternative to hospitalization took place in the United States. Certainly, the results should be replicated in this country before an across-the-board comparison can be made. One such study of 42 clients conducted by the Maine Medical Center and Portland Community Health Services supported home care as a means of preventing or shortening psychiatric hospitalization.[20] Perhaps it is a commentary on the position of hospitals in this country that remaining studies address home care only as a follow-up of hospitalization.

The Visiting Nurses' Association of Cleveland undertook a nine-month study of psychiatric clients referred after hospitalization. Using a two to one ratio of home treatment clients to individuals not receiving VNA services, the findings were explored for 75 home care and 35 control clients. Home care services were delivered by public health and VNA staff nurses, averaging 2.3 visits per month. Only tentative general conclusions were drawn because of methodological difficulties (originally 254 clients were included, but 92 were lost during the study, mostly due to an inability to locate them).

The results at six months after hospital discharge revealed a 14% increase in employment for the treatment group, with no change in the control group. With regard to medication compliance, 57% of the control group reported missing medications, as opposed to 36% of the treatment group. Readmission to the hospital was more frequent for the control group (34%, against 28% for the treatment group). The authors reported no difference between the two groups on socially-expected activities scores, although difficulties with the research design may have influenced this finding.[22]

Admittedly, the preponderance of research cited does not apply directly to the cultural and environmental situations within the United States. It must be noted that replication of the foreign studies could yield different results as a function of these variables. However, the few American studies certainly do not indicate a potential reversal of the findings, and support the need for replication under local conditions.

Future Trends

Psychiatric home care is a challenging new field that makes use of nursing's greatest strengths and skills. Nurses are presently at a juncture of tremendous opportunity. The supporting research already exists, as do the models for further study. Two requirements remain. The first requirement is a vision or concept toward which the field of mental health may move. The nursing profession is primed with this vision, drawing upon its experiences in both psychiatric nursing and home health care. The second requirement is a collaborative effort on the part of all professionals, setting aside self-interests to ensure the most appropriate level of client services. Given the present focus on cost containment in health care services, psychiatric home care may soon become a mandate rather than a choice.

Psychiatric home care nursing is in its infancy. However, isolated programs are growing under the auspices of a variety of agencies. The growth and development will continue until a predominant model emerges. The nursing profession must contribute to the research and clinical skill that will determine the end result.

Summary

1. Psychiatric home care is a new and promising part of the recent trend toward increased home health care. It adapts appropriate milieu concepts to clients' natural environments, capitalizing on the forces that are part of their experience and reality.

2. The nursing process must include additional emphasis on physical health components and case management.

3. Psychiatric home care operates at the primary, secondary, and tertiary levels of prevention. Short-term interventions in psychiatric home care focus on increasing clients' functional adaptation to the independent living environment.

4. Psychiatric home care can be seen as an extension of community mental health care because it takes place in the home environment. The format of home care can vary according to the focus of treatment, the base of operations, and the time allotment.

5. Nurse–client relationships in home care are different than those in other settings. The relationships have both positive and negative effects that result from changes in control and dependency.

6. Psychiatric home care clientele span all age groups and diagnostic categories.

7. Preparation of the psychiatric home care nurse includes experience with intermittent care settings, short-term intervention, and family therapy.

8. Foreign research supports the need for and effectiveness of psychiatric home care. Fewer studies have been done in the United States, and they are less comprehensive, but they offer support. Continued research efforts are necessary.

References

1. Conway-Nicholls K, Elliott A: North Camden community psychiatric nursing service. Br Med J 285:859, 1982

2. Epstein RS: Outpatient psychotherapy in conjunction with a home care nurse. Bull Menninger Clin 46(5):445, 1982

3. Fenton FR, Tessier L, Struening EL: A comparative trial of home and hospital psychiatric care. Arch Gen Psychiatry 36:1073, 1979

4. Granovetter B: The use of home visits to avoid hospitalization in a psychotic crisis. Hosp Comm Psychiatry 26:645, 1975

5. Gurian BS, Scherl DJ: A community-focused model of mental health services for the elderly. J Geriatr Psychiatry 5(1):77, 1972

6. Ham R: Alternatives to institutionalization. Am Fam Physician 22(1):95, 1980

7. Heinrich J: Historical Perspectives on Public Health Nursing. In Pages From Nursing History. New York, American Journal of Nursing, 1984

8. Heymann GM, Stanton LM: A pilot study to evaluate visiting nurses' services to chronic psychiatric patients. Hosp Comm Psychiatry 28(2):97, 1977

9. Johnstone EC, Owens DGC, Gold A et al: Schizophrenic patients discharged from hospital—a follow-up study. Br J Psychiatry 145:586, 1984

10. Niskanen P, Pihkanen TA: A comparative study of home treatment and hospital care in the treatment of schizophrenic and paranoid psychotic patients. Acta Psychiatr Scand 47(3):271, 1971

11. Pai S, Channabasavanna SM, Nagarajaiah et al: Home care for chronic mental illness in Bangalore—an experiment in the prevention of repeated hospitalization. Br J Psychiatry 147:175, 1985

12. Pai S, Kapur RL: Evaluation of home care treatment for schizophrenic patients. Acta Psychiatr Scand 67:80, 1983

13. Pai S, Roberts EJ: Follow-up study of schizophrenic patients initially treated with home care. Br J Psychiatry 143:447, 1983

14. Paykel ES, Mangen SP, Griffith JH et al: Community psychiatric nursing for neurotic patients—a controlled trial. Br J Psychiatry 140:573, 1982

15. Safirstein SL: Psychiatric aftercare, including home visits. NY State J Med 71(20):2441, 1971

16. Selan BH, Gold CA: The late-life counseling service—a program for the elderly. Hosp Comm Psychiatry 31(6):403, 1980

17. Schlosberg A: A model project of comprehensive psychiatry. Int J Soc Psychiatry 29(2):83, 1983

18. Smith FA, Fenton FR, Benoit C et al: Home care treatment of acutely ill psychiatric patients. Can Psychiatr Assoc J 21(5):269, 1976

19. Smith FA, Fenton FR, Benoit C et al: Home care treatment of acutely ill psychiatric patients—a one-year follow-up. Can Psychiatr Assoc J 23(2):73, 1978

20. Soreff SM: New directions and added dimensions in home psychiatric treatment. Am J Psychiatry 140:1213, 1983

21. Spiegel AD: Home Healthcare. Owings Mill, Maryland, National Health Publishing, 1983

22. Vincent P, Price JR: Evaluation of a VNA mental health project. Nurs Res 26(5):361, 1977

23. Wasson W, Ripeckyj A, Lazarus LW et al: Home evaluation of psychiatrically-impaired elderly—process and outcome. Gerontologist 24(3):238, 1984

24. West DA, Litwok E, Oberlander K et al: Emergency psychiatric home visiting—report of four years' experience. J Clin Psychiatry 41(4):113, 1980

25. White DMD: Psychogeriatrics and community care. Lancet 4(1):27, 1975

MARCIA LUNA-RAINES

PSYCHIATRIC LIAISON NURSING

Learning Objectives

Upon completion of this chapter the student should be able to do the following:

1. Define the role and practice setting of the psychiatric liaison nurse.
2. Identify the major developments in the history of liaison nursing.
3. Identify the need for a psychiatric liaison nurse in the general hospital.
4. Describe the relationship between psychiatric liaison nursing and consultation-liaison psychiatry.
5. Relate the functions of the liaison nurse to concepts of mental illness prevention in the general hospital.
6. Identify the major concepts utilized by liaison nurses in their clinical practice.
7. Identify several common clinical problems encountered by liaison nurses.
8. Describe two preventive interventions performed by liaison nurses.
9. Identify when and how to request consultation from a psychiatric liaison nurse for client- or staff-related problems.

Introduction

"Nowhere does an 'ounce of prevention' have a more powerful appeal than in the field of mental health." [24]

Psychiatric liaison nursing, the role the psychiatric nurse fills in the general hospital, is a subspecialty of psy-chiatric/mental health nursing. Within this role, the psychiatric nurse brings mental health expertise into the hospital health care system to improve the psychological care of (1) emotionally or mentally disturbed clients who have a physical illness, and (2) physically ill clients who develop emotional or mental illness brought on by the stress of disability or hospitalization.

The development and current conceptualization of the role are related to the trends in mental health nursing that have produced the psychiatric clinical specialist. Liaison nursing incorporates a body of knowledge, beliefs, attitudes, skills, and activities that represents a dominant trend in psychiatric nursing today. Since the early 1960s, psychiatric/mental health nursing practice has steadily gained recognition as a potent factor in providing comprehensive care to general hospital clients. Its importance may be expected to increase as a result of the scientific, social, and economic forces that presently influence the general hospital as a health care delivery system.

Prevention of mental illness has recently received more attention from general and mental health care planning agencies. This interest has led to greater efforts by mental health practitioners to implement primary prevention programs in their settings. The strategies used in community mental health practice and preventive psychiatry are especially applicable in the general hospital "community." The psychiatric liaison nurse, a key practitioner in the general hospital, makes a unique contribution to the prevention of mental illness in the general hospital's "most-at-risk" populations—clients and their primary care-givers, nurses.

This chapter describes the evolution, scope, and contributions of liaison nursing in the promotion of mental health in the general hospital health care system. It discusses the concepts frequently utilized by liaison nurses, and illustrates how liaison nursing is implemented in various hospital settings.

Definition of Psychiatric Liaison Nursing

Psychiatric liaison nursing has emerged in the past 20 years as a major subspecialty of psychiatric/mental health nursing. *It is practiced in nonpsychiatric settings.* The most common and familiar settings are the general hospital's medical/surgical, pediatric, and gynecologic wards, emergency rooms, or ambulatory clinics. Other settings include convalescent nursing homes, public health, home health care, and visiting nurse agencies. The psychological needs of the clients and families served in these settings, coupled with the consultation needs of their health care providers, are an indication of the enormous potential of the liaison nurse role.

The title "psychiatric liaison nurse" is appropriate for two reasons. Because the practice of liaison nursing is related in theory, history, and setting to liaison psychiatry, it is practical for psychiatric nurses to use the same label in their role description. Also, Webster's dictionary defines "liaison" as "the linking up of or connecting of parts of a whole, intended to bring about proper coordination of activities, especially intercommunication between units." This definition describes the purpose of the liaison role quite well. Using the word "liaison" in their title helps nurses to explain the role, and clients and consultees to understand the role.

Liaison nurses serve as a link connecting the psychological care of clients with physical care. They link psychiatric services in the health care setting with the available medical and nursing services, and apply mental health principles to the common life experiences and stresses that accompany illness and hospitalization. Liaison nurses base their clinical practice on the philosophy that mind and body, or psyche and soma, are linked in both the cause and the treatment of illness.

Historical Development of Psychiatric Liaison Nursing

Psychiatric liaison nursing is a young nursing specialty: it was pioneered in the early 1960s. Documentation by early practitioners laid the foundation for the role's development.[17,37,39] Most of these early practitioners were psychiatric nurses working on psychiatric wards who consulted with medical/surgical nurses requesting their assistance with clients' psychological needs. Before that time, medical/surgical nurses' use of psychiatric nurses as consultants was rare. It was understood by general ward nurses that psychiatric nurse consultants would not work directly with clients, but would help nursing staff to (1) plan appropriate psychological interventions for their clients, (2) increase their sensitivity to clients' emotional concerns, and (3) recognize the impact these concerns had on clients' illness and recovery. Based on their early experiences, successes, and acceptance by general hospital staff, psychiatric nurses expanded the role into a subspecialty—*liaison nursing.*[35]

At about the same time that nurses were experimenting with various aspects of the liaison role (*i.e.,* consultation, teaching, direct and indirect client interventions), psychiatrists in general hospitals began to acknowledge the value of nursing's contributions to their consultation-liaison (C-L) work. Reading nurses' notes, discussing client behaviors with nurses, and having joint meetings to plan psychological interventions on medical wards were recommended if psychiatric consultations were to be comprehensive, appropriate, and successful.[7] The importance of nursing input at every stage of the psychiatrist's consultation (*i.e.,* assessment, diagnosis, and recommendation) was recognized with the help of liaison nurses.[4,13] Soon after this, psychiatric liaison nurses were proclaimed as invaluable members of the C-L psychiatry team. They were asked to participate in teaching psychiatric residents and medical students during their liaison rotations.[52]

Within ten years, the role evolved from experimental nurse-to-nurse consultation to a multifaceted, fully supported service that was well accepted and integrated within the general hospital.[35] This rapid and successful development of the role can be attributed in part to the need of nonpsychiatric nurses for assistance with clients' psychological care. It can also be attributed to psychiatric nurses' desire to integrate their skills in a variety of settings.[41] The move by psychiatric nurses out of psychiatric wards and into other health care settings, especially the general hospital, was a natural consequence of the development of psychiatric/mental health nursing and of the increasing confidence and independence of psychiatric nurses outside traditional psychiatric settings. Both liaison nurses and their consultees easily accepted the expansion of the liaison role to include (1) direct client assessment to aid nursing staff in formulating care plans, and (2) direct intervention with clients and their families when the nature of the problem required their expertise.

As the involvement of psychiatric nurses with the general hospital increased, the complexity of consulting with nonpsychiatric nurses about physically ill clients became more obvious. Liaison nurses became aware of their need for additional knowledge and skills. This desire for more education, as well as a growing interest by graduate nurses in the role, led to the establishment of the first liaison nursing program. It was established in 1971 at the University of Maryland.[40] Yale's School of Nursing has offered a similar graduate track through its Psychiatric/Mental Health Nursing program since 1973; Community Mental Health faculty at UCLA have supervised graduate students in the role since 1975, although UCLA's first official Liaison Nursing course was not offered until 1983.

Liaison nurses have been writing about their diverse consultation and teaching methods in hospital settings for almost 20 years. Although there is still a paucity of literature in the field, a body of liaison nursing knowledge has emerged from the accumulated writings. Two landmark publications should be acknowledged. Each was the culmination of the continual refinement of liaison nursing theory and practice at its respective time. In 1974, Lisa Robinson, a pioneer in developing the role and its first graduate courses, published *Liaison Nursing: A Psychological Approach to Patient Care.*[41] Lewis and Levy completed *Psychiatric Liaison Nursing: The Theory and Clinical Practice* in 1982.[26]

The character of the role continues to be shaped and researched by its current practitioners, as indicated by this sampling of articles. Berarducci and colleagues[5] and Weinstein and colleagues[50] discussed different consultation styles in relation to staff and ward needs, client populations, and staff readiness for group consultation. Baldwin[1] described the attribution process as a method for helping nurses understand their responses to difficult clients. Freeman[10] discussed transactional analysis in resolving staff–client conflict. Barbiaz and colleagues[2] outlined the nursing administrator's role in facilitating the successful functioning of the liaison nurse in the general hospital. Johnson and colleagues[18] explained the importance of a professional support group for psychiatric nurses in general hospitals, because of the particular stresses in the consultant role. Kolson,[23] Wolff,[53] and Stickney and colleagues[45] studied what staff nurses expect from liaison nurses and what types of client problems are referred to them. Davis and Nelson[9] examined how referrals change over time in their specificity, focus, level of sophistication, and kind of liaison involvement requested.

As psychiatric liaison nursing enters its third decade, the scope of its theory base and clinical practice has grown to match the psychological needs of clients, families, nursing staff, and the hospital system.

Components of Psychiatric Liaison Nursing Practice

The clinical practice of psychiatric liaison nursing is multifaceted. The role synthesizes and applies concepts from a variety of nursing areas. These include psychiatric and medical/surgical nursing, general systems theory, consultation and learning theories, and crisis intervention. Liaison implies close and regular contact with clinical staff and their clients to enhance the psychological care of clients and the therapeutic milieu in which care is given. Psychiatric liaison nursing includes participation in ward activities and in mediation among clients, families, and staff. Intervention is designed to prevent disruption of care by inadequate communication or interpersonal conflicts. Sensitizing care-givers to the social, psychological, emotional, and cultural issues that contribute to the illness of clients and to the stress of care-givers is also within the purview of the role.

Most contemporary practitioners have a master's degree in psychiatric/mental health nursing; some have taken graduate-level courses in liaison nursing that are offered in a few graduate programs. Most liaison nurses are hired directly by nursing service departments, as are other clinical nurse specialists. They hold advanced clinical positions rather than administrative or line positions. Most provide a range of services, including individual and group consultation with nursing and other health care staff and direct client and family assessment and intervention. They are also involved in formal teaching and research related to the psychological care of the physically ill. In contrast, a few are hired by hospital departments of psychiatry. Others may be employed as part-time consultants from a psychiatric nursing unit or outside mental health agency.

Although liaison nurses practice in various clinical settings and within different departments, the effectiveness of the role does not depend on either of these; it lies in the individual's ability to integrate the theory and practice of liaison nursing within the particular clinical setting. Some nurses identify themselves as "psychiatric liaison nurses," some as "mental health nurse consultants," and some as "psychiatric clinical nurse specialists."

Theoretical Model

The goals of psychiatric liaison nursing are applicable in all areas of clinical practice, although the consultation model used may differ. Lewis and Levy[26] summarized the goals as follows:

1. To demonstrate and teach mental health concepts and their application to clinical nursing practice
2. To effect appropriate psychiatric and nursing interventions
3. To support nurses in continuing to provide high-quality nursing care
4. To promote and develop the professional and personal self-esteem of the nurse
5. To encourage tolerance among the members of the nursing staff of situations in which immediate and/or effective intervention or resolution is unattainable

A theoretical model for psychiatric liaison nursing has been developed. The model is based on a holistic approach to consultation, and is used to develop guidelines for clinical practice to meet the goals listed above. It contains five basic principles, each dealing with bodies of knowledge related to specific elements of professional practice. All five principles are equally significant and blend with each other in practice, making the model cohesive and applicable through a process called "diagnosing the total consultation."[26] The model's five principles, and a brief explanation of each, follow:

1. *Consultation-liaison theory.* The clinical practice of psychiatric liaison nursing is firmly based on principles inherent in consultation-liaison theory.
2. *The client.* Assessment of the client's psychological status includes history, personality style, defensive structure, culture, societal factors (such as family), and present level of functioning.
3. *The medical illness.* The client's psychological response to illness and hospitalization is assessed in conjunction with the medical illness, its symptomatology, and the client's physical status.
4. *The nurse and the system.* The elements of the medical milieu and its subsystems must be incorporated.
5. *Preventive management.* Therapeutic and prophylactic psychological care is accomplished through the recognition of predictable responses to specific illnesses, along with the application of adult learning theory and crisis theory.[26]

Psychiatric liaison nursing is a complex activity that requires the identification of client, nurse, and system needs. It recognizes the mind–body relationship in health and illness, and emphasizes the importance of the psychological care of the client and the therapeutic milieu in which it is provided. Finally, psychiatric liaison nursing utilizes a broad range of interventions and skills based on the liaison nursing model in meeting its goals.

In order for students to better understand the interventions used by psychiatric liaison nurses to accomplish the fifth principle of liaison nursing identified above—preventive management—students should be able to identify the need for a psychiatric liaison nurse in the general hospital. They should also be familiar with the historical development of the role and be able to de-

scribe the relationship between liaison nursing and consultation-liaison psychiatry.

Consultation-Liaison Psychiatry

Developments in psychiatric nursing in the United States have kept pace with changes in psychiatry.[15] Like most trends in nursing, the psychiatric liaison role developed in a fashion parallel to that of the medical model preceding it, which was the consultation-liaison (C-L) practice in psychiatry.[41] This phenomenon is a result partially of the consumer's need for expanded services and partially of the nursing profession's desire and readiness to understand and use new knowledge and technology. The practice of liaison nursing and the practice of C-L psychiatry rely on the same theory. C-L psychiatry is built on a foundation provided by psychosomatic medicine. Psychosomatic theory stresses mind–body integration in health and illness, and provides a practical framework for participation of psychiatrists in treatment of the physically ill.[27,28]

C-L psychiatry, a subspecialty of psychiatry, is about 30 years older than psychiatric liaison nursing. Current perspectives of C-L psychiatry were fairly well developed before liaison nursing began. Major changes in the field have occurred from the early 1930s, when small C-L services were created in a few general hospitals, to the early 1960s, when Lipowski, the father of C-L psychiatry, solidified its practice in the psychosomatic literature. In its early practice, general hospital psychiatrists focused almost entirely on the diagnosis and treatment of the *client* with a particular psychopathology. Later, the client was assessed and treated *in relation to the family and environment* in which the illness developed. Still later, the client was seen as only a part of a much larger *system.* This system included hospital staff and the hospital milieu itself, all of which influenced the client and the disease process. By the time psychiatric liaison nursing was beginning, the philosophy and practice of C-L psychiatry had expanded from the client-only consultation focus to a general systems, liaison focus. These differences are included in Table 31-1. *Liaison* is defined here as the regular and sustained contact between mental health professionals and the medical/surgical staff. It includes developing working relationships in order to create optimal conditions to help prevent, detect, and manage psychiatric disorders, mediating client–staff conflicts, and teaching. *Consultations* refers here to providing expert opinion as to a client's psychiatric condition and advising on its proper management, at the request of a nonpsychiatric colleague.[30]

With this broader view of their function, "the ultimate aim of consultation-liaison psychiatrists has been described as the optimal care of the sick."[29] This goal is attained by tending to the personal and interpersonal issues involving the client, the family, and the hospital staff that interfere with medical, surgical, or nursing management. This is done largely by the methods defined in

TABLE 31-1.

DIFFERENCES BETWEEN CONSULTATION AND LIAISON FUNCTIONS IN PSYCHIATRY

	CONSULTATION	LIAISON
PURPOSE	At the request of a nonpsychiatric physician, to provide expert psychiatric opinion regarding a client's psychiatric condition and to advise on the client's psychiatric management	To provide regular and sustained contact with nonpsychiatric staff in order to create an optimal working milieu in which to prevent, detect, and manage clients' psychiatric disorders, to mediate staff–client conflicts, and to teach
TARGET POPULATION	The physician referring a client, and the client	All health care staff, clients, clients' family and friends, and any other persons or hospital departments affecting clients or staff
ACTIVITIES AND INTERVENTIONS	Client assessment and diagnosis Providing suggestions for client treatment, including medications and follow-up care arrangements Written documentation of above Little interaction with other care providers Not assigned to specific units	Attendance at ward rounds or conferences with various staff All staff or client-related problems are acceptable for consultation. Any staff member may refer a problem. Frequent staff contact in formal or informal manner Usually assigned to the same unit for several months

Caplan's model of preventive psychiatry and mental health consultation. Today, C-L psychiatry has been called the front line of preventive psychiatry in providing primary prevention to clients in crisis and consulting with their care-givers in nonpsychiatric settings.[3] The preventive goals described here are increasingly striven for in all health care systems.[29]

Where does the liaison nurse fit into this picture of C-L psychiatry? The psychiatric nurse has naturally evolved as the most appropriate health care professional to assume the liaison role described above. This is because of the large numbers of nurses giving direct client care in nonpsychiatric settings who require assistance in meeting the psychological needs of clients.[5] Lipowski[30] suggested: "Let psychiatrists do consultation involving complex medico-psychosocial, diagnostic, and therapeutic problems and let liaison nurses do most of the day-to-day liaison activity on the hospital wards."

Liaison nurses make a unique contribution to C-L psychiatry in several ways:

1. The continual presence of the liaison nurse on medical/surgical wards contributes to the acceptance of psychiatric concepts and integration of them into general nursing and medical care. Through the liaison nurse, psychiatrists become more accessible, acceptable, and useful in patient care management.[6]

2. Liaison nurses are more closely involved with, and aware of, client and staff problems requiring mental health support. Liaison nurses are closest to hospital staff who have the opportunity in their primary care-giver role to reduce the emotional effects of illness for their clients.[26]

3. Liaison nurses reinforce staff nurses' and ward physicians' roles as early problem-finders. The hospital staff learns to make appropriate referrals earlier. On units with liaison nurses, client referrals shift from crisis management and "dumping" to more preventive involvement.[20]

4. Support of the liaison nurse position by hospital and nursing administrators demonstrates the value they place on the psychological care of clients. Meeting client needs is not something done only when there is time; it is a standard of care for which nursing and hospital administration provide expert assistance.[5]

5. Liaison nurses have the knowledge and skills to provide supportive psychotherapy and follow-up management of difficult client cases after psychiatric evaluation. They can screen potential behavioral and emotional problems with clients and staff. Their services assure that clients receive high-quality psychological care without taxing the C-L service.[31]

6. It has been documented that client populations seen by the liaison nurse are different from those seen by the C-L psychiatrist. Nursing referrals tend to include an even distribution of psychological and behavioral patient problems. Psychiatrists are called three times more frequently for psychological problems (e.g., organic brain syndrome, ICU psychosis) than for behavioral problems. Liaison nurses are called much more often than psychiatrists to assist with dying patients and their families, while psychiatrists are called for questions regarding competency and legal matters.[45]

Most referrals for psychiatric consultation fall into five categories:

1. Psychiatric clients with obvious psychopathology in the general hospital

2. Clients with a combination of psychiatric and physical (psychosomatic) disease

3. Clients with personality problems that interfere with medical or surgical treatment

4. Clients with severe emotional reactions to serious medical disease

5. Clients with complicated ethical, moral, and legal cases that require psychiatric evaluation or intervention

The liaison nurse can assist with all of these types of referrals by either direct or indirect intervention. If, as Lipowski believes, "the most common occasion for psychiatric consultation is communication breakdown between the patient and care-givers,"[30] then certainly the role liaison nurses can play is evident. In hospitals where the psychiatrist and liaison nurse collaborate, a method for deciding who will see the client is usually based on the type of client problem and who initiated the referral. Frequently, liaison nurses screen the referral and perform an initial assessment. They call the psychiatrist only after determining a need for further evaluation, for psychotropic medications, or to meet hospital protocol requiring a psychiatrist's direct consultation. Some such circumstances might involve a suicidal client, a drug overdose, or a question about client competency. The availability and visibility of the liaison nurse increase the opportunity for early and appropriate identification of and intervention with clients in all five categories, although the psychiatrist may ultimately become more involved in some cases.

Studies of psychiatric referrals, their initiation and outcome, are extremely important to both C-L psychiatrists and liaison nurses. Wolff[53] concluded that a multitude of factors contribute to the nurse's decision to refer a client. Referred clients tend to exhibit more psychopathology and to evoke more negative reactions in the nurse than do clients who are not referred. Wolff also found, contrary to popular belief, that the nurse's assessment of client behaviors, not the nurse's reactions, is the most significant factor in referral. Davis and Nelson[9] found that referrals from nursing staff change over time. The nature of these changes is viewed as an indication of the direct influence of the psychiatric liaison nurse upon staff nurses. It also reflects the improved psychological care given by staff nurses when a nurse consultant is available. These findings are important in evaluating the effectiveness of past consultation and planning future preventive activities. A stable referral pattern may indicate that staff are not learning or applying the mental health concepts being modeled and taught by the liaison nurse.

Psychiatric liaison nursing is a "discipline which provides a highly skilled level of coordination between the psychiatry department and the general hospital."[41] The goals and methods of the liaison nurse are the same as those of the C-L psychiatrist. Both provide high-quality psychological care for physically ill clients. The roles complement and reinforce each other's unique contributions to providing optimal client care and a therapeutic milieu.

Psychiatric Liaison Nursing in the General Hospital

The general hospital environment can be highly stressful for both clients and staff. The inpatient facilities of today's general hospital are increasingly utilized for only the very ill who must be monitored constantly, require complex surgical procedures, and need prolonged diagnostic work-ups. Outpatient departments are also increasingly stressful: they treat more chronically ill, older, and poorer clients who use the hospital clinics and emergency rooms as their "surrogate physicians." Both settings, because they are specialized, use sophisticated equipment, and serve clients with severe and chronic illnesses, render the hospital stressful for clients and their care-givers.

In addition to the stressful hospital milieu, each technical innovation in the medical field has spawned new human problems. ICU psychosis syndrome has been identified in clients who have been hospitalized in intensive care units.[12] Clients with end-stage renal disease, who would not survive without hemodialysis, require consistent and sophisticated psychological support due to the high incidence of depression and suicide related to their life-long dependence on a "machine."[46]

The "burnout" phenomenon experienced by nurses and other mental health care staff in acute care facilities is another testament to hospital-induced dysfunction. Both clients and staff, although they demand the benefits of increased technology, suffer simultaneously from the resulting depersonalization and fragmentation of care. The modern hospital requires considerable adaptive skill on the part of clients and staff.

All individuals who are admitted to hospitals bring with them not only physical diseases but also expectations, values, coping skills, and illness behaviors that influence both the manner in which they assume their roles as clients and the course of their hospitalizations.[42] How quickly and skillfully clients fit into the social system of the hospital depends on all these factors, as well as on the hospital's ability to provide a milieu that is conducive to treatment. Most clients entering this system have existing emotional and physical stress and are considered at high risk for developing symptoms of mental distress during or following hospitalization. Strain[46] found that 50% of all outpatients and at least 33% of inpatients, had significant psychological reactions accompanying their medical illness or physical condition. Shevitz and colleagues[44] found that almost 70% of the clients referred for psychiatric evaluation during their hospitalization had psychiatrically-related problems, as either a primary or a secondary diagnosis. It is obvious that psychiatric liaison nurses have a role in the general hospital providing psychological care for these clients.

Sometimes called "the nurse's nurse," the liaison nurse's other most important function in the general hospital is providing mental health consultation to the nursing staff. Nurses have the major responsibility for actually carrying out the primary task of caring for ill people who cannot be cared for elsewhere. *Nursing service bears the full, immediate, concentrated, and direct impact of the stress arising from providing this care.* A major goal of nursing services becomes, therefore, to organize itself to reduce this anxiety.[32] Just how successful nursing departments and individual nurses are at minimizing the long-

CLINICAL EXAMPLE

Meghan, the head nurse of the dialysis unit, asked the liaison nurse to help her and her nursing staff with problems related to hospital administration and their own organizational structure. The dialysis programs, pediatric and adult, hemodialysis, and chronic ambulatory peritoneal dialysis, had grown quickly. Staff nurses were overworked and dissatisfied with their head nurse's leadership.

After several meetings with the head nurse, the liaison nurse, known as the mental health nurse consultant to the dialysis staff, began meeting weekly with the different nursing groups to identify problems from their perspectives and to evaluate possible group resources and willingness to change.

About nine months after the consultation groups started, several positive administrative and organizational changes had begun: (1) the staff turnover rate decreased dramatically; (2) the head nurse, after much discussion with the staff, delegated some of her responsibilities and authority to assistant nurses; (3) the medical director of the unit and representative nursing staff met with the hospital administration to outline client and staff needs resulting from the rapid program expansion; and (4) new nurses, hired after consultation began, remarked

how much they enjoy working with dedicated and competent staff in a growing, challenging, and supportive program.

This case describes one of the four types of mental health consultation defined by Caplan.[8] The liaison nurse usually uses client-centered and consultee-centered case consultation methods, as described in the other clinical examples in this chapter. In addition, due to skills in group process, communication, change planning, and organization, the liaison nurse is also asked to consult on program and staff administrative problems.[25,51] These types of mental health consultation also play a role in primary prevention by supporting care-giving professionals in the following ways: (1) increasing their knowledge and confidence in managing difficult, stressful client problems; (2) demonstrating that expert assistance is readily available when an impasse occurs with clients or administration; (3) symbolizing legitimization by the care-givers' institution of the fact that as care-givers they are expected to encounter complex and confusing situations for which consultation is not only provided, but encouraged; and (4) the understanding that requesting assistance with difficult cases casts no reflection on their professional adequacy.

and short-term effects of this inevitable stress on their staffs and on themselves is a prominent concern for more nursing administrators today than ever before. Many look to the benefits of having a psychiatric liaison nurse available to their nurses to allay the stresses they must tolerate in the modern hospital system.[11,41]

Other reasons supporting the presence of psychiatric nurses in the general hospital are related to major changes in the nursing and medical professions since the 1970s. Professional reactions to the public's demands for more personalized, effective, and economical health care have resulted in a more "holistic" approach to clients' needs during hospitalization and other treatment phases. An increased awareness by the general public of client advocacy and consumerism has caused health professionals to focus on clients' rights, health education, and wellness promotion, as well as on the vital part the public plays in shaping health care systems. The general acceptance of research supporting the multicausal theories of disease development and treatment has resulted in increased acceptance and use of psychological and environmental approaches to disease prevention and treatment. The combined influence of these trends has augmented the recognition and appreciation of the psychological aspects of client care.

The psychiatric liaison nurse is a visible reminder of the importance of psychological care of hospital clients, as well as of consultative support for nurses. The presence of a liaison nurse in the general hospital provides an opportunity to fulfill more adequately the hospital's obligation to the community—to apply the mass of psychological knowledge in the prevention and treatment of mental illness in relation to physical illness.

Mental Illness Prevention in the General Hospital

Prevention has been clearly identified as the number one priority for present and future health care systems by both general health and mental health leaders at the federal level.[48] The movement to increase prevention activities in mental health programs has become significant enough to be called "the fourth psychiatric revolution." The impact of these forces has changed the role the general hospital plays in prevention of mental illness.[21]

The logic and urgency of preventive psychiatry in the hospital system are evident when the enormous impact of behavior on general health problems is considered. Statistics repeatedly verify the importance of the general health–mental health connection. At any one time, 15% of the U.S. population has a diagnosable mental disorder.[38] More than half of this group will seek treatment at some time for their mental problems in the ambulatory or inpatient general health care setting. Trend data underscore the significance of these figures: between 1971 and 1975, when overall discharges from general hospitals increased only 16%, individuals with a primary diagnosis of psychiatric disorder increased 42%. Discharges with a secondary diagnosis of mental disorder increased 52%.[47] Research designed to examine the impact of including mental health services in general health care settings has revealed a 20% average reduction in general health service use when mental health services are incorporated.[19] These statistics, combined with factors supporting the need for a liaison nurse in the general hospital, clearly designate the general hospital as an important target area for mental illness prevention.

Levels of Prevention

As has been discussed throughout this text, levels of prevention are divided into three activities. *Primary prevention* is the promotion of optimum health by means of client education and the removal of barriers to health in the environment. *Secondary prevention* includes early detection and treatment of alterations in health. *Tertiary prevention* refers to rehabilitative interventions that restore clients to the optimal possible level of health. Although work with clients in hospitals has traditionally been viewed as secondary and tertiary prevention, there is much that can be done at the primary level to relieve the physical and psychological stresses that accompany hospitalization.

Stress and its Management

The theory underlying the stress-model approach to prevention is based on Selye's work.[43] In adapting stress theory to hospitalized clients and the milieu, liaison nurses and psychiatrists have developed useful strategies. These strategies all rely on stress reduction or adaptation theory for prevention and treatment of hospital- or illness-induced stress. Barton and Abram[3] discussed *psychosocial adaptive failure* on the part of clients who develop emotional or behavioral responses to the stress of illness, surgical procedures, or the hospital milieu. In some situations, failure in adaptation reaches the proportions of "mental disorder." A specific psychopathological state such as an acute schizophrenic episode or a psychotic depression can ensue. The hospital milieu itself may cause adaptive failure when the emotional responses of caregivers interfere with their providing adequate treatment. In this state, the milieu is no longer able to facilitate the client's psychological adaptation. Robinson[41] concluded that "adaptation is the central theme which gives cohesion to liaison practice." The liaison service functions to assist patients in adapting to the stresses caused by illness and hospitalization by attempting to decrease the anxiety accompanying such efforts. Horowitz and Kaltreider[14] presented the *stress response syndrome* as an organizing conceptual model for understanding and planning appropriate primary prevention of stress caused by serious life events and the typical reactions to loss.

Each of these models conceptualizes the development of stress in the hospitalized client and suggests strategies for managing stress. All of their interventions can be categorized under one or more of the four major types of primary prevention identified by Klein and Goldston.[22] A brief explanation of each type, along with sample interventions, is presented below:

1. *Stressor management*—manages the stressors before they have an impact on the client. At the time of admission, the nurse gathers data from the client and others about previous hospital experiences, expectations, and problems. Using this information, the nurse plans interventions to decrease or modify some or all of the stressors identified by the client.

2. *Stressor avoidance*—when stressors are impossible to modify or eliminate, the client is removed from the stressors. If the client cannot tolerate a particular roommate or room assignment, arrangements are made to move the client. If the client has extreme fears of surgery or other invasive procedures that are not diminished through teaching or emotional support, arrangements are made to delay the procedure, if it is not life-threatening, until the client is less anxious.

3. *Stress resistance-building*—mobilizes strength-building experiences that will enable clients more readily to resist or cope with stressors to which they are, or may be, exposed. When clients have been told about a possible diagnosis of cancer or the need for amputation, time is provided for discussion about what the event means to the client. Emotional, intellectual, and social support are built in for the client by including the family in teaching and treatment planning. Client participation in self-help groups is encouraged. Anticipatory guidance is used as a specific strength-building intervention just before exposure to the anticipated crisis.[8]

4. *Stress reaction management*—prevents the client's response to stressors from compounding the problem or becoming more damaging than the stressors themselves. When a client requires postoperative treatment in an intensive care unit, the client is taught before surgery about the ICU, the client's family is informed about visiting, thereby minimizing the effects of sensory deprivation and "ICU syndrome." Desensitization, behavior modification, and relaxation training are also useful interventions in this category.

All of these methods are also applicable to managing stress in hospital staff. Examples will be given in the clinical examples below.

Barton and Abram[3] presented a holistic approach in their model of primary prevention in the general hospital. Their strategies demonstrate the combination of stresses at intrapersonal, interpersonal, and environmental levels that the liaison team must assess in planning preventive actions.

1. Recognition and reduction of psychological stress resulting from the hospital setting and illness
2. Recognition of personality traits and other predisposing factors in clients' environments that make them vulnerable to adaptive failure
3. Appreciation of interactional patterns among clients and those caring for them
4. Recognition and strengthening of the factors in the doctor–client and nurse–client relationships and hospital environment that support the individual's adaptive abilities

CLINICAL EXAMPLE: ROBERT AND ROSE

Robert, a 59-year-old engineer, had been at his wife Rose's bedside in the surgical ICU almost constantly since she lapsed into a coma 10 days earlier. She had been through two abdominal procedures for a perforated bowel about a month before, and since had suffered several major complications including systemic infection, massive abdominal tissue necrosis, and finally renal failure.

The ICU nurses contacted the liaison nurse when Robert refused to go home three nights in a row. He was not eating or sleeping, and had started to complain of chest pain, increased coughing, and dizziness. He was seen "popping" nitroglycerine tablets before and after visiting his wife or talking to her doctors.

Up to this time, the ICU nurses and medical staff had hoped that Rose would recover. They had seen clients with similar "impossible" multiple-system problems leave their unit after weeks of intensive nursing care and come back to thank the staff for believing they could survive. After another week of antibiotics, dialysis, and respiratory therapy with no change in her condition, Robert began to fear her death. He refused to leave the hospital because he had promised to be at her side when she awoke or when she died.

The nurses felt both compassion for and anger toward Robert. They tried to accommodate his need to be with his wife, but his constant presence and worsening physical appearance made them feel helpless and even a bit frightened. How would he react when she died?

The liaison nurse had several goals in planning preventive actions: (1) by using *anticipatory guidance* with Robert, the nurse encouraged his acceptance of, and prepared him for, his wife's death; (2) by reinforcing his trust in the ICU nurses and by building a rapport with him, the liaison nurse decreased his reluctance to leave the hospital to care for his own health needs; and (3) by consulting with the ICU staff, the nurse decreased their stress about his behavior and increased their confidence in managing whatever happened.

Anticipatory guidance, a preventive technique described by Caplan,[8] was used very effectively in Robert's anticipatory grieving as well as with the ICU staff. The technique employs discussion, either in a group or one-to-one, and is led by a mental health specialist. By discussing Rose's impending death with Robert at his request (after her doctors had asked him to consider "Do Not Resuscitate" status), the liaison nurse supported Robert as he moved through the steps of the grieving process. When his wife died, Robert had already planned her funeral with his minister and contacted friends for support. The liaison nurse called him regularly during the following month to monitor his adjustment to life without his spouse of 35 years. Using the same technique with the nursing staff, the liaison nurse helped them identify what they feared most about caring for Rose and her husband, and what interventions would be appropriate if "what they feared most" actually occurred. Although the stresses caused by caring for and grieving for the client could not be avoided, anticipatory guidance provided a method for *stress resistance-building* and *stress reaction-management*. Anticipatory guidance or "emotional inoculation" is most effective when the mental health specialist has already built collaborative relationships with the staff or clients/families involved in the potential crisis. If there was no prior contact or time to implement this technique, the liaison nurse could have used other crisis intervention methods in this case.

5. Appreciation of the disorders resulting in organic dysfunction that predispose the individual to adaptive failure, *e.g.*, post-op organic brain syndrome, or delirium caused by narcotics or sedating medications, especially in the elderly

Other concepts vital to the preventive functions of the psychiatric liaison nurse are crisis intervention, adult learning theory, and general systems theory.

Crisis Intervention

Crisis intervention, discussed in detail in Chapter 13, is an extremely important treatment modality in the general hospital if illness and hospitalization are thought of as potential crises for every client. The situational and developmental crises that occur during these times present care-givers with a unique opportunity to prevent, or at least minimize, unhealthy responses to the stresses caused by the crises. Illness and hospitalization are viewed as a turning point at which the client can either learn new coping behaviors or reinforce maladaptive ones. Prevention is successful when interventions reduce the incidence and severity of emotional distress by helping clients develop new problem-solving or stress-management techniques.

Adult Learning Theory

Adult learning theory assists liaison nurses in identifying potential crises for clients as they experience illness and hospitalization. It also helps in teaching nursing staff to deal with crises for themselves as well as their clients in a manner conducive to positive learning. Knowledge of the process by which adult clients and staff learn is basic to preventive intervention. Ward nurses' success in providing psychological care is related to their ability to recognize and work within clients' learning styles. Nurses need to teach clients to manage their illness and hospitalization. The liaison nurse plays a major role in educating nurse-consultees in the interplay of psychological reactions to illness, stress, and the adult learning process.

For example, when a client who has just had a colostomy for colon cancer and is told that he must learn his own stoma care becomes anxious and declines to participate in any lessons, the nurse can apply adult learning theory. Concepts from adult learning theory, along with basic supportive emotional care, can help nurses guide clients in learning new skills during recuperation. Some of the most useful concepts for nurses include:

1. Assess the client's readiness to learn.
2. Allow the client to set the learning priorities.

CLINICAL EXAMPLE: DIANE

Diane, a 31-year-old divorcee, lived with her disabled mother and teenage son. She was admitted for the third time in two years for treatment of complications resulting from congenital biliary atresia. She had been hospitalized every year since the age of 14, and had had more than 30 surgical procedures to correct her rare anomaly. She was admitted this time for dehydration, abdominal pain, and probable abscess at an old drainage tube site.

The client was known well by the general surgery floor nursing staff who had cared for her before. In anticipation of her third admission, the liaison nurse was called by the head nurse to plan a behavioral program that would minimize the disruption experienced during the client's last hospitalization.

Major problems had resulted in the client's care when she "split" the staff, a common phenomenon with borderline personality patients, so that all her nurses and doctors were angry at each other or at her. Teamwork, pain management, and her overall physical care were jeopardized as all her care-givers reacted to feeling manipulated by her. The liaison nurse met with the nursing staff and head nurse before Diane's admission to plan preventive actions.

When the general surgery nursing staff asked to have the client admitted to another floor due to the high number of acutely ill and terminal clients already on their floor, the liaison nurse arranged to have Diane "boarded" on another surgical floor, and met daily with her nurses there. At the suggestion of the liaison nurse, a pain management consult was arranged soon after admission. The liaison nurse also met daily with Diane to provide support and arbitrate any staff-client con-

flicts. These preventive actions were deemed successful when the client was discharged without any of the prior problems having developed.

Clients with a combined medical and psychiatric diagnosis, such as Diane's are frequently referred to the liaison nurse or psychiatrist. The most successful preventive interventions in these cases are a combination of: (1) visible and frequent support of the staff; (2) informal teaching about the psychiatric condition, its etiology, and its treatment; and (3) supportive treatment, brief psychotherapy if possible, with the client. The net effect is minimal disruption in normal nursing routines, improved communication about the client's care, and, most importantly, uncompromised medical care for the client who has psychological factors affecting a physical condition. The preventive interventions coordinated by the liaison nurse in this case resulted in the nursing staff's readily coping with a difficult client (stressor management) and the client's learning more adaptive hospital behavior (stress resistance-building).

The liaison nurse worked with the staff in applying adult learning principles while working with Diane and her wound care. The nurses felt very competent in wound care, and they discussed with the liaison nurse the possibility of having Diane learn about wound care.

The staff reviewed the principles of adult learning with the liaison nurse. They watched for signals from Diane to indicate that she was ready to learn about wound care. The staff also discussed the importance of a positive attitude in working with the client, to increase the likelihood of Diane's acceptance of the learning program.

---

3. Identify what the client already knows about the new skills.
4. Allow the client to determine learning goals and time-frames, when possible.
5. Encourage the client to identify learning needs and resources for ongoing learning after discharge.

General Systems Theory

General systems theory, introduced to psychiatry by von Bertalanffy,[49] provides an integrating conceptual framework for analyzing the general hospital system. The theory attempts to formulate a set of principles that are flexible and broad enough to encompass a wide variety of phenomena related to mutual interactions. A *system* is composed of matter and energy organized into subsystems and components that constrain, condition, or depend on each other in a common time–space continuum. When this concept is applied to human behavior, it provides a framework within which the content of psychological and social sciences can logically be integrated with that of physical and biological sciences. Miller,[33,34] recognized that the consultant must process a vast amount of data gathered from several sources and levels within the client–hospital system. Miller proposed that

the general systems model can assist in deciding how to select and organize the data, and where to intervene most effectively in the system. Using this framework, the liaison nurse can better decipher the multidimensional problems and plan prudent, preventive actions.

Psychiatric liaison nurses are strong advocates of primary prevention. They work to decrease potential stress in both clients and nurses, and intervene appropriately in situations that might otherwise lead to mental illness for clients or staff. Liaison nurses in general hospitals have assumed responsibility for delivering the mental health support necessary to prevent mental illness.

Behavior Modification

Principles of behavioral theory can be used effectively in clinical practice. This theory describes behavior as "learned." Much of what becomes learned is what is reinforced after a particular desired behavior occurs.

Behavior theory can be effective in working with children. Unfortunately, parents may punish the undesired behavior of a child and not reward the desired behavior (or any approximation of it). The child may perpetuate the undesired behavior because it results in some

---

CLINICAL EXAMPLE: MARIA

Maria, a single 40-year-old woman from central Mexico, had worked in a Los Angeles dressmaker's shop for two years. She lived with friends in a nearby apartment and enjoyed going to church and Spanish-language movies. She was on her way home from work one evening, walking across a street, when a car struck her just as she waved a final goodbye to her friends. She was taken by paramedics to the closest emergency hospital with head wounds, facial cuts, and two mangled legs. The right leg was amputated above the knee in the ER, and the other leg was cleaned and dressed after the bleeding was stopped. X-rays showed that the left tibia and fibula were crushed into multiple small fragments from about four inches below the knee to about three inches above the ankle; soft tissue damage was extensive.

Maria was transferred to the university hospital a few days later. An external fixation device and bone and skin grafting were done. Several times over the next 12 months, Maria had more bone and skin grafts to the severely deformed lower leg. Those surgeries were difficult, of course, but even more traumatic for Maria were the complications and emotional consequences of seemingly minor problems and procedures incidental to her major orthopedic care. For example, Maria had severe pain that normally required frequent doses of narcotics. She was embarrassed to ask for medication because she could not speak English, but also because she thought she should endure the pain. She took a few doses when offered by her nurses, but later refused doses because of the sedation and the "funny feelings" the medication caused. Consistent effective pain management was never really achieved because of the language barrier and Maria's beliefs about the medication. (The liaison nurse tried several times with a translator to answer questions and explain the side-effects of pain medications, but without a translator available more often, the misunderstandings recurred.)

About two months after the accident, Maria began a physical therapy program. During one of these strenuous sessions, she fainted and could not be revived for a few minutes. She later described the incident as a religious experience and refused to participate in physical therapy for several days. The psychiatric liaison nurse contacted a Spanish-speaking psychologist to assess Maria for any serious psychopathology and for consultation with the nursing staff. Staff members were beginning to feel as if they couldn't understand Maria's behavior at all. She had become sullen and withdrawn most of the time, while periodically yelling angrily at almost everyone. The Mexican-American psychologist explained that the change in Maria's behavior was related to the fainting episode a few days earlier. Maria did not believe the explanations about hypotension related to change in position and pain. Rather, she believed that "death" had come to take her at the time of the accident, but she had refused to be taken away and was now "fighting" to stay alive. Apparently, Maria had also been having nightmares and flashbacks related to the accident. All of these stresses, mixed with the effects of chronic pain, poor sleep, and the strain of physical therapy, led to the fainting incident. She had interpreted this as a sign that death was returning for her. She had begun to discuss her fears about never being able to walk again and how ugly she must look to others, especially men—"What man would want me without my legs?"

About five months after her hospitalization, Maria's periods stopped. At about this time, she was also having whirlpool therapy every day for wound debridement. She began refusing to go to the whirlpool, believing that the baths were causing her periods to stop. She also developed lower abdominal cramping and pelvic pain. When her orthopedist asked for a gynecology consult, Maria consented. When the young male doctor arrived and tried to perform a pelvic exam, Maria refused to let him examine her. She sat staring for hours and refused to do any of her own care. The liaison nurse who had been seeing Maria frequently all these months (always with the same translator) discovered that Maria had never had a pelvic vaginal exam before. She thought the gynecologist had broken her hymen intentionally because she had seen several small drops of blood after his partial exam. She thought that she was no longer a virgin, and therefore was not suitable for marriage back in her country. Once she blurted this all out, the liaison nurse attempted to reassure her and discuss, as sensitively as possible, Maria's concerns and fears.

Maria's care over the 12 months she was hospitalized involved many hospital departments. She was seen by dietary, pain management, plastic surgery, dermatology, hematology, and orthopedic staff. She used every ancillary service as well—volunteers who came with diversional therapy projects, the chaplain, hairdressers, and even the housekeeping staff all became involved in her care and emotional support system. The liaison nurse worked with the nursing staff to find ways to ensure productive interaction between Maria and the various departments (each of which is a subsystem within the hospital system).

The nursing staff had many care-planning conferences about Maria. She was alternately a joy and a burden to the staff, an enigma much of the time—at least until they could figure out which of her beliefs or cultural values the medical system had violated. Almost every crisis she experienced was related to medical procedures, or their consequences, that did not match her expectations or values. Each time the staff took time to find out how and why she perceived things, they found a way to work with her.

---

form of parent–child contact, even if it is negative or painful to the child.

An effective behavior modification program can be established with a child by determining the desired behavior and establishing a set pattern of positive reinforcement for that behavior. Positive rewards can include what is pleasurable to the child, such as time spent playing a board game with others, favorite foods, hugs, and so on. Undesired behaviors can be ignored.

Summary

1. Psychiatric liaison nurses use a holistic approach to client care to ensure prevention and treatment of mental illness. Liaison nursing is practiced in the general hospital by providing consultation services to the medical and nursing staff to overcome health care stress.

CLINICAL EXAMPLE: SUSIE

Susie, a seven-year-old girl with encopresis of several years' duration was referred to the pediatric C-L team for psychiatric evaluation and treatment while hospitalized for an abdominal work-up and bowel impaction. The medical and nursing staff were unfamiliar with the usual treatment method used for this childhood problem on the child psychiatric ward, but were willing to learn. As soon as Susie's medical work-up was completed and ruled out any physical cause for her fecal incontinence, the child's care was turned over to the C-L team.

One of the team psychiatrists and the liaison nurse determined that a trial of behavior therapy while the child remained in the hospital was reasonable if the pediatric nursing and play therapy staff could implement a behavior modification program on the ward. After several short teaching sessions on the "basics of behavioral therapy," the nurses and play therapists developed a care plan based on rewarding Susie's use of the toilet and time periods with unsoiled underwear. The liaison nurse met daily with the staff to discuss their attitudes and problems with the reinforcement program and to correct any misunderstandings from the earlier teaching. The team psychiatrist also met daily with the medical staff to check on their acceptance of this type of program on their ward.

Within a week, Susie had decreased her soiling frequency from one or two times per hour to less than once in 12 hours. Her parents were taught how to continue the program at home by the liaison nurse.

Initiating the behavior modification program was difficult: nursing staff were hesitant to start a new type of program because they did not feel they could adequately follow through with the frequent checking for stool and rewarding Susie's desired behavior by spending time with her and recording "stars" on her behavior chart. The liaison nurse made several visits during the first few days (covering all shifts) to explain, encourage and support the staff in their efforts to implement an unfamiliar and complex treatment plan. The child psychiatrist, meanwhile, had frequent discussions with the attending pediatrician to explain the rationale for and expected benefits of treating the child on the general hospital ward rather than on the psych ward. The "dual approach" proved quite effective.

While both doctors and nurses, before their success with Susie, had expected that such a case would require treatment on the psychiatric ward, the next time an encopretic child was admitted they instituted a similar program with minimal direction from the liaison team.

2. The evolution of psychiatric liaison nursing as a separate nursing practice area has paralleled the evolution of the psychiatric medical model of consultation-liaison practice. Advanced educational programs to prepare liaison nurses have been established since the early 1970s.

3. The hospital milieu, with its high technology and increasing severity of client problems, is a stressful environment for both clients and health care team members. The psychiatric liaison nurse provides consultation services to both in order to promote psychological well-being.

4. Consultation-liaison is a subspecialty in psychiatry that uses a general systems liaison focus. Liaison nurses give direct care to clients and nurses in nonpsychiatric settings, keeping communications open and thus preventing psychiatric disorders and reducing staff conflicts.

5. Prevention of mental illness in the general hospital is of primary concern to the liaison nurse. Interventions include stressor management, stressor avoidance, stress resistance-building, and stress reaction-management.

6. Concepts vital to preventive functions of the psychiatric liaison nurse include crisis intervention, adult learning theory, and general systems theory. A holistic approach to consultation guides professional practice.

7. The liaison nurse focuses on overcoming clinical problems that prevent the creation of an optimal working milieu. Staff members may request liaison services for clients or for health care professionals.

References

1. Baldwin CA: Mental health consultation in the intensive care unit: Toward a greater balance and precision of attribution. J Psychiatr Nurs Ment Health Serv 16:17–21, 1978
2. Barbiaz J et al: Establishing the psychiatric liaison nurse role: Collaboration with the nurse administrator. J Nurs Admin 2:14–18, 1982
3. Barton D, Abram HS: Preventive psychiatry in the general hospital. Comp Psychiatry 12:330–336, 1971
4. Barton D, Kelso MT: The nurse as a psychiatric consultation team member. Int Psychiatry Med 2:108–116, 1971
5. Berarducci M, Blanford K, Garant CA: The psychiatric liaison nurse in the general hospital: Three models of practice. Gen Hosp Psychiatry 1:66–72, 1979
6. Bilodeau CB, O'Connor S: Role of Nurse Clinicians in Liaison Psychiatry. In Hackett TP, Cassem NH (eds): Massachusetts General Hospital Handbook of General Hospital Psychiatry. St Louis, CV Mosby, 1978
7. Bursten B: The psychiatric consultant and the nurse. Nurs Forum 2:6–23, 1963
8. Caplan G: Principles of Preventive Psychiatry. New York, Basic Books, 1964
9. Davis DS, Nelson J: Referrals to psychiatric liaison nurses: Changes in characteristics over a limited time period. Gen Hosp Psychiatry 2:41–45, 1980
10. Freeman CK: Transactional analysis: A model for psychiatric consultation in the general hospital. Nurs Forum 28:43–51, 1979
11. Garant CA: The psychiatric liaison nurse—an interpretation of the role. Supervisor Nurse 4:75–78, 1977
12. Hackett TP, Cassem NH (eds): Massachusetts General Hospital Handbook of General Hospital Psychiatry. St Louis, CV Mosby, 1978
13. Holstein S, Schwab JJ: A coordinated consultation program for nurses and psychiatrists. JAMA 194:103–105, 1965

14. Horowitz MJ, Kaltreider NB: Brief therapy of the stress response syndrome. Psychiatr Clin North Am 2:365–377, 1979

15. Huey FL: Psychiatric Nursing 1946 to 1974: A Report on the State of the Art. New York, American Journal of Nursing Company, 1975

16. Jackson HA: The psychiatric nurse as a mental health consultant in a general hospital. Nurs Clin North Am 4:527–540, 1969

17. Johnson BS: Psychiatric nurse consultant in a general hospital. Nurs Outlook 10:728–729, 1963

18. Johnson RM et al: The professional support group: A model for psychiatric clinical nurse specialists. J Psychiatr Nurs Ment Health Serv 20:9–13, 1982

19. Jones KR, Vischi TR: Impact of alcohol, drug abuse, and mental health treatment on medical care utilization: A review of the research literature. Med Care 17(Suppl):1979

20. Kaltreider NB et al: The integration of psychosocial care in a general hospital: Development of an interdisciplinary consultation program. Int Psychiatry Med 5:125–134, 1974

21. Keill SL: The general hospital as the core of the mental health services system. Hosp Comm Psychiatry 32:776–778, 1981

22. Klein DC, Goldston SE (eds): Primary Prevention: An Idea Whose Time Has Come. Proceedings of the pilot conference on primary prevention, April 2–4, 1976. Washington, DC, U.S. Government Printing Office, 1977

23. Kolson G: Mental health nursing consultation: A study of expectations. J Psychiatr Nurs Ment Health Serv 14:24, 31–32, 1976

24. Lamb HR, Zusman J: A new look at primary prevention. Hosp Comm Psychiatry 32:843–848, 1981

25. Lehmann FG: Liaison Nursing: A Model for Nursing Practice. In Stuart GW, Sundeen SJ: Principles and Practice of Psychiatric Nursing. St. Louis, CV Mosby, 1979

26. Lewis A, Levy JS: Psychiatric Liaison Nursing: The Theory and Clinical Practice. Reston, Virginia, Reston Publishing, 1982

27. Lipowski ZJ: Review of consultation psychiatry and psychosomatic medicine. I. General principles. Psychosom Med 29:153–169, 1967

28. Lipowski ZJ: Review of consultation psychiatry and psychosomatic medicine. II. Clinical aspects. Psychosom Med 29:201–221, 1967

29. Lipowski ZJ: Consultation-Liaison Psychiatry: Past, Present, and Future. In Pasnau RO (ed): Consultation-Liaison Psychiatry. New York, Grune & Stratton, 1975

30. Lipowski ZJ: New prospects for liaison psychiatry. Psychosomatics 22:806–809, 1981

31. Luna ML: The Community Mental Health Nurse as a Member of the General Hospital Psychiatric Liaison Team: An Investigation of the Theory and Role. Unpublished manuscript, University of California at Los Angeles, 1977

32. Menzies I: A Case Study in the Functioning of Social Systems as a Defense Against Anxiety: A Report on a Study of the Nursing Service of a General Hospital. In Colman AR, Bexton WH (eds): Group Relations Reader. Sausalito, California, GREX, 1975

33. Miller WB: Psychiatric consultation. Part I. A general systems approach. Psychiatry Med 4:135–145, 1973

34. Miller WB: Psychiatric consultation. Part II. Conceptual and pragmatic issues of formulation. Psychiatry Med 4:252–271, 1973

35. Nelson J, Schilke DA: The evolution of psychiatric liaison nursing. Perspect Psychiatr Care 14:61–65, 1976

36. Pardes HE: Mental health–general health interaction: Opportunities and responsibilities. Hosp Comm Psychiatry 32:779–782, 1981

37. Peterson S: The psychiatric nurse specialist in a general hospital. Nurs Outlook 2:56–58, 1969

38. Regier DA, Goldberg ID, Taube CC: Health services system: A public health perspective. Arch Gen Psychiatry 135:685–693, 1978

39. Robinson L: Liaison psychiatric nursing. Perspect Psychiatr Care 6:87–91, 1968

40. Robinson L: A psychiatric nursing liaison program. Nurs Outlook 20:454–457, 1972

41. Robinson L: Liaison Nursing: A Psychological Approach to Patient Care. Philadelphia, FA Davis, 1974

42. Robinson L: Psychological Aspects of the Care of Hospitalized Patients, 3rd ed. Philadelphia, FA Davis, 1976

43. Selye H: The Stress of Life (rev ed). New York, McGraw-Hill, 1976

44. Shevitz SA, Silberfarb PM, Lipowski ZJ: Psychiatric consultation in a general hospital: A report of 1,000 referrals. Psychosomatics 17:295–299, 1976

45. Stickney SK, Moir G, Gardner ER: Psychiatric nurse consultation: Who calls and why. J Psychiatr Nurs Ment Health Serv 19:22–26, 1981

46. Strain JJ: Psychological Interventions in Medical Practice. New York, Appleton-Century-Croft, 1978

47. Taube CA, Regier DA, Rosenfeld AH: Mental Disorders in Health: United States 1978. Washington, DC, U.S. Government Printing Office, 1978

48. U.S. Government Printing Office: Preventing Disease—Promoting Health: Objectives for the Nation (No. 650–185/3979). Washington, DC, U.S. Government Printing Office, 1979

49. von Bertalanffy L: General System Theory: Essays on its Foundation and Development (rev ed). New York, George Beozilla, 1969

50. Weinstein LJ, Chapman MM, Stallings MA: Organizing approaches to psychiatric nurse consultation. Perspect Psychiatr Care 27:66–71, 1979

51. Wilson HS, Kneisl CR: Consultation in the General Hospital. In Psychiatric Nursing. Menlo Park, California, Addison-Wesley, 1979

52. Wise TN: Utilization of a nurse consultant in teaching liaison psychiatry. J Med Ed 49:1067–1068, 1974

53. Wolff PI: Psychiatric nursing consultations: A study of the referral process. J Psychiatr Nurs Ment Health Serv 16:42–47, 1978

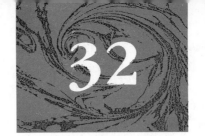

VIVIAN BROWN

THE ROLE OF THE COMMUNITY MENTAL HEALTH SYSTEM

Learning Objectives

Upon completion of this chapter the student should be able to do the following:

1. Describe the historical context of the development of community mental health centers.
2. Identify the major roles of the community mental health center.
3. Identify and discuss the essential services of a community mental health center.
4. Identify six additional roles of the community mental health center within the community.
5. Summarize the major problems that have arisen regarding community mental health centers and their multiple roles.
6. Discuss possible future trends for community mental health centers and community mental health.

Introduction

The trend toward community mental health centers has developed since the turn of the century, when the introduction of reform movements focused on more humane treatment of the mentally ill. By 1950, the state hospital was the primary provider of care for the mentally ill. There were estimates of more than 500,000 hospitalized patients in the United States in 1950. By the mid-1950s, psychoactive drugs were shown to be effective and were introduced into the hospital system. This allowed for a greater push toward treatment of psychotic patients on an ambulatory, close-to-home basis. The new drugs accelerated discharge, and many clients were able to function by continuing to use the medications at home.

Community mental health centers (CMHCs) were designed to fulfill multiple roles, including the following:

1. *Providing comprehensive mental health care,* including prevention, treatment, and rehabilitation services
2. *Coordinating services* within the catchment area
3. *Educating and training* the community
4. *Managing and disseminating information*
5. *Being a linking agency* between research and practice, professionals and paraprofessionals, the mental health system and substance abusers, and the mental health system and other systems
6. *Being innovative* in service delivery systems

This chapter will describe further how CMHCs function. In addition, future directions for community mental health centers will be discussed.

The traditional mental hospital was a highly segregated organization that allowed clients only minimal contact with the communities from which they came. The concept of community mental health today involves a number of significant characteristics that emphasize:[3]

1. Practice in the community rather than in institutional settings
2. The total community or population rather than individuals. The term "catchment area" is used to describe the population of concern to a particular community mental health program
3. Disorder prevention and mental health promotion
4. Comprehensiveness of services and continuity of care
5. A process of rigorous planning of mental health programs, including needs assessment of the communities being served
6. Expansion of the pool of personnel that provide services to include paraprofessional mental health workers

According to Karno and Schwartz,[16] the primary notions underlying the community mental health center are: (1) psychiatric disorders can be improved through treatment or can be prevented from occurring; (2) psychiatric disorders can be prevented or improved by avoiding the separation of clients from their primary relationships and functions in the community; (3) effective prevention and treatment techniques cannot be accomplished by mental health professionals alone; and (4) conditions of social, cultural, and economic environments must be considered at least equal in importance to biological endowment and psychological experience.

As can be seen from these primary characteristics and ideas, the concept of community mental health involves a systems perspective. The client is viewed as a "whole" in interaction with the environment. Individual clients come with certain physical and biological endowments, unique psychological experiences, and specific social, cultural, and economic environmental characteristics. The occurrence of mental illness or disorder is believed to be dependent upon these conditions of individuals, as well as on the larger sociocultural and physical environment.

Historical Development of Community Mental Health Centers

The Joint Commission on Mental Illness and Health[15] was formed to provide a thorough, nationwide analysis of the problems of mental illness. In 1961, the final report of the Commission recommended: (1) immediate and intensive care for acutely disturbed patients in outpatient community mental health clinics (created at the rate of one clinic per 50,000 population), inpatient psychiatric units (located in every general hospital with 100 or more beds), and intensive psychiatric treatment centers (with no more than 1,000 beds each, to be developed by converting existing state mental hospitals); (2) improved and expanded aftercare, partial hospitalization (less than 24 hours a day), and rehabilitation services; and (3) mental health education to inform the general public about emotional disorders and to reduce the potential for the public's rejection of the mentally ill.

After reviewing all the reports and recommendations, President Kennedy stated that a "bold new approach" to mental health care was needed. The new approach proposed included the establishment of comprehensive community mental health centers, grants to improve care in state mental hospitals, and increased funding for research and training.

The full thrust of the federally-funded community mental health center program occurred with the enactment of Public Law 88-164 in 1963, Title 2 of which authorized funds for construction of community mental health clinics, and Public Law 89-105 in 1965, which authorized staffing funds for the new centers. The CMHC Policy and Standards Manual[23] stated that a comprehensive community mental health center was to provide five essential services: outpatient, inpatient, emergency, partial hospitalization, and consultation and education services. Other services to be added were diagnostic, rehabilitative, precare and aftercare, training and research, and evaluation services. These services will be discussed in later sections.

There have been at least 13 amendments to the initial authorizing legislation of 1963, making the CMHC service delivery program increasingly complex. The amendments of 1975 expanded the required services to 12. Some of those services were care for children and the elderly, transitional halfway house services, and programs for the prevention and treatment of alcohol and drug abuse.

The Community Mental Health Amendments of 1975, Section 302, stated that the Congress found that community mental health centers had had a major impact on the improvement of mental health care by:

"(A) Fostering coordination and cooperation between various agencies responsible for mental health care, which in turn has resulted in a decrease in overlapping services and more efficient utilization of available resources;

(B) Bringing comprehensive community mental health care to all in need within a specific geographic area, regardless of the ability to pay; and

(C) Developing a system of care which insures continuity of care for all patients."

Providing Comprehensive Mental Health Care

The community mental health center's primary role is to provide comprehensive mental health care in its catchment area or mental health service area. This care is divided into treatment, rehabilitation, and prevention services. Programs are designed to promote the mental health of the community and prevent specific emotional disorders within the community. The center is also responsible for developing programs of early diagnosis, prompt and effective treatment, and rehabilitation.

Treatment services include a wide variety of programs, from outpatient to day treatment, for a wide variety of clients, from children to seniors. Rehabilitation services are designed to prevent chronic disability, and include programs such as sheltered workshops and transitional living arrangements. Both treatment and rehabilitation services are considered "direct services" because the care-giver works directly with the client. Prevention services, which include consultation and education, often do not involve work directly with clients, and thus

are considered "indirect." Table 32-1 shows the various services of the CMHC.

Outpatient Treatment Services

Treatment services of the community mental health center begin with, or revolve around, the more traditional inpatient/outpatient core, and extend to more flexible and innovative services. Outpatient care for adults, children, and families is a key element in the community system of treatment. It is often the center's entry point for diagnosis and evaluation of problems, and the source of referral to other services outside of the CMHC.

Admission into outpatient services often involves an extensive assessment of the clients. As mentioned in the chapter introduction, this assessment needs to address a number of different aspects of clients in order to give the most complete picture of their functioning. Thus, the assessment includes the physical, psychological, social, environmental, and cultural aspects of the clients. The assessment process helps shape the treatment plan for the clients. The treatment plan answers two basic questions: (1) given the presenting problem and this unique individual, what is the best treatment? and (2) what are the short- and long-term goals for the treatment recommended?

The most common modes of treatment in the outpatient service are individual, family, and group psychotherapy, drug therapy, and children's play therapy. The development of various types of group therapy has enabled CMHCs to reach larger numbers of patients effectively. Therapeutic groups range from group crisis intervention to socialization groups designed for the aftercare and follow-up of clients who have been hospitalized. Many clients who have been discharged from hospitals and are continuing their prescribed medication can be seen in medication groups led by a psychiatrist or psychiatric nurse.

Some clinics have developed programs of home visits or home treatment. These programs allow for extensive casework with the family, and reach clients who may be unmotivated for treatment or fearful of treatment within the CMHC facility. Often, home visits are done by psychiatric nurses or psychiatric social workers.

While most individuals treated in the outpatient ser-

TABLE 32-1.
COMPREHENSIVE MENTAL HEALTH CARE SERVICES

DIRECT		INDIRECT
TREATMENT	REHABILITATION	PREVENTION
Outpatient	Psychosocial rehabilitation	Consultation
Inpatient	Transitional living	Education
Emergency services	Sheltered workshops	Primary prevention projects
Day treatment		
Partial hospitalization		
Drug and alcohol treatment		

vice are young and middle-aged adults, many are children and elderly persons. These latter two groups, which had been neglected, were given special attention in the later amendments of the CMHC Act.

It has been estimated that 10% of all public school children in the United States need psychiatric help.[3] The kinds of problems children and youth present depend largely on their referral sources. Schools predominantly refer children with behavior and learning problems, while courts frequently refer older children and adolescents who have been arrested for juvenile crimes. For children and youth, treatment techniques such as activity therapy and play therapy are being used, and some centers have established therapeutic nursery schools. (See Chapters 22 and 23 for counseling of children and adolescents.)

Often in the past, elderly people were brought to mental health centers only when their behavior became an annoyance to someone else, although they might have been suffering from a psychosis or undergoing organic changes. Some psychiatric problems of aging may respond to psychiatric or medical treatment, or a combination of both. In many CMHCs, if outpatient services are indicated, elderly clients may be visited at home or be transported to the center by the CMHC. Services include activity groups as well as individual, family, and group treatment.

Another underserved population was ethnic minorities, who were not well represented in mental health clinic populations. The community mental health perspective allowed this underrepresentation to be seen as a sign that treatment services might not have been culturally relevant. As a result, many centers began implementing specialized outpatient services for representative ethnic minority groups in their catchment area. Bilingual and bicultural staff members were hired to implement these services in order to respond in more culturally sensitive ways to the needs of the community.

Before this section on outpatient services ends, the role of the nurse needs mention. In a publication by the U.S. Department of Health, Education, and Welfare (now known as the Department of Health and Human Services) that describes outpatient services,[22] there is a description of some of the various nursing roles in outpatient treatment services. These roles include consultation to colleagues in public health, coordination with other nurses and staff of mental hospitals, overseeing medication programs, and home visiting.

Inpatient Treatment Services

Inpatient care must be provided for people who need intensive treatment and care around the clock. If hospitalization is necessary, it should be short-term, and the client should return for continuing care on an outpatient basis as soon as possible. CMHCs provide inpatient treatment directly or through affiliation with a hospital.

Although inpatient services continued to be seen as an essential service in the community mental health cen-

ter, it was clear that this type of treatment was recommended for only a small percentage of clients, and length of treatment was shortened considerably. Sundel, Rhodes, and Ferguson[20] described a 20-bed crisis intervention unit that provided alternatives to admission to state hospital wards. The maximum length of hospitalization in the crisis unit was one week. For more than 40% of the clients referred for admission, long-term hospitalization was avoided. In approximately two thirds of these clients, the crisis unit was not needed and clients were referred to community agencies.

Emergency Services

Emergency psychiatric services within the CMHC were made available 24 hours a day. This was seen as an essential service because to delay treatment of individuals showing indications of mental illness or incapacitating emotional stress lessens the likelihood of successful treatment and increases the probability of long-term illness.

For many decades, communities have had 24-hour emergency services available in local general hospitals. Among the community general hospitals in the United States, fewer than 20% regularly admit clients for the diagnosis and/or treatment of mental illness. Virtually all hospitals that have emergency rooms admit individuals who have injured themselves. However, many hospitals do not have the special facilities or policies requiring a psychiatric evaluation of such persons once the physical condition has been treated. Psychiatric emergency services should be readily available to emotionally disturbed people and their families. These services can help families regain their capacity to tolerate and help the disturbed members.

Most psychiatric emergencies involve suicidal, agitated, intoxicated, and aggressive people. Facilities report that the majority of psychiatric emergencies occur during daytime and early evening hours. However, the emergency service must be readily available at all times. Ideally, a CMHC can operate a walk-in clinic staffed by mental health professionals around the clock. Another model is a 24-hour telephone service, with back-up in the emergency room at a hospital or walk-in capability at the CMHC. In 1965 at the District of Columbia General Hospital, a 24-hour telephone service was established, staffed by experienced nursing assistants who had shown particular skill in dealing with psychiatric patients and who were then given several months of training.

Pisarcik and associates[17] described the role of nurses in a Boston emergency room. The nurses have four main functions: assessment, direct patient care, coordination and collaboration, and teaching and consultation.

Crisis Intervention Services

Crisis intervention services are different from emergency management (ER intervention).[14] In most instances, the logistics of the emergency setting make it impossible for

CLINICAL EXAMPLE

Susan is a 19-year-old woman who was raped in her apartment by an unknown assailant. She was able to get herself to the hospital, and sits silently in an examining room in the hospital emergency room. She is fearful, and unable to respond to the police officer or the physician.

For this young woman, immediate medical treatment and crisis counseling are needed. The following interventions are important:

1. The client is helped to feel safe and protected in the immediate environment. Sensitive, well-trained staff need to be available immediately. It is extremely important to include a woman as part of the treatment team.

2. Medical procedures (examination) are explained before proceeding.

3. A counselor (often a psychiatric social worker or nurse) helps the client to relate what has happened to her. It is also important to help the client understand that what she is feeling is common, and that other feelings and issues may arise after she leaves the emergency room.

4. The counselor can present the resources available to the client. Referral to a rape crisis center and/or crisis intervention service in a CMHC is critical if the hospital does not have a rape treatment service.

5. Follow-up to ensure that the client is functioning adequately and has obtained further assistance (if wanted) is an important step. If the client has not sought further help, additional follow-up contacts are warranted.

the same person to follow a client for several days or weeks in order to assist in the crisis resolution.[9] However, the ideal situation would be that the emergency service have the capability of providing crisis intervention services and suicide prevention services for a maximum of six weeks.

Rape is a problem for which immediate emergency care and crisis intervention services for victims is critical. Burgess and Holstrom[7] established a 24-hour crisis intervention service for rape victims in a Boston hospital emergency room. This service provided immediate medical treatment and counseling. In addition, counseling was offered to family and friends, and follow-up calls were made to the victim/survivor. Their original program has served as the model for other rape crisis intervention programs across the nation.

The author of this chapter has helped to establish crisis intervention services for rape victims in Los Angeles. Services are provided in collaboration with the Los Angeles Commission on Assaults Against Women (LACAAW) and the Didi Hirsch Community Mental Health Center. LACAAW provides telephone hotline services, victim/survivor advocacy services, and counseling. A hotline advocate will accompany the victim to the hospital and/or to court, if wanted. If there is need for additional crisis intervention services, the woman is referred to the CMHC. Crisis services are provided by the CMHC for a maximum of six weeks, and the survivor is often referred back to LACAAW for additional advocacy services and ongoing groups.

Partial Hospitalization Services

Partial hospitalization services are intensive treatment services for less than 24 hours a day. They include day care and treatment for clients who are able to return home evenings and weekends. Services may also include

night care for clients who are able to work but need limited support or who lack suitable home arrangements.

Partial hospitalization services can be seen as an important step in prevention of hospitalization and/or rehospitalization. Becker and colleagues[2] described the day hospital as enabling a "gradual transition from ward to community, the frequency of attendance being 'titrated' to the needs of the patient." In addition, the day hospital was perceived as a strategy for more rational assessment of the patient's need for hospitalization or for more extensive day care. The night hospital, like its daycare counterpart, provides part-time hospitalization for clients who find the transition from hospital to community too stressful. It is described as a "haven for nonhospitalized patients who are experiencing an acute or subacute crisis."[1] It offers clients respite from a stressful home environment, a therapeutic milieu, and an active treatment program without disruption of employment.

The activities in a typical day treatment program include:

1. Group therapy
2. Milieu therapy
3. Recreational activity
4. Occupational therapy
5. Art therapy
6. Social living skill training
7. Assistance in applying for income, medical, and other benefits
8. Family counseling

Drug and Alcohol Treatment Services

In 1975, treatment and prevention services for alcohol and drug abuse were added to the services provided by community mental health centers. Previously, mental health centers did not establish programs for substance abuse because these problems were not seen as primarily psychological, and because treatment by psychiatric or psychological methods had been relatively unsuccessful. Many CMHCs affiliated themselves with existing drug and alcohol treatment programs. The range of services now offered, provided directly or through affiliation, include methadone maintenance programs, detoxification programs, residential treatment programs, and outpatient programs.

These programs attempt to stop the use of the substance (*e.g.,* alcohol, heroin, PCP) while changing the lifestyle of the abuser. In order to stop clients from using the substance, a detoxification program is provided. Clients are given intensive support, a safe environment, and sometimes medication to help them get through the withdrawal. Clients are often referred to a residential treatment program or outpatient program in order to change major aspects of their lives. Often, all of these approaches focus on the social systems in which the substance-abuse behavior is embedded, in an attempt to break the cycle of substance abuse.

Rehabilitation Services

Rehabilitation services are designed to prevent chronic disability. Previously, many mental health services did not focus on social and vocational rehabilitation. A report by the Joint Information Service of the American Psychiatric Association and the National Association for Mental Health,[12] based on a series of field studies of CMHCs, revealed that "several of the centers placed little emphasis on developing community-based rehabilitation and maintenance programs that would attempt to prevent the exacerbation of acute illness in the chronically mentally ill." It appeared at that time that aftercare and rehabilitation should have been considered "essential" services. Later they were added to the list.

The range of rehabilitation services includes halfway houses, transitional living centers, and board-and-care homes. Ex-patient clubs were designed to help with social rehabilitation. Reeducation, job training, and sheltered workshops were also designed to help with vocational rehabilitation. These structured services provide the chronically mentally ill client with a continuum of living arrangements and a range of employment opportunities. The habilitation and rehabilitation programs provide the opportunity to acquire and maintain the life skills that are necessary to cope effectively.

Consultation and Education Services

The placement of consultation and education services among the five essential CMHC services was the most innovative step of the CMHC regulations. Smith and Hobbs[18] stated that the "vanguard of the community approach to mental health seeks ways in which aspects of people's social environment can be changed in order to improve mental health significantly through impact on large groups." They suggested that a CMHC might con-

duct surveys and studies to locate sources of community strains; conduct training programs for managers, teachers, and ministers; and provide consultation to schools, courts, churches, businesses, and state mental hospitals. They stated that one of the major objectives of the CMHC was to help the community's social systems function in ways that develop and sustain the effectiveness of individuals. In this way, the CMHC helps the community systems regroup their forces to sustain and support individuals who run into trouble.

The consultation and education (C&E) services of the CMHC are designed to develop effective mental health programs in the catchment area. This C&E service promotes coordination of mental health services among all the agencies serving the catchment area, increasing awareness of the nature of mental health problems and the types of mental health services available. It also promotes the prevention and control of rape and the proper treatment of rape victims.

Mental Health Consultation

The term *consultation* has been used extensively in medical practice when an outside expert is called in to assist with assessment, diagnosis, and the treatment plan. In mental health, consultation is a process of interaction between two professionals around a work problem.[8] The consultant helps the consultee with the problem, which may concern handling a particular client or the development of a program for serving clients who have a certain problem.

Caplan[8] divided consultation into four categories:

1. *Client-centered case* consultation: the consultant uses specialized skills and knowledge to help the consultee assess the client's problem and to recommend how to deal with it.
2. *Consultee-centered case* consultation: the consultant identifies the consultee's difficulties in handling the client. Those difficulties may involve lack of skill, knowledge, self-confidence, or objectivity on the part of the consultee. The consultant may provide additional data, help the consultee develop skills, provide ego support, or point out (through example or anecdote) how a lack of objectivity may be contributing to the problem.
3. *Program-centered administrative* consultation: the consultant makes recommendations to the consultee in order to develop or modify a program.
4. *Consultee-centered administrative* consultation: the consultant identifies the consultee's difficulties in instituting program changes.

Mental Health Education

Education reaches larger groups or populations than do traditional treatment approaches. It does not require that community residents take on client or patient status. Mental health education builds on the strengths and competencies of people, and has two major goals:[1]

1. Increasing the understanding and knowledge of community residents to help them cope effectively with problems and crises as they arise in daily life
2. Increasing the knowledge and understanding of the community and its subsystems

Adelson and Lurie[1] observed that mental health educators concentrate on three main groups: (1) individuals at risk of developing emotional disorders (*e.g.,* clients who have lost a spouse); (2) individuals who are in positions of power in the community or who have responsibilities for caring for others; and (3) those who are relatively powerless and who can be helped to develop increased control of their own lives.

The most common techniques used in mental health education are lectures, films, and small face-to-face discussion groups. The technique with the widest reach is work with the mass media.

The range of problems under C&E services is wide. Programs include stress management for workers in industry, parenting training for couples contemplating having a child, classroom presentations on coping strategies for elementary school children, consultation to teachers on how to develop nonsexist curricula, and consultation to physicians regarding prescription of certain drugs to women.

While the consultation, education, and prevention services have been the most innovative, they are also the most controversial. Snow and Newton contended that "indirect services" (or consultation and education services) require the greatest degree of change from the medical model, and are therefore never given clear definition or substantial support.[19] Even consultation, they believe, basically reinforces direct clinical service; serious attempts to change social institutions are not encouraged. Moreover, with the lengthening of the list of essential clinical services, consultation and education has been subordinated still further.

Psychiatric nurses, in addition to their treatment role functions, are often involved in consultation and education services. Nurses have always played a psycho-educational role. In addition to providing direct care, they often educate clients and family members to assume responsibility for self-care. For example, nurses can design educational seminars for family members of the chronically mentally ill in the community. These seminars can include information on schizophrenia and/or affective disorders, the role of medications, community resources, prevention of rehospitalization, and the stresses of caring for the mentally ill.

Coordination of Services

One of the major barriers to effective mental health programming is the separation of mental health services from other people-serving agencies. Effective care requires continuity for individuals in their complex involvements with societal institutions.[18] No one system,

however comprehensive, can cover the full range of mental health needs and concerns. Therefore, the CMHC needs to collaborate with the total matrix of community agencies and care-givers. This includes natural support systems such as family groups.

The role of coordinator/collaborator involves a number of activities for the CMHC. First, the CMHC is an integral part of the community network. The CMHC staff needs to understand and be knowledgeable about the other parts of the network, *e.g.,* schools, recreation centers, churches, probation, and health agencies. Next, the CMHC should take an active role in coordinating or "calling together" all of the diverse groups. This will improve service delivery and ensure continuity of care. Finally, in order to sustain the most effective care, the CMHC needs to coordinate "all those agencies out there" in the catchment area.

While the idea of treating "the whole person" is not new, the failure of the mental health system to do so is clear. For example, deinstitutionalization, combined with the lack of integration of human services for the seriously mentally ill, appears to have led to expanding numbers of homeless people. Their disabilities are increased by the lack of affordable housing and insufficient resources. For the elderly, there has been little integration of the many services needed. These services include transportation, housing, nutrition, health care, income maintenance, recreation, social services, and in-house services.[6] The CMHC must take an active role in coordinating these care-giving agencies in order to provide the most effective care.

Education and Training

The *educator* role of the CMHC involves assisting community residents to acquire knowledge of, skills in, and attitudes about their own mental health and the mental health of others. This role involves educating community residents about general mental health concepts. These concepts might include child development, stressful life events, or specific role skills related to special client populations. Helping a family member find the best nursing home for an elderly parent is one example. In the role of educator, the CMHC attempts to raise the level of awareness in the community, destigmatize mental illness, and strengthen and empower the community.

With regard to *training,* the CMHC is involved in training new care-givers, both professional and paraprofessional. Training care-givers already providing services within the catchment area is also a CMHC responsibility. Psychiatrists, psychologists, nurses, and social workers are trained primarily as clinicians. The CMHC can train these care-givers not only in clinical skills but also in community organization and collaboration skills. CMHCs train care-givers to collaborate with other agencies and professional groups. There is much in mental health care professional education that keeps the mental health disciplines separate. The CMHC offers care-givers a real life laboratory for working with other professionals, paraprofessionals, and community residents.

In the field of nursing, Evans[10] advocated, that in addition to the family- and community-centered basic nursing curriculum, a baccalaureate program should offer concepts of epidemiology of mental disorder, community organization, ecology, and care in transitional facilities. The CMHC offers these concepts *in vivo.*

CMHCs need to raise the consciousness of community agencies and policy-makers about cultural and psychological issues relevant to the mental health of the community. In this role, the CMHC acts as a "sensitizer." It helps other key participants understand issues such as the impact of racism, sexism, and ageism on the mental health of the community.

With regard to *training as a sensitizer,* an important study project in the development of affirmative action programs and pluralistic curriculum content was the Western Interstate Commission on Higher Education in Nursing (WICHEN), in 1978.[4] In a later study, Chun and colleagues[9] brought together 64 leading scholars and mental health practitioners to assess the state of the art of integrating into nursing curricula content about people of color. A four-by-four project design was adopted, so that input from the four mental health core disciplines (psychology, social work, psychiatry, and psychiatric nursing) and from each of the four racial–ethnic groups (African-Americans, Asian- and Pacific-Americans, Native Americans, and Hispanic-Americans) would be given. Both studies recommended the following major topics for inclusion in multicultural nursing curricula:

- Historical perspectives and origins
- Migration (past and present)
- Language and communication style
- Nutritional preferences and taboos
- Religious styles and rituals
- Family dynamics and values
- Health and illness belief systems and cultural medicine
- Disease predisposition and resistance related to ethnic background
- Assessments of physical health and mental health
- Community structures and dynamics (*e.g.,* rules, customs)
- Factors affecting health in ethnic communities
- Attitudes, self-awareness, and philosophy

An understanding of these concepts will provide nurses with a more diversified framework for practice. This, in turn, will enable them to provide more holistic mental health nursing care.

Information Management and Dissemination

In its role as *information manager,* the CMHC is involved in a number of important activities. First, it con-

ducts a *comprehensive needs assessment* of its entire catchment area. Utilizing surveys, key informants, community forums, and other assessment techniques, the CMHC identifies the significant human problems in the communities, the gaps in service, and the priorities for mental health programming.

For example, a CMHC may identify an increasing suicide rate among young people in the area. It may reveal a lack of specialized services to address this problem. Both treatment and prevention services can be implemented directly by the CMHC. The CMHC could train a specialized team of child and adolescent mental health professionals in suicide prevention services, and it could also provide separate educational prevention programs in the schools for youth, teachers, and parents.

In another example, the CMHC may identify a dramatic increase in Asian/Pacific Islander populations in the catchment area without specialized mental health services. The CMHC should attempt to hire bilingual, bicultural staff members to plan a specialized needs assessment and provide outreach programs for the new residents. The needs assessment should be updated annually to keep services relevant to community needs.

Second, the CMHC establishes an information *management system* for monitoring and tracking clients within the system. This ensures the continuity of care and the effectiveness of service delivery. Without an internal data system, it is difficult to ensure that the CMHC is delivering services to a representative sample of community residents. An information management system helps to ensure that clients are moving from one service to another with ease and timeliness. It can answer such questions as:

1. Are significant numbers of elderly clients seen at the center?
2. How many clients go from the crisis intervention center to longer-term treatment?
3. What is the average number of sessions for family and child treatment?
4. How many home visits were done by nursing staff?

In addition to monitoring internal data, the CMHC also implements *research programs* in order to generate new knowledge. Research results can have a direct impact on nursing services in CMHCs by suggesting the need for new education programs, different interventions, or additional areas for staff development.

All of the information described above is extremely important to the effectiveness of service delivery within the CMHC. However, the information is also important to others in the catchment area and beyond. In its role as *information-disseminator,* the CMHC provides others, such as community agencies and policy-makers, with the information gathered from its needs assessment, information management system, and research projects. In this way, the information or knowledge is utilized by others to strengthen or modify their service delivery, apply for funding, shift priorities, or generate additional information.

Being a Linking Agency

In its role as information disseminator to other agencies in the catchment area, the CMHC serves as a "linking agency." The literature suggests that innovations spread most effectively when their dissemination is facilitated by a person or group functioning as a linking agent. The linking agent takes new information from one system or subsystem and brings it to another system or subsystem.

There has often been little opportunity for two-way communication between the practitioner/clinician system and the researcher system. Communication includes effective implementation strategies for adapting research results to identified local problems. The CMHC combines both clinicians and researchers interested in these issues. The CMHC is in an excellent position to establish temporary and long-term mechanisms for facilitating communication among practitioners and researchers who hold different value orientations and use different terminologies and technologies.[5]

In addition to providing a link between practitioner and researcher, the CMHCs can serve as links between professional and paraprofessional groups, mental health and substance-abuse systems, and mental health and other systems. Because the CMHC combines these elements within its own delivery system, it can provide the linkage necessary to facilitate communication in and implementation of collaborative efforts.

Innovation

The CMHC is not only the disseminator of innovations, it is also the innovator of service delivery systems. When staff members determine a need in the community, they are in a position to test new kinds of services. In its role as innovator, the CMHC serves as an evolutionary social experiment, testing new techniques and modalities and combinations of these.

Evaluation of Community Mental Health Centers

In their primary role of providing comprehensive mental health care, CMHC programs have been successful in making mental health clinical services more available, accessible, flexible, and culturally sensitive. Tischler and colleagues[21] demonstrated that there is greater representation of socially disadvantaged groups in the client population of a catchmented program than in that of a non-catchmented program (Fig. 32-1). In relation to issues of accessibility and responsiveness, Goldblatt and colleagues[13] found that in the catchmented program intake was briefer, more treatment time per clinician was available, waiting lists were shorter, and more clients started treatment.

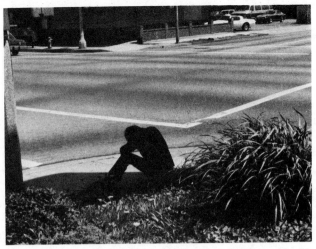

Figure 32-1. The homeless feel the effects of a lack of mental health care resources.

In contrast to the clinical service, the prevention services appear not to be given significant priority. This was reflected in the 1972–73 annual NIMH inventory, which showed that 76.4% of total staff hours was spent in the provision of direct clinical services, while 4.8% went to indirect or preventive services.

The accomplishments of CMHCs have fallen short of the original projections. However, there have been some successes as well as some failures. Table 32-2 summarizes the strengths and weaknesses of the program, as assessed at the beginning of the 1980s.*

Future Trends

In the 1980s, 20 years after the CMHC Act, it is possible to see the problems and the flaws in the vision. However, many of the innovations and successes need to be preserved. The CMHCs of the 1960s and 1970s probably will not continue to exist in their original form. The Mental Health Systems Act, which revised the original act, has been rescinded. States have now assumed responsibility for the provision of community mental health services. Many of the federal regulations governing CMHCs are no longer in effect.

The Omnibus Budget Reconciliation Act of 1982 effectively repealed the 1980 Mental Health Systems Act and provided for block-grant funding of mental health services.[11] This legislation shifted primary responsibility from the federal government back to state governments. Each state is given a specified amount of money for all alcohol, drug-abuse, and mental health services in a "block," and the state determines which programs will be supported. With limited financial resources, the determination of allocations for mental health services is a major political and economic issue. The type of partnership between states and the CMHCs varies as a function of

* References 3, 6, 12, 15, 18, and 24.

TABLE 32-2.
STRENGTHS AND WEAKNESSES OF COMMUNITY MENTAL HEALTH CENTERS

STRENGTHS	WEAKNESSES
1. Many previously unserved and underserved populations began receiving mental health services in the community.	1. CMHCs were not monitored sufficiently, and some did not provide the mandated services.
2. Short-term clinical interventions have increased, reaching many more community residents.	2. Only about 50% of the planned 1500 CMHCs were established, leaving many communities without centers.
3. Innovative community residential facilities are being developed.	3. Prevention services were not given emphasis in the CMHCs.
4. Additional sources and types of personnel have been utilized by CMHCs.	4. CMHCs did not develop strong community involvement in planning and implementation of programs.
5. Specialized services for ethnic minority populations were developed in some CMHCs.	5. CMHCs did not become self-supporting, as had been projected.
	6. CMHCs did not establish sufficient effective alternatives to hospitalization.

state and local leadership. There are some important elements that may determine what the CMHC of the future will look like and what roles it will play.

Catchment Area Concept

With the absence of federal catchment-area regulations or definitions, CMHCs may consider more naturally-occurring community groups or community segments. For example, a CMHC may serve all of the communities in the western area of a city. This avoids splitting communities into different catchment areas and keeps communities that share common bonds together. Because it does not appear that there will be sufficient funds to add new centers, it is also possible that CMHCs of the future will serve larger geographic areas in order to provide services to people living in areas without CMHCs.

Regarding the geographic area of service, unless clients are embedded in their community, it may not be so important to individuals to have services in the community. Thus, in the future we may have two tracks—the CMHC within the community for the "embedded" community resident, and the CMHC or hospital of choice in the geographic area preferred by the "transient" resident who may not feel any tie to a particular community.

Community Mental Health Center Financing

The federal government has provided funds to initiate and develop each CMHC over a period of from eight to twelve years. The funds gradually decline and end during that period. The survival of the CMHC depends on its ability to obtain funds to replace the federal funds.

The expectation that communities would be able to offset the loss of federal funds was not quite realistic. Economically deprived communities could not raise the funds to replace million-dollar budgets. In many instances, inpatient services, the most expensive of the services, paid for other services, which did not help to reduce the number of hospitalizations. The reduction in state hospital beds and reallocation of money to local centers has not been adequate.

Two recent studies examined the "fiscal and programmatic status of CMHCs which had completed their full cycle of federal grant funding."[24,25] The 29 CMHCs studied in both projects were divided into two subgroups. One included "true graduates" of the federal community mental health center program—those that neither sought nor received any further NIMH funds after the end of their eight years. The other group was composed of "quasi-graduates"—those that sought and received additional grant funds after the basic eight years of staffing grants. These studies indicated that systematic long-term differences between the two subgroups, in both sources of funding and patterns of service, began long before the termination of the federal CMHC grants.

The "true graduates" appeared to assure their fiscal viability by maximizing inpatient, outpatient, and emergency services, while cutting back on consultation and education, partial hospitalization, and home visits. During the five years of the study, they relied primarily on third-party reimbursements for increased revenue. The "quasi-graduates" maintained a balanced mix of all the services. However, they remained substantially dependent on government funds, and grew less rapidly than the other group during the five years of the study. One possible cause of this difference, suggested by Woy and colleagues,[25] is the extent to which the centers have strong ties with the medical profession and hospitals.

In a recent report, Larsen and Jerrell (in a presentation at a Mental Health Futures Conference at UCLA, June 1985) presented data on the results of a longitudinal study of the changes in community-based mental health services in 15 states. In more than 65 CMHCs, changes were monitored through questionnaires and interviews over a three-year period. After two years, this study provided the following results:

1. The average amount of total center revenues increased slightly from fiscal year 1982 to 1983.

2. Collections from private fees, insurance, and Champus for the armed services, as well as funding from state and local governmental sources, remained stable or decreased slightly. Medicare and Medi-Cal increased significantly, and funding from non-mental health sources and/or private contracts increased an average of 110%.

3. Compared to 1980 data, CMHC funding from direct governmental sources declined from an average of 85% of total revenues to 65%.

4. At the same time, average revenues from entitlement sources (Medicare/Medicaid and Title XX) increased from less than 10% to approximately 20%.

5. Most centers have attempted to increase the number of private pay clients. Twenty-five percent reported making changes in their corporate legal structure, primarily by spinning off separate corporations to hold real property or to shelter new sources of revenue.

6. Many centers reported increased funding for residential services as a primary impetus for service expansions.

With cutbacks in both federal and state funding, it will be important to study the kinds and amounts of services provided by CMHCs in the future. At present, many CMHCs are exploring methods of increasing treatment fees directly and through third-party payments. Trends include converting consulting activities to produce revenue, taking both treatment and prevention services to industry, and generating income through business ventures. With limited financial resources, the CMHCs may find more creative and innovative ways to utilize their resources.

Commitment to Prevention

As described above, there is a reduction in consultation and education services by some CMHCs as funding is reduced. At the same time, there is a stated commitment by the federal government that prevention services will be given higher status. Whatever the direction of funding and support, the need continues for CMHCs to develop programs aimed at altering social units that interfere with well-being. CMHCs need to continue to create environments that strengthen psychological development. After almost two decades of prevention programming (no matter how small an effort), there appears to be a commitment of some CMHCs to continue prevention services at the same level as treatment services. This requires a strong CMHC leadership committed equally to prevention and treatment, and committed to integrating all the "prevention pieces." Examples include encouraging the integration of drug- and alcohol-abuse prevention projects, juvenile delinquency prevention, rape prevention, child-abuse prevention, and the like, both within the CMHC and external to the CMHC. The accumulated knowledge and experience of these diverse yet similar prevention efforts could be a potent force in designing effective prevention strategies that cut across content areas. If prevention professionals and paraprofessionals cannot collaborate with one another, there is little hope that prevention strategies will work in the community at large.

Collaboration of Services

Even with the ideal of integration, continuity, and collaboration, CMHCs often have continued to be isolated from other agencies that serve people. In an era of fiscal limitations, it is possible that CMHCs in the future will be active partners with other agencies, sharing much-needed resources and expertise. These agencies include drug- and alcohol-abuse treatment facilities, mental retardation centers, and psychosocial rehabilitation centers. The separation into distinct entities of many of the services discussed is relevant only in terms of politics and economics, and has little to do with the real world (*e.g.,* we are seeing an increasing polydrug problem among young people who abuse substances and do not distinguish between drugs and alcohol). It is hoped that the artificial boundaries will be given up as the political and economic picture changes. It could be an extraordinary collaboration if mental health, drug- and alcohol-abuse treatment, health, rehabilitation, and prevention systems were equal partners.

Summary

1. CMHCs provide comprehensive care to the mentally ill through early intervention and outpatient therapy. The Community Mental Health Centers Act, and subsequent amendments, helped to shift the emphasis on mental health care from the hospital to the community.

2. The major roles of the CMHC include assessing catchment needs of the community and early diagnosis and treatment of emotional disturbances.

3. CMHCs offer a diverse range of services that include outpatient, inpatient, emergency, partial hospitalization, drug- and alcohol-abuse treatment, rehabilitation, and consultation and education services. Nurses can provide mental health teaching and promote client well-being in all of these service areas.

4. Additional roles of the CMHC include coordination of services, education and training, information management and dissemination, linking agencies, and innovation. All of these areas need to be addressed in order to provide comprehensive mental health care.

5. CMHCs have a tremendous responsibility to provide comprehensive mental health care to the communities they serve. Success in all areas, such as meeting mandates and emphasizing prevention, has not always been attained.

6. Funding for mental health care has undergone major changes in the 1980s. In order to remain viable, future CMHCs will need to rely on their abilities to generate and utilize resources wisely.

References

1. Adelson D, Lurie L: Mental Health Education: Research and Practice. In Golann SE, Eisdorfer C (eds): Handbook of Community Mental Health. New York, Appleton-Century-Crofts, 1972
2. Becker A, Murphy NM, Greenblatt M: Recent Advances in Community Psychiatry. In Bindman AJ, Spiegel AD (eds): Perspectives in Community Mental Health. Chicago, Aldine, 1969
3. Bloom BL: Community Mental Health: A General Introduction, 2nd ed. Monterey, California, Brooks-Cole, 1984
4. Branch M: Models for Cultural Diversity in Nursing: A Process for Change. Boulder, Colorado, Western Interstate Commission on Higher Education in Nursing, 1978
5. Brown VB, Garnets L, Bickson TK et al: Rationale. In Consensus and Controversy in Sexual Assault Prevention and Intervention: A Delphi Study (Research monograph). Los Angeles, Didi Hirsch CMHC, 1981
6. Brown VB, Fraser M: Planning and shaping of the mental health delivery system of the future. Consultation: An Int J 4(3): 1985
7. Burgess A: Crisis and counseling requests of rape victims. Nurs Res 23:196, 1974
8. Caplan G: Principles of preventive psychiatry. New York, Basic Books, 1964
9. Chunn JC, Dunston PJ, Ross-Sheriff F (eds): Mental Health and People of Color: Curriculum Development and Change. Washington, DC, Howard University Press, 1983
10. Evans FM: The Role of the Nurse in Community Mental Health. New York, MacMillan, 1968
11. Foley H, Sharfstein S: Madness and Government: Who Cares for the Mentally Ill. Washington, DC, American Psychiatric Press, 1983
12. Glasscote RM, Sussex JN, Cumming E et al: The Community Mental Health Center: An Interim Appraisal. Joint Information Service, American Psychiatric Association and National Association for Mental Health. Washington, DC, 1969
13. Goldblatt PD, Berberian RM, Goldberg B et al: Catchmenting and the delivery of mental health services. Arch Gen Psychiatry 28:478, 1973
14. Jacobson G (ed): Crisis Intervention in the 1980s. New Directions for Mental Health Services, No. 6. San Francisco, Jossey-Bass, 1980
15. Joint Commission on Mental Illness and Health: Action for Mental Health. New York, Basic Books, 1961
16. Karno M, Schwartz DA: Community Mental Health: Reflections and Explorations. New York, Spectrum Publications, 1974
17. Pisarcik G, Zigmund D, Summerfield R et al: Psychiatric nurses in the emergency room. Am J Nurs 79:1264, 1979
18. Smith MB, Hobbs N: The Community and the Community Mental Health Center. In Bindman AJ, Spiegel AD (eds): Perspectives in Community Mental Health. Chicago, Aldine, 1969
19. Snow DL, Newton PM: Task, social structure, and social process in the community mental health center. Am Psychol 31:582, 1976
20. Sundel M, Rhodes GB, Ferguson E: The impact of a psychiatric hospital crisis unit on admissions and the use of community resources. Hosp Comm Psychiatry 29:569, 1978
21. Tischler GL, Henisz J, Myers JK et al: Catchmenting and the use of mental health services. Arch Gen Psychiatry 27:389, 1972
22. U.S. Department of Health, Education, and Welfare: Outpatient Services. Publication No. 1578. Washington, DC, U.S. Public Health Service, 1967
23. U.S. Department of Health, Education, and Welfare, National Institute of Mental Health: Community Mental Health Center Program, Operating Handbook. Part 1: Policy and Standards Manual. Washington, DC, NIMH, September 1971
24. Weiner RS, Woy JR, Sharfstein SS et al: Community mental health centers and the "seed money" concept: Effects of terminating federal funds. Comm Ment Health J 15(2):129, 1979
25. Woy JR, Wasserman DB, Weiner-Pomerantz R: Community mental health centers: Movement away from the model? Comm Ment Health J 17:4, 1981

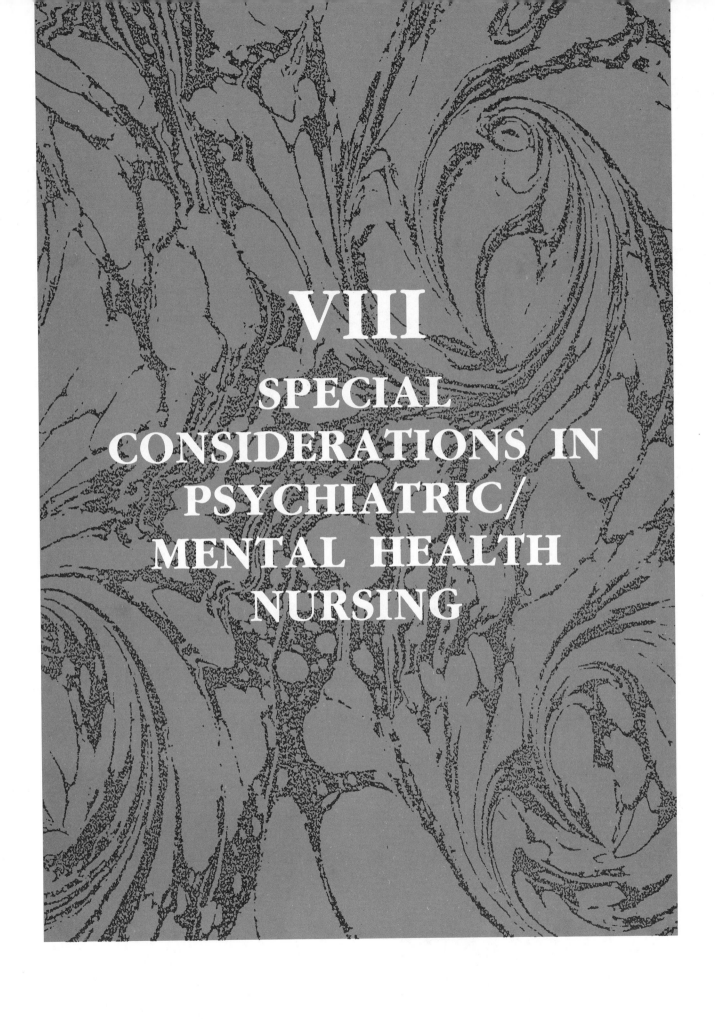

VIII
SPECIAL CONSIDERATIONS IN PSYCHIATRIC/ MENTAL HEALTH NURSING

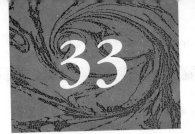

MARGARET L. MITCHELL

SPIRITUALITY IN PSYCHIATRIC/MENTAL HEALTH NURSING

Learning Objectives

Upon completion of this chapter the student should be able to do the following:

1. Define spirituality.
2. Explain the relationship between a systems perspective on a person and spirituality.
3. Identify key questions to ask clients during the psychiatric assessment related to spirituality.
4. List characteristics of each stage of faith in developmental periods.
5. Classify the levels of religious concern.
6. Describe how nurses focus on the spiritual concerns/beliefs of clients within the therapeutic use of self.
7. List examples of spiritual distress at the secondary and tertiary levels of prevention.

Introduction

What is the relationship between spirituality and psychiatric/mental health nursing? At first, it would appear that these subjects have little in common and that they are from different realms. That perspective stems from Western ways of thinking. The Aristotelian and Aquinian philosophies, with their emphasis on logic and order, have shaped Western ways of thinking and looking at things. Rationalism and empiricism, with their emphasis on sensory data and discrete categories, have permeated much of our way of thought. A large part of Western cognition is organized around categorizing ideas in certain conceptual ways.

Spirituality is an aspect of psychiatric nursing that is often overlooked, yet it plays a vital part in the lives of a substantial number of individuals. Statistics indicate that as many as 90% of people in the United States polled profess a belief in God, 40% participate in religious observances regularly, and more than 20% indicate that religion is an important part of their life.[13] Further, studies have shown that some individuals use both mental health

CLINICAL EXAMPLES

Norm, a 40-year-old neurophysiologist, was admitted to the inpatient psychiatric unit with the diagnosis of major depression. His admission followed a suicide attempt in which he had ingested antifreeze. It was apparent from Norm's background that he was very knowledgeable about possible means of suicide. As a result of his suicide attempt, crystals formed in Norm's brain. While he had not killed himself, Norm had sustained significant brain damage, including paralysis and loss of cognitive functions such as seriation (the ability to count) and the ability to read, as well as visual problems. Norm's admission to the psychiatric unit followed several months of medical treatment for injuries sustained as a result of his suicide attempt. After several weeks of hospitalization, it was apparent that Norm's depression was not improving. Norm's family, evangelical Christians, out of a sense of desperation, concluded that Norm's depression must be demonic in origin. Consulting with the psychiatrist and staff, they requested permission for an exorcism to be conducted.

Marcia was from a Mormon family. She came to the city in hope of a career as a singer and an actress. It was not easy for her to get established in her chosen career; the only acting opportunity she found was in pornographic films. This work was not regular enough for her to support herself, so she became a prostitute, and was then arrested. The court referred her for counseling. Marcia began her interview by stating, "I used to believe in God. I don't know what happened."

Geri sought treatment for depression secondary to AIDS. She had contracted the AIDS virus five years previously when she received a blood transfusion following delivery of twins by cesarean section. She was very devoted to her church, and was troubled because her church teaches that AIDS is a curse from God. Although she had been severely ill at times, she had not shared with anyone in her church family the fact that she had AIDS.

Eileen, a 50-year-old Jewish woman, was hospitalized following her son's suicide. She felt that she caused the suicide. She had grown up in a highly-fused family. Her whole mission in life had been to be a mother to her children. During the course of therapy, it was found that she had never emotionally dealt with her divorce, which had occurred ten years earlier. Her daughter lived in another state, yet all the bedrooms in Eileen's home still had ceramic nameplates of the former occupants. Eileen was diagnosed with both major depression and borderline personality. She asked plaintively, "What do I have to live for? It's only going to get worse."

Both of Don's parents were Christian ministers, and he was selected to be their successor in the ministry. Don's childhood revolved around church services. The family moved every year as his parents struggled to find churches to support them. Don attended a seminary for two years, but later completely abandoned his parents' plans for him. Unknown to his parents, Don was homosexual. As an adult, he described himself as "irreligious," and was not comfortable discussing any aspect of religion. His doctor referred him for therapy because of a complaint of loss of memory. After extensive neurological tests, no organic basis was found for his complaints, and it was concluded that his symptoms were a result of depression.

---

professionals and religious practices to cope with emotional problems, while others substitute religious practices for mental health treatment. It is important for mental health nurses to be cognizant of both the range of spirituality in individuals and its potential impact. A crucial aspect of spiritual assessment is the impact beliefs and practices have on the lives of individuals.

Understanding how data are organized and categorized will contribute to an understanding of how the seemingly diverse spheres of spirituality and psychiatric/mental health nursing fit together. For example, whether religion is an independent or a dependent variable is of importance. Mental health is caricatured as viewing religion as "neurotic, immature, or a solace for the mentally disturbed."[13] However, research on the subject indicates a positive correlation between religious activity and mental health.[3,10,13,21] A systems approach (which will be discussed later) allows the possibility that there are positive, as well as negative, aspects of religious involvement.

At the same time, it is important to keep in mind that some individuals do not hold religious beliefs. For some, any association with religious subjects may be a source of pain. Individuals may identify themselves as agnostic, atheist, or holding no formal beliefs. Some individuals may express the idea that they are not religious but they have spiritual concerns. Spirituality takes many different forms, and is not associated with any particular religious belief.

Definition of Spirituality

What is *spirituality?* McFarland and Wasli[17] have defined spirituality as encompassing "all-pervasive needs and forces." As they see it, spirituality leads to:

1. The formulation of a positive personal meaning of and purpose for existence
2. The development of meaning in suffering
3. A positive, dynamic relationship with a deity that is characterized by faith, trust, and love
4. Personal integrity and a sense of self-worth
5. A sense of direction in life that is characterized by hope
6. The development of positive human relationships.

Spirituality is defined as concerning the unseen, the "other-worldly." As such, it cannot be measured or quantified. In this scientific age, it may be difficult to understand the connection between spirituality and psychiatric/mental health nursing.

Spirituality in a Systems Theory Perspective

Each of the vignettes presented above refers to some aspect of spirituality. Spirituality is not a separate part of the person, but one aspect of the whole. Individuals can be viewed as *open systems*. That is, they are composed of interrelated and interdependent parts interacting with their social and physical environments. Von Bertalanffy's[22] general systems theory (discussed in detail in Chap. 7) was drawn from observation of various aspects of biological systems and applying the same framework to nonbiological systems. Biology students are familiar with protective mechanisms of membranes and concepts such as permeability. The biological organism's survival is dependent on allowing certain information or materials to enter the system, having a means of processing or utilizing the materials, and having a means of disposing of the used or unwanted materials.

From a systems perspective, an individual with a psychiatric disorder such as schizophrenia can be viewed as being impaired in communicating with other individuals or systems.[22] It is as if the protective membrane of a cell is so impervious that even materials that would benefit it are not allowed to enter. For example, individuals with schizophrenia may withdraw from others as a result of perceived threats, and may not be able to ask for assistance from others. Systems theory is a means to observe and describe what is happening. Rather than focusing only on the specialized parts of the system, the focus is on interaction among parts of the system.

In this chapter, an additional element, spirituality, is introduced into the systems approach in psychiatric/mental health nursing. A brief review of some terminology from systems theory may help understanding of how spirituality is part of the whole person. *Equifinality,* literally meaning "equal in the end," is a concept that is more congenial to Eastern minds than to Western minds (which have a penchant for categorization). It refers to the ideas that different causes can have similar results and similar causes can yield different results. This suggests that spirituality is not a measurable and predictable element, but rather that it affects individuals differently. This is a shift from a mechanistic framework, such as is found in the Diagnostic and Statistical Manual of Mental Disorders (DSM-III-R), to *circular causality* (the tendency for events to affect each other in a repetitive or circular manner, with no clear cause and effect).

Spirituality is probably best understood in the notion of *non-summativity,* the idea that the whole is different from the sum of the parts. In other words, the whole system is more than simply a list of the composite elements. The parts change in the presence of other elements. It might be possible to isolate and describe spirituality, yet its essence is the impact it has on individuals.

The Nursing Process

Assessment

Assessment of the client is the first phase of the nursing process. Spiritual assessment has some similarities to sexual assessment. In the past, both areas have been considered private, and possibly irrelevant. Only recently have questions about sexuality been included in assess-

ments. The purpose of spiritual assessment is not to glean all the salient details of an individual's belief system, but to assess how they fit into the overall picture of the health–illness continuum.

Several items are of particular importance in the spiritual assessment. These include the relationship between the development of mental illness and religious concern, and the level of religious concern, or "stage of faith." Also important is the similarity or dissimilarity between spiritual beliefs and values learned in the natal family and culture and those held as an adult.

Only through careful assessment and history-taking can the relationship between the development of the mental illness and religious concern be ascertained. Lenters[14] explored dependency issues associated with religion. Field[7] explored the symptom of religiosity in relationship to needs. John[11] developed an assessment tool that can be used to examine the correlation between religious beliefs and mental illness. Some points covered in the assessment tool include the following:

1. Does the person's religious behavior or input seem to create emotional disturbance or contribute in some way to its development?
2. Is the religious aspect of the person's behavior an indirect precipitating factor in the emotional disorder?
3. Is the religious concern a symptom of a deeper conflict?
4. Is the religious concern a defense that is not healthy in the long term, but presently prevents further decompensation?
5. Are the religious behavior and thinking realistic, comforting, and supportive?
6. What part does religion play in the choice of symptoms?
7. Does the religion merely provide the content ideation for the illness or delusion? What is the process beyond the content?[11]

The Nelson-Maloney Religious Status Interview[18] focuses on areas such as awareness of God, relationship to God, response to God in the ethical realm, sense and source of meaning, involvement in organized religion, community participation, ethics and values, open- or closedness in faith, and the ability to communicate. Other studies take note of the degree of commitment to religious beliefs.[21] At present, there are more than 300 tools available for the measurement of religious attitudes and beliefs.[20]

Developmental Aspects

In assessing individuals' spirituality, it is important to keep in mind their overall level of development and maturity. It would be expected that the level of spirituality would not exceed other areas of development. Fowler[8] has studied faith within the context of human development and has developed schemas to measure stages of faith.

According to Fowler, the earliest level, or pre-level, is that of *infancy* or *intuitive faith.* In this stage, "seeds of trust, courage, hope, and love are fused in an undifferentiated way and contend with sensed threats of abandonment, inconsistencies, and deprivations in an infant's environment."[8]

Stage 1, *intuitive-projective faith,* occurs in the child between the ages of three and seven. This stage is characterized by egocentric self-awareness, particularly in the awareness of others. It is at this point that children become aware of cultural and familial taboos surrounding death and sex.

In stage 2, *mythical-literal faith,* children incorporate "stories, beliefs, and observances" that are symbolic of the community to which they belong. In this stage, meaning and coherence are derived through story, drama, and myth. There is an emphasis on literalness, and an insistence on reciprocity.

Stage 3, *synthetic-conventional faith,* coincides with puberty. Individuals' foci extend beyond their family and into the world. As a basis of identity, there is a strong drive toward conformity. Lacking autonomy, individuals at this stage are "acutely tuned to the expectations and judgment of significant others." The ideologies around which individuals have organized their lives are merely a "cluster of beliefs." These beliefs are unexamined and, as with many cultural components, individuals may be unaware of possessing certain beliefs. In this stage, a strong linkage to authority figures persists.

Stage 4, *individuative-reflective faith,* is marked by a sense of responsibility for "his or her own commitments, lifestyle, beliefs, and attitudes."[8] Fowler cogently points out that many adults do not attain this stage, or only reach it much later in life. The influence of the unconscious is minimal at this point. In this stage, individuals are able to take critical self-reflective views of themselves. Finally, it is disillusionment with self that propels the individual out of smug security and on to the next stage.

Stage 5, *conjunctive faith,* may result from defeats and knowledge of "irrevocable commitments." It is highly unusual for individuals to arrive at this point before midlife. Individuals in stage 5 are highly aware of the finite quality of life. In this stage, societal rather than individualistic presuppositions, are examined. Individuals reassess their beliefs in relationship to others and in relationship to their positions in the communal society.

Stage 6, *universalizing faith,* is the final stage in Fowler's framework. He described the few individuals who attain this level of commitment and leadership as being drawn by the "providence of God and the exigencies of history." These individuals, people such as Gandhi, Mother Theresa, Martin Luther King, Jr., and Abraham Heschel, are characterized as embodying qualities of "redemptive subversiveness" and "relevant irrelevance." They demonstrate an

"inclusiveness of community, a radical commitment to justice and love, and a selfless passion for a transformed world, a world made over not in their images, but in accordance with an intentionality both divine and transcendent."[8]

Levels of Religious Concern

Oates[19] classified levels of religious concern in psychiatric clients into five categories. The *superficial level of reli-* *gious concern* is often temporary. It may be a last-ditch "plank grabbing" effort to extricate the individual from a difficult situation. The concern may be manipulative in nature, a convenient game, and used only to find a solution to another dilemma. The religious interest is not genuine.

Conventional religious concern refers to interest in spiritual matters as a matter of conformity rather than of genuine interest. Religion is used primarily to meet needs of belonging. Usually, the spiritual interest is superficial in nature, rather than involving the whole person. Response of the religious community may affect the individual's recovery.

The third area delineated by Oates is *compulsive religious concern.* The unique feature of this level is that religious ritual does not signify a communal bond; rather, it is a highly individualistic and idiosyncratic action. *Religiosity* is found at this level. The compulsively religious person is described as having "a long history of disturbed religious thinking along with a long history of defective religious training and emotional deprivation."[19]

Religious concern in character disorders is the fourth level identified by Oates. Characterized as having the "Elmer Gantry syndrome," these sociopathic individuals rarely seek psychiatric services. They may seek psychiatric services as an alternative to the legal system. Their approach to religion as well as to psychiatric services is one of manipulation.

The last area identified by Oates is *authentic religious concern.* These individuals have a genuine concern about existential issues. Their tasks are monumental as they seek to solve overwhelming life problems, including:

. . . the problem of deliverance from old patterns of existence; the problem of a durable meaning to life in spite of tragedy; the problem of integrity before God in a world that places more value upon appearance than upon reality; the problem of forgiveness for failure and recovery from the shame of never being able to achieve a much cherished goal in life.[19]

Fowler[8] and Oates[19] focused on an external or *etic* assessment that is outside the perspective of the individual. Anthropologists classify assessments or valuations as from an *emic,* or insider's, perspective, or from an *etic,* or outsider's, perspective. It is felt that an *emic* view is valuable because it emphasizes the meaning for the individual.

Self-assessment of spirituality is very useful in obtaining an *emic* viewpoint, and can help individuals explore various facets of spirituality and how they affect their lives. Brallier[5] developed a self-assessment tool composed of two parts. The first part is based on the work of Bolles,[4] who considered beliefs in and relationships with a greater power, the self, others, and the environment. The second part of Brallier's self-assessment focused on ways in which spiritual beliefs affect other areas of life.

A guide for taking a spiritual inventory is included in Table 33-1. As with any assessment tool, it points out various potential areas to be explored. The answers given by individuals determine which areas are of particular

TABLE 33-1.
SPIRITUAL HISTORY AND ASSESSMENT

INTERVIEW SCHEDULE

1. What is your earliest memory of a religious experience or belief?
2. What did your family believe? What was meaningful and important to them?
3. What is your favorite religious story, verse, or character? Why?
4. What does prayer mean to you? If you pray, what do you pray about? When do you pray?
5. What happens when you pray or meditate?
6. Is religion or God important or helpful to you now? How does this affect your personal life?
7. Are there any religious or spiritual practices that are important to you?
8. Are there any religious or spiritual articles that are important to you?
9. Is there any spiritual literature that is important to you?
10. Do you have a special religious leader(s)? How do you view that person?
11. What helps you maintain your spirituality?
12. Has being sick (in the hospital) made any difference in your feelings toward God or in your beliefs?
13. What has bothered you most about being sick (in the hospital)?
14. Who is the most important person to you now? In the past?
15. What is your source of strength and hope?
16. What helps you most when you are afraid or need special help?
17. Is there anything that is especially frightening or meaningful to you?
18. What religious or spiritual idea or concept is most important to you?
19. What is the most religious or spiritual act one can perform?
20. What do you consider the greatest sin one could commit?
21. What is your greatest temptation?
22. Did your religious interests arise gradually, or out of a point of crisis?

SPIRITUAL FINDINGS

1. What exposure, if any, did you have to religious or spiritual beliefs as a child? Has that changed? How?
2. Do religious beliefs conform to or differ from those in your cultural background and family?
3. What is the developmental level of your religious understanding and behavior?

(Stark R: Psychopathology and religious commitment. Rev Rel Res 12:165, 1971.)

concern. It is useful for nurses to be aware of the multidimensional nature of spiritual assessment.

The research box on the next page shows correlations between illness and religiousness.

Nursing Diagnosis

The American Nurses' Association[1] has developed a classification system in order to standardize nursing diagnoses in psychiatric/mental health nursing. The categories related to spirituality include:

60. Alterations in Spirituality
    60.01 Spiritual despair
        60.01.01
    60.02 Spiritual distress
    60.03 Spiritual concerns
    60.99 Alterations in spirituality NOS (not otherwise specified)
61. Alterations in Values
    61.01
        61.01.01 Conflict with social order
        61.01.02 Inability to internalize values
        61.01.03 Unclarified values
    61.99 Alterations in values NOS

A number of diagnostic frameworks have been proposed. They have focused on various aspects of spiritual distress, such as spiritual distress resulting from lack of forgiveness, or spiritual distress resulting in loss of meaning or lack of hope. Other factors, such as biological or physical disorder, may be superimposed on these diagnoses. However, these are important because spiritual manifestations are recognized in addition to better-known physical and psychological disorders.

Planning

Planning is the next phase of the nursing process. Through planning, goals, interventions designed to effect changes, and criteria to measure the effectiveness of the plan are established. Planning is an ongoing process. What are the needed short- and long-term goals related to spirituality? What part will such goals play in the total care of the client?

Intervention

Interventions consist of nursing behaviors designed to accomplish the desired goal. Interventions focused on alleviating spiritual distress are in many ways similar to other interventions in psychiatric/mental health nursing. Interventions focused on spiritual problems are not independent of other nursing behaviors, but are carried out in conjunction with other interventions. Many of the interventions, such as listening, encouraging clients to ventilate disappointments and fears, setting time limits on certain behavior such as obsessing about spiritual matters, or limiting performance of harmful religious rituals, are indistinguishable from other interventions in psychiatric/mental health nursing. Interventions are planned on the basis of the assessment of religious maturity. Maloney[18] suggests the question, can this person's religious faith be used as a resource to call on in working with this person, or will it be a weakness to be overcome or ignored?

Some possible nursing interventions that involve directly assisting the client in carrying out spiritual practices may appear to be exclusively focused on spiritual needs. For example, prayer and spiritual literature have been used in medical/surgical settings, such as oncology units, with the result of decreased anxiety or pain. In viewing the individual from the systems theory perspective, it should be remembered that there is interaction

RELEVANT RESEARCH

Reed examined differences in religiousness and a sense of well-being in terminally ill adults compared to healthy adults. The study was based on the conceptual model of dying as a developmental phase of life. In this model, dying is viewed as the most complicated phase of life, with religion seen as a self-care coping mechanism used during the end of life.

The hypothesis tested in the study was that terminally ill adults describe a greater religiousness than healthy adults. Religiousness was defined as individual expression of beliefs and behaviors that relate to spiritual dimensions or to a power greater than themselves.

The sample consisted of 57 terminally ill adults and 57 healthy adults, matched on the four variables thought to affect religiousness: gender, age, education, and religious affiliation. The terminally ill clients in the sample were ambulatory (not hospitalized), and were identified by their physician as having an incurable form of cancer (Stage III or Stage IV). These clients understood the incurable nature of their disease.

The healthy adult sample had no chronic or serious illnesses. They were included in the study based on referrals from community organizations.

The mean age of the terminally ill group was 54.74, and of the healthy group was 53.81. Both groups had approximately 13 years of education; equal numbers of males and females (17 and 40, respectively); similar religious affiliation (29 individuals were Protestant, 21 were Catholic, 4 were Jewish, and 2 stated no religious affiliation); and similar ethnicity (more than 85% were white).

The Religious Perspective Scale (RPS) was used to assess the extent of religious beliefs and behaviors. The Index of Well-Being (IWB) was used to measure well-being, or satisfaction with life as it was currently experienced by the clients. Both measures were found to be reliable and valid. In addition to being asked to complete the RPS and the IWB, respondents were asked to rate their health status and to estimate their time left to live. The terminally ill group completed the questionnaires while in the clinic or in their home during a visit by the researcher. The healthy group also completed the questionnaires at home or in a community setting.

Responses to the questionnaires indicated that, in self-ratings, terminally ill subjects, compared to the healthy adults, rated as follows: poorer on health status, having a shorter life span, and having greater religiousness, regardless of age. The terminally ill group did not differ from the healthy adult in well-being; both groups indicated a moderately high level of well-being. Female terminally ill clients reported significantly higher RPS scores than males in this group. A similar difference between genders was not found in the healthy group.

The results of this study support a life-span developmental view of terminal illness. The terminally ill group reported greater religiousness, regardless of age, indicating that some of the changes are associated with the final developmental life span stage. Thus, certain health events may influence developmental change in adulthood, rather than age *per se.*

The results of the study concerning gender and RPS scores support examination of religiousness among other women experiencing critical life events. Religiousness may be an issue relevant to women's health care; that needs further investigation. Nurses have frequent contact with clients experiencing critical life events, and can discuss religiousness with these clients. Individuals who are dying appreciate the chance to discuss their experiences.

(Reed P: Religiousness among terminally ill and healthy adults. Res Nurs Health 9:35, 1986.)

among the various parts. While spiritually-oriented interventions affect the spiritual aspect of the person, they also affect other parts, such as changing clients' responses to physical pain, or relieving psychological distress. Similarly, other interventions can affect the spiritual dimension.

The use of spiritual practices, such as prayer, and the use of spiritual literature are among the most controversial nursing interventions. The goal of these interventions is that the client receive comfort, or relief from spiritual distress. When used, prayer and spiritual literature should be included in the treatment plan and documented in the nursing notes.

Cultural Aspects of Spirituality: Ethnocentrism and the Therapeutic Use of Self

When viewing spiritual interventions from the context of a cultural framework, it should be remembered that the purpose of these interventions is to meet the needs of the client rather than of the nurse. It is important for nurses to make a distinction, and separate their own needs and values from the needs, beliefs, and values expressed by the client.

There are times when nurses may feel impotent or overwhelmed by the needs of clients. Responses to patients or clients may be conditioned by the needs of nurses to feel in control, or somehow solve the problem, or escape from the pathos of the situation. It is very important that nurses be aware of their reactions and have a clear purpose in mind in using prayer, religious literature, or any other intervention.

Prayer, combined with the therapeutic use of self, can be a means of meeting and empathizing with the client at the point of spiritual need. It is an intimate form of communication that takes place in a therapeutic relationship in which communication and bonds of trust have already been established. The request for prayer should be initiated by the client. A supportive response may substitute for prayer when the setting or timing is inappropriate, or when this intervention is not congruent with the nurse's own spiritual beliefs.

The therapeutic use of prayer and spiritual literature is based on what is helpful to the client. An awareness of the individual's level of spiritual development is critical.[8,19] The level of the spiritual intervention should not exceed the developmental level of the client. Spiritual concerns often parallel more primitive components of the psyche, and may be involved with basic needs of trust and sustenance. An individual might be intellectually sophisticated and be spiritually simple. It is not that the intellect is abandoned, but rather that spiritual concerns appeal to emotional aspects of the person rather than solely to cognitive aspects.

The content of prayer should be oriented to the expressed needs of the individual. A prayer can consist of a few brief sentences expressing an immediate need or feeling. The nurse can ask the client the specific needs or concerns for which prayer is being requested. The prayer can be related to the expressed feelings of pain, fear, anxiety, stress, helplessness, or anger at God. With disturbed or psychotic individuals, the focus of prayer may be on God's peace, order, or love. Prayer can be an affirmation of God's presence and hope.

As with prayer, the request for spiritual literature should be initiated by the client and should be for the purpose of meeting spiritual needs. Passages should be selected carefully because they may be misinterpreted, be interpreted literally or out of context, or be beyond the level of an individual. Passages can be discussed and their significance to the client can be explored. Lovinger[16] discussed problems with spiritual literature, and is a useful resource. Decisions regarding the use of spiritual literature can be made in staff conferences. It can be helpful to consult with hospital chaplains and other spiritual leaders.

Nurses can convey respect for clients' beliefs when they are different from their own beliefs. Larson and colleagues[13] noted that the beliefs of a mental health professional should not influence the beliefs of clients with whom they work. Further, it is important that spiritual beliefs be approached objectively, rather than from an idiosyncratic ethnocentric view based on the nurse's own beliefs. Use of a cultural framework enables nurses to work with individuals whose beliefs differ from their own. Beliefs and spiritual practices should be considered in the context of the individual's belief system.

In very rare instances, spiritual beliefs or practices may be viewed as harmful. Refusal of a blood transfusion on religious grounds is an example. Too often, evaluation of these situations is from a Western paternalistic (*etic*) view that assumes that the outsider is able to determine what is best for others. It is advisable to discuss these situations in a multidisciplinary conference involving cross-cultural professionals and spiritual consultants. It is critical to recognize that beliefs about health are value-laden and not necessarily shared by others. Awareness of the nurse's own cultural beliefs and assumptions facilitates understanding of the other persons's world view.

Evaluation

Evaluation, the last stage of the nursing process, examines the outcome of nursing interventions to determine whether or not the purpose or goal of intervention was met. The evaluation process is ongoing. Evaluation of spiritual needs takes into account, not only the needs expressed orally by the client, but also what best fits the understanding of the person's belief system.

Primary, Secondary, and Tertiary Prevention

Spirituality is one component of the cultural system. This component can be viewed (as with the environment) as contributing to health or being detrimental to the well-being of the individual. The concept of levels of prevention can be applied to issues of spirituality. It is important that this is not an action that the nurse performs on behalf of the client, but rather that this is explored jointly.

Primary prevention focuses on the promotion of mental health. The nurse may positively reinforce practices that contribute to the person's overall mental health. For example, if meditation has helped a person cope with interpersonal conflict while healthy, then a nursing behavior might be to encourage this health-promoting activity. Prevention is focused, not only on the future, but also on the present. Primary prevention would also include apprising the client of normal developmental changes that take place in the life cycle and their impact on spirituality. Research indicates that there is increasing concern with spiritual matters as individuals age.

Secondary prevention focuses on spotting problems before they become major issues and lead to more difficulties. Spiritual distress related to lack of forgiveness is an example of such a problem. In this situation, nurses might allow clients to ventilate their thoughts and feelings. Together, nurses and clients might explore what events precipitated their subjective experience and their belief that they are beyond forgiveness. The situation might be evaluated as to whether it is a rational or an irrational response. Nurses may explore with clients the actions they might want to take, such as contacting an individual with whom they have had a misunderstanding. Many situations are not resolvable. In these cases, nurses may listen as clients express their feelings. Another nursing behavior associated with secondary prevention might be to refer the individual to a spiritual leader.

Tertiary prevention focuses on rehabilitating the individual to a previous level of peak functioning. An example of this could involve a person who is experiencing spiritual distress related to a lack of meaning and lack of hope. This could be the result of a crisis or loss in which this person's response is to question seriously the beliefs and values around which the person's life had previously been organized. The crisis may be of such a magnitude that change is required in modes of coping or in ways of living. It may be that suppositions on which the individual's life was organized now require revision.

Major crises might include events such as suicide of a family member, loss of a family member through accident, loss of employment, or divorce. Nursing behaviors at this level of prevention focus initially on basic needs, such as prevention of self-injury in the case of the suicidally-depressed individual. Other behaviors include helping clients express feelings of disappointment, rage, helplessness, and grief. As the acute phase is passed, rehabilitation focuses on exploring assumptions clients have held, and helping them to rebuild the framework around which they have organized their life. Another nursing behavior in the recovery phase might be to link the client with community supports, such as Bereaved Parents.

Summary

1. Spiritual concerns and needs of clients are often overlooked in practice, yet they play an important part in the lives of many individuals.

2. Spirituality can provide a sense of well-being and assist in forming positive interpersonal relationships.

3. Two items of particular concern in the nursing assessment are the client's level of religious concern, and the relationship of the development of mental illness and religious concern.

4. Each stage of growth and development is associated with a particular type of faith.

5. Religious concerns of psychiatric clients can be classified into five categories: superficial, conventional, compulsive, manipulative, and authentic.

6. The nurse must consider clients' cultural values regarding spirituality.

7. Spirituality can be addressed in nurse–client relationships at each level of prevention.

References

1. American Nurses' Association: Taxonomy for the Classification of Human Responses of Concern for Psychiatric/Mental Health Nursing Practice. Kansas City, Missouri, American Nurses' Association, 1986

2. American Psychiatric Association: Diagnostic and Statistical Manual of Mental Disorders, 3rd ed, revised. Washington, DC, American Psychiatric Association, 1987

3. Bergin A: Religiosity and mental health: A critical re-evaluation and meta-analysis. Prof Psy: Rsch Prac 14:170–184, 1983

4. Bolles R: The Three Boxes of Life. Berkeley, California, Ten Speed Press, 1978

5. Brallier F: Successfully Managing Stress. Los Altos, California, National Nursing Review, 1982

6. Draper E: On the diagnostic value of religious ideation. Arch Gen Psychiatry 13:202, 1965

7. Field W, Wilkerson S: Religiosity as a psychiatric symptom. Perspect Psychiatr Care 11:100, 1973

8. Fowler J: Stages of Faith. San Francisco, Harper & Row, 1981

9. Gorsuch R: Measurement: The boon and bane of investigating religion. Am Psychol 39:228–236, 1984

10. Himmelfarb H: Measuring religious involvement. Soc For 53:606–618, 1975

11. John S: Assessing Spiritual Needs. In Shelly J, John S (eds): Spiritual Dimensions of Mental Health. Downers Grove, Illinois, InterVarsity, 1983

12. Kleinman A, Good B: Culture and Depression. Berkeley, California, University of California, 1985

13. Larson D, Pattison E, Blazer D: Systematic analysis of research on religious variables in four major psychiatric journals, 1978–1982. Am J Psychiatry 143:329, 1986

14. Lenters W: Sick love and sick religion. J Christian Nurs 3:7, 1986

15. Lindenthal J: Mental status and religious behavior. J Scientif Study Rel 9:143, 1970

16. Lovinger R: Working With Religious Issues in Therapy. New York, Jason Aronson, 1984

17. McFarland G, Wasli E: Nursing Diagnoses and Process in Psychiatric/Mental Health Nursing. Philadelphia, JB Lippincott, 1986

18. Nelson D, Maloney H: The Nelson-Maloney Religious Status Interview (unpublished document). Fuller Theological Seminary, Pasadena, California, 1982

19. Oates W: The Religious Care of the Psychiatric Patient. Philadelphia, Westminster, 1978

20. Silverman W: Bibliography of measurement techniques used in the scientific study of religion. Psych Doc 13:7, 1983

21. Stark R: Psychopathology and religious commitment. Rev Rel Res 12:165, 1971

22. von Bertalanffy L: General Systems Theory. New York, George Braziller, 1968

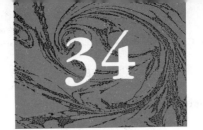

ROSE A. VASTA

PSYCHIATRIC/MENTAL HEALTH NURSING PRACTICE AND THE LAW

Learning Objectives

Upon completion of this chapter the student should be able to do the following:

1. Describe how nursing practice is based on the ANA Standards of Practice and individual state nurse practice acts.
2. Define and describe voluntary treatment for mental health clients.
3. Define and describe involuntary treatment for mental health clients.
4. Summarize various types of consent, and explain the nurse's role in obtaining consent from clients.
5. Discuss the client's right to refuse treatment.
6. Explain the elements of due process and their ramifications for the nursing care of involuntary mental health clients.
7. Discuss client competency and incompetency to make mental health care decisions about treatment.
8. Discuss the nurse's responsibility for the confidentiality of records of mental health clients, especially clients who are dangerous to others.
9. Identify special treatment considerations for nursing care of minors in a mental health setting.

Introduction

In no other type of nursing are the legal and ethical considerations of practice so crucial as in psychiatric nursing. To deal with these demands, psychiatric nurses must be aware of both the laws in the state in which they practice and the common practice of nurses in the area. The nurse must also be aware of current legal decisions at both state and federal levels because these often affect practice. This chapter cannot address the specific laws of each state, but will provide a summary of the types of considerations and the landmark decisions that most often affect the nurse's practice.

Elements of the Law

The United States Constitution guarantees all citizens certain freedoms. For example, it is not possible to deny constitutional freedoms by placing someone in jail for merely having certain thoughts. Criminal plans must be made or a deed must be accomplished before the police power of the state can intervene to restrict a citizen's rights to freedom and privacy.

Under mental health law, however, a person may be removed from home and family and incarcerated because of having thoughts that are judged to be caused by mental illness and to be hazardous to that person or to others. In involuntary hospitalization, constitutional rights are abridged for the welfare of the state and the person. Restriction of rights guaranteed by the Constitution represents a severe impingement on a person's liberty. Sometimes it is necessary to restrict these rights to protect the person or others. However, nurses must always remain sensitive and alert to the ramifications of the loss of freedoms traditionally taken for granted in our society.

The work of psychiatric/mental health nurses is often performed against the wishes of clients. Nurses may administer medications that will alter the brain chemistry of clients against their will. Nurses may be asked to assist in the administration of electroconvulsive therapy to clients who refuse or are unable to consent to this procedure. These procedures, however necessary, are an infringement of clients' constitutional rights to privacy. When administered to clients involuntarily, they must be done with utmost care and regard for the due process rights of clients. *Due process* is the course of legal proceedings that ensures that our laws are enforced fairly. It assures that all citizens are able to follow certain procedures to assert their views.

Nurses must be concerned at all times with the confidential nature of what they hear and are party to in mental health practice. A complicating problem is that psychiatric records are not always subject to the same rules of confidentiality as clients' medical records. These laws also change fairly frequently. Therefore, nurses must remain abreast of changes in the laws of confidentiality that relate to the care of mental health clients.

The Nurse as Part of the Client's System

Effective psychiatric nursing care requires that nurses fully understand the multitude of dynamics operating on a client at a given moment. These include the client's biological make-up, learning history, and family context, and the larger social context in which the client lives and works. The laws that govern and control the person's freedoms have an impact on the client's system. These dynamics include the milieu of the treatment environment and the institution in which it exists. Achieving such an understanding is best accomplished by use of

general systems theory. This theory is more fully developed in Chapter 7.

Clients' Rights: Nurses as Advocates

It is the responsibility of nurses to ensure that their actions promote the welfare of clients. When nurses find that their activities benefit another group, grave questions should be raised about the appropriateness of their actions. Mental health clients are often the least capable of protecting their own rights. Psychiatric problems may cause clients to lack social skills or may cause an inability to make a point clearly understood due to difficulties in concentration. As a result, the rights of mental health clients have been ignored and abused for centuries.

In 1971, a group of mental health care clients prepared a document entitled "The Mental Patient's Bill of Rights."[8] This document stated the rights of every person who is held in a psychiatric hospital. Those rights are summarized in the following box.

THE MENTAL PATIENT'S BILL OF RIGHTS

- The right to be treated as a human being, with decency and respect
- The right to be guaranteed every right given to United States citizens by the Declaration of Independence and the Constitution of the United States of America
- The right to integrity of mind and body
- The right to receive treatment and medication only when administered with informed consent
- The right to have access to one's own legal and medical counsel
- The right to refuse to work in a mental hospital and to receive the minimum wage for any work done there
- The right to decent and prompt medical attention
- The right to uncensored communication by phone or letter and with visitors
- The right to refuse to be locked up involuntarily, and to refuse to give fingerprints and photographs
- The right to decent living conditions
- The right to keep one's own personal possessions
- The right to counsel and a court hearing about any mistreatment
- The right to refuse to be a part of research for experimental drugs or treatments and the right to refuse to be used as a learning experience for students
- The right to protection from defamation of character
- The right to an alternative to commitment in a mental hospital

Various states include in their mental health laws a list of rights that are guaranteed to all mental health care recipients. In California, these rights are read to every client at the time of admission to a facility. The rights are also posted in a prominent spot on each ward, both in English and in the predominant language of the community. Along with these rights are posted the name, address, and telephone number of the local Patients' Rights Office. The rights of hospitalized psychiatric/mental health clients in California are summarized in the following box (Fig. 34-1).

Because of the availability of nurses to mental health clients, they are the professionals most often asked questions about the rights of mental health clients. Informed psychiatric/mental health nurses need to be aware of state laws in order to address client questions. Knowledgeable nurses should maintain awareness in order to protect the rights of clients. One resource that nurses can suggest for clients who express an interest in their rights is *The Rights of Mental Patients,*[5] a guide written in cooperation with the American Civil Liberties Union. Some of the questions frequently asked include:

1. What are the differences between voluntary and involuntary clients?
2. How can individuals be put in mental health facilities against their will?
3. Can clients be forced to take medications?
4. How long can individuals be held involuntarily?
5. What are the rights of an involuntary client?
6. What should individuals do if they want to get out of the hospital?
7. What is a mental health conservatorship or guardianship?
8. Can clients be given shock treatment against their will?

CALIFORNIA PSYCHIATRIC/ MENTAL HEALTH CLIENTS' RIGHTS

1. The right to wear your own clothes
2. The right to keep and use your own personal possessions, including toilet articles
3. The right to keep and be allowed to spend a reasonable sum of your own money for canteen expenses and small purchases
4. The right to have access to individual storage space for your private use
5. The right to see visitors each day
6. The right to have reasonable access to telephones, both to make and to receive confidential calls or to have such calls made for you
7. The right to have ready access to letter-writing materials, including stamps
8. The right to mail and receive unopened correspondence
9. The right to refuse shock treatment and any form of convulsive therapy
10. The right to refuse psychosurgery

---

9. Can individuals be given a lobotomy (psychosurgery) against their will?
10. How can clients complain about their rights?

All of these questions can be answered by nurses who are aware of the laws of the state in which they work, and who are aware and protective of the rights of clients.

Nurse Practice Acts

Before entering into practice in any of nursing's specialty areas, nurses should be aware of the contents of the nurse practice act of the state in which they are licensed. A *nurse practice act* is the law governing the profession of nursing that is adopted by each state. Such laws state the prescribed course of study for professional nurses, require that nurses successfully pass the state board examination, and stipulate the requirements for a license to practice nursing. These laws tell nurses how to obtain a license in each state, as well as regulate and control nursing practice.[3]

The nurse practice act of the state of California is located in the Business and Professions Codes. The section that describes nursing practice reads as follows:

The practice of nursing . . . is the performing of professional services requiring technical skills and specific knowledge based on the principles of scientific medicine, such as are acquired by means of a prescribed course in an accredited school of nursing as defined herein, and practiced in conjunction with curative or preventative medicine as prescribed by a licensed

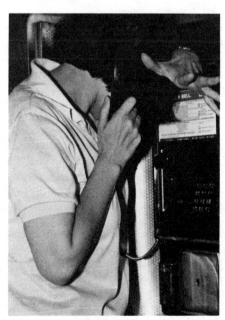

Figure 34-1. A psychiatric client exercising her right to make phone calls.

CLINICAL EXAMPLE

Mr. Jones signed into the Porter Psychiatric Hospital as a voluntary patient at 9 a.m. His problems included severe depression that interfered with his ability to perform well in his position as a vice president of a local bank. During the evening shift, he informed the nurse that he did not like the facility and wanted to leave right away. The nurse was concerned because it was 11 p.m., and Mr. Jones had no transportation.

The nurse was aware that Mr. Jones had the right to leave the hospital at any time because of his voluntary status. She also was aware that she should allow him to leave in a reasonable amount of time. She immediately called Mr. Jones's physician and informed her of Mr. Jones's desire to leave the facility. The nurse also documented on the chart an assessment of Mr. Jones's mental status, including a suicide assessment. After her own assessment of the client, the physician and the nurse agreed that Mr. Jones did not meet the criteria for involuntary hospitalization.

The nurse spoke to Mr. Jones about her concerns over his leaving the hospital at this late hour, and asked if she could be of assistance in obtaining transportation for him. She also asked that he consider remaining in the hospital until morning, when he would be discharged. She informed him that his physician would discharge him against medical advice, since the physician and the rest of the treatment team felt that he could benefit from treatment for his depression. Mr. Jones decided to wait until morning for his discharge, a time when his family could pick him up.

physician and the application of such nursing procedures as involve understanding cause and effect in order to safeguard life and health of a patient and others.[4]

The scope of professional nursing is broad, and continues to change at a rapid pace. Because the practice of nursing develops so rapidly, the definition of nursing practice in an individual state is usually broad and fairly flexible. This lack of specificity means that the nurse practice act in most states does not contain a specific statement of functions that a mental health nurse can perform. It merely defines the general areas of control or the jurisdiction of nursing. To help remedy this problem, the American Nurses' Association, in conjunction with the local state board of nurse examiners, works to establish standards of practice, as well as functions in and qualifications for the practice of professional nursing.[7]

Standards of Practice

The *Standards of Psychiatric and Mental Health Nursing Practice,*[1] introduced in June 1982 by the American Nurses' Association, reflect the various roles of the nurse in outpatient care, long-term care, home settings, and private practice. These standards distinguish between the practice of clinical specialists in psychiatric nursing and the practice of nurse generalists in the field. The standards specifically address psychotherapy, health teaching, daily living activities, somatic therapies, and the therapeutic environment.

These standards help set the general expectations for nurses in psychiatric/mental health nursing. If a nurse's behavior does not compare favorably to the minimal standards set by the state in which the nurse is licensed, the standards of the American Nurses' Association, the standards of the Joint Commission for Accreditation of Hospitals, or any other relevant laws or standards, then it would be very difficult to argue that the nurse was operating within the acceptable limits of the profession.

In addition to these standards, a court of law would also consider the standards of the community of nurses in which the nurse functions. In other words, the judge would be interested in the common practice of the nurse's colleagues. If the nurse's behavior is consistent with the practice of other nurses in the geographic area, the judge may find that the actions of the nurse are within the scope of nursing practice, even if they are not specifically condoned or described by the nurse practice act or other standards.

Voluntary Treatment

Any person admitted to a treatment facility on a voluntary basis or as an involuntary client is entitled to prompt and adequate treatment. In *O'Connor v. Donaldson,*[9] the United States Supreme Court ruled that, if clients are confined for a reason other than dangerousness, they must be given treatment.[12] The goal of inpatient admission of mental health clients is to provide treatment, behavior modification, or rehabilitation to enable individuals to return again to the community. When working in a mental health care setting, nurses must always consider whether their activities are designed to meet this goal. Only when the goal of treatment is to assist the person to regain or develop new levels of functioning is institutionalization justified.

A *voluntary admission* occurs when the client freely consents to enter an institution because of a need for psychiatric care and treatment. Voluntary admission is always made without undue influence, coercion, or duress. Clients who enter a psychiatric hospital on a voluntary basis may leave at any time and may not be held against their will. The only exception to this is when, after voluntarily entering the hospital, the person's condition changes, making involuntary commitment proceedings the appropriate measure.

Involuntary Treatment

Until the early 1960s, it was commonplace in our country to warehouse mentally ill people within a vast system of state hospitals. These individuals were often hospitalized for many years with no real treatment. Indefinite commitments were commonplace, and clients were often unaware of the reason for their admission some 15 to 20 years previously. With few staff willing to work in state hospitals, client care was "streamlined." This meant that clients were often made to wear state-issued clothing, with their hair cut by the hospital in an easily-managed style. It was often difficult or impossible for the long-term client to contact friends or relatives outside the hospital by mail or phone.

With increasing interest in the 1960s in the civil rights of all citizens, there came an interest in the rights of mental health clients. This interest was also spurred by economic considerations because a tremendous portion of public monies was being utilized to warehouse these persons in public institutions.

There was a movement in the early 1960s, culminating in the Federal Community Mental Health Services Act of 1963, toward deinstitutionalization of the mentally ill. Thousands of chronically mentally ill clients were released from state institutions and sent back to the community for treatment in community mental health centers. Later, when the federal funds to support these centers were stopped, communities found themselves with mentally ill clients who had no treatment and were often homeless and in need of emergency psychiatric treatment. These clients were often unable or unwilling to consent to treatment on their own. All of this led to the need for reforms in the laws regarding consent, refusal of treatment, and involuntary hospitalization.

Consent

Laws regarding consent protect people from invasion of bodily integrity and protect their constitutional right to privacy. Adequate information is necessary to make knowledgeable health care decisions. When there is no consent or other type of authorization for treatment, nurses performing procedures with mental health clients can be held liable for battery. *Battery* is defined as harmful or offensive touching. It is the unlawful beating or use of force on a person without the person's consent. *Assault* is an apparently violent attempt or threat to do violence to someone. Battery can occur even when the procedure is properly performed and can be proved to be helpful for the client. For example, the administration of electroconvulsive therapy to a client who refuses, and then later improves with the treatment, can be considered battery. This is true even if there are no negative effects of the treatment. It is the unapproved touching alone that leads to liability.[12]

Simple and Informed Consent

There are two general types of consent: simple consent and informed consent. *Simple consent* implies no consent other than authorization for the procedure or treatment. It is currently held that the physician, nurse, or other practitioner responsible for a procedure has a separate legal duty to give the client enough information so that the consent can be based on an informed decision. If full information is not disclosed to the client, the performance of the procedure is not considered battery. However, the failure to disclose information about the procedure may be considered negligence. To get a client's consent without providing complete information is called *uninformed consent*. Obtaining uninformed consent protects the nurse from criminal prosecution for battery, but only adequate informed consent by the client protects the nurse from civil liability for negligence.[12]

Express or Implied Consent

Express consent is given when the client gives consent either orally or in writing. In most states, electroconvulsive therapy and psychosurgery require express consent. The state of California requires express consent for the use of psychotropic medications with voluntary adult clients. With those general exceptions, most states require only oral consent for authorization of procedures. Because oral consent is often difficult to prove, most mental health facilities have internal policies that require written consent.[12]

Implied consent is always presumed to exist in medical emergencies unless there is a particular reason for the nurse to think it would be refused, as in psychiatric emergencies. In such situations, when a person's life is endangered, express consent is not required to carry out measures to reduce the danger to the person or others.

Refusal of Treatment

The right to give consent for treatment implies a right to refuse treatment. There are three legal bases for the right to refuse treatment: (1) the right to freedom from nonconsensual invasion of bodily integrity, (2) the constitutional right to privacy, and (3) the constitutional right to freedom of religion.[12]

It is usually considered the physician's responsibility to give clients adequate information regarding the use of psychotropic medications and other procedures that require the order of a physician. In the state of California, where clients must give informed consent for the administration of psychotropic medications, this is considered to be a nontransferable responsibility. This means that nurses cannot take upon themselves the sole responsibility of informing clients of the risks of psychotropic medications. Written documentation of informed consent is usually required to be kept on clients' charts. Nurses are responsible for knowing that clients have given adequate informed consent before they follow a physician's order that requires consent. If nurses administer a psychotropic medication without informed consent in the state of California, they can be held criminally liable for assault and battery even if the client never suffers any side-effects from the medication.

CLINICAL EXAMPLE

Mrs. Colby, a very depressed, elderly woman, was given electroconvulsive therapy for three weeks after she had signed a written consent for the treatment. On three mornings each week, the nurse assisted Mrs. Colby in her morning hygiene and then walked her to her treatment. As the treatments progressed Mrs. Colby became increasingly mute and regressed. One morning when the nurse tried to walk her to her treatment, Mrs. Colby shook her head "no," and refused to leave her room. It appeared that Mrs. Colby was silently refusing her treatment.

The nurse explained to Mrs. Colby that she was due for another electroconvulsive treatment and that the treatment team had decided that these treatments would be beneficial to her. She also explained the use and effectiveness of the treatments. When Mrs. Colby continued to refuse to leave for the treatment, the nurse documented on the chart that Mrs. Colby had withdrawn her consent for the treatment and immediately called Mrs. Colby's physician to inform him of the development. The physician then began legal proceedings to evaluate Mrs. Colby's competency to decide against electroconvulsive treatment, and attempted to get a court order for the treatment.

The right to refuse treatment continues even after the client has given oral or written permission for a treatment. Clients and their conservators or the parents of a minor can withdraw consent by simply objecting to the continuation of treatment. This is true even if the client has consented to an ongoing procedure for weeks or months. As soon as the nurse becomes aware that consent has been withdrawn by the client, the procedure should be discontinued, without endangering the client, and the attending staff member should be informed of the change as soon as possible. The nurse may make a reasonable effort to convince the mental health client to continue to accept treatment. For example, it is permissible to explain to the client the purpose and use of the medication as well as problems that may develop if treatment is stopped.[12]

However, there are times when the client's right to refuse treatment is outweighed by the interests of the state. Interests of the state can vary. They include protection of the rights of others as well as protection of the welfare of the client when the client is found to be a danger to self or to be gravely disabled. *Grave disability* is defined as a condition in which a person is unable to provide for the elements of food, clothing, and shelter due to mental illness. This can sometimes present a problem for nurses who believe in the right of clients to commit suicide, yet work in institutions in which they must actively work to prohibit suicide. Nurses may find themselves working in a social system that cannot or refuses to provide adequate continuing care for mentally ill clients, yet insists that clients remain alive.

Involuntary Hospitalization

Each state has certain provisions within its mental health law for the involuntary admission of clients (Fig. 34-2). Involuntary admissions are permitted when individuals meet certain criteria. The standards for involuntary admission are similar in all states, although there are variations in procedure and interpretation of the required criteria. Current practice in all states is to hospitalize clients without consent only when the client's behavior is such that there is a threat of harm to the client or to others that is due to a mental illness.

Clients are not usually hospitalized for behavior that is merely eccentric or that varies from the norm. This does not mean that all voluntary clients are always *entirely* voluntary in practice. Many clients are voluntary only because a health care worker or family member has made it clear to them that if they do not cooperate with treatment they will be placed on an involuntary hold, and hospitalized anyway, placing another impediment in the way of discharge. This sort of coercion is unethical and does not allow clients their due process rights.

Minors may be placed in a psychiatric facility because of the wishes of their parents. In addition, clients placed on a conservatorship or guardianship may be hospitalized because of the judgment of their conservator or guardian. *Conservatorship* occurs when a person is found to be in-

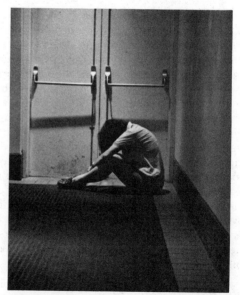

Figure 34-2. A psychiatric client who is being held on a psychiatric unit involuntarily.

competent to the extent that the court appoints someone to take over and protect that person's rights.

Thus, there exists an entire class of clients commonly known as *involuntary-voluntary clients*. Many of these clients, however, could not actually be held on involuntary holds because their behavior, while not entirely normal, does not endanger anyone.[6]

Commitment

Commitment is the legal act of certifying that a person requires involuntary treatment for a mental disorder. This is usually done only when the person is found to be (1) a danger to self, (2) a danger to others, or (3) gravely disabled.

Most states allow emergency commitment of an individual after certification by two physicians that the person meets at least one of the above criteria. Both physicians need not be psychiatrists. In California, nurses, psychologists, social workers, police, and park rangers, when properly designated by the state, may also perform the evaluation and sign the "hold" or commitment. The person signing the certification must have examined the individual and believe that person to be mentally ill and a danger to self or others or gravely disabled.[7]

Commitment is not the same as a court determination of incompetency. Under the law, individuals who have been committed involuntarily to a treatment facility are still considered sufficiently competent to be involved in some or all of their personal medical decisions. Commitment laws authorize involuntary treatment that is necessary to preserve the client's life or avoid permanent injury to the client or to others. An incompetency ruling by a judge declares the need for a guardian or conservator who will be given authority to make certain decisions for the client.

States vary in the extent to which the commitment laws authorize the use of antipsychotic drugs or electroconvulsive therapy for nonemergency treatment of mental illness. A federal judge in New Jersey ruled in *Rennie v. Klein*[11] that psychotropic medications could not be forcibly administered to an involuntarily-committed client. Another landmark decision[13] was made when a judge agreed that a group of patients in Massachusetts who were held against their wills had the same rights as others to give or withhold consent for medical treatment. Because laws and opinions vary greatly from state to state, it is very important for nurses to be familiar with their own state laws regarding involuntary treatment.

Several states have ruled that, except in an emergency, the constitutional rights to privacy and due process are violated if medication or electroconvulsive therapy is given on an involuntary basis without a judicial finding of incompetency. In some states, the issue has been resolved by requiring the judicial officer to find the person unable to make treatment decisions as part of the commitment process. A few states have even required a judicial determination of the need for antipsychotic medications when an incompetent client refuses the medication in a nonemergency situation.[12]

Due Process

When individuals are hospitalized against their will, it is due to the imposition of the police power of the state. The most severe restrictions on state power are written in the Fourteenth Amendment. It states that no state shall "deprive any person of life, liberty, or property without due process of law; nor deny to any person within its jurisdiction the equal protection of the laws."[16] This is referred to as the "due process" or "equal protection" clause. *Due process* is the course of legal proceedings carried out regularly and in accordance with established legal rules and principles. This ensures that our laws are enforced fairly, and that all citizens are able to follow certain procedures to assert their views.

The due process clause is applied to any action of the state that would deprive a person of "life, liberty, or property." The process that is due the mentally ill client varies, but includes two primary elements: (1) the rules applied must be reasonable and not vague; and (2) fair procedures must be followed in enforcing the rules. State mental health laws that are too arbitrary or vague violate the due process clause and are not enforceable. Clients must be offered notice of the fact that they are about to be hospitalized against their will and given an opportunity to present information about why this should not occur.[12]

The U. S. Constitution requires that due process must be given before deprivation of liberty can take place. This means that clients must be notified of the allegations made about their behavior before being taken to the hospital. Clients must be given an opportunity to rebut the charges and be given the opportunity to be heard by an impartial party who will listen to all sides of the issue. In an emergency, it is considered sufficient if the person making the decision has reasonable grounds to believe that the individual is mentally ill and a danger to self or others. This emergency commitment protects clients and others for a specific time period, until a full judicial hearing and involuntary commitment can be arranged.

The right to due process means that each person is entitled to a day in court. After involuntary hospitalization, the person has the right to petition for a Writ of Habeas Corpus. A *Writ of Habeas Corpus* is the process through which clients are permitted to demand a hearing before a judicial body that will question the right of the state to detain them involuntarily. This right is part of the due process rights of involuntary mental health clients. At the time of this court hearing, the client is able to meet with an impartial judge who listens to the facts about the situation, hears testimony from the client and physician, and makes a decision about whether the client should remain in the hospital.[7]

Competence

Adults are considered competent if the court has not already declared them incompetent and if they are gener-

CLINICAL EXAMPLE

Mrs. Driscol is an elderly woman who has been living as a "bag lady" for five years on the streets of a large city. Recently, Mrs. Driscol began shouting at people outside a neighborhood grocery store. The store owners placed a complaint with the county department of mental health and asked that she be placed in a conservatorship and sent to a psychiatric hospital for the treatment that she obviously needed. Mrs. Driscol had obvious hallucinations and delusions, but refused to take the medications prescribed for her at the local mental health center.

Mrs. Driscol was picked up for evaluation at the area hospital by the police. She was held for three days for observation, during which time she received a major tranquilizer. At the end of the three days, Mrs. Driscol asked to go to court for a Writ of Habeas Corpus. By the time of the court hearing, a week later, Mrs. Driscol's mental state had significantly improved from the medications and the hospital environment. The judge released her from her involuntary hold on the grounds that she was no longer gravely disabled and that her choice to live on the street was one of lifestyle rather than due to mental illness.

ally capable of understanding the consequences of alternatives that they may choose. The law always assumes that an individual remains competent unless steps have been taken to prove otherwise. It is not necessarily the function of anyone on the treatment team to determine whether a client continues to be competent. When it is difficult to assess competency, the courts are often asked to make the determination. When a person expresses wishes concerning psychiatric treatment before becoming incompetent, those wishes should be considered seriously in making decisions about treatment.[12]

When a court finds that a person is incompetent to make health care decisions, including decisions that affect mental health care, it will designate someone as a guardian or conservator. That person is then given legal authority to make specific decisions regarding the incompetent individual's care. The specific range of permissible choices that the guardian or conservator can make is determined by the court that appointed the guardian or conservator.[12] Some of those choices include the right to hospitalize the client in an acute care psychiatric hospital, in a state hospital, in a nursing home or long-term treatment facility, and in an unlocked residential facility. Occasionally, judges give the guardian or conservator the right to place the client in an acute care psychiatric hospital while requiring that placement within a state hospital necessitates returning to court for a further decision by the judge. For this reason, it is imperative that nurses, and the facilities in which they work insist that a copy of the guardianship or conservatorship papers be placed with the chart at admission. This ensures that nurses and others on the treatment team are not treating or holding a client without proper consent.

It often happens that a person who is actually incompetent has never been determined to be so by a court. Therefore, the incompetent person does not have a legally appointed guardian or conservator to make decisions for him or her. This is a very difficult and precarious situation for nurses and all others involved in treating clients. It is often unclear that proper consent has been received for certain procedures such as the administration of psychotropic medication or electroconvulsive therapy. It is best to attempt to foresee such situations, but it is not always possible to do so. In a situation in which the client appears to be unable to give consent and no guardian or conservator has been appointed by the court, common practice is for the physician to seek approval from the next of kin. If this is not possible, consent is sought from others who have unofficially assumed supervision of the client. In many states, this practice is supported by local laws or court decisions, while in other states the propriety of this arrangement is in question and the procedure should be postponed until a conservatorship has been obtained.[12]

Confidentiality

Mental health records are held to a much higher level of confidentiality than are general medical records. In New York State, a court held in 1982 that a spouse cannot be given information from mental health records even when the couple is not separated. The only time the information can be released to a spouse is when the client authorizes it or when there is a danger to the client, spouse, or another person that can only be reduced by disclosure of information. In other states, the laws may be more or less stringent.

In 1974, the California Supreme Court made a landmark decision that greatly affected mental health care workers all over the country. In the case of *Tarasoff v. Regents of the University of California,*[15] a female college student was murdered by a fellow student. The student who killed her had told his therapist of his desire to kill the woman, and the court later found the therapist liable because he did not warn her or the police about the danger that existed. Nurses who receive information from a client indicating that the client may present a danger to others are required to inform the intended victim and/or the police as soon as possible.[14]

There are certain situations in which confidentiality is very difficult to maintain and necessitates particular care on the part of psychiatric/mental health nurses. Nurses who conduct group therapy are responsible for the confidentiality of the material discussed by the mem-

CLINICAL EXAMPLE

Abigale Doral was admitted as a voluntary patient by her parents because she was exhibiting strange behaviors at home, refused to eat, and had not slept for several days. Abigale was 15 years old. After two days in the hospital, a family conference was held in which Abigale's parents announced that they were getting divorced. Abigale left in an upset state and returned to the unit, where she attempted to slash her wrists with a coat hanger. Abigale's parents became upset with the hospital staff when they learned of the incident, and demanded that their daughter be discharged immediately to their home. It was the firm opinion of the entire treatment team that Abigale's life would be in danger if she were allowed to leave the hospital, because of her severe suicide potential and the current chaotic situation at home.

Abigale's physician evaluated her, found that she met the criteria for involuntary hospitalization, and placed her on an involuntary hold because she was a danger to herself. Mr. and Mrs. Doral were told that they did not have the right to remove her from the hospital until the evaluating physician was assured that Abigale no longer presented a danger to herself.

bers of the group. Nurses should caution groups that all material mentioned during sessions should remain confidential and should not be repeated outside the group.

Telephones present a particular problem for confidentiality on the psychiatric unit. Nurses and other professionals should never respond to the question, "Is Mr. Jones (or anyone) there?" when asked over the phone. If answered in either the affirmative or the negative, the answer gives an unknown caller information about an individual's psychiatric treatment. The nurse's correct response to that question is to tell the caller that the nurse cannot give out that information over the telephone because of confidentiality laws. The nurse may then ask for the name and number of the caller, and inform the caller that if that person is a client at the facility and chooses to return the call, the client may do so through the patient phone. Telephone calls are usually placed through a "patient phone" or pay phone because this gives clients the opportunity to screen their own calls.

Minors

The age at which a person is considered an adult and legally capable of making decisions about health care or marriage is decided by the legislature of each state. In most states, the age is set at 18. In some states, a person can be declared an adult before the established age by having the court declare the person an emancipated minor.[12]

Emancipated minors may consent to their own medical and mental health care. Minors become emancipated when they are no longer subject to parental control or regulation and are not financially supported by their parents. Emancipation must be established in a specific manner, and these procedures vary from state to state. In some states, the parent and child must both agree on the emancipation so the child cannot become emancipated by simply running away from home.[12]

In most states, parents may place their child in a psychiatric hospital or treatment center without the child's consent. In the case of *Parham v. J. L. and J. R.,*[10] the Supreme Court ruled that states could allow parents to admit minors involuntarily for mental health treatment without court authorization if the admission is approved by a qualified physician. In *Barley v. Kremens,*[2] the federal court decided that minors have the right to due process and that parents or guardians cannot waive this right. This means that the minor has the right to a court hearing to determine if the involuntary hospitalization is necessary. The state has an interest both in preserving the authority of the parent and the family unit and in the physical and mental health of the child. The state must also be concerned with the potential danger to society from activities of children with mental disorders.[7]

When the mental health nurse is involved in the treatment of a minor, it is usually wise to involve both of the parents and the client in decisions about treatment. Either parent can give consent for treatment of a minor, unless there is a legal separation or divorce and one or the other parent has been given custody of the child. It is usually best to know if the other parent objects to treatment and to attempt to obtain authorization from that parent or withhold treatment if necessary.[12]

Issues of confidentiality become very complex in the treatment of minors. Often parents feel that by placing their son or daughter in a psychiatric facility they have the right to know everything that transpires in that child's treatment. While this is understandable from the parents' point of view, this type of disclosure does not allow for adequate development of a trusting relationship between client and therapist. Minors have the right to expect that their therapist will respect their right to confidentiality. Conflicts over confidentiality can be avoided through frequent family conferences and a treatment approach that includes the system in which the minor client lives.

The Nurse and the Law

The legal basis for the mental health care of clients is complex and dynamic. Several issues must often be weighed at once. It is not uncommon for nurses to consider together clients' rights to privacy, to treatment, and to protection from dangerous impulses, before making treatment decisions. Answers are often vague, determined by institutional policy and a desire to serve the best interests of clients. Nurses who work in the psychiatric/mental health setting should be aware of changes and trends in the mental health laws at federal and state levels.

Summary

1. Nursing practice should be based on sound theoretical standards of care. Nurse practice acts govern the profession of nursing in each state.

2. Voluntary admission requires client consent. The goal of admission is to enable individuals to return to the community.

3. Involuntary treatment may be deemed necessary for clients requiring mental health care. Commitment is necessary if the individual needs to be protected from self or others.

4. Consent can be either simple or informed. Awareness of client consent will enable the nurse to avoid situations of negligence, or those involving battery or assault.

5. Constitutional rights ensure privacy and freedom of religion. The right to freedom from nonconsensual invasion of bodily integrity completes the three legal bases for a client's right to refuse treatment.

6. Due process guarantees that laws are enforced fairly for each citizen. The nurse has a responsibility to assure that all mental health clients receive due process.

7. Competence means the ability to understand consequences. Guardianship and conservatorship may be necessary to meet the incompetent person's needs for mental health care.

8. Mental health care records have higher standards of confidentiality than general medical records. The mental health care team is responsible for maintaining confidentiality except under circumstances endangering the life of the client or others.

9. Decision-making is very complex in the case of minors. Nurses have a responsibility to provide adequate mental health care to minors.

References

1. American Nurses' Association: Standards of Psychiatric and Mental Health Nursing Practice. Kansas City, Missouri, American Nurses' Association, 1982
2. *Barley v. Kremens,* 402 F. Supp. 1039 (E.D. Pa. 1975), reversed on other grounds, 429 U.S. 882 (1977)
3. Bullough B: Law and the Expanding Nursing Role. Norwalk, Connecticut, Appleton-Lange, 1975
4. California Board of Registered Nursing: Laws Relating to Nursing Education Licensure—With Rules and Regulations. California Department of Consumer Affairs, 1980
5. Ennis BJ, Emery RD: The Rights of Mental Patients, 2nd ed. New York, Avon Books, 1978
6. Fenner K: Ethics and Law in Nursing: Professional Perspectives. New York, van Nostrand Reinhold, 1980
7. Hemelt M, Mackert M: Dynamics of Law in Nursing and Health Care, 2nd ed. Reston, Virginia, Prentice-Hall, 1982
8. Mental Patients' Alliance of Central New York: The Mental Patient's Bill of Rights. Syracuse, New York, 1971
9. *O'Connor v. Donaldson,* 422 U.S. 563 (1975)
10. *Parham v. J. L. and J. R.,* 422 U.S. 584 (1979)
11. *Rennie v. Klein,* 462 F. Supp. 1131, 1145 (1978)
12. Rhodes A, Miller R: Nursing and the Law, 4th ed. Rockville, Maryland, Aspen Systems, 1984
13. *Rogers v. Okin,* 478 F. Supp. 1342 (1979)
14. Simmons S et al: California court ruling on dangerousness stirs controversy. APA Monitor 6:12, 1975
15. *Tarasoff v. Regents of the University of California,* 13 Cal. 3d 177, 529 P. 2d 553, 118 Cal. Rptr. 129 (1974)
16. U.S. Constitution: 5th and 14th amendments

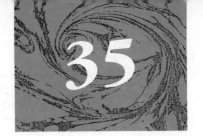

JANE A. RYAN AND VIVIAN BROWN

POLITICAL, ECONOMIC, AND SOCIAL INFLUENCES ON PSYCHIATRIC/MENTAL HEALTH NURSING

Learning Objectives

Upon completion of this chapter the student should be able to do the following:

1. Identify the social, political, and economic forces that affect the mental health care system.
2. Discuss the historical changes in mental health practice in relation to client population, mental health settings, and types of services.
3. Describe the role of nurses in contemporary mental health nursing practice.
4. Analyze the impact of citizen participation and consumerism on mental health care services and community mental health centers.
5. Summarize how new federalism and block grant programs have changed the delivery of mental health care services.
6. Discuss the forces for competition as a cost-containment strategy in health care.
7. Describe the reimbursement program implemented by the federal government to curb the spiraling costs of health care.
8. Identify contemporary trends in mental health care practice, and hypothesize their impact on the future.

Introduction

Contemporary psychiatric/mental health nurses are challenged with providing a broad spectrum of mental health services, in a cost-effective manner, to a heterogeneous client population, in a variety of settings. These compo-
nents are an integral part of the mental health system, which undergoes continual change because of its interactions with the political, economic, and social factors present in society. Psychiatric/mental health nurses must therefore understand these political, economic, and social factors if they are to continue to expand their scope of

practice and influence the future direction of the mental health care system in the United States.

A Systems Theory Perspective on the Client

Johnson defined the individual person as a behavioral system comprising a complex of observable features and actions that determine and limit the interaction between the individual and the environment. Behavior functions as a set of responses, and serves as a mechanism for communication between the person and the surrounding environment. The factors in the external environment that have great impact on the person are called "regulators".[22] They represent the current and historical experiences that influence and modify the individual's response to environmental stimuli. The physical environment and sociocultural factors are *external* regulators of behavior, while the physiological and psychological factors constitute *internal* regulators of behavior. Their functions are to limit and direct behavior.

The goal of mental health intervention in clinical practice is to help the individual restore, maintain, or attain a balance. Psychiatric/mental health nurses, therefore, act as *external* regulators by promoting fulfillment of unmet needs and assisting individuals to change their behavior.

Mental Health System Components

As stated in the chapter introduction, the major components of mental health care include (1) heterogeneous clients; (2) a broad spectrum of cost-effective mental health programs; (3) a variety of service settings; and (4) mental health care providers. Based on general systems theory, these four components are viewed as "subsystems" of the mental health system. The subsystems are *interdependent,* since a change in one part affects the other parts. The four subsystems must be protected, nurtured, and stimulated if they are to maintain a steady state or level of adaptation. Each subsystem has specific functions and roles that must be maintained if the mental health system is to remain open to change and meet its goal of providing mental health care for clients.

This chapter will analyze the impact of political, social, and economic factors on the mental health system. For the purposes of this chapter, "social" includes environmental and cultural issues. A time perspective—from the 19th century to the present—is used in order to trace the significant changes in mental health practice.

The historical development of the mental health system, as influenced by the above factors, will be discussed. This will help psychiatric/mental health nurses to understand the interactive nature of these factors in defining the client, the setting, the type of service provided, and the role of the nurse. The practice settings of psychiatric/mental health nursing—the psychiatric hospital, a nonhospital or community mental health center, and private practice—will be included.

The Historical Development of the Mental Health System

19th Century

During the 18th century, the United States experienced the Age of Understanding or Enlightenment, when attempts were made to replace mystical and religious explanations of phenomena with "reason" and rational inquiry.[12] This era led people to question human nature and capability, which led to a reexamination of the nature of mental illness. Views of the cause of mental illness were polarized around two opposing themes: individuals were viewed as genetically defective in mind or will, *or* individuals were believed to be born with a clean mind but subjected to immoral and dehumanizing life experiences that produced disorder.[24]

The most celebrated approach of this period was "moral management" or "moral treatment." Moral treatment was developed in the late 18th century by Philippe Pinel in France, Vincenzo Chiarugi in Italy, William Tuke in England, and Benjamin Rush in the United States. Several broad ideals characterized this system and are well documented by Caplan.[11] While the movement was short-lived, many of the practices of moral treatment resembled those of the progressive community mental health programs of today. Insanity was believed to be a readily-curable physical disease. Treatment of the disease included manipulation of the physical and social environment, which is an early version of milieu therapy. The insane were taken to hospitals, where they received individualized programs of recreation and work as well as religious and education services. They were well cared for by a disciplined staff.

Practitioners of moral treatment tried to reach their objectives by directing educational programs toward the general population (prevention). The hospital environment was organized to offer a corrective experience to the insane (treatment). In the institution, all aspects of the client's life could be regulated in order to provide the optimum chance of recovery.[11]

The essence of moral treatment can be seen most clearly in the social organization of the institutions. Early practitioners recognized that (1) the classic "madhouse" environment damaged patients; (2) restraints produced violence; and (3) idleness and sensory deprivation produced other problems. Unlike institutions created before and after it for custodial care, the asylum was designed as a setting to provide the protection, privacy, and insulation of clients. A program of recreational, occupational, and social activities was provided. Therefore, the setting provided the mentally ill with a buffer, of time and space, from the mainstream of life. It was a retreat.

These developments occurred simultaneously with a dramatic population increase from urban immigration, resulting in an increase in the numbers of mentally ill needing treatment. A lack of psychiatric facilities, combined with the humanitarian spirit of the times and the presence of "moral treatment," motivated a few rich, powerful men to become philanthropists for the mental health system. This social movement resulted in the building of private psychiatric facilities such as Friends' Asylum in Pennsylvania (1817), McLean Asylum in Massachusetts (1818), and Hartford Retreat in Connecticut (1824). The clients, the settings, and the health care providers were not significantly different from those found at the first public hospital established in Virginia in 1773. What did change was the type of service provided—*moral treatment* was used.

Because moral treatment was based on the fostering of a corrective social experience, it was easily disrupted by an influx of criminal patients, alcoholics, and immigrants, who did not share the values and characteristics of the "average patients." In addition, moral treatment evoked a large body of legislation governing insanity. Before its advent, the insane were considered under the poor laws if they were destitute or under criminal law if they were disruptive to the peace of the public. The efforts of reformers and legislators made the insane a new and distinct legal category.

The poor mentally ill were confined in almshouses and jails without treatment because there were not enough psychiatric facilities. Dorothea Dix, an outstanding social activist of the time, spent many years lobbying with state legislatures to provide facilities for the poor mentally ill so they could be removed from the penal system. Her efforts, combined with the results of moral treatment in private psychiatric hospitals, resulted in the appropriation of funds by the legislatures of various states to build large public psychiatric institutions.

A number of factors combined in the mid-19th century to make the asylum system ineffectual in relieving the problems of the insane. Caplan stated that the prime factor in the growth of custodial care was not the replacement of a humane and progressive regimen by cruelty, neglect, and a repressive institution. Rather, asylums could no longer be devoted to the active therapy and cure of recent cases, but had to provide a sheltered environment for chronic misfits. By the mid-1860s and the 1870s, treatment in the asylums was poor by any standards; overcrowding had become the norm.[11]

By the end of the 19th century, the formal mental health system, which would endure for many decades, was firmly established. Clients who had sufficient income would receive moral treatment in private psychiatric hospitals, and indigent clients would receive custodial care in public state psychiatric hospitals.

While hospitals increased in size and number, commitment procedures continued to show a lack of concern for the individual's right to freedom. In the late 19th century, regulatory agencies were established by states to prevent abuses in commitment procedures. Monitoring practices were established. The emphasis in the legislation enacted during the 1870s was on preventing the commitment of sane persons. Clients' rights after commitment were not considered.

Nursing was not introduced in the United States until the early 1870s. The first school for psychiatric nurses was started in 1882 at McLean Asylum. Because there were large numbers of clients in hospitals and so few nurses to provide care, the early role of psychiatric/mental health nurses was custodial. The main goal was the provision of a safe, clean environment.

Table 35-1 summarizes the political, economic, and social forces of the 19th century that were responsible for changes in the mental health care system. Other forces and variables are also included.

Early 20th Century

The predominant mental health practice of the first four decades of the 20th century continued to be custodial care. However, there were significant forces attempting to alter this practice. The mental hygiene movement is generally regarded as the next turning point in psychiat-

TABLE 35-1.
MENTAL HEALTH CARE CHANGES IN THE 19TH CENTURY

POLITICAL
- Shift from use of poor laws and criminal laws for the insane to specific legislation governing insanity
- State regulatory agencies established
- Legislation enacted to prevent commitment of the sane

ECONOMIC
- Legislature-appropriated funds to build public psychiatric facilities

SOCIAL
- Nature of mental illness reexamined
- Treatment for the insane that attempted to manipulate social and physical environment
- Dramatic population shifts due to immigration

CLIENT POPULATION
- Better definition of clients
- Large influx of immigrants

SETTING
- Shift in responsibility from family to state
- Mentally ill moved from homes, poorhouses, and jails to hospitals
- Large public hospitals implemented

TYPES OF SERVICES
- From chains to custodial care with emphasis on physical care and clean environment
- Moral treatment implemented for a short period of time

NURSES' ROLE
- Custodial care in hospitals

ric history. Community forces made a concerted attack on institutional management, and psychiatry began to move out of asylums and into schools, child guidance and outpatient clinics, and the military. The growth of outpatient care in close-to-home treatment programs proceeded after the emergence of the first psychiatric outpatient clinics in the 1880s. The further developments of psychological clinics, settlement houses, juvenile courts, and child guidance clinics were all important roots of today's community mental health movement.

Two scientific developments that occurred during this time were the introduction of psychoanalysis and the somatotherapies. Psychoanalysis, as defined by Freud, was responsible for a major change in the practice of psychiatry because it introduced the concept of a psychological genesis of mental illness.[23] Unfortunately, it did not lead to any remarkable change in the practice of public hospital psychiatry; clients continued to receive only custodial care and remained in public hospitals for extended periods of time. Psychoanalysis did give practitioners insight into the functioning of the mind, and an understanding of both the relationship between physical and psychological illness and the impact of environment on behavior.

In the 1930s, three somatic therapies were introduced into the psychiatric hospital setting. Sakel developed insulin shock therapy in 1932, as a way to induce hypoglycemic coma through the administration of progressively increased doses of insulin. The coma was viewed as the essential therapeutic factor in the remediation of symptoms of mental illness.[21]

Electroconvulsive therapy (ECT) was introduced in 1935 by Meduna. This treatment induced convulsions through the administration of pharmacologic agents. Bini changed the procedure in 1938 by replacing the pharmacological agent with an electrical stimulus to the brain to produce a seizure.[5] Empirical observations revealed improvements in clients' mental status with the utilization of insulin therapy and ECT, but the etiology of how they work is still unknown.

Psychosurgery was introduced in 1935 by Moniz. The usual form of psychosurgery was a prefrontal lobotomy. The procedure involved drilling a hole through the skull, inserting a leukotome, and cutting the white nerve fibers connecting the frontal lobe with the thalamus. The client's postoperative course frequently included a blunting of the personality, along with apathy and irresponsibility.[18] These somatic therapies were used initially as treatments for schizophrenia, and were viewed as enlightened psychiatric practice at the time.

Table 35-2 summarizes the political, economic, and social forces of the early 20th century that were responsible for changes in the mental health care system.

Mid-20th Century

A significant series of social, political, and economic forces were set in motion during the mid-20th century. These factors ultimately shifted the responsibility for the

TABLE 35-2.
MENTAL HEALTH CARE CHANGES IN THE EARLY 20TH CENTURY

POLITICAL
- The United States Army consulted with psychiatrists during World War I to assist with war neuroses, thereby bringing psychiatry more into consideration as with other medical specialties.
- Writings in forensic psychiatry began to describe the relationship between psychiatry and the law.

ECONOMIC
- Governmental agencies and philanthropic foundations devoted money to establishing centers to do research on mental illness and treatment.

SOCIAL
- Mental hygiene movement pointed out abuses in the mental health system.
- Children began to be considered and treated.

CLIENT POPULATION
- Client population expanded, includes children.

SETTING
- Outpatient clinics implemented
- Growth of community-based programs, including child guidance clinics and settlement houses

TYPES OF SERVICES
- Primarily custodial care
- Introduction of psychoanalytic treatment
- Introduction of somatic therapies (ECT)

NURSES' ROLE
- Began to expand into outpatient clinics

mentally ill from the state to the federal government. Public awareness of mental illness was raised in the 1940s when almost two million men were rejected by the Army and Navy because of mental problems. During World War I, the rejection of large numbers of men by the Armed Services attracted attention, but did not lead to significant reforms. The experience of World War II, however, revealed even larger numbers of mentally disturbed men who were rejected from service or who were discovered among the troops.

The magnitude of the problem led Congress to pass the National Mental Health Act of 1946, which authorized the National Institute of Mental Health (NIMH) and the National Advisory Mental Health Council. NIMH proposed developing a mental health delivery system that would provide treatment in the community rather than in large, isolated state hospitals. To achieve this goal, grants-in-aid were given to a number of states to develop community services. The number of psychiatric outpatient clinics grew from approximately 450 in 1945 to 1,234 by the end of 1954. In addition, funds were made available for research and training. These efforts moved the federal government into a position of prominence in mental health.[24]

After World War II, the commitment laws were again altered. In 1952, the Draft Act Governing Hospitalization of the Mentally Ill, which advocated voluntary admissions, was published by NIMH. It served as a model to be adapted by state legislatures according to local needs and conditions.

The renewed interest in mental health was reinforced when Congress passed the Mental Health Study Act of 1955. This act authorized the first national study on mental illness. The study was carried out by the Joint Commission on Mental Illness and Health. They reported their recommendations in 1960 for a new, comprehensive approach towards mental health. Congress put this recommendation into action in 1963 with the passage of the Mental Retardation Facilities and Community Mental Health Centers Construction Act, which established a mental health system with an emphasis on community psychiatry. This movement was also supported by the publication of *Social Class and Mental Illness,*[20] *Midtown Manhattan Study,*[36] and *Stirling County Study.*[28] These three important investigations of psychiatric disorder in the natural community reflected a far greater incidence of disorder than had previously been believed to exist. These investigations studied the sociocultural aspects of mental disorder.

Hollingshead and Redlich[20] conducted a study in New Haven, Connecticut, attempting to link social class and mental illness. Data were collected on identified psychiatric clients and on a sample of New Haven residents. Social class was assessed, using a formula that included area of residence, occupation, and education. This study documented that the poor were more often coerced into entering treatment than the affluent, that psychotic disorders were more common among the lower socioeconomic classes, and that neurotic disorders were found more frequently in higher social classes.

The Midtown Manhattan study by Srole and his associates[36] used community surveys rather than known psychiatric clients. A large sample (1,600) of residents in Manhattan, New York, was studied. Ten stress factors were studied as possible causal factors of the mental disorder in three socioeconomic groups. The stress factors included broken homes in childhood, economic deprivation, parental conflict, and inadequate interpersonal relationships. The study found that these factors had an additive effect on subsequent mental disorder with decreasing socioeconomic status. Nearly one quarter of the sample was judged to be significantly impaired.

The Stirling County study[28] was undertaken by Leighton and his associates. It was conducted in a rural area in Nova Scotia, with a sample of about 1,000 residents in both socially-integrated and socially-disintegrated communities. Social disintegration included factors such as lack of membership in associations, broken homes, overt hostility, and few sanctions against deviant behavior. This study found that half of the adults were suffering from some psychiatric disorder. The authors also concluded that disintegrated social systems produced disintegrated personalities.

Another significant piece of legislation that affected the mental health system was the 1965 Medicare and Medicaid amendments to the Social Security Act. Massive amounts of money were authorized for treatment of the elderly and indigent mentally ill. This legislation firmly established the federal government as the new primary funding source for the treatment of mental illness, and the state as the secondary source. To help to convey the implications of this legislation for the mental health system, a review of the changes in hospital psychiatry during the same time period will be presented.

Hospital Psychiatry

The decade of the 1950s experienced the highest number of hospitalized mentally ill clients in the history of the United States. The 1950 census revealed a resident rate (number of persons in a hospital on a given day) of 512,501, while the number of admissions totalled 152,286. In contrast, the 1970 census showed a resident rate of 337,619, with the number of admissions totalling 384,511.[25] These 1970 data reflect a higher admission rate, a shorter length of stay, and fewer people in a hospital on a given day. These changes were achieved through *deinstitutionalization,* or the discharge of mentally ill clients from the traditional state hospitals to community-based mental health services. Deinstitutionalization (DE) has played such a significant role in changing public hospital psychiatry that it deserves a detailed explanation. The experience of the state of California will be presented because it has been considered one of the leading states in implementing deinstitutionalization.[29]

Deinstitutionalization

California reached an all-time high of 37,489 hospitalized mentally ill clients in 1959.[29] Although psychotropic drugs were introduced in the mid-1950s, they did not have an appreciable immediate impact on decreasing the number of clients in hospitals. The Short-Doyle Act was effected in 1957. This legislation served as the blueprint for community mental health practice in California. The act provided for an emphasis on nonhospital, community-based treatment services. It encouraged education of and consultation to care-giving agencies in the community. The state was required to reimburse 50% of the funds spent by local governments for developing and maintaining local mental health services. Cost-sharing between participating counties and the state, on a 50–50 basis, proved to be a problem, and was later revised.

The move of clients from hospitals to community mental health services was made possible by new federal legislation such as Medical Assistance for the Aged (MAA), a precursor to Medicare.[7] MAA provided funds to subsidize needy elderly clients in general chronic care hospitals and to pay for medical services for the elderly in nursing homes. These funds were used to discharge some of the elderly from state hospitals into nursing homes. In 1962, the Department of Health, Education, and Welfare (DHEW) issued new regulations which, for the first time, permitted clients other than old-age benefit recipients to claim federally-supported welfare payments while on "convalescent leave" from a hospital. These regulations were responsible for a large emigration of clients out of state hospitals.

In addition, in 1963 the Department of Mental Hygiene persuaded the California state legislature to authorize funds for a geriatric screening program at the Langley Porter Institute in San Francisco. The program was designed to reduce the number of admissions of elderly clients to state mental hospitals. During its first four years of operation, geriatric commitments dropped from 486 per year to 18 per year. The reduction was possible through the use of the various financial aid programs such as old-age assistance, Medical Assistance to the Aged, and general relief. These programs allowed older people to use nursing homes, general hospital care, and private physicians. When deinstitutionalization in California is compared to that in the rest of the nation, it appears that the massive deinstitutionalization was accomplished by concentrating on older mental clients. From 1962 to 1968, California showed a decrease of 64.4% in the state mental hospitals' population of individuals 65 and older, while the national average only decreased by 21.6%.[29]

In 1963, the California Short-Doyle Act was amended so that county-administered mental health programs received 75% of their funding from the state, rather than the previous 50%. Later, counties were designated to provide community mental health services, subject to state reimbursement. The formula became 90% state–10% local for all programs. By July 1966, Short-Doyle programs were operating in counties that encompassed 96% of the total state population. Greater use was being made of local services as alternatives to state institutionalization.[29] This was occurring at the same time as federal monies were being put into community mental health centers. These efforts were responsible for a 19% reduction in the California mental hospital population between 1959 and 1965.

The next significant development in deinstitutionalization was the 1965 Medicare and Medicaid legislation. A California Medi-Cal program was developed to obtain new federal funds. These funds included payments for inpatient and outpatient services provided by general hospitals; for services provided by skilled nursing facilities (SNFs); and, after 1967, for services provided by intermediate-care facilities (ICFs). This led to a further exodus of clients from state hospitals, so that, by 1977 only 5,715 clients remained.[29] From 1959 to 1977, the California mentally ill population in public hospitals had been reduced by 85%.

While there are fewer clients in California mental hospitals, there are not fewer mentally ill clients in California. The outcome of deinstitutionalization is that clients are scattered in many settings, such as nursing homes, general hospitals, board-and-care homes, halfway houses, and group homes. Clients are receiving mental health services in the community. Unfortunately, many mentally ill individuals are part of the homeless population and receive no mental health care.

In the 1950 census, two types of nontraditional institutions were mentioned—commercial boarding homes for the aged and dependent, and commercial nursing, rest, and convalescent homes. These types of homes began to assume major social importance following the passage of the Social Security Act. Today, the nontraditional institutions also include alcohol- and drug-abuse treatment centers, residential treatment centers for children, halfway houses, group homes, board-and-care homes, and homes and schools for the emotionally disturbed.

The nursing-home industry and the board-and-care industry have been supported by welfare programs, which resulted in a rapid growth of for-profit facilities. However, individual owners were not the only beneficiaries of the shift to new institutions. As can be seen in the California experience, states also were offered an opportunity to gain fiscal advantages by deinstitutionalization. The expansion of the federal welfare state helped to effect an integration of anti-institution ideology, private-profit motivation, and state fiscal expediency.[29]

Community Mental Health Movement

The federally-funded community mental health centers (legislated in 1963) were designed to provide comprehensive mental health care in a defined catchment area or mental health service area. The care involves treatment, prevention, and rehabilitation services. In addition to this comprehensive care, community mental health centers (CMHCs) foster coordination and cooperation among agencies responsible for mental health care and the development of a system that ensures continuity of care.

The community mental health center was thought to have played a major role in reducing the number of mental hospital admissions by providing community alternatives for treatment. Connery[13] reflected that the dichotomy seen between the "disease" concept of mental illness associated with hospitalization and the "environmental" concept of such illness associated with community mental health services was too simplified.

First, there is the issue of whether CMHCs have reduced hospitalizations. Since 1967, the Division of Biometry and Epidemiology in NIMH has collected inpatient data on the federally-funded community mental health centers. Of the 528 CMHCs existing in 1976, 127 were hospital-based, 338 were hospital-affiliated, and the remainder were free-standing.[25] In January 1976, there were 10,193 CMHC designated inpatient beds. A total of 246,900 inpatient-care episodes occurred in 1975 in the CMHCs, accounting for about 13.8% of all specialty inpatient care.[29]

It appears that the CMHCs may have helped reduce the number of state hospitalizations. However, the CMHCs have picked up a significant proportion of inpatient-care episodes. It also appears that the CMHCs have had an impact on the length of hospitalizations. Data indicate shorter lengths of stay in state hospitals and in CMHCs. However, there is much work to be done to build strong community-based treatment alternatives to hospitalization. This issue is discussed further in later sections.

In addition to the reduction in hospitalizations, CMHCs were projected to attract new categories of the "mentally ill." It appears that CMHCs have served significant numbers of new categories of clients, such as ethnic minorities, abused children, and sexual assault victims. However, with fiscal limitations, services may not continue to be available to all who need or request them. At the present time, there is a strong mandate to treat only the seriously disturbed.

The emphasis on community psychiatry, combined with the infusion of federal funds into nursing education during the 1960s, led to expanded role development of the psychiatric/mental health nurse. With the increasing need for mental health personnel and the expansion of services within the community mental health system, federal training money became available. Nurses could apply for federal traineeships, but access to graduate education was limited. As more nurses applied to graduate school, the number of graduate programs increased from 8 in 1947 to around 90 by the early 1980s.[30]

In addition to the availability of training funds, two events had a great impact on the development of psychiatric nursing. In 1952, Peplau published *Interpersonal Relations in Nursing,* a classic text on psychiatric nursing. In 1956, at the National Working Conference on Graduate Education in Psychiatric Nursing, the concept of the clinical specialist in psychiatric nursing was firmly established.[30] By 1962, psychiatric nursing was based on the interpersonal process.

Graduate programs redesigned their curricula to replace the functional focus of administration and education with a new focus on clinical specialization. The graduates of the 1960s programs pioneered the development of the role of the nurse psychotherapist with a variety of clients in outpatient settings such as the CMHCs. These new areas of concentrated study received professional validation when the American Nurses' Association established Psychiatric/Mental Health Nursing Standards (1973), a certification program in Psychiatric/Mental Health Nursing (1975), and a Statement on Psychiatric/Mental Health Nursing Practice (1976). Psychiatric/mental health clinical specialists were hired as psychotherapists in large numbers during the 1970s to provide a broad range of mental health services in a variety of settings. A series of legislated actions to change nurse practice acts were sought and obtained in many states. These new laws reinforced the view by psychiatric/mental health clinical specialists that psychotherapy was a component of nursing practice.

Validation of the expanded scope of practice for the psychiatric/mental health nurse by clients, legislatures, the professional association (ANA), and employers (hospitals, CMHCs) resulted in many clinical specialists' seeking autonomy in their practice. In 1974, a group of pioneer nurses established the ANA Council of Specialists in Psychiatric/Mental Health Nursing. Their goal was to advance the opportunities for nurses to engage in independent private practice. The lack of third-party insurance reimbursement for services provided by clinical specialists limited opportunities for private practice to clients who were able and willing to pay for their own therapy.

Table 35-3 summarizes the political, economic, and social forces of the mid-20th century that were responsible for changes in the mental health care system.

Late 20th Century

The late 20th century has seen an increasing focus on specific client populations such as women, ethnic minorities, drug and alcohol abusers, and the elderly. New client groups receiving attention include the victims of violence, such as rape victims, battered women, abused children, and elder-abuse/parent-abuse victims. The setting for care expanded its community base. The predominant hospital setting shifted from the public (not-for-profit) hospital to the private (for-profit) hospital and psychiatric units in general hospitals. Types of services expanded to include self-help groups, preventive/educational groups, and employee assistance programs in industry. In the late 1970s, NIMH also developed a program

TABLE 35-3.
MENTAL HEALTH CARE CHANGES IN THE MID-20TH CENTURY

POLITICAL
- Commitment laws altered; voluntary admissions advocated
- Short-Doyle Act (California) passed; emphasis on community-based treatment
- CMHC and mental retardation legislation

ECONOMIC
- NIMH established; grants-in-aid given to states to develop community services, and funds for research and training made available
- Appropriations made for CMHC construction and staffing
- Growth of the federal welfare state

SOCIAL
- Public awareness raised by mental health casualties in the armed forces and large-scale epidemiological studies
- Research conducted related to social issues and mental health

CLIENT POPULATION
- Client population continued to expand; included armed forces and less severely disturbed clients.

SETTING
- Expansion of outpatient programs
- Military programs initiated
- Community mental health centers (CMHCs) implemented
- Shift from state to federal government responsibility

TYPES OF SERVICES
- Community-based services, including partial hospitalization, day and night hospitals, crisis intervention
- Deinstitutionalization began

NURSES' ROLE
- Continued to expand; included individual psychotherapy
- Development of clinical nurse specialist role

to meet the needs of clients released from hospitals: the *Community Support System,*[38] which will be discussed in more detail below.

Role of the Nurse

Differentiation of levels of psychiatric/mental health nursing occurred in 1975 when the American Nurses' Association introduced its certification program. Certification became available for psychiatric/mental health nurses and clinical nurse specialists in adult or child and adolescent psychiatric/mental health nursing.[2]

Certified psychiatric/mental health nurses understand theories concerning personality development and the behavior patterns involved in the treatment of mental illness. Their practice also requires knowledge of the expected effects of treatment on client behavior and its relationship to nursing care.[2] These nurses base their practice on the nursing process and the ANA Standards of Psychiatric and Mental Health Nursing.[3] They provide nursing care to a variety of clients in multiple settings. They do not engage in nursing psychotherapy, because therapy is included in the expanded role of the clinical nurse specialist.

Certified clinical nurse specialists (CNS) in adult or child and adolescent psychiatric/mental health nursing possess a high degree of proficiency in therapeutic and interpersonal skills. They not only influence and modify attitudes and behaviors of clients, but also assume responsibility for the advancement of nursing theory and therapy. In addition to therapy, the role of the CNS includes teaching, research, consultation, supervision, management, and coordination of client care.[2]

As of March 1987, there were 8,214 certified psychiatric/mental health nurses; 2,756 certified clinical nurse specialists in adult psychiatric/mental health nursing, and 317 certified clinical nurse specialists in child and adolescent psychiatric/mental health nursing.[2] These 9,459 certified nurses represent 18% of the reported 51,564 psychiatric nurses in 1978.[34] Although no current percentage figures are available, the percentage is known to have increased since 1978, and can be anticipated to increase still more in the future.

During this period, psychiatric/mental health nursing roles expanded as nurses became involved in individual, group, and family psychotherapy. These roles, and their development, are discussed in Chapters 10, 11, and 12 respectively. Psychiatric/mental health liaison nursing also emerged as another nursing role, as is discussed in detail in Chapter 30.

The scope of practice of psychiatric/mental health clinical nurse specialists expanded during this period to include the provision of all mental health services except for those restricted by law to the practice of medicine, such as prescribing medications. Psychiatric/mental health nurses practiced in any setting where there were clients, such as hospitals, outpatient clinics, homes, and prisons. The role of the psychiatric/mental health nurse received further clarification when the ANA Standards of Psychiatric and Mental Health Nursing were revised in 1982.

While the majority of psychiatric/mental health nurses continued to be employed by hospitals, an increased number of clinical nurse specialists chose to work in private practice. This trend gained momentum with the advent of third-party reimbursement for services provided by certified clinical nurse specialists. The ANA Council on Psychiatric and Mental Health Nursing established Guidelines for Private Practice of Psychiatric and Mental Health Nursing in 1987. These guidelines identify professional expectations for nurses in private practice. They include criteria for expected nurse behavior in the areas of (1) identification process, (2) credentialing and standards, (3) client relationships, (4) interprofessional relationships, and (5) financial guidelines.[4]

Consumerism/Citizen Participation

In the mental health field, there is almost half a century of history of citizen participation through volunteer programs. More recently, volunteer involvement has moved away from the hospital setting and into the community. The volunteer groups that once included only the wealthy and powerful in the community have expanded to include all citizens. Citizen participation involves the consumers of services (clients), professionals, and volunteers.

In the 1960s, a large number of "constituencies" began to emerge as power groups. Participants in the civil rights movement, the war on poverty, the drive for black power, and the revolt of university students staged sit-ins, demonstrations, and marches to exert power. Political action became high drama, viewed by millions with the aid of the media. Added to the explosion of power movements were "flower" power, youth power, the women's movement, the gay and lesbian movement, and the elder power. The emergence of these advocacy groups has led to a number of significant changes—citizen participation in decision-making, training of indigenous nonprofessionals or paraprofessionals, and development of community support systems.

During the past two decades, a number of large-scale programs, supported by federal funds, have helped delineate the problems and issues of consumer participation in health and mental health services. These programs include the President's Committee on Juvenile Delinquency, the Office of Economic Opportunity, and projects initiated under the CMHC Act. Among the most significant elements in this context approach were: the decision to designate and provide services to specific target populations; the decentralization of programs, with neighborhood-based facilities; direct funding in response to the appraisal of need; and participation of target-area residents in advisory and employment roles. The federally-funded community mental health center program allowed for consumer participation on boards and advisory committees, as well as in planning for and evaluation of service.

Citizen participation is an integral part of a participatory democracy that involves people in making decisions that affect their lives. The consumer movement emerged, not only to allow all people to claim their right to decision-making, but also as a protection against fraud and exploitation. Resource allocation is a constant problem. To change the distribution of resources always involves opposition by or resistance from groups that are satisfied with and/or that benefit from the established pattern. "The oppressed are groups denied substantial participation or power in societal decision-making, which typically reduces their share of the resources essential for their well-being."[20] The decision-making system of any group may include laws, norms, and social intelligence systems, all of which favor groups with high power over those with low power. A key prerequisite for the gaining of power by oppressed groups is that members of these groups recognize their low-power position, and see themselves as possessing objectively-related interests ("consciousness-raising"). The elite group will increase communication among elite members and retain control over utilization of scientific knowledge.

Citizen participation in the decision-making process is most frequently seen on citizen boards. For the CMHCs, the citizen board was to be representative of the catchment area served by the center. The citizen board members were expected to be the "links" between the community and the center, expressing the needs of the community to the CMHC staff and sharing the center's ideas, constraints, and guidelines with community groups.

This citizen board is the ideal. While citizen participation is widespread in human service organizations, the ideal has not been met. Many centers do not have truly representative boards. It is often seen as too threatening to give power or decision-making authority to community residents who are different from the "average" board member. Often the board and/or the agency staff feel uncomfortable with or threatened by the idea that the poor, ethnic minorities, young, and elderly should have an equal say about allocation of resources and setting program priorities. In addition, turf struggles are quite common during the decision-making process. Citizens may feel that they should be able to make decisions about every center issue, including organizational structure, program, policy, and budget. Center professional staff often feel that citizens cannot make decisions about type of services and programs because they do not have the necessary professional education.

At the same time in which the CMHCs were being implemented, the "new careers" movement was emerging. In order to implement the "maximum feasible participation" called for in the Economic Opportunity Act of 1964, there was a need for the development of nonprofessionals to participate in the antipoverty programs. Within the mental health agencies, it was clear that there were not enough professionals to meet the expanding needs of the CMHCs. In addition, "paraprofessionals" or nonlicensed mental health workers, have been shown to be competent assistants. This is based on perceptions and values shared with the community, practical experience, and sensitivity to cultural issues. The client now had an advocate within the mental health system.

Related to the use of nonprofessionals, natural support systems emerged as another important focus. These support systems include neighbors, bartenders, family members, pharmacists, local healers, and other informed care-givers and self-help groups. Caplan[10] believed that there is a characteristic attribute of support systems that acts as a buffer against disease. That attribute is a relationship in which the person is dealt with as a unique individual and is cared about in a personalized way. The support consists of three elements. Significant others help the individual mobilize psychological resources and master emotional burdens; they share the individual's tasks; and they provide the individual with money, material, tools, skills, and cognitive guidance to improve handling of situations. Self-help groups have developed within the last two decades. Alcoholics Anonymous (AA) has been considered the primary model for other groups. Recovery, Inc., provides mutual support for former mental health care clients.

In a recent study of long-term severely disabled clients in the community, more than 50% were found to be living with relatives.[27] Advocacy organizations have emerged to offer support to families with a disturbed member, such as the National Alliance for the Mentally Ill (NAMI). This group, with a membership that increases every week, has become an important national force in sensitizing mental health professionals to issues and needs that have been ignored. At the present time, one of these issues is substance abuse among the chronically mentally ill. In addition, NIMH developed the Community Support System (CSS) program to meet the needs of discharged clients more adequately. CSS is defined as "a network of caring and responsible people committed to assisting a vulnerable population to meet their needs and develop their potential without being unnecessarily isolated or excluded from the community."[38] The major functions of the support system are: (1) to identify clients and reach out to offer appropriate services; (2) to assist clients in applying for income, medical, and other benefits; (3) to provide 24-hour crisis assistance in the least restrictive setting possible; (4) to provide psychosocial rehabilitation services; (5) to provide supportive services of indefinite duration; (6) to provide adequate medical and mental health care; (7) to provide back-up support to family, friends, and community members; (8) to involve concerned community members; (9) to protect client rights, both in the hospital and in the community; and (10) to provide case management services.[38] The system, established separately from the CMHCs, has been developing across the country. One of the issues to be addressed is the integration of the CMHC and the Community Support Systems.

Client Rights

Patient or client rights has been an important theme and has sensitized mental health professionals to possible abuses in their own system. Helping professions, by the very nature of their policies, often deprived clients of their rights as consumers. For example, by deciding who was entitled to help and under what conditions, by rationing services, and by not giving clients the opportunity to judge professional competence, clients were deprived of their rights. In addition to the concepts of consumer participation and empowerment discussed above, clients as consumers were given the rights by legislation in most states to: (1) consent to or refuse treatments under conditions in which they were fully informed of the treatments to be utilized, as well as the possible risks, benefits, and alternatives; (2) evaluate the services given to them; (3) be paid minimum wage for institutional labor; and (4) retain civil rights, such as the rights to communication, visitation, and medical self-determination.

New Federalism

By the late 1970s, the country had entered an "era of fiscal limitation." Two major goals of the "new federalism" were to reduce the role of the federal government in the lives of its citizens by giving control back to the states and to reduce the federal budget by cutting its share of spending for social and health care programs. These goals were part of the platform espoused by Ronald Reagan during his campaign for the Presidency of the United States. His resounding election victories in 1980 and 1984 were viewed as justification for seeking legislation to accomplish these goals.[17]

The Reagan administration immediately recommended a 25% reduction in spending. This was combined with changing the funding of mental health services from categorical funding to one single block grant. *Categorical funding* provided a specified amount of money for a particular category, such as programs for the elderly, whereas a *block grant* contained a specified amount of money for all alcohol- and drug-abuse and other mental health services. Each state was allowed to determine which programs would be supported with specified funds.

The Omnibus Budget Reconciliation Act of 1981 effectively repealed the 1980 Mental Health Systems Act, which would have continued direct funding for CMHCs, and provided for block-grant funding of mental health services.[17] This legislation shifted the primary responsibility for the mentally ill from the federal government back to state governments. With financial resources limited, the determination by each state of the percentage of its budget to be allocated to mental health services is a major political, as well as economic, issue.

The community mental health centers have been affected directly by cutbacks in funding. The federally-funded CMHCs were expected to receive increased local/community funding as the federal funds declined. However, given the era of fiscal limitation, this plan did not prove feasible for many of the CMHCs, particularly those that were nonhospital-based. When plans for increased ongoing funding (Mental Health Systems Act)

were stopped, "graduate" centers needed to find new sources of revenue. They also had to increase fee collection from clients and third-party payments from insurance providers. The concern is that centers will place priority on the services that can bring money, such as inpatient services, and priority on serving clients who can afford to pay fees.

The new federalism and the block grant program in the 1980s will have serious consequences for mental health practice in the next decades. One of the authors of this chapter was an appointed member of the California Block Grant Task Force (AB 2185); a description will be given of the process of decision-making in the task force.

The amount of change stemming from the federal Omnibus Budget Reconciliation Act and the timetable for this change were unprecedented in history. Many states assumed program responsibility in October 1981, without knowing how much money they would receive. It appeared that the federal government was planning to withdraw completely from funding and management of health, education, welfare, and other social and community services. Income maintenance programs such as Medicaid, Aid for Dependent Children, and Food Stamps were also under scrutiny.

The consolidation of categorical programs into a block grant has been discussed since the 1940s, as a way to streamline federal assistance programs. Between 1966 and 1974, five block grants were enacted: the Partnership for Health Act of 1966, the Omnibus Crime Control and Safe Streets Act of 1968, the Comprehensive Employment and Training Act of 1973, the Housing and Community Development Act of 1974, and the Title XX Amendments to the Social Security Act of 1975. The arguments used to support block grants are that more efficient and responsive delivery of services will occur at the state and local level, and that federal red tape and duplication of services will be reduced. The experience with the five early block grants mentioned, however, does not support these arguments.[1]

For the Preventive Health, Health Services, and Social Services Block Grants combined, there was an average reduction of 21% to 22% in actual federal dollars for all states in the country. (If inflation were taken into account, the reduction would be approximately 40%.) For California, there was a reduction of 21.1% from 1980 levels. Sugarman[37] attempted to provide a comprehensive description of legislation that would be repealed if the block grant proposals were adopted. Approximately fifteen sections of legislated acts (*e.g.,* Title II, CMHC Act) would be repealed or eliminated.

Another important concern is the removal of all targeting and need-related requirements in human service programs. This turns the allocation process into a political struggle in which the most vulnerable groups may lose the ground gained in the past 20 years. The block grant proposals eliminated dozens of specific federal requirements that helped to safeguard the rights of disadvantaged and minority citizens.[1]

In California, the Block Grant Task Force held public hearings in order to advise the legislature and the governor on how and under what conditions the state would assume the eight block grants enacted under the Federal Omnibus Reconciliation Act of 1981.[8] Determining the amount of federal funds actually available to California under each block grant for State FY 1982–83 was nearly impossible due to the fact that Congress, up until April 1, was budgeting for programs in four-month continuing resolutions. In general, the Task Force recommended: (1) a July 1, 1982 assumption date for all of the block grants, with the exception of Primary Care, Community Services, and Community Development Grants; (2) no additional funds for administrative costs for state and local agencies; (3) no transfer of funds during the transition year, except those already authorized; and (4) that all existing projects should receive some funding during the transition year, but not at their prior funding level.

There were specific issues defined for the Alcohol, Drug Abuse, and Mental Health Block Grant. In FY 1982, this block grant was to be used to fund existing community mental health centers and for drug- and alcohol-abuse services. In FY 1982, federal funds for mental health services in California were reduced by 26%; approximately $13.72 million in federal funds was available for California. There was no requirement to continue consultation and education grants in FY 1983. No inpatient services were to be funded with the federal block grant dollars.

The Task Force debated the issue of whether to integrate the community mental health centers into the county Short-Doyle program, as was recommended by the State Department of Mental Health, or whether a parallel system should be maintained. There was considerable concern expressed that CMHCs not be disadvantaged or discriminated against in competition with county programs. The Task Force recommended that "whatever distribution system is utilized," it should "guarantee the rights of community mental health centers to make program determinations as specified under federal law."[8] The Task Force also recommended that the consultation and education grants be maintained on a limited basis.

Competition

As an integral component of the new federalism, the Reagan administration advocated the utilization of competition as a cost-containment strategy in the health care industry. California took the lead in 1982, when it became the first state to enact legislation that allowed the public and private sectors to engage in competition. This was done by contracting for discounted rates with hospitals and health care providers. AB 799/3480 allowed the public sector to decrease its budget for Medi-Cal (California's Medicaid program). It created the California Medical Assistance Commission and authorized it to negotiate per diem contracts with hospitals for inpatient hospitalization of Medi-Cal clients.

AB 799/3480 was unique because it also provided for contracting by the private sector. After observing the con-

tractual agreements achieved by the state with reduced spending, the insurance industry decided to enter the arena of contracting to save money for its clients or purchasers of health insurance plans. Its competitive approach was to contract with hospitals or groups of providers for discounted rates through a structural arrangement known as *preferred provider arrangements (PPAs)*. Hospitals in California have contractual agreements with multiple insurance plans because the clients or enrollees in the insurance plans are expected to use the plan's participating hospitals. PPAs benefit clients because their "out-of-pocket" expenses are reduced when they elect to receive their health care from authorized hospitals and providers.

The concept of contracting with PPAs is rapidly developing in all parts of the country as a measure to contain health care costs. Insurance industry executives predict that, in the future, they will contract with 25% of the hospitals in most metropolitan areas, or 2,000 to 3,000 hospitals nationwide.[6]

Competition has also promoted the proliferation of *health maintenance organizations (HMOs)* as alternative health care delivery systems. HMOs are prepaid health plans that offer total health care to their enrollees for a fixed monthly premium that is paid by the client or the client's employer. Whereas clients with private health insurance can elect to see the provider of their choice and pay the difference if the provider is not in an authorized PPA, clients in HMOs are restricted to seeing providers employed by the HMO; to be seen by a nonHMO provider, they pay the full charges.

Nearly 10% of the total population, or 23.7 million persons, were enrolled in HMOs in 1986.[31] A recent study of 149 HMOs providing services to 813,712 Medicare enrollees revealed that extended mental health care was provided by 52 (34.9%) HMOs to 137,192 enrollees (16.9%).[31] It is projected that 50 million individuals will be enrolled in HMOs by 1995.[19] Whether these alternative delivery systems will provide accessible and appropriate mental health care services to their clients is unknown at this time due to the limited experience with HMOs.

Deinstitutionalization combined with competition resulted in changing the location and ownership of psychiatric inpatient beds. There were 524,900 beds in 1970, with 78% located in state and county mental hospitals. In 1982, there were 249,600 beds, with 56% located in public hospitals. During this same period, the number of beds in private psychiatric hospitals increased from 14,300 to 19,000.[34] The significance of the increase in beds owned by private psychiatric hospitals is that a majority of these beds are owned by multinational corporations. These private hospitals tend to offer only profitable mental health services, such as those for clients with eating disorders or alcohol or substance abuse.[14]

Federal Prospective Payment System

In addition to a reduction in funding of state mental health services via block grants, the federal government also reduced its funding of the Medicare hospitalization program through the Social Security Act amendments of 1983. This legislation provided a new reimbursement structure, called a *prospective payment system* (PPS). Under this system, payment for Medicare costs was changed from a retrospective cost reimbursement basis. Payments are now made at a predetermined specific rate for each client at discharge, by diagnosis. All discharges are classified according to a list of *diagnosis-related groups (DRGs)*. The list currently contains 470 specific categories of diagnostic groupings, of which there are 15 psychiatric and substance-abuse DRGs.[32]

DRGs were developed as a way to determine the cost of care by diagnosis. The provision of care was conceptualized as the consumption of resources by the client. Using a large data base to analyze the cost of all resources commonly used by clients with a specific diagnosis has resulted in payment being fixed at a set fee per diagnosis.[35,39]

Very limited data were available on hospital use by diagnosis in psychiatric hospitals. Therefore, these hospitals were allowed to request an exemption from PPS for a two-year period and to continue to be paid on a limited-cost basis. A recent study by the National Association of Private Psychiatric Hospitals concluded that the 15 psychiatric and substance-abuse DRGs have only a 4% ability to predict the cost of providing care for the average psychiatric client, whereas the entire DRG system for general hospitals has a 30% ability to predict resource consumption and the average cost of care.[16] Psychiatric hospitals are hoping to receive continued exemptions from Congress in order to develop a PPS that is workable for psychiatry.

The changes in health care financing previously described are attempts to curb the inflationary spiral in health costs of the last decade. The rapidity of the changes has resulted in a health care revolution. The relationships among clients, providers, and health delivery systems can be described as chaotic. Clients say they want high-quality care at a lower price; providers say they can't provide high-quality care at a lower price, and health care systems are telling their employees to "do more with less" in order to survive with less revenue.

As with any revolution, some groups can gain in power. Psychiatric/mental health nurses have an opportunity to expand their practice settings and become revenue-generators in the hospital industry. Psychiatric/mental health nurses need to become providers in HMOs and PPAs, or psychiatric/mental health nursing will be taken over by other disciplines in ambulatory settings. With the advent of DRGs in the hospital industry, psychiatric/mental health nurses need to do studies to determine the cost of providing psychiatric nursing care. This will help ensure that the cost is firmly built into the system of payment that is finally decided on for the psychiatric industry. When the cost of psychiatric nursing care is known, then psychiatric nursing will be in a position to demonstrate that it is revenue-producing rather than expense-draining.

As with any revolution, some groups can lose in power. One such group is the homeless mentally ill. With decreased welfare support, decreased emphasis on civil rights, and a reduction in mental health service, this group of clients is literally living on the streets and hoping to survive each day. The abdication of responsibility, by all sectors of society, for its dysfunctional, disturbed citizens is unacceptable. Krauthammer[26] aptly described the plight of these clients in relationship to retention of their civil rights when he stated, "In the name of a liberty that illness does not allow them to enjoy, we have condemned the homeless mentally ill to die with their rights on." The issue of the homeless mentally ill needs to be resolved with additional financing and adequate planning by both the public and the private sectors of society.

Table 35-4 summarizes the political, economic, and

TABLE 35-4.
MENTAL HEALTH CARE CHANGES IN THE LATE 20TH CENTURY

POLITICAL
- Clients' rights emerged as a central issue.
- Laws passed safeguarding clients' rights to treatment, least restrictive environments, and privacy
- Commitment laws better defined

ECONOMIC
- Era of fiscal limitations; welfare state seen as too great a burden
- "New federalism" shifted responsibility back from federal to state and local governments
- Reductions in funding for mental health care

SOCIAL
- "Power" movements emerged as important forces for ethnic minorities, women, and the elderly.
- Advocacy, empowerment, and citizen participation issues emerged
- Support systems emerged as important buffers to prevent rehospitalization.

CLIENT POPULATION
- Specific client populations were targeted, including women, ethnic minorities, and the elderly.
- Focus on victims of crime

SETTING
- Expansion of community-based programs, including community support systems and employment setting
- Shift from public hospitals to proprietary and psychiatric units of general hospitals

TYPES OF SERVICES
- Expansion to include self-help groups, preventive/educational groups, and community networking
- Deinstitutionalization continued.

NURSES' ROLE
- Expanded to include community organization, consultation, liaison, and family and group psychotherapy
- Nurses established as therapists in private practice.

social forces of the late 20th century that were responsible for changes in the mental health system.

The Future

Given the interactive nature of political, economic, and social factors and the prevailing attitudes of limitation and reduction, we cannot predict the exact future of psychiatric/mental health nursing practice, or the mental health system. In a recent study, Brown and Fraser[9] asked key informants to envision the needs, issues, and trends affecting the mental health delivery system in the year 2000, and to describe trends and innovations in service delivery for meeting these needs. The most significant issues discussed by respondents were the future financing of mental health services, increasing aging populations, increasing ethnically and culturally diverse populations, and the need for an integrated system. With regard to future financing, respondents envisioned a continued increase in for-profit providers, with an associated impact on the types of services provided. Another issue was the public policy question of who will pay for the treatment of the chronically mentally ill and the indigent. Related to the issue of financing and a possible widening gap in our existing two-tiered system of care (*i.e.,* one for the poor and another for the affluent), respondents discussed the need for a future system that integrated all providers. Respondents envisioned some innovative mix of for-profit, not-for-profit, private, and public providers.

The report of another future study, the Future Mental Health Services Project,[33] coordinated by the National Mental Health Association and the Institute for Alternative Futures, lists four goals with implementing strategies that are intended to guide the development of mental health services over the next several decades. The goals include: (1) make mental health a national priority; (2) provide services for all who need them; (3) eliminate the causes of mental illnesses; and (4) eradicate prejudice and discrimination.

The status of deinstitutionalization as continuing public policy for the mental health system is undergoing needed scrutiny. Social and political pressures are being exerted on politicians to do something about the mentally ill homeless and the absence of available community mental health services. How they respond will be greatly influenced by the advocacy efforts of the mental health constituency. Elpers[15] has identified reinstitutionalization or a return to hospitalization as one possible response. How reinstitutionalization would be made operational is unknown, given the current high costs of health care. On one hand, it could provide opportunities for the development of a new type of community-based facility. This facility would be rehabilitative in nature and integrated into the larger continuum of mental health services. On the other hand, it could lead to the development of inadequate, independent, and mostly-locked facilities that would make the 1950s wards look good by comparison.[15]

Future nursing practice will depend, in part, upon psychiatric/mental health nurses' assuming active roles in influencing legislation and funding policies, and raising social consciousness about society's continuing responsibility to care for its mentally ill. The potential danger is that mental health practice could revert to custodial care or "non-care." This is conceivable because the supportive mental health structure may be reduced to a minimum. During adverse times, the opportunity exists to design and implement new, innovative mental health settings and services.

Summary

1. Legislation throughout the 19th and 20th centuries reflects a growing concern for protecting mental health clients. Economic and societal factors altered the delivery of mental health care in the United States as a result of increased awareness of, and concern for, psychiatric clients.

2. The client population in the mental health care system continually has expanded due to the increasing mental health needs of citizens. Settings and types of services provided also expanded with deinstitutionalization and considerable emphasis on community-based mental health practice.

3. The nurse's role was first defined by the active role of Dorothea Dix during the Civil War. Custodial care was later replaced by expanded nursing roles that include clinical nurse specialists, certified psychiatric/mental health nurses, and private practice.

4. Participatory democracy lays the foundation for consumerism. Citizen participation includes involvement in decision-making on CMHC boards, as well as nonprofessional support systems such as community support systems.

5. New federalism and block grant programs are the federal government's attempt to delegate responsibility to state governments for designing, implementing, and funding mental health care programs. Mental health care is now under the auspices of each individual state and, therefore, varies considerably.

6. Spiraling health care costs mandated implementation of a program that would curb spending on health care. Preferred Provider Arrangements (PPAs) and Health Maintenance Organizations (HMOs) were implemented as viable cost-containment alternatives.

7. The Medicare hospitalization program is largely funded by the federal government. In order to cut health care costs, a prospective payment plan superseded retrospective cost reimbursement.

8. Mental health care needs to be a national priority, providing services to all who need them. Prevention

of mental illness, funding for adequate services, and future planning for provision of services are vital to meeting the mental health care needs of society.

References

1. Ad Hoc Coalition on Block Grants: Block Grant Briefing Book. Washington, DC, Ad Hoc Coalition on Block Grants, 1981

2. American Nurses' Association: The Career Credential—Professional Certification. Kansas City, Missouri, American Nurses' Association, 1987

3. American Nurses' Association, Division on Psychiatric and Mental Health Nursing Practice: Standards of Psychiatric and Mental Health Nursing Practice. Kansas City, Missouri, American Nurses' Association, 1982

4. American Nurses' Association, Council on Psychiatric and Mental Health Nursing: Guidelines for Private Practice of Psychiatric and Mental Health Nursing. Kansas City, Missouri, American Nurses' Association, 1987

5. American Psychiatric Association: Task Report 14: Electroconvulsive Therapy. Washington, DC, American Psychiatric Association Press, 1978

6. Anderson G, Studnicki J: Insurers competing with providers. Hospitals 54:64, 1985

7. Aviram U: Mental health reform and the aftercare state service. Unpublished doctoral dissertation. Berkeley, California, University of California, 1972

8. Block Grant Advisory Task Force: Report to the Governor and the Legislature of the State of California. Sacramento, California, April 12, 1982

9. Brown VB, Fraser M: Planning and shaping of the mental health delivery system of the future. Consultations: An Int J, in press.

10. Caplan G: Support Systems and Community Mental Health. New York, Behavioral Publications, 1974

11. Caplan RB: Psychiatry and the Community in Nineteenth Century America. New York, Basic Books, 1969

12. Church OM: From custody to community in psychiatric nursing. Nurs Res 1:48, 1987

13. Connery R: The Politics of Mental Health. New York and London, Columbia University Press, 1968

14. Demand is huge for inpatient eating disorders programs. Hospitals 59:92, 1985

15. Elpers JR: Are we legislating reinstitutionalization? Am J Orthopsychiatry 3:441, 1987

16. Fackelmann KA: Group contends study proves DRGs won't work in psychiatric hospitals. Mod Healthcare 15:38, 1985

17. Foley AF, Sharfstein SS: Madness and Government. Washington, DC, American Psychiatric Association Press, 1983

18. Freeman W: Psychosurgery. In Arieti S (ed): American Handbook of Psychiatry, vol 2. New York, Basic Books, 1959

19. Graham J: Corporatively managed healthcare will dominate 1990s, experts say. Mod Healthcare 15:34, 1985

20. Hollingshead AB, Redlich FC: Social Class and Mental Illness: A Community Study. New York, Spectrum, 1974

21. Horwitz WA: Insulin Shock Therapy. In Arieti S (ed): American Handbook of Psychiatry, vol 2. New York, Basic Books, 1959

22. Johnson DE: The Behavioral System Model of Nursing. In Riehl J, Roy C (eds): Conceptual Models for Nursing Practice, 2nd ed. New York, Appleton-Century-Crofts, 1980

23. Jones E: Sigmund Freud: Four centenary addresses. New York, Basic Books, 1954

24. Karno M, Schwartz DA: Community Mental Health: Reflections and Explorations. New York, Spectrum Publications, 1974

25. Kramer M: Analytic and special study reports. U.S. Government Printing Office Series B, No 12. Washington, DC, National Institute of Mental Health, 1977

26. Krauthammer C: When liberty really means neglect. Time 126: 38, 1985

27. Lamb HR, Goertzel V: Discharged mental patients—are they really in the community? Arch Gen Psychiatry 24:29, 1971

28. Leighton AH: My Name Is Legion: The Stirling County Study of Psychiatric Disorder and Sociocultural Environment, vol 1. New York, Basic Books, 1959

29. Lerman P: Deinstitutionalization: A Cross-Problem Analysis. U.S. Government Printing Office, DHHS No. (ADM) 81-987. Washington, DC, Department of Health and Human Services, 1981

30. Lewis A, Levy JS: Psychiatric liaison nursing. Reston, Virginia, Reston Publishing, 1982

31. McMillan A, Lubitz J, Russell D: Medicare enrollment in health maintenance organizations. Health Care Financing Rev 3:87, 1987

32. Medicare program: Changes to the inpatient hospital prospective payment system and fiscal year 1986 rates. Federal Register 60:35646, 1985

33. National Mental Health Association: Blueprint for the Future of Mental Health Services—Report of the Future Mental Health Services Project. Alexandria, Virginia, National Mental Health Association, 1986

34. NIMH Division of Biometry and Epidemiology: Hospital Statistics. Chicago, American Hospital Association, 1983

35. Pointer D, Ross M: DRG cost-per-case management. Mod Healthcare 14:109, 1984

36. Srole L, Langner TS, Michael ST et al: Mental Health in the Metropolis—The Midtown Manhattan Study. New York, McGraw-Hill, 1962

37. Sugarman J: State Reaction to Changes in Human Services Programs. Paper presented at the National Issues Seminar on Block Grants, October, 1981

38. Turner JEC, Shifren I: Community Support Systems: How Comprehensive? In Stein LI (ed): Community Support Systems for the Long-Term Patient. New Directions for Mental Health Services, no 2. San Francisco, Jossey-Bass, 1979

39. Young DA: Prospective payment assessment commission: Mandate, structure, and relationship. Nurs Econ 2:309, 1984

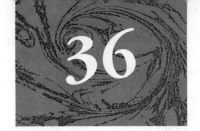

36

JACQUELYN H. FLASKERUD

EVALUATION OF THE IMPACT OF PSYCHIATRIC/ MENTAL HEALTH NURSING THROUGH RESEARCH

Learning Objectives

Upon completion of this chapter the student should be able to do the following:

1. Describe the development of psychiatric/mental health nursing research.
2. Identify the parameters of psychiatric nursing practice.
3. Describe three contributions nursing has made to the study of psychiatric patient problems.
4. List at least one study that has made a contribution to the psychiatric/mental health nursing field in each of these practice arenas: inpatient and outpatient treatment of the psychiatric patient.
5. List the criteria for evaluating the applicability of research findings to practice.
6. List three barriers to research in psychiatric/mental health nursing.
7. Identify two current trends in psychiatric nursing research.
8. Identify three types of studies needed to advance psychiatric/mental health nursing practice.

Introduction

Nursing is usually described as a process. It begins with an assessment of client problems that are specified in nursing diagnoses. Goals are then prioritized and specific interventions and outcome criteria are identified. An evaluation of the interventions determines whether the problem has been solved or modified. The purpose of this chapter is to evaluate the impact of psychiatric nursing on the mental health problems of clients through the research process.

This chapter provides a review of research that examines the impact of psychiatric nursing interventions on client outcomes. When research is not available, impressionistic reports of the impact of nursing on psychiatric/mental health problems are included. The quantity of research in this area is limited. Studies on the relationship between the process of psychiatric nursing care and client outcomes is of recent origin. Prior to the mid-1970s, most of the research in nursing focused on nurses rather than on nursing practice. Furthermore, many of the investigations in client care done since that time have not been replicated or sufficiently substantiated. For these reasons, many of the findings in early studies cannot yet be fully accepted as accurate data on nursing practice.

Historical Developments in Psychiatric/Mental Health Nursing Research

The development of research in psychiatric/mental health nursing has paralleled the development of nursing research in general (see Table 36-1). In the first half of the 20th century, nursing research focused on educational and occupational problems.[29] Early studies concentrated on the quality of educational programs and later on the functions and roles of nurses as characterized by different educational levels. Studies of occupational and administrative problems in nursing focused on surveys of nurse manpower, methods of increasing the numbers of nurses, and better utilization of nursing personnel.[26,29] Nursing research was influenced by its relationships with education and the social sciences. Much of the research was conducted in collaboration with these disciplines.

In psychiatric nursing, studies focused on the basic preparation of students, on upgrading client care by increasing psychiatric nursing personnel, and on integrating concepts from the social and behavioral sciences into psychiatric nursing. Studies derived from the social sciences concentrated on the function of psychiatric nurses and the role of the nurse with the mental health client.[26]

From 1955 to 1975, many individuals and groups continued their involvement in studies of students in all types of educational programs in nursing. Studies also focused on curriculum development and evaluation. Stud-

TABLE 36-1.
DEVELOPMENT OF PSYCHIATRIC/MENTAL HEALTH NURSING RESEARCH

1900–1950	Educational problems
	Occupational problems
1950–1970	Identifying nursing's role and function
	Evaluating nursing's role and function
1970–1985	Nursing's role
	Nursing education
	Clinical practice/patient care problems

ies of the nurse outnumbered practice studies by ten to one, and more than half of the doctoral theses were carried out in the field of education.[26] However, a growing concern began among nurses that nursing research should become practice-related. Nursing leaders noted that the functions of nursing research are to provide a sound basis for practice and to determine what action has significant consequences for client well-being. They endorsed as a priority research that focused on the effects of nursing acts on client outcomes. The term "patient care research" became synonymous with an emphasis on clinically relevant studies.[26]

Since the 1970s, there has been a progressive increase in the investigation of clinical problems. However, the number of studies related to the nurse's role and nursing education still remains large. Practice-related studies began as descriptions of nursing care plans and case studies. In the last ten years, client care studies have been conducted using descriptive, analytical, and experimental methods, and have gained increasing sophistication.

Several summaries of psychiatric nursing research have been published in the last ten years.* Some of these have concentrated on specific aspects of psychiatric nursing research such as compliance,[15] the community,[48,55] or barriers to research,[44] while others have given a more general overview.[10,54] Sills[54] examined research in the field of psychiatric nursing, looking at the changes that have occurred over three decades.

Each decade emphasized a different area for investigation and research. In the 1950s, psychiatric nursing was concerned with the move from custodial care to therapeutic care. Research focused on assumptions within the person. Personality was viewed as the explanatory variable, and it was hypothesized that therapeutic nursing care would decrease anxiety, increase ego strength, improve communication skills, improve attitudes toward mental illness, and so forth.

In the 1960s, psychiatric nursing emphasized the role and function of the nurse. Research focused on assumptions within the relationship. Role was considered the explanatory variable. The nurse–client relationship, client–family relationships, and perceptions of, attitudes toward, and opinions about the nurse's role were studied.

In the 1970s, research focused on assumptions within the social system. The social system (families, cultures, organizations, groups) was viewed as the explanatory variable. Research examined the effects of nursing on changes in system states.

The changes in psychiatric nursing research identified by Sills[54] are similar to the changes in nursing research in general. Changes have also reflected the research emphasis in the other mental health and social service disciplines. These research emphases have, over the last decades, taken on more of a social and psychological focus. Psychiatric nursing research has shared that focus, and researchers have shied away from studying the effects of psychiatric nursing interventions on the mental

* References 10, 15, 44, 48, 54, and 55.

health of clients.[51] In a review of psychiatric consultation-liaison nursing, Robinson noted that the literature has dealt with the role and function of the psychiatric liaison nurse, but not with the effectiveness of the nurse's practice. Recommendations for future studies focus on the effectiveness of practice as measured by client outcomes.

Davis[10] in 1981 reviewed trends in psychiatric nursing research and categorized them according to topic, methods used, and relationships among practitioners, policy-makers, and researchers. Psychiatric nursing research was focused on two topics: definition of the nurse's role, and evaluation of the nurse's role. The first topic can be subdivided into: (1) identifying or specifying the role, and (2) acquiring the role. Major roles identified were those that nurses could play in communication and relationships, and as therapists, behavior modifiers, behavior assessors, and community workers. In the second category, evaluation of the nurse's role, the same subcategories of role appear, with the addition of the nurse as manager and change agent. Research focused on the willingness of nurses to assume an extended role, the training of psychiatric paraprofessionals, staff functioning, and relaxation training. Research that evaluated nurses' roles in terms of their impact on mental health problems was included in this category, but there was not enough of this kind of research to justify categorizing it as a major trend.

The second trend reviewed by Davis[10] was in the methods that nurses used in research. Most research in psychiatric nursing was descriptive. Many of these studies related to the roles specified for nurses, and demonstrated attempts to have these roles implemented in practice. Methods appeared to be changing slowly, from descriptive approaches to comparative, experimental, and action approaches. The latter two categories require the identification of criteria, indicators, and outcomes against which judgments can be made on practicability and effectiveness of treatment. Very few studies have achieved this or even attempted it.

The third trend, relationships among practitioners, policy-makers, and researchers, is in a developmental stage. Sills[54] has stated that research questions ought to arise from the practice arena. However, often the answers sought by practitioners are not the ones found by researchers. This indicates that the wrong answer was expected, or that the question was not carefully asked. Research is essential to nursing practice, and provides the body of knowledge from which policy is drawn, and upon which practice is based. In psychiatric/mental health nursing, there is only the very beginning of a trend of relating research to practice and policy-making.

The Parameters of Psychiatric/ Mental Health Nursing

In order to evaluate the impact of psychiatric nursing interventions on the mental health problems of clients, it is necessary first to examine the dimensions of psychiatric nursing practice. This is done here by focusing on a major aspect of practice: psychiatric nursing interventions in the various settings in which they occur. (see Table 36-2). Admittedly, the parameters of psychiatric/mental health nursing practice encompass more than just psychiatric nursing interventions. Assessment, monitoring, planning, and coordinating are other aspects of practice that readily come to mind. However, to evaluate the impact of nursing on the psychiatric/mental health problems of clients, it is most productive to focus on interventions. The dimensions of psychiatric/mental health nursing practice interventions can be approached theoretically, historically, and practically.

Nurse theorists have conceptualized nursing interventions broadly as management of the interaction between the client and the environment to promote health.[18] From a *theoretical* perspective, the distinctiveness of psychiatric nursing derives from its congruence with the general framework for nursing provided in the nursing practice models. The characteristics of psychiatric nursing include a total-person orientation, an expertise in the physical and social environment and management of that environment, an acknowledgement of the importance of the social system, and a systems approach to care.[17]

Psychiatric nursing intervention has been described more specifically as: constructive management of the physical and social environment in the client setting, primary therapy in a one-to-one relationship, and primary therapy in a group interaction.[2,16] Fagin[16] described seven distinguishing characteristics of psychiatric nursing interventions, including: (1) varying amounts of time spent with clients, (2) varying spatial areas in which intervention occurs, (3) the variety of clients related to simultaneously, (4) the focus on physical as well as emotional aspects of care, (5) rapid adjustments from one-to-one interventions to group interventions and vice versa, (6) the varying and shifting composition of groups interacted with, and (7) the on-the-spot decision-making that occurs. These characteristics suggest a versatility in psychi-

TABLE 36-2.
PARAMETERS OF PSYCHIATRIC/MENTAL HEALTH NURSING

1. *Theoretical perspective*
   Total person orientation
   Expertise in managing the social and physical environment
   Social systems approach
2. *Historical perspective*
   Milieu management
   Total client care in home and community
3. *Practice perspective*
   Monitoring behavior and pharmacotherapy
   Coordinating services to clients
   Primary therapy
   Secondary therapy

atric nursing interventions that encompasses a variety of settings (hospital, home, community), a total client approach, and an expertise in use of the social and the physical environment.[2,16]

Historically, psychiatric nursing interventions have consisted of providing a therapeutic milieu, or managing the social and physical environments, and secondary therapy, or working with clients' here-and-now problems and providing social and recreational activities.[21] Psychiatric nursing interventions added through the years included primary therapy for individuals, groups, and families as a direct nursing intervention, and education and consultation as indirect interventions. These additions moved psychiatric nursing interventions into homes and community settings, as well as hospital settings.

From a *practical* point of view, psychiatric nursing interventions can be identified from what mental health nurses do in practice. Psychiatric nursing practice involves monitoring behavior and pharmacotherapy, coordinating total services provided for clients, and supervising staff, as well as direct nursing interventions. Aspects of psychiatric nursing practice that can be identified as nursing interventions include: milieu management in the hospital, primary and secondary therapy in the community and the hospital, and precare and aftercare in the community and the home.[7,57]

There is a remarkable amount of agreement among the theoretical, historical, and practical approaches to delineating the dimensions of psychiatric nursing practice. All three perspectives demonstrate that psychiatric nursing interventions take place in the hospital and in the community, both in agencies and in homes. In the hospital, psychiatric nursing interventions include both direct and indirect care in the forms of milieu management, primary therapy, secondary therapy, and consultation-liaison. In community agencies, psychiatric nursing interventions include both direct and indirect care in the forms of primary and secondary therapy and consultation-liaison. In the home, precare and aftercare are included. These involve client and family education in social milieu management.

Psychiatric/Mental Health Nursing Interventions in the Hospital

The impact of nursing on mental health problems can be determined by reviewing the research done on each of the psychiatric nursing interventions identified. In the hospital setting, these are milieu management, primary therapy, secondary therapy, and consultation-liaison.

Milieu Management

Milieu therapy has been defined as a careful structuring of the social and physical environments of a psychiatric treatment program.[13] The creation and management of a therapeutic milieu is the responsibility of nurses.[5,13] Milieu therapy includes behavior modification techniques

to effect behavior change and to deal with here-and-now problems. It also includes secondary therapy consisting of recreational, educational, and work activities. Nursing staff are considered the most crucial personnel involved in any behavior treatment program.[27] Milieu therapy, which encompasses behavior modification, has been shown to lead to a decrease in symptoms and abnormal personality characteristics, an increase in social skills, and earlier discharge.[13]

Most studies of the effects of milieu therapy on client outcomes have involved long-term psychiatric patients, such as schizophrenics, who were exposed to behavior modification through token economy programs.[19,28,37] In these studies, nurses were the chief agents of therapy. When experimental groups of clients who were exposed to a behavior modification token economy program were compared with control groups receiving custodial care, the experimental groups were shown to have experienced significantly less social withdrawal behavior, less socially embarrassing behavior, and improved physical appearance. Clients who improved most were those who were initially most deteriorated.[19,28] These studies demonstrated that treatment carried out by nurses within the social milieu resulted in positive client outcomes.[37] When milieu therapy was combined with pharmacotherapy in a controlled clinical situation, the experimental group experienced improved socialization and increased conversation. The pharmacotherapy resulted in a decrease in head-banging, unprovoked attacks on others, and dribbling saliva.[63]

Looking at milieu therapy from another perspective, a transcultural study of schizophrenics examined the effects of the physical and social milieu (considered to be part of conventional nursing care) on rehospitalization. The study found that the effects varied with social class and urban–rural differences. A physical and social milieu that was congruent with the client's own social and cultural patterns was determined to be a positive aspect of total treatment. An important outcome noted that any particular form of physical and social milieu is not helpful to all clients; to enforce a particular kind of milieu indiscriminately was considered a disservice.[38]

To illustrate this finding further, another study described the changes that were needed when manic clients were treated with milieu therapy. In this study, nurses implemented a modified program that involved strict limit-setting on physical and social activities and an authoritarian administrative position. Clients in the program, when compared with clients not in such a program, showed a significant decrease in motor activities and social acting out, and an increase in sleeping and eating.[5]

These studies illustrate that milieu therapy is an effective nursing intervention. Nurses are successfully implementing milieu management. It is an intervention that has an impact on the mental health problems of clients. As a psychiatric nursing intervention, milieu management is effective in changing client behavior when the diagnosis, social class, and culture of the client are taken into consideration and when milieu therapy is combined with pharmacotherapy. It is not a single-theory intervention. It encompasses theories from the biological, social, and health sciences. It is being implemented carefully, based on a number of client variables. As such, it demonstrates nursing's attention to both the client and the environment, and to the interaction between them.

Primary Therapy

Primary therapy is the client's foremost treatment and, in some instances, is considered total case management. Primary therapy can be individual, group, or family treatment. In the hospital setting, primary therapy can include taking a history, administering a mental status exam, recommending diagnostic tests, making a diagnosis, identifying presenting problems, interviewing the family, providing individual, group, or family interventions, recommending pharmacotherapy, planning discharge referrals, charting data, and writing summaries. The impact of any one or a combination of these components on the mental health problems of the client can be studied.

In most cases, the impact of interventions (individual, group, or family therapy) on client outcomes is not studied directly. Instead, an emphasis is placed on roles and functions of various professionals. Vander Zyl and colleagues[61] compared client and therapist expectations of therapy. In this study, clients expected directive therapy involving advice and approval. Nurse therapists were more reflective, and expected self-direction from the clients. The authors suggested that incongruent expectations of therapy can affect outcomes, and identified two options for dealing with incongruent expectations. One alternative was that the nurse therapist modify treatment to approximate patient expectations. This option was rejected by the investigators because they believed it encouraged patient dependence. The second option was to spend therapy time educating clients to the benefits of self-directed therapy. This option was supported.[61]

The question of whether nurses have a unique orientation to primary therapy can legitimately be asked. Although the study described above found that nurse therapists expect therapy to be self-directive, other studies have shown an opposite orientation. Studies have also shown a range of distinguishing characteristics of primary therapy by nurses in hospital settings. Probably the most common characteristic of therapy conducted by nurses is an emphasis on here-and-now problems and current life situations.[1,23] Using a total-person approach that attends to physical and emotional problems is another distinguishing characteristic.[23,58] When primary therapy is done in combination with traditional psychiatric nursing practice, such as observing, reporting, and carrying out secondary therapy, a characteristic emerges that clients identify as important to their care. This is the immediacy and constancy of nursing care, in contrast to psychiatric care or social work care.[58] In addition, nurses have identified their therapy as coming from an interactional and communications framework,[1] and as being directive and supportive in nature.[41]

Nurses are as individual in their approaches to primary therapy as are professionals in other disciplines.

Overriding individual differences, however, are the nursing emphases on the total person in the context of the person's social and physical milieu and the on here-and-now problems.[17] These approaches to primary therapy have produced positive client outcomes.

In a study of individual primary therapy in a psychiatric unit of a general hospital, the roles of nurse therapists were compared to those of a control group of non-nurse therapists in relation to several outcome measures. Nursing intervention consisted of primary therapy plus traditional psychiatric nursing practices such as observing, recording, monitoring pharmacotherapy, and coordinating services. Therapy included total case management, with a medical consultant to countersign requests for diagnostic tests and medications. Client outcomes were compared with those of the control group. In a follow-up of clients' rates of improvement one year post-discharge, no difference based on the discipline of the therapists was found. Other differences *were* found. The mean length of hospital stay for clients with nurse therapists was less than for clients with non-nurse therapists. With nurse therapists, hospital training costs decreased. Clients described therapy by nurses as excellent. They found nurse therapists less threatening than non-nurse therapists, and commented favorably on the immediacy and constancy of nursing care as opposed to the brief and intermittent care given by physicians and social workers.[58]

A similar study compared diploma and baccalaureate-degree nurse therapists with psychiatric resident therapists. Several measures were used to rate clients at admission, at discharge, and at one year post-admission. Ratings for these measures were given by the psychiatric staff, the nursing staff, the client, and the family. The study found no differences in client outcomes between the two groups on symptom and behavior ratings or on satisfaction with care ratings.[41]

Establishing that there is no difference in client outcomes of primary therapy done by nurse therapists and that done by non-nurse therapists is important, because it will encourage acceptance of primary therapy as a nursing intervention by other psychiatric disciplines. More important to nursing, however, is demonstrating that primary therapy by nurses produces a more positive outcome, *i.e.,* behavior change and symptom reduction, for clients who experience it than for control groups of those who do not. There are few studies of this kind.

Gelperin[23] used two psychological tests that are sensitive to behavior and emotional changes to measure the differences between control groups and experimental groups of elderly patients with organic brain syndrome. Members of the experimental groups were exposed to three contact hours per week of individual primary therapy by a nurse therapist over a two-month period. Control groups were exposed to the normal hospital routine that did not include primary therapy. Therapy consisted of a supportive, reflective approach to client problems that focused on current life situations and included attention to physical problems. In addition, experimental group clients were required to take part in recreational activities. At the end of two months, the experimental groups showed improvement significantly greater than that of the control groups in both emotional and behavioral changes. Their symptoms subsided, and their behavior became more socially acceptable.

In a similar study, Beard and Scott[1] examined the effects of group therapy on chronically regressed clients. One hundred clients were randomly assigned to five control groups and five experimental groups. Group therapy consisted of two one-hour sessions per week for three months. The nurse therapists used an interpersonal and communications framework, and focused on here-and-now problems such as family, staff, and other patients. Control groups received no group therapy but were exposed only to regular hospital routines. The Nurses' Observation Scale for Inpatient Evaluation was used to measure changes in social competence, social interest, personal neatness, irritability, manifest psychosis, and retardation (regression). The only improvement in behavior was a significant decrease in irritability for the experimental group. However, the control groups experienced a deterioration in behavior, indicated by significantly higher manifest psychosis and retardation scores and significantly lower social competence and social interest scores.

These studies demonstrate that primary therapy is a legitimate nursing intervention, and that it has a positive effect on client outcomes. Primary therapy is an advanced psychiatric nursing intervention and is not a skill possessed by entry-level nurses. However, the therapeutic nurse–client relationship in many ways mirrors primary therapy. It is a skill that entry-level nurses can practice. It is effective in changing patient behaviors and reducing symptoms. All nurses can incorporate the therapeutic nurse–client relationship into their patient care. The character of that relationship can take direction from the primary therapy practiced by nurses.

From studies reviewed, the distinguishing characteristics of primary therapy as a nursing intervention begin to emerge. Nurses are effective primary therapists when compared with non-nurses; their interventions can result in positive behavioral changes in clients; and their therapy is characterized by a total client approach, an emphasis on here-and-now problems, and attention to the social and the physical milieu.

Secondary Therapy

Secondary therapy is an adjunct to, or one component of, primary therapy. It consists of psychiatric nursing activities such as monitoring and evaluating behavior and pharmacotherapy, reporting, involving the client in social and recreational activities, coordinating services, tests, and treatments, and relating to family and friends of clients. Secondary therapy involves the majority of activities that psychiatric nurses practice at the entry level or without a master's degree. It is also the least investigated of the psychiatric nursing interventions.

Routines that fall into the category of secondary therapy, or are part of conventional psychiatric nursing care, were examined in one study to determine their effects on rehospitalization.[38] Routines that affect personal hygiene, clothing, sleep, food, privacy, social and recreational ac-

tivities, and religious activities were found to vary in their relationship to rehospitalization according to subculture and class. When nurse-directed hospital routines were congruent with cultural and social norms, they were related to a decrease in rehospitalization. The greater the incongruence of client cultural patterns and routines with hospital patterns and routines, the greater the chance of rehospitalization.

More studies can be found on secondary therapy as a psychiatric nursing intervention when it is defined as one component of total treatment. Primary therapists rely on ongoing monitoring, evaluation, and reporting of client behavior outside the therapy situation. Nurses are considered reliable observers and evaluators of behavior as well as valuable sources of information about clients' behavior.[14,49] As observers and evaluators of behavior, first-level nurses are relied upon to determine which clients are ready for therapy or rehabilitation, to determine the effects of pharmacotherapy on clients, and to predict behavior changes.

Psychiatric nurses can usually accurately assess social and illness-related behaviors of long-stay psychiatric patients and can predict which patients will be amenable to rehabilitation.[49] Nurses' ratings of psychotic behavior correspond with psychiatrists' ratings on anxiety, tension, depression, hostility, preoccupation with hypochondriasis, grandiosity, self-depreciation, hallucinations, thought disorders, mannerisms, retardation, emotional withdrawal, hypomania, and uncooperative behavior.[14] Nurses' ratings of client behaviors have also been used to gather data in research. Studies of various therapeutic protocols have used nurses to observe and record client behaviors.[20,31,56]

In a study of side-effects of antidepressant drugs, it was found that the client was the best source of evaluating mood, the psychiatrist was the best source of evaluating physical symptoms, and the nurse was the best source of observing and evaluating behavior. The study recommended that nurses' observations and evaluations of behavior should play a major part in determining drug therapy.[50]

Secondary therapy is a valued part of patient treatment. Nurses at beginning levels can and do implement it successfully. Nurses should continue their practice of monitoring and evaluating behavior and pharmacotherapy and documenting the conditions and situations that affect behavior. In addition, nurses should begin working on operationalizing the rest of their secondary therapy functions, such as involving clients in social and recreational activities, coordinating services, and developing relationships with clients' families and friends. Once these are carefully defined, nurses can begin documenting the effects of these activities on client behavior and begin to identify the variables that might intervene in behavior outcomes, such as culture, socioeconomic status, age, sex, and so forth.

Psychiatric Consultation-Liaison Nursing

At least three models of nursing consultation in the general hospital have been identified.[3] Nursing consultation in the general hospital is considered a liaison service, involving liaison between psychiatric nursing and the other nursing specialties, between nurses and physicians, between nurses and clients, and between nurses and administrators. Psychiatric consultation-liaison nursing is generally considered an advanced psychiatric nursing skill. The three models of its use in the general hospital are shown in Table 36-3.

Studies of consultation using the indirect service model revealed an initial resistance on the part of nursing staff because of a lack of knowledge about the service. This is the model in which consultation is provided to nursing staff for problems in interactions with clients after staff have initiated a request for it. In a descriptive study of 248 referrals over a one-and-one-half-year period, Davis and Nelson[11] reported a change in general hospital nurses' receptivity to a consultation service. Initially, nurses were uncertain as to how to use the service. With in-service education, time, and experience with the service, referrals became more client-specific, more client-focused, more psychology-related, and more comprehensive. Furthermore, nurses became more informed about client problems, more sensitive, and more psychologically sophisticated in client care. These changes in the nurses can be considered an indirect intervention in the mental health problems of clients. They can be expected to have a positive influence on client outcomes.

The direct service model uses a team approach to consultation. Both psychiatric nurses and physicians are members of the consultation team, and both provide client assessments and interventions. A study comparing calls for psychiatric nurses and those for physicians in a general hospital using this approach to consultation revealed significant differences.[59] In this hospital, requests for consultation could be made to a specific nurse or physician rather than being randomly assigned. The study compared 100 consecutive calls for a nurse to 100 consecutive calls for a physician. Physicians were called to evaluate psychotic behavior, to prescribe psychotropic medications, to evaluate organic brain syndrome, and to evaluate abnormal behavior of Critical Care Unit clients.

TABLE 36-3.
MODELS OF CONSULTATION-LIAISON IN THE GENERAL HOSPITAL

MODEL	SERVICES PROVIDED
Indirect service	Psychiatric nurses consult with nursing staff about client interactions and provide suggestions for approaches to client problems. Psychiatrists conduct diagnostic assessments and provide interventions.
Direct service	Psychiatric nurses and physicians provide client assessments and interventions in a team approach.
Client-centered service	Psychiatric nurses consult with nursing staff about their clients' problems (indirect service) *and* provide client care through primary therapy (direct service). Physicians are not involved in the delivery of services in this model.

In comparison, nurses were called to give client and family support when death and dying were issues, to evaluate and intervene in manipulative behavior, and to deal with client management problems that were disrupting the smooth functioning of wards. Both nursing staff and physician staff requested consultant referrals, and there were no differences in who initiated the request except in the case of ward management problems. Most of the requests for consultation with clients who were creating ward management problems originated with the nursing staff.

This study suggests that nurses and physicians, while seeming to share the use of a psychiatric intervention, have different areas of expertise within the broad category of consultation. These areas of expertise seem to be congruent with generally accepted definitions of nursing and medicine. Nurses manage the interaction between the client and the psychological, social, and physical environments. Physicians diagnose and treat disease.

In addition to the study above, Severin and Becker[53] also looked at the direct service model, and found similar results. Both of the studies of consultation using the direct service approach demonstrated that psychiatric nursing consultation has an impact on the mental health problems of clients. The studies did not measure that impact in terms of outcome, but they did reveal important differences in the psychiatric consultation of physicians and nurses. In both studies, these differences were congruent with the definitions of nursing and medicine.

Two impressionistic reports of psychiatric nursing consultation using the client-centered model revealed general acceptance of a psychiatric nurse consultant service, and general satisfaction with the results of the service.[35,65] In this model, psychiatric nurses provide indirect service to nursing staff for problems they might have in interacting with clients and direct service to clients through primary therapy. Psychiatrists were not involved in providing consultation services.

In the general hospital situation described by Issacharoff and colleagues,[35] psychiatric nursing consultation included, in addition to client-centered services, assessments and dispositions or referrals to physicians in the outpatient clinic and the emergency room. Consultation services also included resolving problems among staff members. The author's overall impressions were that the services provided by psychiatric nurse consultants were heavily used, and that both clients and staff were satisfied with the service. The report by Wise[65] also claimed general acceptance of and satisfaction with a client-centered approach to psychiatric consultation. In addition to the other services offered in this approach, the report described another aspect of psychiatric nursing consultation: teaching liaison psychiatry to physicians and nurses. This aspect of psychiatric nursing consultation appeared to be well-accepted and valued also.

Based either on research or on impression, reports of the results of psychiatric nursing consultation are usually construed as positive for clients. One report of negative results did not fit conveniently into any of the three consultation models.[30] This impressionistic account was a situation involving a 14-bed surgical treatment unit for clients with intractable pain. In addition to their surgical treatment, which was provided by a single surgeon, clients were to receive psychological treatment as part of their care. Staff nurses were expected to provide the psychological, as well as postoperative, care. Through a combination of resistance to providing the psychological care and lack of knowledge about how to provide it, nurses were responsible for negative outcomes for the clients and for a deterioration of staff relationships. A psychiatrist consultant rectified the situation through application of systems theory, group process theory, and organizational theory. The authors concluded that staff nurses *per se* are not adequately prepared for an expanded liaison role because they do not have knowledge of the theories behind the role.

This case suggests that psychiatric liaison nursing is an advanced skill. Entry-level nurses can provide valuable assistance to the liaison nurse by identifying problems, observing and evaluating behavior, and reporting outcomes of therapeutic intervention. They can also carry out interventions under the direction and supervision of the liaison nurse. However, nursing liaison services themselves appear to be advanced psychiatric nursing skills.

The literature demonstrates that consultation as a psychiatric nursing intervention has a positive influence on the mental health problems of clients. Furthermore, it shows that there is a distinctly nursing character to the consultation done by psychiatric nurses that is in keeping with definitions of nursing. The distinctive character complements psychiatric consultation and the services offered by the physician consultant. A combination of physician and nurse consultation, as offered in the direct and client-centered models, probably provides the greatest impact and has the most positive influence on the mental health problems of clients.

Psychiatric/Mental Health Nursing Interventions in the Community

The impact of nursing on mental health problems can be assessed in community and home settings as well as in hospital settings. This assessment can be made by examining the different psychiatric nursing interventions that are delivered in community agency and home settings. The main forms of intervention practiced by nurses in the community are primary therapy, consultation, and transitional care.

Primary Therapy

Primary therapy in the community setting is similar to that in the hospital setting. It is the predominant therapy that the client receives, and in most cases involves total case management. Primary therapy involves the total nursing process, beginning with an intake interview and progressing through planning, treatment, evaluation, referral, placement, and documentation. It includes the modalities of individual, group, couples, and family treatment. Primary therapy is generally considered an advanced psychiatric nursing skill.

The most extensive study of primary therapy as a psychiatric nursing intervention was done by Ginsberg and Marks.[24] In this study, multiple outcome measures were used to determine the effects of individual behavioral therapy. Clients diagnosed as neurotic were seen for nine sessions (16 hours). They were pre-tested, and post-tested one year after treatment ended. At the one year post-treatment test, clients experienced a reduction in psychopathology, as evidenced by a decrease in fear and anxiety and an improvement in mood. On a second outcome measure, clients experienced an increase in social activities, as measured by dating, going out with a spouse, visiting friends and relatives, and going to dances and parties. In addition, there was a 35% mean reduction in use of mental health services, a 59% mean reduction in use of general practitioners, and a 43% mean reduction in use of specialists. Clients experienced reduced expenses for such items as taxis and help at home. Finally, clients recorded a gain in employment or ability to work. A cost–benefit analysis of this program was done. The costs of clients, relatives, and the training program, and wages and materials for teaching, were compared to the benefits at yearly follow-ups for four years. After three years, the internal rate of return was 39%, and at four years it was 62%. The cost decrease was due to clients' using health care sources less after treatment. Decreases also resulted from clients' and relatives' taking less time off work and incurring fewer additional expenses.

Client satisfaction with nurses as individual primary therapists was studied by Oozeer and colleagues.[47] Five groups of interviewers were compared: nurses, psychiatric residents in their first and third years, medical students, and clinical psychologists. Client satisfaction was measured at the conclusion of cumulative intake interview sessions in which a psychological history was taken and a mental status exam administered. The study found no significant differences in clients' evaluations of their interviewers. No important biases against nurse therapists were discovered. The investigators concluded that the public is less concerned with professional role distinctions than professionals may have suspected.

Two studies compared client outcomes of individual nurse primary therapy to those of psychiatrist and psychologist primary therapy.[4,43] Both studies concluded that primary therapy as a nursing intervention was clinically effective. Client outcomes were at least as good as those obtained by psychiatrists and psychologists; selection and management decisions matched those of psychiatrists; and nurse primary therapy was cost-effective: costs to clients decreased and training costs were less. Nurse therapists differed from non-nurse therapists in their appreciation of clients' day-to-day problems and of their home environment.

Psychiatric/mental health nurses have made a major impact on the care of the chronically mentally ill client in the community.[40,52,56,64] Nurses have detailed the problems of the deinstitutionalized chronically mentally ill in the community, developed models of care, and tested the effects of care with several client outcome measures. In addition, they have demonstrated that nurses are the primary care givers for this client population, and that they are uniquely qualified to provide such care.

In their landmark studies of treatment of the chronically mentally ill in the community, Slavinsky and Krauss[56] demonstrated the efficacy of an individually-oriented medication clinic over a group social support program for chronically ill psychiatric outpatients (65% psychotic, 13% neurotic, 7% personality disorder, 15% other). After one and two years of treatment, the medication clinic group improved more than the social support group in socialization and satisfaction with care ratings and in lowered depression and agitation ratings. These findings substantiated those of researchers in other psychiatric disciplines who, in several longitudinal studies, demonstrated the efficacy of medication management over sociotherapy (which included home visits and problem-solving in therapy sessions). To add to the significance of this work, Krauss and Slavinsky[40] carefully distinguished the types of chronically ill clients who would benefit most from medication clinics, medication groups, supportive individual therapy, or supportive group therapy. This was done according to the clients' ability to tolerate intimacy, interaction, transference, and stimulation. They also distinguished levels of insight that can be expected with this client population, and modified therapy techniques according to client needs for contact, support, advice, and problem-solving. Their work demonstrated that the care of the chronically mentally ill in the community is complex and multifaceted, and could provide rewarding research and clinical challenges to nurses for some time.

Wilson's work[64] had a different perspective, focusing on a population with the potential for chronic illness. This study demonstrated the effectiveness of a residential care treatment program for a population of clients experiencing their first psychotic episode. This program, which used a democratic approach to residential care, resulted in a reduction of symptoms without the accompanying isolation and withdrawal usually associated with institutional care.

Both Rowan[52] and Krauss and Slavinsky[40] believe that psychiatric nurses should take the lead in the care of the chronically ill psychiatric outpatient. In many instances, nurses are already the primary care-givers. They are uniquely qualified to become experts in the care of the chronically ill population because of their traditional background in physical and mental health problems, pharmacology, community nursing experience, and working with clients' families and social systems.

Individual and group primary therapy in a community agency setting is an effective nursing intervention. Client outcomes on a variety of measures indicate that nursing has an impact on mental health problems. In addition, nurse primary therapy compares well to that provided by psychiatrists and psychologists, again on a variety of measures. Primary therapy delivered by nurses is cost-effective for both the agency and the client. A distinguishing characteristic of nurse primary therapy (unlike non-nurse therapy) is the attention paid to the patient's physical and social environments. This characteristic of nursing intervention was noted in the hospital setting as well.

A special case of the advanced psychiatric (master's-prepared) nurse as primary therapist in the community is provided by nurses in private practice. Goodspeed[25] demonstrated that primary therapy as a nursing intervention has distinguishing characteristics. Independent practitioners described their therapy as family-centered, dealing with here-and-now problems, and using the home as the setting for therapy.

Nurses in private practice provide individual, group, and family therapy as well as consultation services and educational opportunities. In one case, nurses ran a psychiatric nursing outpatient clinic that provided primary therapy, consultation, and clinical placement for graduate psychiatric nursing students. In all cases, private practitioners reported that, after some early difficulties in getting established, their nursing practice was well-accepted by both the lay and the professional communities. Clients were satisfied with their care, and physicians and nurses were giving them referrals.[46]

Client outcomes of primary therapy by private practitioners have not been established through research. Impressionistic accounts report that both the public and professionals are satisfied with the nurses' practice. A more important aspect of these accounts is their validation of the distinguishing characteristics of primary therapy as a nursing intervention. The emphasis, again, is on a total client approach and an understanding of and appreciation for the client's physical and social environments.

Primary therapy in the community is almost always an advanced psychiatric nursing skill. Entry-level nurses are often not employed in community mental health centers and not involved in private practice. In situations in which entry-level nurses work in community facilities, they are usually involved in medication clinics, medication groups, or substance-abuse programs. In these instances, they work under the supervision and direction of other psychiatric personnel, including psychiatric nurse specialists. Entry-level nurses can provide valuable services in these settings through their monitoring, evaluating, and reporting of behavior and responses to pharmacotherapy and other treatments. In addition, they can further develop, define, and document the effects of the secondary therapy services they provide in these settings, just as they would in hospital settings.

Psychiatric Consultation-Liaison Nursing

Consultation in the community setting is almost always an indirect service similar to the indirect service model in the hospital setting. It is generally considered an advanced psychiatric nursing skill. Intervention is aimed directly at the staff of agencies and indirectly, through staff, at agency clients. Consultation can be general theme-centered or client case-centered, depending on the needs of the agency. However, it does not involve taking on a client case load and intervening directly with clients, as it can in the hospital setting.

Psychiatric nurses in community settings are involved in consultation as one of several interventions that include individual, group, and family therapy and crisis intervention. A descriptive account of 44 nurses who worked in urban community mental health settings found that half of them worked as primary therapists, one quarter worked in crisis intervention, slightly more than half worked with families, and one third worked as consultants.[12] Consultation was provided to community organizations, agencies, and key individuals. Consultation clients included social service agencies, the police, clergy, and teachers.

One nurse's account of her duties working in an urban anti-poverty agency described the various aspects of liaison nursing.[33] She provided a liaison service between clients and health or social service agencies, and in-service education for members of the anti-poverty agency staff and the lay staff of other agencies. She also provided case-centered or theme-centered consultation to community agencies. Her role at the agency was one she developed in response to agency needs and staff expectations of the services she could provide. Once this role was established, both staff and clients valued her services.

Consultation as a nursing intervention does exist in a community setting, and is usually provided by advanced psychiatric nurses. It can be assumed that entry-level nurses would be involved in liaison services through their identification of problems and monitoring of the outcomes of intervention strategies. However, evidence of the impact of psychiatric nursing consultation on mental health problems is scarce. Furthermore, there is a dearth of information on the character of nurse consultation in the community. It is presumed that consultation by nurses would not continue if it were considered ineffective. It is possible also to speculate that there would be distinguishing characteristics of consultation as a psychiatric nursing intervention.

Transitional Care

Transitional care is usually given between the client's leaving the hospital and discharge from the health care system, although it can include care given before a treatment program begins. In many cases, "transitional care" signifies home care. With the exception of the house calls made by the old-fashioned physician general practitioner, home care has traditionally been a nursing intervention. Its goals have always been to decrease hospitalization by providing health care in the home. At times, decreasing hospitalization means preventing readmission; at other times, it means early discharge. Home care can include monitoring a pharmacotherapy regimen, detecting drug side-effects, detecting relapse, and organizing admissions and discharges. It can also include preventing adverse environmental effects through crisis intervention, one-to-one nurse–patient relationships, patient and family support and counseling, and, in residential homes, group therapy. Home care nursing interventions involve a total client approach and an expertise in management of the client's physical and social environments. The client's home can be a traditional single-family home or a residential care facility.

Transitional care can also signify pre-care in the home. This includes treatment of clients prior to admission and/or support services for outpatients placed on a waiting list. Finally, transitional care can mean partial hospitalization. In this context, it includes the treatment of clients who have not been discharged but are living outside the hospital. In many cases, home care is provided by entry-level nurses under the supervision of an advanced psychiatric nurse specialist.

In a descriptive study of home care by community mental health nurses, Corrigan and Soni[8] found the nurses involved in providing comprehensive client care. This included assessing and monitoring behavior and medication use, intervening with supportive counseling and crisis intervention, and coordinating and administering admissions, discharges, and relationships with other agencies. These services were believed to be essential to client welfare as well as to other health professionals.

The impact of home visits on discharged mental health system clients has been to decrease readmission. Whether or not therapy was part of the treatment during a home visit, clients are believed to benefit from home care provided as a nursing intervention. Maisey[42] reported that home visits by community nurses that focused on medication monitoring and education and on general support for the client and family decreased readmission to the hospital. Keener[36] compared a control group who did not get follow-up care in the home with an experimental group who did. Follow-up care consisted of general support and medication monitoring. It resulted in a significant decrease in readmission and in a significant increase in family and community functioning. It did not affect whether clients were seen as less of a burden by their families, however. These two studies demonstrate that home- and family-centered nursing intervention can significantly reduce readmission to the hospital.

Home care can also include pre-care. A common problem when clients come to an agency is that they are placed on a waiting list. Many patients placed on waiting lists do not follow through on therapy. Hildebrandt and Davis[32] studied the effects of nursing pre-care on decreasing the pre-intake dropout rate. A control group who did not receive pre-care were compared to an experimental group who did. The experimental group received a home visit by a nurse, who listened to their problems and conveyed information about the agency, procedures, and directions. As a result of this pre-care nursing intervention, there was a significant decrease in the pre-intake dropout rate. This intervention indirectly prevents hospitalization through encouraging treatment, if it is assumed that lack of treatment could lead to hospitalization. Again, it is demonstrated that supportive family- and home-centered nursing care is an effective intervention for clients' mental health problems.

Partial hospitalization is another approach to follow-up care or transitional care. With this approach, clients are allowed to return home but are not discharged from the hospital. They make periodic returns to the hospital for treatment. Day hospitalization and night hospitalization are forms of partial hospitalization. In a study of the effects of this type of transitional care, partial hospitalization consisted of one evening per week of nursing care for 10 to 12 weeks.[22] Nursing care included a staff meeting that clients attended as observers, a team meeting of clients and staff that utilized a behavioral approach, and a community meeting of clients and staff. Nursing staff led the treatment team, evaluated patient progress, modified the treatment program, recommended medications, and planned discharges. Clients were followed for one-and-one-half years after discharge. During that time period, none of the 52 clients treated in the first six months of the program had been rehospitalized. In addition, clients had favorable comments about the program.

Transitional care provides a good example of the characteristics that distinguish psychiatric nursing intervention. Its comprehensiveness exemplifies the total client approach; the setting in which it occurs most often (the home) demands attention to the physical and social environments, including the client's family. Furthermore, it is an effective nursing intervention. Research reports consistently demonstrate that transitional care decreases hospitalization, which is obviously a goal of nursing intervention. In addition, transitional care can be carried out effectively by entry-level nurses (baccalaureate-prepared) who have community and psychiatric nursing skills. Working under the supervision of advanced psychiatric nurse specialists, entry-level nurses can extend nursing care into the community through transitional care services. They have the necessary skills, and their services have been demonstrated to have an impact on the care of clients at home.

Evaluation of Research for Nursing Practice

Thus far, this chapter has focused on identifying psychiatric nursing interventions and determining whether they have positively affected client outcomes. The next step is to decide whether there is enough evidence of the effectiveness of psychiatric nursing interventions to guide nursing practice.

Before nurses can apply the results of research in psychiatric/mental health nursing to their practice, they must evaluate the merit of research findings (Fig. 36-1). As noted earlier in this chapter, most studies have not been replicated or substantiated to the point at which they can be applied in practice. Marram[44] identified criteria for evaluating the applicability of research findings to practice. These include an evaluation of the study design as well as its feasibility, fit, and congruence with nurses' theoretical basis for practice.

The first step in evaluating research findings consists of examining the adequacy of the study design and appro-

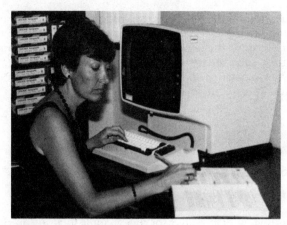

Figure 36-1. A nurse researcher examines clinical research data.

priateness of the conclusions. Included in this step is an assessment of the sample size, sample selection process, operational definitions, validity and reliability of the instruments, and statistical procedures. Attention should also be given to the author's discussion of the findings, their limitations, and their applicability to practice. If the study design is rigorous and the conclusions appear to be appropriate, the nurse can continue on to the next step.

The second step in evaluating research findings consists of examining the results for applicability in the setting in which the nurse works. This step involves looking for substantiating evidence in other empirical studies. Often, an investigator will include in the discussion of findings a comparison of the study's results with those of other investigators. The nurse can check these references and make a determination of agreement of the findings with those of other studies. This is also a good time to check whether the findings were obtained in settings similar to those in which the nurse works. The fit of the findings to a particular work setting can be assessed by asking how similar the sample population is to the nurse's client population and how similar the study's environment is to the hospital or agency in which the nurse works. A study conducted in a natural (clinical) setting often has a better chance of fitting with the nurse's workplace than does a study conducted in a laboratory.

The nurse must also examine the feasibility of applying the findings in a specific setting. Appropriate questions include: Do the findings require additional resources? Does this hospital or agency encourage change? Does the nurse have the authority and/or autonomy to introduce change? What are the potential legal or ethical risks? A final aspect of this step is to determine whether the findings are congruent with the nurse's theoretical basis for practice. It is possible that the findings will validate the nurse's current practice or can be integrated easily into a current approach or intervention. On the other hand, they may be incongruent. If the nurse's practice in this area is effective, it may not be desirable to change a particular approach.

The final step in evaluating research findings is to decide whether or not to apply them to practice. If the study findings do not meet the above criteria, they should not be applied. If they do meet the criteria, the nurse has the option to gather more data on this approach in the work setting, apply the findings directly, or test the results and further substantiate them. This final option gives all nurses in practice an opportunity to participate in the development of nursing research and nursing science.

The State of Research in Psychiatric/Mental Health Nursing

The review of research for this chapter focused on the topic of the impact of nursing on the mental health problems of clients. More specifically, whenever possible, it focused on the effect of psychiatric nursing interventions on client outcomes. The volume of research on this topic was small. When psychiatric nursing is identified in terms of specific interventions, there are few studies on the impact of particular interventions on mental health problems. Many more studies are needed to verify that each psychiatric nursing intervention has an impact on mental health problems. Studies are needed also that identify both the distinguishing characteristics of psychiatric nursing interventions and further interventions in clients' mental health care that might be considered nursing interventions.

When studies on the impact of nursing on mental health problems are being reviewed, it might be assumed that nurses are conducting the research. At least half the studies reviewed in this chapter were conducted by non-nurses. If nurses are conducting research in psychiatric nursing, they are not focusing on the effects of their nursing interventions, which would seem to be the heart of nursing research. Instead, non-nurses are involved in identifying nursing interventions and documenting their effects. In addition, most of the research that does examine the impact of psychiatric nursing interventions on client mental health outcomes is being done in Great Britain. Nurses in the United States do few of these studies, seeming to prefer psychosocial research instead.

In an overview of nursing research in the United States, Gortner and Nahm[26] noted that nursing problems have rarely been formulated as questions of practice, but rather as questions of social science. The proper testing of scientific principles in nursing has been retarded by the lack of relevancy of research problems to practice and by a lack of knowledge of sound experimental design. These limitations are a barrier to the development of psychiatric nursing practice theory.

Barriers to Nursing Research

There are other barriers to conducting psychiatric nursing research that become apparent when studies are reviewed. Perhaps the most important of these is the difficulty encountered by the psychiatric disciplines in

specifying what the outcomes of their interventions should be and how these should be evaluated.[44,45] Another problem is that of finding sensitive measures of outcomes in a psychiatrically ill population.[56] Controlled clinical studies in natural settings attempting to use experimental methods encounter other problems. These include whether the treatment under study is delivered under optimal conditions, and ethical considerations such as the morality involved in withholding the experimental treatment from the control group.

These problems are not unique to psychiatric nursing. They plague all of psychiatry, and are evident in the dearth of outcome studies in all psychiatric disciplines (with the notable exception of the behaviorists in psychology and psychiatry). However, they appear to be more of a barrier in psychiatric nursing because nursing has not carefully identified its interventions. It becomes increasingly difficult to test the outcome of interventions when they have not been identified. Although all psychiatric disciplines share the problem, nursing experiences it to a greater degree.

However, these are not insurmountable problems. Nursing is moving toward identifying its interventions. Outcomes can be specified, and tools are available or are being developed to measure outcomes. Miller[45] reported a review and evaluation system for psychiatric patient care developed by the interdisciplinary staff of a large teaching hospital. Nurses, psychiatrists, psychologists, social workers, and secretaries were all involved in building the system, which obtains data on clients' presenting problems, demography, number of visits, medications, methods of treatment, discipline of the evaluator, and outcome of treatment based on presenting problem and a general assessment.

The Nurses' Observation Scale for Inpatient Evaluation (NOSIE) is another outcome measure that has been used successfully by nurses to measure behavior change as the result of varying interventions.[1,49] This instrument has been used to measure social and illness behaviors of inpatients. Other valid and reliable measures of behavior change are also in use. Downing and Brockington[14] used a rating scale of psychotic behavior with inpatients. Raskin and Crook[50] used a rating scale to measure antidepressant drug effects, and Wilkinson[63] used a checklist to measure the effects of medication and behavior modification as interventions with inpatients. Other tools used by nurses with inpatients are the Ward Behavior Rating Scale,[6] the Modified Wing Ward Behavior Scale,[28] and the Short Clinical Rating Scale.[20,31] Slavinsky and Krauss[56] used this same rating scale with outpatients. Another measure used with chronic mentally ill outpatients was the Psychological Mental Health Index, which assesses psychological well-being and distress.[60]

Many studies use a variety of instruments to measure outcome. Lieb and colleagues[41] reported the use of seven different instruments to measure social and illness behaviors from the perspectives of the client, the family, and the nurse. Likewise, Bird and colleagues[4] and Ginsberg and Marks,[24] in a series of studies, reported the use of measures of psychopathology, social activities, use of services, and cost of services. Table 36-4 provides a list of the studies cited in this chapter that identified instruments to measure outcomes with a psychiatric client population. Many other instruments are also in use and available to nurse researchers. Of particular interest to nurses is the book *Instruments for Measuring Nursing Practice and Other Health Care Variables* by Ward, Lindeman, and Bloch.[62]

A final barrier to psychiatric nursing research is the attitude of nurses. Negative attitudes of nurses toward themselves and each other could be preventing the specification or identification of psychiatric nursing interventions. For example, there was evidence in the studies reviewed that, when nursing was defined as primary therapy or consultation, the biggest barrier to this definition was other nurses.[34,53] Objections by other nurses were about the legitimacy as nursing interventions of the actions studied, but the underlying theme was that nursing was overstepping its boundaries or getting an inflated sense of itself. This interpretation is supported by Hocking and colleagues,[34] who found that the majority of nurses were unwilling to assume an extended role. Only young nurses, those in nursing a short time, and those with few children were willing to learn or perform additional nursing skills.

It is common for nurses to fault physicians' resistance as the reason for their not being able to extend their practice. The studies reviewed here showed the opposite. In these studies, other psychiatric professionals were supportive of nurses in extended roles. Only one negative case was discovered. In addition, a study that focused specifically on physician attitudes reported that physicians not only had positive attitudes toward nurse therapists, but were utilizing the nurses' services and making referrals to them.[9] Clients were also found to accept nurses in a therapist role.[47] Although it is possible that many nurses in practice may not have encountered this kind of support, it is also possible that nurses may limit themselves and each other. This would be a serious barrier to psychiatric nursing practice and the research that develops it.

The Future of Nursing Research

Research into the impact of nursing on mental health problems is limited. Much more is needed before nurses can make predictive statements about the outcomes of their interventions. Despite this, much of the research that does exist provides direction and guidance for psychiatric nursing practice. It provides direction for defining practice, for distinguishing it from other disciplines, and for measuring its impact on mental health problems. It should encourage the development of psychiatric nursing practice through further research (Fig. 36-2).

The trend in psychiatric nursing research is away from studies that focus on nurses, nursing education, and social problems and toward studies that are related to nursing practice and are client-oriented. Finding alterna-

TABLE 36-4.
STUDIES THAT IDENTIFY INSTRUMENTS USED TO MEASURE OUTCOMES

Beard and Scott[1]	"The Efficacy of Group Therapy by Nurses for Hospitalized Patients"
Bird and others[4]	"Nurse Therapists in Psychiatry: Developments, Controversies, and Implications"
Burdock and others[6]	"A Ward Behavior Rating Scale for Use With Mental Hospital Patients"
Downing and Brockington[14]	"Nurse-Rating of Psychotic Behavior"
French and Heninger[20]	"A Short Clinical Rating Scale for Use by Nursing Personnel: Part 1. Scale Development"
Gelperin[23]	"Psychotherapeutic Intervention by the Nurse Clinical Specialist"
Ginsberg and Marks[24]	"Costs and Benefits of Behavioral Psychotherapy: A Pilot Study of Neurotics Treated by Nurse Therapists"
Hall and others[28]	"A Controlled Evaluation of Token Economy Procedures With Chronic Schizophrenic Patients"
Heninger and others[31]	"A Short Clinical Rating Scale for Use by Nursing Personnel: Part 2. Reliability, Validity, and Application"
Lieb and others[41]	"The Staff Nurse as Primary Therapist: A Pilot Study"
Miller[45]	"A Multidimensional Problem-Oriented Review and Evaluation System for Psychiatric Nursing Care"
Philip[49]	"Prediction of Successful Rehabilitation by Nurse Rating Scale"
Raskin and Crook[50]	"Sensitivity of Rating Scales to Antidepressant Drug Effects"
Slavinsky and Krauss[56]	"Two Approaches to the Management of Long-Term Psychiatric Outpatients in the Community"
Ulin[60]	"Measuring Adjustment in Chronically Ill Clients in Community Mental Health Care"
Wilkinson[63]	"The Problems and the Values of Objective Nursing Observations in Psychiatric Nursing Care"

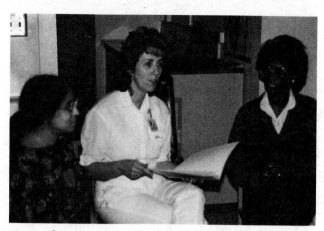

Figure 36-2. A nurse discusses data gathering procedures with other nurses on her unit.

tive means for assuring the quality of nursing practice is one of the most cogent research issues of the 1980s. Perhaps most characteristic of the current research activity is the diversity of approaches. These include the use of client outcomes for chart audit, the development of a valid and reliable process measure of quality of care, experimentation with different health care delivery structures, and the search for direct cause-and-effect relationships between the process of nursing care and client outcomes.[26]

Several types of studies are needed to advance psychiatric/mental health nursing practice.[10,26,54] These studies can be categorized according to their focus:

1. Studies that focus on building a science of psychiatric/mental health nursing practice through the systematic identification of various characteristics, health problems, and health needs of clients and potential clients
2. Studies that focus on evaluating psychiatric nursing techniques, procedures, and methods, including technical, physical, verbal, psychosocial, and interpersonal interventions
3. Studies that focus on the effects of the physical and social environments on client outcomes
4. Studies that focus on the development of methodologies or measurement tools specific to outcomes
5. Studies that focus on single replications as well as wide-scale demonstrations in order to apply research findings to psychiatric nursing practice

Major research focused on practice must continue to address improvements in client health status and the efficacy of nursing procedures and therapies. These findings must be applied in practice and must influence policy-makers in nursing care delivery in order to advance psychiatric/mental health nursing practice.

Summary

1. Psychiatric/mental health nursing research since the 1970s shows an increased focus on investigation of clinical problems, the nurse's role, clinical practice, and nursing education. The developments of research in psychiatric/mental health nursing parallel those in nursing research in general.
2. Theoretical, historical, and practical approaches delineate the dimensions of psychiatric/mental health nursing practice. Psychiatric nursing interventions take place in the hospital, in the community, and in the home.
3. Psychiatric/mental health nursing interventions have a positive effect on the mental health problems of clients. Positive client outcomes can be found by investigating psychiatric nursing care through research.
4. Evaluation of research for adequacy, usefulness, and applicability is vital. Psychiatric/mental health nursing that is scientifically based requires systematic studies that assess the efficacy of nursing procedures and therapies.
5. The current trend in psychiatric nursing research emphasizes studies related to nursing practice interventions and client problems. Quality assurance advancement is a valid research topic for nursing investigation in the 1980s.
6. Knowledge of sound experimental design, identification of appropriate nursing interventions, and the positive attitude of nurses can all help to eliminate barriers to nursing research. A useful definition of psychiatric/mental health nursing will help to encourage practice that is motivated by research.
7. The advancement of psychiatric/mental health nursing practice depends on the ability to scrutinize research for evidence of effectiveness of nursing interventions. The ability to replicate and substantiate investigations will further enhance nursing practice.

References

1. Beard M, Scott P: The efficacy of group therapy by nurses for hospitalized patients. Nurs Res 24:120, 1975
2. Benfer B: Defining the role and function of the psychiatric nurse as a member of the team. Perspec Psychiatr Care 18:166, 1980
3. Berarducci M, Blandford K, Garant C: The psychiatric liaison nurse in the general hospital: Three methods of practice. Gen Hosp Psychiatry 1:66, 1979
4. Bird J, Marks I, Lindley P: Nurse therapists in psychiatry: Developments, controversies, and implications. Br J Psychiatry 135:321, 1979
5. Bjork D, Steinberg M, Lindenmayer J: Mania and milieu: Treatment of manics in a therapeutic community. Hosp Comm Psychiatry 28:431, 1977
6. Burdock E et al: A ward behavior rating scale for use with mental hospital patients. J Clin Psychol 16:246, 1960
7. Cormack D: Psychiatric nursing in the U.S.A. J Adv Nurs 1:399, 1976
8. Corrigan J, Soni S: Community psychiatric nursing. J Adv Nurs 2:347, 1977
9. Davidson K et al: A descriptive study of the attitudes of psychia-

trists toward the new role of the nurse therapist. J Psychiatr Nurs Ment Health Serv 16:24, 1978

10. Davis B: Trends in psychiatric nursing research. Nurs Times 77: 73, 1981

11. Davis D, Nelson J: Referrals to psychiatric liaison nurses. Gen Hosp Psychiatry 2:41, 1980

12. Davis A, Underwood P: Role, function, and decision-making in community mental health. Nurs Res 25:256, 1976

13. Devine B: Therapeutic milieu/milieu therapy: An overview. J Psychiatr Nurs Ment Health Serv 19:20, 1981

14. Downing A, Brockington I: Nurse-rating of psychotic behavior. J Adv Nurs 3:551, 1978

15. Ecock-Connelly C: Patient compliance: A review of the research with implications for psychiatric/mental health nursing. J Psychiatr Nurs 16:15, 1978

16. Fagin C: Psychotherapeutic nursing. Am J Nurs 67:298, 1967

17. Flaskerud J: Distinctive characteristics of nursing psychotherapy. Issues Ment Health Nurs 6:1, 1984

18. Flaskerud J, Halloran E: Areas of agreement in nursing theory development. Adv Nurs Sci 3:1, 1980

19. Fraser D et al: Against the odds: The results of a token economy programmed with long-term psychiatric patients. Int J Nurs Stud 13:55, 1976

20. French N, Heninger G: A short clinical rating scale for use by nursing personnel: Part 1. Scale development. Arch Gen Psychiatry 23:233, 1970

21. Fried A, Fried F: Hospital and community psychiatric nursing. J Psychiatr Nurs Ment Health Serv 14:31, 1976

22. Furedy R, Crowder M, Silvers F: Transitional care: A new approach to aftercare. Hosp Comm Psychiatry 28:122, 1977

23. Gelperin E: Psychotherapeutic intervention by the nurse clinical specialist. J Psychiatr Nurs Ment Health Serv 14:16, 1976

24. Ginsberg G, Marks I: Costs and benefits of behavioral psychotherapy: A pilot study of neurotics treated by nurse therapists. Psychol Med 7:685, 1977

25. Goodspeed H: The independent practitioner: Can it survive? J Psychiatr Nurs Ment Health Serv 14:33, 1976

26. Gortner S, Nahm H: An overview of nursing research in the United States. Nurs Res 26:10, 1977

27. Hall J, Baker R: Token economy systems. Behav Res Ther 11: 253, 1973

28. Hall J, Baker R, Hutchinson K: A controlled evaluation of token economy procedures with chronic schizophrenic patients. Behav Res Ther 15:261, 1977

29. Henderson V: Development of Research in Nursing. In Simmons L and Henderson V (eds): Nursing Research: A Survey and Assessment. New York, Appleton-Century Crofts, 1964

30. Hendler N, Wise T, Lucas M: The expanded role of the psychiatric liaison nurse. Psychiatr Quart 51:135, 1979

31. Heninger G et al: A short clinical rating scale for use by nursing personnel: Part 2. Reliability, validity, and application. Arch Gen Psychiatry 24:241, 1970

32. Hildebrandt D, Davis J: Home visits: A method of reducing the pre-intake dropout rate. J Psychiatr Nurs Ment Health Serv 13: 43, 1975

33. Hitchcock J: An innovative use of the nurse's evolving role. Comm Ment Health J 7:3, 1971

34. Hocking I, Hassanein R, Bahr R: Willingness of psychiatric nurse to assume the extended role. Nurs Res 25:44, 1976

35. Issacharoff A et al: Psychiatric nurses as consultants in a general hospital. Hosp Comm Psychiatry 21:361, 1970

36. Keener M: The public health nurse in mental health follow-up care. Nurs Res 24:198, 1975

37. Kelleher M: Reappraisal of nurse's role in the treatment of schizophrenia. Int J Nurs Stud 11:197, 1974

38. Klein H et al: Transcultural nursing research with schizophrenics. Int J Nurs Stud 15:135, 1978

39. Kolson G: Mental health nursing consultation: A study of expectations. J Psychiatr Nurs Ment Health Serv 14:24, 1976

40. Krauss J, Slavinsky A: The Chronically Ill Psychiatric Patient and the Community. Boston, Blackwell Scientific, 1982

41. Lieb A, Underwood P, Glick I: The staff nurse as primary therapist: A pilot study. J Psychiatr Nurs Ment Health Serv 14:11, 1976

42. Maisey M: Hospital-based psychiatric nurse in the community. Nurs Times 71:354, 1975

43. Marks I et al: Nursing in Behavioral Psychotherapy (book for research series). London, Royal College of Nursing, 1977

44. Marram G: Barriers to research in psychiatric/mental health nursing: Implications for preparing the nurse researcher. J Psychiatr Nurs 14:7, 1976

45. Miller S: A multidimensional problem-oriented review and evaluation system for psychiatric nursing care. Med Record News 48:9, 1977

46. Offer P: Professional action through positive thinking: A case in point. Am J Nurs 80:1454, 1980

47. Oozeer I, Trauer R, Watson J: A role for a nurse therapist in a psychiatric outpatient clinic. J Adv Nurs 3:47, 1978

48. Parnell J: Community Psychiatric Nurses (abridged version of the report of a descriptive study). London, Queen's Nursing Institute, 1978

49. Philip A: Prediction of successful rehabilitation by nurse rating scale. Br J Psychiatry 134:422, 1979

50. Raskin A, Crook T: Sensitivity of rating scales to antidepressant drug effects. J Psychiatr Res 13:31, 1976

51. Robinson L: Psychiatric liaison nursing 1962–1982: A review and update of the literature. Gen Hosp Psychiatry 4(2):139, 1982

52. Rowan F: The Chronically Distressed Client. St Louis, CV Mosby, 1980

53. Severin N, Becker R: Nurses as psychiatric consultants in a general hospital emergency room. Comm Ment Health J 10:261, 1974

54. Sills G: Research in the field of psychiatric nursing. Nurs Res 26:201, 1977

55. Sladden S: Psychiatric Nursing in the Community: A Study of the Working Situation. London, Churchill Livingstone, 1979

56. Slavinsky A, Krauss J: Two approaches to the management of long-term psychiatric outpatients in the community. Nurs Res 31:284, 1982

57. Sloboda S: What are mental health nurses doing? J Psychiatr Nurs Ment Health Serv 14:24, 1976

58. Smith S, English J: The training and role of nurse therapists in a general hospital's psychiatric unit. Hosp Comm Psychiatry 26: 21, 1975

59. Stickney S, Hall R: The role of the nurse in a consultation-liaison team. Psychosomatics 22:224, 1981

60. Ulin P: Measuring adjustment in chronically ill clients in community mental health care. Nurs Res 30:229, 1981

61. Vander Zyl S, Ernst C, Salinger R: Role expectations: A significant concern for the nurse therapist. J Psychiatr Nurs Ment Health Serv 17:23, 1979

62. Ward M, Lindeman C, Bloch D (eds): Instruments for Measuring Nursing Practice and Other Health Care Variables. Washington, DC, U.S. Government Printing Office, 1978

63. Wilkinson T: The problems and the values of objective nursing observations in psychiatric nursing care. J Adv Nurs 4:151, 1979

64. Wilson H: Deinstitutionalized Presidential Care for the Mentally Disordered. New York, Grune & Stratton, 1982

65. Wise T: Utilization of a nurse consultant in teaching liaison psychiatry. J Med Ed 49:1067, 1974

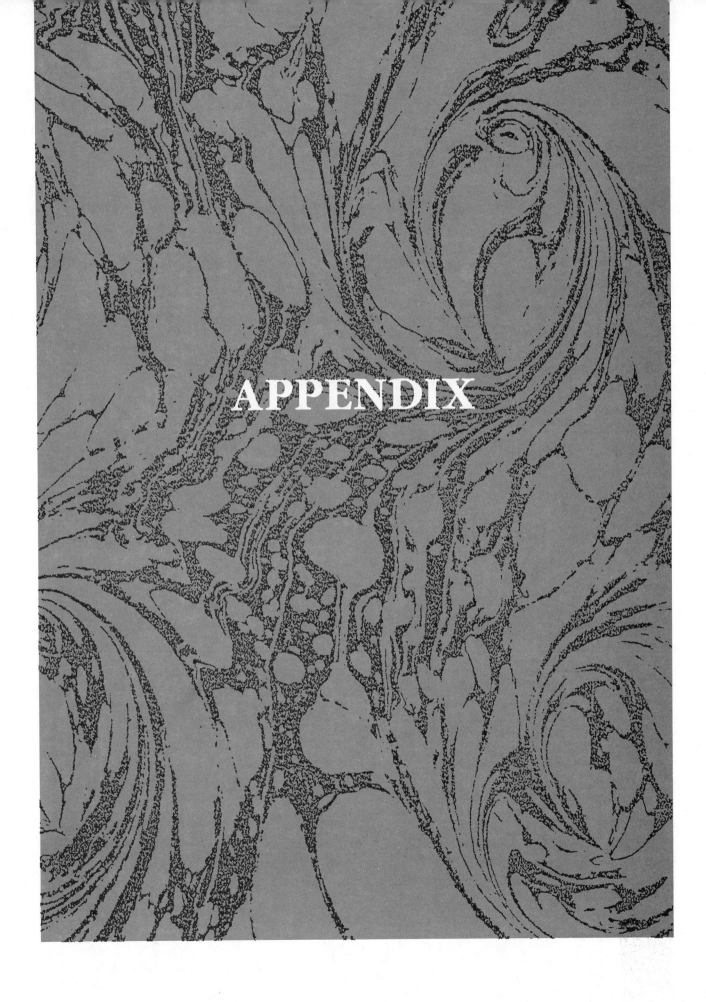

APPENDIX

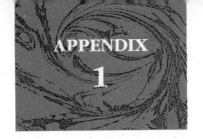

GLOSSARY

accountability The fulfillment of a formal obligation to disclose to referent others the purposes, principles, results, income, and expenditures for which one has authority.

acetaldehyde The chemical compound produced by the liver's oxidation of alcohol.

acting out Inappropriate behavior in which an individual reacts to a current situation based on maladaptive patterns learned in the past. These patterns develop from unresolved conflict between internal demands and frustration while trying to meet demands in the external world.

action research Studies in which the research process becomes part of the situation being studied. There is a cycle of implementing changes, monitoring, evaluating, and changing again.

action responses of communication Responses of clinicians that help clients change.

addiction A behavioral pattern of drug use characterized by overwhelming involvement with the use of a drug, compulsive drug-seeking behavior, and a high tendency to relapse after withdrawal (WHO definition).

adjustment disorder A DSM-III-R diagnosis in which the essential feature is a maladaptive reaction to an identifiable psychosocial stressor. This reaction occurs within three months after the onset of the stressor.

advocacy The process of pleading the cause of another.

affect The observable component of an emotion.

aftercare The total treatment program for the psychiatric client after discharge from the hospital.

ageism Discrimination based on age.

agitated depression A depression with psychomotor agitation that takes the form of an inability to sit still (*e.g.,* pacing; handwringing; pulling of hair, skin, or clothing; pressure of speech).

altruism The personally-experienced benefit derived from being of help to another.

analogic communication Verbal or nonverbal communication that involves degrees of a characteristic of that quality of communication. Can be noted in the following qualities: posture; gesture; facial expression; voice inflection; speech sequence, rhythm, cadence.

anhedonia Chronic inability to experience pleasure.

antagonist A drug that counteracts the effects of another drug.

antidepressants Drugs used for relief of symptoms of depression. The two major groups are tricyclics and monoamine oxidase (MAO) inhibitors, but various other forms are also now in use.

antidote A substance that counteracts the effects of another or prevents harmful effects.

anxiety An acute feeling of fear or dread that includes apprehensiveness, tenseness, fearfulness, and feelings of guilt, inadequacy, personal worthlessness, shame, self-loathing, eerie personality change, and all other forms of emotional distress.

anxiolytic A drug that diminishes or removes anxiety.

appearance Size, stature, mannerisms, dress, physical characteristics, handicaps, and age-appropriate behavior.

apprenticeship A method of instruction wherein a learner observes and listens to the teacher, often in unquestioning fashion, in order to obtain knowledge of a particular field. This method of learning occurred in the early days of psychiatric/mental health nursing (around 1882), when nurses observed physicians in order to understand the practice of psychiatric/mental health nursing.

assault An apparently violent attack on or threat of violence to another person.

attachment A longing-for the presence of the Other on the part of the Self and a need to integrate an alliance with the Other that will fulfill the particular characteristics of the attachment experience of the Self. The Self needs to be with the Other to the extent that, when the Self is deprived of the Other, the well-being of the Self is affected (decreased).

attitude therapy A psychoanalytically-based model of milieu organization around a set of predetermined approaches to clients. Staff adopt specific attitudinal responses to the client depending on the needs indicated by the client's diagnosis and behavior. Such attitudes include active friendliness, passive friendliness, matter-of-factness, watchfulness, kind firmness, indulgence, and reality encouragement.

authority The rightful power to fulfill a responsibility.

autism A tendency toward fantasy and withdrawal from reality. The behavior displayed by the client has meaning to the client, but this meaning is not understood by others.

autogenic training A technique of deep relaxation. A systematically designed practice in which clients place themselves in a hypnotic state for self-determined periods of time. This helps clients to achieve unusual states of consciousness and a marked degree of autonomic control.

autonomy The freedom to make discretionary and binding decisions consistent with one's scope of practice, and the freedom to act on those decisions.

avoidance A defense mechanism by which the ego avoids having any level of awareness of, and therefore bypasses, a situation, object, or activity that would be anxiety-producing.

awareness The process of the cognizance of the meaning of Truth.

BAC Blood alcohol concentration, or the amount of alcohol present in the blood, defined as grams of alcohol per milliliter of blood.

"bad-me" Individuals' perceptions of themselves as doing something that is wrong or being a "terrible" person.

barriers to effective communication Aspects of the nurse, the client, the relationship of the nurse and client, or the environment that prohibit effective communication.

battery The unlawful beating of or use of force on a person without that person's consent.

behavior One's thoughts, feelings, or actions.

biogenic amines Organic substances that act as neurotransmitters.

bipolar affective disorder A DSM-III-R diagnosis that is made when there is a manic episode, whether or not there has been a depressive episode.

bisexual An individual who becomes erotically aroused by people of both sexes and/or engages in sexual behavior with people of both sexes.

Bleuler, Eugene (1857–1930) Described the symptoms of schizophrenia (language and thought disorder).

bonding An alliance of Self and Other(s) in which the Truth of the Other is confirmed (from the perspective of the Self). Confirmation involves understanding the Truth of the Other.

case management Term derived from social work; means being responsible for moving the client through various systems to meet the client's needs.

catchment area A defining geographical area where mental health program services are provided.

child abuse Nonaccidental physical injury or neglect, with resultant cognitive, psychological, and/or maturational damage, inflicted upon a person under the age of 18 years by any family or surrogate family member.

circumstantiality Deviation into irrelevant details without communicating the central idea.

clarifying Statements made by clinicians to clients to correct ambiguities in what clients have said.

client outcome measures Measures of changes in the status, health, behavior, or function of the client as the result of a nursing intervention.

clinical specialist in psychiatric/mental health nursing A nurse with a master's degree in psychiatric/mental health nursing who uses advanced clinical skills in the field. Clinical specialist roles may include the private practice clinician, clinician in an inpatient psychiatric unit, teacher, researcher, consultant, or manager.

co-behaviors Patterns of behavior that develop in response to an addicted individual's behavior.

cognitive process The mental process of comprehension, judgment, memory, and reasoning, as contrasted with emotional and volitional processes.

cohesiveness The sense of bonding among group members that reflects mutual acceptance.

command aspect The imbedded portion of any communication that addresses the relative relationship between or among the participants. Elements of the message indicate the degree of power or control exercised by each participant. Also known as the **relationship aspect.**

commitment The legal act of certifying that a person requires involuntary treatment for a mental disorder. This is usually done only when the person is found to be a danger to self or others, or is gravely disabled.

commitment aspect of communication Communication from one to another that implies the nature of the relationship between them. Typically in troubled relationships the nature of the relationship is not defined openly and clearly.

communication The interchanges among individuals through which they define and change their awareness of Self and their relationships with Others.

communication theory A theoretical framework that details the manner in which communication operates to maintain or change an individual's perceptions and behavior.

community meeting A joint meeting of patients and staff in which issues may be addressed, including unit business, patient feedback, privilege increases, and unit conflicts. The meeting serves as a vehicle for patient government.

comparative research Studies in which characteristics of two or more groups of subjects, methods, facts, behaviors, or events are examined in relationship to each other.

competencies Intellectual and interpersonal skills that individuals need in order to maintain a sense of well-being.

complementary communication Communication in which each participant is in a position different from that of other participants, yet each participant provides rationale for the positions of the others.

compulsive religious concern Highly individualistic and idiosyncratic actions related to religion that are performed in ritualistic fashion in order to deal with intrapsychic anxiety.

conceptualization (or **abstraction**) The ability to interpret appropriately the meaning of what occurs.

concrete thought A literal thought that lacks depth of meaning.

confronting Caring and empathic statements made by clinicians to clients to point out discrepancies in clients' thoughts, feelings, or actions.

conjugal violence Severe, deliberate, and repeated physical violence inflicted on one partner by another with whom the former has or has had an intimate relationship.

conservatorship The court appointment of someone to take over and protect an incompetent person's interests.

consultation Providing expert opinion about a client's psychiatric condition and advising on its proper management, at the request of a nonpsychiatric colleague.

content aspect Communication that transmits information. Also known as the **report aspect.** The spoken words or overt messages exchanged in an interaction.

continuity theory A theory of aging that posits that successful adjustment to old age is based on the continuity of previous life patterns.

contracting A technique used to institute changes in an individual's lifestyle. The contract is an agreement with one's self or between an individual and another person to accomplish a specific goal in a set period of time.

control group The group that does not receive the experimental treatment, condition, or intervention in an experimental or quasiexperimental study.

conventional religious concern Interest in spiritual matters as a matter of conformity rather than genuine interest.

conversion reaction The manifestation of anxiety as functional symptoms in organs or parts of the body inervated by the sensory–motor nervous system, rather than being consciously experienced either diffusely as in anxiety reactions or by displacement as in phobias.

coping ability An individual's method of dealing with anxiety and problem-solving, including the type of defenses used.

coping skill An adaptive method or capacity developed by a person to deal with or overcome a psychological or social problem.

counseling A therapeutic process characterized by the giving of advice or counsel.

countertransference The conscious or unconscious effects on a clinician's understanding of clients or on the techniques of clinicians precipitated by clients' behavior.

cross-tolerance Adaptation at a cellular level such that tolerance developed for one type of drug is also experienced for the pharmocologic action of a drug in the same general class.

curandera Latino term for a female folk healer.

curandero Latino term for a male folk healer.

custodian/controller role Psychiatric/mental health nursing practiced in the period from 1906 to 1932, when nurses were expected to observe patients, enforce rules, and manage patients' behavior.

cyclothymic disorder Chronic mood disturbance of at least two years' duration involving numerous periods of depression and hypomania, but not of sufficient severity and duration to meet the criteria for a major depressive or manic episode.

defense mechanisms Automatic, primarily unconscious coping devices used by the ego as a means of protecting itself against unwanted thoughts, feelings, or external reality.

delusion An inadequate conclusion about or explanation of an experience in which panic was experienced. The idea is elaborate, and remains despite another's disconfirmation of the delusional idea.

dementia Losses of brain functioning, typically occurring in old age, that result in impaired intellectual functioning, memory, judgment, and orientation. These changes result in a person's inability to function in social and occupational roles.

denial A defense mechanism used by the ego to shut out external reality that is too frightening or threatening to tolerate; conscious awareness is blocked.

dependency needs Needs of children for mothering, love, affection, shelter, protection, security, food, and warmth.

dependent variable A factor or condition that changes based on the action of an independent variable.

depersonalization A lack of a sense of identity or realness about one's own person.

depression Feelings of sadness, despair, and unhappiness used to describe mood. As a specific psychiatric diagnosis, behaviors such as slowed thinking, alterations in purposeful physical activity, and mood change are included.

derealization The denial of reality of experiences or events.

descriptive research Studies in which characteristics, opinions, attitudes, or behaviors are identified and/ or described.

detoxification programs Treatment programs for chemically dependent individuals that aim to help clients withdraw from the drug.

development Physiological processes whereby an individual progresses from an undifferentiated state to a highly organized and functional capacity. Development implies an increase in skill and in complexity or function. Increased psychological specialization accompanies physiological growth and development.

Diagnostic and Statistical Manual of Mental Disorders (DSM-III-R) A classification of mental disorders developed by the American Psychiatric Association in 1987.

digital communication Specific words used to name things.

disqualifications of communication Communication behaviors wherein messages from others are invalidated, such as by switching the subject to avoid a topic.

dissemination The process of distributing or sharing information and new knowledge.

dissociation The separation of the mind or consciousness by a splitting off of one (or more) component or system of ideas. The personality or remainder of the mind is unable to exert any control over the split-off portion.

distortion A misunderstanding or misinterpretation of an event, caused by anxiety about the event, that leads to behaviors that do not facilitate the client's current state of well-being. A distortion is a thought or feeling that reflects one's own Truth rather than the Truth of the Other.

Dix, Dorothea (1802–1887) Crusaded for improvements in the care of the mentally ill.

double bind A form of miscommunication in which an individual states one message while at the same time stating another message that contradicts the first message. The person receiving the contradictory messages is usually unaware of the dilemma, and is unable to respond appropriately. For instance, a parent may say "I love you" to a child, but in an angry tone of voice.

dual addiction The simultaneous dependence on psychoactive drugs that have similar effects, such as alcohol and sedatives (heroin).

due process The course of legal proceedings carried out regularly and in accordance with established legal rules and principles. This ensures that laws are enforced fairly and that each citizen is able to follow a certain procedure to assert his or her views and rights.

dynamic psychiatry The theory and practice of psychiatry that emphasizes an understanding and resolution of past intrapsychic trauma and its effect on the person's current relationships.

dysthymic disorder Chronic disturbance of mood, of at least two years' duration, involving either a depressed mood or loss of interest or pleasure in all, or almost all, usual activities and pastimes. This disturbance is not severe enough to meet the criteria for a major depressive episode.

ego The part of the personality that establishes a relationship with the environment through conscious perceptions, feelings, and emotions, as defined in the psychoanalytic model.

ego psychology A theoretical perspective that emphasizes the ego in psychotherapy. The ego is viewed as existing at birth and developing from a primitive, undifferentiated core to an independent and separate ego. The ego is also seen as having its own psychic energy and instincts, separate from the id.

electroconvulsive therapy (ECT) The use of electric current to induce a convulsive seizure to treat the course of some mental illnesses.

elopement escape precautions Specific measures implemented for clients restricted to psychiatric units for their own safety when they are considered at risk to elope.

emotion An experience composed of affect and mood.

emotional distancing Movement away from the expression of a response to feelings and emotional involvement.

empathy The ability to be aware of the emotions of another in the pursuit of altruistic purposes.

enabling Actions by which individuals unintentionally support the behavior of an addicted individual.

endogenous depression Well defined, biochemically transmitted disease.

energy transference The transfer of energy from one person to another with intent to heal or promote an energy level capable of assisting the recipient to restructure his or her whole person—physical, psychological, mental, and spiritual.

entropy The tendency of a system to become random in its organization and to dissipate its energy.

envelopment The extent to which a residential facility limits the number of life choices that residents are free to make for themselves.

epidemiology The study of the distribution and determinants of diseases or disorders in order to identify possible causal factors.

Esquirol, Jean-Etienne (1772–1826) Established that there is an emotional basis for mental illness.

ethics The system or code of morals of a particular philosophy, religion, group, or profession.

euphoria A feeling of well-being not necessarily related to realistic circumstances.

eustress Stress that serves some positive or conditioning function for one's health.

existentialism A school of thought that stresses the way in which individuals (1) experience the phenomenological world around them and (2) take responsibility for their existence.

exogenous depression A conditional state dependent upon environmental stressors.

experiences of Self, Other, or Relationship Aspects of daily life awareness that have a high potential for arousing a sense of anxiety or well-being in individuals.

experimental group The group that receives the experimental treatment, condition, or intervention in an experimental or quasi-experimental study.

experimental research Studies that attempt to demonstrate causal relationships among facts, behaviors, and events and thus allow prediction of these. The investigator controls the independent variable and the assignment of sample members to a control or an experimental group.

family life cycle The sequential pattern of change through which families progress.

family myths Beliefs shared by all family members about each other that are not altered, despite evidence of their falsehood.

family rules Organized and repetitive behavioral patterns that are established, modified, and maintained by family members and that direct members to behave in predictable ways.

family schism A family pattern in which the parents are in continuous conflict and compete for children's loyalty. There is general, overall disruption in the family.

family therapy Treatment of more than one member of the family simultaneously in the same session. The assumption is that a mental disorder of one family member may be a manifestation of a disorder in the family.

fear An effect of apprehension that has an identified source.

feedback The element of communication in which information given by one participant prompts a response by the recipient in direct reaction to the original message. Hence, every message that is transmitted creates an impact, and the sharing of that impact with the original sender constitutes feedback.

fetal alcohol syndrome (FAS) Characteristics of infants exposed to alcohol in utero that include growth deficiencies, structural anomalies, and signs of central nervous system dysfunction.

flight of ideas A severe rapidity of ideas expressed in speech. The ideas flow without a logical connection between the ideas.

Freud, Sigmund (1856–1939) One of the foremost clinicians and theoreticians who developed many of the ideas of psychoanalysis.

gender identity An individual's sense of himself or herself as a man or woman.

general adaptation syndrome (GAS) The state that occurs as a response to prolonged stress and includes the stages of alarm, resistance, and exhaustion.

genuineness Being oneself without being phony or playing a role.

"good-me" Individuals' perceptions of themselves as secure and free from anxiety. Self-esteem accompanies a sense of the "good-me."

grave disability The condition in which a person is no longer able to utilize the elements of food, clothing, and shelter due to a mental disorder.

grief Normal, appropriate emotional response to an external and consciously recognized loss. It is self-limited and gradually subsides within a reasonable time.

group process What is "really going on" (the "real" issue) in a group but is not discussed. The term may also be used to indicate a description of what has gone on in a group or the cause of events that have happened in a group.

growth The physiological process through which humans assimilate or transform essential, nonliving nutrients into living protoplasm.

halfway house A family-like group living unit of mentally disturbed individuals who do not require full hospitalization but need the support of a social community that can help them with problems. The living unit represents a bridge between the hospital and complete community living.

hallucination An untrue or abnormal perception that is not based on objective sensory data.

heterogenous group A group in which members are unlike in one or more central aspects (such as problem area, sex, age).

heterosexual The sexual orientation of individuals who become erotically aroused by people of the opposite sex and/or engage in sexual behavior with people of the opposite sex.

holistic A concept used in therapy or treatment that takes into consideration the client's whole mind, body, spirit, emotions, and environment.

holistic medicine A method of practicing medicine that treats not only illness-specific process, but all aspects of individuals as a whole and as part of all that comprises their life-style and life choices.

homeostasis The maintenance of a system's internal stability through the coordinated responses of the system's components to compensate for ongoing change.

homogeneous group A group in which members are alike in some central aspect (such as all being female).

homosexual Individuals who become erotically aroused by people of the same sex and/or engage in sexual behavior with people of the same sex.

honesty The ability to relate one's perception of what is true in an experience or situation.

ho'opono pono Problem-solving process engaged in by Hawaiian culture in order to restore harmony.

hypomania A psychopathological state and abnormality of mood that falls somewhere between normal euphoria and mania.

id The reservoir of the instinctual and unconscious drives, as defined in the psychoanalytic model.

illusions Misinterpreted perceptions of an actual external stimulus.

immediacy The demonstrated intent of the clinician to provide assistance when it is needed and as soon as possible.

inadequate reality testing An inability to differentiate between reality and fantasy.

incest All forms of sexual contact, sexual exploitation (*e.g.,* pornography), and sexual overtures initiated with a child by any one who is related to the child by family ties or surrogate family ties.

independent variables Conditions or factors that precede measurement of dependent variables or are manipulated by the investigator.

individual relationship intervention A psychotherapeutic intervention by a nurse with an individual client in which: the nurse and client consider ways whereby a client can attain a sense of well-being while considering the client's societal, psychological, cultural, environmental, and physical circumstances; the nurse and client consider conscious memories of past experiences of the client, but only as such experiences relate to the client's present life; the nurse uses the learning process as a method of working with clients; the nurse makes use of the problem-solving manner of delivering care (the nursing process); the nurse views the client as one with strengths, regardless of the extent of illness; the nurse considers all the components of the person as a system in providing care. These components include the cultural, the societal, the psychological, the environmental, and the physical.

individuation The child's development of unique and special characteristics.

information-giving Statements made by the clinician to the client to provide the client with needed data.

instinct, psychological An innate psychological disposition originating from within the organism. Instincts have an aim, an object, a source, and an impetus.

instrument Device, technique, or tool that an investigator employs to collect data.

interactionist perspective of communication The theory of communication that emphasizes the shared symbols involved in communication, the ability of individuals to assume the perspective of others, and the ability to form shared meanings so that understanding can occur.

interdisciplinary team A group composed of members from different disciplines who determine what functions are needed from individual members.

interpretation A summary statement, made by the clinician, that indicates the meaning of the experiences of the client or a connection or reason behind a thought, feeling, or action of the client.

intimacy The experience of the Self and the Other of the presence of bonding and attachment.

intoxication A substance-induced state of temporarily diminished control of physical and mental powers.

kinesics The study of body movements in communication.

King, Imogene Developed the King systems model of nursing which emphasizes the concepts of systems, adaptation, perception, interpersonal relations, and health/illness.

kinship network Family structure in which two or more reciprocal households (related by birth or marriage) live in close geographic proximity.

Kraepelin, Emil (1856–1926) Established a system of psychiatric (medical) diagnoses.

latent content Group members' covert behavior, which may be implied from manifest content.

learning process Steps of understanding through which clients progress in order to understand themselves and their relationships with others.

learning theories Psychological theories that include stimulus–response learning, social learning theory, and observational learning. Some principles of learning theories include the effect of reward and punishment on behaviors, and the contingency of the reactions of others to behavior with what behavior continues to be demonstrated.

least restrictive alternative An environment that provides the minimum supervision necessary, in the smallest living unit possible, with the maximum integration of clients into the mainstream of the community.

listening responses of communication Responses of clinicians that help clients fully describe what they are thinking and feeling.

lithium carbonate A lithium salt usually used in the treatment of acute manic states and in the prevention of future episodes in individuals with recurrent affective disorders.

love The experience of intimacy in which both bonding and the need for attachment occur.

malpractice A failure of professional skill or learning, or a neglect of professional duty.

management information system An internal data system that allows the monitoring and tracking of clients within a system in order to ensure effective service delivery and to allow for the study of relevant treatment issues.

manifest content Group members' observable behavior.

manipulation Purposeful behaviors designed to get one's needs met at the expense of other people.

McLean Hospital A private psychiatric hospital in Waverly, Massachusetts; the first school for psychiatric nursing.

mechanistic perspective of communication A theory of communication that describes communication as a behavioral transfer from one person to another; the transfer of a word or gesture clearly to another person without any "noise" or unintended feature.

medical model A health care perspective that assumes an organic cause of an illness or symptom, a lack of responsibility by the individual for the symptom, and the presence of an ordered classification of disorders.

mental health education A prevention approach aimed at assisting community residents to acquire knowledge, skills, and attitudes that directly contribute to their mental health and to their impact on the mental health of others.

metacommunication Communication about communication; the process of communication that addresses how individuals communicate. Metacommunication focuses on the command or relationship aspect of communication rather than merely on the exchange of information.

methadone A synthetic narcotic used to treat heroin addicts. Methadone eliminates the heroin withdrawal syndrome and blocks the euphoric effects of heroin. It is itself an addicting drug.

milieu Any program or setting that manipulates any part of the environment in a systematic manner for therapeutic purposes.

mixed addiction Psychological and/or physiological dependence on more than one substance.

monoamine oxidase (MAO) inhibitor One group of antidepressants used to treat depression by inhibiting certain brain enzymes and raising the serotonin level.

mood The internal experience of emotion.

multidisciplinary team A group of clinicians from different disciplines; each member provides services learned in his or her discipline.

National Institute of Mental Health (NIMH) Founded by the federal government in 1949 to dis-tribute funds for research and training in the mental health sciences. It also provides public education about mental health/illness concerns.

needs assessment The process of identifying significant problems, gaps in services, and priorities for programs in a community or catchment area.

negative feedback Information given to the sender of communication which indicates to the sender not to change what the sender is doing.

negentropy The evolution of a system toward higher levels of complexity.

negligence Conduct that falls below acceptable legal standards of nursing practice; failure to exercise the prudent care that professionals are usually expected to exhibit.

neurogenic stress Stress reactions arising from physical sources.

nonverbal communication Bodily actions and non-word utterances that have meaning in communication. Nonverbal communication includes sound patterns such as voice tone, facial gestures, and space between communicating individuals.

"not-me" Individuals' perceptions of themselves as decompensating. The "not-me" is experienced in moments of insecurity and panic.

nuclear family A family in which husband, wife, and children live together.

Nurse Practice Act Legislated activities of the nurse determined by each state government.

nursing The diagnosis and treatment of human responses to actual or potential health problems.

nursing notes A shift-by-shift (or other scheduled) account of the client's status and progress toward resolution of the client's problems or needs.

nursing rounds Meetings of the nursing staff, either exclusively or with the client, in which client status is discussed.

object relations theory A theory of psychological processes that considers the formation of, and relationship of, self-representations and object-representations.

occupational therapists Professionals who provide activities for clients that encourage the use of art materials to produce products that are meaningful, are representative of the client's artistic abilities, and promote self-esteem.

old age A developmental stage categorized into four age groups: the young-old (55–64 years); the middle-old (65–74 years); the old-old (75–84 years); and the very old (85 years and over).

operational definition In research, specifies what a researcher does to make a concept measurable.

Orem, Dorothea Developed the Orem self-care model which emphasizes the person's environment, self-care, and health. According to this model, nursing intervention is needed when individuals need assistance with self-care activities in order to maintain integrity.

Other Another person in the environment of the Self with whom the Self bonds and/or attaches.

overvalued ideas An excessive or unrealistic emphasis on, and preoccupation with, a particular set of ideas to the exclusion of a critical examination of the ideas.

panic Intense anxiety wherein an individual experiences distortions in perception and meaning and the inability to learn.

paranoia Suspiciousness that is not based on reality.

parentification The assumption of a parent-like (or adult) role by the child.

Peplau, Hildegard The founder of modern psychiatric nursing, whose clinical and theoretical writings provide a basis for psychiatric/mental health nursing. Peplau founded the interpersonal theory of psychiatric/mental health nursing.

phobia An unrealistic fear that promotes withdrawal of the individual from an event or experience.

Pinel, Philippe (1745–1826) Physician in Chief of Bicetre Hospital in Paris; removed the chains from the mentally ill and began the era of humane treatment.

play therapy A mode of intervention with children wherein play is used as a form of symbolic communication. Through the use of play materials, children symbolically express themselves in the play materials they choose and the ways in which they use the materials. Through the use of play, children give evidence of their underlying thoughts, feelings, and needs.

positive feedback Information given to the sender of communication that indicates to the sender the need to change what the sender is doing.

positive regard The ability to value a client as a person with worth and dignity.

poverty of thought A restriction of what is included in thought.

primary prevention Planning and carrying out programs to reduce the incidence in the community of mental disorders of all types.

privilege/step system Hierarchical system in the milieu setting in which patients earn increased privileges and freedom of movement by exhibiting improved degrees of appropriate behavior.

probing Statements made by the clinician to the client to encourage the client to elaborate or provide examples to further clarify content.

problem-oriented charting Statements entered into a client's clinical record according to stated problems.

process Actual occurrences in an interaction. The "process" of communication is important because what is said may not be congruent with nonverbal expressions.

professionalism The art and science of psychiatric/mental health nursing wherein the needs of the client are the primary focus of care.

proxemics The study of space in communication.

pseudodementia A group of depressive symptoms of older adults similar to symptoms of dementia. Pseudodementia can be distinguished from dementia on the basis of history, appearance, affect, and cognitive functioning.

psychiatric home care The provision of psychiatric services in the home of the client.

psychiatric liaison nursing A psychiatric nursing role in the general hospital wherein the psychiatric nurse assists in providing psychological care of (1) emotionally or mentally disturbed clients who have a physical illness, and (2) physically ill clients who develop emotional or mental illness as a result of the stress of disability or hospitalization.

psychiatric/mental health nurses Individuals who may have a baccalaureate degree (the psychiatric/mental health nurse) or a master's degree (the clinical specialist). Nurses with a baccalaureate do individual relationship intervention, and may also work with groups and families. Nurses with a master's degree can provide psychotherapy for clients with mental health/illness concerns. Psychiatric/mental health nurses also emphasize (1) the dignity and right to treatment of the individual regardless of cultural background, socioeconomic status, or diagnosis; (2) a systems perspective on the client; (3) crisis intervention; and (4) working with clients on here-and-now concerns in living. The master's degree typically is the advanced clinical degree. Clinical specialists with a doctoral degree obtain their degree usually in preparation for research.

Psychiatric Nursing Diagnoses I (PNDI) A taxonomy of nursing diagnoses developed in 1986 by the Council of Psychiatric/Mental Health Nursing of the American Nurses' Association.

psychiatrists Medical doctors who provide psychotherapy for clients with mental health/illness concerns. Psychiatrists also emphasize the use of medications to decrease symptoms of mental disorders and the role of clients' biological nature in promoting mental illness.

psychoactive compounds Drugs that alter the level of consciousness and/or the mood of the user.

psychoanalysis A type of therapy originated by Sigmund Freud in which understanding of personality is sought through in-depth exploration of events that occurred during growth and development. The clarification, with the therapist, of the repetition of conflicts originating in the client's early life facilitates change in the client.

psychoanalytic model A definition of mental functioning and cure in which an individual recalls traumatic experiences and works through, or comes to understand, the meaning and effects of the experiences.

psychogenic stress Stress reactions arising from psychological sources.

psychological perspective of communication The theory of communication that emphasizes the mental processes of communication, the attribution of meaning to communication, and the choice involved in deciding what communication to send to another.

psychologists Individuals with an advanced degree in psychology who provide psychotherapy for clients with mental health/illness concerns. Psychologists may also emphasize the use of psychological testing and behavior modification techniques in working with clients.

psychomotor excitement Generalized physical and emotional overactivity in response to internal and/or external stimuli, as in hypomania.

psychomotor retardation A generalized slowing of physical and emotional reactions.

psychotherapists Mental health clinicians who have attained skills through education and clinical practice (usually a master's degree and supervised clinical practice).

quasi experimental research Studies that attempt to demonstrate causal relationships among facts, behaviors, and events and thus allow prediction of these. In contrast to what happens in experimental research, the investigator lacks control of one of the characteristics of an experimental design—for instance, random assignment of subjects to groups.

rapprochement A subphase of growth and development, described by Margaret Mahler, that occurs during the period from 14 to 24 months of age. It is a chaotic period in which the child wants both togetherness with the mother and separateness. Feelings of anger are common as the child realizes the mother cannot meet all demands of the child.

rating scale A measuring instrument composed of several items that have a logical or empirical relationship to each other. Subjects are asked to rate the items.

reactive alcoholism A cluster of symptoms of dysfunctional alcohol use in response to life events that results in significant life change.

recreational therapists Professionals who work with clients on strengthening individual and group skills during physical activity and exercise.

reflecting A listening response wherein a rephrasing or summary of what the client has said or implied is made to the client.

regenesis training A process for discovering the limiting patterns of the past and transforming them into freer, healthier, and more fulfilling ways of being. Regenesis uniquely integrates deep relaxation, trance induction, visualization, autonomic control, age regression, trauma release, and psychophysiological reprogramming.

regression A coping mechanism by which a person reverts back to an earlier pattern of behavior. Regression occurs naturally in some growth and development periods, such as adolescence.

rehabilitation The methods and techniques used in a program that seeks to achieve maximal function and optimal adjustment for the client and to prevent relapses or recurrences of the client's problem. The focus is on the client's assets and recoverable functions.

relaxation response The physiological and emotional effect of an attempt by an individual (intended or not) to achieve a sense of well-being.

relaxation training A series of practical exercises

comprising four essential elements: (1) a quiet environment, (2) a comfortable position, (3) suggestions or statements describing mental and physical calmness and balance, and (4) a gradual separation from the environment. Results are an increased sense of self-knowledge and decreased physiological stress.

resistance A reluctance by the client to engage in therapeutic work, manifested by various feelings and behaviors during therapy; the process wherein the client avoids the Truth about Self or Other, or the Relationship of Self and Other.

responsibility A charge or duty for which one is held accountable.

risk factors Constitutional and social traits that alter the individual's vulnerability to disease.

Rogers, Carl (1902–1987) A psychologist whose ideas included focusing less on a client's past and unconscious forces than on a person's capability to value and decide questions on his or her own. He valued feelings and genuineness.

Rogers, Martha Developed the unitary man model of nursing, which focuses on the changing nature of the person–environment interaction.

role A pattern of behavior or a regular way of acting that is expected of all persons who occupy a given position in the social order and who confront others; the actual and intangible forms that the self takes (such as the role of nurse); the structurally given demands, including norms, expectations, responsibility, and taboos, associated with a given social position.

role conflict The difficulty that occurs when a person is subjected to two or more contrary expectations that the person cannot satisfy simultaneously.

role overlap The experience of various professionals from different disciplines working together and sharing many of the same functions.

role-playing A therapeutic technique wherein the client and/or clinician act out a specific scenario that is either similar to a situation experienced by the client or designed to facilitate the client's learning of a new behavior.

Roy, Sister Calista Developed the Roy adaptation model of nursing, which focuses on the health–illness continuum, adaptation of the person, and the person–environment system. The function of nursing care is to promote effective adaptation responses.

sample A microcosm of the population, or the participants or respondents selected to be studied.

scapegoat A person or object who is blamed for the actions of others.

seclusion areas Specific rooms on a psychiatric unit set up for the safe containment of acutely disturbed or destructive clients.

secondary gain The support, sympathy, and attention that are unconsciously and consciously sought and received by a person. It is frequently associated with illness.

secondary prevention Clinical practices that seek to decrease the duration of a significant number of mental disorders that occur.

selective inattention A psychological mechanism of individuals wherein certain real experiences are not awarded awareness in order to avoid the experience of anxiety.

Self The Self is the process of awareness of experiences of the Self, Other, and Relationship of Self and Other.

Self–Other Relationship A conceptual framework developed by Loretta Birckhead in which three basic phenomena are seen as the core of psychological life: the Self, the Other, and the Relationship of Self and Other. The model emphasizes the idea of a dialectic because balance is needed in each of the three components for psychological health. The model focuses on the need to understand simultaneously both one's personal identity (Self) and one's Relationship to Others. The idea of Self in this model is one of awareness of present experience.

senile dementia of the Alzheimer's type (SDAT) A disease characterized by changes within the brain such as senile plaques, neurofibrillary tangles, granulovacuolar structures, and loss of neurons. Possible causes of SDAT include genetic, viral, biochemical, immunological, or toxic factors.

separation–individuation The process of psychological development in which major aspects of behavioral and intrapsychic life are formed. Mahler emphasized separation–individuation, and described growth and development as representing ways in which a person differentiates experiences relating to the "self" or to an "other."

sexual orientation The individual's physical and emotional preference for other individuals.

sexual response cycle Conceptualization of sexual response by Masters and Johnson into four phases: excitement, plateau, orgasm, and resolution.

short-term therapy Psychotherapeutic intervention designed to last for a limited time, usually for fewer than 12 hours of therapy.

sick role Societal expectation of how a person should behave when ill.

Simonton technique A therapy for cancer and other serious diseases developed by Drs. O. Carl and Stephanie Simonton. Self-help techniques, which successfully reinforce usual medical treatment, include learning positive attitudes, relaxation, visualization, goal-setting, managing pain, exercise, and building an emotional support system.

single-parent family A family in which only one parent and children live together as a result of divorce, separation, or death of the other parent.

skewed family A family in which one parent is psychiatrically disturbed and the other parent does not acknowledge the emotional problems of the disturbed spouse. One parent attempts to form excessively close emotional bonds with his/her child to the exclusion of the other parent.

socialization A complex process by which an individual acquires skills to adapt to the demands and restrictions of society.

social services Professionals (usually social workers) who are actively involved with the families of clients, and who help in discharge planning.

social workers Individuals with an advanced degree in social work who provide psychotherapy for clients with mental health/illness concerns. Social workers may also emphasize the social network of services used by clients.

somatic treatments The use of medical treatments such as medications and electroshock therapy to decrease symptoms of mental illness.

spirituality The formation of a positive, personal meaning and purpose for existence; frequently developed through a positive, dynamic relationship with a deity. The relationship is characterized by faith, trust, hope, and love.

splitting The externalization onto others by a client of the client's own internal conflict, such that the others are considered by the client to be acting out polarities of the conflict (such as ''good'' and ''bad'').

Statement on Psychiatric and Mental Health Nursing A publication of the American Nurses' Association that defines the role of the nurse within the mental health system. It also defines the role of the psychiatric/mental health nurse and the scope of practice.

steady state The state of a system in which there is relative adaptation.

stress The nonspecific response of the body to any demand made upon it. When an organism is called upon to readjust or adapt in order to maintain normal functioning, it is under stress.

stress management The practice of activities that individuals personally initiate and perform to stay within healthful stress limits.

stress resistance-building Mobilizing strength-building experiences that will enable clients to more readily resist or cope with stressors to which they are or may be exposed.

structure of a system The arrangement of parts of a system.

structure, psychiatric inpatient unit A formal plan for a psychiatric inpatient unit, detailing the ages served on the unit, the diagnoses, whether or not the unit has an ''open door'' or a ''closed door'' policy, the floor plan, and the schedule of activities.

suicide precautions Specific measures implemented to ensure the safety of clients who actively wish to harm themselves.

Sullivan, Harry Stack (1892–1949) One of the foremost U.S. psychiatrists; developed the interpersonal theory of psychiatry.

summarizing Statements made by the clinician to the client to pull together a theme or topic mentioned by the client.

superego An internalized moral arbitrator, as defined in the psychoanalytic model. The main functions of the superego are to strive for perfection, to inhibit the impulses of the id, and to persuade the ego to substitute moralistic goals for realistic ones.

superficial religious concern Religious interest that is not genuine. It is often temporary and may be manipulative.

susto (fright) Anxiety state caused by a frightening or traumatic experience; symptoms include excessive nervousness, loss of appetite, and loss of sleep. If not resolved immediately it can become *susto pasad* (passed fright).

symmetrical communication Communication in which the equality of participants is emphasized.

sympathy The existence of feelings identical to those of another person without accompanying behaviors or understanding the experience of the other.

system A set of relationships between objects and their properties or attributes.

tangentiality A wandering of speech in which an idea does not relate to those preceding it.

teratogenic A substance that induces birth defects or deformities.

tertiary prevention Fostering improvement in individuals, groups, and families with mental illness concerns.

testing behavior Expectations of others that, when not met, indicate the absence of trustworthiness of others. Testing is an expected part of relationships.

therapeutic community Specific type of milieu therapy that fosters behavioral change through emphasis on social interactions.

therapeutic interviewing Communication between a professional person and a client wherein the focus of the communication is on the needs, behaviors, conflicts, and psychological growth and well-being of the client rather than on the life of the interviewer.

therapeutic touch The transfer of energy with the intent to heal; viewing all living systems as energy fields, and thus open fields where a continuous exchange of energy, matter, and information is possible.

''Third-force'' theorists/clinicians Individuals in the mental health/illness field who do not believe in the theories of psychoanalysis or behaviorism, but rather follow a third belief system that emphasizes the person's ability to deal with feelings and experiences in the present. Examples of third-force clinicians/theorists include Carl Rogers, Fritz Perl (gestalt therapy), and Abraham Maslow.

thought disturbance A disorder caused by the parent–child relationship (including biochemical causes) in which anxiety was experienced. Such experiences result in an inability to maintain accurate perceptions of reality. This inability, in turn, causes the production of symptoms that are most prominent when the person is confronted with the stresses of interpersonal relationships.

thoughts Internal cognitions.

time out A therapeutic technique in which a client is allowed time away from the excitable stimulus of the psychiatric unit and placed in a secluded area with staff available to work through disturbing issues.

token economy A technique of behavior modification in which clients earn negotiable tokens in exchange for appropriate behavior. The tokens act as positive reinforcement to produce desired changes in behavior.

tolerance A state characterized by the need for increased amounts of a substance to produce the desired effect.

transference   The process of the client wherein the clinician is transposed into being a person from the client's past with whom the client has had difficulty.

transpersonal spiritual counseling   Counseling techniques that promote dialogue with a highly evolved expression of self, for insight, healing, and growth.

triangulation (in substance abuse)   A process wherein an individual forms emotional bonds with an individual, activity, or substance that is external to relationships within the family.

unidisciplinary team   A group of clinicians, all of whom are members of the same discipline (such as nursing).

unipolar disorder   An affective disorder with one or more major depressive episodes and no manic episodes.

universality   The realization that other group members have similar problems which, in turn, decreases one's sense of aloneness.

variable   Factor or condition that varies and has different values that can be measured. Variables result from operationally defining a concept.

verbal communication   Spoken and written words transmitted between people.

warmth   A clinician's attitude that denotes the clinician's wish to comfort the client.

well-being   An individual's experience of feeling secure; what promotes security is individually determined.

wellness   A state of being in which an individual's attitudes, physical functions, and social interactions demonstrate a positive sense of self and the ability to respond to one's needs assertively.

wholeness of a system   The quality of a system wherein the total system is more than the mere sum of its parts.

withdrawal   (1) (in substance abuse) A substance-specific syndrome that occurs following the cessation of or reduction in intake of a substance regularly used by the individual to induce a physiological state of intoxication; (2) pathological retreat from people or the world of reality, often seen in depression.

word salad   A mixture of words that lack apparent connection in meaning.

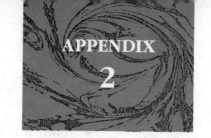

NANDA-APPROVED NURSING DIAGNOSTIC CATEGORIES

This list represents the NANDA-approved nursing diagnostic categories for clinical use and testing (1988). Changes have been made in 15 labels for consistency.

Pattern 1: Exchanging

1.1.2.1	Altered Nutrition: More than body requirements
1.1.2.2	Altered Nutrition: Less than body requirements
1.1.2.3	Altered Nutrition: Potential for more than body requirements
1.2.1.1	Potential for Infection
1.2.2.1	Potential Altered Body Temperature
**1.2.2.2	Hypothermia
1.2.2.3	Hyperthermia
1.2.2.4	Ineffective Thermoregulation
*1.2.3.1	Dysreflexia
#1.3.1.1	Constipation
*1.3.1.1.1	Perceived Constipation
*1.3.1.1.2	Colonic Constipation
#1.3.1.2	Diarrhea
#1.3.1.3	Bowel Incontinence
1.3.2	Altered Patterns of Urinary Elimination
1.3.2.1.1	Stress Incontinence
1.3.2.1.2	Reflex Incontinence
1.3.2.1.3	Urge Incontinence
1.3.2.1.4	Functional Incontinence
1.3.2.1.5	Total Incontinence
1.3.2.2	Urinary Retention
#1.4.1.1	Altered (Specify Type) Tissue Perfusion (Renal, cerebral, cardiopulmonary, gastrointestinal, peripheral)
1.4.1.2.1	Fluid Volume Excess
1.4.1.2.2.1	Fluid Volume Deficit (1)
1.4.1.2.2.1	Fluid Volume Deficit (2)
1.4.1.2.2.2	Potential Fluid Volume Deficit
#1.4.2.1	Decreased Cardiac Output

* New diagnostic categories approved 1988.
** Revised diagnostic categories approved 1988
\# Categories with modified label terminology

1.5.1.1	Impaired Gas Exchange
1.5.1.2	Ineffective Airway Clearance
1.5.1.3	Ineffective Breathing Pattern
1.6.1	Potential for Injury
1.6.1.1	Potential for Suffocation
1.6.1.2	Potential for Poisoning
1.6.1.3	Potential for Trauma
*1.6.1.4	Potential for Aspiration
*1.6.1.5	Potential for Disuse Syndrome
1.6.2.1	Impaired Tissue Integrity
#1.6.2.1.1	Altered Oral Mucous Membrane
1.6.2.1.2.1	Impaired Skin Integrity
1.6.2.1.2.2	Potential Impaired Skin Integrity

Pattern 2: Communicating

2.1.1.1	Impaired Verbal Communication

Pattern 3: Relating

3.1.1	Impaired Social Interaction
3.1.2	Social Isolation
#3.2.1	Altered Role Performance
3.2.1.1.1	Altered Parenting
3.2.1.1.2	Potential Altered Parenting
3.2.1.2.1	Sexual Dysfunction
3.2.2	Altered Family Processes
*3.2.3.1	Parental Role Conflict
3.3	Altered Sexuality Patterns

Pattern 4: Valuing

4.1.1	Spiritual Distress (distress of the human spirit)

Pattern 5: Choosing

5.1.1.1	Ineffective Individual Coping
5.1.1.1.1	Impaired Adjustment
*5.1.1.1.2	Defensive Coping
*5.1.1.1.3	Ineffective Denial
5.1.2.1.1	Ineffective Family Coping: Disabling

5.1.2.1.2	Ineffective Family Coping: Compromised
5.1.2.2	Family Coping: Potential for Growth
5.2.1.1	Noncompliance (Specify)
*5.3.1.1	Decisional Conflict (Specify)
*5.4	Health-Seeking Behaviors (Specify)

Pattern 6: Moving

6.1.1.1	Impaired Physical Mobility
6.1.1.2	Activity Intolerance
*6.1.1.2.1	Fatigue
6.1.1.3	Potential Activity Intolerance
6.2.1	Sleep Pattern Disturbance
6.3.1.1	Diversional Activity Deficit
6.4.1.1	Impaired Home Maintenance Management
6.4.2	Altered Health Maintenance
#6.5.1	Feeding Self-Care Deficit
6.5.1.1	Impaired Swallowing
*6.5.1.2	Ineffective Breastfeeding
#6.5.2	Bathing/Hygiene Self-Care Deficit
#6.5.3	Dressing/Grooming Self-Care Deficit
#6.5.4	Toileting Self-Care Deficit
6.6	Altered Growth and Development

Pattern 7: Perceiving

#7.1.1	Body-Image Disturbance
#**7.1.2	Self-Esteem Disturbance
*7.1.2.1	Chronic Low Self-Esteem
*7.1.2.2	Situational Low Self-Esteem
#7.1.3	Personal Identity Disturbance
7.2	Sensory/Perceptual Alterations (Specify) (Visual, auditory, kinesthetic, gustatory, tactile, olfactory)
7.2.1.1	Unilateral Neglect
7.3.1	Hopelessness
7.3.2	Powerlessness

Pattern 8: Knowing

8.1.1	Knowledge Deficit (Specify)
8.3	Altered Thought Processes

Pattern 9: Feeling

#9.1.1	Pain
9.1.1.1	Chronic Pain
9.2.1.1	Dysfunctional Grieving
9.2.1.2	Anticipatory Grieving
9.2.2	Potential for Violence: Self-directed or directed at others
9.2.3	Post-Trauma Response
9.2.3.1	Rape-Trauma Syndrome
9.2.3.1.1	Rape-Trauma Syndrome: Compound Reaction
9.2.3.1.2	Rape-Trauma Syndrome: Silent Reaction
9.3.1	Anxiety
9.3.2	Fear

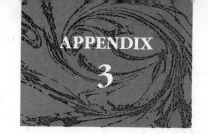

APPENDIX
3

NURSING DIAGNOSES DEVELOPED BY THE AMERICAN NURSES' ASSOCIATION

Taxonomy for the Classification of Human Responses of Concern for Psychiatric/Mental Health Nursing Practice*

Response Class

A. Biological Human Response Patterns
10. Alterations in Circulation
10.01
  10.01.01 Bradycardia
  10.01.02 Dizziness
  10.01.03 Drug-related blood dyscrasias
  10.01.04 Hypertension
  10.01.05 Hypotension
  10.01.06 Palpitations
  10.01.07 Tachycardia
10.99 Alterations in circulation NOS (Not Otherwise Specified)
11. Alterations in Elimination
11.01 Bowel excess/deficit
  11.01.01 Constipation
  11.01.02 Diarrhea
  11.01.03 Encopresis
  11.01.04 Incontinence
11.02 Urinary excess/deficit
  11.02.01 Enuresis
  11.02.02 Frequency
  11.02.03 Incontinence
  11.02.04 Retention
11.03 Skin excess/deficit

  11.03.01 Diaphoresis
  11.03.02 Anhidrosis
11.99 Alterations in elimination NOS
12. Alterations in Endocrine/Metabolic Functioning
12.01
  12.01.01 Atypical growth and development
  12.01.02 Hirsutism
  12.01.03 Hypoglycemia
  12.01.04 Impaired temperature regulation
  12.01.05 Premenstrual stress syndrome
12.99 Alterations in endocrine/metabolic functioning NOS
13. Alterations in Musculo/Skeletal Functioning
14. Alterations in Nutrition/Metabolism
14.01 Less than body requires
  14.01.01 Anorexia
  14.01.02 Hyperthyroidism
14.02 More than body requires
  14.02.01 Bulimia
  14.02.02 Hypothyroidism
  14.02.03 Obesity
14.99 Alterations in nutrition/metabolism NOS
15. Alterations in Neurological/Sensory Functioning
15.01 Impaired level of consciousness
  15.01.01 Alcohol-related impairment
  15.01.02 Comatose
  15.01.03 Drug-related impairment
15.02 Impaired sensory acuity
  15.02.01 Impaired auditory acuity
  15.02.02 Impaired gustatory acuity
  15.02.03 Impaired olfactory acuity

* American Nurses' Association, Division on Psychiatric and Mental Health Nursing Practice, 1986

15.02.04   Impaired tactile acuity
15.02.05   Impaired visual acuity
15.03   Impaired sensory processing
     15.03.01   Headaches
     15.03.02   Seizures
     15.03.03   Tremors
15.04   Impaired sensory integration
     15.04.01   Delirium
     15.04.02   Extreme temperament
     15.04.03   Hyperirritable
     15.04.04   Hypoirritable
     15.04.05   Learning disabilities
     15.04.06   Pupil changes
     15.04.07   Startle response
     15.04.08   Tics

16.   Alterations in Oxygenation
     16.01   Ineffective breathing patterns—excess/deficit
     16.02   Respirations
         16.02.01   Breath-holding
         16.02.02   Dyspnea
         16.02.03   Hyperventilation
         16.02.04   Hypoventilation
         16.02.05   Shallow breathing
         16.02.06   Shortness of breath
     16.99   Alterations in oxygenation NOS

17.   Alterations in Reproductive/Sexual Functioning
     17.01
         17.01.01   Amenorrhea
         17.01.02   Dysmenorrhea
         17.01.03   Dyspareunia
         17.01.04   Impaired sexual functioning
         17.01.05   Infertility
         17.01.06   Malformation
         17.01.07   Unwanted pregnancy
     17.99   Alterations in reproductive/sexual functioning NOS

18.   Alterations in Physical Integrity
     18.01   Skin impairment/injury
         18.01.01   Abrasions
         18.01.02   Contusions
         18.01.03   Dryness/scaling
         18.01.04   Lacerations
         18.01.05   Lesions
     18.99   Alterations in physical integrity NOS

B.   Socio/Behavioral Human Response Patterns
20.   Alterations in Communication
     20.01   Impaired nonverbal
         20.01.01   Incongruent
         20.01.02   Inappropriate
     20.02   Impaired verbal
         20.02.01   Aphasia
         20.02.02   Bizarre content
         20.02.03   Circumstantial
         20.02.04   Confabulation
         20.02.05   Dysarthria
         20.02.06   Dysphasia
         20.02.07   Echolalia
         20.02.08   Elective mutism
         20.02.09   Incoherent
         20.02.10   Mute
         20.02.11   Neologisms
         20.02.12   Nonsense/word salad
         20.02.13   Overelaboration
         20.02.14   Perseveration
         20.02.15   Pronoun reversal
         20.02.16   Rate accelerated
         20.02.17   Rate retarded
         20.02.18   Severe delay
         20.02.19   Stuttering
         20.02.20   Volume too loud
         20.02.21   Volume too soft
     20.99   Alterations in communication NOS

21.   Alterations in Conduct/Impulse Control
     21.01   Aggression/violence toward environment
         21.01.01   Destruction of property
         21.01.02   Fire-setting
     21.02   Aggression/violence toward others
         21.02.01   Abuse—physical
         21.02.02   Abuse—sexual
         21.02.03   Abuse—verbal
         21.02.04   Assaultive
         21.02.05   Homicidal
         21.02.06   Temper tantrums
     21.03   Aggression/violence toward self
         21.03.01   Head-banging
         21.03.02   Self-mutilation
         21.03.03   Substance abuse
         21.03.04   Suicidal
     21.04   Bizarre behavior
     21.05   Compulsive behavior
     21.06   Disorganized behavior
     21.07   Age-inappropriate behavior
         21.07.01   Pseudomature behavior
         21.07.02   Regressed behavior
     21.08   Unpredictable behavior
     21.99   Alterations in conduct/impulse control NOS

22.   Alterations in Motor Behavior
     22.01
         22.01.01   Bizarre gesturing
         22.01.02   Catatonia
         22.01.03   Coordination impaired
         22.01.04   Dystonias
         22.01.05   Echopraxia
         22.01.06   Extrapyramidal symptoms
         22.01.07   Hyperactivity
         22.01.08   Hypoactivity
         22.01.09   Mobility impaired
         22.01.10   Muscular rigidity
         22.01.11   Psychomotor retardation
         22.01.12   Restlessness
         22.01.13   Toe-walking
     22.99   Alterations in motor behavior NOS

23.   Alterations in Role Performance
     23.01   Impaired family role
         23.01.01   Dependence deficit

23.01.02 Dependence excess
23.01.03 Enmeshment
23.01.04 Role loss/disengagement
23.01.05 Role reversal
23.02 Impaired social/leisure role
23.02.01 Withdrawal/social isolation
23.03 Impaired work role (play/academic/occupational)
23.03.01 Dependence
23.03.02 Lack of direction
23.03.03 Overachievement
23.03.04 Truancy
23.03.05 Underachievement
23.99 Alterations in role performance NOS
24. Alterations in Self-Care
24.01 Impairment in activity/rest
24.02 Impairment in elimination
24.03 Impairment in nutrition/feeding
24.05 Impairment in solitude/social interaction
24.99 Alterations in self-care NOS
25. Alterations in Sleep/Arousal
25.01
25.01.01 Bruxism
25.01.02 Early morning waking
25.01.03 Hypersomnia
25.01.04 Insomnia
25.01.05 Narcolepsy
25.01.06 Nightmares/night terrors
25.01.07 Sleep-walking
25.01.08 Somnolence
25.99 Alterations in sleep/arousal NOS
26. Alterations in Sexuality
26.01
26.01.01 Excess in masturbation
26.01.02 Excess seductiveness
26.01.03 Excess sex play/talk/activity
26.01.04 Exhibitionism
26.01.05 Impaired sexual activity
26.01.06 Impaired sexual desire
26.01.07 Inappropriate sexual objects
26.99 Alterations in sexuality NOS
C. Emotional Human Response Patterns
30. Excess of or Deficit in Dominant Emotions
30.01 Impaired emotional experience
30.01.01 Anger/rage
30.01.02 Anxiety
30.01.03 Disgust/contempt
30.01.04 Distress/anguish
30.01.05 Envy/jealousy
30.01.06 Fear
30.01.07 Grief
30.01.08 Guilt
30.01.09 Helplessness
30.01.10 Hopelessness
30.01.11 Joy/elation/happiness
30.01.12 Loneliness
30.01.13 Sadness
30.01.14 Shame/humiliation
30.01.15 Surprise/startle
30.02 Impaired appropriateness of emotional expression
30.03 Impaired congruence of emotions, thoughts, behavior
30.04 Impaired range of expression
30.05 Impaired range of focus
30.99 Excess of or deficit in dominant emotions NOS
D. Defensive Human Response Patterns
40. Excess of or Deficit in Defenses
40.01 Impaired functioning of defenses
40.01.01 Denial
40.01.02 Displacement
40.01.03 Fixation
40.01.04 Introjection (identification/incorporation)
40.01.05 Isolation
40.01.06 Projection
40.01.07 Rationalization
40.01.08 Reaction formation
40.01.09 Regression
40.01.10 Repression
40.01.11 Sublimation
40.01.12 Turning against the self
40.01.13 Undoing
40.02 Impaired appropriateness of defenses
40.03 Impaired focus of defenses
40.04 Impaired range of defenses
40.99 Excess of or deficit in defenses NOS
E. Perceptual/Cognitive Human Response Patterns
50. Alterations in Perception/Cognition
50.01 Alterations in attention
50.01.01 Distractibility
50.01.02 Hyperalertness
50.01.03 Inattention
50.01.04 Selective attention
50.02 Alterations in intelligence
50.02.01 Impaired intellectual functioning
50.02.02 Knowledge deficit
50.03 Alterations in judgment
50.03.01 Blocking of ideas
50.03.02 Circumstantial thinking
50.03.03 Constructional difficulty
50.03.04 Flight of ideas
50.03.05 Impaired abstract thinking
50.03.06 Impaired concentration
50.03.07 Impaired judgment
50.03.08 Impaired learning
50.03.09 Impaired logical thinking
50.03.10 Impaired problem-solving
50.03.11 Impaired thought processes
50.03.12 Indecisiveness
50.03.13 Loose associations
50.04 Alterations in memory
50.04.01 Amnesia
50.04.02 Distorted memory
50.04.03 Forgetfulness
50.04.04 Impaired long-term memory

50.04.05   Impaired short-term memory
50.04.06   Selective memory
50.05   Alterations in orientation
50.05.01   Autism
50.05.02   Confusion
50.05.03   Delirium
50.05.04   Disorientation
50.06   Alterations in perception
50.06.01   Delusions
50.06.02   Hallucinations
50.06.03   Illusions
50.06.04   Impaired comfort/pain
50.06.05   Impaired self-awareness
50.07   Alterations in self-concept
50.07.01   Impaired body image
50.07.02   Impaired gender identity
50.07.03   Impaired personal identity
50.07.04   Impaired self-esteem
50.07.05   Impaired social identity
50.08   Alterations in thought content
50.08.01   Ideas of reference

50.08.02   Illusions
50.08.03   Impaired insight
50.08.04   Magical thinking
50.08.05   Misinterpretation
50.08.06   Obsessions
50.08.07   Suicidal/homicidal ideation
50.99   Alterations in perception/cognition NOS

F.   Value/Belief Response Patterns
60.   Alterations in Spirituality
60.01   Spiritual despair
60.02   Spiritual distress
60.03   Spiritual concerns
60.99   Alterations in spirituality NOS
61.   Alterations in Values
60.01
60.01.01   Conflict with social order
60.01.02   Inability to internalize values
60.01.03   Unclarified values
60.99   Alterations in values NOS

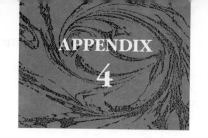

DSM-III-R CLASSIFICATION: AXES I AND II CATEGORIES AND CODES

All official DSM-III-R codes are included in ICD-9-CM. Codes followed by a * are used for more than one DSM-III-R diagnosis or subtype in order to maintain compatibility with ICD-9-CM.

A long dash following a diagnostic term indicates the need for a fifth digit subtype or other qualifying term.

The term *specify* following the name of some diagnostic categories indicates qualifying terms that clinicians may wish to add in parentheses after the name of the disorder.

NOS = Not Otherwise Specified

The current severity of a disorder may be specified after the diagnosis as:

> mild ⎤
> moderate ⎬ currently meets diagnostic criteria
> severe ⎦
> in partial remission
>   (or residual state)
> in complete remission

Disorders Usually First Evident in Infancy, Childhood, or Adolescence

Developmental Disorders
Note: These are coded on Axis II.

Mental Retardation

317.00	Mild mental retardation
318.00	Moderate mental retardation
318.10	Severe mental retardation

© Copyright 1987, American Psychiatric Association

318.20	Profound mental retardation
319.00	Unspecified mental retardation

Pervasive Developmental Disorders

299.00	Autistic disorder *Specify* if childhood onset.
299.80	Pervasive developmental disorder NOS

Specific Developmental Disorders

	Academic skills disorders
315.10	Developmental arithmetic disorder
315.80	Developmental expressive writing disorder
315.00	Developmental reading disorder
	Language and speech disorders
315.39	Developmental articulation disorder
315.31*	Developmental expressive language disorder
315.31*	Developmental receptive language disorder
	Motor skills disorder
315.40	Developmental coordination disorder
315.90*	Specific developmental disorder NOS

Other Developmental Disorders

315.90*	Developmental disorder NOS

Disruptive Behavior Disorders

314.01	Attention-deficit hyperactivity disorder
	Conduct disorder,
312.20	group type
312.00	solitary aggressive type
312.90	undifferentiated type
313.81	Oppositional defiant disorder

Anxiety Disorders of Childhood or Adolescence

309.21 Separation anxiety disorder
313.21 Avoidant disorder of childhood or adolescence
313.00 Overanxious disorder

Eating Disorders

307.10 Anorexia nervosa
307.51 Bulimia nervosa
307.52 Pica
307.53 Rumination disorder of infancy
307.50 Eating disorder NOS

Gender Identity Disorders

302.60 Gender identity disorder of childhood
302.50 Transsexualism
    Specify sexual history: asexual, homosexual, heterosexual, unspecified.
302.85* Gender identity disorder of adolescence or adulthood, nontranssexual type
    Specify sexual history: asexual, homosexual, heterosexual, unspecified.
302.85* Gender identity disorder NOS

Tic Disorders

307.23 Tourette's disorder
307.22 Chronic motor or vocal tic disorder
307.21 Transient tic disorder
    Specify: single episode or recurrent.
307.20 Tic disorder NOS

Elimination Disorders

307.70 Functional encopresis
    Specify: primary or secondary type.
307.60 Functional enuresis
    Specify: primary or secondary type.
    Specify: nocturnal only, diurnal only, nocturnal and diurnal.

Speech Disorders Not Elsewhere Classified

307.00* Cluttering
307.00* Stuttering

Other Disorders of Infancy, Childhood, or Adolescence

313.23 Elective mutism
313.82 Identity disorder
313.89 Reactive attachment disorder of infancy or early childhood
307.30 Stereotypy/habit disorder
314.00 Undifferentiated attention-deficit disorder

Organic Mental Disorders

Dementias Arising in the Senium and Presenium

Primary degenerative dementia of the Alzheimer type, senile onset
290.30 with delirium
290.20 with delusions
290.21 with depression
290.00* uncomplicated
(Note: code 331.00 Alzheimer's disease on Axis III.)

Code in fifth digit: 1 = with delirium, 2 = with delusions, 3 = with depression, 0* = uncomplicated.

290.1x Primary degenerative dementia of the Alzheimer type, presenile onset, _____
(Note: code 331.00 Alzheimer's disease on Axis III.)
290.4x Multi-infarct dementia, _____
290.00* Senile dementia NOS
    Specify etiology on Axis III if known.
290.10* Presenile dementia NOS
    Specify etiology on Axis III if known (*e.g.,* Pick's disease, Jakob-Creutzfeldt disease).

Psychoactive Substance-Induced Organic Mental Disorders

Alcohol
303.00 intoxication
291.40 idiosyncratic intoxication
291.80 uncomplicated alcohol withdrawal
291.00 withdrawal delirium
291.30 hallucinosis
291.10 amnestic disorder
291.20 dementia associated with alcoholism

Amphetamine or similarly acting sympathomimetic
305.70* intoxication
292.00* withdrawal
292.81* delirium
292.11* delusional disorder

Caffeine
305.90* intoxication

Cannabis
305.20* intoxication
292.11* delusional disorder

Cocaine
305.60* intoxication
292.00* withdrawal
292.81* delirium
292.11* delusional disorder

Hallucinogen
305.30* hallucinosis
292.11* delusional disorder
292.84* mood disorder
292.89* posthallucinogen perception disorder

Inhalant
305.90* intoxication

Nicotine
292.00* withdrawal

Opioid
305.50* intoxication
292.00* withdrawal

Phencyclidine (PCP) or similarly acting
arylcyclohexylamine

305.90*	intoxication
292.81*	delirium
292.11*	delusional disorder
292.84*	mood disorder
292.90*	organic mental disorder NOS

Sedative, hypnotic, or anxiolytic

305.40*	intoxication
292.00*	uncomplicated sedative, hypnotic, or anxiolytic withdrawal
292.00*	withdrawal delirium
292.83*	amnestic disorder

Other or unspecified psychoactive substance

305.90*	intoxication
292.00*	withdrawal
292.81*	delirium
292.82*	dementia
292.83*	amnestic disorder
292.11*	delusional disorder
292.12	hallucinosis
292.84*	mood disorder
292.89*	anxiety disorder
292.89*	personality disorder
292.90*	organic mental disorder NOS

Organic Mental Disorders associated with Axis III physical disorders or conditions, or whose etiology is unknown

293.00	Delirium
294.10	Dementia
294.00	Amnestic disorder
293.81	Organic delusional disorder
293.82	Organic hallucinosis
293.83	Organic mood disorder
	Specify: manic, depressed, mixed.
294.80*	Organic anxiety disorder
310.10	Organic personality disorder
	Specify if explosive type.
294.80*	Organic mental disorder NOS

Psychoactive Substance Use Disorders

Alcohol

303.90	dependence
305.00	abuse

Amphetamine or similarly acting sympathomimetic

304.40	dependence
305.70*	abuse

Cannabis

304.30	dependence
305.20*	abuse

Cocaine

304.20	dependence
305.60*	abuse

Hallucinogen

304.50*	dependence
305.30*	abuse

Inhalant

304.60	dependence
305.90*	abuse

Nicotine

305.10	dependence

Opioid

304.00	dependence
305.50*	abuse

Phencyclidine (PCP) or similarly acting
arylcyclohexylamine

304.50*	dependence
305.90*	abuse

Sedative, hypnotic, or anxiolytic

304.10	dependence
305.40*	abuse
304.90*	Polysubstance dependence
304.90*	Psychoactive substance dependence NOS
305.90*	Psychoactive substance abuse NOS

Schizophrenia

Code in fifth digit: 1 = subchronic, 2 = chronic, 3 = subchronic with acute exacerbation, 4 = chronic with acute exacerbation, 5 = in remission, 0 = unspecified.

Schizophrenia

295.2x	catatonic, _____
295.1x	disorganized, _____
295.3x	paranoid, _____
	Specify if stable type.
295.9x	undifferentiated, _____
295.6x	residual, _____
	Specify if late onset.

Delusional (Paranoid) Disorder

297.10	Delusional (paranoid) disorder

Specify type: erotomanic
grandiose
jealous
persecutory
somatic
unspecified

Psychotic Disorders Not Elsewhere Classified

298.80	Brief reactive psychosis
295.40	Schizophreniform disorder
	Specify: without good prognostic features or with good prognostic features.
295.70	Schizoaffective disorder
	Specify: bipolar type or depressive type.
297.30	induced psychotic disorder
298.90	Psychotic disorder NOS (Atypical psychosis)

Mood Disorders

Code current state of Major Depression and Bipolar Disorder in fifth digit:

1 = mild
2 = moderate
3 = severe, without psychotic features
4 = with psychotic features (*specify* mood-congruent or mood-incongruent)
5 = in partial remission
6 = in full remission
0 = unspecified

For major depressive episodes, *specify* if chronic and *specify* if melancholic type.

For Bipolar Disorder, Bipolar Disorder NOS, Recurrent Major Depression, and Depressive Disorder NOS, *specify* if seasonal pattern.

Bipolar Disorders

Bipolar disorder
296.6x	mixed, _____
296.4x	manic, _____
296.5x	depressed, _____
301.13	Cyclothymia
296.70	Bipolar disorder NOS

Depressive Disorders

Major Depression
296.2x	single episode, _____
296.3x	recurrent, _____
300.40	Dysthymia (or Depressive neurosis)
	Specify: primary or secondary type.
	Specify: early or late onset.
311.00	Depressive disorder NOS

Anxiety Disorders (or Anxiety and Phobic Neuroses)

Panic disorder
300.21	with agoraphobia
	Specify current severity of agoraphobic avoidance.
	Specify current severity of panic attacks.
300.01	without agoraphobia
	Specify current severity of panic attacks.
300.22	Agoraphobia without history of panic disorder
	Specify with or without limited symptom attacks.
300.23	Social phobia
	Specify if generalized type.
300.29	Simple phobia
300.30	Obsessive compulsive disorder (or Obsessive compulsive neurosis)
309.89	Post-traumatic stress disorder
	Specify if delayed onset.
300.02	Generalized anxiety disorder
300.00	Anxiety disorder NOS

Somatoform Disorders

300.70*	Body dysmorphic disorder
300.11	Conversion disorder (or Hysterical neurosis, conversion type)
	Specify: single episode or recurrent.
300.70*	Hypochondriasis (or Hypochondriacal neurosis)
300.81	Somatization disorder
307.80	Somatoform pain disorder
300.70*	Undifferentiated somatoform disorder
300.70*	Somatoform disorder NOS

Dissociative Disorders (or Hysterical Neuroses, Dissociative Type)

300.14	Multiple personality disorder
300.13	Psychogenic fugue
300.12	Psychogenic amnesia
300.60	Depersonalization disorder (or Depersonalization neurosis)
300.15	Dissociative disorder NOS

Sexual Disorders

Paraphilias

302.40	Exhibitionism
302.81	Fetishism
302.89	Frotteurism
302.20	Pedophilia
	Specify: same sex, opposite sex, same and opposite sex.
	Specify if limited to incest.
	Specify: exclusive type or nonexclusive type.
302.83	Sexual masochism
302.84	Sexual sadism
302.30	Transvestic fetishism
302.82	Voyeurism
302.90*	Paraphilia NOS

Sexual Dysfunctions

Specify: psychogenic only, or psychogenic and biogenic. (Note: If biogenic only, code on Axis III.)
Specify: lifelong or acquired.
Specify: generalized or situational.

Sexual desire disorders
302.71	Hypoactive sexual desire disorder
302.79	Sexual aversion disorder

Sexual arousal disorders
302.72*	Female sexual arousal disorder
302.72*	Male erectile disorder

Orgasm disorders
302.73	Inhibited female orgasm
302.74	Inhibited male orgasm
302.75	Premature ejaculation

Sexual pain disorders

302.76	Dyspareunia
306.51	Vaginismus
302.70	Sexual dysfunction NOS

Other Sexual Disorders

302.90*	Sexual disorder NOS

Sleep Disorders

Dyssomnias

Insomnia disorder

307.42*	related to another mental disorder (nonorganic)
780.50*	related to known organic factor
307.42*	Primary insomnia

Hypersomnia disorder

307.44	related to another mental disorder (nonorganic)
780.50*	related to a known organic factor
780.54	Primary hypersomnia
307.45	Sleep–wake schedule disorder
	Specify: advanced or delayed phase type, disorganized type, frequently changing type.

Other dyssomnias

307.40*	Dyssomnia NOS

Parasomnias

307.47	Dream anxiety disorder (Nightmare disorder)
307.46*	Sleep terror disorder
307.46*	Sleepwalking disorder
307.40*	Parasomnia NOS

Factitious Disorders

Factitious disorder

301.51	with physical symptoms
300.16	with psychological symptoms
300.19	Factitious disorder NOS

Impulse Control Disorders Not Elsewhere Classified

312.34	Intermittent explosive disorder
312.32	Kleptomania
312.31	Pathological gambling
312.33	Pyromania
312.39*	Trichotillomania
312.39*	Impulse control disorder NOS

Adjustment Disorder

Adjustment disorder

309.24	with anxious mood
309.00	with depressed mood
309.30	with disturbance of conduct
309.40	with mixed disturbance of emotions and conduct
309.28	with mixed emotional features
309.82	with physical complaints
309.83	with withdrawal
309.23	with work (or academic) inhibition
309.90	Adjustment disorder NOS

Psychological Factors Affecting Physical Condition

316.00	Psychological factors affecting physical condition
	Specify physical condition on Axis III.

Personality Disorders
Note: These are coded on Axis II.

Cluster A

301.00	Paranoid
301.20	Schizoid
301.22	Schizotypal

Cluster B

301.70	Antisocial
301.83	Borderline
301.50	Histrionic
301.81	Narcissistic

Cluster C

301.82	Avoidant
301.60	Dependent
301.40	Obsessive compulsive
301.84	Passive aggressive
301.90	Personality disorder NOS

V Codes for Conditions Not Attributable to a Mental Disorder that Are a Focus of Attention or Treatment

V62.30	Academic problem
V71.01	Adult antisocial behavior

V40.00	Borderline intellectual functioning (Note: This is coded on Axis II.)

V71.02	Childhood or adolescent antisocial behavior
V65.20	Malingering
V61.10	Marital problem
V15.81	Noncompliance with medical treatment

V62.20   Occupational problem
V61.20   Parent–child problem
V62.81   Other interpersonal problem
V61.80   Other specified family circumstances
V62.89   Phase of life problem or other life
         circumstance problem
V62.82   Uncomplicated bereavement

| V71.09* | No diagnosis or condition on Axis II |
| 799.90* | Diagnosis or condition deferred on Axis II |

Additional Codes

300.90   Unspecified mental disorder (nonpsychotic)
V71.09* No diagnosis or condition on Axis I
799.90* Diagnosis or condition deferred on Axis I

Multiaxial System

Axis I	Clinical Syndromes
	V Codes
Axis II	Developmental Disorders
	Personality Disorders
Axis III	Physical Disorders and Conditions
Axis IV	Severity of Psychosocial Stressors
Axis V	Global Assessment of Functioning

SEVERITY OF PSYCHOSOCIAL STRESSORS SCALE: ADULTS

| | | EXAMPLES OF STRESSORS | |
CODE	TERM	ACUTE EVENTS	ENDURING CIRCUMSTANCES
1	None	No acute events that may be relevant to the disorder	No enduring circumstances that may be relevant to the disorder
2	Mild	Broke up with boyfriend or girlfriend; started or graduated from school; child left home	Family arguments; job dissatisfaction; residence in high-crime neighborhood
3	Moderate	Marriage; marital separation; loss of job; retirement; miscarriage	Marital discord; serious financial problems; trouble with boss; being a single parent
4	Severe	Divorce; birth of first child	Unemployment; poverty
5	Extreme	Death of spouse; serious physical illness diagnosed; victim of rape	Serious chronic illness in self or child; ongoing physical or sexual abuse
6	Catastrophic	Death of child; suicide of spouse; devastating natural disaster	Captivity as hostage; concentration camp experience
0	Inadequate information, or no change in condition		

SEVERITY OF PSYCHOSOCIAL STRESSORS SCALE: CHILDREN AND ADOLESCENTS

| | | EXAMPLES OF STRESSORS | |
CODE	TERM	ACUTE EVENTS	ENDURING CIRCUMSTANCES
1	None	No acute events that may be relevant to the disorder	No enduring circumstances that may be relevant to the disorder
2	Mild	Broke up with boyfriend or girlfriend; change of school	Overcrowded living quarters; family arguments
3	Moderate	Expelled from school; birth of sibling	Chronic disabling illness in parent; chronic parental discord
4	Severe	Divorce of parents; unwanted pregnancy; arrest	Harsh or rejecting parents; chronic life-threatening illness in parent; multiple foster home placements
5	Extreme	Sexual or physical abuse; death of a parent	Recurrent sexual or physical abuse
6	Catastrophic	Death of both parents	Chronic life-threatening illness
0	Inadequate information, or no change in condition		

GLOBAL ASSESSMENT OF FUNCTIONING SCALE (GAF SCALE)

Consider psychological, social, and occupational functioning on a hypothetical continuum of mental health–illness. Do not include impairment in functioning due to physical (or environmental) limitations.

Note: Use intermediate codes when appropriate, *e.g.,* 45, 68, 72.

CODE

90 ⎤ 81 ⎦	**Absent or minimal symptoms** (*e.g.,* mild anxiety before an exam), **good functioning in all areas, interested and involved in a wide range of activities, socially effective, generally satisfied with life, no more than everyday problems or concerns** (*e.g.,* an occasional argument with family members)
80 ⎤ 71 ⎦	**If symptoms are present, they are transient and expectable reactions to psychosocial stressors** (*e.g.,* difficulty concentrating after family argument); **no more than slight impairment in social, occupational, or school functioning** (*e.g.,* temporarily falling behind in school work).
70 ⎤ 61 ⎦	**Some mild symptoms** (*e.g.,* depressed mood and mild insomnia) **OR some difficulty in social, occupational, or school functioning** (*e.g.,* occasional truancy, or theft within the household), **but generally functioning pretty well, has some meaningful interpersonal relationships**
60 ⎤ 51 ⎦	**Moderate symptoms** (*e.g.,* flat affect and circumstantial speech, occasional panic attacks) **OR moderate difficulty in social, occupational, or school functioning** (*e.g.,* few friends, conflicts with co-workers)
50 ⎤ 41 ⎦	**Serious symptoms** (*e.g.,* suicidal ideation, severe obsessional rituals, frequent shoplifting) **OR any serious impairment in social, occupational, or school functioning** (*e.g.,* no friends, unable to keep a job)
40 ⎤ 31 ⎦	**Some impairment in reality testing or communication** (*e.g.,* speech is at times illogical, obscure, or irrelevant) **OR major impairment in several areas, such as work or school, family relations, judgment, thinking, or mood** (*e.g.,* depressed man avoids friends, neglects family, and is unable to work; child frequently beats up younger children, is defiant at home, and is failing at school)
30 ⎤ 21 ⎦	**Behavior considerably influenced by delusions or hallucinations OR serious impairment in communication or judgment** (*e.g.,* sometimes incoherent, acts grossly inappropriately, suicidal preoccupation) **OR inability to function in almost all areas** (*e.g.,* stays in bed all day; no job, home, or friends)
20 ⎤ 11 ⎦	**Some danger of hurting self or others** (*e.g.,* suicide attempts without clear expectation of death, frequently violent, manic excitement) **OR occasionally fails to maintain minimal personal hygiene** (*e.g.,* smears feces) **OR gross impairment in communication** (*e.g.,* largely incoherent or mute)
10 ⎤ 1 ⎦	**Persistent danger of severely hurting self or others** (*e.g.,* recurrent violence) **OR persistent inability to maintain minimal personal hygiene OR serious suicidal act with clear expectation of death**

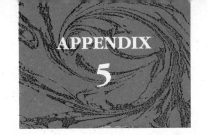

MENTAL HEALTH RESOURCES

Abuse

Clearinghouse on Child Abuse and Neglect
P.O. Box 1182
Washington, DC 20013

Emerge (a men's group that works with batterers)
25 Huntington Avenue, Room 324
Boston, MA 02116

National Clearinghouse on Child Abuse and Neglect
    Information
P.O. Box 1182
Washington, DC 20013
(800) 251-5157

Parents Anonymous (a support group of parents who
    share concerns about child abuse and neglect)
Call (800) 421-0353 for a local chapter.

Addictions

Addicts Anonymous
P.O. Box 2000
Lexington, KY 41001

Narcotics Anonymous
P.O. Box 622
Sun Valley, CA 91352
(818) 997-3822

National Clearinghouse for Drug Abuse Information
P.O. Box 416
Kensington, MD 20795

National Nurses' Society on Addictions (NNSA)
2506 Grosse Point Road
Evanston, IL 60201
(312) 475-7300

Pills Anonymous
184 East 76th Street
New York, NY 10021

Alcoholism

Alcoholics Anonymous
P.O. Box 459
Grand Central Station
New York, NY 10163
Call (212) 686-1100 or look in the telephone directory
    for a local number.

Alcohol Hotline
(800) ALC-OHOL (252-6465)

Al-Anon Family Groups
P.O. Box 182
Madison Square Station
New York, NY 10010

Children of Alcoholics Foundation
540 Madison Avenue
New York, NY 10022

National Institute on Alcohol Abuse and Alcoholism
National Clearinghouse for Alcohol Information
P.O. Box 2345
Rockville, MD 20852
(301) 468-2600

Women for Sobriety, Inc.
P.O. Box 618
Quakertown, PA 18951
(215) 536-8026

Alzheimer's Disease

Alzheimer's Disease and Related Disorders Association,
    Inc.: National Headquarters
360 North Michigan Avenue, Suite 601
Chicago, IL 60601
(800) 621-0379; in Illinois (800) 572-6037

Autism

Autism Society of America
1234 Massachusetts Avenue, NW, Suite 1017
Washington, DC 20005
(202) 783-0125

Dying—Death

Concern for Dying
250 W. 57th Street, Room 831
New York, NY 10107
(212) 246-6962

National Hospice Organization
1311-A Dolly Madison Boulevard
McLean, VA 22101
(703) 356-6770

Eating Disorders

The American Anorexia Nervosa Association, Inc.
133 Cedar Lane
Teaneck, NJ 07666

Anorexia Nervosa and Related Eating Disorders, Inc.
P.O. Box 5102
Eugene, OR 97405

National Association to Aid Fat Americans, Inc.
P.O. Box 43
Bellerose, NY 11426
(516) 352-3120

Elderly Concerns

American Association of Retired Persons
Program Department
1909 K Street, NW
Washington, DC 20049
(202) 872-4922

Gerontological Society of America
1411 K Street, NW, Suite 300
Washington, DC 20005
(202) 393-1411

Gray Panthers: National Office
3635 Chestnut Street
Philadelphia, PA 19104
(215) 382-3300

Widowed Persons' Service
K Street, NW
Washington, DC 20049

Health-Related Organizations and Information

American Nurses' Association
Council on Psychiatric and Mental Health Nursing
2420 Pershing Road
Kansas City, MO 64108

National Alliance for the Mentally Ill
1901 Fort Myer Drive, Suite 500
Arlington, VA 22209
(703) 524-7600

National Center for Health Statistics
Department of Health and Human Services
Public Health Service
3700 East-West Highway
Hyattsville, MD 20782

National Citizens' Coalition for Nursing Home Reform
1424 16th Street, NW, Suite 204
Washington, DC 20036
(202) 797-8227

National Health Information Center
P.O. Box 1133
Washington, DC 20013-1133
(800) 336-4797

The National Information System for Health-Related Services
University of South Carolina
1244 Blossom Street
Columbia, SC 29208

National Institute of Mental Health
Public Inquiries Branch
Parklawn Building, Room 15C05
Rockville, MD 20857
(301) 443-4517

National Mental Health Association
1021 Prince Street
Alexandria, VA 22314

Self-Help

National Self-Help Clearinghouse
33 West 42nd Street
New York, NY 10036

Sexuality—Sexually Transmitted Diseases

AIDS Hotline
(800) 342-AIDS (342-2437)

Gay Men's Health Crisis
Box 274
132 West 24th Street

New York, NY 10011
(212) 807-6655

National Gay Task Force
80 Fifth Avenue
New York, NY 10011
(212) 741-5800

Sex Information and Education Council of the United
  States (SIECUS)
New York University
32 Washington Place
New York, NY 10003
(212) 673-3850

Sexually Transmitted Disease Information
(800) 227-8922

Suicide

Youth Suicide National Center
1811 Trousdale Drive
Burlingame, CA 94010
(415) 877-5604

Womens' Issues

Older Women's League: National Office
1325 G Street, NW, Lower Level B
Washington, DC 20005
(202) 783-6686

Working Women's Institute (Provides information concerning sexual harassment)
593 Park Avenue
New York, NY 10021

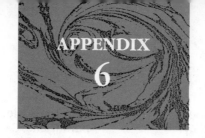

STANDARDS OF PSYCHIATRIC AND MENTAL HEALTH NURSING PRACTICE*

Standard I. Theory

The nurse applies appropriate theory that is scientifically sound as a basis for decisions regarding nursing practice.

Standard II. Data Collection

The nurse continuously collects data that are comprehensive, accurate, and systematic.

Standard III. Diagnosis

The nurse utilizes nursing diagnoses and/or standard classification of mental disorders to express conclusions supported by recorded assessment data and current scientific premises.

Standard IV. Planning

The nurse develops a nursing care plan with specific goals and interventions delineating nursing actions unique to each client's needs.

Standard V. Intervention

The nurse intervenes as guided by the nursing care plan to implement nursing actions that promote, maintain, or restore physical and mental health, prevent illness, and effect rehabilitation.

Standard V-A. Intervention: Psychotherapeutic Interventions

The nurse uses psychotherapeutic interventions to assist clients in regaining or improving their previous coping abilities and to prevent further disability.

Standard V-B. Intervention: Health Teaching

The nurse assists clients, families, and groups to achieve satisfying and productive patterns of living through health teaching.

Standard V-C. Intervention: Activities of Daily Living

The nurse uses the activities of daily living in a goal-directed way to foster adequate self-care and physical and mental well-being of clients.

Standard V-D. Intervention: Somatic Therapies

The nurse uses knowledge of somatic therapies and applies related clinical skills in working with clients.

Standard V-E. Intervention: Therapeutic Environment

The nurse provides, structures, and maintains a therapeutic environment in collaboration with the client and other health care providers.

Standard V-F. Intervention: Psychotherapy

The nurse utilizes advanced clinical expertise in individual, group, and family psychotherapy, child psychotherapy, and other treatment modalities to function as a psychotherapist, and recognizes professional accountability for nursing practice.

---

* American Nurses' Association: Standards of Psychiatric and Mental Health Nursing Practice. Kansas City, Missouri, American Nurses' Association, 1982.

Standard VI. Evaluation

The nurse evaluates client responses to nursing actions in order to revise the data base, nursing diagnoses, and nursing care plan.

Professional Performance Standards

Standard VII. Peer Review

The nurse participates in peer review and other means of evaluation to assure quality of nursing care provided for clients.

Standard VIII. Continuing Education

The nurse assumes responsibility for continuing education and professional development and contributes to the professional growth of others.

Standard IX. Interdisciplinary Collaboration

The nurse collaborates with other health care providers in assessing, planning, implementing, and evaluating programs and other mental health activities.

Standard X. Utilization of Community Health Systems

The nurse participates with other members of the community in assessing, planning, implementing, and evaluating mental health services and community systems that include the promotion of the broad continuum of primary, secondary, and tertiary prevention of mental illness.

Standard XI. Research

The nurse contributes to nursing and the mental health field through innovations in theory and practice and participation in research.

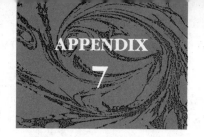

PSYCHOTROPIC DRUGS

Important Notice

Pharmacology is a rapidly changing science. In the psychiatric field, new drugs are continually being formulated and drug therapies continue to change to meet client needs. Therefore, information regarding acceptable methods of pharmacologic intervention with clients is constantly evolving. The author and editors of this book have made every effort to ensure that the information provided in this Appendix is accurate, complete, up-to-date, and in accordance with present, commonly acceptable standards. However, readers are advised to consult product manufacturers' information, packaged with each drug, to determine whether contraindications, dosage instructions, or warnings have been changed or updated. This information is particularly important with new drugs or drugs that are prescribed infrequently.

Antianxiety Drugs

Benzodiazepines

Actions

Although the exact mechanism is unknown, these agents act at the limbic, thalamic, and hypothalamic levels of the CNS, producing all levels of CNS depression, from mild sedation to hypnosis to coma.

Uses

Indicated for relief of tension, anxiety, and fear. Different benzodiazepines have varying anticonvulsant, hypnotic, sedative, and skeletal muscle-relaxant effects. Also used in management of delirium tremens following alcohol withdrawal. Mild analgesia and some appetite stimulation have been noted.

Contraindications

Benzodiazepines should not be used in clients with known hypersensitivity, acute narrow-angle glaucoma, or

Acknowledgement is given to Bruce D. Clayton, Pharm. D., University of Arkansas, for his assistance in reviewing this Appendix.

psychoses. Use is not recommended during pregnancy and lactation.

Side-Effects

Sedation, drowsiness, lethargy, and ataxia are common. Other side-effects include nausea, vomiting, diarrhea, constipation, urinary retention, rashes, urticaria, and pruritis. Psychiatric side-effects include paradoxical reactions (anxiety, hallucinations, hyperexcitement, and depression). Prolonged use of hypnotic agents may produce vivid dreams and/or nightmares.

Drug Interactions

Additive effects result from use of benzodiazepines with other sedative-hypnotics. Serious toxic effects result from use with MAO inhibitors, alcohol, antihistamines, analgesics, anesthetics, narcotics, and cimetidine. Metabolism of benzodiazepines is enhanced by smoking; larger doses may be needed in clients who smoke.

Warnings

Clients can develop a tolerance for (or dependence upon) benzodiazepines. Withdrawal symptoms may appear following abrupt discontinuation after using high dosages for prolonged periods. Decrease dosage gradually to avoid possibility of withdrawal symptoms. When depression accompanies anxiety, suicide precautions should be instituted.

Overdosage

Symptoms include somnolence, diminished or absent reflexes, confusion, hypotension, impaired coordination, and coma. Treatment includes gastric lavage, administration of IV fluids, maintenance of an adequate airway, and monitoring of vital signs. Do **not** administer barbiturates.

Client Education

Instruct clients as follows: Take medication as ordered; do not change dosage; do not stop taking this medication abruptly. Do not take this drug with other CNS drugs or alcohol. Consult a health care provider before taking any other prescription or nonprescription drugs. If side-effects appear, consult a health care provider immediately. Benzodiazepines can cause drowsiness, dizziness,

ANTIANXIETY DRUGS

GENERIC NAME; BRAND NAME	FORMS AVAILABLE	DOSAGES	COMMENTS
ALPRAZOLAM			
Xanax	Tabs: 0.25, 0.5, 1 mg	0.25-0.5 mg, 3 times/day; maximum dose, 4 mg/day	
CLORAZEPATE DIPOTASSIUM			
Tranxene	Tabs and caps: 3.75, 7.5, 15 mg Tabs: 11.25 mg	For anxiety: 30 mg/day in 3 divided doses; gradually increase to 15-60 mg/day; may be given as single dose of 15 mg at bedtime. Elderly: initial dose is 7.5-15 mg/day.	Also used for relief of alcohol withdrawal symptoms and partial seizure management
Tranxene-SD Half Strength Tranxene-SD	Tabs: 22.5 mg		
CHLORDIAZEPOXIDE			
Librium	Caps and tabs: 5, 10, 25 mg Inj: 100 mg	Adults: 5-25 mg, 3 or 4 times/day Elderly: 5 mg, 2-4 times/day Children: 5 mg, 2-4 times/day (not recommended for children under 6 years of age)	Various combination products also available; also used for alcohol withdrawal symptoms
Libritabs			
* A-poxide			
* Medilium			
* Novopoxide			
* Solium			
DIAZEPAM			
Valium	Tabs: 2, 5, 10 mg Inj: 5 mg	Adults: 2-10 mg, 2-4 times/day Elderly: 2-2.5 mg, 1 or 2 times/day Children: 1-2.5 mg, 3 or 4 times/day	Dosages may be increased gradually as needed and tolerated; also used as an anticonvulsant and muscle relaxant
Valrelease	Caps: 15 mg timed release		
* D-Tran			
* E-Pam			
* Meval			
* Stress-Pam			
* Vivol			
FLURAZEPAM			
Dalmane	Caps: 15, 30 mg	Adults: 15 or 30 mg, at bedtime Elderly: 15 mg, at bedtime initially	Hypnotic
* Somnol			
HALAZEPAM			
Paxipam	Tabs: 20, 40 mg	Adults: 20-40 mg, 3 or 4 times/day Elderly: 20 mg, 1 or 2 times/day	
LORAZEPAM			
Ativan	Tabs: 0.5, 1, 2 mg Inj: 2, 4 mg/ml	Adults: 2-6 mg/day, in divided doses, largest dose at bedtime Elderly: initial dose of 1-2 mg/day, in divided doses; increase as needed and tolerated	
OXAZEPAM			
Serax	Tabs: 15 mg Caps: 10, 15, 30 mg	Adults: for mild to moderate anxiety, 10-15 mg, 3 to 4 times/day; for severe anxiety, 15-30 mg, 3 to 4 times/day Elderly: 10 mg, 3 times/day; increase gradually to 15 mg, 3 to 4 times/day	Also used for alcohol withdrawal symptoms
PRAZEPAM			
Centrax	Tabs: 10 mg Caps: 5, 10, 20 mg	Adults: 30 mg/day in divided doses; may be increased gradually to 20-60 mg/day Elderly: 10-15 mg/day in divided doses May be given as a single dose at bedtime; initial dose is 20 mg; optimum dose is 20-50 mg/day	
TEMAZEPAM			
Restoril	Caps: 15, 30 mg	Adults: 15-30 mg, at bedtime Elderly: initial dose is 15 mg	Hypnotic

(Continued)

ANTIANXIETY DRUGS (CONTINUED)

GENERIC NAME; BRAND NAME	FORMS AVAILABLE	DOSAGES	COMMENTS
TRIAZOLAM Halcion	Tabs: 0.125, 0.25, 0.5 mg	Adults: 0.25 or 0.5 mg at bedtime Elderly: initial dose is 0.125 mg; may be increased to 0.25 mg.	Hypnotic

* Available only in Canada.

and lightheadedness. Use caution while driving or operating machinery until effects of drug are known.

Barbiturates

Actions

Barbiturates cause central nervous system depression as a result of a reduction in nerve impulses to the cerebral cortex. Respiratory and muscular function are also depressed by barbiturates. Barbiturates used in psychiatric settings are classified as short-, intermediate-, or long-acting according the duration of their depressive actions.

Duration of Action	Drugs	Onset (P.O.)
Short (3–6 hours)	Pentobarbital	15–30 minutes
	Secobarbital	10–15 minutes
Intermediate (4–10 hours)	Amobarbital	20–30 minutes
	Aprobarbital	20–60 minutes
	Butabarbital	30–60 minutes
	Talbutal	20–60 minutes
Long (10–16 hours)	Mephobarbital	60 minutes
	Phenobarbital	60 minutes

Uses

Indicated for short-term relief of insomnia and anxiety. Because they raise the seizure threshold, selected barbiturates (*e.g.,* phenobarbital) are also used in anticonvulsant therapy.

Contraindications

Barbiturates should not be used in clients with known hypersensitivity, previous history of addiction, hepatic or respiratory impairment, or porphyria.

Side-Effects

Sedation, drowsiness, hangover, and dizziness are common. Other side-effects include nausea, vomiting, rashes, urticaria, asthma, and Stevens-Johnson syndrome. Elderly and debilitated clients occasionally demonstrate marked excitement and confusion rather than sedation.

Drug Interactions

Use with other central nervous system depressants including alcohol, antihistamines, benzodiazepines, methotrimeprazine, narcotics, and other sedative/hypnotics produces additive sedative effects. Since barbiturates are enzyme inducers, they may decrease the effects of other drugs. MAO inhibitors potentiate the CNS depression of barbiturates. Valproic acid and chloramphenicol enhance the sedative/hypnotic effects of barbiturates, apparently by inhibiting the metabolism of the barbiturates.

Warnings

Avoid abrupt withdrawal. Dependence and tolerance can occur with misuse. Extended use can produce sleep pattern disturbances, particularly rebound insomnia. Avoid use of alcohol because of additive CNS depression.

Overdosage

Symptoms include depressed respiration, extreme CNS depression, pupillary constriction, diminished or absent reflexes, shock or coma. Treatment includes removal of drug by emesis in conscious clients or gastric lavage in unconscious clients. Initiate supportive therapy to maintain vital signs, including respiration and blood pressure.

Client Education

Instruct clients as follows: Take medication as ordered; do not change dosage; do not stop taking this medication abruptly. Do not take this drug with other CNS drugs or alcohol. Consult a health care provider before taking any other prescription or nonprescription drugs. Consult a health care provider immediately if any of the following side-effects are noted: abdominal pain, bruising, uncommon bleeding, fever, jaundice, rashes, or sore throat. Barbiturates cause drowsiness; use caution while driving or operating machinery until effects of drug are known.

Other Antianxiety and (Non-Barbiturate) Sedative/Hypnotic Drugs

A variety of other non-barbiturate drugs are used for sedation and insomnia. In general, these drugs are more closely related to the barbiturates than to the benzodiazepines, and have potential for development of tolerance, dependence, abuse, and withdrawal symptoms.

Because contraindications, side-effects, drug interactions, and warnings vary widely, students and practition-

OTHER ANTIANXIETY AND (NON-BARBITURATE) SEDATIVE/HYPNOTIC DRUGS

GENERIC NAME; BRAND NAME	FORMS AVAILABLE	DOSAGES	COMMENTS
ACETYLCARBROMAL			
Paxarel	Tabs: 250 mg	Sedation: 250–500 mg, 2 or 3 times/day	Short-acting
CHLORAL HYDRATE			
Aquachloral Supprettes Chloral Hydrate Noctec * Chloralvan * Novochlorhydrate * Oradrate	Suppos: 324, 500, 648 mg Caps: 250, 500 mg Elix: 500 mg/5 ml Syrup: 250, 500 mg/ml	Sedation: 250 mg, 3 times/day, with food Insomnia: 500 mg–1 g, at bedtime	
ETHCHLORVYNOL			
Placidyl	Caps: 200, 500, 750 mg	Insomnia: 500 mg at bedtime; may be increased to 750–1000 mg for severe insomnia	Do not use for more than 1 week; excitability may precede sedation.
ETHINAMATE			
Valamid	Caps: 500 mg	Insomnia: 500–1000 mg, at bedtime	Do not use for more than 1 week.
GLUTETHIMIDE			
Doriden Glutethimide	Tabs: 250, 500 mg Caps: 500 mg	Insomnia: 250–500 mg, at bedtime	
HYDROXYZINE			
Atarax Anxanil Atozine Durrax Hydroxyzine HCl Hydroxyzine Pamoate Hy-Pam Vamate Vistaril	Tabs: 10, 25, 50, 100 mg Syrup: 10 mg/5 ml Inj: 25, 50 mg/ml Caps: 25, 50, 100 mg Elix: 25 mg/5 ml Susp: 25 mg/5 ml	Anxiety: PO: 50–100 mg, 4 times/day IM: 50–100 mg, every 4–6 hours	Also used as an antiemetic, for alcohol withdrawal symptoms, and as a preoperative sedative
MEPROBAMATE			
Equanil Meprobamate Miltown Meprospan Neuramate * Meditran * Quietae	Caps: 200, 400 mg Tabs: 200, 400, 600 mg	Anxiety: 1200–1600 mg/day, in 3–4 doses Children: 100–200 mg, 3–4 times/day	
METHYPRYLON			
Noludar	Caps: 300 mg Tabs: 50, 200 mg	Insomnia: 200–400 mg, at bedtime	Intermediate-acting
PARALDEHYDE			
Paral Paraldehyde	Liquid: 30 ml (for oral use) Liquid: 1 g/ml (for inj, oral, or rectal use)	Sedation: 5–10 ml orally or rectally IM: 2–5 ml IV: 5 ml diluted	Used primarily in delirium tremens; give orally in milk or juice to mask taste and odor

* Available only in Canada.

BARBITURATES

GENERIC NAME; BRAND NAME	FORMS AVAILABLE	DOSAGES	COMMENTS
AMOBARBITAL AND AMOBARBITAL SODIUM			
Amytal	Caps: 65, 200 mg	Sedation: 30-50 mg, 2-3 times/day	Intermediate-acting; also used as a[n]
Amytal Sodium	Inj: 250, 500 mg	Hypnosis: 100-200 mg, at bedtime	anticonvulsant
* Isabec	Tabs: 30, 100 mg	IM/IV: 65-500 mg, per dose	
APROBARBITAL			
Alurate	Elix: 40 mg/5 ml	Sedation: 40 mg, 3 times/day	Intermediate-acting
		Mild insomnia: 40-80 mg, at bedtime	
		Severe insomnia: 80-160 mg, at bedtime	
BUTABARBITAL SODIUM			
Buticaps	Caps: 15, 30 mg	Sedation: 15-30 mg, 3-4 times/day	Intermediate-acting
Butisol Sodium	Tabs: 15, 30, 50, 100 mg	Insomnia: 50-100 mg, at bedtime	
	Elix: 30 mg/ml		
MEPHOBARBITAL			
Mebaral	Tabs: 32, 50, 100 mg	Sedation: 32-100 mg, 3-4 times/day	Long-acting; also used as an anticonvulsant
PENTOBARBITAL AND PENTOBARBITAL SODIUM			
Nembutal	Elix: 18.2 mg pentobarbital (= to 20 mg	Sedation: 30 mg, 3-4 times/day	Short-acting
Nembutal Sodium	pentobarbital sodium)/5 ml	Insomnia: 100 mg at bedtime	
	Caps: 50, 100 mg		
	Supp: 30, 60, 120, 200 mg		
	Inj: 50 mg/ml		
PHENOBARBITAL AND PHENOBARBITAL SODIUM			
Barbita	Caps: 16 mg	Sedation: 30-120 mg, in 2 or 3	Long-acting; also used as an
Luminal Sodium	Elix: 15, 20 mg/ml	divided doses	anticonvulsant
Phenobarbital	Inj: 30, 60, 65, 130 mg/ml	Insomnia: 100-320 mg, at bedtime	
Phenobarbital Sodium	Tabs: 8, 16, 32, 65, 100 mg		
Solfoton			
* Gardenal			
SECOBARBITAL AND SECOBARBITAL SODIUM			
Secobarbital Sodium	Caps: 50, 100 mg	Insomnia: PO: 100 mg, at bedtime	Short-acting; also used as an
Seconal Sodium	Tabs: 100 mg	IM: 100-200 mg, at bedtime	anticonvulsant; not recommen[ded]
* Novosecobarb	Inj: 50 mg/ml		for long-term sedation
	Rectal inj: 50 mg/ml		
TALBUTAL			
Lotusate	Tabs: 120 mg	Insomnia: 120 mg, at bedtime	Intermediate-acting

* Available only in Canada.

ers should refer to one of the references listed at the end of this appendix.

Antidepressant Drugs

Monoamine Oxidase Inhibitors (MAOI)

Actions

Monoamine oxidase inhibitors (MAOI) block inactivation of biogenic amines, causing an increase in naturally-occurring epinephrine, norepinephrine, and serotonin.

Uses

Indicated for relief of exogenous depression; gene[rally] used in clients who have not responded to other ant[ide]pressant therapy.

Contraindications

MAO inhibitors should not be used in clients with kn[own] hypersensitivity; hepatic or renal failure; congestive h[eart] failure; cerebrovascular disorders; or pheochrom[ocy]toma; in children; or in elderly clients.

Side-Effects

Common side-effects include insomnia, dizziness, agitation, headaches, hypotension, constipation, nausea, vomiting, diarrhea, and abdominal pain. Other side-effects include confusion, edema, urinary retention, and rashes. Serious side-effects include severe hypertension.

Drug Interactions

CNS depressant effects of MAOI may be potentiated by alcohol, hypnotics and sedatives, anesthetics, and narcotics. Severe hypertension may result from concurrent administration with adrenergics, amphetamines, levodopa, methyldopa, reserpine, or vasoconstrictors. MAOI should not be administered with tricyclic antidepressants. Severe hypertension may also result from ingesting foods that are high in tyramine. (See Client Education.)

Warnings

Carefully monitor blood pressure; hypertensive crises can arise within hours after ingestion, and can be severe or fatal. Hypertension is generally first noted as a headache. Benefit to risk must be carefully evaluated in pregnant or nursing women; safety for use during pregnancy and lactation has not been established. Not recommended for use in children under 16.

Overdosage

Symptoms may develop slowly and last for one to two weeks, and may include confusion, excitement, flushing, hyper- or hypotension, convulsion, and coma. Treatment includes gastric lavage and supportive measures to maintain vital signs.

Client Education

Instruct clients as follows: Take medication as ordered; do not change dosage; do not stop taking this medication abruptly. Effects of drug may not be seen for up to four weeks, and continue for two weeks after dosages stop. Do not take this drug with other CNS drugs or alcohol. Consult a health care provider before taking any other prescription or non-prescription drugs. If side-effects appear, consult a health care provider immediately. MAO inhibitors can cause drowsiness, dizziness, and light-headedness. Use caution while driving or operating machinery until effects of drug are known.

Certain foods and beverages contain tyramine and/or other substances that can cause dangerous reactions. Avoid the following while taking MAO inhibitors:

Alcohol: beer, red wine (especially Chianti), sherry
Caffeinated beverages: coffee, tea, cola
Dairy products: cheese (especially aged cheeses), sour cream, yogurt
Fish: caviar; pickled, salted, or smoked fish
Fruits: bananas, figs, raisins
Meats: liver, bologna, pepperoni, salami, tenderized meats
Other: avocado, chocolate, soy sauce, yeast

Antidepressant Drugs

Tricyclic Antidepressants

Actions

Tricyclic antidepressants block the reuptake of norepinephrine and/or serotin at the presynaptic neurons. Other actions include anticholinergic and sedative effects.

Uses

Indicated for treatment of endogenous depression. Not indicated for drug-induced or reactive depression, and seldom used for bipolar (manic–depressive) disorders.

Contraindications

Tricyclic antidepressants should not be used in clients with known hypersensitivity; during the acute recovery phase after myocardial infarction; in hepatic or renal failure; or in narrow-angle glaucoma.

ANTIDEPRESSANT DRUGS: MAO INHIBITORS

GENERIC NAME; BRAND NAME	FORMS AVAILABLE	DOSAGES	COMMENTS
ISOCARBOXAZID			
Marplan	Tabs: 10 mg	Initial: 30 mg/day in divided doses Maintenance: 10–20 mg/day in single or divided doses	Slow-acting; may take several weeks to take effect
PHENELZINE SULFATE			
Nardil	Tabs: 15 mg	Initial: 15 mg, 3 times/day; increase rapidly to 60 mg/day, and then reduce dosage slowly	Slow-acting; may take 4 weeks (at 60 mg/day) for full effect
TRANYLCYPROMIDE SULFATE			
Parnate	Tabs: 10 mg	Initial: 20–30 mg/day in divided doses Maintenance: 10–20 mg/day	Can be used concurrently with ECT; reduce slowly to maintenance dosage

ANTIDEPRESSANT DRUGS: TRICYCLIC ANTIDEPRESSANTS

GENERIC NAME; BRAND NAME	FORMS AVAILABLE	DOSAGES	COMMENTS
AMITRIPTYLINE HYDROCHLORIDE			
Amitril Elavil Emitrip Endep Enovil * Levate * Meravil * Novotriptyn	Inj: 10 mg/ml Tabs: 10, 25, 50, 75, 100, 150 mg	Initial: 25 mg, 2–4 times/day Maintenance: 40–100 mg/day in one or divided doses; or 20–30 mg, 4 times/day	Has a strong sedative effect; may be administered at bedtime; do not administer IV; use IM route only for parenteral administration
AMOXAPINE			
Asendin	Tabs: 25, 50, 100, 150 mg	Initial: 50 mg, 2–3 times/day; increase to 100 mg, 2–3 times/day during first week Maintenance: up to 300 mg, at bedtime Elderly: 25 mg 2–3 times/day, up to 50 mg, 2–3 times/day	Not recommended for children under 16
DESIPRAMINE HYDROCHLORIDE			
Norpramin Pertofrane	Caps: 25, 50 mg Tabs: 10, 25, 50, 75, 100, 150 mg	Initial: 75–200 mg/day, in single or divided doses Maintenance: up to 300 mg/day Adolescents and elderly: 25–100 mg/day	Not recommended for children under 12
DOXEPIN HYDROCHLORIDE			
Adapin Sinequan	Caps: 10, 25, 50, 75, 100, 150 mg Concen: 10 mg/ml	Initial: 25 mg 3 times/day Maintenance: 75–150 mg/day in divided doses or in single dose at bedtime	Not recommended for children under 12
IMIPRAMINE HYDROCHLORIDE/PAMOATE			
Janimine Tipramine Tofranil * Impril * Novopramine	Caps: 75, 100, 125, 150 mg Inj: 25 mg/2 ml Tabs: 10, 25, 50 mg	Initial: 25 mg, 3 times/day; up to 50 mg, 3 times/day Maintenance: 50–150 mg/day, at bedtime Adolescents and elderly: 30–40 mg/day	Also used for childhood enuresis
MAPROTILINE HYDROCHLORIDE			
Ludiomil	Tabs: 25, 50, 75 mg	Initial: 75 mg/day in single or divided doses; increase slowly to 150 mg/day Maintenance: 75–150 mg/day Elderly: 50–75 mg/day	Not recommended for clients under 18
NORTRIPTYLINE HYDROCHLORIDE			
Aventyl HCl Pamelor	Caps: 10, 25, 75 mg Liquid and sol: 10 mg/5 ml	Adults: 25 mg, 3–4 times/day; do not exceed 150 mg/day Adolescents and elderly: 30–50 mg/day in divided doses	Not recommended for children
PROTRIPTYLINE HYDROCHLORIDE			
Vivactil * Triptil	Tabs: 5, 10 mg	Adults: 5–10 mg, 3–4 times/day, up to 60 mg/day Adolescents and elderly: 5 mg, 3 times/day	Not recommended for children
TRIMIPRAMINE MALEATE			
Surmontil	Caps: 25, 50, 100 mg	Initial: 25 mg, 3 times/day, up to 150 mg/day at bedtime Adolescents and elderly: 50–100 mg/day	Not recommended for children

* Available only in Canada.

Side-Effects

Common side-effects include sedation and anticholinergic effects (including blurred vision, confusion, constipation, dry eyes and mouth, and urinary retention).

Drug Interactions

Tricyclic antidepressants are generally not indicated for concommitant use with monoamine oxidase inhibitors (MAOI); use can result in severe hyperpyrexia and hypertension. Use with caution in clients taking guanethidine, anticholinergic drugs, oral contraceptives, and thyroid medications. The depressant actions of alcohol and other CNS depressants are potentiated by tricyclic antidepressants.

Warnings

Use with caution in clients with a history of seizure disorders, since tricyclic antidepressants lower the seizure threshold. Cardiovascular problems, including arrhythmias, increased anginal pain frequency, and orthostatic and postural hypotension may result from use of tricyclic antidepressants. Benefit to risk must be carefully evaluated in pregnant or nursing women; safety for use during pregnancy and lactation has not been established. Not recommended for use in children under 12. Tricyclic antidepressants may cause manic–depressive clients to shift to the manic phase. Paranoid or schizophrenic clients may show increased symptoms. Carefully monitor clients with depression for suicidal ideation or attempts. Limit access to drugs.

Overdosage

Initial symptoms include CNS stimulation, exhibited by agitation, delirium, irritability, hallucinations, hypertension, and seizures. Symptoms progress to CNS depression, including drowsiness, hypotension, respiratory depression, cardiac arrhythmias, and cardiac arrest. Treatment includes gastric lavage and supportive measures to maintain vital signs.

Client Education

Instruct clients as follows: Take medication as ordered; do not change dosage or stop taking this medication abruptly. Effects of drug may not be seen for days or weeks. Do not take this drug with other CNS drugs or alcohol. Consult a health care provider before taking any other prescription or non-prescription drugs. If side-effects appear, consult a health care provider immediately. Use caution while driving or operating machinery until effects of drug are known.

Antipsychotic Drugs

Actions

The method by which antipsychotic agents work is not completely understood. However, some of the actions of antipsychotics include receptor blockade of dopamine in the basal ganglia, brain stem, hypothalamus, limbic system, and medulla, as well as decreased release of dopamine.

Uses

Indicated for control of symptoms of psychotic disorders including, in some cases, schizophrenia. Others are used as antiemetics, and occasionally for the relief of non-psychotic anxiety. See "Comments" below for individual drugs for additional uses.

Contraindications

Antipsychotic drugs should not be used in clients with: known hypersensitivity; bone marrow depression; drug-induced CNS depression; Parkinson's disease; hyper- or hypotension; renal or hepatic disease; circulatory collapse; or blood dyscrasias.

Side-Effects

Antipsychotic drugs can cause extrapyramidal symptoms; tardive dyskinesia; drowsiness; agranulocytosis; hemolytic anemia; increased pulse rates; hyper- or hypotension; ocular changes, including blurred vision; contact dermatitis; photosensitivity; and adverse behavioral changes.

OTHER ANTIDEPRESSANTS

GENERIC NAME; BRAND NAME	FORMS AVAILABLE	DOSAGES	COMMENTS
FLUOXETINE HYDROCHLORIDE			
Prozac	Caps: 20 mg	Initial: 20 mg/day in the morning; doses above 20 mg/day should be divided on a 2 times/day schedule of morning and noon; do not exceed 80 mg/day	Chemically unrelated to other antidepressants
TRAZODONE HYDROCHLORIDE			
Desyrel	Tabs: 50, 100, 150 mg	Initial: 150 mg/day, in divided doses; increase gradually to 600 mg/day maximum Maintenance: use lowest possible dose.	Non-tricyclic, non-MAO inhibitor

ANTIPSYCHOTIC DRUGS

CLASS—GENERIC NAME; BRAND NAME	FORMS AVAILABLE	DOSAGES	COMMENTS
BUTYROPHENONE—HALOPERIDOL			
Haldol * Novoperidol * Peridol	Concen: 2 mg/ml Inj: 5 mg/ml Tabs: 0.5, 1, 2, 5, 10, 20 mg	Adult, moderate symptoms: 0.5–2 mg, 2 or 3 times/day Severe symptoms: 3–5 mg, 2 or 3 times/day, up to 100 mg/day IM: 2–5 mg every 4–8 hours (up to 10–30 mg every 30–60 minutes) Children: 0.5 mg/day, initially, increasing in 0.5-mg increments at 5- to 7-day intervals; dose may be divided and given 2 or 3 times/day	Also used as an antiemetic in small doses
DIBENZOXAZEPINE—LOXAPINE			
Loxitane Loxitane C * Loxapac	Caps: 5, 10, 25, 50 mg Concen: 25 mg/ml Inj: 50 mg/ml	Initial: 10 mg, 2 times/day, up to 50 mg/day Maintenance: usually 20–60 mg/day Severe symptoms: do not exceed 250 mg/day IM: 12.5–50 mg, every 4–6 hours	
DIHYDROINDOLONE—MOLINDONE HYDROCHLORIDE			
Moban	Concen: 20 mg/ml Tabs: 5, 10, 25, 50, 100 mg	Initial: 50–75 mg/day; gradually increased to 100 mg/day within 3 to 4 days; up to 225 mg/day for severe symptoms Maintenance: 5–25 mg, 3 or 4 times/day Elderly: 1/3 to 1/2 adult dose	
PHENOTHIAZINE, ALIPHATIC—CHLORPROMAZINE HYDROCHLORIDE			
Chlorazine Ormazine Promapar Promaz Sonazine Thorazine Thor-Prom * Chlorpromanyl * Largactil	Caps sust rel: 30, 75, 150, 200, 300 mg Concen: 30, 100 mg/ml Inj: 25 mg/ml Suppos: 25, 100 mg Syrup: 10 mg/5 ml Tabs: 10, 25, 50, 100, 200 mg	Initial: PO 10 mg, 3–4 times/day, or 25 mg 2–3 times/day IM: 25 mg; then give 25–50 mg in 1 hour, if needed Maintenance: 200–800 mg/day, in divided doses Children: 0.5 mg/kg every 4–6 hours	Also used in hyperactive children; for relief of preoperative apprehension; for control of intractable hiccoughs
PHENOTHIAZINE, ALIPHATIC—PROMAZINE HYDROCHLORIDE			
Prozine Sparine * Promanyl	Inj: 25, 50 mg/ml Tabs: 25, 50, 100 mg Syrup: 10 mg/5 ml	Initial adult: IM, 50–150 mg PO: 10–200 mg, every 4–6 hours; do not exceed 1000 mg/day Children over 12: 10–25 mg, every 4–6 hours	
PHENOTHIAZINE, ALIPHATIC—TRIFLUPROMAZINE HYDROCHLORIDE			
Vesprin	Inj: 10, 20 mg/ml Tabs: 10, 25, 50 mg	Adult, IM: 60–150 mg/day PO: 100–150 mg/day Children over 2 1/2 years: 0.2–0.25 mg/kg up to 10 mg/day Adult with nausea and vomiting: 5–15 mg, IM, every 4 hours	Also used to control nausea and vomiting
PHENOTHIAZINE, PIPERAZINE—ACETOPHENAZINE MALEATE			
Tindal	Tabs: 20 mg	Adult: 20 mg, 3 times/day; optimum dosage range 80–120 mg/day	

ANTIPSYCHOTIC DRUGS

CLASS—GENERIC NAME; BRAND NAME	FORMS AVAILABLE	DOSAGES	COMMENTS
PHENOTHIAZINE, PIPERAZINE—FLUPHENAZINE HYDROCHLORIDE			
Permitil Prolixin * Modecate * Moditen	Concen: 5 mg/ml Inj: 2.5 mg/ml Tabs: 1, 2.5, 5, 10 mg	Adults IM: 1.25 mg increasing to 2.5-10 mg/day in 3 to 4 doses PO: 0.5-10 mg/day, in 3 to 4 doses Elderly: 1-2.5 mg/day, increased gradually according to response	
PHENOTHIAZINE, PIPERAZINE—PERPHENAZINE			
Trilafon * Phenazine	Concen: 16 mg/5 ml Inj: 5 mg/ml Tabs: 2, 4, 8, 16 mg Tabs sust rel: 8 mg	Adults, PO: 4-8 mg, 3 times/day for outpatients; 8-16 mg, 2 to 4 times/day for hospitalized clients; do not exceed 64 mg/day IM: 5-10 mg, every 6 hours; do not exceed 15 mg/day in outpatients and 30 mg/day in hospitalized clients Children over 12: use lowest adult doses	Also used to control nausea, vomiting, and intractable hiccoughs
PHENOTHIAZINE, PIPERAZINE—PROCHLORPERAZINE			
Compazine * Stemetil	Caps: 15, 30 mg Inj: 5 mg/ml Suppos: 2.5, 5, 25 mg Syrup: 5 mg/ml Tabs: 5, 10, 25 mg	Adult PO: 5 or 10 mg, 3 or 4 times/day IM: 10-20 mg, every 2 to 4 hours Children over age 2 years and 20 lbs: 2.5 mg, 2 or 3 times/day (oral and rectal) IM: 0.06 mg/kg, initial dose, and then switch to oral doses Elderly: give lowest adult doses	Also used to control nausea and vomiting
PHENOTHIAZINE, PIPERAZINE—TRIFLUOPERAZINE HYDROCHLORIDE			
Stelazine Suprazine * Novoflurazine * Solazine * Terfluzine	Concen: 10 mg/ml Inj: 2 mg/ml Tabs: 1, 2, 5, 10 mg	Adult PO: 2-5 mg, 2 times/day; usual dose is 15-20 mg/day IM: 1 or 2 mg, every 4-6 hours; do not exceed 10 mg/day Children over 6 years: individualize dosages by weight and symptoms; PO or IM: 1 or 2 mg, 1 or 2 times/day	Also used to control non-psychotic anxiety
PHENOTHIAZINE, PIPERADINE—MESORIDAZINE			
Serentil	Concen: 25 mg/ml Inj: 25 mg/ml Tabs: 10, 25, 50, 100 mg	Adult PO: 10-50 mg 2 or 3 times/day. Raise up to: 400 mg/day in schizophrenia; 300 mg/day in chronic brain syndrome and behavioral problems; 200 mg/day in alcoholism; 150 mg/day in psychoneurotic problems IM: initial dose of 25 mg; repeat in 30-60 minutes, if necessary	Also used for alcohol withdrawal symptoms, hyperactivity and behavioral problems, and chronic brain syndrome
PHENOTHIAZINE, PIPERADINE—THIORIDAZINE HYDROCHLORIDE			
Mellaril Mellaril-S Millazine * Novoridazine	Concen: 30, 100 mg/ml Susp: 25 mg/5 ml Tabs: 10, 15, 25, 50, 100, 150, 200 mg	Adults: 50-100 mg, 3 times/day up to 800 mg/day, divided in 2-4 doses Children over 2 years: 0.5-3 mg/kg/day in divided doses Elderly: dosages range from 10 mg, 2-4 times/day to 50 mg, 3-4 times/day	Also used to control anxiety, depression, and insomnia in the elderly
THIOXANTHENE—CHLORPROTHIXENE			
Taractan * Tarasan	Concen: 100 mg/ml Inj: 12.5 mg/ml Tabs: 10, 25, 50, 100 mg	Adult PO: 25-50 mg, 3 or 4 times/day, up to 600 mg/day in divided doses IM: 25-50 mg, 3 or 4 times/day Children over 6 years: 10-25 mg, 3 or 4 times/day Elderly: 10-25 mg, 3 or 4 times/day	

ANTIPSYCHOTIC DRUGS

CLASS—GENERIC NAME; BRAND NAME	FORMS AVAILABLE	DOSAGES	COMMENTS
THIOXANTHENE—THIOTHIXENE HYDROCHLORIDE			
Navane	Caps: 1, 2, 5, 10, 20 mg Concen: 5 mg/ml Inj (powder): 5 mg/ml Sol (IM): 2 mg/ml	Adult PO: initial dose of 2 mg, 3 times/day; up to 15 mg/day in divided doses IM: 4 mg, 2 to 4 times/day; do not exceed 30 mg/day	

* Available only in Canada.

Drug Interactions

Additive CNS depression can result from use of antipsychotic drugs with alcohol, anesthetics, barbiturates, or narcotics. Antacid medications can decrease absorption. Antihypertensive effects of guanethidine are inhibited.

Warnings

Because antipsychotic therapy can result in possibly irreversible symptoms of tardive dyskinesia, clients should be cautioned to report any signs immediately. Many antipsychotic drugs have an antiemetic effect, which can suppress cough reflexes; use caution to prevent aspiration of vomitus. Cardiovascular side-effects include increased pulse rate and hypertension; use with caution.

Overdosage

Symptoms of overdosage include CNS depression, ranging from somnolence to coma, hypotension, and extrapyramidal symptoms. Treatment includes maintaining adequate respiration and blood pressure by administration of IV fluids. Do not administer epinephrine.

Client Education

Inform clients of symptoms of tardive dyskinesia and tell them to report any appearance of signs immediately. Also advise clients to report any signs of fever, sore throat, or malaise. Instruct clients as follows: Take medication as ordered; do not change dosage; do not stop taking this medication abruptly. Antipsychotic medications can cause drowsiness and/or dizziness, especially at the beginning of therapy. Use caution while driving or operating machinery until effects of drug are known. Do not take antipsychotic medications with alcohol or other CNS depressants. Avoid contact with liquid forms of these drugs. Clients should avoid direct sunlight and high temperatures. The full effect of these drugs may not be felt for several weeks.

Antimania Drugs

Lithium

Actions

Lithium alters sodium transport in muscle and nerve cells and changes catecholamine metabolism.

Uses

Indicated for clients experiencing manic phases of manic-depressive illness. Also used to prevent recurrence of manic episodes.

Contraindications

Lithium should not be used in clients with known hypersensitivity, cardiovascular disease, debilitation, dehydration, sodium depletion, or concurrently with diuretics.

Side-Effects

Side-effects and adverse reactions are related to serum levels. At lower levels nausea, hand tremors, thirst, and

ANTIMANIA DRUGS

GENERIC NAME; BRAND NAME	FORMS AVAILABLE	DOSAGES	COMMENTS
LITHIUM CARBONATE Cibalith-S Eskalith Lithane Lithium Carbonate Lithium Citrate Lithobid Lithotabs	Caps: 150, 300, 600 mg Syrup: 8 mEq/5 ml Tabs: 300 mg Ext rel tabs: 300, 450 mg	Adult: 600 mg, 3 times/day; or 900 mg, 2 times/day of ext rel tabs Maintenance: 300 mg, 3 or 4 times/day	Monitor serum levels carefully.

polyuria may occur. At toxic levels side-effects may include arrhythmias, hypotension, ataxia, dizziness, drowsiness, seizures, blurred vision, and coma.

Drug Interactions

Administration with haloperidol may cause encephalopathic syndrome. Diuretics, indomethacin, methyldopa, probenecid, and other nonsteroidal anti-inflammatory agents may raise plasma levels and the possibility of toxicity. Use with thiazides may increase lithium toxicity. Use with substances containing iodine may cause hypothyroidism.

Warnings

Therapeutic serum lithium levels are very close to toxic levels. Monitor clients closely for signs of lithium toxicity. Lithium can cause sodium depletion and lithium retention. Advise clients to maintain normal diet and salt intake. Use with caution in clients with cardiovascular or renal disease. Benefit to risk of use in pregnant and lactating mothers must be weighed, since lithium crosses the placenta and is excreted in breast milk. Congenital anomalies and neonatal effects have been reported.

Overdosage

Signs include ataxia, drowsiness, diarrhea, slurred speech, and muscle weakness. Treatment includes gastric lavage, restoration of fluid and electrolyte balance, and monitoring of kidney function.

Client Education

Instruct clients as follows: Take medication as ordered; do not change dosage. Report immediately any incidence of vomiting, diarrhea, or anorexia. Maintain a normal diet and salt intake, while avoiding caffeine and excessive exercise.

References

Abrams A: Clinical Drug Therapy, 2nd ed. Philadelphia, JB Lippincott, 1987

Clayton BD: Mosby's Handbook of Pharmacology in Nursing, 4th ed. St Louis, CV Mosby, 1988

Drug Facts and Comparisons. St Louis, JB Lippincott, 1988

Irons PD: Psychotropic Drugs and Nursing Interventions. New York, McGraw-Hill, 1978

Malseed R: Pharmacology: Drug Therapy and Nursing Considerations, 3rd ed. Philadelphia, JB Lippincott, 1989

Physicians' Desk Reference. Oradel, New Jersey, Medical Economics, 1988

Scherer J: Lippincott's Nurses' Drug Manual. Philadelphia, JB Lippincott, 1985

United States Pharmacopeia Dispensing Information. Rockville, Maryland, United States Pharmacopeial Convention, 1988

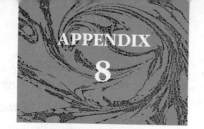

JOANNA SHEAR

PSYCHIATRIC EMERGENCIES AND NURSING INTERVENTIONS

SUICIDAL IDEATION

RELATED NURSING DIAGNOSES: Alterations in perception/cognition (50.)
Alterations in thought content (50.08)
Suicidal ideation (50.08.07)

DEFINING CHARACTERISTICS	NURSING INTERVENTIONS	RATIONALE
• Clients may present with physical or emotional symptoms.	1. Obtain medical evaluation for physical symptoms.	Rule out physical causes for suicidal ideation.
• Auditory command hallucinations ("A voice is telling me to jump off a building.")	2. Stay with client.	Provide support for client and prevent self-injury.
• Psychotic clients, with impaired reality testing and low impulse control, who hear command hallucinations are at highest risk for suicide.	3. Perform psychiatric assessment and mental status exam. 4. Question client in a calm, nonjudgmental manner.	Determine degree of client's self-control. Promote client's confidence in the nurse and establish a trusting nurse–client relationship.
• Factors that place clients in a high risk category include:	5. Perform a suicide risk assessment. Questions to ask include:	
(a) A history of multiple, high lethality suicide attempts, such as shooting, stabbing, hanging, and poisoning	(a) Have you attempted to harm yourself in the past? When? How? What precipitated the events?	Clients with a history of suicide attempts are at higher risk.
(b) Alcoholism	(b) What method would you use?	Level of risk can be determined from method chosen (*e.g.,* attempting to overdose on aspirin is far less lethal than an attempt by shooting).
(c) Lack of a support system	(c) Is the method available?	Risk increases as the availability, specificity, and lethality of the method increase.
(d) Chronic pain or illness		
(e) Psychosis	(d) Have you established a plan? (How specific is the plan?)	
(f) Depression	(e) How lethal is the method?	
	6. Refer client for hospitalization or psychotherapy.	Protect client from self-harm and facilitate client's understanding of the nature of the problems.

SUICIDE THREAT

RELATED NURSING DIAGNOSIS: Suicide threat

DEFINING CHARACTERISTICS	NURSING INTERVENTIONS	RATIONALES

• Clients may use suicide threats as a method of manipulating significant others or health care providers (*e.g.,* "If you don't _____, I'll kill myself").	1. Take all suicide threats seriously, even if they seem manipulative.
	2. Perform psychiatric assessment and mental status exam.
	3. Question client in a calm, nonjudgmental manner.
	4. Perform a suicide risk assessment. Questions to ask include:
	  (a) Have you attempted to harm yourself in the past? When? How? What precipitated the events?
	  (b) What method would you use?
	
	  (c) Is the method available?
	  (d) Have you established a plan? (How specific is the plan?)
	  (e) How lethal is the method?
	5. Refer client for hospitalization or psychotherapy.
		Suicide threats may indicate client's intent to inflict self-harm or commit suicide. Determine degree of client's self-control.
		
		Promote client's confidence in the nurse and establish a trusting nurse–client relationship.
		
		Clients with a history of suicide attempts are at higher risk.
		
		Level of risk can be determined from method chosen (*e.g.,* attempting to overdose on aspirin is far less lethal than an attempt by shooting). Risk increases as the availability, specificity, and lethality of the method increase.
		
		Protect client from self-harm and facilitate client's understanding of the nature of the problems.

SUICIDE GESTURE

RELATED NURSING DIAGNOSIS: Suicide gesture

DEFINING CHARACTERISTICS	NURSING INTERVENTIONS	RATIONALE

• A self-destructive act with low lethality (*e.g.*, superficial wrist lacerations, self-inflicted cigarette burns)
• An experience of extreme anxiety accompanied by a loss of cognitive/perceptual abilities and an urgency to obtain resolution of the panic
	1. Take all suicide gestures seriously.
	2. Refer client for medical evaluation as soon as possible.
	3. Perform psychiatric assessment and mental status exam.
	4. Question client in a calm, nonjudgmental manner.
	5. Perform a suicide risk assessment. Questions to ask include:
	  (a) Have you attempted to harm yourself in the past? When? How? What precipitated the events?
	  (b) What method would you use?
	
	  (c) Is the method available?
	  (d) Have you established a plan? (How specific is the plan?)
	  (e) How lethal is the method?
	6. Refer client for hospitalization or psychotherapy.
		Suicide gestures can precede suicide attempts. Ensure physical safety of client.
		
		Determine client's present mental and emotional status.
		Promote client's confidence in the nurse and establish a trusting nurse–client relationship.
		
		Clients with a history of suicide attempts are at higher risk.
		
		Level of risk can be determined from method chosen (*e.g.*, attempting to overdose on aspirin is far less lethal than an attempt by shooting). Risk increases as the availability, specificity, and lethality of the method increase.
		
		Protect client from self-harm and facilitate client's understanding of the nature of the problems.

SUICIDE ATTEMPT

RELATED NURSING DIAGNOSIS: Suicide attempt

DEFINING CHARACTERISTICS	NURSING INTERVENTIONS	RATIONALE
• A self-destructive act with the intent to die by methods such as shooting, stabbing, hanging, jumping, drug overdose, or asphyxiation	1. Refer client for medical evaluation and treatment as quickly as possible.	Suicide attempts represent medical and psychiatric emergencies. Life-threatening conditions must be treated immediately. Ensure staff compliance with accepted procedures and protocols. Ensure client safety, and protect client from additional attempts at self-harm.

• Suicidal behavior is a symptom of a variety of DSM-III-R[2] diagnostic categories, including:
   Affective disorders
   Depression
   Schizophrenia
   Psychoses
   Personality disorders
	2. Institute suicide precautions according to institutional protocols
	3. Provide safe environment for client:
	  (a) Remove all dangerous objects from client's surroundings.
	  (b) If agitated, client should be restrained.
	  (c) Observe client closely.	

• Individuals with high-risk potential for suicide attempts generally have poor impulse control and exhibit self-destructive behaviors, (*e.g.,* suicide threats or gestures).	4. Perform psychiatric assessment, mental status exam, and further suicide risk assessments.	Determine degree of client's self-control.

• Alcoholism is frequently seen in clients who attempt suicide.	5. Determine risk for additional suicide attempts:
	  (a) Did client believe that the method would work?
	  (b) Was the suicide attempt planned in such a way that it was unlikely to be discovered or prevented?
	  (c) Is client unhappy or surprised to be alive?
		Affirmative answers to any of these questions place the client in a high-risk category. Suicide potential is determined on a low- to high-risk continuum, with clients who are in danger of attempting suicide at the high-risk end of the continuum. High-risk clients usually require hospitalization; low-risk clients can be treated on an outpatient basis as an alternative to hospitalization.

PANIC

RELATED NURSING DIAGNOSIS: Panic[3]

DEFINING CHARACTERISTICS	NURSING INTERVENTIONS	RATIONALE

• The client is out of control.
• The perceptual field is focused on a very small detail.
• The client loses a sense of self or personal identity.
• Rising anxiety precedes panic.
• Motor behavior is disorganized (*e.g.,* client can be observed pacing restlessly, rocking, or the like).
• Panic always precedes psychosis.
• Panic, when accompanied by hallucinations, can relieve loneliness, although anxiety is a factor.
• Panic is relieved by psychotic behavior. For example, delusional beliefs may resymbolize various pre-panic experiences, or the panic experience itself (*e.g.,* if an individual has been degraded or humiliated, as in rape or incest, denial of these emotional experiences and compensation for them is inherent in delusions).
• Panic is most readily observed in the following DSM-III-R categories:
    Anxiety disorders
    Delusional disorders
    Dissociative disorders
    Schizophrenia
• Panic as described above should be differentiated from the type of panic seen in Panic Disorders. The latter panic is not associated with psychosis, and frequently manifests with somatic symptoms such as shortness of breath, palpitations, and tachycardia.
	1. Stay with client; if client is pacing, nurse should pace with client.
	2. Do not touch client.
	
	3. Use short, directive phrases in a calm tone of voice (*e.g.,* "I'll stay with you," "Tell me what is happening," "Are you anxious?").
	4. Reduce stimuli around client.
	
	5. Since anxiety is contagious, nurses should be aware of their anxiety levels.
		Provide reassurance and help calm client.
		
		Client may misinterpret the gesture, which may escalate the panic.
		Enable client to focus on specific responses.
		
		Reduction in stimuli facilitates decrease in client's level of panic.
		Nurses' increased anxiety can escalate client's level of panic.

AGGRESSION

RELATED NURSING DIAGNOSES: Alterations in conduct/impulse control (21.)
Aggression/violence toward environment (21.01)
Destruction of property (21.01.01)
Aggression/violence toward others (21.02)
Abuse—verbal (21.02.03)
Alterations in conduct/impulse control NOS (21.99)
Alterations in motor behavior (22.)
Muscular rigidity (22.01.10)
Restlessness (22.01.12)

DEFINING CHARACTERISTICS	NURSING INTERVENTIONS	RATIONALE
• Verbally threatening, swearing, spitting • Psychomotor agitation with increased pacing, tension • Body language indicating rigidity in posture or clenched fists • Angered facial expressions • Direct and hostile eye contact or direct aversion of gaze • Paranoia and delusions—believing that others want to harm the client • Command hallucinations telling client to hurt others • Destruction of objects • Invasion of others' interpersonal space • Nurses' feelings about impending assault or violence • Panic (see Panic)	1. Prevent assaultive behavior and deescalate threatening behavior. 2. Be aware of behavioral cues, and respond accordingly (*e.g.*, if client is yelling, nurse remains calm and speaks softly). 3. Provide verbal interaction with client. 4. Attempt to get client to verbalize feelings (*e.g.*, "Tell me how you feel," or "Are you anxious?"). 5. Reassure client that help will be provided (*e.g.*, "While you are here, I'm going to help you stay in control"). 6. Set firm limits with client (*e.g.*, "You may not pace in the waiting room, but you may pace in the hall"). 7. If client has a weapon, it must be surrendered before interview can proceed; if client refuses, leave interview and contact hospital security or police. 8. Determine whether any medications have been helpful for client in the past; inform physician. 9. Stay with client; if client is pacing, nurse should pace with client. 10. Do not touch client. 11. Use short, directive phrases in a calm tone of voice (*e.g.*, "I'll stay with you," "Tell me what is happening," "Are you anxious?"). 12. Reduce stimuli around client. 13. Since anxiety is contagious, nurses should be aware of their anxiety levels.	Prevent harm to client and health care providers Provide a role model for client; diffuse client's aggressive behavior. Help decrease client's frustrations and sense of threat. Demonstrate nurse's concern for client. Assist client in feeling safe. Reduce anxiety by providing client with expectations for behavior. Ensure staff and client safety. Medications may assist in calming client. Provide reassurance and help calm client. Client may misinterpret the gesture, which may escalate the panic. Enable client to focus on specific responses, and not to be overwhelmed by stimuli. Reduction in stimuli facilitates decrease in client's level of panic. Nurses' increased anxiety can escalate clients' levels of panic and aggression.

RAPE

RELATED NURSING DIAGNOSES: Excess of or deficit in dominant emotion (30.)
Impaired emotional experience (30.01)
Anger/rage (30.01.01)
Anxiety (30.01.02)
Disgust/contempt (30.01.03)
Distress/anguish (30.01.04)
Fear (30.01.06)
Guilt (30.01.08)
Helplessness (30.01.09)
Shame/humiliation (30.01.04)

DEFINING CHARACTERISTICS	NURSING INTERVENTIONS	RATIONALE

• Rape is an aggressive, violent assault; it has medical, legal, and psychological implications.
• Legally, three elements must be present to define an act as rape:
  (a) Use of force, threat, or duress
  (b) Vaginal penetration (oral or anal sodomy is included in some states)
  (c) Lack of consent of the victim[4]
• Most victims believe that they are going to be murdered, resulting in acute, complex emotional reactions that have been identified in the DSM-III-R[2] as *Post-traumatic Stress Disorder* (PTSD). Victims may experience intense fear, terror, helplessness, anger, rage, shock, embarrassment, guilt, disbelief, denial, or a desire for revenge.
	1. Obtain immediate medical attention for injuries.
	2. Strictly follow legal statutes and protocols for collection of evidence.
	3. Act as client advocate and liaison with other members of the health care team, the family, and the police.
	4. Approach client in a nonjudgmental manner; avoid:
	  (a) Blaming the victim
	  (b) Suggesting that the victim enjoyed the experience of the rape
	  (c) Casting doubt on the victim's claim of rape
	5. Remain with client during the gynecological exam.
	6. Explain all procedures, and request consent from client.
		Provide for physical needs and comfort of client.
		Evidence gathered during the examination corroborates the charge of rape at a trial. Assist in obtaining cooperation of client, family, and others.
		
		Facilitate in the development of a trusting nurse–client relationship.
		
		Be aware of the impact of the exam on client.
		
		Client has recently endured a flagrant disregard for her consent.

(Continued)

RAPE (CONTINUED)

DEFINING CHARACTERISTICS	NURSING INTERVENTIONS	RATIONALE

• The *acute phase* begins at the time of the rape and may last for several weeks.
• Symptoms of PTSD include:
  (a) Persistent reexperiencing of the event
  (b) Numbing of responsiveness to outside stimuli
  (c) Sleep disturbances
  (d) Outbursts of anger and irritability
  (e) Difficulty in concentrating
(Note: symptoms must persist for at least one month to warrant this diagnosis.)
• Somatic symptoms may include: fatigue, headache, GI or GU disturbances, physical trauma from the assault.
• Victims who appear under control may be coping by masking painful and confused feelings.
	7. If client has difficulty describing the incident, nurse can ask: "What happened when he assaulted you?", "Where were you when the assault occurred?", "Did he have a weapon?", "Did you feel that your life was in danger?".
	8. Assess client's emotional state.
	
	9. Determine whether client feels guilt or blames herself for the rape; if so, reassure client that she was a *victim*, and that the rapist acted out of a desire to degrade, humiliate, and dominate her.
	10. Offer anticipatory guidance about the physical and emotional consequences of rape.
	11. Offer referral to crisis intervention services for counseling.
	
	12. Document thoroughly all observations, assessment findings, and interventions.
		Considerate questions from nurse may facilitate client's recollection of details.
		
		Nursing responses at client's level of ability and understanding facilitate nurse–client relationships.
		Clients frequently blame themselves or feel "guilty" for rape incident.
		
		By understanding probable consequences, client will be better able to cope with physical and emotional problems.
		Rape victims have a higher chance of developing PTSD, and should be provided with crisis intervention as well as the opportunity for long-term counseling.
		Medical and nursing records are frequently used in court proceedings, which may not take place for months to years after the incident.

ASSAULTIVE BEHAVIOR

RELATED NURSING DIAGNOSES: Alteration in conduct/impulse control (21.)
Aggression/violence (21.02)
Assaultive (21.02.04)

DEFINING CHARACTERISTICS	NURSING INTERVENTIONS	RATIONALE

• Client experiences frustration and an inability to cope with intense internal feelings.
• Events are perceived as threatening.
• Inhibitions are weakened and impulsivity is heightened.
• Assaultive behavior occurs, including hitting, kicking, biting, and scratching.
• One (or more) of the characteristics of Agitated Threatening Behavior is usually evident before the assault.
• DSM-III-R disorders that are sometimes associated with loss of control of aggressive impulses include:
  (a) Psychotic Disorder
  (b) Organic Personality Syndrome
  (c) Antisocial Personality Disorder
  (d) Borderline Personality Disorder
  (e) Conduct Disorder
  (f) Intoxication with a psychoactive substance
• A rare diagnostic criterion for Intermittent Explosive Disorder is "several discrete episodes of loss of control of aggressive impulses resulting in serious assaultive acts or destruction of property."[2]
	1. Consult physician to determine whether medications are necessary; parenteral administration may be necessary if client remains out of control.
	2. Restrain client or place client in seclusion.
	3. If physical restraint is necessary, it is best accomplished by 4–6 staff members, who restrain both wrists and ankles and place client in four-point leather restraints.
	4. Carefully document all seclusion or restraint procedures according to institutional procedure.
	
	See chapter 14, Milieu Therapy, for additional discussion of restraint and seclusion procedures.
		Medications can assist in alleviating symptoms of restlessness, combativeness, hallucinations, or delusions.
		
		When a client cannot establish internal control, external controls are necessary. A show of force may help client gain internal control and cooperate with the restraint procedure.
		
		Medical and nursing records are frequently used in court proceedings, which may not take place for months to years after the incident. Records provide a way to review client progress.

HOMICIDAL IDEATION

RELATED NURSING DIAGNOSES: Alterations in perception/cognition (50.)
Alterations in thought content (50.08)
Homicidal ideation (50.08.07)

DEFINING CHARACTERISTICS	NURSING INTERVENTIONS	RATIONALE

<ul><li>A client attempting to cope with violent and homicidal thoughts may seek assistance from health care providers.</li><li>The presenting complaint may be, "I'm thinking of killing my wife," but more likely the complaint will be somatic symptoms of "marriage problems."</li><li>The individual with homicidal thoughts is usually isolated, and has difficulty establishing meaningful interpersonal relationships.</li><li>The individual feels powerless and helpless.</li><li>Paranoia may be evident.</li></ul>	1. Obtain a medical evaluation.
	
	2. If client is intoxicated with drugs or alcohol, keep client on the unit until client is sober.
	
	3. Use a direct, nonjudgmental approach with client, particularly when client is relating anxiety-producing or repugnant information.
	
	4. Be aware of legislative statutes governing confidentiality and exceptions to confidentiality between clinicians and clients.
	
	5. Perform a psychiatric assessment and mental status exam.
	
	6. Assess for the presence of psychoses, paranoia, or command hallucinations. Questions nurse might ask include:
	  (a) Do you think anyone wants to harm you?
	  (b) Are you hearing voices?
	  (c) What are the so-called voices saying?
	
	7. Determine whether there is a family history of violence, abuse, or suicide attempts. Questions nurse might want to ask include:
	  (a) Have you ever been violent?
		Rule out neurological or other organic disorders.
		Homicidal ideations should be evaluated when client is sober.
		
		Promote client's confidence in nurse and establish a trusting nurse–client relationship.
		
		Legislative statutes vary from state to state.
		
		Determine degree of client's self-control; a mental status exam may reveal mental states that carry a high risk for violence.
		A client who is psychotic, particularly with paranoia or command hallucinations, is at increased risk for acting on homicidal thoughts and should be hospitalized on a locked unit.
		
		A previous history of family violence or abuse places client at a higher risk for being violent.

(Continued)

HOMICIDAL IDEATION (CONTINUED)

DEFINING CHARACTERISTICS	NURSING INTERVENTIONS	RATIONALE
	(b) Have you ever killed or injured another person? (c) Were you or anyone else in your home abused as a child? (d) Have you ever been arrested? (e) Have you used weapons? (f) Have you had homicidal thoughts, threats, or plans in the past?	
	8. Assess the current situation to determine the nature of client's homicidal ideation. Questions nurse might want to ask include: (a) Do you want to kill someone? (b) Who is that person? (c) Where is that person? (d) Do you have a plan? (e) How would you do it? (f) Are weapons available or accessible? (g) Do you feel that others will view you with more respect if you kill that person?	The level of risk increases as the availability, specificity, and lethality of the plan increase; client may feel that homicide will "solve" a longstanding emotional conflict; the nature of the thoughts must be judged in relation to client's internal and external controls.
	9. Determine whether client should be referred for hospitalization.	
	10. Refer client for psychotherapy. and/or medication, if needed.	Hospitalization is indicated if client is likely to act on the homicidal thoughts. Long-term psychotherapy and medication therapy may be indicated.
	11. Request advice and support from other staff members; have access to good supervision.	Working with violent or potentially violent clients produces anxiety in nurses, who need a method to cope with it.

HOMICIDAL THREAT

RELATED NURSING DIAGNOSES: Alterations in conduct/impulse control (21.)
Aggression/violence toward others (21.02)
Homicidal (21.02.05)

DEFINING CHARACTERISTICS	NURSING INTERVENTIONS	RATIONALE
• Homicidal threats represent an escalation from homicidal thoughts. • Threats may be verbal or behavioral. • The individual may be brought to health care providers by the family or police. • Violence may have already occurred, or the individual may be agitated, with imminent potential for violence. • Homicidal threats and thoughts can occur in most of the DSM-III-R diagnostic categories.	1. Take all homicide threats seriously. 2. If client is out of control, restrain or place client in seclusion. 3. Notify security personnel or police if additional assistance is required to control client. 4. Obtain a medical evaluation. 5. If client is intoxicated with drugs or alcohol, keep client on the unit. 6. Use a direct, nonjudgmental approach with client, particularly when client is relating anxiety-producing or repugnant information. 7. Be aware of legislative statutes governing confidentiality and exceptions to confidentiality between clinicians and clients. 8. Perform a psychiatric assessment and mental status exam. 9. Assess for the presence of psychoses, paranoia, or command hallucinations. Questions the nurse might ask include: (a) Do you think anyone wants to harm you?	Homicide threats may indicate that client intends to harm or kill another person. When a client cannot establish internal control, external controls are necessary. Ensure the safety of staff members, client, and other clients. Rule out neurological or other organic disorders. Homicidal threats should be evaluated when client is sober. Promote client's confidence in nurse and establish a trusting nurse–client relationship. Legislative statutes vary from state to state. Determine degree of client's self-control; a mental status exam may reveal mental states that carry a high risk for violence. A client who is psychotic, particularly with paranoia or command hallucinations, is at increased risk for acting on homicidal thoughts, and should be hospitalized on a locked unit. *(Continued)*

HOMICIDAL THREAT (CONTINUED)

DEFINING CHARACTERISTICS	NURSING INTERVENTIONS	RATIONALE
	(b) Are you hearing voices?	
	(c) What are the so-called voices saying?	
	10. Determine whether there is a family history of violence, abuse, or suicide attempts. Questions nurse might want to ask include:	A previous history of family violence or abuse places client at a higher risk of attempting homicide.
	(a) Have you ever been violent?	
	(b) Have you ever killed or injured another person?	
	(c) Were you or anyone else in your home abused as a child?	
	(d) Have you ever been arrested?	
	(e) Have you used weapons?	
	(f) Have you had homicidal thoughts, threats, plans, or attempts in the past?	
	11. Assess the current situation to determine the nature of client's homicidal threat. Did client have a plan? How specific and lethal was the plan? Did client have the ability to carry out the threat?	The level of risk increases as the availability, specificity, and lethality of the threat increase.
	12. Determine whether client should be referred for hospitalization or legal action.	If client poses a threat to others, hospitalization or legal action is necessary.
	13. Refer client for psychotherapy and/or medication, if needed.	Long-term psychotherapy and medication may be the treatment of choice.

References

1. American Nurses' Association: Taxonomy for the Classification of Human Responses of Concern for Psychiatric/Mental Health Nursing Practice: A Model for Identification of Psychiatric Nursing Phenomena. Kansas City, Missouri, American Nurses' Association, 1986

2. American Psychiatric Association: Diagnostic and Statistical Manual of Mental Disorders, 3rd ed, revised. Washington, DC, American Psychiatric Association, 1987

3. Fields W (ed): The Psychotherapy of Hildegard E. Peplau. New Braunfels, Texas, PFS Productions, 1979

4. Foley T, Davies M: Rape: Nursing Care of Victims. St Louis, CV Mosby, 1983

INDEX

Page numbers followed by *f* indicate figures; numbers followed by *t* indicate tabular material.

ISBN 0-397-54412-X

90000
9 780397 544127